FUNDAMENTALS OF NURSING
A Nursing Process Approach

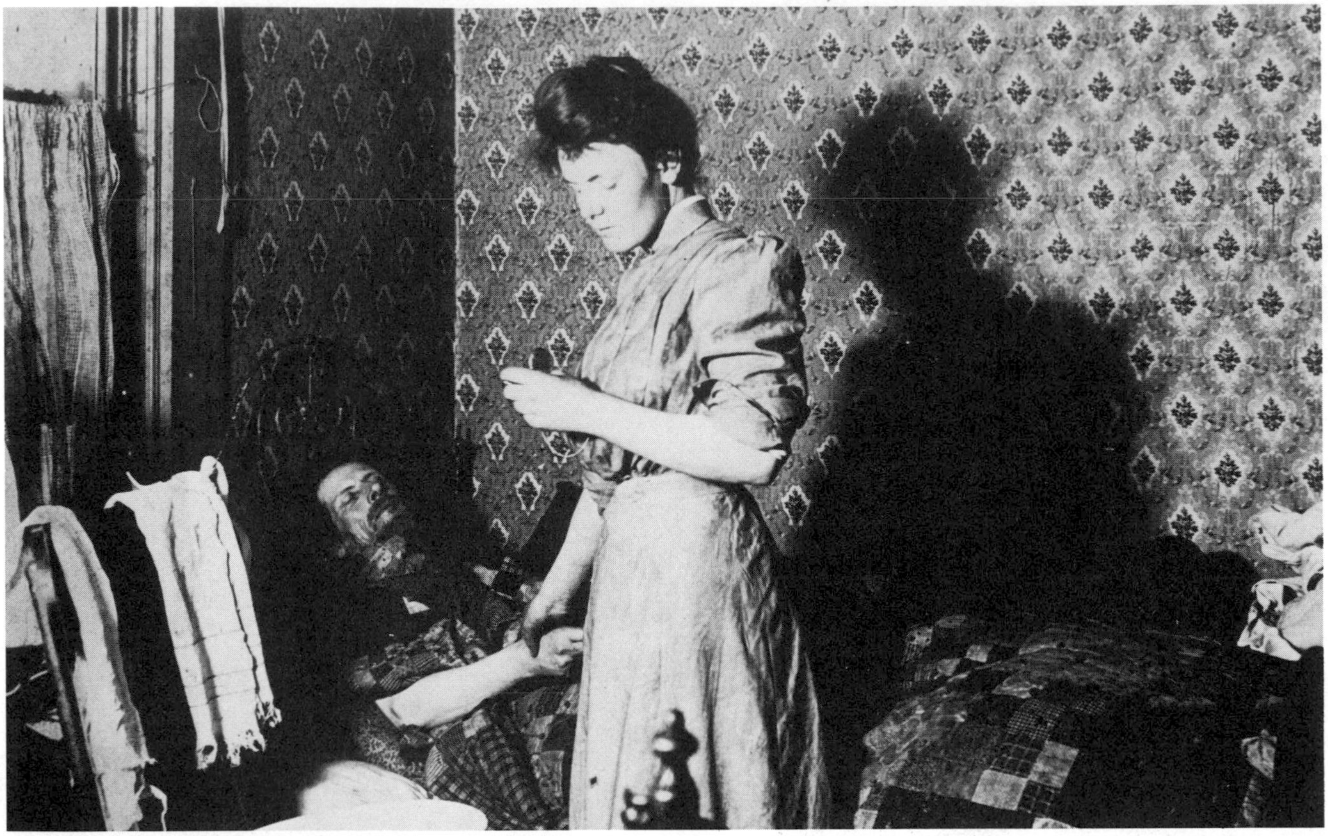

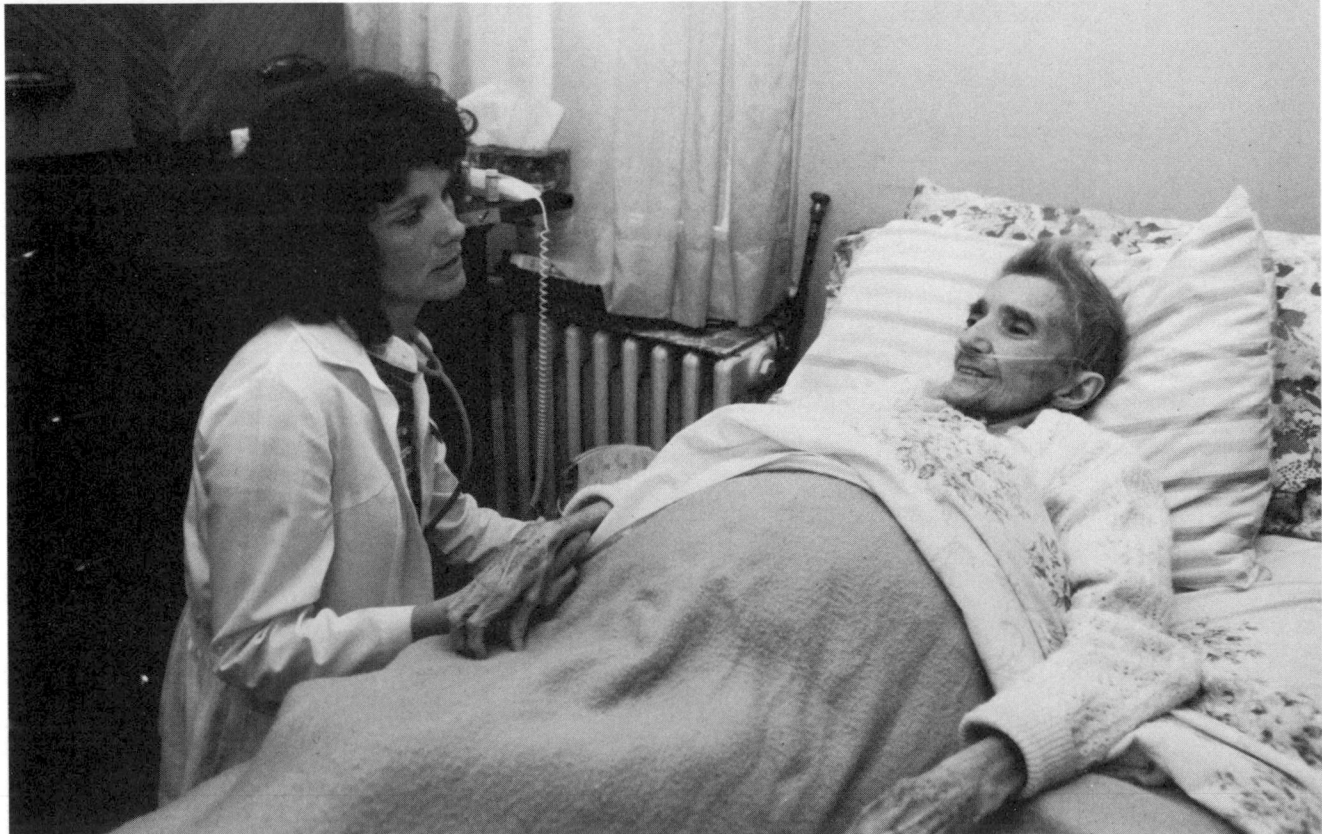

FUNDAMENTALS OF NURSING
A Nursing Process Approach

Leslie D. Atkinson, R.N., M.S.
Instructor, Nursing Program
Normandale Community College
Bloomington, Minnesota

Mary Ellen Murray, R.N., M.S.
Assistant Professor
Raymond Walters College
University of Cincinnati
Cincinnati, Ohio

MACMILLAN PUBLISHING CO., INC.
NEW YORK

COLLIER MACMILLAN CANADA, INC.
TORONTO
COLLIER MACMILLAN PUBLISHERS
LONDON

Macmillan Publishing Company
866 Third Avenue, New York, New York 10022

Collier Macmillan Canada, Inc.
Collier Macmillan Publishers • London

Library of Congress Cataloging in Publication Data

Atkinson, Leslie D.
  Fundamentals of nursing.

  Includes bibliographies and index.
  1. Nursing.   I. Murray, Mary Ellen.   II. Title.
[DNLM: 1. Nursing Process.   WY 100 A876f]
RT41.A8   1985   610.73   84–21311
ISBN 0–02–304590–6

Printing: 1 2 3 4 5 6 7 8   Year: 5 6 7 8 9 0 1 2 3

To marriages, families, and friendships
that have survived
the writing of this text.

PREFACE

A Process Approach

This text has been designed for the beginning student in nursing in any of a variety of educational programs. The authors believe that all students "begin at the beginning", and share the need for a common knowledge base, regardless of academic program. *Fundamentals of Nursing: A Nursing Process Approach* is designed to be a nursing fundamentals text which focuses on presenting methods, strategies, and processes the student may use to plan and provide nursing care. Because contemporary students function in rapidly changing environments, this text will deemphasize student memorization of a specific body of knowledge, while strongly emphasizing process skills of self-assessment, communication, change, problem solving, teaching-learning, and the developmental process. These processes are viewed as tools of the profession which enable the nurse to cope with a constantly increasing data base.

Organization

This text has six units which reflect various processes in nursing:

Unit I. The Process of Evolution in Nursing

This unit describes the present state of nursing, as well as summarizing the past and forecasting the future.

The following concepts are discussed and related to nursing: health, disease, illness, basic human needs, ethics, problem solving (nursing process), change. The legal regulation of nursing practice is presented. The issues of malpractice in nursing, patients' rights, ethical-legal dilemmas, and documentation are discussed in detail.

Unit II. The Communication Process

The process of communication is presented with several applications: individual, group, professional, and technological (computer based). Self-awareness based on self-assessment is introduced and carried throughout the remainder of the book.

Unit III. The Developmental Process

Growth and development from conception through death are presented in a basic human-needs framework. Each of the basic human needs is discussed for each of the ten stages of development. Common health problems and implications for nursing care are identified. The process of growth and development is extended to families, and family-centered nursing care is introduced.

Unit IV. The Nursing Process

The nursing process is presented as an approach fundamental to the nursing role. Care plans are discussed as one application of the nursing process and appear in all the following chapters to illustrate nursing interventions related to basic human needs.

Unit V. The Process of Environmental Management

Nursing interventions to establish and maintain a biologically and chemically safe environment are explained. Nursing skills related to medical and surgical asepsis are included. Medication administration is presented as a form of chemical safety.

Unit VI. Basic Human Needs: A Framework for Nursing Intervention

Each human need is discussed, and the normal means for meeting the need are explained. Alterations in the need or the patient's ability to satisfy the need are included. Assessments and interventions related to need satisfaction are emphasized in each chapter and illustrated with a care plan. A self-assessment section related to each need is included for the student in each chapter.

A *Teachers' Guide* is available with the textbook to summarize content and suggest teaching strategies.

Innovative Characteristics

Features of this book include:

A strong nursing process orientation throughout the book, in addition to a detailed nursing process chapter.

A self-assessment section in each chapter to help the student recognize aspects of self related to basic needs and how these may affect the ability to give nursing care. Self-assessment of learning through review questions and terms is available at the end of each chapter. Answers are provided for questions.

Safety considerations for both nurse and patient are integrated into the nursing care of each chapter.

The interrelated nature of basic human needs is presented in each need chapter, showing how one unmet need may affect many other needs.

Several chapters are devoted to individual psychosocial needs and related nursing interventions in an effort to emphasize an often neglected area of patient care at the fundamentals level.

An entire chapter is devoted to computer application to patient care. Use of computers is viewed as a communication skill. Advantages and disadvantages of computer use are discussed.

A chapter detailing the increasingly problematic issue of nurses' involvement in malpractice. Specific examples involving nurse defendants illustrate potential legal problem areas in nursing practice and how to avoid them.

Chapters by eight contributing authors have been carefully integrated to broaden the range of clinical expertise provided.

The nursing care of preoperative and postoperative patients is integrated throughout the text since it is felt that this care is the application of general nursing skills in a specialized area.

Use of Terms

Every attempt is made to avoid referring to the nurse as a specific sex since both men and women are nurses.

The authors have selected the use of the word "patient" to indicate the recipient of nursing care. This term is consistent historically with the primary care role of nursing. The alternative term "client" may be more appropriate when persons contract individually for nursing services.

L.D.A.
M.E.M.

ACKNOWLEDGMENTS

We wish to acknowledge the assistance of the following persons:

- Our colleagues at Normandale Community College
- Typists: Peggy Whitlock, Ann Trumm
- Readers: Gary Atkinson, Peter Murray
- Reviewers: Pam Reierson, Learning Resource Specialist, Normandale Community College; Frank J. Varga, Assistant Professor of Biology, University of Cincinnati
- Photograph models: Wilma Atkinson; Sheila Cohen, R.N.; Leslie Courseau; Victor Courseau, J.D.; Patti DeMay; Craig Gilbertson; Marianne Gilbertson, R.N.; June Mason; Lester Mason
- Gerald Nidich, and the library staff of Raymond Walters College
- Kay Barthel, R.N. and Tim O'Brien, photographer; Bethesda North Hospital, Cincinnati, Ohio
- Helen Jameson, R.N. and Sharon Tennis, R.N.; Rochester Methodist Hospital, Rochester, Minnesota
- Susan Forstrom, R.N., University of Minnesota Hospitals, Minneapolis, Minnesota
- Carol Wolfe, Senior Editor–Nursing and Toni Ann Scaramuzzo, Editorial Supervisor; Macmillan Publishing Company

CONTRIBUTORS

Stephen R. Bergerson B.A., J.D.
Associate Professor, Metropolitan State University, Minneapolis, Minnesota; Consultant, Continuing Education for Nurses

Linda Edmunds R.N., M.S.
Practice Editor, *Computers in Nursing*; Nursing Systems Consultant with Travenol Laboratories, Inc., and was formerly Systems Nurse and Clinical Assistant Professor in Adult Health Nursing at University Hospital, State University of New York at Stony Brook, New York

Delores E. Johnson R.N., M.S.
Instructor, Nursing Program, Normandale Community College, Bloomington, Minnesota; Clinical Nursing Specialist in Mental Health, Esse Associates, Incorporated, Minneapolis, Minnesota

Barbara J. Leonard R.N., P.N.A., Ph.D.
Assistant Professor, Program in Maternal Child Health, School of Public Health, University of Minnesota, Minneapolis, Minnesota

Tom Olson R.N., M.S.
Clinical Nursing Specialist, Hennepin County Mental Health Center, Minneapolis, Minnesota, and is currently a faculty member of the College of the Virgin Islands

Mary E. Schuler Richards R.N., M.S.
Instructor, Nursing Program, Normandale Community College, Bloomington, Minnesota

Jan Davis Schluter R.N.
Minnesota Regional Sleep Disorder Center, Hennepin County Medical Center, Minneapolis, Minnesota

Alexandra Wright R.N., M.S.
Clinical Oncology Nurse Specialist, North Carolina Baptist Hospital, Winston-Salem, North Carolina

CONTENTS
in Brief

CONTENTS
in Detail

NURSING SKILLS

NURSING CARE PLANS

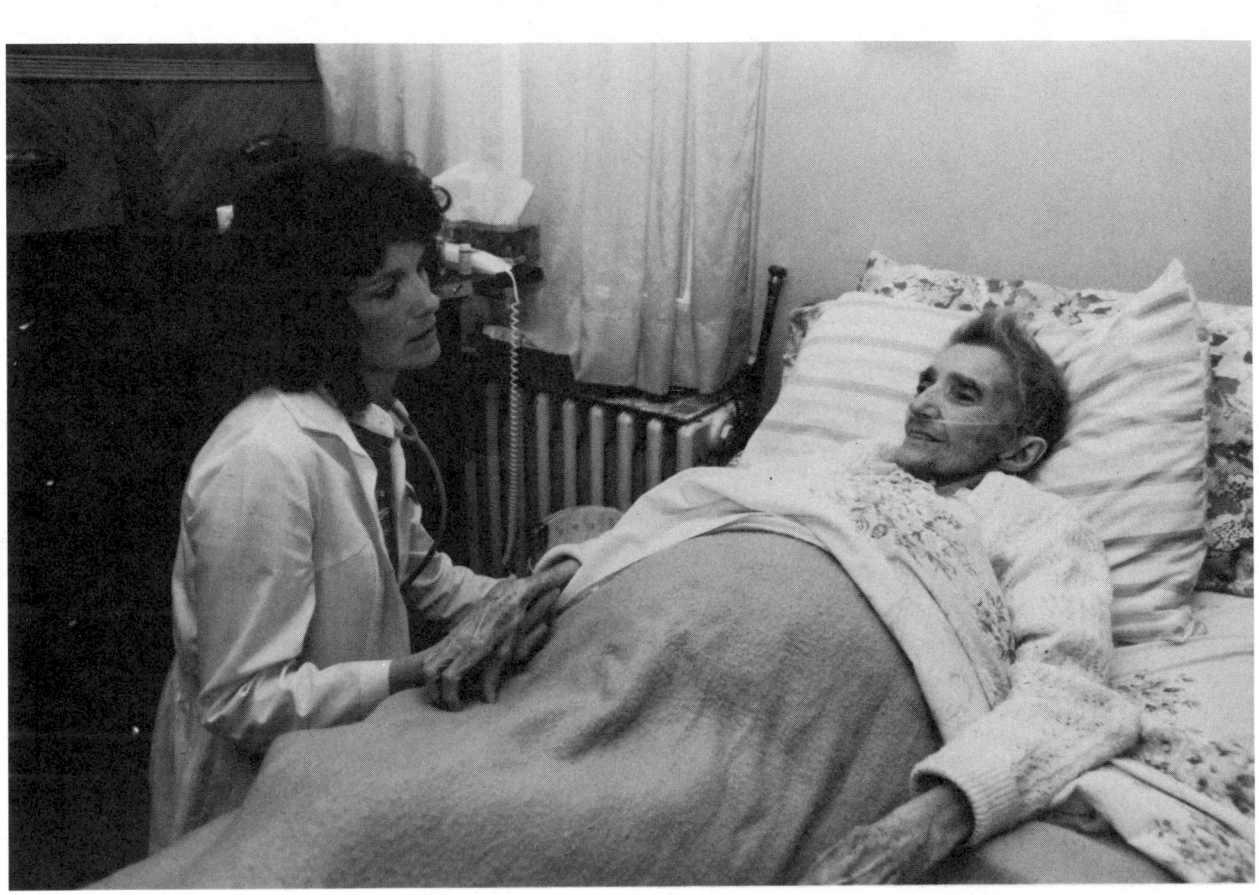

UNIT **I**

THE PROCESS OF EVOLUTION IN NURSING

CHAPTER 1

NURSING: PAST—PRESENT—FUTURE

Nursing Student Life in the 1870s and 1880s
The History of the Nurse's Uniform
Historical Developments in Nursing Education

The Beginning of Modern Nursing
Nursing Student Life in 2085
Nursing in the Future

Objectives

1. Describe the life of the nursing student in the hospital setting in the late 1870s.
2. Describe the work of graduate nurses in the late 1870s and 1880s.

3. Trace the evolution of nursing education from its beginning in the 1870s to the present.
4. Identify nursing skills for the future.

Nursing Student Life in the 1870s and 1880s

As a person interested in the healing arts, you are considering a career in nursing. It is 1875 and the first schools of nursing in the United States are now available on the East Coast. These schools are new, and you wonder what your chances of being accepted are since they have almost three times the applicants for each student position available. Becoming a trained nurse would be a very good way to support yourself since nurse's wages are two to three times the average woman's salary (by the late 1880s). Graduate nurses are earning 10 to 30 dollars a week compared to 4 to 6 dollars for the average working woman.

You send a letter to several schools asking for more information and learn the following information about nursing education and student requirements.
Students must be:

Between the ages of 25 and 35 years (considering the average male life expectancy in 1875 was 40 years, these early schools were not looking for young women!)
Single (married or divorced students were unacceptable)
Able to see and hear perfectly (as measured by the standards of the time)
Examined for healthy feet prior to acceptance, since the student would be on her feet most of the time

Of good moral character attested to by submission of several character witnesses
Willing to live in the rooms assigned to nursing students in the hospital (often between patient wards)
Female (schools of nursing for men began in 1888)

Your nursing education will be two years in length but classes are only presented during the first year. The entire second year is spent giving patient care in the hospital. Classes are held in the evenings to enable the students to give the hospital a full day of service. Students receive one-half day off every week. Classes and hospital service are part of the student's life seven days a week. As a nursing student in 1875, you have no tuition requirements but instead are paid approximately 10 dollars each month by the hospital for your personal and educational needs.

It is a wonder that anyone entered the field of nursing during these early years. The work was long and hard. There was no time for the nursing student to have any outside interests or relationships. Nursing was indeed a career of service and sacrifice in the early years. But by the late 1880s, nursing was emerging as a career for intelligent, devoted people rather than solely the occupation for religious orders or "paroled women convicts, convalescing patients and illiterate persons of low morals'' (Kalisch and Kalisch, 1978) who were the hospital nurses in the 1860s.

Students in the early schools literally had every hour of their life filled for two years. There was no such thing as an eight-hour workday for students. Students in nursing did not receive this luxury until 1913 in California (by state law) and much later in most other states. The first-year student in nursing was responsible for her patients 24 hours a day. She received two hours off duty each day and was often awakened during the night to attend to her patient's needs. Each student was responsible for six or more patients, day and night. There were no hours set aside in the day for the student to study or for recreation. There was no time off on Sunday for attending religious services. Students in the first schools of nursing had no textbooks on nursing since the first textbook on nursing in the United States was not written until 1879, six years after the first trained nurse graduated. Many schools had no examinations, and those that did only had tests the first year when the student was receiving a few hours each week of formal instruction. There was no state licensing examination to take at the end of the training program, and the idea of registering nurses and bestowing the title of RN did not begin until 1903, and then, only in a few states. National tests for licensing nurses began in 1944 to reduce the differences among the widely varying state standards then in use. By 1950, almost all states in the United States and provinces of Canada were using these national tests to license registered nurses. Each state was still establishing its own passing score until a few years later when a standard passing score was recommended for all states. Today, all states use a nationally developed licensing examination with the same passing score.

Students in nursing were called ''probationers'' for approximately one month until they proved their ability to handle the work and the hours. By the second week of training, they were often responsible for the care of 6 to 15 patients. The hospitals at this time were staffed almost exclusively by nursing students. No graduate nurses worked in the hospitals. The students were completely in charge of the patient wards with a senior nursing student filling the role of head nurse.

All graduate nurses at this time were employed as private duty nurses. People needing nursing care would contact private duty nurses to provide care in the home for everything from surgery to tuberculosis. (See Figure 1-1.) People who could afford private duty nurses avoided hospitals whenever possible, since the death rates in hospitals in this era were extremely high. Patients often died of infections they contracted after being admitted to the hospital since the germ theory had not been discovered, and no effort was made to wash hands between caring for different patients or to steril-

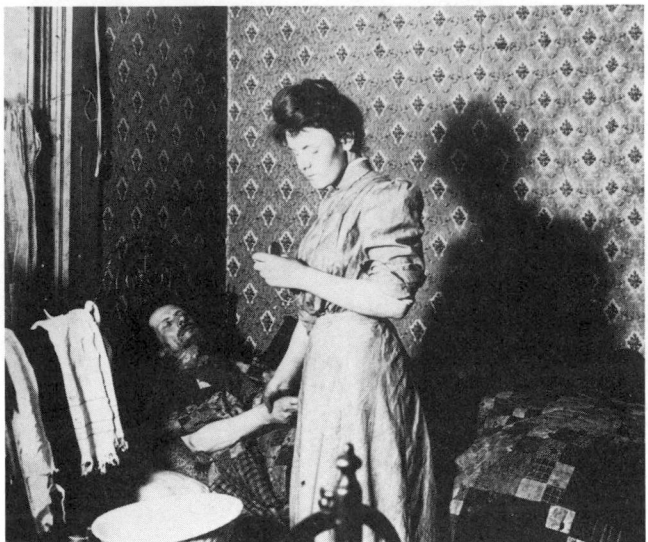

Figure 1-1. A visiting nurse in a patient's home around 1900. (Minnesota Historical Society.)

ize instruments. Surgery during the 1870s and 1880s was done by physicians in street clothes without gloves and with questionable handwashing. (See Figure 1-2.) By 1904, sterile linen and gowns were used in addition to sterile gloves, but no masks were used until later. After graduation, the nurse would advertise her services on printed cards left in doctors' offices, hospitals, and drug stores. The nurse would usually live with the family until her services were no longer needed. She received two hours off each afternoon and worked seven days a week. For this 24-hour daily service, she was paid approximately fifteen dollars a week. By 1919, the private

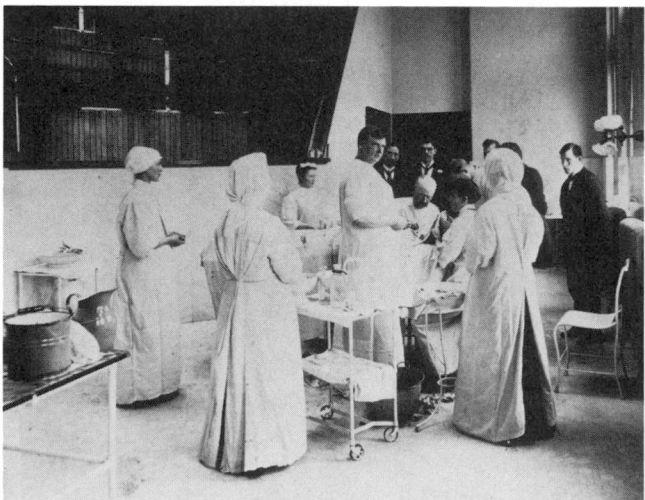

Figure 1-2. An operating room in 1890. Note the bare hands, lack of masks, and the street clothes on the observers. (Minnesota Historical Society.)

duty nurse received five hours off duty each day. In 1930, the eight-hour workday was established for the private duty nurse, for which she was paid five dollars for each day she worked. The depression in 1933 reduced this salary to four dollars, which returned to five dollars by 1936. Private duty nursing remained the primary source of employment for graduate nurses well into the 1930s, with nursing students still responsible for total care of the hospitalized patients.

In the first schools of nursing, the students were permitted to work only on the female wards. Men and women patients were not permitted to be on the same wards regardless of the similarity of their medical and nursing needs. It was considered very improper for "lady nurses" to care for men. However, the health status and recovery rates of the women patients improved so remarkably when nursing students were introduced into hospitals to replace untrained nurses that the physicians soon began to request that students be assigned to the male wards. When the nursing students began caring for the male patients, their recovery rates improved to become comparable to those of the women's wards.

Nursing students were graded on such things as "quietness, trustworthiness, punctuality, cleanliness, personal grooming, ward management and technical skills" (Bullough and Bullough, 1969). Students during their probationary period were not permitted to leave the dormitory unless accompanied by another student.

Nursing duties for the student included ward cleaning, cooking and serving patients' meals, washing soiled linen and bandages, ironing patients' linen, folding linen and keeping a neat linen closet, providing ventilation for the rooms, providing heat, which often involved keeping the wood-burning stove on the ward supplied with wood, washing dishes and giving ordered patient treatments. Treatments in the 1880s included medication administration as is true today, however, the nurses were not to know the name of the medications they dispensed. Each bottle was labeled and ordered by number so that only the physician and pharmacist knew what the patient received. Other nursing treatments included applying leeches to the patient's skin to treat a variety of illnesses. The leeches were alive and active

and left in place until they were so full of blood that they fell off. This usually took about one teaspoon of blood from the patient per leech. Several leeches were often put on at once, and it was the nurse's responsibility to count carefully the number of leeches applied to ensure that the same number were removed and accounted for since they were often reused on the same or a different patient. The nurse was also careful not to apply the leech too close to any body orifice such as the rectum, vagina, nose, ear, or mouth. If a leech was needed to treat such areas, it was watched more closely by the nurse and removed if it came close to entering the body. Actions were identified for use in the event the leech entered the body through any of these orifices, which makes the author believe this was not a totally unusual occurrence.

The use of counterirritants also was commonly ordered during this era. These were substances designed to irritate the skin in one area of the body to varying degrees, from slight redness, to deep redness, or blisters and, in some severe cases, tissue destruction. The belief of the time held that irritation in one body area would relieve the disease or pain in another body area. Poultices, which were watery mixtures of various substances from charcoal to oatmeal, were spread on paper or cloth and applied to the skin until the desired degree of irritation or skin damage was achieved. Tissue destruction was caused by passing an extremely hot piece of metal near the patient's skin to burn but not sear it. Tuberculosis, pneumonia, heart disease, and diarrhea (in children under 2 years) were the leading causes of death. Counterirritants were used to treat many of these ailments. They also were used to treat narcotic overdoses, depression, and inflammation (Kalisch and Kalisch, 1978).

The student spent several months in various specialties such as pediatrics, obstetrics, medical, surgical, and skin diseases. Often two first-year students, one second-year student, and one second-year student head nurse cared for an entire ward of 30 patients. In hospitals that had nursing students on night duty, the average student could expect to spend six months throughout the two-year training course on night duty. A night shift was usually 14 hours.

The History of the Nurse's Uniform

By the 1890s, most students were required to wear uniforms which they made themselves. At first, there was much resistance to the whole idea of uniforms because uniforms were associated with servants. The first uniforms were health hazards. The skirts were long, just

a few inches off the floor, and had long, stiff sleeves and cuffs. (See Figure 1–3.) This prevented any thorough handwashing and served as a medium for the transmission of microorganisms from one patient to another. Common sense would have told the nurse to roll

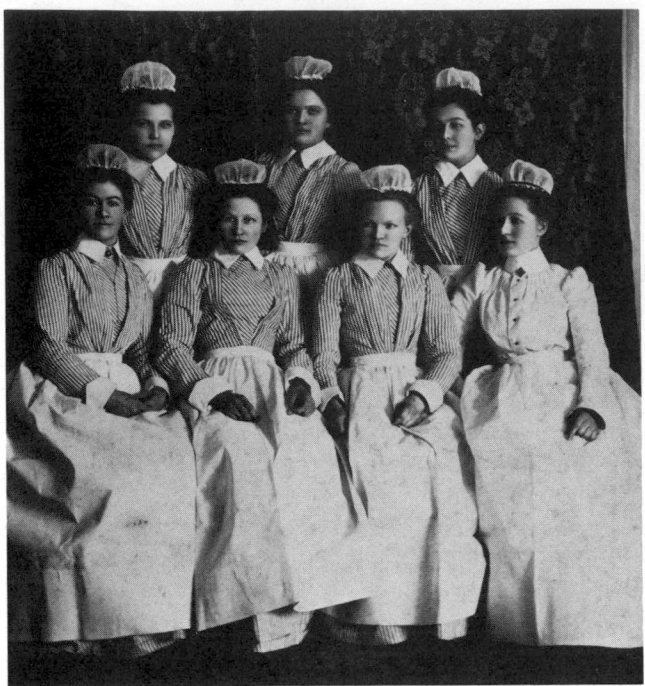

Figure 1-3. Graduating classes of 1901 and 1902 in nursing school uniforms. Note the long sleeves and the functional use of the cap to cover upswept hair. (Photograph by Petri and Svenson, Minneapolis. Courtesy of Metropolitan Medical Center and Minnesota Historical Society.)

up her sleeves during direct patient care, but customs of the time prevented this since it was done only by scrub-women of the lowest class. Any student caught with her sleeves rolled up, no matter how contaminated or messy the treatment or duty in which she was engaged, was chastised by a more experienced student or the supervisor of students. With the introduction of the germ theory, the skirts and sleeves were made shorter to permit handwashing and prevent microorganism transfer by the hem of the skirt touching the floor and by the sleeves touching the patients.

The nurse's cap came into existence for very practical reasons. Most women of the time had very long hair (almost to the waist). The rigorous schedule of the nursing student did not allow much time for personal grooming, especially hairwashing which was often a lengthy process. Therefore, most students had dirty hair. To keep this long, dirty hair out of the way, a dust cap was used, and the student was to tuck all hair under this cap. It also added to the plain look of the nurse since there was essentially no individual hairstyling possible. Makeup also was prohibited.

A utility apron was also part of the original uniforms. In this apron, the nursing student kept matches, pencils, scissors, and a thermometer. Black shoes and stockings completed this uniform.

Historical Developments in Nursing Education

After the 1890s, the training courses in the hospitals gradually expanded from one or two to three years, with a reduction in the number of hours students worked each day. For 40 years, these two- and three-year hospital training programs were the only form of nursing education available, and they raised nursing to being a respected health care profession. Schools for black nurses opened in the 1880s, with the first black trained nurse graduating in 1879 from an integrated school in Boston. In 1930, the first school opened specifically for American Indian women in Arizona. (See Figure 1-4.) By 1945, this school was training 40 women from 25 different tribes. In 1909, the first complete university school of nursing began at the University of Minnesota and required three years of training (Canedy, 1983). Graduates received a graduate of nursing diploma. This program was unique for the time because the students were required to meet the same admission requirements as all other university students (except that they had to be female) and were given the same rights and privileges as other students. The five-year courses leading to a bachelor of science degree in nursing were initiated around 1916. The first two years were devoted to general education courses, and the last three years to nursing educa-

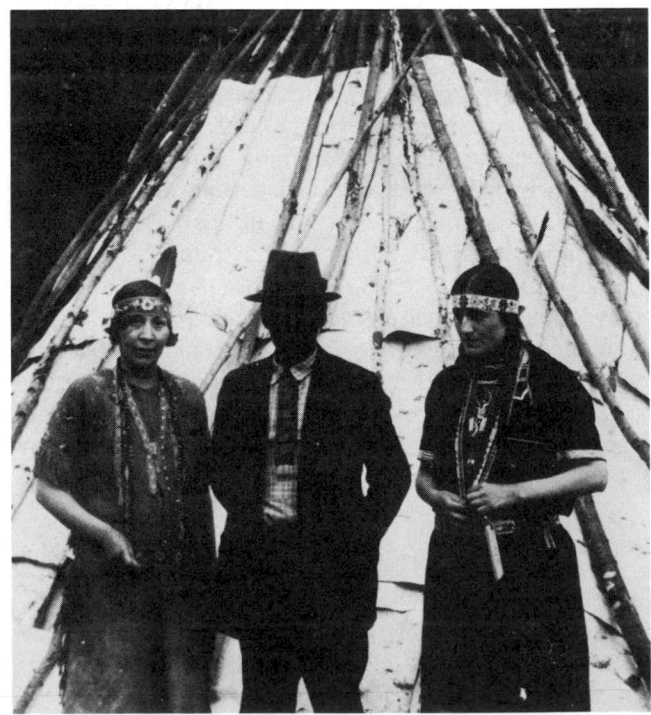

Figure 1-4. Two Indian nurses making a home visit in the early 1900s. (Minnesota Historical Society.)

tion courses. Most of these five-year courses changed to four-year programs in the 1950s and 1960s.

A recent addition to the nursing education scene was the associate degree course in nursing offered in junior or community colleges. This was a two-year nursing program which began in seven junior colleges in a 1952 experiment. Today, the majority of nurses receive their nursing education through the three-year hospital-centered diploma program or the two-year associate degree program in a community college.

Postgraduate education in nursing is available at the master's degree and doctoral level. Education is also available in specialized clinical fields, such as intensive care nursing, pediatric nurse practitioners, nurse midwifery, and operating room nursing. After completing this type of specialized education and passing an examination on the content, the nurse is certified and receives the credentials associated with the specialty area, such as PNP (pediatric nurse practitioner) or CNM (certified nurse midwife).

The Beginning of Modern Nursing

Florence Nightingale is considered to be the founder of modern nursing. She was born in 1820 but did not enter nursing until she was 31 years old because of objections from her wealthy English family who felt that nursing was totally inappropriate for a well-bred English lady. After much persistence, her family consented to her entrance into a nurse's training program run by a pastor and his two wives in Germany. In 1860, Florence Nightingale opened the first nurse's training school in England. Since the discovery of the germ theory was not to come for another ten years, Florence Nightingale did not understand the concept of microorganism transfer, but she did believe in meticulous attention to environmental and personal cleanliness, fresh air and light, adequate warmth, good nutrition, and rest with conservation of the patient's strength for healing. During the Crimean War, Florence Nightingale's nursing efforts reduced the death rate among British soldiers from 40 to 2 percent and proved the effectiveness of trained nurses in improving recovery. Prior to this time, only women and men from religious orders were allowed to care for the soldiers in the army.

The philosophy of Florence Nightingale's schools was based on four key ideas:

1. Training for nurses should be considered as important as any other form of education and be supported by public funds.

2. The training schools for nurses should have close affiliation with hospitals but retain financial and administrative independence from them.

3. Professional nurses should be responsible for the education of nursing students rather than persons not involved in nursing.

4. Nursing students should be provided with a residence during their training which offered them pleasant, comfortable surroundings close to the hospital.

Training at the first Nightingale schools in England was one year in length and later expanded to two years. The first schools in the United States and Canada copied the Nightingale schools of England very closely. The

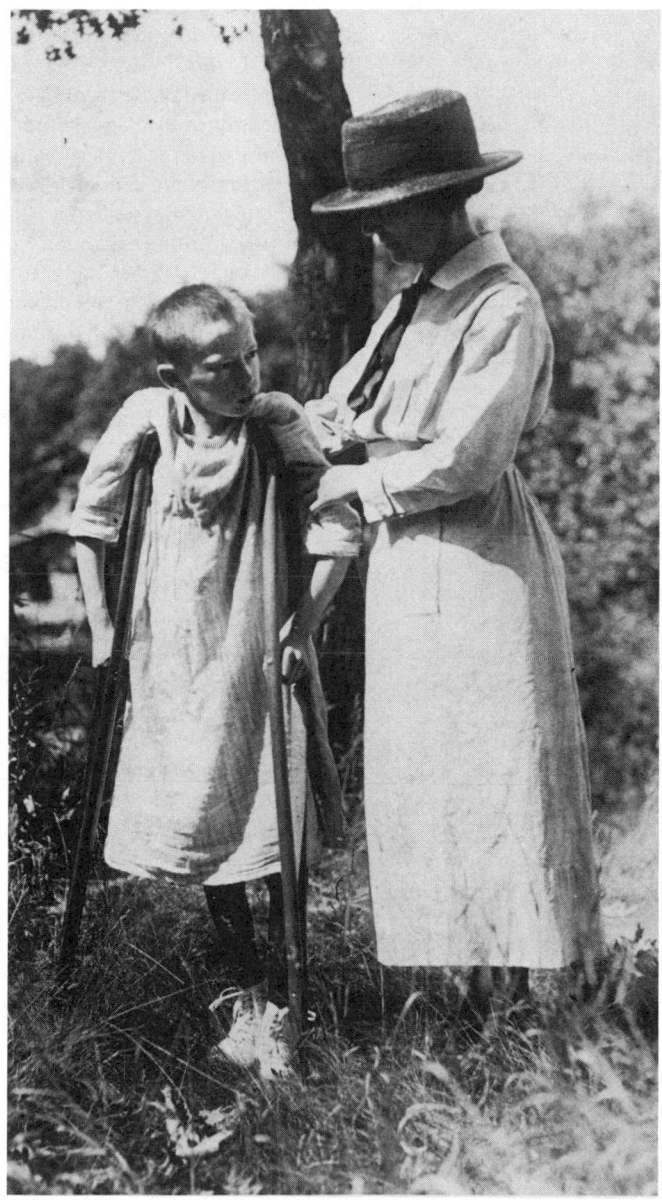

Figure 1-5. A visiting nurse in 1925 assisting a young boy on crutches. (Minnesota Historical Society.)

United States training schools failed to remain separate from the hospitals as Florence had recommended, which resulted in a form of educational abuse of nursing students by the hospitals who virtually had free nursing labor.

Written physician's orders originated with Florence Nightingale, who insisted that her nurses accompany the physician on patient visits "to prevent mistakes, misunderstood directions and forgotten or ignored instructions and orders" (Palmer, 1983). She believed health teaching was a critical responsibility of the nurse if national health was to improve. She felt health was "not only to be well, but to be able to use well every power we have." Florence Nightingale felt the purpose of nursing was "to put us in the best possible condition for nature to restore or to preserve health, to prevent or to cure disease or injury" (Palmer, 1983).

Table 1–1 presents some historical events in the development of nursing. The progress made in nursing in the United States and Canada over the last 100 and

Table 1–1. **Historic Events in the Development of Nursing**

1859	First Nightingale school of nursing opened in England
1873	First Nightingale schools of nursing opened in the United States; first trained nurse in the United States graduates (Linda Richards)
1877	First trained nurses begin giving care in patients' homes in New York
1879	First trained black nurse graduates (Mary P. Mahoney); first nursing textbook published in the United States, *The New Haven Manual of Nursing*
1888	Mills Training School for Male Nurses opened
1890	Private duty nurses had a 22-hour workday, seven days a week
1890–1900	Nurses' training expanded from two to three years
1893	First organized meeting of nurses held on a national scale in Chicago (eventually became the National League for Nursing)
1897	First Canadian school of nursing opened
1898	School of nursing for men opened by Alexian Brothers in Chicago
1900	First issue of the *American Journal of Nursing* published
1902	School nursing began in New York, reducing absent days from 10,567 to 1,101 in one year
1903	First nurse's registration law passed
1909	First training school for nurses established as part of a university curriculum at the University of Minnesota
1910	7 percent of graduate and student nurses were men
1911	Formation of the American Nurses' Association
1912	National League for Nursing developed from the former American Society of Superintendents of Training Schools for Nursing
1916	Five-year bachelor degree programs in nursing introduced in universities
1919	Private duty nurses received five hours off duty each day
1930	First school of nursing for American Indian women opened in Arizona; eight- and ten-hour workday established for nurses
1940	Male Nurses' Section of American Nurses' Association organized; first class of nurse's aides started as ten-week hospital course
1942	Nursing aides became paid hospital employees
1944	National tests for registering nurses began in six states
1950	Practical nursing curriculum developed; beginning of practical nurse licensing in many states; all states using national tests for nursing registration
1951	National Association of Colored Graduate Nurses (42 years old) merged with American Nurses' Association
1952	First two-year associate degree in nursing programs opened
1954	First male nurse in army given rank appropriate to nursing education as second lieutenant (prior to this, male nurses were drafted into the army as privates and not allowed to practice nursing or to join the army or navy nursing corps)
1965	American Nurses' Association Position Paper stating "education for those who work in nursing should take place in institutions of learning within the general system of education"

Source: *Am. J. Nurs.*, 65, p. 106, Dec. 1965.

more years is truly remarkable. Consider that as late as 1860 there were no trained nurses in the country and by 1900 the first issue of the *American Journal of Nursing* was published by and for trained nurses, who were graduating from nurses' training at the rate of approxi-

mately 3,500 a year. Nursing has been needed since earliest recorded history. Where the profession of nursing will be in the next 100 years is difficult to foresee. The need for nursing care will continue to be a human need as long as the race survives.

Nursing Student Life in 2085

As a student interested in health, you are considering a career in nursing. The year is 2085, and several very good schools are now available on the outlying space stations and planet colonies. As is true with all of the health professions, a doctoral degree is now the minimum educational preparation for professional nursing. Back in 2025, the entry level into the profession of nursing required a master's degree, but just ten years ago this was changed to the full doctoral requirement. Your title after completing your doctoral program and passing the interplanetary licensing examination will be NCS (nursing care specialist). The RNT (registered nurse technician) will be under your direction if you choose to work in any of the varied hospital settings on earth, space satellites, or hospital space cruisers. You also may choose employment as a public health nurse specialist where you are in charge of local health clinics and where home health care is the primary focus.

You have chosen a school of nursing on planet Earth. Reciprocal arrangements between educational institutions of various countries make it possible for students to select a school anywhere on the planet or satellites for the same basic tuition costs. This cooperation, especially among medical institutions throughout the world, came about as a result of a planetwide effort to halt the epidemic of AIDS strain III which occurred in the late 2010s as a variant strain of the original strain of virus labeled AIDS in the 1980s and 1990s. The planetwide illnesses in susceptible individuals (much like the polio epidemic in ancient history) necessitated a coordinated effort among all medical research and educational facilities on the planet. This cooperative effort continued in medical education and research after a cure was found.

Your postgraduate study and research in nursing will focus on one of many fields in nursing, such as communicable disease control of alien organisms on the various space colonies, psychiatric nursing, rehabilitation nursing on the low-gravity or zero-gravity orbiting health centers, health care mangement, nursing education, and the biggest field of current practice, home health maintenance.

Nursing in the Future

As a home health maintenance nurse at the NCS level, you will be visiting clients in their homes and assisting them to maintain their optimum health level. People are living to an average age of 95 years, and there are often three or more generations within each household (the expense and scarcity of private housing makes it difficult for people to afford a separate residence until their late 50s or 60s). The visiting NCS has the experience and knowledge to understand the health needs of all age groups. The NCS carries a health computer terminal on family visits and uses this to assess individual's health status based on the results of blood, urine, retina visualization tests, and heat-emitting levels from all body surfaces. Vaccinations for diseases such as cancer, arthritis, and AIDS III are administered to families periodically, but most immunization to disease is accomplished by genetic engineering shortly after conception. Birth and death now are handled commonly in the home with the assistance of the NCS. Only the rare

individual who has no friends or family enters or leaves the world in the unfamiliar hospital setting. Hospitals are staffed by RNTs under the direct supervision of the admitting NCS, physician, or pharmacist.

The pharmacist gained a dominant role in the direct care of patients as the professional responsible for ordering, administering, and regulating medication administration. Between 1990 and 2000, there was such an explosion of the number of drugs as the result of genetic engineering and space exploration that physician education was unable to include both drug therapy and medical technology. The pharmacist's professional organization was successful in convincing the international health professional licensing and regulation board that total drug therapy was the appropriate function of pharmacists. This removed the function of drug prescribing from physicians and drug administration from nursing.

As a graduate of any nursing care specialist program, you will have developed your communication skills far beyond those of any other professional group. The entire health care system will be based on professional nurses' ability to communicate effectively with the families they visit as they accurately diagnose, treat, or refer their client's health problems. Part of your communication skills involves computer expertise, using the most advanced telecommunication health systems available. Based on the information your patient gives you on life-style, personal habits, and health problems, along with the data you obtain from physical examination and specimen collection, the computer will assist you in identifying each client's optimum health maintenance behavior. Computer communication with the main district health terminal will enable the visiting nurse to consult with physicians, pharmacists, nutrition-

ists, physical therapists, and other NCSs from the client's home. Consulting with other professionals involved in the family case, the nurse will initiate treatments and monitor the health progress of each family member. A family's primary health professional is the nursing care specialist who is employed in their geographic area. Physicians are centered in the regional hospitals dealing with complex medical problems where cure through surgery, medication, transplantation, regeneration, energy fields, or biofeedback is the focus. Most of the physician's patients are referrals from other professionals, especially the nursing care specialist.

The nurse handles births in the client's home much as the midwives of ancient history had done. Hospitalizing healthy women for the birth of a baby became too costly in the 1990s, and nurse-attended home births be-

Table 1–2. **Future Events in Health Care**

YEAR	COMMUNICATION AND COMPUTER TECHNOLOGY	BIOMEDICINE AND THERAPEUTICS	EDUCATION AND OCCUPATIONS	MISCELLANEOUS
By 2000	"Teleprescriptions" commonly used Wristwatch TV commonly available Wide availability of computers that "learn" from experience	Moderate chemical control of senility Effective transplantation of all organ systems except for CNS Development of electronic sensors enabling blind people to "see" Laboratory demonstration of regeneration or repair of destroyed neurons	Pharmacists primarily trained for research careers Robots with sensory feedback performing routine household chores in hospitals	World population: 6 billion First clinic or hospital on the moon Periodic polling of public health care issues by computer
By 2005	Wide use of "pharmaceutical automats"	Demonstration of way to decrease time between birth and maturity Development of drugs from substances originating on other planets or the moon Human parthenogenesis	15 percent of medical schools devoted totally to training medics	
By 2010	Automatic reprogramming of medical computers	Wide use of artificial insemination to produce genetically superior offspring Use of highly complex chemical simulation models of the human body for use in drug experimentation *In vivo* renewal of worn-out hearts by stimulating natural growth processes Most forms of mental retardation are cured	Virtual cessation of pharmacy schools Reliable tests available to predict interpersonal skills of medics which are used as admission criteria	Breeding of new animals and plants to alter man's ecosystem for his benefit

Table 1–2. **Future Events in Health Care** (*Cont.*)

YEAR	COMMUNICATION AND COMPUTER TECHNOLOGY	BIOMEDICINE AND THERAPEUTICS	EDUCATION AND OCCUPATIONS	MISCELLANEOUS
By 2015	Demonstration of man-machine symbiosis, enabling people to extend their intelligence by direct electromechanical interaction between their brains and a computer "Telemedicine" services widely delivered in homes	Use of drugs or altered prenatal conditions to raise IQ of normal individuals by 10 to 20 points Laboratory demonstration of biochemical processes that stimulate growth of new organs and limbs Extrauterine development of human fetus Replacement of human organs with those derived from specially bred animals	Virtual obsolescence of the pharmacist Virtual cessation of MDs providing clinical services, except for surgery	AMA disbanded Average U.S. life expectancy, 95 years, with commensurate prolongation of vigor Effective weather control, thereby enhancing global food production
By 2020	Nationwide automated continuous clinical feedback to allow for perpetual updating of computer-rendered medical decisions 95 percent of population has medical records stored in computers	Electrical control of mood disorders available Demonstration of long-duration human hibernation; allows for prolonged space travel Moderate use of genetic engineering in humans by chemical substitution of DNA chains	Enormous expansion of medic training programs	Wide use of self-contained dwellings using life-support systems that recycle water and air to provide independence from external environment 5,000 hospitals in U.S. (down from 6,000 in 1995)
By 2025	Inexpensive high-capacity worldwide, regional, and local (home, hospital, business) communication (using satellites, lasers, light pipes, etc.)	Development of man-machine chimeras *In utero* genetic modification First subject using cryogenic preservation "unfrozen" without success Maintenance of human brain extracorporeally for one month	Frequent international health care seminars conducted via computer satellite communication	Researchers rather than surgeons (MDs) conduct most operations

Source: J. Maxmen: *The Post-Physician Era*. Wiley, New York, 1976. Reproduced with permission.

gan to gain popularity. With the advent of the OSC (ossification structure controller) in 2030, a woman planning a near-future pregnancy was given as many treatments as were needed to alter the pelvic bone structure to ensure the passage of the full-term fetal head for home delivery. Development of this device eliminated the need for surgical delivery of the fetus. Table 1–2 presents some future events in health care as viewed by Maxmen (1976).

The future of nursing will be affected by changes in the composition of the population with more people in the group above age 65 years. Life expectancy will increase gradually, but the quality of life will also improve as people remain active mentally, physically, and socially well into what is now considered the retirement years. There will be fewer and fewer young people moving in to replace retiring persons as the population continues to decline. People will delay childbearing until their late 30s which will result in an increasing infertility rate among families and fewer children. Only the families able to afford technological fertility augmentation will be able to have as many children as they desire when natural fertility fails with advancing maternal age. Financial considerations also will serve to limit the number of children in families as the cost of large, single-family homes moves farther and farther above the financial resources of most families. Most families will have both parents in the work force as a financial necessity to maintain current standards of living. This will reduce the number of children each couple decides to have. More effective birth control measures virtually will eliminate the current unplanned teenage pregnancy rate which now is reaching epidemic proportions. The strong move against induced abortions in this country will add impetus to mandatory vaccination for birth control for all dependent children until the age of 21 years.

Gerontology will become a major nursing focus in the future, as will the expanded public health role. Health maintenance will become the primary responsibility of the nurse, with cure for diseases and trauma remaining the focus of the physician. Functions of the bedside nurse within the hospital setting will remain much as we know them today. The registered nurse technician will be trained in using and interpreting the continuous progression of new medical equipment to assess and treat patients with various diseases and trauma. This nurse (RNT) will be responsible directly to the physician, pharmacist, and nursing care specialist. Health maintenance research will be an expected part of the professional nurse's (NCS) role in all fields. If nursing changes just half as much in the next century as it has changed from its inception approximately a century ago with the opening of formal training schools, nurses' technical skills can be expected to become outdated very rapidly, requiring a life of continued learning and change. What will endure are nurses' "people skills" of communication and the fostering of caring, health-promoting relationships. The skills of listening, talking, teaching, and comforting never will become outdated in the nurse-patient (client) relationship.

References and Bibliography

Aydelotte, M.: The future of health care delivery system in the United States. In Chaska, N. (ed.): *The Nursing Profession: A Time to Speak*. McGraw-Hill, New York, 1983.

Bullough, V., and Bullough, B.: *The Emergence of Modern Nursing*, 2nd ed. Collier-Macmillan Limited, London. 1969.

Christman, L.: The future of nursing is predicted by the state of science and technology. In Chaska, N. (ed.): *The Nursing Profession: A Time to Speak*. McGraw-Hill, New York, 1983.

Canedy, B.: *Remembering Things Past: An Heritage of Excellence*. Biomedical Graphic Communications Dept., University of Minnesota, 1983.

Dock, L., and Stewart, I.: *A Short History of Nursing*, 4th ed. Putnam, New York, 1983.

Fasano, N., and White, M.: Futurism scenario—Commencement address to the class of 2010. *J. Nurs. Educ.,* **21**:20-25, Mar. 1982.

Fitzpatrick, M.: *Prologue to Professionalism*. Robert J. Brady, Bowie, Md., 1983.

Goostray, S.: *Memoirs: Half a Century in Nursing*. Nursing Archive, Division of Special Collection, Boston University Library, Boston, 1969.

Kalisch, P., and Kalisch B.: *The Advance of American Nursing*. Little, Brown, Boston, 1978.

Lesse, S.: The preventive psychiatry of the future. *The Futurist,* **10**:228–33, Oct., 1976.

Maxmen, J.: *The Post-Physician Era: Medicine in the 21st Century*. Wiley-Interscience, New York, 1976.

Palmer, I.: From whence we came. In Chaska, N. (ed.): *The Nursing Profession: A Time to Speak*. McGraw-Hill, New York, 1983.

Rosenfeld, A.: Prolongevity: The Extension of the Human Life Span. *The Futurist,* **1**:13–17, Feb., 1977.

Schlotfeldt, R.: Nursing in the future. *Nurs. Outlook,* **29**:295–301, May, 1981.

Talbot, D.: Public health nursing: Now and as it might be. In Chaska, N. (ed.): *The Nursing Profession: A Time to Speak*. McGraw-Hill, New York, 1983.

NURSING PRACTICE: FOUNDATIONS AND ETHICS

Objectives

1. State one definition each of nursing, health, illness, and disease.
2. Discuss what is meant by the care and cure roles of nursing.
3. Explain how the nursing process is used in the practice of nursing.
4. State and describe the four steps of the nursing process.
5. Describe the relationship between physiological stress and psychosocial stress.
6. Describe the local adaptation syndrome.
7. Describe the general adaptation syndrome.
8. Discuss the responsibilities of the nurse as identified in the International Council of Nurses' Code for Nurses.
9. Describe what is meant by Maslow's hierarchy of basic needs and how it applies to patient care.
10. List and define the basic needs.
11. Name and state the purpose of an international and a national nursing organization.

What Is Nursing?

There are probably as many definitions of nursing as there are individual nurses. *Nursing* has been defined as:

Giving assistance to persons who are unable to meet their own health care needs (Orem, 1980)

Promoting a positive adaptation to changing internal and external environments (Roy, 1976)

Nursing is the caring and nurturing of the physical, social, spiritual, cultural and emotional well-being of an individual, family, or community (De-Young, 1981).

Each of these definitions by nurse leaders is a statement of how individuals have viewed nursing. Each definition has been studied, debated, and researched. Individual schools of nursing and health care institutions each select a definition that seems to best reflect the purpose of their unique organization.

Other definitions of nursing which have widespread acceptance are put forth by the American Nurses' Association (ANA), the Canadian Nurses' Association (CNA), and the International Council of Nurses (ICN). The ANA defined nursing practice as "a direct service, goal oriented, and adaptable to the needs of the individual, the family, and the community during health and illness." The CNA offers this definition: "Nurses direct their energies toward the promotion, maintenance, and restoration of health, the prevention of illness, the alleviation of suffering and the ensuring of a peaceful death when life can no longer be sustained." The ICN states: "The unique function of the nurse is to assist the individual, sick or well, in the performance of those activities contributing to health or its recovery (or to a peaceful death) that he would perform unaided if he had the necessary strength, will or knowledge."

From these definitions, it is possible to identify four main areas of nursing:

1. Maintenance of health
2. Promotion of health
3. Restoration of health
4. Care of the dying

Health, like nursing, has many different meanings and is probably best defined by the individual. Health is more than the absence of disease. Any definition of health must consider that human beings are composed of both mind and body. These parts are inseparable and interdependent. This indivisability of the human being is the basis of *holistic health,* an approach that considers the physical, mental, and social well-being of the individual.

Health is the state of a fully functioning human being, a person using mind and body to live in a way that is personally satisfying and acceptable. A person with a handicap, such as blindness, is capable of attaining this state of health. Moreoover, health is not an all-or-none proposition but rather exists on a scale that ranges from acute illness to optimal health. At any given time, an individual is someplace on this scale. Over time, the individual's place on the scale changes because health status changes and fluctuates.

Maintenance of Health

Nurses work in many settings where the goal of health care is the maintenance of health. Residents of nursing homes utilize the skills of nurses to continue maximum functioning. On college and university campuses, nurses provide a variety of educational programs focused on health maintenance as part of a student health service. This aspect of the nurse's role makes good sense economically. It has been well documented that it is less expensive to maintain health than it is to treat illness. For example, nurses teach young schoolchildren to cover their mouths when coughing and to wash their hands carefully after using the toilet. These simple measures can stop the spread of some contagious diseases, thereby eliminating the costs of related physicians' visits, medications, and days missed from school.

Promotion of Health

When promoting health is the goal of nursing, the person is already in an acceptable state of health but is seeking an improved state of health, a higher level on a continuum between illness and health. The individual who begins running to improve physical fitness is an example of a person seeking health promotion. The individual may seek nursing help in determining that it is safe to begin an exercise program. After assessment of health history and a physical examination, which includes a physician's evaluation, the nurse may work with the person to plan a diet and exercise program.

Restoration of Health

Most of the public expectations of nurses have to do with the nurse caring for sick persons, and the majority of nurses do function in this setting. Nurses who work in hospitals and in medical clinics spend most of their time working to restore the health of patients.

Care of the Dying

Because cure and the restoration of health are not always possible, another goal of nursing is to provide care for dying patients. Many persons will die in hospitals, but others, depending on circumstances, cultural practices, or disease conditions, choose to die at home. Two nurse-author-researchers worked with families of dying children to teach them to care for the child at home. They write about the comfort that both the child and the family gained from this experience when adequate support from nurses was available (Moldow and Martinson 1980). Other nurses work in agencies that plan programs of care for dying patients. Some agencies provide a place where dying patients are cared for until their death. This is called a hospice after the inns of the Middle Ages where weary travelers could find rest and refreshment. The goal of hospice programs is to assist patients and their families to prepare for death and to live as comfortably and fully as possible until death.

What Is Illness?

Like nursing, illness is defined in many ways. Some nurses view *illness* as an inability of the individual to function physically, mentally, or socially at a level that is both individually satisfying and appropriate to the stage of growth and development of the individual (Hadley, 1974). Thus, illness in a seven-year-old child may be defined in terms of an inability to attend school or play with friends. A new mother may define illness in terms of being unable to care for her infant.

Disease is the diagnosis of a particular physiological or psychological malfunction as diagnosed by a professional, usually the physician. The diagnosis of disease depends both on the *symptoms* reported by the individual and on the results of objective measurements and diagnostic tests (called *signs*).

A consideration of disease versus illness also helps to clarify the role of nursing in contrast to the role of medicine. The difference in the two professions may be thought of as the "care versus cure" dichotomy. Nursing has as its primary focus the *caring, nurturing role,* while medicine focuses on the *cure role.* Both roles overlap. Excellent nursing care includes many duties that are ordered by the physician and are directed toward cure. Similarly, physicians are dependent upon nurses to carry out the care role which is essential to the success of the physician cure role. For example, the physician makes the diagnosis that the patient has diabetes and prescribes that the patient be taught to administer a daily dose of insulin. This is the cure role. The nurse then works with the patient to assess feelings about giving self-injections, to help the person cope with the stress of self-injection, to teach injection technique, and to observe response to the medication. These activities are within the care role of nursing. Both care and cure roles are mutually supportive. The care role of nursing is seen within all four areas of nursing: maintenance of health, promotion of health, restoration of health, care of the dying.

The Experience of Stress

Psychologist Hans Selye, often called the father of stress research, gave a simple definition of stress: the rate of wear and tear on the human body (1956). A broader definition considers *stressors* to be all of those factors, either internal or external to the body, that require a response from the human being. Stressors produce the experience of stress for the individual. It is believed that all human beings need a certain amount of stress for well-being. An excess of stress creates illness and disease. *Time* magazine comments that stress is so epidemic in present society that the three best-selling drugs are an ulcer medication (TAGAMET), a drug to reduce high blood pressure (INDERAL), and a tranquilizer (VALIUM) (*Time,* 1983). There are some stressors that are shared by all human beings. Examples of these might be extreme cold, food deprivation, or the death of a loved one. Other stressors are highly individualized. One person may enjoy the experience of a mathematics examination, finding it a satisfying experience, while another person may find it difficult and emotionally draining. Another person may enjoy public speaking, while a second person dreads the occasion, becoming physically ill before the event. Individuals respond to stress both physiologically and psychologically.

Physiological Response to Stress

When a stressor affects the body, the response may be confined to a small area of the body or the response may be throughout the body. The local response is called the local adaptation syndrome (*LAS*), that is, a group of responses that confine the effects of the stressor to a small area of the body. An example of a localized adaptation response is the inflammatory response in which the body destroys or weakens the effect of the stressor. If the stressor is a bacteria that causes an infection, the body attempts to kill the bacteria and to wall off the infection, preventing its spread throughout the body. The mechanisms of this response are discussed in Chapter 18.

The general adaptation syndrome (*GAS*) is the name given to the total body response of the organism as described and defined by Selye (1956). This response has three stages. In the first stage, the alarm reaction, the body recognizes the stressor and produces body hormones essential for readying the body for action, for a "fight or flight" response. (See Figure 2–1 for a summary of the major physiological responses to severe stress.) It is during this stage that human beings have been known to perform remarkable feats of strength and courage. Stories are told of persons being able to lift a car from a trapped child, or of dragging unconscious victims long distances through a burning building. In explanation, the person will usually say, "I never even thought about it. I just did it," or "The old adrenalin was really pumping." The latter explanation is probably most accurate since increased hormones account for many of the responses. During this stage, the individual may experience increased heart rate, increased blood sugar which makes energy available, dilated pupils, slowed digestion, increased mental alertness, increased muscle strength, and increased blood clotting. This is a brief, all-out, total body effort to meet the demands of the stressor.

In the second stage, called the adaptation or resistance stage, the body attempts to return to a normal state, to repair the damage done by the stressor, and to replace the defenses used by the body in the alarm stage. If successful the symptoms of the first stage begin to lessen. If the body is unsuccessful in reversing the changes of the alarm stage, the stress response progresses.

In the final stage, the stage of exhaustion, the body is no longer able to maintain the demands of the stressor, and the body must either rest and return to normal or death may ensue. An example of exhaustion is the situation that occurs when a patient has a greatly elevated temperature which does not drop in response to medications or treatments. Ultimately neuroregulation of vital functions is destroyed and death occurs. In this case, there has been a failure of the body to adapt to a stressor.

Psychosocial Stress

Stressors that are primarily physiological in nature also have a psychosocial component. The reverse is also true. A person who suffers the pain of a stomach ulcer has a physiological condition caused by an "excess of acid and pepsin for the amount of local tissue resistance" (Robinson, 1982). Increased acid in stomach ulcers may be associated with worry over a very high-pressure job with a great demand to meet deadlines and produce maximum results. Individuals cope with psychosocial stress in many ways. There is a group of responses called defense mechanisms which the individual uses primarily to protect self-esteem. (See Chapter 31.) One example of the use of a defense mechanism is called rationalization, a technique used by everyone at some time. This is an attempt to explain or justify one's behavior without risk to one's self-esteem. The student nurse who does not pass an examination may protest, "I really knew the material, but the instructor asked such insignificant detailed questions. It really was a poor test that didn't let me show how much I really knew."

Stress also has a social component in that human beings can be stressors for each other, just as the absence

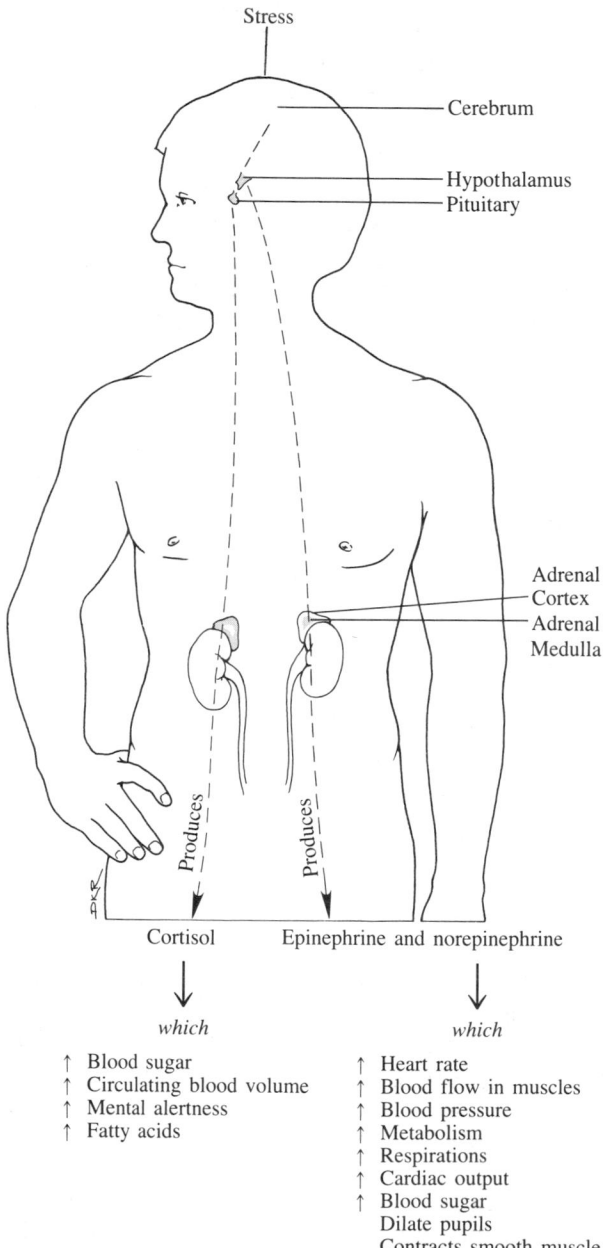

Figure 2–1. Summary of major physiological responses to severe stress.

of human beings can be a stress. The patient whose condition requires placement in a private room with no visitors soon reports loneliness and a "need for someone to talk to." Occasionally two patients who share a hospital room are incompatible. One prefers staying up late, while the other retires early. One hates the noise of televised football games, and the other patient never misses the chance to watch a game. When this situation occurs, the nurse intervenes to reduce the stress, by moving the patients, if necessary, in order that the recovery of each patient is enhanced. In planning nursing care, the nurse collects information about the stress the patient is experiencing, as well as the methods the patient is using to cope with the stress.

Who Is the Recipient of Nursing Care?

The person who receives nursing care is a unique individual, a human being who is not exactly the same as any other person. For this reason, nursing care must be designed specifically for each person, to meet the needs of a particular set of circumstances. Within the acute care setting of the hospital, the recipient of nursing care is most often called a patient. This term comes from the Latin verb *pati*, meaning to suffer, and has historically been used to mean the recipient of nursing care. Some nurses now prefer to use the term "client" because they feel that it reflects more independence and decision-making power on the part of that person. It has been suggested that the term "client" be used to denote the individual seeking health-promotion assistance from nurses. Because this textbook will focus primarily on the care of hospitalized persons, the term "patient" will be used.

By whatever term the recipient of care is designated, the important element to nursing is the individuality and uniqueness of the human being. In addition to the direct recipient of nursing care (patient), nurses also consider the needs of other people who are affected by the patient's illness or injury—the other people who love the patient and are loved by the patient. These persons are called the "primary group." For many persons the primary group consists of family members. For another person, the primary group might be several nonrelated friends at a nursing home where the patient lives. For a college student, the primary group may be several friends who share an apartment. Since human beings do not often live in isolation, it is important for the nurse to consider the effect that the illness of an individual will have on the support group. The hospitalization of the mother in a single-parent family, for example, may create additional problems that require nursing assistance.

The recipient of nursing care is also a consumer of a service with all the rights and responsibilities of a consumer. As a consumer, the patient has the right to make decisions related to care. The patient has the right to refuse nursing care, a situation that creates real difficulty for nurses who feel that they are in a position to "know what is best" for the patient. Nursing must provide a service that is of high quality, that is valued by the consumer, and that meets the needs of the public if the public is going to continue to "purchase" nursing care.

Who Is the Health Team?

As the complexity of health care has increased, many professionals, paraprofessionals, and technicians have become involved with providing health care services to patients. The group of workers providing these services is called a *health care team*. Health team members might include chaplain, dietitian, inhalation therapist, medical technologist, nurse, occupational therapist, pharmacist, physical therapist, and physician. Each of these disciplines also may have auxiliary or technical workers to support the work of the professional staff. Because the number of individuals caring for one patient is so great and is likely to increase in the future, coordination becomes a crucial function in health care. And who coordinates the work of health team members? Frequently this depends upon the nature of the need or the problem that has brought the individual into the health care system. If the major problem is within the realm of nursing, as is, for example, teaching parents to care for a chronically ill child at home, then nurses coordinate the work of health team members. At another time, such as when teaching self-care skills to a patient who recently has had a stroke, the physical therapist may coordinate health team efforts.

The Nursing Process

The practice of professional nursing requires the skills of observation, communication, thinking, applying knowledge from physical and behavioral sciences, and making decisions and judgments. The nurse uses all of these skills when applying the scientific method or the problem-solving method to planning nursing care. This is called the nursing process. It is essentially a four-step process (assessment, planning, implementation, and evaluation) which nurses use to plan the nursing care of an individual patient. Some nurses choose to break the nursing process down into five steps, separating analysis as a distinct step. It is the same process regardless of how the steps are labeled. (See Table 2–1.) It is the way one thinks and acts as a nurse. After the nurse completes the steps of the process, one result is a plan of care for a particular patient. Because the care plan is available to all members of the health team, the patient does not have to repeat the same information for several professionals. Efficiency is increased because the care plan includes the care the particular patient is to receive, as well as any modifications of the care that have been necessary or desired by the patient. Chapter 17 discussed this process in detail.

Steps in the Nursing Process

Assessment.   Assessment is the first step in the nursing process, and it consists of the activities of data collection and determining nursing diagnoses. The nurse begins data collection by gathering all relevant information about the patient. When this is completed, the nurse carefully analyzes the data and attempts to identify problems that require nursing intervention. The nurse then makes a statement of the problem and the cause, if known. This problem statement is called a nursing diagnosis.

Planning.   Having identified patient problems, the nurse determines which of the problems require immediate nursing intervention and which are less critical. This is called setting priorities. It helps the nurse to make decisions and to know where to begin nursing care. Next, the nurse sets goals related to the problems identified as nursing diagnoses. For example, if the nursing diagnosis was "pain related to surgical incision," the nurse would set a goal having to do with relief from pain within a given time period. Having established the goal, the nurse then selects a series of nursing actions that will accomplish the goal.

Implementation.   During this step of the nursing process, the nurse writes out the care plan and, if necessary, checks it with a nurse colleague for safety and appropriateness. Student nurses may request the assistance of a nursing instructor to review a care plan. The nurse is now ready to give the planned care to the patient. While giving care, the nurse continues to collect data about the patient. This data will be used to modify or add to the care plan as the patient's condition changes or as additional facts become known.

Evaluation.   The final step in the nursing process is evaluation. This involves making a judgment as to whether the stated goal was achieved. If the goal has been met, it may not be necessary to continue certain nursing actions. If the goal has not been met, it may be necessary to revise the care plan. At this time, the nurse may have additional data, or the patient's condition may have changed. These situations also may require a change in the care plan.

Table 2–1. **Comparison of Four- and Five-Step Nursing Process Formats**

Four-Step Format	Nursing Activities	Five-Step Format
1. Assessment	Collecting patient data	1. Assessment
	Writing nursing diagnosis	
2. Planning	Setting priorities	2. Analysis
	Writing patient care goals	
	Planning nursing actions	3. Planning
3. Implementation	Giving nursing care	4. Implementation
4. Evaluation	Evaluating goal achievement	5. Evaluation
	Reassessing plan of care	

Source: L. Atkinson and M. E. Murray: *Understanding the Nursing Process*, 2nd ed. Macmillan, New York, 1983.

A Framework for the Nursing Process

When the nurse begins the data collection activity of the nursing process, a systematic approach is used. Without this, the end result of data collection could be a random assortment of unrelated facts which is of little help to the nurse. There are many approaches nurses use to begin data collection. All are useful and beneficial. This book is organized around the work of psychologist Abraham Maslow. The framework of basic human needs that Maslow (1968) described is widely accepted because it can be used with many different theories of nursing without any conflict. Maslow views human beings as all sharing *basic needs* (a need is the lack of something desirable). Maslow stated that something is a basic need if:

1. Its absence breeds illness
2. Its presence prevents illness
3. Its restoration cures illness
4. Under certain conditions, it is preferred by the deprived person over other satisfactions
5. It is inactive, minimally active, or not operating in a healthy person

There are two additional characteristics that must be reported by the person experiencing the need: there is a feeling of something lacking when the need is unmet and a feeling of satisfaction when the need is met.

Although Maslow views all of the needs as existing for all human beings, he arranges the needs in hierarchical order. Needs at the lower level consist of survival needs, those basic physical needs which must be met if life and the human species are to continue. Higher level needs begin with safety and security needs and continue to higher values. (See Figure 2-2.) Maslow maintains that although some of the needs are of a higher level, they are still basic to every human being. He states, "It would not occur to anyone to question the statement that we need iron or vitamin C. I remind you that the evidence that we need love is of exactly the same type" (Maslow, 1968). Maslow views satisfaction of lower needs as facilitating growth and movement toward satisfaction of higher needs.

Physiological Needs

These are the needs that must be met, at least minimally, for survival of the body or the species. They include food, oxygen, water, temperature, elimination, rest, pain avoidance, sexual activity, mobility, and stimulation, with oxygen being the most critical of the sur-

vival needs. When a patient is first admitted to the emergency room after being in an automobile accident, medical care first centers on meeting survival needs. This may mean providing an adequate oxygen supply by giving cardiopulmonary resuscitation, giving oxygen by face mask, and stopping blood loss. After these needs are met, emergency room staff can begin to consider other needs.

Safety and Security Needs

Actions that make the person feel safe and comfortable fulfill safety and security needs. For the patient in the automobile accident, the presence of a family physician and information about the extent of personal injuries may be ways of meeting this need.

Love and Belonging Needs

To give and receive love and affection as well as to feel a part or a valued member of groups or relationships are love and belonging needs. They include such things as affection, sexual love, friendship, maternal love, and self-love. Without satisfaction of these needs, persons may feel lonely and alienated from family and friends.

Self-Esteem Needs

A person has a need to feel good about self, to feel a sense of pride in one's abilities and accomplishments. Frequently, this need is fulfilled through careers as evidenced by the fact that, upon first meeting, adults often ask each other, "What do you do?" The need for self-esteem is a powerful motivator of behavior.

Self-Actualization Needs

Self-actualization is the need to continue to grow and change, to work toward future goals, to develop talents, to develop one's potentials. When the lower needs of an individual are satisfied, the person can progress toward self-actualization. This rarely is achieved before maturity. The self-actualized adult is satisfied with accomplishments and how life has been spent. There is a sense of fulfillment and contentment.

The nurse uses the categories of human needs as a

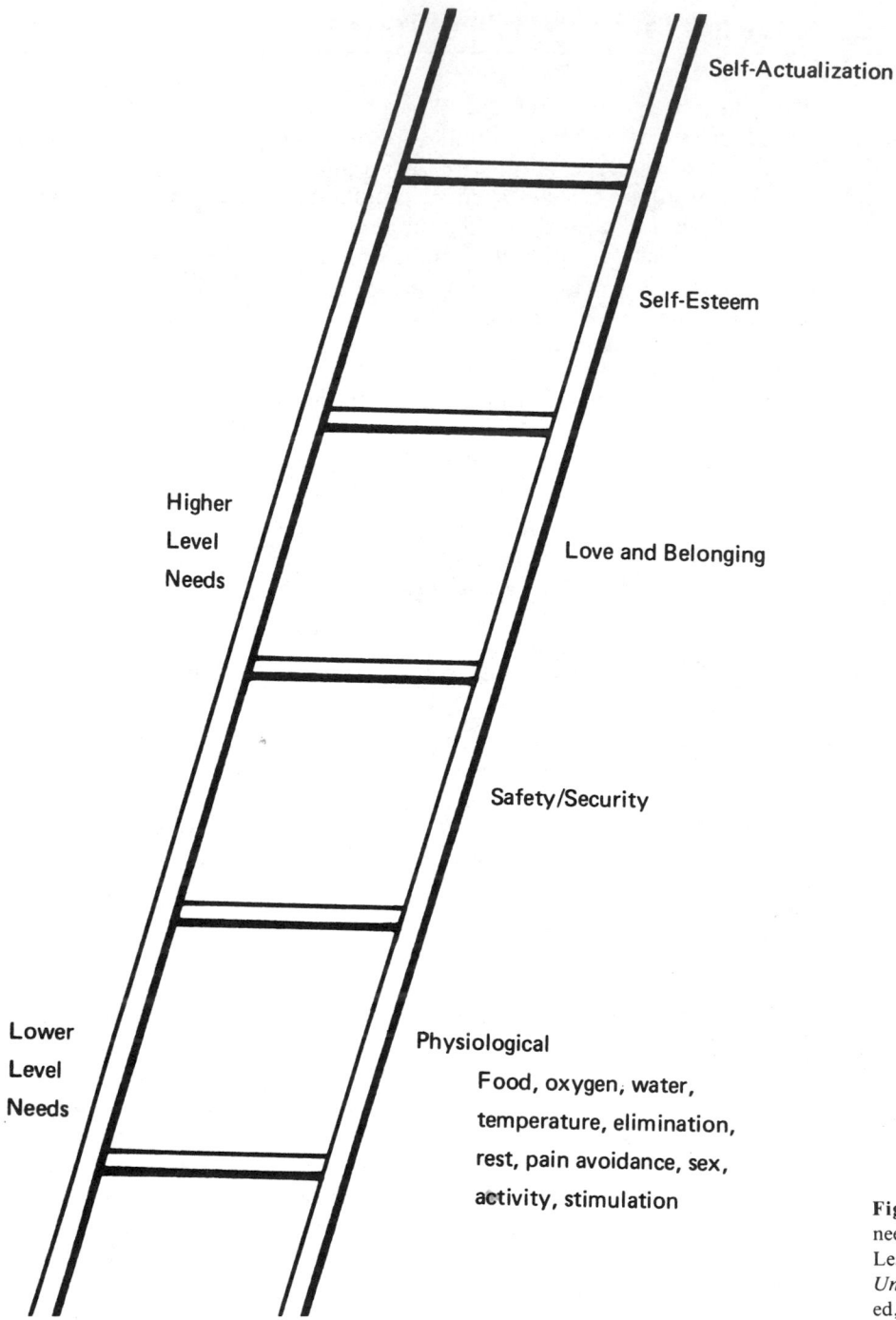

Figure 2–2. Maslow's basic human needs. (Reproduced with permission from Leslie Atkinson and Mary Ellen Murray: *Understanding the Nursing Process*, 2nd ed, Macmillan, New York, 1983, p. 14.)

guide to collect, organize, and analyze data about the patient. Then, using the ranking of needs, the nurse sets priorities for nursing care. For example, if the patient is in pain, the nurse seeks to provide pain relief before encouraging visitors to enter the room. The nurse seeks to meet lower needs at least to a minimal degree before considering higher level needs. Often a higher need af-fects a lower need (or vice versa) such that nurses must consider both needs simultaneously. In the example above, the patient may be very worried about a spouse traveling alone to the hospital. The concern for the spouse increases the pain the patient is feeling. Thus, both the need for pain relief and the need for love and belonging must be met.

Guides to Nursing Intervention

Certain guidelines must be followed no matter what type of nursing care is given to a patient. Some of the guidelines provide for the comfort and safety of the patient; others, such as documentation, in addition to contributing to patient care, serve to protect the nurse.

1. The nurse introduces self to the patient and provides an explanation of purpose, of what the nurse will be doing. In this manner, the patient has an understanding of who is responsible for care and what to expect.

2. The nurse washes hands before and after giving care to each patient. In addition to protecting both the nurse and patient from germs which are spread by the hands, the time spent handwashing provides a brief moment for the nurse to think. It may be used as time to mentally review a certain procedure, to make a schedule for a busy time, to set priorities, or to take a moment to regroup after a stressful time.

3. The nurse maintains the confidentiality of the nurse-patient relationship. The nurse does not discuss the patient or hospital situations with people who are not direct care providers in need of the information.

4. The nurse documents all nursing care and observations in the patient's permanent record. This is a legal requirement. Once written, these records are not to be changed.

5. Nursing care must be given in accordance with institutional policy. If a nurse does not agree with a certain policy, the nurse is still bound by the policy. However, the nurse may work to change the policy.

6. When in doubt—ask! And ask the appropriate person! It has been said that the only dumb question is the one you don't ask. Many lawsuits could have been avoided if the nurse had asked questions. For example, if the nurse is unsure about a medical order due to illegible handwriting, if the patient questions receiving a medication that "looks different than the one I got yesterday," if the nurse is uncertain how to operate a particular machine, *ask*! Often the best source of information or clarification is another nurse or the professional responsible for a certain aspect of the patient's care. Asking may take courage because people may respond with irritation under stress, but this is done to safeguard the patient. It is better to ask than to risk causing injury to a patient.

7. A nursing student giving patient care is held to the same legal standards as a registered nurse. The purpose of this is to guarantee the patient's safety. Any errors made while giving care or documenting care must be reported to the responsible nurse and your nursing instructor. They will help initiate any corrective measures safely and rapidly for maximum patient safety.

8. The patient has the legal right to refuse any care and may not be forced physically or threatened mentally into accepting any particular treatment.

9. The nurse has an obligation to provide optimum nursing care for the patient regardless of race, color, sex, age, or medical problem.

The Ethical Basis of Nursing

"Nurses are concerned with doing what is right when faced with the complexities of today's medical care system. Doing what is right is what ethics is all about" (Greenlaw, 1980). A nurse has an obligation to practice within the rules of moral behavior established by the profession. This collection of moral guidelines is called a code of ethics. It includes statements of good/bad, right/wrong, duty, obligation, and responsibility. The code requires that nursing practice is carried out in accordance with the provisions of the code. Failure to comply with the code may result in disciplinary actions.

In the nursing profession there are several codes of ethics that are broadly accepted. The American Nurses' Association, The Canadian Nurses' Association, and The International Council of Nurses have all published codes of ethics. The codes are intended to guide both the individual and the profession in the practice and development of nursing. Application of code statements to

difficult decisions in nursing may assist the nurse in making choices that are morally consistent with the goals of the profession and personal values.

Frequently within the practice of nursing, situations arise that place the personal values of the nurse in conflict with professional ethics. This situation is called a dilemma because the nurse is forced to make a choice that involves some action the nurse perceives as negative. There is no clear-cut right or wrong. Dilemmas occur in various forms:

- The nurse on the night shift may observe a co-worker reporting for duty while intoxicated. The person has been reported previously for the same offense, and another report will probably mean dismissal. The nurse, a single parent, begs not to be reported and promises it will not happen again.

- In another situation, a patient tells of being sexually molested by a physician but refuses to give permission to the nurse to report the incident because the patient does not want to cause trouble.

- In another instance, on a unit that is frequently understaffed, one nurse often is observed to have completed assignments well ahead of other staff and to be consistently off duty on time. A second nurse discovers that, although the duties of the first nurse are recorded as completed in patients' charts, they have not been done in fact. The first nurse argues that most of the duties were not really necessary anyway.
- In another situation, a nurse is asked to assist and provide nursing care for a patient who is about to have an abortion. The nurse believes that abortion is morally wrong and to assist and provide care is wrong.

Other ethical dilemmas may have to do with questions about the nurses' right to inform patients about alternative treatment, the exploitation of patients for the sake of learning, the alteration of notations on a patient's chart, telling the truth to patients in response to direct questions, or the observation of health team members engaged in unprofessional behavior.

In order to resolve a situation that presents a dilemma, the nurse uses a problem-solving process, similar to the nursing process applying both personal and professional codes of ethics to guide action.

Assessment. First the nurse collects all relevant data. The nurse is careful to see that all the facts are free of interpretation or judgment. Next, the nurse makes a statement of the dilemma. This statement identifies the values that are in conflict and to whom the values belong.

Planning. The nurse then identifies several possible solutions to the dilemma and attempts to anticipate the outcome of each solution. At this point, the nurse may wish to consult a colleague for professional advice, much as the nurse requests the assistance of other nurses in planning patient care. This type of consultation between nurses is of a confidential nature, and both nurses respect this. The nurse determines who is the person who must make the decision. In some cases, the best solution might be to present a responsible superior with all the facts; at other times, the physician may need to make a decision; but the nurse also may be required to make a decision alone. The nurse considers the alternative solutions and selects a course of action.

Implementation. The nurse implements the preferred solution. In some cases, a written record of the situation should be kept. This may be necessary if there is a possibility that the incident may involve lawsuits. The neces-

sity of documentation is discussed in Chapter 8, and the legal issues in Chapter 3.

Evaluation. Finally, the nurse judges the results of the action to determine if the action produced the desired results and if further action is necessary. The nurse also learns from this experience and may be able to use the experience in a similar situation at a later date.

Resolving an ethical dilemma is a difficult stressful situation for the nurse. It is helpful if the nurse has a professional support system, persons who subscribe to the same code of ethics and who will respect the need for confidentiality. However, in many situations the nurse must be prepared to make an independent decision and to accept the responsibility for the decision.

In the situation above which involved abortion, the nurse believes that abortion is morally wrong and to participate in this care is morally wrong. The additional fact is that the patient requires nursing care. The personal value of the nurse is the belief that the fetus is human life and that abortion is wrong. The code of ethics requires the nurse to provide services unrestricted by the nature of the health problem. The dilemma is a conflict between the value of the nurse that to assist in abortion is wrong and the demand of the code to provide care without regard to the nature of the health problem. There is no dilemma if the nurse is able to resolve the issue by assigning the care of the patient to an equally competent registered nurse who does not hold the same values. The dilemma results when the nurse must choose between personal values which conflict with the professional code. Because values are ranked in order of importance, one resolution the nurse might consider is reasoning that the patient is most importantly a human being entitled to safe care as a human right. The humanity of the patient may be a value that takes precedence over all else for this nurse. The nurse would then give the required care in order to respond to a higher value. Finally, the nurse evaluates the outcome of the solution. In this case, the nurse may decide that employment in this particular nursing position is likely to cause the same conflict in the future and may request a transfer to another area of the hospital. The nurse alternatively may decide that abortion is a decision that can be judged only by the individual involved, and the nurse provides care and does not judge the decision of the patient. If the latter is the evaluation, the nurse may have no difficulty working in the area in the future.

Ethical dilemmas, in varying degrees, arise in the day-to-day practice of nursing. In the future, as medical technology increases the possibility of maintaining human life under extreme conditions, even more difficult ethical decisions will face the health care professions. A very real current dilemma is the financial consideration in transplant surgery. In some instances, patients who

Exhibit 2–1. **An Ethical Dilemma**

"Gift of Life" Too Costly for Heart Patient

Jim Rohrer

A dying man finds little comfort in being at the center of a great moral issue.

Joseph Montgomery of Westwood is 35 years old, his heart is failing rapidly and unless he gets a new one he will soon die. He is another example in an expanding list of similar cases.

If his story ends happily, Montgomery could easily be little Brandon Hall of Mississippi, who needed a new liver to survive. When the first liver failed, he got a second one.

He could be Jamie Fiske of Massachusetts, whose father successfully appealed to a convention of pediatricians for the gift of life in the form of a liver donor.

He could be Apryl Graham of Alabama, who received the gift of life last December from 10-year-old Julie Hoffman of Fort Thomas, Ky. Within hours of Julie's death from a brain tumor, Apryl had received her heart in a transplant operation.

He could be Christopher Seiler, the local infant who needed a bone-marrow transplant to survive. It was accomplished with more than $100,000 in donated funds.

Montgomery has a rapidly deteriorating heart. He suffers from cardiomyopathy, a degenerative disease which affects the heart muscle. He has, at best, three to six months to live.

Only one thing can save him—a heart transplant.

Therein lies the moral issue.

"It just doesn't seem right, somehow, that only a rich person could be saved," said his wife, Deborah. "It was hard enough for me to comprehend that my husband had to have a heart transplant just to survive. Then, to realize that there is no chance for a heart transplant unless we can come up with $60,000 up front. This has sent me into outer space."

Montgomery's physician, Dr. Ali Razavi, could not be reached Thursday, but Ron Dreffer, transplant coordinator for the University of Cincinnati Medical Center, called Montgomery's plight "probably the greatest moral issue in medicine today.

"I know of no hospital insurance which will cover heart transplant because it is classed as experimental surgery. And yet, a new antirejection drug has been found to reduce rejection of most organs dramatically.

"So what is happening, not only here in Cincinnati, but across the nation, is that the same questions are being asked that were asked years ago about kidney transplants.

"Who gets the transplant? What about the others who need them? Should somebody step in and help pay for this? Should less money be spent on costly, experimental procedures, and more on preventative medicine?"

The Montgomerys have medical insurance, through Deborah's employment at the UC College of Medicine. The policy would pay up to $500,000 for related medical expenses in the event of a heart transplant, but the operation itself would not be covered.

The couple has been referred to the University of Pittsburgh Hospital for the transplant procedure. Officials there said it would require a $60,000 deposit before Montgomery could be placed on a waiting list.

"As far as we know, there are no insurance programs commonly available which cover such surgery," said David Hillman of CORVA, the regional health planning agency.

"The issue has developed into a sticky one," he said. "The cost of medical care is rising terribly. A moral question—the right to health care—has become entangled with economics. It's crazy."

Dreffer said community fund-raising efforts (which occurred in the Brandon Hall case, and locally in the Christopher Seiler case) are often the only solution. "It's starting to happen more and more," he said.

"In the case of kidney transplants, the federal government stepped in about 10 years ago and provided funding through Medicare. That has not happened for heart and liver transplants, though there has been a lot of pressure on Congress recently for similar action."

Some of that pressure was applied recently by Billie Hall, Brandon's mother, who appealed to Congress to allow federal medical programs to cover the enormous cost of organ transplants.

Montgomery has not worked in more than a year as his condition worsened.

"He's in Good Samaritan hospital now, and it's the fourth time he's been in since January," his wife said. "He's getting weaker and he feels a lot of pain. The crazy thing is, the insurance has already paid about half what we wanted for the heart transplant in the first place. Sometimes, it just doesn't make sense."

Dr. Thomas Peters, a Cincinnati native, is a member of the three-person transplantation team from the University of Tennessee Center for the Health Sciences which performed the two liver transplants on Brandon Hall in Memphis, Tenn.

"A heart transplant is one of three or four transplant operations which are literally life-saving operations," he said. "While the government and the insurance companies regard them as experimental, the fact is, if a patient doesn't get a heart transplant, or a liver transplant, he dies. There is no other way to keep them alive.

"Denying such operations by not making funds available is often more expensive than permitting them to proceed with funding," he said.

"Then, there is an enormous amount of strain on the transplant teams, too," he said. "How would you like to be the surgeon who tells a dying patient he can't have a transplant operation?"

"What is needed," he said, "is more recognition by the public that every person is a walking bundle of spare parts. It will take an educational effort to alert people that when they can no longer use their hearts, or livers, other people can use them."

Source: *Cincinnati Enquirer,* April 29, 1983. Reprinted with permission.

require an organ transplant are required to demonstrate their ability to pay or "put down" thousands of dollars before they will be considered as a recipient. A very real ethical question is: Is the right to highly expensive care determined by who can afford to pay? (See Exhibit 2–1.)

It is important that nurses understand both their own value system and the code of ethics in order to prepare for this type of decision making. Much of the legal aspects of the practice of nursing is inseparably related to ethical behavior. This is further discussed in Chapter 3.

Education for Nursing Practice

A student selecting a nursing career may choose among several types of educational programs. Each of the following programs prepares a person to become a "registered nurse," although their education may be very different. Each type of educational program prepares a statement of the skills of the graduate of that

---

Exhibit 2–2. Competencies of the Associate Degree Nurse on Entry into Practice

Assumptions Basic to the Scope of Practice

The practice of graduates of associate degree nursing programs:

• Is directed toward clients who need information or support to maintain health

• Is directed toward clients who are in need of medical diagnostic evaluation and/or are experiencing acute or chronic illness

• Is directed toward clients' responses to common, well-defined health problems

• Includes the formulation of a nursing diagnosis

• Consists of nursing interventions selected from established nursing protocols where probable outcomes are predictable

• Is concerned with individual clients and is given with consideration of the person's relationship within a family, group, and community

• Includes the safe performance of nursing skills that require cognitive, psychomotor, and affective capabilities

• May be in any structured care setting but primarily occurs within acute- and extended-care facilities

• Is guided directly or indirectly by a more experienced registered nurse

• Includes the direction of peers or other workers in nursing in selected aspects of care within the scope of practice of associate degree nursing

• Involves an understanding of the roles and responsibilities of self and other workers within employment setting

Roles of Practice

Five interrelated roles have been defined for graduates of the associate degree nursing program based upon the above assumptions underlying the scope of practice. These roles are provider of care, client teacher, communicator, manager of client care, and member within the profession of nursing. In each of these roles, decisions and practice are

determined on the basis of knowledge and skills, the nursing process, and established protocols of the setting.

Role as a Provider of Care. As a provider of nursing care, the associate degree nursing graduate uses the nursing process to formulate and maintain individualized nursing care plans.

Assessment

• Collects and contributes to a data base (physiological, emotional, sociological, cultural, psychological, and spiritual needs) from available resources (e.g., client, family, medical records, and other health team members)

• Identifies and documents changes in health status which interfere with the client's ability to meet basic needs (e.g., oxygen, nutrition, elimination, activity, safety, rest and sleep, and psychosocial well-being)

• Establishes a nursing diagnosis based on client needs

Planning

• Develops individualized nursing care plans based upon the nursing diagnosis and plans intervention that follows established nursing protocols

• Identifies needs and establishes priorities for care with recognition of client's level of development and needs, and with consideration of client's relationship within a family, group, and community

• Participates with clients, families, significant others, and members of the nursing team to establish long- and short-range client goals

• Identifies criteria for evaluation of individualized nursing care plans

Implementation

Carries out individualized plans of care according to priority of needs and established nursing protocols

Participates in the prescribed medical regime by preparing, assisting, and providing follow-up care to clients undergoing diagnostic and/or therapeutic procedures

Uses nursing knowledge and skills and protocols to assure an environment conductive to optimum restoration and maintenance of the client's normal abilities to meet basic needs

- Maintains and promotes respiratory function (e.g., oxygen therapy, positioning, etc.)
- Maintains and promotes nutritional status (e.g., dietary regimes, supplemental therapy, intravenous infusions, etc.)
- Maintains and promotes elimination (e.g., bowel and bladder regimes, forcing fluids, enemas, etc.)
- Maintains and promotes a balance of activity, rest, and sleep (e.g., planned activities of daily living, environmental adjustment, exercises, sensory stimuli, assistive devices, etc.)
- Maintains an environment that supports physiological functioning, comfort, and relief of pain
- Maintains and promotes all aspects of hygiene
- Maintains and promotes physical safety (e.g., implementation of medical and surgical aseptic techniques, etc.)
- Maintains and promotes psychological safety through consideration of each individual's worth and dignity and applies nursing measures that assist in reducing common developmental and situational stress
- Measures basic physiological functioning and reports significant findings (e.g., vital signs, fluid intake and output)
- Administers prescribed medications safely

Intervenes in situations where:

- Basic life support systems are threatened (e.g., cardiopulmonary resuscitation, obstructive airway maneuver)
- Untoward physiological or psychological reactions are probable
- Changes in normal behavior patterns have occurred

Participates in established institutional emergency plans

Evaluation

- Uses established criteria for evaluation of individualized nursing care
- Participates with clients, families, significant others, and members of the nursing team in the evaluation of established long- and short-range client goals.
- Identifies alternate methods of meeting client's needs, modifies plans of care as necessary, and documents changes

Role as a Communicator. As a communicator, the associate degree nursing graduate:

- Assesses verbal and nonverbal communication of clients, families, and significant others based upon knowledge and techniques of interpersonal communication
- Uses lines of authority and communication within the work setting
- Uses communication skills as a method of data collection, nursing intervention, and evaluation of care

- Communicates and records assessments, nursing care plans, interventions, and evaluations accurately and promptly
- Establishes and maintains effective communication with clients, families, significant others, and health team members
- Communicates client's needs through the appropriate use of referrals
- Evaluates effectiveness of one's own communication with clients, colleagues, and others

Role as a Client Teacher. As a teacher of clients who need information or support to maintain health, the associate degree nursing graduate:

- Assesses situations in which clients need information or support to maintain health
- Develops short-range teaching plans based upon long- and short-range goals for individual clients
- Implements teaching plans that are specific to the client's level of development and knowledge
- Supports and reinforces the teaching plans of other health professionals
- Evaluates the effectiveness of client's learning

Role as a Manager of Client Care. As a manager of nursing care for a group of clients with common, well-defined health problems in structured settings, the associate degree nursing graduate:

- Assesses and sets nursing care priorities
- With guidance, provides client care utilizing resources and other nursing personnel commensurate with their educational preparation and experience
- Seeks guidance to assist other nursing personnel to develop skill in giving nursing care

Role as a Member Within the Profession of Nursing. As a member within the profession of nursing the associate degree nursing graduate:

- Is accountable for his or her nursing practice
- Practices within the profession's ethical and legal framework
- Assumes responsibility for self-development and uses resources for continued learning
- Consults with a more experienced registered nurse when client's problems are not within the scope of practice
- Participates within a structured role in research (e.g., data collection)
- Works within the policies of the employee or employing institution
- Recognizes policies and nursing protocols that may impede client care and works within the organizational framework to initiate change

Source: Competencies of the associate degree nurse on entry into practice. © 1978 by the National League for Nursing. Pub. no. 23-1731.

Exhibit 2–3. **Role and Competencies of Graduates of Diploma Programs in Nursing**

The graduate of the diploma program in nursing is eligible to seek licensure as a registered nurse and to function as a beginning practitioner in acute, intermediate, long-term, and ambulatory health care facilities. In order to fulfill such roles, graduates should demonstrate the following competencies.*

Assessment

- Establishes a data base through a nursing history including a psychosocial and physical assessment
- Utilizes knowledge of the etiology, pathophysiology, usual course, and prognosis for the prevalent illnesses and health problems
- Establishes priorities when providing nursing care for one or more patients
- Recognizes the significance of nonverbal communication

Planning

- Formulates a written plan of nursing care based on the assessment of patient needs
- Includes in the nursing care plan the effects of the family or significant others, life experiences, and socio-cultural background
- Involves the patient, family, and significant others in the development of the nursing plan of care
- Incorporates the learning needs of the patient and family into an individualized plan of care
- Applies principles of organization and management in utilizing the knowledge and skills of other nursing personnel

Implementation

- Meets the health needs of individuals and families
- Utilizes concepts, scientific facts, and principles when providing nursing care
- Performs technical nursing procedures
- Initiates appropriate intervention when environmental and safety hazards exist
- Initiates preventive, habilitative, and rehabilitative nursing measures according to the needs demonstrated by patients and families
- Performs independent nursing measures and/or seeks assistance from other members of the health team in response to the changing needs of patients

- Collaborates with physicians and members of other disciplines to provide health care
- Documents nursing interventions and patient responses
- Utilizes effective verbal and written communication
- Communicates pertinent information related to the patient through established channels
- Assists the physician in implementing the medical plan of care
- Applies knowledge of individual and group behavior in establishing interpersonal relationships
- Teaches individuals and groups to achieve and maintain an optimum level of wellness
- Utilizes the services of community agencies for continuity of patient care
- Protects the rights of patients and families

Evaluation

- Evaluates the effectiveness of nursing care and takes appropriate action
- Initiates and cooperates in efforts to improve nursing practice

Professionalism

- Recognizes the legal limits of nursing practice
- Demonstrates ethical behavior in the performance of nursing
- Practices nursing in a nondiscriminatory and non-judgmental manner
- Respects the rights of others to have their own value systems
- Accepts responsibility and accountability for professional practice
- Pursues independent study and continuing education
- Demonstrates flexibility in functioning in a changing society
- Adjusts with minimal difficulty to the role of employee

This revised statement by the Council of Diploma Programs in Nursing, National League for Nursing, was approved at the Council's April 1978 meeting.

Source: Role and competencies of graduates of diploma programs in nursing. Copyright 1978 by the National League for Nursing. Pub. no. 16–1735.

*Competency, as used in this document, is the ability to apply in practice situations the essential principles and techniques of nursing and to apply those concepts, skills, and attitudes required of all nurses to fulfill their role, regardless of specific position or responsibility.

program. These are called competencies. The competencies of three types of programs are included in Exhibits 2-2 to 2-4.

Associate Degree Nursing Program.   This program is approximately two academic years in length and is offered in community colleges and universities. Course work consists of about one-half nursing courses and one-half supportive courses in the arts and sciences. Upon graduation, an associate degree is awarded by the college.

Diploma Nursing Program. This program is approximately three years in length and is offered by a hospital-based nursing school, frequently in cooperation with a university or community college. This program is under

---

Exhibit 2–4. Characteristics of Baccalaureate Education in Nursing

The baccalaureate program in nursing, which is offered by a senior college or university, provides students with an opportunity to acquire (1) knowledge of the theory* and practice of nursing; (2) competency in selecting, synthesizing, and applying relevant information from various disciplines; (3) ability to assess client needs and provide nursing interventions; (4) ability to provide care for groups of clients; (5) ability to work with and through others; (6) ability to evaluate current practices and try new approaches; (7) competency in collaborating with members of other health disciplines and with consumers; (8) an understanding of the research process and its contribution to nursing practice; (9) knowledge of the broad function the nursing profession is expected to perform in society; and (10) a foundation for graduate study in nursing.

Nurses are prepared as generalists at the baccalaureate level to provide within the health care system† a comprehensive service of assessing, promoting, and maintaining the health of individuals and groups. These nurses are prepared to (1) be accountable for their own nursing practice; (2) accept responsibility for the provision of nursing care through others; (3) accept the advocacy role in relation to clients; and (4) develop methods of working collaboratively with other health professionals. They will practice in a variety of health care settings—hospital, home, and community—and emphasize comprehensive health care, including prevention, health promotion, and rehabilitation services; health counseling and education; and care in acute and long-term illness.

Baccalaureate nursing programs are conceptually organized to be consistent with the stated philosophy and objectives of the parent institution and the unit in nursing. These programs provide the general and professional education essential for understanding and respecting people, various cultures, and environments; for acquiring and utilizing nursing theory upon which nursing practice is based; and for promoting self-understanding, personal fulfillment, and motivation for continued learning. The structure of the baccalaureate degree program in nursing follows the same pattern as that of baccalaureate education in general. It is characterized by a liberal education at the lower division level, on which is built the upper division major. In baccalaureate nursing education, the lower division consists of foundational courses drawn primarily from the scientific and humanistic disciplines inherent in liberal learning. The major in nursing is built upon this lower division general education base and is concentrated at the upper division level. Upper division studies include courses that complement the nursing component or increase the depth of general education.

Consistent with the foregoing characteristics and directly related to the Criteria for the Appraisal of Baccalaureate and Higher Degree Programs in Nursing, the graduate of the baccalaureate program in nursing is able to:

• Utilize nursing theory in making decisions on nursing practice

• Use nursing practice as a means of gathering data for refining and extending that practice

• Synthesize theoretical and empirical knowledge from the physical and behavioral sciences and humanities with nursing theory and practice

• Assess health status and health potential; plan, implement, and evaluate nursing care of individuals, families, and communities

• Improve service to the client by continually evaluating the effectiveness of nursing intervention and revising it accordingly

• Accept individual responsibility and accountability for the choice of nursing intervention and its outcome

• Evaluate research for the applicability of its findings to nursing actions

• Utilize leadership skills through involvement with others in meeting health needs and nursing goals

• Collaborate with colleagues and citizens on the interdisciplinary health team to promote the health and welfare of people

• Participate in identifying and effecting needed change to improve delivery within specific health care systems

• Participate in identifying community and societal health needs and in designing nursing roles to meet these needs

These characteristics were developed by the professional nurse membership of the Council of Baccalaureate and Higher Degree Programs and are an expression of professional accountability to the consumer, both student and client. This statement by the Council of Baccalaureate and Higher Degree Programs is a revision of a 1974 statement and was approved at the Council's November 1978 meeting.

*Throughout this statement, theory is used in the universal sense as it applies to all disciplines.

†The health care system includes social, cultural, economic, and political components. It can be conceptualized from an individual perspective of nurse and client/family to the broad, national health care scene. For the most part, the graduates of baccalaureate programs in nursing work within the local health care system although fully aware of the regional and national health care scenes. The master's graduates in nursing are proficient in working within the local health care system and have learned to extend their influence and effectiveness to and through the regional and national levels.

Source: Characteristics of baccalaureate education in nursing. Copyright 1978 by the National League for Nursing. Pub. no. 15-1758.

the support of a hospital organization where students take clinical nursing courses. Upon successful completion of the program, a diploma in nursing is awarded.

Baccalaureate Degree Nursing Program.   This program is approximately four academic years in length and is offered in colleges and universities. Course work is divided between nursing and the arts and sciences. A baccalaureate degree is awarded by the college upon graduation.

Upon successful completion of one of the above programs, the student may apply to take the examination for licensure to become a registered nurse. It is an important distinction to make that licensure is a function of the state or government and is not conferred by the educational program.

Graduate Study.   Nurses who have completed a baccalaureate degree may choose advanced academic preparation which results in a master's or doctoral degree in nursing. This student may choose a clinical specialty such as pediatric or mental health nursing, or may prepare for nurse faculty positions, leadership, or administrative careers within nursing.

Nursing Organizations

Nursing organizations have united the efforts of individual nurses to advance the profession of nursing and to safeguard the rights of nurses. Some of the activities of nursing organizations include initiating and supporting health care legislation, establishing and interpreting ethical codes for the profession, expanding nursing knowledge by supporting nursing research, setting standards for nursing care, promoting the economic welfare of nurses.

International Council of Nurses

The ICN was founded in 1899 and today has a membership of 95 nations. The purpose of the ICN is to provide an organization through which the national nursing associations can work together. The headquarters of the ICN is in Geneva, Switzerland.

American Nurses' Association

The ANA is the professional organization for nurses in the United States. It was founded in 1896. It is made up of the state nursing associations from all 50 states and Guam, the Virgin Islands, and Puerto Rico. It has approximately 160,000 nurse members. The purposes of the ANA are to:

Work for the improvement of health care standards and the availability of health care for all people
Foster higher standards of nursing
Stimulate and promote the professional development of nurses
Advance the economic and general welfare of nurses

Canadian Nurses' Association

The CNA is the professional nursing association of Canada. It has both provincial and local organizations and has a membership of about 132,000 nurses. The CNA is a federation of ten provincial associations and the Northwest Territories Nurses' Association. The objectives of the CNA are concerned with:

Quality and quantity of nurses available to the health team
Standard of preparation and performance of professional nurses
Social and economic welfare of nurses
Advancement of knowledge within the profession
Representing the nursing profession

National League for Nursing

The membership of the NLN is composed of both nurses and non-nurses. It was founded in 1952. The purpose of the NLN is to promote the development of both nursing service and nursing education. The NLN accredits nursing schools as one way of developing and maintaining quality nursing education. This accreditation is voluntary and is not a requirement of the state.

Nursing Student Organizations

Both the United States and Canada have national nursing student associations. These are organized in much the same manner as the nurses' organizations. They seek to represent the student nurses of the country and focus on the needs of nursing students.

Summary

The unique function of nursing, as described by the International Council of Nurses, is "to assist the individual, sick or well, in the performance of those activities contributing to health or its recovery (or to a peaceful death) that he would perform unaided if he had the necessary strength, will or knowledge." The activities of the nursing role focus around the maintenance of health, promotion of health, restoration of health, and care of the dying.

Stress, the "wear and tear on the human body" is an experience common to all persons. Human beings respond to stress at both a local level (local adaptation syndrome) and at a total body level (generalized adaptation syndrome). Stress has both physiological and psychosocial components.

The nursing process is a systematic method of using the problem-solving process in providing patient care. It consists of four steps: assessment, planning, implementation, and evaluation. The nurse uses the nursing process to plan nursing care for individual patients. When planning nursing care, the nurse uses a systematic approach to data collection. One such approach uses the theory of basic human needs of psychologist Maslow. The human needs identified by Maslow are survival or physiological needs, safety and security, love and belonging, self-esteem, self-actualization. The nurse collects data in each of the categories whenever possible and appropriate.

The nursing process also can be applied to the resolution of ethical dilemmas in nursing. The nurse's ethical behavior is guided by a professional code of ethics.

Education for nursing practice occurs in a variety of programs: diploma, associate degree, and baccalaureate. Competencies for the graduate of each program are included within the chapter.

Nursing organizations, national and international, exist to advance the profession of nursing and to safeguard the rights of nurses.

Terms for Review

basic need	GAS	illness	patient
care versus cure role	health	LAS	signs
code of ethics	health care team	nursing	stressor
disease	holistic	nursing process	symptoms

Learning Activities

1. State your own definition of nursing, health.
2. State the term you will use to designate the recipient of nursing care, and give the reasons for your choice.
3. State your reasons for selecting your nursing educational program, and reasons why you did not select the alternatives.
4. Attend a local meeting of a national nursing students' organization, and find out the benefits and responsibilities of membership.

Review Questions

1. Most of the public's expectation of nursing has been
   a. Health promotion
   b. Illness care
   c. Care of the dying patient
2. Licensure to practice nursing as a registered nurse is conferred:
   a. By the state
   b. By the university upon graduation
   c. By the academic program upon successful completion of requirements
3. The nursing process is best described as:
   a. A written care plan
   b. Synonymous with the scientific method
   c. The way one thinks and acts as a nurse
4. The physician role is to cure as the nursing role is to:
   a. The nursing process
   b. Care
   c. Assessment
   d. Adaptation
5. The purpose of a Code of Ethics is to:
   a. Provide disciplinary measures against nurses who do not adhere to it
   b. Form the foundations of national nursing associations
   c. Identify values and attitudes appropriate to the nursing profession
   d. Guide nurses in making moral choices in the practice of nursing

Answers

1. b
2. a
3. c
4. b
5. d

Suggested Readings

Dillon, A.: Reducing your stress. *Nurs. Life,* **3**(3):17–24, May/June, 1983. Six experts tell how to recognize stress and describe several strategies for dealing with it.

Lee, A.: A celebration of life. *RN,* **44**(8): 25-28, Aug., 1981. Nurses from the United States tell what is right about nursing.

References and Bibliography

American Nurses' Association: *Bylaws.* Kansas City, Mo., 1980.

Atkinson, L., and Murray, M. E.: *Understanding the Nursing Process,* 2nd ed. Macmillan, New York, 1983.

Canadian Nurses' Association: *The Canadian Nurses' Association.* Ottawa, Ontario, Canada, 1982.

DeYoung, L.: *Dynamics of Nursing,* 4th ed. Mosby, St. Louis, 1981.

Greenlaw, J.: To whom is the nurse accountable. *Nurs. Law and Ethics.* **1** (1):3, Jan. 1980.

Hadley, B.: Current concepts of wellness and illness; Their relevance for nursing. *Image,* 6(2):24, 1974.

Henderson, V.: *The Nature of Nursing.* Macmillan, New York, 1978.

International Council of Nurses. Geneva, Switzerland.

Maslow, A.: *Toward a Psychology of Being.* Van Nostrand, New York, 1968.

Mitchel, P., and Loustau, Anne: *Concepts Basic to Nursing,* 3rd ed. McGraw-Hill, New York, 1981.

Moldow, D., and Martinson, I.: *From Research to Reality—Home Care for the Dying Child, Matern. Child Nurs. J.,* **5**:139-60t, 1980.

Murray, R., and Zentner, J.: *Nursing Concepts for Health Promotion,* 2nd ed. Prentice-Hall, Englewood Cliffs, N.J., 1979.

Orem, D.: *Concepts of Practice,* 2nd ed., McGraw-Hill, 1980.

Riehl, J., and Roy, Sister Callista: *Conceptual Models for Nursing Practice,* 2nd ed., Appleton-Century-Crofts, New York, 1980.

Robinson, C., and Lawler, M.: *Normal and Therapeutic Nutrition,* 16th ed. Macmillan, New York, 1982.

Roy, C.: *Introduction to Nursing: An Adaptation Model.* Prentice Hall, Englewood Cliffs, N.J., 1976.

Selye, H.: *The Stress of Life.* 2nd ed. McGraw-Hill, New York, 1978.

Thompson, J., and Thompson, H.: *Ethics in Nursing.* Macmillan, New York, 1981.

Wallis, C.: Stress: Can we cope. *Time,* **121**:48–54 June 6, 1983.

LEGAL ISSUES IN NURSING PRACTICE*

Objectives

1. Identify the reasons malpractice litigation against nurses has increased.
2. Enumerate and distinguish the three types of torts for which nurses can be held liable by patients.
3. Describe the five elements of negligent nursing practice that a plaintiff must prove to establish liability for negligence.
4. Discuss the four types of intentional torts for which nurses are most often found liable.

*Written by Stephen R. Bergerson, B.A., J.D., an Associate Professor and past president of the faculty at Metropolitan State University, and an Adjunct Professor of Law at William Mitchell College of Law in St. Paul, Minnesota. He practices law with Kinney and Lange, P.A., in Minneapolis. He is a contributing author of nursing law articles to nursing magazines and journals, and is a consultant on nursing law to many universities and hospitals. He frequently conducts workshops throughout the country.

5. Describe how a jury determines the appropriate standard of care in a malpractice trial.
6. Differentiate between the function of an expert witness and other witnesses in a malpractice trial.
7. List areas of practice where nurses are most vulnerable to charges of malpractice.
8. Specify the six elements of a nursing malpractice prevention program.

Malpractice: The Need to Recognize and Deal Effectively with It

Malpractice law is not something that nurses care to think about, much less study. But malpractice is an unavoidable fact of life. It is a word which has become embedded in the fabric of the delivery of health care. This chapter is designed to demonstrate the need to understand the law of malpractice. The principles of malpractice law will be explained, examples offered, and suggestions made as to how nurses can constructively use the law to safeguard the interests of patients and themselves. Guidelines for creating an effective malpractice prevention program also will be identified and discussed.

Malpractice: What Is It?

Not only is malpractice quite new to nurses, it is a relatively new word in the history of the law itself. It has quickly become an important area of law. Simply put, *malpractice* is negligence.

But it is not just *any* negligence. It is negligence on the part of a professional. When society relies on people with special training and education and those people practice their profession "badly" (negligently), they are liable for their bad (*mal*) practice. Such liability results in the legal duty to pay money damages to a person who has been injured because of the malpractice.

Malpractice and the Nursing Student

It is important to understand that nursing students who perform nursing tasks and procedures are legally responsible for their own acts of negligence. When acting under the direction of a licensed nurse, they are held to the same standard of care as the licensed nurse who normally would perform the function. In other words, even though nursing students are not licensed to practice, the law nonetheless holds them to a standard which assumes they are. The rationale is based on the notion that the patient should not be required to expect less simply because a task or procedure has been delegated to an unlicensed person. Thus, the principles of malpractice are directly applicable to the nursing student. Furthermore, nursing students are deemed to be employees of the hospital at which they work. This is true even though they are working at the hospital on affiliation and not, in fact, as employees. Again, the rationale is to protect the patient. Since the hospital is considered the employer, it is liable, along with the student nurse, for any patient injury caused by the student nurse's negligence.

Most hospitals that permit nursing students to work require that the students maintain their own personal malpractice insurance coverage.

Malpractice: Why Nurses Are Being Sued

Malpractice reflects our society's response to, among other things, changes that have taken place in the health care industry. Understanding the reasons health care practitioners are being sued with increasing frequency not only helps put the problem in perspective, but clearly identifies opportunities for the individual nurse to deal effectively with it.

Greater Expectations

The many considerable advances in health care—new technology, surgical techniques, treatment procedures, and medications—along with attendant exposure by the news and entertainment media, have led the public to expect much of its health care providers—perhaps too much. What do these expectations have to do with lawsuits? As expectations increase, so does the likelihood of disappointment. As disappointment increases, so does the likelihood of anger. And as the likelihood of anger increases, so do the chances of a lawsuit. Nurses, therefore, should take care not to encourage unrealistically high expectations on the part of the patient.

New Rights-Oriented Patients

Patients are consumers. They learned from the massive social revolution of the 1970s, called consumerism, that they have *consumer rights*. They feel entitled to quality health care and good results. They are often pre-occupied with getting what is theirs and getting revenge if they don't. The consumerism movement taught them that they are entitled to relevant information, reasonable precautions to protect their safety, the right to express themselves, and the right to choose from among reasonable options.

New Litigation-Oriented Patients

Increasingly, patients have not gotten what they expect and feel entitled to. Their dissatisfaction has brought about the ultimate patient rebellion: malpractice suits. They want to "get even." And getting even in our society has increasingly meant bringing a lawsuit. Until recent times, Americans viewed courts as a last resort. Now, litigation is one of the first thoughts to enter an unhappy consumer's mind. Today's consumers are no longer willing to show physicians, nurses, and other professionals the deference they have enjoyed historically.

New and Greater Risks

Innovative technology, medicines, and surgical and treatment procedures have done more than increase performance expectations. They have also introduced new and greater risks. Inevitably, some of these risks materialize and contribute to patient dissatisfaction. Innovative care has also introduced another important factor into the malpractice equation: dramatically increased costs. When consumers pay more, they demand more. The cost of health care has become a visible and controversial public issue.

Perceived Lack of Sufficient Interest

Today's nurse is busier than ever. The time available to spend on a per-patient basis has decreased as the nurse's role has expanded. Consider that patients come into the hospital with a set of feelings no one enjoys: anxiety, fear, pain, disorientation, and the knowledge that they are expected to relinquish a large part of their independence to a group of total strangers. They know that they are supposed to be a "good patient." They feel entitled, therefore, to expect certain things in return. They expect a technically competent nurse who knows what to do and how and when to do it. But they also expect a nurse who cares, who is interested and concerned. They expect to be treated as an individual, not just as a medical problem.

Often, however, because of staffing shortages, work load, and increased responsibilities, today's nurse may not *appear* to be as interested or care as much as the patient expects. And there is no difference, from the patient's perspective, between a nurse who appears not to care and a nurse who does not care. Many hospitals have effectively incorporated the idea of the nurse who cares into advertising campaigns. Their marketing information has identified an issue their consumers feel strongly about: how nurses would treat them.

Just as some patients are more inclined than most others to sue, some nurses are more likely than others to get sued. Against whom is a patient more likely to seek revenge if they are disappointed with the results: a nurse who is friendly, patient, open and honest, concerned, and interested? Or the nurse who is impersonal, abrupt, guarded, insensitive, and distant? Which of the two is most likely to be the cause of disappointment, the target of anger, and the defendant in a malpractice suit?

Simply put, patients tend not to sue people they perceive as friends. They are inclined to forgive rather than seek revenge, even when a mistake has been made. The nurse who regularly makes an effort to *show* interest and concern is serving not only the patient's best interest, but the nurse's as well. It is the least expensive, yet most effective malpractice insurance a nurse can get. It is important to remember that, just as there are *suit-prone patients,* there are *suit-prone nurses.*

Malpractice Publicity

The early lawsuits against nurses were new and newsworthy. The media coverage of those suits served to identify nurses as legitimate litigants in malpractice proceedings. It served to encourage others to name nurses as defendants. Large, well-publicized awards of damages, coupled with the news that many nurses were carrying malpractice insurance, made a previously disregarded class of health care professionals a more visible and vulnerable group to dissatisfied patients and their attorneys.

More Malpractice Lawyers

As malpractice suits were brought and won, more and more attorneys have been attracted to this area of practice. There are now more attorneys with the interest and requisite expertise in malpractice litigation than ever before. Although this is a factor in the increase in the number of suits brought against nurses, it is not the cause of the problem. Lawyers do not cause the incidents nor create the dissatisfaction that provokes a patient to sue. Lawyers can only take the facts as they find them and present them to a jury, which also hears testimony from expert witnesses before deciding whether the nurse met or fell short of the standards of nursing care.

Expanded Nursing Roles

Nurses in recent years have been challenging the physician's traditional role as controller of health care delivery. They have gained, for a variety of reasons, a more significant role as members of the health care team.

As nursing's role has expanded, nurses have become professionals in their own right. They have become responsible for exercising their own professional judgment and discretion. This autonomy has been accompanied by accountability. Accountability carries with it the prospect for liability (the legal duty to be answerable for one's own conduct and judgment). No other single reason has played a greater role in the increase of nursing malpractice litigation than the expanded role of the nurse.

Malpractice Law: Where it Comes from

The Criminal Law

Laws are one of two general types: criminal or civil. Criminal laws are those that are enacted by elected public bodies. They identify types of conduct that are so wrong that they are deemed injurious not only to the immediate victim, but to the public as a whole.

The offender is prosecuted by the government through the appropriate law enforcement office, such as the city or county attorney, and punished according to the law. Malpractice is not a part of the criminal law. Nurses are seldom involved with criminal charges arising from their nursing responsibilities. Criminal laws do require certain conduct of nurses, however, and carry penalties for noncompliance. They will be discussed later in this chapter.

The Civil Law

Civil law is not designed to protect the public interest. It is designed to protect individuals. When a person fails to meet a legal responsibility and violates another's civil (private, as distinguished from public) rights, the wrongdoer must compensate the other for any resulting injury. Malpractice is a part of the civil law. When professionals negligently injure someone, they have violated that person's civil rights.

The amount of damages due in such an event is usually dependent on the loss that the plaintiff (person bringing a lawsuit) can prove. Such loss may be in the form of wages, medical bills, expected loss of future earnings, or, more difficult to evaluate, pain and suffering, loss of reputation, or embarrassment. The amount of damages that the defendant (person being sued) owes the plaintiff is the amount needed to compensate the plaintiff for the loss attributable to the injury. Civil law seeks to reimburse the plaintiff. Criminal law, on the other hand, seeks to punish the defendant. Many kinds of conduct may violate both the criminal law and an individual's private civil rights. In such instances, the wrongdoer is subject to criminal proceedings brought by the government and to separate civil proceedings brought by the victim.

All laws, whether criminal or civil, come from one of three sources: constitutions, legislation, or the common law.

The Constitution

Neither the United States Constitution or the various state constitutions provide patients with a legal basis for suits against nurses. Although they create important legal rights and responsibilities and provide the foundation for our government and system of justice, the rights created are not of the type that directly pertain to the nurse-patient relationship. Constitutions, whether state or federal, do not provide the legal basis for malpractice suits.

Legislation

The second source of laws is legislation. Such laws, which can be either civil or criminal, are enacted by publicly elected bodies like Congress or state legislatures and assemblies. Laws so enacted must not be inconsistent with constitutional law. When a legislative body enacts a law, it does so in the form of a statute. Nurse practice acts, Good Samaritan laws, and abused child and adult laws are examples of statutes that directly affect nurses.

Only occasionally do statutes provide the basis upon which a former patient relies when suing a nurse for malpractice. Although the preponderance of our laws today originate from legislative bodies, quite the opposite is true with respect to malpractice law.

The Common Law

The common law is the third source of laws. It is a large body of law which has developed as the result of court decisions. Although courts are frequently called upon to interpret and/or apply constitutional or statutory law, they are also frequently asked to resolve disputes between two parties, neither of whom can point to a statutory or constitutional provision to support their case. Common sense, it might be said, must be applied to the facts of the case in order to resolve the dispute.

In the process of making its decision, the court will be inclined to follow earlier precedents (decisions), if any exist, or set a precedent, if none exists. If a compelling argument can be made to overturn an earlier precedent because it no longer is good law, a court will do so. The ebb and flow of these decisions by courts across the country comprise what we call the common law.

Although the common law is less visible, definite, and certain than constitutions or statutes, the problems that malpractice law deals with do not lend themselves well to exactness or precision. The legislator who is asked to draft a statute detailing every possible combination of facts and circumstances within which a nurse and patient might someday interact (and which might give rise to a malpractice claim) could spend an entire career working on the language of that statute alone.

Nonetheless, the law must provide a unifying principle that can be fairly applied to each and every claim of malpractice that may arise, irrespective of the facts and circumstances from which the claim arose. It is the common law, then, that provides the principles of malpractice law.

Negligence Through Fault: The Law of Torts. Although the common law cannot provide an all-inclusive list of what nurses can, cannot, and must do in order to avoid liability to patients, it has established a unifying principle that is used to resolve malpractice claims on a case-by-case basis. It is called the fault principle. The fault principle, and all of malpractice law, is part of the law of torts (one of the many categories of the civil law). (See Figure 3–1.)

Generally, before someone can be held liable for another's injury, it must be shown that the defendant was "at fault." The mere fact that a patient has been injured, in and of itself, is not sufficient cause to hold a nurse liable for the injury. The patient has a legal obligation to prove that the injury is the nurse's fault.

The word *tort* is derived from the Latin language. Loosely translated, it means "bad" or "wrong." It is used to describe, within the context of the civil law, conduct that the law deems "bad" or "wrong." Nearly all litigation against nurses alleges that the nurse has violated a patient's civil rights by committing a tort.

Types of Torts. There are three types of torts. Put another way, there are three legal theories that can be used

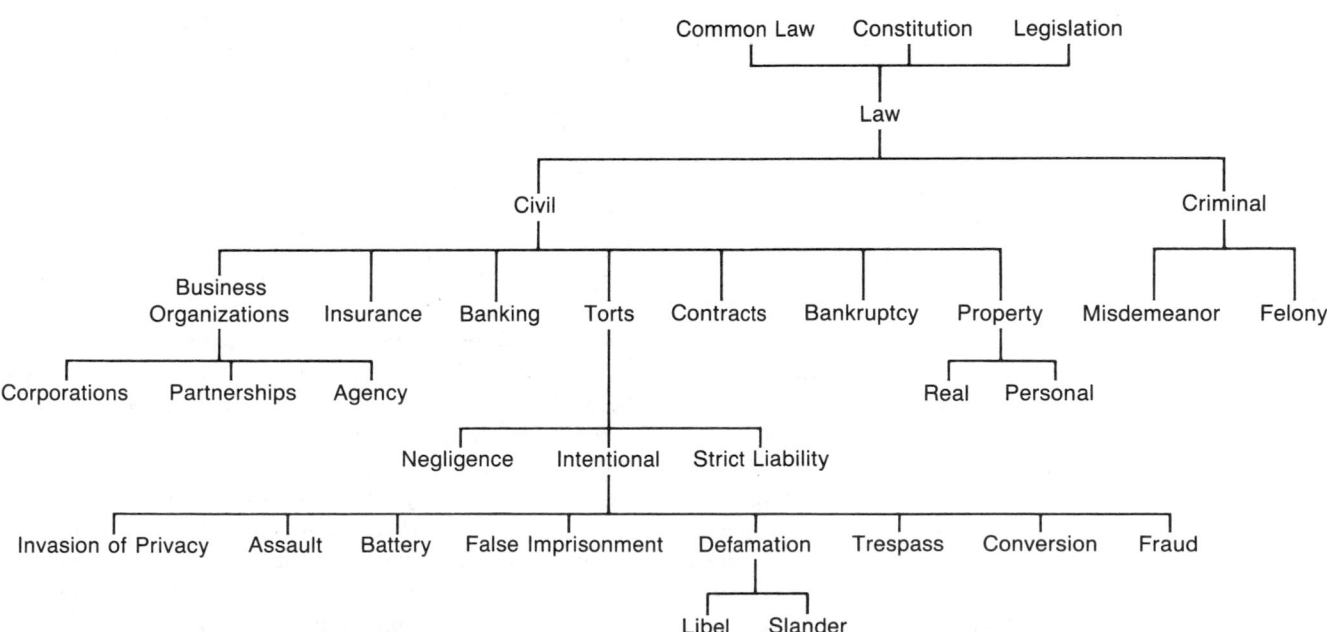

Figure 3–1. Categories of the Law.

to establish liability for having committed a tort. They are strict liability, negligence, and intentional torts. Figure 3-1 shows the three types of torts and some examples of intentional torts.

STRICT LIABILITY. The strict liability theory is an exception to the fault principle. In certain, very limited situations, professionals can be held liable without fault. Even though they have not been negligent or committed an intentional tort, they are said to be strictly liable for any injury caused by their conduct.

Since the rule is so strict and harsh in its consequences, the courts have been careful to limit the situation to which it applies. The only cases in which it is applied to nurses are those in which it is proven that the nurse-defendants have exceeded the scope of practice for which they have been licensed and have engaged in the practice of medicine. If that is established, the nurse is in no position to argue that the patient's injury was not the result of nursing negligence or an intentionally committed tort. The law simply says that if a nurse engages in a practice for which a required license has not been obtained, the nurse does so at the risk of standing strictly liable for any injury caused while so doing. Never mind, for example, that the nurse performed the procedure in question as ably as a licensed physician would have.

Although that may seem a most troublesome doctrine, it should be kept in perspective. Very few suits have actually been brought on the basis of a strict liability theory. The reason, simply put, is that the line between the practice of nursing and the practice of medicine has become increasingly difficult to draw precisely. In view of past and emerging practices and very generally worded nurse practice acts, it would be difficult, except in the obvious cases, to convince a jury that a nurse crossed the line. And nurses stay away from the obvious practice of medicine.

NEGLIGENCE. The second type of tort provides the most common basis for suits brought against nurses. It is malpractice in the truest sense and rests squarely upon the fault principle. Without fault, there can be no liability for negligence.

PROVING NEGLIGENCE: THE ROLE OF THE EXPERT WITNESS. Proof of negligence is a two-step process. First, the plaintiff must persuade the jury of the standard of care against which they should measure the nurse-defendant's conduct. Since jurors are unfamiliar with the standards of nursing practice, expert witnesses who have no direct interest in the outcome of the case are used to help the jury understand these standards. They offer their professional opinions, subject to cross-examination by the attorney who did not call them as a witness, as to what the commonly accepted, generally recognized standard of nursing care in instances such as those surrounding the alleged incident is.

Expert witnesses typically base their testimony and opinion on such things as standards adopted by professional groups (such as the American Nurses' Association), accrediting agencies (such as the Joint Commission for the Accreditation of Hospitals), hospital policies and protocols, customary practice, or perhaps something as seemingly unlikely as information contained in a medication-package stuffer. Since the parties to the suit may disagree on which standard is appropriate to the facts of the case, or agree on the standard, but differ as to its interpretation, each side will offer different experts with differing opinions to support their rspective positions. The jury, whose responsibility it is to determine the applicable standard, is not bound by the testimony of experts, but is free to choose which of their opinions is more credible and persuasive. The selection and presentation of expert witnesses is, therefore, a critical part of malpractice litigation. While the attorneys choose the experts they wish to present, the judge determines whether the *expert witness* presented possesses the requisite knowledge, skill, experience, or training in the area of dispute to qualify as an expert for purposes of the trial.

In addition to offering opinion testimony on the standard of care, experts are also permitted to give their opinion on what is called the ultimate question of fact: did the nurse in this case *meet* the standard of care. They do this in response to what is known as a hypothetical question. The question, asked by the attorney who has called them to testify, asks the expert to decide, on the basis of the evidence which that attorney has introduced, whether the nurse-defendant was negligent. Again, the jury is not bound by the answer given. It is important to remember that the expert witness's purpose is not to help "win" the case for either of the parties, but to assist the jury by providing information from which they may make fair and realistic conclusions.

PROVING NEGLIGENCE: THE ROLE OF THE CHART. The second step through which the plaintiff seeks to show that the defendant was at fault is to convince the jury that the defendant departed from, or failed to meet, the standard of care that the plaintiff hopes the jury will adopt when it retires to reach a verdict. This stage requires that the alleged incident be *reconstructed*. As will be discussed, the patient's chart plays a crucial role—one way or the other—in convincing the jury what did or did not happen. For purposes of reconstructing events, regular, as distinguished from expert, witnesses are called to offer their recollections and factual observations. They are typically not permitted to offer conclusions or opinions, even though they may possess sufficient expertise to qualify as an expert.

At the close of the trial, after all evidence has been introduced, all the witnesses examined and cross-examined, and all closing arguments made, the judge instructs (charges) the jury on the law that they must apply to the facts as they find them to be. For example, as to the credibility of witnesses, the Court's instructions will include the following:

> You are the sole judges of whether a witness is to be believed, and of the weight to be given this testimony. In determining believability and weight, you should take into consideration for each witness the following:
>
> 1. The witness's interest or lack of interest in the outcome of the case
> 2. The witness's relationship to the parties
> 3. The witness's ability and opportunity to know, remember, and relate the facts
> 4. The witness's manner and appearance
> 5. The witness's age and experience
> 6. The witness's frankness and sincerity
> 7. The reasonableness of the witness's testimony in light of all other evidence
> 8. Any impeachment of the witness's testimony
> 9. Your own experience, good judgment, and common sense

Impeachment is evidence of some prior conduct or statement of a witness which is inconsistent with the testimony given, or other indications, such as confusion or bad memory, that the testimony is unreliable.

The jury is given these additional instructions for evaluating expert testimony.

> In determining the believability and weight to be given expert, opinion evidence, you may consider, among other things:
>
> 1. The education, training, experience, and knowledge of the witness
> 2. The reasons given for their opinion
> 3. The sources of the information
> 4. Factors already given you for evaluating the testimony of a witness
>
> Such opinion evidence is entitled to neither no more nor less consideration by you than other fact evidence presented.

As to the question of fault, the jury is instructed, in part, as follows:

> The mere fact that an incident or injury has occurred does not of itself mean that anyone has been negligent. Negligence is the failure to use reasonable care. Reasonable care is that care which a reasonable person would use under the same or similar circumstances. It is the doing of something which a reasonable person would not do, or the failure to do something which a reasonable person would do under the same or similar circumstances.

It is important to note that nurses are not required to act perfectly or ideally. Nurses owe patients a legal duty to act *reasonably*. Reasonableness is both a relative and a subjective standard. It is relative to the facts and circumstances that existed at the time of the alleged incident. It is subjective in that what one person may believe reasonable, another may not. We have seen that expert witnesses may reasonably differ in their opinions on the appropriate standard of care and over whether the nurse met the standard.

NEGLIGENCE AND THE REASONABLY PRUDENT NURSE. Nurses and nursing students must act as a reasonably prudent (careful) nurse would have acted under the same or similar circumstances. The reasonably prudent nurse is a legal fiction, a mythical character the law has created to serve as a guide to the jury in its deliberations. The *reasonably prudent nurse* is a person who practices according to commonly accepted, generally recognized standards of nursing practice. The court will instruct the jury that such a nurse is a person of average:

* Perception
* Memory
* Skill
* Foresight
* Judgment
* Intelligence

The standard of care required is *objective* rather than subjective. It is immaterial that the nurse thought she/he was acting carefully. The jury must decide, in view of testimony and evidence offered, what it feels *should* reasonably have been done and what *was* done.

PROVING NEGLIGENCE. Negligence is more than failing to practice according to the appropriate standards of care, at least for purposes of determining whether a nurse is liable to a patient. Negligence consists of five *elements*, each and every one of which must be proven by the plaintiff in order to be entitled to damages. They are:

* Duty
* Breach of duty
* Reasonable foreseeability of injury
* Causation of injury
* Actual injury

Duty. Whether a nurse owed a patient a duty to exercise reasonable care to protect the patient's safety is rarely a point of contention in nursing malpractice cases. Once a nurse-patient relationship exists, the law imposes a duty on the nurse to exercise reasonable care to protect the patient from injury.

Breach of Duty.   The second element of negligence, and a frequent issue between the parties to a malpractice suit, is whether the nurse fulfilled the duty owed the patient: did the nurse fail to exercise reasonable care under the circumstances? Even if the answer is yes, the plaintiff must prove more in order to be entitled to damages.

Reasonable Foreseeability.   One can be held liable for negligent conduct only for those injuries that are reasonably foreseeable. The rationale is that people should not be expected to guard against those injuries that are not reasonably foreseeable. People have a legal duty to exercise reasonable care only to the extent that an injury is reasonably foreseeable. The law does not require that the defendant actually have foreseen, or anticipated, that such an injury might have occurred in the absence of certain precautions, but that a reasonable person in a similar situation *should* have foreseen it. Again, the standard is objective, not subjective. It is for the jury to decide.

Foreseeability is often an issue in cases involving suicides or suicide attempts by patients, when it is alleged that nurses did not exercise sufficient precautions in attending to such patients. One case, for example, involved a professional football player who was admitted to a hospital on the advice of his friend, a physician, to have a biopsy done on a small growth on his arm. The patient hired a private duty nurse, who left the room without being excused when the physician came to tell the patient of the result of the biopsy, which was positive. After the physician left the room, the patient jumped to his death from the hospital window. His widow sued the nurse, alleging that her unexcused absence from the room was negligent and was a direct contributing cause of her husband's death. Since the evidence showed that the patient had exhibited no signs of despair, depression, or unusual concern, the suicide was not reasonably foreseeable. Although the nurse had a legal duty to be in the room and had breached that duty, nonetheless, she was not liable for the patient's death.

The opposite result was decided in a case where a nurse was sued for injuries sustained by a patient who tripped over an electrical cord from an inhalator which the nurse had placed on his nightstand and plugged into a wall outlet between the bed and the adjacent bathroom. When the patient got up during the night to use the bathroom, he tripped and fell. Did the nurse owe the patient a duty to exercise reasonable care? Of course. And the duty extended to those events that were reasonably foreseeable. Was it foreseeable that if she left the cord extended between the bed and the bathroom, the patient might get out of bed during the night and trip over it? The jury said yes. Both cases clearly demonstrate the need to anticipate the consequences of one's actions (or inactions) and conduct oneself accordingly.

Causation of Injury.   Even when a plaintiff can prove that the nurse breached an acknowledged duty and that the patient suffered an injury that was foreseeable as resulting from such a breach, the plaintiff must still show that the injury was, in fact, caused by the breach. There must be a cause-and-effect relationship between the injury and the breach of duty. The jury must be able to conclude that, but for the defendant's negligence, the injury would not have occurred.

In one case, for example, a patient who was admitted for a hysterectomy brought suit for infection, internal adhesions, and other abnormalities that required subsequent surgery and removal of her fallopian tubes and ovaries. During the preoperative procedure, a nurse had inserted a catheter into the patient's rectum instead of her bladder, which was contrary to established practice. During the surgery, the surgeon noticed the catheter, removed it, rinsed the surgical field with a strong antiseptic solution, and inserted the catheter in the patient's bladder. Nonetheless, the complications resulted and precipitated the suit against the surgeon, hospital, and nurse. The jury found that the nurse had breached her duty and that it was reasonably foreseeable that such a breach would cause harm to the patient. The jury concluded, however, that it was not the nurse's negligence that caused the injury. Instead, it found that the surgeon's negligence in removing the catheter during surgery was the cause. The surgeon was liable. The nurse was not.

In another case, a patient who had attempted to commit suicide by leaping from a hospital window shortly after being admitted and diagnosed as paranoid schizophrenic sued the nurses and the hospital. He alleged that the nurses were not sufficiently alert or attentive, given his diagnosis, and that their inattention was a contributing cause of his injuries. The jury agreed that the nurses were not paying sufficient attention to the patient, and that it was reasonably foreseeable that he might try to harm himself. Nonetheless, because of the timing of events (approximately 30 seconds) and expert testimony that such patients sometimes injure themselves despite all precautions, the jury concluded that it could not be said that there was a causal connection between the nurse's negligence and the patient's injury. The nurses therefore, were not, liable.

Actual Injury.   The fifth element of negligence says if no one is injured by a nurse's negligence, there is no one to be liable to. It should be mentioned, however, that the negligent practice of nursing is typically grounds for disciplinary action (reprimand, censure, suspension, or revocation of a license to practice) by state nursing boards. This is true even though no actual injury to patients has occurred.

One should conclude that proving that a nurse is at

Table 3–1. **The Most Common Claims of Nursing Negligence**

Burns

From smoking, heating pads, inhalators, sitz baths, and solutions that are too hot or of improper concentration

Falls

By patients who are elderly, sedated, preoperative and postoperative, dizzy, disoriented, blind, or semiconscious, and people who slip on wet or waxed floors

Failure to Observe

As ordered, as policy, nursing standards, or circumstances require. Result: the failure to recognize in time the patient's deteriorating condition or the need for action

Failure to Communicate

As ordered, as policy, nursing standards, or circumstances require. Result: important patient information is not (1) passed along (2) noticed (3) understood

Medication Errors

Administration of wrong medicine, wrong dosage or concentration, or at improper intervals or site. The reasonably prudent nurse must know the (1) medicine's nature and purpose, (2) symptoms of probable adverse reactions, and (3) recommended corrective measures

Negligent Following of Orders

From physician, supervisor, administrator, or any other. Every person is responsible for personal acts of negligence and has an individual responsibility to act reasonably and exercise judgement

Use of Defective Equipment

It is negligent to use equipment that the nurse knows or should know is defective

Patient Mix-Ups

When one patient is given another patient's medicine, treatment, or surgery

fault and should be held liable for a patient's injury is not a matter of routine. The plaintiff must prove, by a preponderance of the evidence, that each individual element is supported by evidence. A preponderance of the evidence means that the jury must find the plaintiff's allegations more likely than not to be true. See Table 3–1 for examples of the most frequent types of claims of nursing negligence.

Defenses to Claims of Negligence

Even assuming that a nurse's negligent conduct has caused a reasonably foreseeable injury to a patient, the law provides a number of defenses which the nurse can use in a malpractice case. Depending on the defense used, the nurse who convinces the jury that the defense is valid will either reduce or eliminate liability to the patient.

Statutes of Limitations

Every state has a statute of limitations for negligence suits. Some have special statutes for malpractice suits. In either event, the applicable statute sets a period of time within which a plaintiff must commence a lawsuit. If the lawsuit is not begun before the statutory time runs out, the plaintiff is barred from bringing the suit.

The statutory period varies from state to state, but is typically in the two- to six-year range. An important question is when the statutory period begins to run. That, too, varies from state to state, depending on the legislation itself and on judicial interpretations of it. The general rule is that the time begins to lapse when the negligence or injury occurs. However, in instances where the injury may not be immediately apparent to the patient, the time may not begin to run until the patient should have discovered it. Many states put a maximum number of years "cap" on even those instances. And some states allow minor's the full statutory period after they reach the age of adulthood, which itself varies from state to state.

Since malpractice suits are of more recent origin for nurses than physicians, many states that passed statutes of limitations especially for malpractice suits did not specifically include nurses in their language. In those states where the courts have not interpreted the statute to cover nurses by implication, nurses are left to the protection of the general negligence statute of limitations, which typically gives the plaintiff a longer period of time within which to file suit.

Contributory Negligence

The defense of contributory negligence is another defense that nurses can raise after a suit has been brought against them. Like the statute of limitations, it results in no liability to the patient if it is successfully argued. Instead of barring the lawsuit itself, however, it results in a favorable verdict for the nurse.

A patient may be barred from recovering for an injury when it is shown that his own negligence contributed to his injury. Thus, a jury is asked to determine the respective amounts, or degrees, that the plaintiff's and nurse's negligence played in causing the injury. In those states that use the contributory negligence rule, a finding of any degree of negligence at all on the patient's part will bar any recovery whatsoever (irrespective of how negligent the nurse was when compared to the patient). Only a few states recognize the defense of contributory negligence.

Since negligence is determined in light of the circumstances under which it allegedly occurred, it should be pointed out that the effects of old age, disease, injuries, disabilities, anesthesia, confusion, dependence, and medications would all be mitigating factors in determining a patient's negligence. They are not held to the same standard of care in protecting themselves from injury as a person who is not subject to such effects. The burden of proving contributory negligence is on the nurse, and the same elements of negligence that must be proven by

the plaintiff against the nurse must be proven by the nurse against the plaintiff in order for the contributory negligence defense to succeed.

Comparative Negligence

Since the contributory negligence rule acts as a complete bar to recovery, irrespective of the proportional degrees of negligence of the plaintiff and defendant, most states have found the rule to be a harsh one. As a result, most states have adopted a modified version of the rule. The comparative negligence rule also permits the nurse to defend a malpractice claim by alleging that the plaintiff's injury was caused, at least in part, by the patient's own failure to act reasonably under the circumstances.

The difference lies in the outcome. If the nurse is able to convince the jury that the plaintiff was negligent, the jury again compares the degrees of negligence of the respective parties. But instead of the plaintiff's negligence barring any recovery, it results in reducing the amount to which the plaintiff is entitled. Instead of eliminating the nurse's liability, it minimizes it. Each party bears the financial burden of their own proportional and respective degree of negligence. For example, if the jury determines that the total damages attributable to the injury are $100,000, but finds that the plaintiff was 20 percent at fault in causing the injury, the court would award the plaintiff $80,000. Some states have specified that if the plaintiff's negligence exceeds a certain point, such as 50 percent, the plaintiff is then totally barred from recovering.

Because of the nurse's legal duty to the patient, it is especially important to monitor patients closely whom the nurse knows or should know are unable to exercise reasonable judgment in caring for themselves. The standard of care for nurses caring for such patients increases, while the standard of care expected of patients in protecting themselves from injury decreases.

The Use of the Chart in Proving Contributory or Comparative Negligence.   Because of the doctrines of contributory and comparative negligence, it is especially important to document actions of patients who are not impaired when those actions are contrary to the patient's best interests. For example, if a patient is not following medical orders, the nurse should chart that fact, as well as any discussions or warnings that take place or are given that point out the risk associated with the patient's conduct. The documentation may prove invaluable as a basis for alleging patient negligence in a subsequent suit in which the patient seeks to pass blame to the hospital or staff.

Assumption of Risk

In instances where a competent patient knowingly and voluntarily assumes a risk, the patient has no legal grounds to complain when that risk materializes. For example, when a patient refuses to consent to a recommended procedure, insists on discharge against medical advice, or slips in a water puddle that had been warned of, the assumption-of-risk defense might be applicable. Not all states make the defense available, and those that do differ in whether the defense eliminates or only minimizes the defendant's liability.

Good practice requires that the nurse warn patients of risks that they might not reasonably be expected to recognize for themselves and to document that the warning was given. In appropriate cases, the patient should be asked to sign a release, such as in the first two of the above examples. If the patient should refuse to sign the release, then the request and refusal should be documented. Preferably the explanation, request, and refusal should take place with another witness present so that the likelihood of using the defense is enhanced should the patient be unwilling or unable to acknowledge the conversation during subsequent litigation.

Good Samaritan Acts

Most states have enacted Good Samaritan statutes which also provide a defense to claims of negligence in limited circumstances. Few states require citizens to come to the aid of people in distress. Although there may be a moral duty to do so, there is no legal duty, at least for most members of the public. Until the early 1960s, however, people who chose to stop at the scene of an emergency to render aid did so at some legal risk. If they were negligent in their efforts, the accident victim could hold them liable for any resulting injury. Since that time, the District of Columbia and nearly every state has enacted legislation to encourage citizens to be "Good Samaritans" and stop to render aid. These statutes did so by providing that a Good Samaritan could not be held legally liable for injuries caused under such circumstances even if they resulted from the negligence of the person rendering the emergency assistance.

A few states, however, have enacted legislation that does require that people trained in health care actually stop, and the legislation creates both civil and criminal liability in the event that such persons fail to stop.

The statutes are varied insofar as who is protected. Some protect only the general public; others identify health practitioners by category; some limit the protection only to professionals licensed in that state; and others extend protection to any licensed professional, irrespective of the licensing state. Still others define, in varying detail, what constitutes an emergency or add the qualification that the emergency aid was not rendered with the expectation of payment.

No Good Samaritan statute extends protection to within the walls of a health care facility, even if an emergency exists and even if a nurse volunteers to help. Some statutes specifically make such an exclusion, while others have been so interpreted by courts on the rationale that the statutes were passed to encourage help where none is usually available.

In one case, for example, a nurse who worked in pediatrics on the fifth floor of a hospital had made arrangements to meet another who worked in the emergency department on the first floor at the end of their shifts. When the pediatric nurse arrived in ER to meet her friend, she found that her friend was occupied by a sudden influx of patients and had been asked to stay on. The pediatric nurse volunteered her services and, in the process of attending to a patient, left that patient unattended and unsecured on a cart. The patient later sued, alleging that she was injured when she fell off the cart, and that her injuries were caused by the nurse's negligently leaving her unattended and without proper restraints. The nurse raised the Good Samaritan law as a defense, alleging that she volunteered her assistance at the scene of an emergency without any expectation of compensation. The court disagreed that she fell within the intent of the legislation.

It might also be noted that the hospital's insurance carrier denied coverage to the nurse on the grounds that her actions were not within the scope of her employment, since she had not been asked nor was she expected to help out under such circumstances. In her suit against the insurance company, the court agreed that her actions were not within the employer's policy coverage.

When nurses stop to render emergency assistance, they do not lose their status as nurses. Their education and experience as a nurse will be one of the important factors in determining the standard of care expected of them. What can be considered reasonable for a nonnurse under such circumstances can be quite different than what can reasonably be expected of a nurse. However, since the situation is an emergency, that will be taken into account. And what can be expected of a nurse in an emergency could be different than what is to be expected in a nonemergency.

Nurses will not be protected if their negligence exceeds what the law considers to be ordinary negligence. If their conduct can be considered *gross negligence*, the statutes afford no protection. Gross negligence is a term that defies exact definition but usually involves conduct that exhibits reckless, willful, or wanton disregard for the safety of another. In one case, for example, a nurse came across the scene of a nighttime one-car roadside accident. After dragging the victim to the edge of the road, giving first aid, and covering the victim with a dark raincoat, the nurse left to get help. She returned to find that the patient had been struck by another vehicle while lying unconscious where she had left him. The jury found that the nurse's conduct constituted more than ordinary negligence, and the court rejected the nurse's contention that she was deserving of protection as a Good Samaritan.

No Negligence

The most frequently used defense is that the nurse was not negligent. As has been discussed, the plaintiff has the burden of proving that each element of negligence exists. When the plaintiff is unable to do that, no finding of negligence can be made, and no liability imposed.

The Doctrine of *Respondeat Superior*

Respondeat Superior and the Health Care Employer

A hospital, or other employing institution, is legally liable for the negligent acts of its employees. The doctrine of *respondeat superior* (let the superior respond) was created long ago by the courts in an effort to increase the likelihood that a person whose legal rights had been violated could collect the damages to which they were entitled.

Courts recognized that employees are sometimes unable to pay judgments granted against them. Since employers are able to decide whom they wish to hire, how they wish to train and supervise them, and whom they wish to retain as employees, it is reasonable to expect that they be ultimately responsible in the event of employee negligence. This "deep pockets" theory also is based on the employer's ability to build the cost of such a risk into their cost of doing business.

Respondeat Superior and the Nurse

The purpose of the doctrine is not to relieve the person whose negligence actually caused the injury of liability for it. The *principle of personal liability* requires that every person be liable for personal acts of negligence. In the event that the nurse cannot pay some or all of the required judgment, the plaintiff is entitled to enforce the judgment against the employer, which is said to be vicariously liable (liable on behalf of another). But, because of the principle of personal liability, the hospital has the right to seek a judgment requiring the nurse to reimburse the hospital for any amounts it is required to pay because of the nurse's negligence.

The hospital (or its insurer) is entitled to file a cross-claim against the nurse seeking such reimbursement, and that matter becomes a part of the main trial. However, if the hospital has secured insurance coverage for both itself and the nurse, neither it nor the insurance company is entitled to any reimbursement from the nurse.

***Respondeat Superior* and Intentional Torts.** The doctrine of *respondeat superior* does not apply to intentional torts, unless it can be shown that the employer had reason to know that the employee was likely to commit the intentional tort in question. And even in negligence cases, the doctrine has limitations.

***Respondeat Superior* and Negligent Torts.** The courts apply the doctrine only when it can be shown that (1) an employer-employee relationship actually existed and (2) the negligence was committed within the scope of the nurse's employment. If, for example, the nurse is on private duty (hired by the patient or family) or is under the direct supervision and control of a nonhospital employee (such as a surgeon in the operating room) at the time of the negligence, the employer-hospital is not liable. The same would be true if the nurse's negligence occurs at a time when the nurse is doing something unrelated to employment responsibilities.

The liability for patient injury is imputed to the employer, irrespective of its degree of fault. The doctrine of *respondeat superior*, like the doctrine of strict liability, is an exception to the fault principle.

Respondeat Superior and the Supervisor

Nursing supervisors are liable for their *own* acts of negligence. They are not, however, responsible for the negligent acts of those they *supervise*. It is important to distinguish the supervisor's responsbility to supervise from the supervisor's liability for the negligence of those they supervise. The former exists; the latter does not. The doctrine of *respondeat superior* does not apply to supervisor-supervisee relationships. The doctrine is limited in its application to employer-employee relationships. Supervisors are not considered to be employers.

Often an incident that provides the basis for a lawsuit against both the supervisor and supervisee will involve a common set of facts. Nonetheless, each is being sued for personal respective negligent acts or omission.

Those with supervisory authority and responsibility, whether they have a supervisory title or not, are required to act as reasonably prudent supervisors would act under similar circumstances.

If, for example, a nurse came to work impaired and the supervisor failed to notice the nurse's impaired condition, it could be alleged that the supervisor was negligent for not being as observant and attentive as a reasonably prudent supervisor should have been. If the impaired nurse injured a patient, both might be liable to the patient, and a jury would have to apportion the damages between the two. But each would be liable for personal negligence, not for one another's.

If, as a further example, the supervisor did notice the impaired nurse, but chose to do nothing about it in order to avoid unpleasantries or to show some deference to a colleague who had no previous related history, both could again be held liable for their separate acts of negligence if it caused a patient to be injured.

In one case, two nurses requested permission to leave the recovery room and take a coffee break. At the time, there were two patients in the room. The supervisor granted permission. Within minutes after the nurses left, three additional patients arrived. Because the supervisor was unable to tend to all five of the patients, one suffered brain damage as a result of lack of oxygen. The patient brought suit against the supervisor for negligence in granting the nurses' request and the nurses for having left their station. The jury found all three liable, since an operating room schedule was reasonably available which would have revealed, if checked, that the new patients could have been expected.

Malpractice Insurance

The Need for Insurance

Neither practicing nurses nor student nurses should be without malpractice insurance coverage. With the likelihood of a patient's bringing suit higher than ever, it is imprudent to "go bare" as the phrase is used. The phrase is apt: it conjures up an image of one who is exposed and vulnerable.

The Purpose of Insurance

In addition to paying any judgment (or settlement) up to the limit stated in the policy, a malpractice policy also pays for costs of defending, including attorney's fees, against a malpractice suit. Such costs are covered even if the suit is unmeritorious, and whether the suit is won or lost. If uninsured, a nurse must finance the costs of defending a suit from personal resources. It is small consolation to "win" a lawsuit under such circumstances. Malpractice insurance can be obtained quite inexpensively through nurses' associations or through independent insurance agents.

Individual needs, the risk associated with the particular area of nursing practice, and the geographic area of practice determine what kind and amount of insurance coverage should be purchased.

Types of Insurance

There are two types of coverage. *Occurrence* policies will cover liability arising out of any incident that occurred while the policy was in effect, even though the suit is brought after the policy has lapsed. *Claims* policies, on the other hand, will cover liability for any claim (lawsuit) that is filed while the policy is in effect, even though the incident itself may have occurred before the policy went into effect. Since the latter policy requires the insurance company to assume a great risk, it is considerably more expensive. Each type of policy covers liability for negligence. Neither provides coverage for intentional tort liability.

Coverage by an Employer

Nurses should never assume that they are covered individually by the policy of the institution for which they work. They should request written confirmation of such coverage, as well as information as to type and amount of coverage. Too often a nurse who has made such an assumption or who has been given a casual (and inaccurate) verbal assurance that coverage is in effect has learned the truth after a suit has been commenced. Institutions, as a rule, do have insurance coverage for malpractice liability, but it often extends no further than institutional liability that may arise under the doctrine of *respondeat superior* or because of actual administrative or corporate negligence.

Individual Coverage. Even nurses who are covered for personal liability by an employer's policy should consider carrying a personal policy of their own. Nurses who volunteer their services to community agencies or activities, for example, are liable for their negligence in many states even if they were doing so on a volunteer basis. Similarly, nurses who exercise their professional judgment or discretion in giving advice which is relied upon by friends or neighbors may be held liable when negligent in doing so. And very few employer's policies will extend to liability for negligence that occurs beyond the scope of the nurse's employment.

No Coverage, No Lawsuit? No Way!

Some nurses feel that carrying a malpractice policy increases the chances that a patient who learns of that will decide to sue. Although that may be true occasionally, the opposite is not. The fact that a nurse does not carry insurance will not result in a patient who has a meritorious claim deciding not to sue. As has been seen, if an employee is negligent, the employer will be sued under the doctrine of *respondeat superior*. The negligent nurse will still be interviewed, subjected to pretrial proceedings such as depositions (the answering of questions under oath), and called as a witness as part of the plaintiff's case against the employer. It is clear that if the plaintiff's attorney must deal with the nurse to that

extent, the nurse can be dealt with as an actual defendant with only minimal additional effort. Further, unless the employer has insurance coverage which extends to and also protects the employee, we have seen that the employer (or its insurer) has the right to cross-claim against the nurse for any liability it may subsequently incur caused by the nurse's negligence.

Insurance is something people buy when they recognize that an appreciable risk exists that they can afford to protect themselves against. The risk of malpractice is an appreciable one. And the cost of malpractice insurance is affordable.

It should be understood that a judgment remains enforceable for many years, typically in the 15- to 20-year range and usually can be renewed, if it remains unsatisfied, for a similar period. So, even though a nurse is asset- and income-free (a most unlikely event) at the time a plaintiff obtains a judgment, subsequently obtained assets and income are subject to the legal reach of a judgment creditor for the purposes of satisfying (collecting) the judgment.

Intentional Torts

The Difference Between Negligence and Intentional Torts

Although most suits against nurses are based on negligently committed torts, a nurse also may be liable for intentionally committed torts.

Intentional torts can be distinguished from negligence in three important ways. First, negligence can result from either an act or an omission. An intentional tort cannot exist unless certain prohibited acts are committed. Second, for an intentional tort to be committed, the act in question must have been willful and deliberate (intentional). Negligence does not involve the intentional conduct, as such, but a failure to use due care. Third, negligent conduct cannot be reduced to an all-inclusive list, but intentional torts can be. Certain specific types of conduct, when intentionally done, have been identified as "bad" and "wrong" in that they injure a person's reputation, property, or personal interests. It is important to note that a nurse can be liable for an intentional tort even though there was no intent to harm the patient. For that matter, it is not even necessary that the patient be injured. All that is required is that the nurse have intentionally done an act that is classified as an intentional tort.

Many intentional torts are of marginal concern to nurses. For example, conversion (the unauthorized use of another's personal property), trespass (going onto

another's real property without permission), or libel and slander (damaging another's reputation by speaking or writing factual inaccuracies about that individual). Four intentional torts, however, are particularly relevant to nursing practice. (Refer to Table 3-2.)

Types of Intentional Torts

The Intentional Tort of Battery. Battery is the unconsented touching of another person in a socially unacceptable way. The touching itself constitutes the offense. No injury need result, although the presence or absence of an actual injury will affect the amount of damages to which the plaintiff is entitled. For example, if a nurse administers a hypodermic injection to a competent, nonconsenting patient, a battery would occur (physician's orders notwithstanding). Or if a nurse, trying to ambulate a competent and unconsenting patient, pulls the patient up in bed, the patient could properly sue for battery. Any medical or surgical procedure that is carried out without proper consent from the patient or implied consent (to be discussed) provided by law would likely result in a battery. Since the basis of the protection from battery is the patient's right to self-determination and to be free from invasions of person, the law recognizes a compensable injury even if the patient has benefited from the touching.

The Intentional Tort of Assault. The words "assault" and "battery" are often used together, even though they are two separate torts. An assault often precedes a battery. It is an act that causes the person to reasonably believe a battery is about to occur. It is the threat of doing something that, if carried out, would result in a battery. The threat can be expressed by words or conduct. Thus, before the nurse actually administers the unwanted hypodermic injection, it usually appears to the patient that the nurse is about to administer it. The appearance in such an instance constitutes an assault.

The Intentional Tort of Invasion of Privacy. Invasion of privacy is a tort that has been recognized with increasing frequency by the courts. It reflects aroused sensitivity to personal and private matters and affairs and to being dealt with discreetly and with respect. Liability usually results from one or the other of two general kinds of conduct: passing along confidential patient information or intruding into a patient's protected private domain.

Information that comes to the nurse as a result of the nurse-patient relationship is considered confidential. It cannot be shared, in the absence of the patient's consent, with anyone who is not directly involved with the patient's care, irrespective of good faith or intentions. This includes, but is not limited to, the information on the patient's chart.

For example, in one invasion-of-privacy suit, a nurse was sued successfully for using a patient as a case history. She and a group of colleagues regularly met once each week to share experiences that they felt would be mutually educational and would further their professional development. The nurses had discussed the patient's dramatic improvement following a hysterectomy after the nurse was able to gain the patient's confidence by spending a considerable amount of time offering support to the patient. The patient learned that the many embarrassing, intimate details she had related to the nurse had been discussed when a maintenance person found the notes the nurse had used for the discussion and returned them to the patient's room. Even though all nurses had the best of intentions and meant no harm, they had no direct involvement with the patient and, therefore, no lawful right to information relating to her. Table 3–2 contains representative examples of patient's privacy cases that have been brought before courts in recent years.

In some instances, nurses have not only a right but a duty to act in a way that would constitute an invasion of privacy under normal circumstances. For example, when a nurse believes that a patient is concealing contraband such as cigarettes, alcohol, or other drugs that are contrary to the patient's best interests, a failure to make

Table 3–2. **Patient's Privacy Cases**

Court decisions have interpreted the right of privacy to include:

The right to refuse to see any visitors.

The right to refuse to see anyone not officially connected with the hospital.

The right to refuse to see anyone who is officially connected with the hospital but who is not directly involved in the patient's care and treatment.

The right to refuse to see social workers and to deny them access to patient records.

The right to wear personal bedclothes when they do not interfere with treatment.

The right to wear religious and other expressive medals.

The right to have a member of the patient's own sex present during a physical examination.

a reasonable inquiry, even a search, could be negligent, particularly if the patient is unable to recognize and appreciate the danger involved. The nurse, in such situations, should document the facts relied on in concluding that a need for action exists. If the patient denies the existence of the contraband and refuses to consent to a search, the nurse is entitled to make a reasonable search if a reasonable factual basis can be shown to justify it. It does present somewhat of a dilemma: an unjustified search could result in liability for invasion of privacy, while a failure to make the inquiry and search could result, in appropriate cases, in liability for negligence in caring for the patient. Whether or not the search actually produces the object of the search is not determinative of whether the search was justified. Similarly, all states have a variety of statutes that impose a duty to report certain otherwise confidential patient information. Although such statutes vary from state to state, they typically require reporting of gunshot wounds, suspected abuse of children or the elderly, venereal and certain other contagious diseases, and out-of-wedlock births. The statutes also provide immunity from liability for libel, slander, or invasion of privacy when the disclosures are made in good faith.

From time to time, nurses are asked to testify in court cases as witnesses and are faced with the need to decide whether they can lawfully relate information to a jury or attorney concerning a former patient. The laws that protect privileged communications in this regard are very complex and differ from state to state. Before a nurse offers information either in court, in a formal or informal statement, or in response to interrogatories or depositions in pretrial proceedings, an attorney should be consulted at the first indication that such information is being requested.

The Intentional Tort of False Imprisonment. False imprisonment is the unconsented, unreasonable interference with a person's right to move about freely. Its relevance to the practice of nursing is clear. The key considerations are whether the interference has been *consented* to, either expressly (verbally or in writing by a competent patient or an appropriate other in the case of an incompetent patient) or impliedly (by the actions and conduct of the patient or by the law itself in appropriate cases), and whether the form and extent of the interference is *reasonable* under the circumstances.

The right of self-determination is again apparent when discussing the patient's right to decide whether restrictions on movement are lawful. A competent patient may refuse such restrictions even though health practitioners feel they are necessary for the patient's well-being. In such an event, the risks should be explained to the patient, the explanation documented, and the patient asked to sign a release or waiver acknowledging a voluntary assumption of the risk.

When dealing with incompetent patients who are unable to appreciate the consequences of their decisions, the same principles apply, except that another person, such as a guardian or next of kin, should be consulted. In emergency situations, when it is not reasonable to seek consent from the patient or others, the law provides implied consent to do what is reasonably necessary to save the patient's life or prevent further injury or complications. As a general rule, the law permits the use of restraints when it is necessary to protect the patient from himself, or to protect others, including staff, from the patient in such emergency situations.

The use of restraints presents the nurse with another

Table 3–3. **False Imprisonment**
Courts have held the following to constitute false imprisonment:
Restraining a mentally ill patient who presents no danger to self or others.
Refusing to permit a patient to leave the hospital because a bill is unpaid.
Refusing to let a competent patient discharge self against medical advice.
Threatening patients with disciplinary consequences if they get out of bed or leave the room.
Restraining a competent and unwilling patient while administering medication (also an assault and battery).
The use of excessive restraint appliances in an instance where more moderate devices are customarily called for.

dilemma. Failure to use an appropriate restraint could constitute negligence. The inappropriate use of restraint, or the use of an excessive restraint, could constitute false imprisonment and perhaps assault and battery. Decisions about restraints clearly require the sound exercise of discretion and judgment. The nurse must consciously weigh the options and balance the interests in making such decisions.

Since the matter is often a close call and does require professional judgment, juries typically show the nurse a considerable amount of deference in these cases. But when it is shown that the nurse failed to exercise professional judgment or abused the discretion, juries are not forgiving. (See Table 3–3 for representative illustrations of false imprisonment.)

Informed Consent

A patient who has properly consented to conduct on the part of a nurse cannot hold the nurse liable for what would have been an intentional tort in the absence of that consent. For years, the practice was to have patients sign consent forms, which they usually did not read, that gave the hospital and physician authority to do whatever they felt necessary. In more recent times, as patients have become more aware of their rights and more assertive in pursuing them, the courts have been asked to define more particularly the meaning of consent. The result has been the creation of the concept of informed consent.

The Purpose and Meaning of Informed Consent

The courts have made it clear that all adults of sound mind have the right to determine what, if anything, shall be done to their person and body. All competent patients have the right to choose whether they shall be treated, and if so, how. No matter how necessary medical practitioners believe treatment to be, no matter how serious the risk to life or health is in the absence of treatment, patients are legally entitled to determine their own destiny.

Court decisions have repeatedly held, moreover, that the right to self-determination is a meaningless right unless the patient is put in a position to *knowledgeably* exercise it. So, even though the patient has signed a consent form, or otherwise indicated a willingness to go along with a recommended procedure, the consent may be treated by the patient, and the court, as *apparent* but not *real*. In such an instance, for legal purposes, the effect is the same as if there were no consent at all. In order for the consent to be real, it must be informed. In order for it to be *informed consent*, it must be (1) voluntary and (2) knowledgeable.

Consent is voluntarily given when patients give it of their own free will, absent of any coercion or deception. It also must be given by a patient who understands, or is in a position to understand, the significance and effect of consenting. Patients who, for example, are sedated, senile, under the influence of alcohol, disoriented, or otherwise not able to function mentally cannot be said to freely and voluntarily consent.

Consent is knowledgeably given when the patient has been given a reasonably understandable explanation of the *alternatives* and the *probable results* and *risks* that accompany each. Although no rules exist to exhaustively detail when such explanation is required, or what should be explained when one is, it is expected that the patient be given the information that a reasonable person could be expected to want before deciding whether to go forward with the procedure.

Generally, the more elective the procedure, the more important informed consent becomes. Even when *informed* consent is not required, it should be remembered that ordinary consent must be obtained for even the most routine procedures. That is usually done by obtaining the patient's signature on a general consent form at the time of admission, by the patient's verbal consent as the care plan is implemented, or by the patient's acquiescence to particular treatment procedures.

Informed Consent and the Nurse.

It is the responsibility of the person who will *perform* the procedure to obtain the patient's informed consent. Although that is usually the physician, the responsibility may be delegated to the nurse. Nurses should be careful not to accept a responsibility that is beyond their ability to perform. The nurse should, for example, understand the alternatives and risks that must be explained to the patient.

There is a difference between being asked to obtain the patient's signature on a consent form and obtaining the patient's informed consent. Nurses are regularly asked to do the former. In so doing, they are also usually asked to witness the signature. Their signing as a witness is not considered to be a verification that the patient understands what has been consented to. It merely affirms that the nurse saw the patient sign the form and believes the patient to have been of sound mind when signing it. Nurses should not, however, permit a patient to sign the form when it appears that the patient has not been given or understood the requisite explanation. Nor should the nurse permit a procedure to be carried out if a competent patient has a change of mind and revokes a previously given consent. In either event, the physician or other appropriate person should be notified. Nurses should remember that patients can revoke their consent verbally, even though it may have been initially in writing.

Informed Consent and the Patient.

Not all patients are able, even if they wish, to consent to treatment procedures. Patients who are mentally incompetent, whether a court has so found or not, are unable to give effective legal consent. They are considered to lack the legal capacity to do so. Since consent is nonetheless required, it must be obtained from someone who is entitled to act on their behalf. If the person has been declared incompetent in a legal proceeding, the person who was named guardian is entitled to give or withhold consent.

When a patient's capacity to consent is in doubt, even though not adjudged incompetent, the consent of the nearest reasonably available relative should be sought. If consent is withheld, particularly in life-threatening cases, the hospital or physician will consider seeking permission to proceed from a court, at least if time permits. If time does not permit, the policy is often to treat now and worry about legal liability later. The other choice is often to withhold treatment and worry about legal liability later.

Minors present another instance in which questions of legal capacity to give or withhold consent are raised. Generally, a minor's consent is not legally effective. The result is that any treatment given a minor, even if with consent, is deemed to have been given without consent. The policy should be to obtain consent from a parent. If the parents wihhold consent, the same procedures as described for mental incompetents should be followed.

Many states have statutes that create exceptions to the general rule, although the exceptions can differ from state to state. For example, minors who are emancipated (living independently from their parents), whether married or not, are often given legal capacity to consent for themselves. Other statutes permit minors to consent for such procedures as obstetrical care, blood donations, and treatment for venereal disease and drug dependency.

The Role of the Chart in Malpractice Litigation

Remember that proving negligence is a two-step process. The patient must prove to a jury that (1) a particular standard of care should be applied to the case, and that (2) the nurse failed to meet that standard. The second step requires that the alleged incident be reconstructed by presenting evidence that tends to show what did (or did not) happen.

The Chart Is the Best Evidence . . . For Someone

Since the trial of a malpractice case usually occurs several years after the incident that prompted the litigation, it is difficult for a witness to recall details with sufficient clarity to be effective. Further, since the nurse-defendant has a personal interest in the outcome of the case, a jury may be reluctant to take the nurse's testimony at face value, especially if it is not supported by, or is inconsistent with, other evidence in the case.

The chart is introduced routinely as evidence in malpractice cases. It is viewed by juries as the most reliable indicator as to what really happened. As such, it plays a crucial role in reconstructing the alleged incident. What *is* documented, the *manner* in which it is documented, and what *is not* documented, along with the inferences that the plaintiff's attorney can persuade the jury to draw from that, will weigh heavily in the outcome of the verdict. It will have the same effect on settlement discussions. Simply put, the chart is often the hinge upon which a case turns.

If the nurse was not negligent, the nurse's defense should be able to rely on the chart to rebut the plaintiff's claim. Unfortunately, that is often not the case. Even though the nurse was not *actually* negligent, the chart, especially in the hands of a skilled plaintiff's attorney, might make it *appear* that the nurse was. Since juries must deal with appearances and perceptions, there is no difference at the end of a trial between appearing to have been negligent and actually having been negligent. If it appears that the nurse was negligent, then, for purposes of the verdict, a jury will find accordingly.

Nurses who realize that the chart is increasingly likely to be used as evidence in malpractice litigation are more likely to chart in ways that do not permit a plaintiff's attorney to suggest that jurors draw inferences that are not consistent with the nurse's testimony. They will recognize that charting is an *opportunity* that gives them considerable protection against malpractice liability.

Although a definitive, all-inclusive list cannot be assembled, a considerable number of practices can be identified that affect the likelihood of a jury determining that a nurse was negligent. They comprise an important part of a malpractice-prevention program. They demonstrate that, as the chart becomes increasingly unreliable, the nurse's case becomes decreasingly defensible.

A Legal Perspective: Things to Think About

The Failure to Make an Entry. Often, the failure to make an entry raises questions as to whether care that the nurse was required to give, and that the nurse testifies was given, was in fact given. For example, one case involved the patient's allegation that the nurse had failed to follow the physician's order to "watch condition of toes" after the patient's leg had been put in a cast to set a fracture. During the second night of hospitalization, the nurse made no entries regarding the condition of the toes until 6:00 A.M., at which time the nurse documented an abnormal observation and called the physician. Subsequent treatment was unsuccessful, and the patient's leg was amputated because of irreversible ischemia, allegedly caused by the cast's interference with blood circulation for too long a time before the physician was notified.

The nurse testified that she had observed the toes on a regular basis but made no entries because observations were normal. The patient's attorney was able to persuade the jury that the absence of entries between 11:00 P.M. and 6:00 A.M. was sufficient evidence that the nurse's testimony was not reliable. Even though hospital policy did not require that entries be made for normal observations, the jury was aware that nurses on earlier shifts had made such entries.

In another case, a nurse was sued for allegedly failing to reduce the amount of oxygen administered to a premature baby from 6 to 4 liters per minute after the first 12 hours, as ordered by the physician. The infant was blinded by retrolental fibroplasia, allegedly caused by excessive quantities of oxygen. The nurse testified that she had followed the order, but the chart was devoid of any entries reflecting her testimony that 4 liters had been given after 12 hours. There were, however, several entries reflecting the 6-liters-per-hour administration during the first 12 hours. The jury concluded, on the basis of the inferences they drew from indirect, circumstantial evidence, that 6 liters had been administered throughout.

In each case the nurse's testimony was not supported by entries in the chart, and the jury chose to believe the chart. No absolute rules can be created for deciding what to chart, but it is beneficial to anticipate the effect not charting might have on a jury if a lawsuit were brought.

Inaccurate Entries. In other cases, inaccurate entries, whether intentionally or inadvertently made, have diminished the reliability of the records, consequently, the strength of the nurse's case. In one case, for example, a nurse was accused of having been negligent in observing a pregnant patient and failing to call her physician in time to deliver the baby. The nurse claimed that there were no indications that should have caused her to call the doctor earlier than she had. During the trial, evidence was produced that the nurse had actually delivered the baby. The notes, however, indicated that another physician had performed the delivery (which was not the issue). Nonetheless, the inaccuracy undoubtedly affected the jury's decision in finding that the nurse had been negligent in calling the patient's physician. The nurse, who was convinced that she had not been negligent, appealed the verdict on the grounds that there was insufficient evidence to support it. The appellate court's opinion, in upholding the verdict, is instructive:

> . . . the records are still subject to the jury's scrutiny in light of all the evidence. The evidence in this case showed that the nurse performed the delivery of the baby and that she had been instructed by her supervisor never to state in the hospital records that she had delivered a baby. The jury might have been persuaded that if the records were erroneous in one respect, they were erroneous in other respects also.

In another case, where records had been falsified after a patient had suffered severe and permanent brain damage by wedging her head between a wall and a metal bed frame which was supposed to have been removed from the schizophrenic patient's room, the consequences were even more immediate. Although the hospital maintained that its staff was not negligent in causing the patient's injury, the judge instructed the jury that they were entitled to consider the falsification of records as evidence that there was "a consciousness of negligence" by those who changed the records.

The case makes it clear that very often the consequences of a cover-up are worse than what it seeks to conceal. Even though the nurses may not have been legally negligent in allowing the bed to remain in the room, the jurors were undoubtedly influenced by the falsification of records.

It should also be noted that falsification of records can result in criminal liability and professional disciplinary proceeding as well as civil liability.

Apparent Alterations. Records that appear to have been tampered with or altered can have the same consequences as those that, in fact, have been. Even though the nurse acts in good faith and without any wrongful motive, a plaintiff's attorney can suggest quite the contrary. Consider the inferences a jury might draw from the following questions and answers:

Attorney: Please read your first entry on January 3.

Nurse: I'm sorry, I can't.

Attorney: You can't?

Nurse: No.

Attorney: And the reason you can't is because you have completely whited it out, haven't you?

Nurse: Yes.

Attorney: You have completely obliterated it, haven't you?

Nurse: Yes, but it was just a mistaken entry.

Attorney: Could it be that instead of a mistaken entry you were really trying to conceal a nursing error?

Nurse: No. It was just a mistaken entry.

Attorney: You would deny then, that, in anticipation of this lawsuit you felt the need to cover up an entry which would have shown you deviated from the standards of nursing practice?

Nurse: Yes. That is untrue. I wouldn't do that.

Attorney: You are the defendant in this suit, are you not?

Nurse: Yes.

Attorney: And you do admit whiting out that entry, do you not?

Nurse: Yes, but. . . .

Attorney: And instead of simply drawing a line through what you say was merely a mistaken entry, which is the practice in such cases as I understand it, you completely obliterated the entry didn't you? Completely and permanently concealed the meaning of that entry?

Nurse: Yes, but it's not what it seems. . . .

Attorney: Thank you.

A similar inference could be suggested to a jury from such practices as writing in the margins or between lines, or from the discovery of late entries that are not clearly identified as late entries. Although late entries themselves can raise questions, they should be made and so labeled. The problem is worsened when the plaintiff's attorney discovers that an entry was late but not disclosed as such. It only adds to the appearances of a cover-up. For similar reasons, records should not be thrown away, even for what seem to be good reasons. It may be difficult to explain that you had a good reason from the witness stand in a malpractice trial, especially after it has been suggested that you have destroyed evidence that would have been incriminating.

Charting at the End of the Shift. The practice of waiting until the end of a shift to chart, while not uncommon, is a risky one. Again, it raises questions about the accuracy and reliability of the chart. Consider the effect on a jury of the following dialogue:

Attorney: About these entries which you have been reading, may I ask when during your shift they are made?

Nurse: I don't understand the question.

Attorney: Do you make your entries as the developments to which they refer occur, or do you wait until the end of your shift to do your charting?

Nurse: Usually the end of the shift, but. . . .

Attorney: And how long is your shift?

Nurse: Eight hours.

Attorney: And during these eight hours, how many patients do you normally have contact with?

Nurse: About 20.

Attorney: Twenty. And how many times, on average, do you see each of these 20 patients?

Nurse: It varies. But I would say from five to seven.

Attorney: So it is fair to say that you have up to 140 patient-contacts, maybe more, on a given day?

Nurse: Yes.

Attorney: Are you sometimes, at the end of your shift, a little tired?

Nurse: Sometimes.

Attorney: And are you, at the end of your shift, sometimes in a hurry to leave to go elsewhere?

Nurse: Sometimes.

Attorney: And would you agree that the patient's chart is an important part of the care that the patient receives? That others rely on it for purposes of determining the patient's progress and prognosis?

Nurse: Yes.

Attorney: And that it is important, therefore, that the chart be accurate, complete and reliable?

Nurse: Yes.

Attorney: And is it true that you are sometimes distracted from things that you were planning on doing by unexpected developments?

Nurse: Yes.

Attorney: And that you may, by the end of your shift, chart something that you had planned on doing but didn't do because of a distraction? Or forget to chart something that you did do?

Nurse: It's possible . . .

Attorney: So, at the end of an eight-hour shift, during which you have had, perhaps, 140 patient contacts and been distracted different times, and at a time when you are sometimes tired or in a hurry, you are trying to recall in detail everything which is significant to the well-being of each of your patients?

Nurse: Yes, but . . .

Attorney: Thank you. That is all.

It should be apparent that the practice of waiting until later to chart can be used to raise serious questions about the reliability of the chart, and, if the chart is perceived to be unreliable, the nurse's credibility also suffers.

Subjective Versus Objective Charting. Facts, accurately recorded, give the plaintiff's attorney much less room to maneuver than subjectively reached opinions or conclusions. To the extent that charting procedures permit, nurses should limit their entries to the facts they observe. They should use their senses like a camera and record what the camera "sees."

It is tempting and easy to chart conclusions based upon what you observe. It also may offer a plaintiff's attorney an opportunity to discredit the reliability and accuracy of the chart, as the following dialogue shows:

Attorney: Would you read your entry from October 5 to the jury, please.

Nurse: Yes. It begins, "Patient fell out of bed . . ."

Attorney: Thank you. By the way, did you see the patient fall out of bed?

Nurse: No.

Attorney: Did the patient tell you he fell out of bed?

Nurse: Not that I remember.

Attorney: Did the patient have a roommate?

Nurse: I'm not sure.

Attorney: You don't remember a roommate telling you that the patient fell out of bed either then, I assume?

Nurse: No.

Attorney: Please read that entry again.

Nurse: "Patient fell out of bed . . ."

Attorney: Thank you. Now that is stated as a fact, is it not?

Nurse: Yes.

Attorney: If you did not actually see the patient fall out of bed, and no one else saw or told you they saw the patient fall out of bed, how do you know, in fact, that he did?

Nurse: I guess I don't.

Attorney: But you charted it as if you did.

Nurse: Yes.

Attorney: So what you have charted as a fact is nothing more than a guess. It is only speculation and conjecture?

Nurse: I guess so.

Attorney: Yes or no please.

Nurse: Yes.

Attorney: So you are charting guesses as facts. Would you agree that the chart is relied upon by other members of the health care team for purposes of caring for the patient?

Nurse: Yes.

Attorney: And that it should be accurate and reliable in all respects?

Nurse: Yes.

Attorney: And would you agree that it is not accurate or reliable in this respect?

Nurse: Yes.

Attorney: Thank you.

Whether or not this particular entry is germane to the case, it has been effectively used to damage the believability of the chart upon which the nurse is most likely basing the defense of the case. Further, such cross-examination often has the effect of "shaking" the nurse-witness, thus decreasing the likelihood that the testimony will be effective. And it has the additional potential for "diluting" the nurse's testimony and distracting the jury from more important points that might have been made or creating confusion in jurors' minds. Table 3–4 contains other examples that distinguish objective and subjective entries.

The use of objective statements also minimizes use of the word "apparently" or the phrase "it appears that. . . ." Neither is advisable from a legal perspective, and neither is as effective, descriptive, or communicative as facts. Remember to chart what you *see, hear, smell,* and *feel.*

Table 3–4. Examples of Subjective and Objective Chart Entries

SUBJECTIVE STATEMENTS	OBJECTIVE STATEMENTS
Patient is drunk.	Patient's pupils are dilated and speech is slurred; patient is unsteady on his feet and has alcohol-like odor on breath.
Patient slept all night.	Checked on patient every two hours, eyes closed, respirations regular.
Patient's diet taken fair.	Half of diet consumed.
IV running well.	IV site clear, infusing at 60 gtt per minute.
Patient had a good day!	No C/O pain or discomfort.

Neatness Counts. Writing must also be legible and neat. Entries that are not legible are less likely to be read by others, thus resulting in a failure of communication that can lead to patient injury. They are more likely to be misunderstood by others who do read them, which can lead to the same result. Furthermore, a jury might conclude that a nurse who is a sloppy charter is a sloppy nurse. Neatness does more than look nice. Use good penmanship and concise phrases. Begin each phrase with a capital letter, and each new topic on a separate line.

Proper Use of Terms. Nurse should be familiar with and use terminology that is commonly accepted by others in the institution. Such consistency enhances communication among members of the health care team and reduces the possibility of miscommunication. On the other hand, nurses should not use terms with which they are unfamiliar. Use only those that you are certain you understand to mean what others understand them to mean.

Proper Use of "White Space." Nurses should not skip lines between entries. Every entry should be "snugged up" to the previous entry. The plaintiff's attorney could suggest that a "margin for error" has been deliberately left for "late entries," "clarifications," or other self-serving "corrections." Furthermore, such space may be used by other health care personnel for such entries. And, when an entry is completed with space left on the line, good practice calls for the nurse to draw a line from the end of the entry to the end of the right-hand margin.

Similarly, space should not be left between the last entry and the nurse's signature. And be sure to sign each entry and postscript.

Patient Quotes and Activities.   Whenever appropriate, direct patient quotes should be made a part of the patient's chart. Be sure to use quotation marks to indicate exactly what the patient said, e.g., patient said, ''I must have fallen out of bed while asleep.''What the patient says is an objective observation, a fact, and should be documented as such when it bears on the patient's health or care plan.

If a patient does not comply with instructions reasonably related to his best interests or otherwise fails to conduct himself in a reasonably prudent manner, such activities should be objectively reported. A competent patient has a responsibility to exercise reasonable care to prevent injury to himself. As previously discussed, a patient is responsible for any injury to himself caused by his own negligence. Such negligence is more easily proven and used as a contributory or comparative negligence defense in a subsequent suit against the nurse, if it has been objectively, accurately, and completely documented at the time it occurred. When appropriate, more detailed information should be included in an incident or variance report.

The Chart as Friend or Foe: The Nurse Decides

Since the chart is considered by juries to be the most reliable indicator of patient care, and since it is, for the most part, the nurse who decides what is charted, how it is charted, and what is not charted, the chart should be viewed as an opportunity to accurately, factually, and completely document the good care that a patient receives. It can be an important factor in a malpractice prevention program. Table 3–5 recaps the various other elements of a malpractice program.

Table 3–5. **A Malpractice-Prevention Program**

There are a number of opportunities that nurses can capitalize on to minimize effectively the likelihood of being sued or of losing the suit if they are. These are the key elements in a malpractice-prevention program:

The nurse's concern for the patient should be *apparent*, as well as real.

The nurse's knowledge of nursing standards should be complete and current.

The nurse's delegation or acceptance of delegated responsibility should be selective.

The nurse's chart should be accurate, complete, and factual, and entries should be made in a timely manner.

The nurse should carry an individual malpractice insurance policy.

The nurse must exercise professional discretion and judgment.

Incident Reports

As has been indicated, the purposes of incident reports and charts are different. Therefore, the information included in each is different. The chart is a vehicle through which members of the health care team communicate information that has a direct bearing on the care of the patient. The *incident report* is used by administrators to identify problems with procedures, personnel, equipment, and so forth, that need to be dealt with. It is also used to preserve important evidence for possible use by hospital or insurance company attorneys in any subsequent litigation. Unless specifically referred to in the chart, incident reports are generally not available for use by the plaintiff's attorney. Each hospital or other institution has a policy on when an incident report should be filed. Such policies generally require that incident reports be completed when there has been an ''unusual occurrence.'' Unusual occurrences are typically defined as including, but not being limited to, events such

Table 3–6. **Guidelines for Completing Incident Reports**

1. Describe whether person is a patient, visitor, volunteer, or staff person.
2. State your involvement with the incident (caring for patient, witness, found the patient, recipient of complaint, etc.).
3. Describe how you became aware of the situation.
4. Describe the names, locations, and roles of others who saw or were otherwise involved in the incident, including information on how they can be reached.
5. Describe remarks made by the patient and others before, during and/or after the incident. Who said what?
6. State your opinion on cause, effects, seriousness, future health and/or legal implications.
7. Add whatever other information you feel important, including suggestions on avoiding similar future incidents.

UNIVERSITY OF MINNESOTA HOSPITALS & CLINICS
INCIDENT REPORT

NAME OF PERSON INVOLVED (LAST, FIRST, M.I.)	AGE	SEX	INCIDENT DATE	INCIDENT TIME ☐ AM ☐ PM	INCIDENT LOCATION (AREA AND ROOM#)

CATEGORY OF PERSON INVOLVED		
☐ PATIENT →	UH#	CONDITION ☐ AMBULATORY ☐ UP WITH HELP ☐ BEDREST ☐ SEDATED
☐ EMPLOYEE →	JOB TITLE	DEPARTMENT
☐ OTHER →	SPECIFY (E.G.,VISITOR, VOLUNTEER, ETC.)	HOME PHONE (AREA CODE) ( )

GENERAL TYPE OF INCIDENT			
☐ INJURY / FATALITY	☐ PROPERTY /FACILITY DAMAGE	☐ MEDICATION ERROR	☐ ADVERSE DRUG REACTION
☐ THEFT (CALL SECURITY IMMEDIATELY)	☐ PATIENT PROPERTY OR VALUABLES	☐ DEFECTIVE PRODUCT ☐ POTENTIAL HAZARD	OTHER (SPECIFY) ☐

DESCRIPTION OF INCIDENT - PLEASE OBJECTIVELY DESCRIBE ALL INCIDENTS IN THIS SPACE. IN ADDITION, A CHECKLIST HAS BEEN PROVIDED FOR MEDICATIONS, FALLS AND LABORATORY-RELATED INCIDENTS FOR YOUR CONVENIENCE. CONTINUE ON REVERSE IF NECESSARY.

CHECK HERE IF CONTINUED ON BACK ☐

MEDICATION RELATED INCIDENTS	TYPE (CHECK ALL THAT APPLY)	STEPS WHICH MAY HAVE CONTRIBUTED TO INCIDENT (CHECK ALL THAT APPLY)	INTRAVENOUS FLUIDS (CHECK ALL THAT APPLY)
	☐ DIFFERENT MED/DOSE/SOLUTION ARRIVED ON STATION	☐ ORDERING MEDICATION	☐ TOO FAST
	☐ DIFFERENT MEDICATION GIVEN	☐ TRANSCRIBING ORDER	☐ TOO SLOW
	☐ DIFFERENT DOSAGE GIVEN	☐ LABELING MEDICATION	☐ DIFFERENT SOLUTION
	☐ MED. GIVEN TO DIFFERENT PATIENT	☐ READING MEDICATION LABEL	☐ DIFFERENT ADDITIVE
	☐ MED. GIVEN AT DIFFERENT TIME	☐ COMPARING LABEL W/MED KARDEX	☐ DIFF. ADMINISTRATIVE APPARATUS
	☐ MED. GIVEN BY DIFFERENT ROUTE	☐ CHECKING PATIENT I.D. BAND	☐ I.V. INFILTRATED
	☐ MEDICATION OMITTED	☐ GIVING MEDICATION	☐ OTHER
	☐ OTHER	☐ PATIENT DISREGARDED INSTRUCTIONS	
		☐ OTHER	

INCIDENTS INVOLVING FALLS	TYPE OF FALL	ACTIVITY AT TIME OF INCIDENT	CIRCUMSTANCES (CHECK ALL THAT APPLY)
	☐ FROM COMMODE	☐ WALKING ALONE	☐ SLIPPERY WALKING SURFACE
	☐ FROM WHEELCHAIR	☐ WALKING ASSISTED	☐ TRIPPED
	☐ FROM CHAIR	☐ TRANSFER ALONE	☐ FAINTED
	☐ FROM BED	☐ TRANSFER ASSISTED	☐ LOSS OF BALANCE
	☐ OTHER	☐ SITTING UP	☐ SEIZURE
		☐ LYING DOWN	☐ DISREGARDED INSTRUCTIONS
		☐ OTHER	☐ OTHER

LABORATORY RELATED INCIDENTS	TYPE OF INCIDENTS		
	☐ RESULTS REPORTED INCORRECTLY	☐ RESPONSE TIME	☐ OTHER
	☐ SPECIMEN HANDLED IMPROPERLY	☐ MISLABELED SPECIMEN → ☐ UNLABELED SPECIMEN →	STATION/CLINIC SENDING SPECIMEN WAS / PHLEBOTOMIST WAS

PHYSICIAN NOTIFIED? ☐ YES ☐ NO	IF YES, NAME SIGNATURE X	PHYSICIAN'S FINDINGS CHECK HERE IF CONTINUED ON BACK ☐		
PERSON COMPLETING	SIGNATURE X	TITLE	DATE	PHONE

UH 1038, APR 81

Please forward to Box 708 Mayo within 24 hours.

Figure 3–2. An example of an incident form. (Courtesy of the University of Minnesota Hospitals and Clinics, Minneapolis, MN.)

as accidents, injuries, thefts, burns, assaults, damage to property, confrontations, medication errors, defective products, mistakes or failures in delivering health care services, or subsequent complaints or expressions of concern about any of these by patients or personnel.

Responsibility for filing incident reports rests with the individual who perceives that an incident has occurred. The report should be made on the form generally provided for that purpose and should be made as soon as possible after the incident occurs. (See Figure 3–2.) Routing procedures are usually established by institutional policy and often vary, depending on the type of incident. If not all information is available at the time the report is completed, a follow-up report, on a separate incident-report form should be made. The follow-up report should be marked as an addendum, and the initial report clearly referred to and identified. Policy usually also determines whether copies should be made and, if so, to whom they should be distributed. Table 3–6 contains guidelines for completing incident reports.

Patients' Rights

As the foregoing discussion on malpractice has shown, the health care professions and industry have not been immune from the sweeping effects of the consumerism movement and its focus on consumer rights. Since 1972, when the American Hospital Association adopted its "A Patient's Bill of Rights," a wide variety of other such statements of patients' rights have been promulgated. They include separate statements for the old, the young, the dying, the handicapped, the pregnant, the mentally ill, the retarded, and the disabled patient.

They are instructive reading. Although sometimes

Exhibit 3–1. A Patient's Bill of Rights

1. The patient has the right to considerate and respectful care.

2. The patient has the right to obtain from his physician complete current information concerning his diagnosis, treatment, and prognosis in terms the patient can be reasonably expected to understand. When it is not medically advisable to give such information to the patient, the information should be made available to an appropriate person in his behalf. He has the right to know, by name, the physician responsible for coordinating his care.

3. The patient has the right to receive from his physician information necessary to give informed consent prior to the start of any procedure and/or treatment. Except in emergencies, such information for informed consent should include but not necessarily be limited to the specific procedure and/or treatment, the medically significant risks involved, and the probable duration of incapacitation. Where medically significant alternatives for care or treatment exist, or when the patient requests information concerning medical alternatives, the patient has the right to such information. The patient also has the right to know the name of the person responsible for the procedures and/or treatment.

4. The patient has the right to refuse treatment to the extent permitted by law, and to be informed of the medical consequences of his action.

5. The patient has the right to every consideration of his privacy concerning his own medical care program. Case discussion, consultation, examination, and treatment are confidential and should be conducted discreetly. Those not directly involved in his care must have the permission of the patient to be present.

6. The patient has the right to expect that all communications and records pertaining to his care should be treated as confidential.

7. The patient has the right to expect that within its capacity a hospital must make reasonable response to the request of a patient for services. The hospital must provide evaluation, service, and/or referral as indicated by the urgency of the case. When medically permissible a patient may be transferred to another facility only after he has received complete information and explanation concerning the needs for and alternatives to such a transfer. The institution to which the patient is to be transferred must first have accepted the patient for transfer.

8. The patient has the right to obtain information as to any relationship of his hospital to other health care and educational institutions insofar as his care is concerned. The patient has the right to obtain information as to the existence of any professional relationships among individuals, by name, who are treating him.

9. The patient has the right to be advised if the hospital proposes to engage in or perform human experimentation affecting his care or treatment. The patient has the right to refuse to participate in such research projects.

10. The patient has the right to expect reasonable continuity of care. He has the right to know in advance what appointment times and physicians are available and where. The patient has the right to expect that the hospital will provide a mechanism whereby he is informed by his physician or a delegate of the physician of the patient's continuing health care requirements following discharge.

11. The patient has the right to examine and receive an explanation of his bill regardless of source of payment.

12. The patient has the right to know what hospital rules and regulations apply to his conduct as a patient.

No catalogue of rights can guarantee for the patient the kind of treatment he has a right to expect. A hospital has many functions to perform, including the prevention and treatment of disease, the education of both health professionals and patients, and the conduct of clinical research. All these activities must be conducted with an overriding concern for the patient, and, above all, the recognition of his dignity as a human being. Success in achieving this recognition assures success in the defense of the rights of the patient.

Source: Reprinted with permission. The American Hospital Association. *Nurs. Outlook*, Feb., **21**:82, 1973.

imprecise, they are comprehensive. In effect, they outline the parameters of nursing responsibility and provide the context within which most malpractice litigation occurs. To a large extent, they reflect the principles that the common law of malpractice has developed; and, since they have been adopted by professional groups, they can be introduced as evidence in a trial and used as evidence of what a nurse in any given case should have done. A growing number of states have enacted legislation that substantially duplicates some of these statements, thus giving them the full force and effect of law.

Included here are the American Hospital Association's statement on patients' rights (Exhibit 3–1) the American Nurses' Association's "Code for Nurses," most recently revised in 1976 (Exhibit 3–3), the Canadian Nurses' Association's "Code of Ethics" (Exhibit 3–4), and the Minnesota legislature's "Patients' Bill of Rights" (Exhibit 3–2), most recently amended in 1983.

Exhibit 3–2. Patients' Bill of Rights (Statutory)

**144.651 Patients and residents of health care facilities:
bill of rights**

It is the intent of the legislature and the purpose of this section to promote the interests and well being of the patients and residents of health care facilities. No health care facility may require a patient or resident to waive these rights as a condition of admission to the facility. Any guardian or conservator of a patient or resident or, in the absence of a guardian or conservator, an interested person, may seek enforcement of these rights on behalf of a patient or resident. It is the intent of this section that every patient's civil and religious liberties, including the right to independent personal decisions and knowledge of available choices, shall not be infringed and that the facility shall encourage and assist in the fullest possible exercise of these rights.

For the purposes of this section, "patient" means a person who is admitted to an acute care inpatient facility for a continuous period longer than 24 hours, for the purpose of diagnosis or treatment bearing on the physical or mental health of that person. "Resident" means a person who is admitted to a non-acute care facility including extended care facilities, nursing homes, and board and care homes for care required because of prolonged mental or physical illness or diability, recovery from injury or disease, or advancing age.

It is declared to be the public policy of this state that the interests of each patient and resident be protected by a declaration of a patients' bill of rights which shall include but not be limited to the following:

(1) Every patient and resident shall have the right to considerate and respectful care;

(2) Every patient and resident can reasonably expect to obtain from his physician or the resident physician of the facility complete and current information concerning his diagnosis, treatment and prognosis in terms and language the patient can reasonably be expected to understand. In cases in which it is not medically advisable to give the information to the patient or resident the information may be made available to the appropriate person in his behalf;

(3) Every patient and resident shall have the right to know by name and speciality, if any, the physician responsible for coordination of his care;

(4) Every patient and resident shall have the right to every consideration of his privacy and individuality as it relates to his social, religious, and psychological well being;

(5) Every patient and resident shall have the right to respectfulness and privacy as it relates to his medical care program. Case discussion, consultation, examination, and treatment are confidential and should be conducted discreetly;

(6) Every patient and resident shall have the right to expect the facility to make a reasonable response to his requests;

(7) Every patient and resident shall have the right to obtain information as to any relationship of the facility to other health care and related institutions insofar as his care is concerned;

(8) Every patient and resident shall have the right to expect reasonable continuity of care which shall include but not be limited to what appointment times and physicians are available;

(9) Every resident shall be fully informed, prior to or at the time of admission and during his stay, of services available in the facility, and of related charges including any charges for services not covered under medicare or medicaid or not covered by the facility's basic per diem rate;

(10) Every patient and resident shall be afforded the opportunity to participate in the planning of his medical treatment and to refuse to participate in experimental research;

(11) No resident shall be arbitrarily transferred or discharged but may be transferred or discharged only for medical reasons, for his or other residents welfare, or for nonpayment for stay unless prohibited by the welfare programs paying for the care of the resident, as documented in the medical record. Reasonable advance notice of any transfer or discharge must be given to a resident;

(12) Every resident may manage his personal financial affairs, or shall be given at least a quarterly accounting of financial transactions on his behalf if he delegates this responsibility in accordance with the laws of Minnesota to the facility for any period of time;

(13) Every resident shall be encouraged and assisted,

throughout his period of stay in a facility, to understand and exercise his rights as a patient and as a citizen, and to this end, he may voice grievances and recommend changes in policies and services to facility staff and outside representatives of his choice free from restraint, interference, coercion, discrimination or reprisal;

(14) Every resident shall be free from mental and physical abuse, and free from chemical and physical restraints, except in emergencies, or as authorized in writing by his physican for a specified and limited period of time, and when necessary to protect the resident from injury to himself or to others;

(15) Every patient and resident shall be assured confidential treatment of his personal and medical records, and may approve or refuse their release to any individual outside the facility, except as otherwise provided by law or a third party payment contract;

(16) No resident shall be required to perform services for the facility that are not included for therapeutic purposes in his plan of care;

(17) Every resident may associate and communicate privately with persons of his choice, and send and receive his personal mail unopened, unless medically contraindicated and documented by his physician in the medical record;

(18) Every resident may meet with representatives and participate in activities of commercial, religious, and community groups at his discretion; provided, however, that the activities shall not infringe upon the right to privacy of other residents;

(19) Every resident may retain and use his personal clothing and possessions as space permits, unless to do so would infringe upon rights of other patients or residents, and unless medically contraindicated and documented by his physician in the medical record;

(20) Every resident, if married, shall be assured privacy for visits by his or her spouse and if both spouses are residents of the facility, they shall be permitted to share a room, unless medically contraindicated and documented by their physicians in the medical record; and

(21) Every patient or resident shall be fully informed, prior to or at the time of admission and during his stay at a facility, of the rights and responsibilities set forth in this section and of all rules governing patient conduct and responsibilities.

Source: Minnesota Statutes, Chapter 144.

Exhibit 3-3. American Nurses' Association—Code for Nurses

1. The nurse provides services with respect for human dignity and the uniqueness of the client unrestricted by considerations of social or economic status, personal attributes, or the nature of health problems.

2. The nurse safeguards the client's right to privacy by judiciously protecting information of a confidential nature.

3. The nurse acts to safeguard the client and the public when health care and safety are affected by incompetent, unethical, or illegal practices of any person.

4. The nurse assumes responsibility and accountability for individual nursing judgments and actions.

5. The nurse maintains competence in nursing.

6. The nurse exercises informed judgment and uses individual competence and qualifications as criteria in seeking consultation, accepting responsibilities, and delegating nursing activities to others.

7. The nurse participates in activities that contribute to the ongoing development of the profession's body of knowledge.

8. The nurse participates in the profession's efforts to implement and improve standards of nursing.

9. The nurse participates in the profession's efforts to establish and maintain conditions of employment conducive to high-quality nursing care.

10. The nurse participates in the profession's efforts to protect the public from misinformation and misrepresentation and to maintain the integrity of nursing.

11. The nurse collaborates with members of the health professions and other citizens in promoting community and national efforts to meet the health needs of the public.

Source: Reproduced with permission of the American Nurses' Association, Pub. No. G-56.

Exhibit 3–4. **Canadian Nurses' Association—Code of Ethics**

Statements of Ethical Responsibility

1. Caring demands the provision of helping services that are appropriate to the needs of the client and significant others.

2. Caring recognizes the client's membership in a family and community and provides for the participation of significant others in his or her care.

3. Caring acknowledges the reality of death in the life of every person, and demands that appropriate support be provided for the dying person and family to enable them to prepare for, and to cope with death when it is inevitable.

4. Caring acknowledges that the human person has the capacity to face up to health needs and problems in his or her own unique way, and directs nursing action in a manner that will assist the client to develop, maintain or gain personal autonomy, self-respect and self-determination.

5. Caring, as a response to a health need, requires the consent and the participation of the person who is experiencing the need.

6. Caring dictates that the client and significant others have the knowledge and information adequate for free and informed decisions concerning care requirements, alternatives and preferences.

7. Caring demands that the needs of the client supersede those of the nurse, and that the nurse must not compromise the integrity of the client by personal behavior that is self-serving.

8. Caring acknowledges the vulnerability of a client in certain situations, and dictates restraint in actions which might compromise the client's rights and privileges.

9. Caring involving a relationship which is, in itself, therapeutic, demands mutual respect and trust.

10. Caring acknowledges that information obtained in the course of the nursing relationship is privileged, and that it requires the full protection of confidentiality unless such information provides evidence of serious impending harm to the client or to a third party, or is legally required by the courts.

11. Caring requires that the nurse represent the needs of the client and that the nurse take appropriate measures when fulfillment of these needs is jeopardized by the actions of other persons.

12. Caring acknowledges the dignity of all persons in the practice or educational setting.

13. Caring acknowledges, respects and draws upon the competencies of others.

14. Caring establishes the conditions for the harmonization of efforts of different helping professionals in providing required services to clients.

15. Caring seeks to establish and maintain a climate of respect for the honest dialogue needed for effective collaboration.

16. Caring establishes the legitimacy of respectful challenge and/or confrontation when the service required by the client is compromised by incompetency, incapacity or negligence, or when the competencies of the nurse are not acknowledged or appropriately utilized.

17. Caring demands the provision of working conditions which enable nurses to carry out their legitimate responsibilities.

18. Caring demands resourcefulness and restraint—accountability for the use of time, resources, equipment, and funds, and requires accountability to appropriate individuals and/or bodies.

19. Caring requires that the nurse bring to the work situation in education, practice, administration or research, the knowledge, affective and technical skills required, and that competency in these areas be maintained and updated.

20. Caring commands fidelity to oneself, and guards the right and privilege of the nurse to act in keeping with an informed moral conscience.

Source: The Canadian Nurses' Association, 1980, Ottawa. Reproduced with permission.

Beyond Liability for Malpractice

Although tort law, particularly negligence, constitutes the one area of law that has the most noticeable effect on nurses, there are other laws with which the nurse should be familiar. Even more than the law of torts, these areas of law overlap with and raise questions of ethics and conscience for the nurse; and, in addition to civil liability, they represent the prospect of criminal liability. Furthermore, like tort law, they also set standards that can be used in disciplinary proceedings which can affect the nurse's license to practice.

These areas of law deal with the scope of legal nursing practice, euthanasia and the right to die, induced abortions, and dealing with incompetent colleagues.

The Regulation of Nursing Practice

Since the early 1900s, the respective states have sought to protect the public by regulating who is entitled to practice nursing and by defining the parameters of nursing practice. Since each state has authority to make these determinations, the language and effects of legislation have varied considerably from state to state.

One method of exercising this authority is to set standards that a nursing educational institution must meet in order to receive state approval, and to require that graduation from a state-approved school be a prerequisite for taking the examination the graduate must pass in order to obtain the required license to practice nursing.

State legislatures also have enacted nurse practice acts in an attempt to limit the scope of practice for those who do obtain their license. A recent development has been to establish certification mechanisms that permit licensed nurses to obtain a certificate that recognizes their expertise in various nursing specialty areas, such as nurse practitioners, midwives, and anesthetists. In nearly every state, the responsibility and authority for administering and carrying out the purpose of these statutes are delegated to a board of nursing or nurse examiners. These boards adopt criteria that nursing schools must meet to attain and maintain approval and regulations for use in examining nursing candidates, issuing licenses, and, when necessary, disciplining licensed nurses who violate the rules, regulations, and statutes that regulate nursing practice.

At one time these boards were dominated by nonnurses, especially physicians. Today, most boards are comprised of registered and practical nurses. In many states, board members are selected from a pool of candidates recommended by the state nurses' association. The most notable recent development is the requirement that board membership include consumer representatives. Nearly half the states now have such a requirement. Physicians now hold seats on boards in only half a dozen states.

Mandatory licensure now exists in all but a few states. In states where licensure remains permissive, unlicensed nurses can practice, but they cannot refer to themselves as an RN or LPN. As a practical matter, unlicensed nurses in those states find it difficult to work professionally, as many health care institutions limit their hiring to licensed nurses. The mandatory licensure requirements, however, are not all that they seem. They contain exceptions, for example, for nursing by domestic servants, friends, nurse-maids, out-of-state nurses accompanying patients or awaiting registration, new graduates, student nurses, federal employees, and nurses attending graduate school. The exceptions, of course, differ from state to state.

In the last decade, the need to expand the role of nursing has led to the revision of most states' nurse practice acts. These changes have taken different forms, but all have dealt with the authority of nurses to diagnose and treat, both of which were previously prohibited. The model definitions of professional and practical nursing, adopted by the American Nurses' Association in 1976, are often incorporated into rules adopted by state boards or statutes passed by legislative bodies. Note the absence of a restriction on diagnosis.

Practice of Nursing by a Registered Nurse
The practice of nursing as performed by a registered nurse is a process in which substantial specialized knowledge derived from the biological, physical, and behavioral sciences is applied to the care, treatment, counsel, and health teaching of persons who are experiencing changes in the normal health processes, or who require assistance in the maintenance of health or the management of illness, injury, or infirmity or in the achievement of a dignified death, and such additional acts as are recognized by the nursing profession as proper to be performed by a registered nurse.

Practice of Nursing by a Licensed
Practical Vocational Nurse
Practical vocational nursing means the performance under the supervision of a registered nurse of those services required in observing and caring for the ill, injured, or infirm, in promoting preventive measures in community health, in acting to safeguard life and health, in administering treatment and medication prescribed by a physician or dentist, or in performing other acts not requiring the skill, judgment, and knowledge of a registered nurse.
[American Nurses' Association, 1976]

In over half of the states, the task of drafting guidelines to permit the expanded roles has been delegated to either the nursing board, acting alone, or to the nursing and medical boards acting in concert. In the dozen or so states where several boards are to write the guidelines together, the process has been especially slow and progress difficult, caused largely by political problems created by those who see an expanded nurse's role as unwanted competition.

Some legislatures have, instead of leaving the matter to a regulatory board, enacted legislation that defines the practice of nursing by a registered nurse as including diagnosis. That has created more problems than it has solved. Again, political influences have led to efforts to distinguish between medical and nursing diagnosis, with unsatisfactory results. Rather than clarify, they have confused, and left nurses asking exactly where, from a legal point of view, nursing ends and the practice of medicine begins. A definitive, exacting answer is not determinable. The answer will be forthcoming as actual practice evolves, as further attempts are made to add true meaning and clarity to the statutes and regulations, and as courts are called upon to deal with individual cases in each state.

Still other states have dealt with the need to broaden the parameters of nursing practice by developing certification procedures. In these states, the nursing boards have adopted regulations that define advanced registered nurses and specialized registered nurses. These definitions typically use education as a basis and provide for the granting of a certificate to nurses who demonstrate the appropriate advanced preparation.

Other states have responded with legislated protocols and standardized procedures that nurses are either entitled or obligated to follow. Others have revised the nurse practice acts to permit diagnosis and treatment to be done when delegated by and done under the supervision of a physician. In these states, a continuing question is how direct the supervision must be to comply with the intent of the statutes.

Although it is natural for nurses to want to know, with some certainty, the legal boundaries of practice, it must be recognized that nursing has undergone, and is undergoing, change of enormous proportions. Nursing is in a transition period, and the question is in the process of being answered.

Euthanasia, the Right To Die, and the Nurse

- Is it ever right not to aggressively treat a disease or condition known or expected to be fatal if not treated?
- Is it ever right to withdraw life support?
- Is it ever right to withhold life support?

Such questions are stirring heated controversy in hospitals and nursing homes. As technology has given the medical profession the ability to sustain life almost indefinitely, and as the public increasingly considers the meaning of quality of life, the ethical and legal issues are becoming increasingly urgent. For now, firm ethical and legal guidelines can only be said to be developing. Nonetheless, certain principles do exist to serve as guides to the nurse who must deal with these questions; and the answers are important, as they could raise the prospect of civil or criminal liability.

Compassionate as it may sound, euthanasia is not consistent with the law. Mercy killing, as it is sometimes called, is nonetheless killing. It is homicide within the meaning of the criminal law. It constitutes the civil tort of wrongful death, for which one is answerable in damages. Affirmatively terminating life, irrespective of good intentions or moral convictions, is legally wrong.

The question of when life ceases to exist is itself in a state of change. Death was traditionally considered to occur when respiratory functions ceased. But medicine's capability of artificially maintaining respiratory functions has prompted some state legislatures, and some courts, to adopt a "brain death" standard. The first was adopted in 1977. It should be emphasized that this standard has not met with universal acceptance, but is in effect in about half the states.

It is also important to distinguish between *withholding* and *terminating* artificial life-support measures, such as respirators. It is difficult to find legal support anywhere for the physician or nurse who turns off life-sustaining equipment being used on a living patient, even if the patient has executed a living will. Living wills, which are legislatively recognized in approximately 14 states are generally thought to permit *withholding* of "heroic measures," but not *terminating* them once they have begun. A prosecutor and grand jury could easily conclude such conduct to constitute murder or attempted murder, no more legal than administering a lethal injection. In the much-publicized Quinlan case, in fact, the New Jersey Attorney General promised to prosecute any physician who "pulled the plug." The case, brought by Quinlan's father, eventually resulted in a ruling that the question of whether to withdraw the artificial life-support system from a patient whom doctors agreed had no reasonable possibility of recovery was a matter for the patient or her guardian (father) to decide. If the guardian decided to withdraw consent (on the basis of the patient's constitutional right to privacy), the physicians would be relieved of any legal duty to continue the treatment.

It should be remembered that the Quinlan decision was novel, that it was based on a constitutional interpretation of an issue not yet addressed by the U.S. Supreme Court, and is not legally binding on the courts of any other jurisdiction in the country.

Where statutes do exist that authorize living wills, they also spell out procedures that must be adhered to when following the patient's written expression of the wish to be allowed to die if reasonable hope for recovery is gone. They include, for example, obtaining a court order, or the agreement of an ethics panel, a medical committee, the family, or a confirming medical opinion, or some combination of these. The statutes also usually grant civil and criminal immunity to those who carry out living-will requests.

"No Code" and "Slow Code" Orders

Another dilemma nurses often face is presented by a "no code," "slow code," or "code blue" order. It is not uncommon, particularly in intensive care units and nursing homes, for physicians to order that no effort to resuscitate (no code) or half-hearted efforts to resuscitate (slow code) be made for certain patients. Nonetheless, few cases have actually dealt with the legal propriety of such orders (and those that have cannot be relied upon beyond their own unique facts or state boundaries). It is an issue that the professions are reluctant to formally address, legislators avoid, and courts are rarely asked to consider. The result is that such decisions are made in a political and legal vacuum. Efforts are now underway, however, by many states' professional associations to develop guidelines, but they are impeded by the ethical, religious, emotional, and political considerations that weigh heavily when dealing with the issue. Similarly, some hospitals have formal protocols to be followed. Since they have supposedly been carefully thought through and reviewed by legal counsel, they should serve to substantially minimize the risk of legal liability when followed.

The American Heart Association and the National Academy of Science's National Research Council have adopted "Standards for Cardiopulmonary Resuscitation and Emergency Cardiac Care." While the standards, like those of any professional organization are not legally binding on a judge or jury, they are often persuasive. They indicate that, in appropriate cases, no CPR is an acceptable medical option. An appropriate case exists, according to the standards, "in cases of terminal irreversible illness or where death is not unexpected." In other words, CPR is intended to prevent *unexpected* death. Again, however, one must keep in mind that standards are not law, that courts may decide that acceptable medical practice is not acceptable legally, and that the standard speaks only to the use or nonuse of CPR.

In any event, when a physician determines that such an order is appropriate, the nurse should insist that the order be in writing, both on the order sheet and the patient's progress note (the standard referred to above in fact so requires). Although many physicians prefer such orders to be oral, nurses must be mindful that oral orders are much more easily misunderstood and disclaimed. Both can lead to serious problems for the nurse. If a physician refuses to write out no/slow code orders, the nurse should seek support from the hospital administration and the nursing department. If the nurse finds the administration recalcitrant or unsympathetic, a legal opinion should be sought through the hospital attorney. If none is forthcoming, the nurse has a personal and difficult decision to make.

These are wrenching issues that have caused much agonizing. They raise questions for which there seem to be few universally accepted answers. It is unrealistic to expect neat guidelines or tidy formulas. But since the questions will not go away, nurses must face them, armed not so much with the law, but with their own consciences, moral courage, and sense of humanity.

Induced Abortions and the Nurse

Although for abortion the law provides much more guidance on what is legally permissible, the extent to which a nurse wishes to participate in an induced abortion unavoidably requires personal, ethical, and perhaps legal considerations be taken into account.

Since 1973, when the *Roe v. Wade* and *Doe v. Bolton* cases were decided, the U.S. Supreme Court has considered a number of abortion cases. Most of these cases have dealt with the issue of the extent to which state government has a right to legislatively interfere with a pregnant woman's decision to have an abortion.

As a result of these rulings, it is constitutionally impermissible for a state to restrict or regulate abortions during the first trimester of pregnancy, except to require that they be performed by a licensed physician. The Court has held that the state has no compelling interest that could justify overriding the woman's right to privacy (which the Court found extended to a woman's decision to abort a pregnancy).

During the second trimester, from the fourth to sixth months of pregnancy, the state has a legitimate interest in the health of the mother. Accordingly, the mother's privacy rights must yield to *reasonable* restrictions designed to protect the mother's health. Such restrictions include, for example, licensure requirements for the facility in which the abortion is performed.

During the third trimester, according to the Supreme Court's decisions, the state has the right to completely restrict a woman's decision to abort. The rationale is that by this stage of the pregnancy, the state has gained a compelling interest in the product of the conception, the viable but unborn child, which outweighs the woman's right to privacy. According to the *Roe* opinion:

> For the stage subsequent to viability, the State, in promoting its interest in the potentiality of human life, may, if it chooses, regulate and even proscribe abortion, except where it is necessary, in appropriate medical judgment, for the preservation of the life or health of the mother.

Many states, of course, have enacted statutes since these decisions. They regulate, to varying degrees and in various ways, the matters involved in the abortion process. Many also include what are known as "conscience clauses," the validity of which have been upheld by the Supreme Court. The clauses specify that hospitals have the right to turn abortion patients away, and nurses and other personnel have the right to refuse to participate in abortions. The statutes also protect them from discrimination or retaliation if they exercise that right.

The Court has, since its initial rulings, struck down legislation which required that the parents of a pregnant minor consent to the abortion, that the father of a woman's child (whether he is her husband or not) consent, and that physicians performing an abortion of a potentially viable fetus attempt to assure its survival (since it was during the second trimester and not reasonably related to the mother's health).

The Nurse and Incompetent Colleagues

What does the nurse who is aware of an incompetent or unprofessional colleague do? The "Code for Nurses," reprinted earlier, speaks directly to the question: "The nurse acts to safeguard the client and the public when health care and safety are affected by incompent, unethical, or illegal practices of any person."

The Code reinforces the notion that the nurse's foremost concern is to protect the health, safety, and best interests of the patient. The interpretive statements (3.2–3.3) detail the recommended action. Essentially and minimally, the person whose conduct is in question should be talked with and, when appropriate, reported. The report may be made to appropriate administrative staff and/or the state board of nursing. Surveys have shown that most nurses would take some action, but would not report the matter to a peer review committee or licensing board. There are somewhat understandable reasons for this reluctance, but they are not consistent with the intent of the Code or the nurse's professional, ethical, or legal responsibilities. If a patient were injured by an incompetent nurse, the patient could bring a malpractice suit against the incompetent nurse, of course. But the patient could also sue the nurse who knew of another's incompetence but failed to take reasonable measures, such as reporting, to protect the patient from it.

A jury would not be favorably impressed with a defense based on the rationale that the nonreporting nurse "didn't want to create a scene," "didn't want to be the subject of resulting harassment," or "didn't want to risk losing my job." The patient's interests are the priority, even when difficult decisions and choices present themselves.

Some states have laws, in fact, which require that such conduct be reported to the licensing board under penalty of being cited for unprofessional conduct if such a report is not made, and nearly every state has a law that grants immunity from civil liability for reporting. Some nurses are afraid that they will be sued for libel or slander by the person whom they report. Although one cannot literally prevent another person from bringing a lawsuit, such a suit, because of the immunity and because of exceptions contained in the libel and slander laws themselves, can usually be dismissed early in the proceedings. Most likely, however, an attorney would not agree to bring such a suit on behalf of the disgruntled colleague in the first place.

Nurse practice acts provide for disciplinary action if, after a hearing in which all parties have an opportunity to present their views, a nurse is found to have engaged in unprofessional conduct. Such conduct is specified in the acts themselves. Typical examples include practicing while impaired by alcohol or drugs, practicing negligently or incompetently, and being convicted of a crime involving moral turpitude (immoral or dishonest conduct). Unprofessional conduct is often further defined as including, for example, failing to properly supervise the practice of a person who is authorized to practice only under supervision, abandoning, harassing, or intimidating a patient, failing to maintain accurate patient records, and failing to make a patient's records (or copies) available upon request.

Disciplinary action can result in (1) official reprimand, or (2) suspension, or (3) revocation of the nurse's license. Although much of the attention of reporting laws and requirements have, in the past, focused on physicians, the expanded role of the nurse, as well as an ever-increasing professional self-image among nurses, is expected to cause considerable change for nurses in this regard.

Future Prospects

American society is undergoing dramatic change. Among these changes are the ones previously discussed as reasons for the increase in malpractice litigation against nurses. Nurses and nursing are affected by and affecting that change. Nursing itself is undergoing revo-

lutionary change. Those changes have raised a considerable number of questions, the answers for many of which remain unclear. Only with the passage of time and accompanying debate, both within and without the nursing and medical arenas, will the questions, issues, dilemmas, and disagreements among nurses and between nurses and other health practitioners begin to be resolved.

One thing, however, seems clear. The autonomy and accompanying accountability discussed in this chapter are not likely to be temporary, nor is it likely that they will diminish. On the contrary, it is more likely that the professional nurse's role will continue to expand. As it does, it can be expected to be accompanied by at least a proportional increase in public demand for accountability. Increased responsibilities are typically accompanied by increased responsibility.

Summary

Nurses have stepped out from behind the shadow of the physician as members of the health care team. As their role has expanded and they have assumed increased responsibility, they have become both more visible and accountable to the consuming public they serve.

As the consuming public has become increasingly dissatisfied with the health care industry (along with other previously highly regarded institutions), they have also become more aware and assertive of their rights. The result has been the ultimate expression of patient rebellion: lawsuits.

Courts have been willing to hold nurses liable for the consequences of their actions. Like everyone, nurses have an obligation to avoid engaging in conduct that has been defined as constituting intentional torts when dealing with patients. Like everyone, nurses also have an obligation to conduct themselves reasonably when exercising judgment and discretion. They must act as reasonably prudent nurses would have acted under the same or similar circumstances or be prepared to compensate an injured patient.

Although the number of lawsuits gives nurses good cause for concern, there is no cause for paranoia. Many opportunities are available to nurses who are interested in minimizing the likelihood that a patient will bring a suit or, if they do, that they will prevail. While it may not be a pleasant thought, the nurse who is willing to "think litigation" will realize the value and ease of incorporating the elements of a malpractice-prevention program into the day-to-day practice of nursing.

The nurse who understands the law also realizes that an injury to a patient does not automatically result in liability to the nurse. The fault principle of the law of negligence requires that a plaintiff meet strict and often difficult standards of proving the claim. And, just as the plaintiff has access to highly skilled malpractice attorneys, so do nurses.

The principle of personal liability makes every person liable for individual negligence—physicians, administrators, supervisors, patients, and nurses. Someone else's negligence does not serve as a legal excuse for the individual nurse's negligence.

Nurses are not expected to react, as if they were programmed, in neatly predictable ways to every given set of circumstances. They are expected to deliberate and weigh, to the extent circumstances reasonably permit, the probable outcomes of their actions. Such weighing may identify the single most reasonable action or, more likely, alternative reasonable courses of action. In the latter case, the nurse must, in choosing among these alternatives, be guided by a standard of care that acts as a baseline.

There is no avoiding the need to exercise professional judgment and discretion. The ability to do so cannot be taught, bought, or inherited. It is the product of education, maturity, experience, and enlightened recognition and acceptance of professional responsibility.

Terms for Review

civil law	expert witness	malpractice	reasonably prudent nurse
claims policy	gross negligence	malpractice prevention program	respondeat superior
common law	incident report	negligence	suit-prone nurse
consumer rights	informed consent	occurence policy	suit-prone patient
criminal law	intentional tort	principle of personal liability	tort

Evaluation Questions

1. List the three sources of law, and indicate the one from which most nursing law principles come.
2. What, in negligence or malpractice cases, is the standard of care against which nurses' performance is measured? Briefly explain.
3. May nurses, by their individual negligence, cause the hospital and/or doctor for whom they work to be liable to the injured patient?
4. Distinguish negligence, intentional torts, and strict liability. Give an example of each.
5. From a legal point of view, of what value is charting? Does thorough and complete charting ensure a successful defense if sued for malpractice? Explain.

Answers

1. The three sources of law are:
   Constitutions (state and federal)
   Legislation (state and federal)
   Common law (from court decisions)
   Most nursing law principles are established on a case-by-case approach in litigation. Thus, the common law is by far the greatest source of law for nursing malpractice cases.
2. In malpractice cases, a nurse is measured against the standard of care that a reasonably prudent nurse would have given. That standard is determined by the jury in view of testimony given by expert witnesses as to what a reasonably prudent nurse, in view of generally recognized and accepted standards of practice, would have done under the same or similar circumstances.
3. Yes. Under the doctrine of *respondeat superior* a nurse can create liability on the part of the institution or physician by whom employed. A nurse cannot, however, avoid personal liability for personal negligent actions. The doctrines only serve to expand, not shift, liability.
4. Negligence is the failure to act as a reasonably prudent nurse would have acted under the same or similar circumstances. It is "accidental" or "inadvertent."

   An intentional tort is not inadvert, but, by definition, intentional. When a person intentionally does an act that can be reasonably expected to cause a type of harm that the law protects individuals from, an intentional tort has been committed (whether or not the actor knew that the type of harm was one the law sought to protect against). Examples are assault, battery, invasion of privacy, false imprisonment, libel, and slander.

   The doctrine of strict liability is applied in nursing malpractice cases only after it has been shown that the nurse did an act that constitutes the practice of medicine. In that event, there can be no defense to any liability for harm caused thereby.
5. The chart is the most important evidence of what was or was not done by the nurse. It carries great weight with a jury. Assuming that the nurse's care met all appropriate

standards, the chart will be a valuable defense tool. The opposite, of course, is also true.

Review Questions

Place a check mark beside the appropriate response(s).
1. An injured patient could successfully bring a malpractice suit against a nurse on the basis of *negligence* if:
   a. The nurse had used unreasonable force in controlling the uncooperative patient.
   b. The nurse had forgotten to do something that is customarily done by other nurses in such instances.
   c. The nurse had done something that is not customarily done by other nurses in such instances.
   d. The patient had been injured even though the nurse had followed another's order.
2. Negligence in nursing situations:
   a. Is a statutorily defined standard of care under a categorized series of circumstantial situations.
   b. Is determined by comparing the nurse's conduct to a standard of perfection embodied in the character of the reasonable person who is capable of doing no wrong in his or her chosen occupation or profession.
   c. Is determined on a case-by-case basis by whomever is the "finder of fact" in a trial.
   d. Is rarely at issue, since most malpractice suits involve intentional torts.
   e. Can usually be proved without the expert testimony of other nurses.

Match the following sets of terms with the appropriate definitions.

_____ 1. Civil law	a. Laws derived from court decisions
_____ 2. Criminal law	b. Laws enacted by legislation
_____ 3. Common law	c. Laws that control the legal actions between an individual and government
_____ 4. Statutory law	d. Laws that control the legal actions between individuals

_____ 1. Assault	a. "Offensive" touching
_____ 2. Battery	b. The person being sued
_____ 3. Defendant	c. The person bringing a lawsuit
_____ 4. Plaintiff	d. Threat to do battery

_____ 1. Liability	a. An act on the part of the patient, concurring with the negligent act of the nurse
_____ 2. Contributory negligence	b. A legal wrong committed against the person, property, or reputation of another
_____ 3. Negligence	c. Negligence on the part of a professional

_____ 4. Malpractice

_____ 5. Tort

_____ 6. *Respondeat superior*

d. Legal responsibility to account for one's own actions

e. The failure to do something that a reasonable person would do, or doing something that a reasonable person would not do

f. A legal concept in which the principal (hospital, employer) is legally liable for the acts of the agent (nurse) committed during employment. Both parties become liable for the acts of the agent

Answers

Multiple Selection

1. b, c
2. c

Matching

1. d
2. c
3. a
4. b

1. d
2. a
3. b
4. c

1. d
2. a
3. e
4. c
5. b
6. f

Discussion Question—Case Study

Read the following hypothetical situation and identify the possible lawsuits that could be brought. Be sure to identify the plaintiff and defendant for each suit and to discuss the legal basis upon which each claim would be made.

A nurse who had worked in the emergency room of a hospital for eight years was asked by the nursing supervisor to work in labor and delivery for a shift. Two of the three nurses ordinarily covering that area were out sick, and the patient load was rapidly increasing. The ER nurse agreed and, on entering the obstetrics area, asked the already overworked nurse there how often she should check fetal heart tones. The answer was, "With all that's going on, we'll be lucky to get them every half hour." Deciding to be on the cautious side, the ER nurse set about making the patient comfortable, noting new orders, and managed to check fetal heart tones every 20 minutes. There were now five patients in active labor and a call to the supervisor for more help had not been returned. A few minutes after her fetal-heart-tone check, one patient, whose labor was being induced by oxytocin drip, began having tetanic contractions. She complained of severe pain, so the helpful ER nurse administered an analgesic prescribed by the admitting physician. However, she did not recheck the fetal heart tones at that time, discontinue the IV, or report to the regular obstetrics nurse. The fetal monitor which would ordinarily have been used on this patient was a new one and, even with the most careful application of the monitor lead, it did not register fetal heart tones. The manufacturer's representative had been called the day before and had not delivered another monitor and picked up the defective one as promised. The representative had been called three times.

Twenty minutes after the last check, the ER nurse checked the fetal heart tones again and found that the fetus was obviously in great distress. The admitting physician was called immediately but did not arrive for 40 minutes. When he did arrive, the patient delivered rapidly, but the infant was pale, flaccid, had low Apgar scores, and had to be intubated immediately. The child was maintained on life-support systems for four days but had massive brain damage and died.

Answers

1. The ER nurse was working outside the area of her expertise and could be held to as high a standard of care as the nurse regularly assigned to the unit. Further, this was a nurse with many years of experience who should have been able to foresee the element of risk to the fetus involved when labor is being induced by oxytocin. The nurse must consider the potential for injury and base frequency of the checks on that potential.

2. The experienced obstetrics nurse on duty was working beyond her capacity, but she still should have been able to foresee the possibility of harm to the patients from the understaffing problem. She was aware that the ER nurse needed supervision when she asked how often to check fetal heart tones. The forseeable risk began there, but the OB nurse chose to give a casual answer and ignore the problem.

3. The nursing supervisor for the shift may be liable, too, for understaffing the units. The supervisor is responsible for being aware of qualifications and experience of the staff and for making appropriate staff changes. Even if the hospital has a chronic understaffing problem, the supervisor is responsible for reporting the problem and to reasonably

follow through on the solution to it. When a supervisor is reporting a problem, such as understaffing, which has the potential for patient harm, it is advisable to submit the report in writing and to retain a personal copy of the report. Personal notes should also be kept of efforts to follow through and to obtain a satisfactory and safe solution to the problem.

4. The hospital also has a duty to protect the patients from harm by providing adequate staffing and equipment. The hospital shares in the liability of the nurses because it is the employer of both the nurses and the supervisor. This is the doctrine of *respondeat superior*. This doctrine, "let the master answer," involves the hospital in the negligence of the nurse and extends the liability but does not dilute it. The supervisor can still be held personally responsible for negligence as a supervisor. The individual nurses could also be held liable for not foreseeing the risk and taking action to prevent it. The nurse also has a duty to inform the physician of any condition endangering the patient. The ER nurse in this hypothetical example did notify the physician and carefully documented in the record the time of the notification, but the duty did not end there. When the doctor did not respond, prudence would dictate that the nurse notify a supervisor, call another physician, or report the problem to an appropriate administrator.

5. The physician may share legal responsibility for the problems in this case. Leaving the hospital while the patient was being induced by oxytocin drip may have been negligent. The physician was aware of the risks and dangers to both mother and child in this situation and should have remained in the hospital. The physician also was aware of the malfunctioning fetal monitor.

6. This hypothetical case also is an example of product liability. If the nurse had read and understood the manufacturer's instructions for the fetal monitor and was using it properly, the manufacturer could be liable for its allegedly defective product, as well as the negligence of its representative (who would also be liable). So, five individuals, the hospital, an equipment manufacturer, and all of their respective insurance companies and attorneys are involved in a long, complicated legal battle.

THE NURSE AND THE PROCESS OF CHANGE

Objectives

1. Identify the nurse's role in promoting change in a patient's behavior.
2. Describe various types of change.
3. Describe three basic steps in the process of change.
4. Relate the activities involved with making a change to the nursing process.
5. Identify various responses people may have to proposed change.
6. Describe the relationship between stability and change in a person's life.
7. Identify factors that facilitate change.
8. Identify factors that interfere with change.
9. Contrast leaders and managers in the area of change.
10. Describe strategies to help the individual cope successfully with change.
11. Describe strategies useful in helping others accept and implement change.
12. Describe traits associated with effective change agents.
13. Describe activities of the nurse for planning and implementing change in a patient care setting.

Introduction

Without change, there is no growth, no excitement, no challenge. With too much change, there is fear, confusion, and failure. Change is inevitable, yet many people fail to accept this fact. Our internal body environment is different today than it was yesterday. Dramatic changes in technology will change all our lives for as long as we live. Nurses have a great potential to help people make needed changes in their behavior to improved health. Knowledge of possible reactions to pro-posed change, change theory, and factors involved in planning and implementing change will be helpful to the nurse, both professionally and personally. This chapter is designed to help the student in nursing understand and utilize information about change.

New students in any academic program are faced with tremendous amounts of change. They are taking on the student role which may be very different from their roles over the past years. The changes made in individual's lives by returning to school will affect them directly. Students feel the anxiety most people experi-ence when they change from the known to the un-known. There is some loss of predictability in life, yet students are willing to risk this uncertainty because of their commitment to nursing. By becoming a student in nursing, you are also causing change for those around you, especially close family members. Within any given nursing class over the course of the nursing program, there may be births, deaths, marriages, separations,

abuse, and divorce as students struggle to balance the requirements of the nursing program with the demands of family, friends, finances, and the day-to-day changes to which we are all exposed. Too many changes, occur-ring too rapidly, with inadequate planning and re-sources may mean failure or delay in attaining your goal of graduation.

Nursing education is difficult enough without the new information and skills required to deal with the rapid technological advances that are occurring today. Yet these advances will continue for as long as people are capable of creative thought. There are times as a nurse (or a student in nursing) when you will want to call a halt to accepting more change. It is at this point, when change is resisted, that you will become progres-sively more and more unfit to give safe, effective nurs-ing care to your patients. A nurse who stops learning and changing after graduation is unsafe to practice nursing in a very short time.

Definition of Change

A change is an act or process that makes something or someone different in some way. A change may be mi-nor or radically different from current behavior or prac-tices. A change may involve totally new behavior or skills necessitated by application of new discoveries in research. A change may also involve reinstituting old policies, beliefs, and behavior as the pendulum of change swings away from the progressive to the conserv-ative. An example of this is the renewed interest in breastfeeding. Years ago, it was the obvious method for feeding. Gradual change put breastfeeding out of favor with most families and health care professionals, as bot-

tle-feeding was encouraged. Now, once again the value of breast milk for the infant is being recognized, and health professionals encourage breastfeeding. A change involves moving from the familiar to the unfamiliar and altering behavior, feelings, or ways of thinking.

A *change agent* is a person who actively seeks to in-fluence other people to change their behavior in a prede-termined manner. This may involve change in one indi-vidual, change in a group, or change in an institution. The change agent may come from within the group or institution or from the outside.

Changing Nature of Human Society and Health Care

People are continually changing, both physically and psychologically. From the time of conception to the time of death, the human organism is constantly in the process of cellular growth and cellular destruction. Peo-ple change physically without any conscious control as children grow into adults and as body systems gradually deteriorate over the course of sixty, seventy, maybe even ninety years of life. Human bodies repair themselves and fight off foreign bacteria and viruses. People change their bodies through overeating, dieting, exercis-ing, or reproduction. Psychological changes occur as people interact with their environment. The unending variety of experiences that life on this planet and beyond

offers is a challenge for change if individuals are to reach their potential.

Because people are constantly changing, society is also in a constant state of flux. People empowered to run governments are continually being replaced or guided by new people and ideas or by new information and advancing technology. Economic prosperity and depression are recurring themes that drastically alter people's lives. Loss of a job and income forces extensive changes in individuals' life-styles.

Medicine is advancing into the future faster than most other professions. Preventive health care is the fo-cus for the future. The changes that today's graduate nurses will see in the course of their professional careers are innumerable. The changes in health care as computers take over more and more of the data gathering and tasks analysis will alter the roles of all health care providers. The nurse entering today's health care field must be capable not only of coping with change instituted by others, but of assisting others to cope with change and possibly grow from the experience. The nurse of the future will be active in implementing change and evaluating the effectiveness of change as it relates directly and indirectly to improving health care. Costs, in terms of personnel, resources, time, and energy, are crucial issues in the management and delivery of health care. They will continue to be important motivators for future change. A patient's ability to pay for medical care is affecting length of hospitalization, elective surgery, and even the ability to obtain certain services. If a patient's insurance will not pay for desired medical procedures or treatments, that patient may not be able to obtain those services. For example, advances in medical technology make *in vitro* fertilization a viable option for some infertile couples. However, most insurance companies refuse to pay for this procedure, and the couple must either be able to pay for these services independently, remain childless, or adopt. Heart and liver transplants are available after prospective patients demonstrate an ability to pay the bills, which may approach $250,000.

Ethical Considerations in Change

The decision to change or not to change is the right of the individual. The medical professional does not have the right to force a patient to change against that person's will. As health professionals, nurses are expected to help patients understand the risks of maintaining the status quo, while identifying the benefits and risks the individual patient may gain if change is selected. The patient's decision to change is based on information, not on fear of reprisal from the nurse or other health professionals. For example, a patient may be a cigarette smoker with some form of long-term breathing difficulty. The patient, the nurse, and the physician are aware of the fact that smoking is causing this patient's respiratory status to slowly and progressively deteriorate. Neither the nurse nor any other health professional has the right to physically restrain this patient from smoking by taking away the cigarettes. Unless the patient is posing a threat to others, the decision on changing smoking habits is the choice of the patient. When working with a patient who is a minor, changing behaviors of the child against the will of the parents is unethical. Educating parents, so they are able to understand any definite risks to their child's health if current behavior continues, is part of the nurse's role.

Types of Change

People encounter many different types of changes throughout their lives. Most changes will fall into the following seven categories:

1. Physical changes
2. Affective or attitudinal changes
3. Cognitive or informational changes
4. Behavioral changes
5. Procedural changes
6. Environmental changes
7. Technological changes

Some changes involve change in only one of the above categories while other changes involve several categories.

Physical Changes

Physical changes involve changes in structure, integrity, and appearance of the human body. Normal growth and maturation are examples of ongoing physical change processes as the human structure is altered in appearance. Conception and death are dramatic physical changes that all people experience. Deterioration in the acuity of the senses of taste, vision, and hearing are physical changes related to aging. Injuries and inadequate or lost functioning of body parts are physical changes reflecting lost integrity which nurses encounter in many patients. Changes in appearance related to illness and treatment are often difficult physical changes for patients and their families to accept, especially if these changes occur rapidly. Physical changes can also be the result of various medical treatments. Surgery creating scars, and radiation and chemotherapy resulting in hair loss, are examples. Physical changes can be caused by injury to the body as occurs in burns, fractured bones, blows to the head, and accidental amputation. The nurse trys to help the patient and family adapt to these physical changes on a temporary or permanent basis, depending on the severity of the injury.

Affective or Attitudinal Changes

Affective or attitudinal changes are those changes related to a person's feelings or emotions toward something or someone. These affective changes are very difficult to assess yet they are a vital element to consider when changes in a person's behavior are the desired goal. Almost all people who drive automobiles are aware of the facts associated with the use of seat belts and the decreased incidence of deaths and severe injuries in an automotive accident. Yet many people choose not to wear seat belts. To change behavior, people must have an attitudinal change and begin to value the protective function of seat belts. Facts or information may not be sufficient to cause attitudinal changes. People change their attitudes when their emotions are brought into an experience. A certain degree of empathy seems to be necessary for attitudinal changes to occur.

When nurses are trying to change a patient's behavior to improve health status, there is a risk of neglecting the patient's feelings related to the behavioral change. The patient may change behavior temporarily, but long-lasting changes may require supportive changes in the way the patient feels about the old behavior and the new behavior the nurse is encouraging. The nurse who ignores the patient's feelings associated with change may meet resistance. Assisting patients to value changes designed to improve their health status is often an early step in changing behavior. This applies to changes involving co-workers, other members of the health team, fellow students, and academic instructors. It also applies to the student in nursing. If an instructor cannot assist the student in making the appropriate attitudinal changes associated with performing a skill correctly, the student may temporarily comply and perform the skill as the instructor wishes. Later, when that instructor is no longer evaluating performance, the student may revert to previous ways of performing the skill.

Cognitive or Informational Changes

Cognitive or informational changes are changes in which there is an increase in knowledge or a correction of inaccurate information. Much of formal education is involved in making cognitive changes in students. Cognitive changes may be evaluated by asking people to recall the new information or to use it in a way that shows a change from previous thought or behavior patterns. As a nurse, you will be helping your patients increase their knowledge about health, illness, and specific treatments and medications appropriate to their individual needs. The first step in helping individuals change their behavior may involve cognitive changes as people become knowledgeable about their health problems.

Cognitive changes may also involve a loss of intellectual ability or knowledge. For example, patients experiencing a stroke (cerebrovascular accident or CVA) are often confronted with devastating changes to their cognitive functions. The changes in memory and thought processes imposed by a CVA may necessitate a great deal of relearning, depending on the area of the brain affected. Cognitive changes that involve a loss of information and cognitive ability may be extremely frustrating for the patient, family, and hospital or nursing home staff. The patient may be unable to recognize spoken or written words or be unable to speak.

Behavioral Changes

Behavioral changes may be thought of as changes in physical abilities and functioning that require some degree of neuromuscular coordination. Changes in this area, as in most others, may involve a loss or gain in physical ability. As individuals mature physically, their strength and coordination improve. Rapid behavioral changes occur in the first two years of life. The child is able to sit, crawl, stand, walk, and run as neuromuscular coordination continues to develop. Individuals may develop new physical abilities through practice and repetition. Behavioral changes involve some alteration from previous patterns of behavior. Life-style modifications for improved health such as altering inappropriate eating habits, reducing alcohol consumption and cigarette smoking, and increasing physical activity are all examples of behavioral changes. People usually need a good reason to change behavior, and cognitive and affective changes may be prerequisite to behavioral changes. As nurses, a consideration of how a patient thinks and feels about a proposed change in behavior is an integral part of planning.

Illness and trauma may result in behavioral changes. The patient after a CVA is an example of someone experiencing a loss of normal behavior patterns. Loss of ability to speak, control bowel and bladder function, and perform self-care activities such as shaving, eating, and dressing are common behavioral losses after a stroke. Another example is a person with trauma to the spinal cord which may result in almost total paralysis and drastic behavioral changes as new ways of meeting even the most basic physical needs are learned.

Students in nursing are continually required to make behavioral changes as they advance through a nursing curriculum. The coordination necessary to perform required nursing skills may be difficult to learn. The first bed bath may take a long time to complete. Another area that exemplifies behavioral changes for many students is in the area of communication. Effective communication skills are learned by people who are willing to take the risk of altering their familiar communication patterns and to try new techniques.

Procedural Changes

Procedural changes are those changes that involve policy, laws, regulations, and other formal and informal statements of appropriate behavior. Procedural changes are usually imposed on the individual from people in a superior power position or by the agreement of the majority of individuals in a group. In a hospital or extended care facility, procedural changes may come from the administration with the individual nurse having minimal involvement in decision making. Changes directly affecting the delivery of nursing care are most effective when a combination of nurses and other health team members are involved in planning and implementing the change. Examples of procedural changes would be changing from traditional eight-hour shifts to ten-hour shifts with three days off each week. Instituting new chart forms is another procedural change. Procedural changes related to nursing are designed to improve or maintain the overall quality of patient care while maintaining or reducing expenditures in the form of time, energy, resources, and personnel.

Environmental Changes

Environmental changes are those changes involving some alteration in the physical setting. Environmental changes may involve equipment, office space, number and size of rooms, location of bathrooms, and other similar physical layout changes. Changes in such things as heat, light, noise and air quality are also considered environmental changes. Addition or deletion of supportive health services and community resources may also be considered environmental changes in a broader sense.

Illness or disability will sometimes require alterations in the environment if patients are to function independently in the community. Environmental changes occurring in architectural design are enabling people with handicaps to reach their maximum level of independence. Large bathroom stalls, ramps, and automatically opening doors are architectural changes in buildings that make them more accessible.

As a student in nursing you may have found it necessary to make some environmental changes to enable you to reach your maximum level of achievement. Converting a den or bedroom into a study room is one example. Child care in another person's home is an environmental change the children of many students encounter.

Technological Changes

Technological changes are those changes that incorporate advances in computers, medical research, pharmacology, and various other fields into the individual's environment. Technological changes affect the way we work, the way we play, the way we learn, and the way we maintain or regain our health. Transplants, genetic engineering, and artificial and bionic parts are just the

Table 4–1. **Categories of Change**

TYPES OF CHANGE	EXAMPLES
1. Physical changes	1. Weight gain of 30 lb
2. Affective or attitudinal changes	2. Intolerant of current overweight status
3. Cognitive or informational changes	3. Knowledge of weight reduction diet
4. Behavioral changes	4. Eats only 900 calories/day; walks 2 miles/day
5. Procedural changes	5. Use of scales measuring kilograms rather than pounds
6. Environmental changes	6. Opening of a local weight reduction clinic
7. Technological changes	7. Development of medication to decrease appetite

tip of the iceberg as more and more people are touched by the possibilities of changing medical technology.

To briefly summarize, there are many different types of change. Consideration of aspects of several different categories of change is often necessary when planning for any one type of change. The following categories may be helpful as you consider personal change, the role of the nurse in helping others adapt to change, and in adapting to a profession in change as nursing is today. A review of change categories is presented in Table 4–1.

The Process of Change

Using the three-step framework of Kurt Lewin from the 1950s, change can be thought of as the process of unfreezing, moving, and refreezing. In the stage of *unfreezing,* motivation for change is the primary focus. Cognitive or information changes are occurring during this stage as people are made aware of problems or of an unsatisfactory gap between the actual situation or behavior and that which is desired. The next stage, of *moving,* involves actual changing of behavior. This stage begins with collecting data from various resources and planning the actual strategy for change. The change is then initiated following the chosen strategy. In the last stage of *refreezing,* the changed behavior becomes stable and is the new status quo. The initial resistance to change has been overcome, and the individual's changed behavior does not revert to previous behavior patterns.

Almost any proposed change will meet with some degree of resistance. In order for the change to occur, the resistance must be overcome by the forces desiring the change. There are three general ways this may be accomplished. First, and least effective, is to increase the forces pushing for the change. This method is authoritarian and uses power over others as a necessary element. Behavior may change, but changes made against people's wills or without their support seldom endure.

In fact, what may happen is that people will increase their resistance to the change if they feel it is being forced upon them. Their increased resistance may make it impossible for them to consider the positive aspects of the change.

A second approach to promote change involves decreasing the resistance, thus allowing change to occur. When the change has the support of the individual, group, or institution, overcoming the barrier is enough motivation for the change without any increase in the driving force. Barriers may be such things as inadequate finances, personnel, time, or resources. Individuals in key power positions may be effective barriers to the change desired by the majority. It may not be necessary to have these people in full agreement with the desired change, but it will be necessary to have them stop actively resisting the change for it to occur.

The third approach involves both of the above approaches by increasing the driving force for change and simultaneously decreasing the resistance. This method would be most appropriate when some of the people are desiring a change but many people are unsure or against the proposed change. Table 4–2 compares Lewin's three-stage change framework to that of several other more current frameworks. Table 4–3 shows the steps in the nursing process adapted to the process of change.

Table 4–2. **Frameworks of Change**

Lippitt's Stages	Lewin's Stages	Reinkemer's Stages
1. Diagnosis of the problem		1. Recognition of a need and desire for change
2. Assessment of the individual's, group's, or institution's motivation and ability to change	1. Unfreezing	2. Establishment of relationship between change agent and client system
3. Assessment of the change agent's motivation and resources		3. Clarification or diagnosis of client system's need, problem, or objective
4. Selection of progressive change objectives	2. Moving	4. Examination of alternative routes and tentative goals and intentions of actions
5. Identification of the most effective role for the change agent		5. Transformation of intentions into actual changed behavior
6. Maintenance of the change once started	3. Refreezing	6. Stabilization
7. Termination of change agent's role in the change		7. Termination of the relationship between the change agent and the client system

Table 4–3. **The Process of Change Adapted from the Steps of the Nursing Process**

CHANGE ACTIVITIES	NURSING PROCESS	CHANGE ACTIVITIES	NURSING PROCESS
Collection of data related to the problem area	Assess	Implementing the selected strategies and changing behavior	Implement
Identification of the specific problem		Evaluating the achievement of the selected goals during the course of the change	Evaluate
Setting specific goals for the type of change desired that will improve the problem	Plan		
Selecting actions to reach each identified goal in the process of change		Reassessing the change and determining the effectiveness in improving the problem identified initially	

Responses to Proposed Change

Change may be viewed by some people as a challenge with a potential for growth and increased rewards. Change may also be viewed as a threat with the potential for failure and loss of current rewards, whether those be money, power, prestige, or any of the many other things valued by individuals. Regardless of whether a change is viewed as positive or negative, there is often some degree of resistance experienced by the people who will be affected. This resistance is not always a negative thing. Resistance to a proposed change in the form of critical analysis of the problem and the proposed change may be helpful. Without a variety of individuals examining the proposed change from different perspectives, the success of the change is in jeopardy. One person, planning for change in isolation, cannot anticipate all of the problems that may arise as the change is instituted. Without critical review by others, the best solution to a problem may never be considered. People who offer constructive criticism to proposed change help the individuals planning the change to clarify and modify various aspects of the change to give it the best chance to succeed. Resistance to change decreases the incidence of random change and promotes change having positive outcomes and a good chance of succeeding in a particular situation.

Fears Associated with Change

Resistance to change may be designed to block change completely. Individuals who feel threatened by a proposed change are attempting to protect themselves from the real or imagined losses they anticipate with a particular change. Many people fear change. This is especially true of people with a low self-esteem. People who continually underestimate their ability will tend to hold firmly to what is, rather than risk failing at what might be. The list below presents examples of the types of concerns some people may experience when change is considered.

Fear of the Unknown. Loss of predictability in people's lives can be quite threatening. How will new people accept me? Where will I live? How will I find my classes? What will be expected of me? What are the new rules? The phrase, "I don't care much for what I'm doing, but at least I know what I'm doing," expresses the hesitancy some people experience when a change is associated with too many unknowns.

Fear Related to Loss of Competence, Skill, or Proficiency Associated with a Job or Activity. These types of fears are associated with job changes and role changes. A nursing student previously employed as a nursing assistant may have been very competent in that role. Is the individual willing to risk the temporary lack of competence associated with learning the skills for a new job or career? Being able to do a particular skill very well can be a source of pride. New learning, which supports changing the way one does a skill or replacing the outdated procedure with a new one, demotes the individual to an unskilled level of performance, at least initially.

Fear Related to Loss of Power. Procedural changes that alter the chain of command may leave some individuals with less autonomy and control over others. For some people this may be a positive aspect of change, making others more responsible for their own actions. Other people enjoy directing others and value the power to manage things as they choose. These people will resist change if it means a personal loss of power.

Fear Related to Loss of Rewards. This type of loss may be monetary if salary is reduced, or it may be loss of an office, benefits, or personal possessions. Patients entering the hospital or a nursing home face this type of loss. For many, the losses will always outweigh the benefits derived from such a change, especially if it is a permanent change.

Fear of Losing Respect, Support, and Love from Others. Changes that affect our families may involve risking some of our basic human needs for close contact with loved ones. Individuals making large changes in their life, such as returning to school, may find that their family cannot accept the change. The disruption in family life may exceed the family's ability to adapt. Divorce, separation, or reversal of the change may result. Making changes is difficult enough when an individual's support system favors and encourages the change. Consider how much more difficult a change would be to make if family and friends were opposed to it. Patients are often faced with these types of losses as health professionals ask them to accept changes in their lives for heatlh-related reasons. The woman facing a decision on having mastectomy surgery for cancer may feel the change in her physical appearance will result in rejection by her sexual partner and friends. Another example is people who have the perseverance to change their life-style and lose large amounts of excessive weight. Sometimes they find they are risking the loss of spouses or friends who cannot adjust to their new slender form. Friends who choose to remain overweight may also be lost as an individual adjusts to life as a person of normal weight.

Fear of Failure. Many changes carry the risk of failure. The student role is a good example of this. Failure in the literal sense is a reality for a certain percentage of students. When nurses ask patients to try new skills or relearn behavior lost from illness or trauma, they are asking them to risk failure. For some people, the risk is too great, and they prefer not to try at all, rather than discover they are unable to perform an activity. If the change can be broken down into a series of simple activities where success is more likely, the risk of failure can be diminished. A newly diagnosed diabetic may be completely overwhelmed by the changes in life-style required for optimal management of the diabetes. Learning and implementing diet changes, urine and blood testing, skin care, and injection of insulin may overload the person initially. The fear of failure may be very realistic, and the patient may go through a time of denying that the disease exists. Giving the patient time to accept and adjust to the idea of having diabetes is important before attempting to change behavior. Breaking down activities, such as insulin administration, into simple steps the patient is able to master will help overcome the initial fear of failure and the accompanying resistance to change. People who have tried to make changes in the past and have met with failure will often experience more fear of failure and increased resistance when they are again confronted with a need to change.

The more people who favor a change, the more difficult it will be for an individual to resist changing with the group. Resistance to change against the pressure of others for a change requires energy. An individual may become so exhausted fighting a change that continued resistance is impossible.

Balancing Change with Stability

It may at first seem as though change and stability are opposing concepts. People taking risks and attempting to make changes are using a great deal more physical and psychological energy than they would by maintaining the status quo. Disruptions and problems encountered in areas other than the change focus seem disproportionately difficult because of the energy drain created by the change. For change to proceed with a minimum amount of frustration and disruption, other areas of a person's environment should be held as stable as possible. Trying to do too much too quickly can mean failure for a change project. People can only focus their attention and energy on a certain number of things at one time without becoming overwhelmed. Take care of people's physical needs; reassign work loads; delay as many distracting concerns or extraneous issues as possible when initiating change. As a student, the demands of family, work, and other activities can lead to a total overload where the individual becomes unable to perform satisfactorily at anything. To have available the energy needed to adjust successfully to change, people need to set priorities and delay or reassign other activities.

Factors Encouraging and Discouraging Change

Why do people change? Sometimes people are unaware of gradual changes. When the individual and the majority of people in the immediate environment are slowly changing, change is often unrecognized. There is no "before" and "after" contrast. Married couples who grow apart over the childbearing and childrearing

Table 4–4. **Factors Encouraging Change**

Change is viewed as being better by the affected individual, group, or institution.

Change is compatible with the values and norms of the people involved.

The change agent or group planning and implementing change is viewed with confidence.

Change is possible within the roles and structure of the current individual, group, or institution.

Change is simple and concrete. Specifics are understood by the people affected.

People involved in the change know that others have succeeded with similar changes.

Change is run on a small scale initially to work out any unanticipated problems before it is attempted on a large scale.

Change is initially attempted in a controlled, managed environment to increase the likelihood of success.

Change projects involving many smaller changes are spread out over time to give people the opportunity to adjust to one new activity at a time.

Leaders and superiors within the group or institution are involved and support the change.

People instituting the change are coordinated and are all providing similar information and direction.

People affected by the change have been involved in planning.

Problems are the focus for change rather than blaming individuals.

Open, nonthreatening communication is maintained among people initiating the change and those affected or doing the actual changing.

Evaluation is part of the change project.

years may not be aware of personal changes until the children leave the home. It is at this time they find they have no common interests as they did when they were newly married. A patient may make such slow improvement over time that progress is imperceptible. A reminder, using photographs or visits to other patients just beginning the recovery phase of similar illnesses, reveals the progress to a patient and can be very rewarding. The phrase, "You've come a long way, baby," has little meaning unless people are aware of where they started and where they are now. In contrast, very rapid change is easily recognized and may discourage people from changing if it is viewed as a radical and frightening departure from their familiar behavior.

Table 4–5. **Factors Interfering with Change**

An authoritarian or controlling approach is used to change people's behavior; various forms of punishment or withdrawal of rewards are threatened.

Change involves complex activities or abstract concepts.

Change is viewed as equal to, or worse than, present status.

Individuals meet unanticipated problems related to change.

Inadequate support and guidance are available when change is initiated.

There is disagreement or lack of coordination among people guiding the change.

Radical changes or multiple changes are initiated over a short time.

Poor communication leads to rumors and inaccurate information.

Excessive work pressure is related to change.

Fears of individuals related to change are not considered and dealt with.

The problem associated with a need to change is not clearly identified.

There is inadequate planning for change; lack of attention to details, lack of consideration of the effect change may have on other people, groups, departments, or the institution as a whole.

Input from people who will be asked to change is not solicited.

Support or approval from superiors in the early stages of planning for change is not obtained.

Table 4–4 describes some factors that tend to encourage people to change. Table 4–5 describes some factors that may interfere with people's willingness or ability to change.

People will begin to consider change when a problem is recognized. Kron (1981), defines a problem as "a discrepancy between a present situation and a desired condition or outcome, indicating that some action must be taken." Individuals who are experiencing negative feedback related to their behavior may be motivated to change. Guilt and anxiety can also be motivators for change. Sometimes it takes a tragedy or near tragedy to make people change their behavior.

Leaders, Managers, and Power in the Process of Change

A *leader* may be thought of as someone who initiates, sets precedent, guides less experienced people, and is given the recognition of superior ability by a group. Leaders stimulate people to consider new ideas and develop new skills. They are able to influence the behavior of a group because their opinion is valued. Leaders tend to disrupt the steady state of things. They are frequently initiators of change and, if not initiators, then their support to a change project encourages others to support it. Leaders are given power by their peers because of their demonstrated abilities in particular areas. Trying to initiate change without involving the leaders in a group makes it very difficult to achieve widespread support for the project. If the people desiring change can involve the leaders of various groups and get their support, these leaders will be the best people to convince others in the groups of the project's merit.

Managers, in contrast, tend to be involved with maintaining the efficient functioning of the status quo. A competent manager may not be an effective leader, and the reverse is also quite true. Managers receive their power from people higher in the institutional chain of command. Head nurses on clinical stations are viewed more and more as nurse managers, reporting to supervisors and having the power associated with hiring, firing, and maintaining an efficient hospital unit. Managers must be involved in any change project, at least to the point of agreeing to let others plan and implement the change. Convincing people in management positions of the need for change is an early step in any successful project. Management people can arrange time, personnel, and needed resources to make change occur as easily as possible. Managers who are completely opposed to a project often have the power to block it. The reason a head nurse or a nursing supervisor is against a proposed change may be very different from the reasons staff nurses are opposed to that same change. Identifying all the specific reasons that people have for opposing a change is one step toward decreasing resistance.

Coping with Change

Coping with change is an ongoing process in which an individual attempts to restore the sense of physical and psychological security and well-being experienced prior to the change. Some people will achieve a higher level of well-being following a successful change. Others may never achieve the level of satisfaction they had prior to the change. Many strategies are used by people who cope successfully with change. Some are listed in Table 4–6. People who adapt well to change seem to be able to set realistic expectations for themselves and others and to ask for help when needed. They set priorities based on what is most important to accomplish and then deal with one problem or change at a time. This is more likely to result in a positive outcome. Achieving a balance between activities associated with a change and other responsibilities that are important is a way of avoiding problems that can occur when all time and energy are spent on one concern to the neglect of other important areas. A person adapting to the student role may devote all energies to academic excellence and achieve an A for the course, but at what price to family, friends, and personal health? Perhaps a B or C instead of all A grades would indicate more of a balance between academic and outside life, allowing the individual to grow as a person with important family and social responsibilities. Consider the fact that individuals coping with change always have options they can use if things get too difficult: lighten outside responsibilities; request help from people who seem to be coping well with change; get out of the situation for a while and regroup.

Table 4–6. **Strategies for Coping with Change**

- Obtain complete and accurate information about the problem and proposed change.
- Keep lines of communication open; talk with others about your feelings and concerns; talk with peers and superiors; ask for clarification of conflicting information.
- Remember that you are not alone; there is always help available.
- Form helping relationships with others experiencing similar change; develop task-oriented support groups and help each other through stressful times.
- Set realistic expectations for yourself based on your abilities, resources, and additional commitments.
- Reward yourself; do something nice for yourself.
- Take care of yourself physically—rest, exercise, adequate nutrition, and relaxation are all critical to maintaining energy levels and a sense of well-being.
- Approach proposed change with a critical, yet positive, attitude.
- Involve yourself in the planning phase of change.
- Answer the following questions very carefully: "Does the change have the potential for making things better?" "Is it worth the effort?" If the answers are "yes," then support and work for the change. If the answers are "no," then work with the people who are urging the change and ask them to reevaluate the situation for a more positive outcome. Be specific about the reasons you feel the change is not beneficial or realistic. If this is impossible, then either resign yourself to the change and hope the outcome will be more rewarding than you anticipated or remove yourself from the environment affected by the change.
- Delete or reassign work to others during change.
- Get organized. Work on tasks until complete and move on.
- Anticipate problems and plan solutions or ways to avoid them before they become insurmountable.

Helping Others Cope with Change

As students in nursing, you will be helping two major groups cope with change. One group is the patients you will be working with during your education. The other group is made up of families, both the patient's family and your own family. When one member of a family changes, all members of the family are affected

Table 4–7. **Helping Others Cope with Change**

Provide people with complete and accurate information at their level of understanding related to the problem and the proposed changes to improve it.

Help people identify resources in their environment to assist with the change.

Help people set realistic goals for making changes with realistic time frameworks.

Help people accurately assess their ability to change and chances for being successful.

Reduce external energy drains as people begin to change their behavior.

Involve the individual's support system (friends, family) as early as possible in planning and implementing change.

Provide people with evidence of the success they have achieved in some aspects of the change.

Support and encourage the individual's repeated efforts to make the desired change.

Inform and coordinate efforts among other people providing help for the individual so the direction and goals of change are supported by others.

Involve individuals in planning the desired changes in their behavior.

Give the individual the ultimate decision-making power when it comes to accepting or rejecting the change. Help the person understand the consequences, both positive and negative, of accepting or rejecting change.

in some way. Change places stress on family function and structure. It may cause the family to organize and become more efficient. Conversely the family may fail to deal with change and become disorganized and ineffective. Other individual family members taking on the activities of another member is a positive method of handling the problems created when one member chooses to or is forced to change. Families who can pick up the slack when illness forces changes on one member seem to cope well with change. Families in which each person has rigid roles and activities to perform within the family often have a very difficult time adjusting to change. The individual trying to change may find no one in the family is willing or able to take some of the family roles and responsibilities from them to free some of their energy for change. The lack of support by the family can be enough to result in an unsuccessful outcome to attempted change. Take, for example, a mid-

dle-aged man of 45 years who is suddenly hospitalized with a heart attack (myocardial infarction or MI). The very real fear of dying from this or a repeated heart attack may motivate this individual to make some drastic changes in his life. Is his job too stressful? Are the working hours to long? How will he incorporate progressive exercise, weight loss, and no smoking into his life? Will his sexual relationship with his wife be altered for fear of another MI? Can the family adapt to his temporary absence? Is he indispensable in the type of family functions he performs, or is the family flexible enough to take over some responsibilities temporarily or permanently? The nurse has a major role in helping the individual patient cope with the various changes and fears associated with illness, poor health, and recovery. Table 4-7 lists some suggestions to consider when helping patients and their families adjust to change.

The Changing Nature of Nursing

The history of nursing is a story of ongoing change. The future of nursing can be expected to contain many changes from nursing as we know it today. Both the length and setting for different levels of nursing education are unresolved issues today, and movement toward changes in this area can be seen in various states. Roles and responsibilities of the nurse will continue to change.

Changes in medications, treatments, equipment, and setting should all be anticipated by people entering nursing today. Patients' needs may also change as medical advances make transplants, mechanical parts, and new vaccines available to alter the course of what we now view as terminal illness. The ages of patients will change as more people live on into their 80s and 90s.

The Nurse as a Promoter of Change

The nurse of today is an agent of change both in the care given to patients and in guiding the direction of the profession for the future. Nurses are using professional organizations such as the American Nurses' Association (ANA) to voice their opinions about problems in nursing and directions for change. Nurses are becoming active in government and are exerting their influence on laws affecting nursing and health care. The nurse's primary role, however, involves the nursing care provided to patients and their families. Nurses are continuously improving the quality of patient care by making changes in techniques or procedures based on application of research. Research in nursing is one way of investigating a problem and generating alternative solutions to improve the quality of patient care. The individual staff nurse spends a good deal of time in helping patients cope with physical and psychological changes in their lives created

Table 4-8. **Skills Associated with Effective Change Agents**

Communication skills, ability to relate to people
Knowledge of change theory
Problem-solving skills
Decision-making skills
Ability to take risks
Persistence
Flexibility
Realistic expectations of self and others
Ability to predict actions/reactions of others
Knowledge of the structure and functioning of the setting in which the change is to occur
Power or influence within the setting for change
Ability to attend to details
Ability to envision the change and its outcome

Table 4–9. **Advantages and Disadvantages of an Insider and Outsider as an Agent of Change**

ADVANTAGES	DISADVANTAGES
Insider	*Insider*
Knows people, power structure, and lines of communication	May have tunnel vision and see problem from only one view
Understands norms and values	Inadequate power in the system
Committed to group, institution	Inadequate experience as change agent; unsure how to proceed
Accepted by people in system	Past behavior may affect acceptance by others as capable change agent
Viewed as one who understands the problems and constraints	
Continuing support of change as an employee of system	
Outsider	*Outsider*
Has support of power structure yet independent of it	Lack of commitment over time
Broader base of knowledge and skills	Financial issues, fee for service
Able to view problem and possible solutions in a new way	Viewed as a stranger who may not understand
Viewed as an expert	Time is required to become familiar with system, people, and problems
Familiar with role as change agent and practice with activities associated with role	May have inadequate clinical skills to assess and help implement change in a highly specialized area
	May lack support of insiders

by illness, trauma, and sometimes just normal aging. The knowledge, skill, and empathy that nurses offer to patients is a very significant resource for them as they attempt new behavior to improve their health and independence.

There are several skills that are important to the nurse who hopes to be successful in promoting change. These are described in Table 4–8. Most important of these is communication and an ability to relate well to people. As a change agent, or one who is attempting to influence others to alter behavior in a predetermined direction, the nurse must also be a very careful planner with attention to detail. This is crucial to a smooth and successful change. If the nurse acting as a change agent is viewed by others as a competent nurse who understands the problems of the patients, staff, and the institution, change is facilitated. A nurse considered an expert may be brought in from outside the group or institution to assist in planning and implementing change. A nurse from within a group or institution may also emerge to fill this role. Advantages and disadvantages to either of these options are presented in Table 4–9.

Planning and Implementing Change

Kron (1981) suggests there are seven questions to answer in planning for change. The following descriptions are adapted from her recommendations:

1. *What*? Specifically, what is the problem and proposed change?
2. *Why*? Why is the change desirable or better than current behavior; what is gained; what is lost; why should people support it?
3. *Who*? Who will be involved and affected by the change?
4. *How*? How, specifically, will the change be implemented?
5. *When*? This involves designing a time framework for planning and implementing the change.
6. *Where*? Where will the change take place or be tried first?

7. *Can*? Is the change feasbile? Can this group or individual change? Does the individual have the cognitive, physical, and emotional ability to change? Are resources adequate?

In planning for change, it is usually important to obtain the approval of superiors. Written requests for change, identifying the problems and proposed solutions, are one way of beginning this process. Resources needed for change and the benefits of change in terms of patient care and savings in time and energy are important to include. Cost considerations, staffing, equipment, and needed support services from other departments are also discussed in the written proposal to supervisors and administration. The change agent considers and documents potential effects on other departments and people within the larger system that may be affected by change in one area.

Another step in planning for change is to define the problem specifically. Involving others in clarifying the problem, as they see it, helps this process. Define the scope of the problem. Is it unique to me, to our staff, to our type of patients, or is the problem more widespread? Involve the experts within the larger setting in identifying the problem. Nurse clinicians, head nurses, supervisors, nursing directors, and articles from the professional nursing journals may all offer valuable information and potential solutions from similar problems.

After the problem is clearly identified, try to involve people in meetings to generate potential solutions to the problem. The technique of ''brainstorming'' in which any solution is considered, no matter how unusual, can effectively involve many people. It may also generate creative solutions. Contrasting an ideal situation with the real situation can be an interesting approach to help people look at different solutions to a problem. Along with this goes a contrast of the ideal solution to a minimally acceptable solution. After this is done, the group can begin working toward a compromise which may be the best solution, given the circumstances in which the change is to occur, the particular individuals involved, and the constraints of the situation. Identify what things can be changed and what things must remain constant in the planning phase. Combine ideas or parts of ideas to make creative new solutions that are agreeable to more people. Examine the implications for gains, losses, and cost for each of the most workable solutions that emerge from the group planning the change.

The next step is to make a decision. Select the solution to the initial problem that seems to be the most economical over time and has the potential for the most improvement in the current status. Set progressive goals to produce the change identified in the chosen solution to the problem. Set realistic deadlines for the progressive goals in the change that allow people time to adjust to each new activity. Identify specific activities that will lead to accomplishment of each of the goals in the change project. Decide who will be responsible for doing what, and set time limits for completion of these tasks. Then implement the change.

The nurse, as a change agent, can create an atmosphere of trust and cooperation by respecting the opinions and fears of people affected by the change. They may identify problems with the proposed change that the change agent has failed to consider. The nurse can use communication skills to encourage individuals to participate in the planning. By helping the group set up ground rules for discussions, the change agent can keep people from negating opinions expressed before actually considering them. The nurse may be able to involve the natural leaders of a group and make allies in the change project. Identify specific ways that individuals can communicate problems and concerns to the change agent as the change is implemented.

Try the change out on a small scale first. It is much easier to deal with confusion and unanticipated problems on a small scale. Work the problems out before implementing a large-scale change. Provide adequate leadership and reinforcement as change is implemented. People benefit from knowing they are doing things correctly and that they have some back-up problem-solvers if the need arises. Encourage some individual flexibility and decision making as the change is adapted to particular individuals, families, groups, and institutions. Develop written policy or procedure statements for reference by various areas affected by change.

Evaluating Change

Develop a plan for ongoing evaluation of the change and the original problem. Provide support and encouragement over time until people have incorporated the change into their behavior and value the results. Evaluation of the change may lead to further changes or even to a reversal of the change, if too many undesirable outcomes develop. People involved in the change should also be involved in its evaluation. If change was effective, it will endure. In an effective change, the nurse–change agent is able to become less and less active in supporting the change and finally has no role at all in maintaining the change.

Summary

This chapter defines change as a process that results in someone or something being different in some way. The student in nursing is affected personally by changes associated with reentering school. In the nurse-patient role, change may improve an individual's current health status and future quality of life. The practice of imposing change on others against their will or the wishes of their legal guardian is unethical.

Various types of changes are discussed which include physical, affective, cognitive, behavioral, procedural, environmental, and technological.

The process of change involves unfreezing or motivating people for change, moving or actually changing, and refreezing when the chance becomes accepted as the norm. The forces of resistance must be less than the forces pushing for change if change is to occur. Removing barriers to change, decreasing people's resistance to change, or increasing the forces pushing the change are ways to promote change.

Activities involved with making a change are compared to the nursing process:

1. Diagnosis of the problem
2. Assessment of the individual's, group's, or institution's motivation and ability to change
3. Assessment of the change agent's motivation and resources
4. Selection of progressive change objectives
5. Identification of the most effective role for the change agent
6. Maintenance of the change once started
7. Termination of change agent's role in the change

The responses people may have to change can be helpful to the change project if they are in the form of constructive criticism. Resistance to change in some degree is an almost universal response and should be anticipated. Without this resistance, people would change randomly, often leading to lost efficiency and other negative outcomes. People change when they are convinced the change will improve things, and personal risks of failure or lost rewards are minimal. Loss of power, competence, respect, love, and the familiar are all reasons that individuals may resist change.

Stability in other areas of a person's life increases the energy available for changing. Arranging for stability prior to change will add to the chances that the individual will make a successful change with a minimum of stress. Other factors encouraging successful change include compatibility with personal values, confidence in a change agent, identifying concrete and specific activities for changing, personal involvement, open communication in a nonthreatening atmosphere, ongoing evaluation of change, support from other people, and a reasonable rate of change.

Strategies for coping with change in one's personal life are discussed, as well as ways of helping others change. These focus on the following activities:

Involvement and expression of fears, concerns

Accurate, complete understanding of change and effect on individual

Asking for help from others when needed to reduce outside stress, clear up unexpected problems, and provide encouragement to continue

Having realistic expectations of self and others

Anticipating problems and planning solutions before they occur

Organizing goals and working on one task with maximum energy until completed, rather than trying to do too much at one time

The skills and roles of the change agent are discussed, with involvement of others and detailed planning being essential for successful change.

Terms For Review

change	change (*cont'd*)	leader
affective change	physical change	manager
behavioral change	procedural change	moving
cognitive change	technological change	refreezing
environmental change	change agent	unfreezing

Self-Assessment

Consider your immediate family and its flexibility and ability to support a member going through change.

1. Are family members in favor of the change you are going through as a student in nursing?

2. Do certain people always do certain tasks, or is there flexibility for tasks, depending on who has the time?

3. Are you being asked to continue to perform all activities you performed prior to entering school?

4. Are family members taking some of your responsbilities away from you to provide more time and energy for the changes you are encountering as a nursing student?

5. Can men in your family be responsible for stereotypical female activities in the home such as cooking, child care, housecleaning, and chauffeuring?

6. Can women in your family be responsible for some of the stereotypical male activities such as financial management, car maintenance, family discipline, lawn work, and other tasks that may take needed time away from schoolwork?

7. Is your family life fairly stable or in turmoil?

8. Can your family act as a buffer to protect you from additional outside stress and problems as you cope with the changes related to your education?

9. Are you asked to handle additional problems and stress in a work setting where supervisors and co-workers are unwilling or unable to give you the flexibility in scheduling to balance work and school?

10. What factors acted to "unfreeze" you from previous roles and encouraged you to return to school in the nursing area?

11. What type of personal and interpersonal resistance did you encounter as you considered returning to school?

12. What type of obstacles were overcome, and what was helpful in accomplishing this?

Self-Test

Answer the following questions and rate yourself on your potential to assume the change-agent role.

	T	F
1. I enjoy taking risks, even if there is little chance of success.	___	___
2. I will take a risk and try something new when I feel reasonably sure the outcomes can be positive if adequate preparation is made beforehand.	___	___
3. I usually prefer to maintain my current behavior until others have tested new methods and worked out all the problems.	___	___
4. I am able to continue to work on a project I feel is worthwhile, even when repeated problems develop.	___	___
5. If problems develop when I am learning a new way of doing something, I prefer to go back to previous known methods of performance.	___	___
6. I enjoy working out the details of a project.	___	___
7. I enjoy planning general directions for changing things but lose interest when working out the specifics.	___	___
8. I am usually unable to visualize what things will be like after a change project is complete.	___	___
9. Once I understand the specific change I want to make, I can visualize how it may affect me and other people.	___	___
10. The people in my peer group often look to me for help in making decisions.	___	___
11. I am never the first person to suggest a specific change, even if I know one is needed.	___	___
12. Once I have the details of a plan worked out, I am very reluctant to change them, even though a few other people suggest change.	___	___
13. I like to consider the advantages and disadvantages of my choices and make my own decisions.	___	___
14. I am uncomfortable making serious decisions and prefer others with more ability to make them for me.	___	___
15. I tend to overestimate people's ability.	___	___
16. I tend to underestimate my ability.	___	___
17. I was completely surprised when my decision to go to school for nursing affected all other aspects of my life.	___	___
18. I feel comfortable talking with people.	___	___
19. I have a way of making people feel at ease.	___	___
20. People frequently confide in me.	___	___

Answers

1. F — This attitude frequently leads to failure.
2. T — Calculated risks are taken by change agents after considering potential for success.
3. F — This person is more of a manager than a leader or change agent.
4. T ⎫ Persistence with a change project is needed if it is to
5. F ⎭ succeed.
6. T ⎫ Ability to attend to the details of a plan for change is
7. F ⎭ a trait of an effective change agent.

8. F   The ability to visualize (conceptualize) change will
9. T   help the change agent understand the advantages and details of a potential change.
10. T   Decision-making skills are required.
11. F   This answer reflects an inability to take risks.
12. F   This answer indicates a tendency toward rigidity which may prevent the "best" plan for change from being used in different situations.
13. T   Decision-making skills
14. F   Lack of decision-making skills
15. F   Change agent needs realistic expectations of self and
&   others.
16.
17. F   Reflects inability to visualize effects of change before it occurs.
18. T   Indicates good communication skills and ability to
19. T   deal with people.
20. T

Learning Activities

1. Discuss how other students in your study group are coping with the changes associated with returning to school. Identify activities that could help ease your adjustment or that of your family or employer.
2. Contrast your feelings when changes are forced upon you to when you actively choose to change. What type of feelings are associated with forced change?
3. Discuss changes that illnesses have imposed on patients in the clinical area. Talk with patients and their families about their initial reactions and how they rearranged family roles and responsibilities. What are they able to identify as helpful in adapting to change associated with illness. What unanticipated problems were experienced?
4. Discuss the potential reactions a patient and family may have to the physical changes resulting from physical disfigurement. What type of reactions might you have as a new staff nurse or student to a patient's physical disfigurement? What things would be helpful to you in working with this patient and family? What type of support will the patient need in accepting and adapting to permanent physical change? What behavioral changes may be related to a patient experiencing disfiguring physical changes?

Review Questions

1. Stability is important to people as they begin to change their behavior. Which of the explanations is the best description of this relationship?
    a. Stability in other areas of a person's life requires a minimum energy expenditure so the individual can concentrate maximum effort on the change.
    b. Most people resist stability in their lives, therefore, stability is an important motivator for change.
    c. By reducing the stability in a person's environment, stress is created which make problems more apparent and change more acceptable.
    d. Stability is in conflict with change. Total instability leads to the most effective change.

2. True or False
    _____ Managers tend to be initiators of change.
    _____ Resistance to change can affect a change project, both positively and negatively.
    _____ Loss of hair from chemotherapy is an example of a behavioral change.
    _____ Behavioral changes frequently have prerequisite cognitive, and affective changes.

3. Which of the following activities is *not* helpful in coping with change?
    a. Obtaining accurate information about the proposed change
    b. Keeping your feelings and concerns about the change to yourself
    c. Omitting or reassigning work to others during change
    d. Identifying where to go for help if problems arise

4. All of the following tend to increase resistance to change *except*:
    a. Fear of failure
    b. Anticipated loss of power
    c. Fear of rejection by family, friends
    d. Anticipated losses outweighed by anticipated gains

5. One *disadvantage* of an "expert" change agent brought in from outside the group is that:
    a. There is unlimited time commitment made by the "expert."
    b. The expert has a fee for service.
    c. The expert is familiar with the role of the change agent.
    d. The expert is able to view a problem from many perspectives.

6. Which of the following skills are associated with an effective change agent?
    a. Ability to use power to force changes in other people's behavior
    b. Ability to take risks

c. Rigid persistence in following a course of action

d. Implements change with broad goals and a general plan

7. All of the following factors encourage change *except*:

   a. Confidence in the change agent

   b. Open communication

   c. An abstract and complex plan for change

   d. Support of natural leaders within the group

Answers

1. a
2. F, T, F, T
3. b
4. d
5. b
6. b
7. c

References and Bibliography

Barbossi, K.: Hidden resistance: When "yes" means "no." *RN* **42**:89–96, Sept., 1979.

Holle, M., and Blalchley, M.: *Introduction to Leadership and Management in Nursing.* Wadsworth, Belmont, Calif., 1982.

Kramer, M.: *Reality Shock—Why Nurses Leave Nursing.* Mosby, St. Louis, 1974.

Kron, T.: *The Management of Patient Care.* 5th ed. Saunders, Philadelphia, 1981.

Lewin, K.: Field Theory in Social Science. Harper and Row, New York, 1951.

Lippitt, G.: *Visualizing change: Model Building and the Change Process.* University Associates, La Jolla, Calif., 1973.

Mitchel, P., and Loustau, A.: *Concepts Basic to Nursing.* McGraw-Hill, New York, 1981.

Moskowitz, R.: Got problems that won't go away? Solve them creatively! *Nurs. Life,* **2**:25–31, Sept./Oct. 1982.

Olson, E.: Strategies and techniques for the nurse change agent. *Nurs. Clin. North Am.,* **14**:323–36, 1979.

Rapoport, L.: The state of crisis: Some theoretical considerations. In Parad, H. (ed.): *Crisis Intervention: Selected Readings.* Family Service Association of America, New York, 1965.

Reinkemer, A.: Nursing's need: A commitment to an ideology of change. *Nurs. Forum,* **9**:341–55, 1970.

Welch, L.: Planned change in nusring: The theory. *Nurs. Clin. North Am.,* **14**:307–21, 1979.

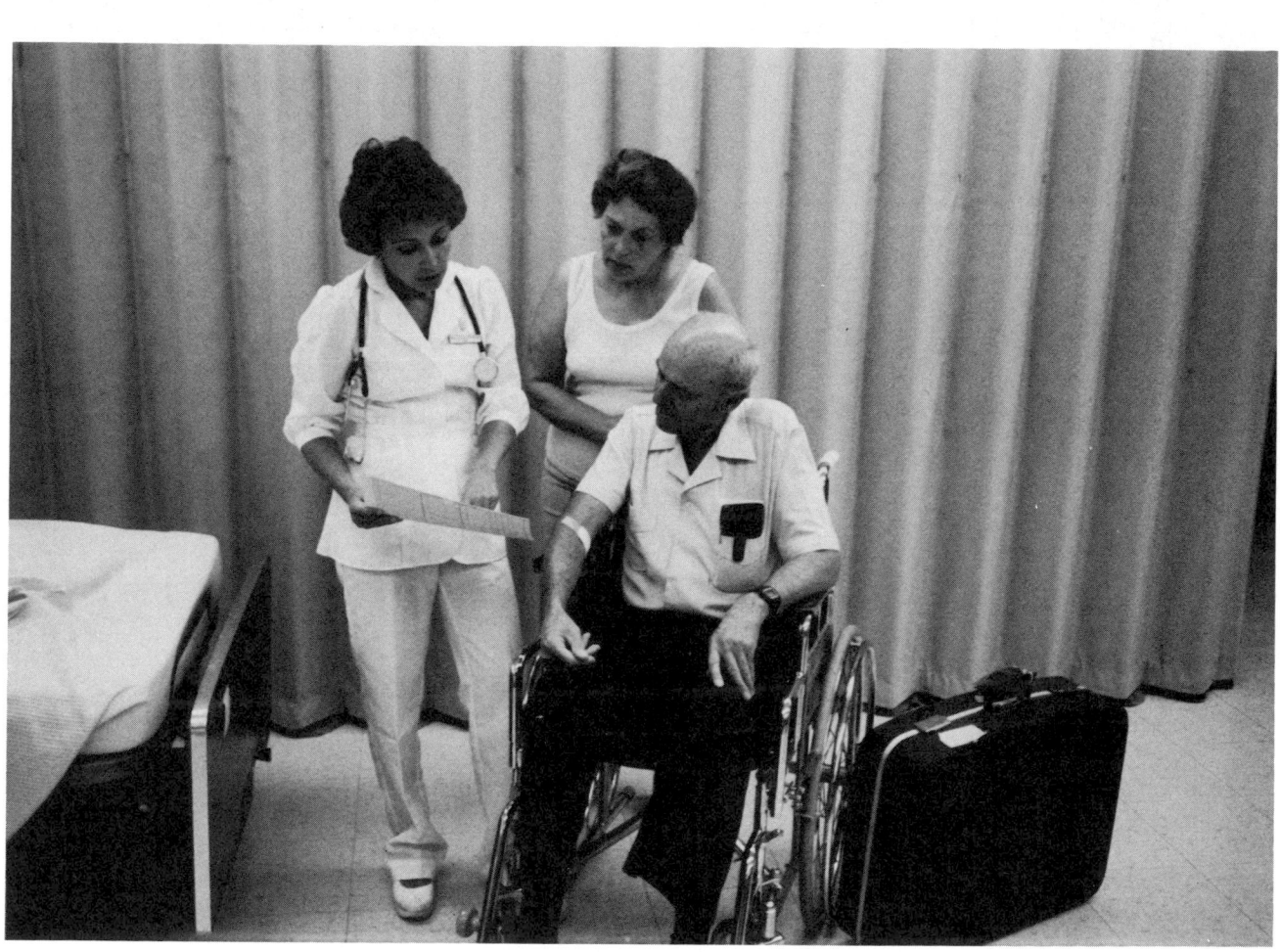

UNIT II
THE COMMUNICATION PROCESS

CHAPTER 5

SELF-AWARENESS AND THE SELF-ASSESSMENT PROCESS

Objectives

1. Discuss the importance of an accurate self-assessment to nursing.

2. Complete self-assessment of:
   Wellness
   Learning style
   Feelings
   Attitudes
   Values
   Transcultural knowledge

3. Define what is meant by a philosophy of nursing.

4. Make two statements of belief that are the beginning of a personal philosophy of nursing.

The Self-Assessment Process

The Importance of the Self-Assessment Process to Nursing

The self-assessment process may be thought of as the process of developing self-awareness or even the process of internal communication since the person begins to look at and describe self. Many aspects of the individual's personality are brought to awareness during self-assessment. The goal of self-assessment is to provide the individual, in this case the student in nursing, with an understanding of personal behavior and, to some degree, an understanding of what motivates that behavior. If this is lacking, the nurse may be unable to perceive patient needs due to interference from personal unmet needs. For example, a nurse whose brother died in a motorcycle accident as a teenager may have difficulty pro-

viding nursing care for young men in this age group. The nurse is able to meet all the physical needs of these patients, but remains distant and aloof, unable to offer personal support or warmth. The nurse may be unaware of a personal need to talk about the brother and express pent-up grief. This personal need is affecting the nurse's ability to provide care.

In addition, accurate self-perception is essential if growth is to occur.

Self-assessment is a process of collecting both subjective and objective data about oneself. *Subjective data* refer to that information the individual is able to provide about self and is unobservable to others. *Objective data* comprise that information that can be observed or noted by a second observer. Physical characteristics and behavior such as height, weight, and hair color are examples of objective data. "Physiology is the subject I like best" or "It is difficult for me to meet new people" are examples of subjective data. The student beginning self-assessment considers both types of data, although subjective data comprise the major portion of self-assessment.

The process of self-assessment may be uncomfortable or perhaps even painful for some individuals. Each human being has an image of the self, a *self-concept*, that is the sum total of how the individual sees self. The self-concept is formed as a result of past experience, interaction with both the interpersonal and physical environments, culture, and education. For some individuals the self-concept can be a protective device which helps to maintain self-esteem. This is especially true if the self-concept held by the individual differs significantly in a positive direction from the evaluation of other observers. Consider, for example, the student nurse whose self-concept is that of a very warm and caring individual, while feedback from patients indicates that the student is abrupt and "too busy to listen." Conversely, the individual who has a very negative self-concept, despite much feedback to the contrary, may never reach personal potential because of untrue beliefs held about self.

It is also recognized that one can never know the self with complete accuracy. Luft (1963) describes four parts of each individual:

> Part 1—The part that is known to both the self and others
> Part 2—Those parts of the self known to others of which the person is largely unaware
> Part 3—A private self of which the individual is aware but chooses not to share with others
> Part 4—The aspects of self unknown to both the individual and others

The process of self-assessment helps the individual to learn more about each of these aspects of self.

As the level of trust established with other human beings increases, more can be learned about the self without risk to the self-concept. An accurate and effective self-assessment process requires trust that those contributing to the process are sincerely interested in the well-being and development of the other. Confidentiality must be established and maintained. The term "constructive criticism" is often used when one individual helps another improve an aspect of behavior by increasing self-awareness of actual behavior.

Beginning the Process

The purpose behind the assessment will determine the type of data collected. The head nurse in a hospital unit, for example, may wish to focus on time utilization in order to increase the time spent on patient care. The head nurse might then collect data related to the amount of time nurses spend on nonnursing duties. In this text, the purpose of self-assessment is to assist the nursing student develop an accurate self-perception that will facilitate growth and safety in the practice of nursing. At the end of each chapter of this text, materials are provided that enable the nursing student to begin self-assessment as it relates to specific content and skills. The student is provided with review terms and questions related to chapter content. Answers are given to provide feedback and to evaluate learning. This chapter provides the student with materials to help assess personal wellness, learning style, attitudes, feelings, values, and cultural knowledge. Because wellness influences every aspect of life, self-assessment begins with a consideration of one's own state of health. Next, in recognition of the student role, the self-assessment process will focus on learning style and the adult learner before moving on to more abstract assessments of attitudes, feelings, and values.

It is important for the student to realize that self-assessment is not to be equated with an evaluative process. The self-assessment process is intended to be a *nonjudgmental* process. The individual does not say, "I know I should not feel like this, but . . . or "I know it is wrong to have this attitude, but. . . ." The self-assessment process does not yield a "good person/bad person" score. There is no right or wrong; no good, better, or best situation. The process of self-assessment merely yields data that enable the individual to make decisions or choices. It may be thought of as including a potential for action or change. Self-assessment is also never complete and probably never would be the same at two points in time due to the continuously changing nature of human beings.

Self-assessment may be a difficult task for some individuals because of a cultural prohibition against what may seem to be bragging. Typically, research in the behavioral sciences has indicated that individuals find it is much easier to identify weaknesses or perceived faults than to list capabilities or strengths. It is necessary, however, to have a realistic appraisal of both aspects of self if growth is to occur and if the nurse is to be successful in meeting the needs of patients.

Self-Assessment of Wellness

In their professional role, nurses consider the promotion of wellness a major function. Yet, one need only to walk through a hospital or spend a few minutes in a hospital coffee shop or cafeteria to realize that many nurses do not model good health behavior. Although nurses know and teach good health habits, like much of the rest of the general population, some nurses avoid exercise, smoke excessively, and are overweight. One nurse author put it even stronger when she wrote, "Wellness is the goal of nursing care. Wellness should also be the goal of nurses" (Carlin, 1982).

Table 5-1 presents a brief health-assessment tool that will help to identify obvious poor health habits. Having identified potential threats to health, the nurse can use this information to set personal health goals. This may involve an independent plan which the individual can design, or it may require that the individual seek professional assistance. Because the educational program of nursing is mentally and physically demanding, it makes sense to begin an academic program with all the assets of good health.

Table 5-1. **Self-Assessment of Wellness**

Respond to the following questions. Score one point for each yes answer, deduct one point for each negative answer.

YES No

1. _____ __ Do you wear seat belts regularly?
2. _____ __ Do you fall asleep easily and without medication?
3. _____ __ Are you in control of your own fertility?
4. _____ __ Do you feel you are reasonably attractive and intelligent?
5. _____ __ Do you have as much energy as most people have?
6. _____ __ Are you satisfied with how you spend your time?
7. _____ __ Do you exercise vigorously for at least one-half hour, three times per week?
8. _____ __ Are you within 10 lb of your ideal weight?
9. _____ __ Do you have a close friend?
10. _____ __ Have you eaten a raw vegetable or a whole-grain product or a cup of milk within the last 24 hours?

Score

10–9. You model wellness.
8–7. Room to improve.
6 or less. Start learning about wellness today.

Nursing Students as Adult Learners

Nursing students are adult learners and this fact has important implications for both faculty and students. Rosendahl (1974) described several characteristics of the adult learner:

1. Adults see themselves as self-directed and mature people . . . and resist situations in which they are treated with disrespect.
2. Adults have a broader basis of experience to relate to new learning.
3. Adults are more inclined to acquire practical results from learning.
4. Adults have a different quality of experience and different developmental tasks than those of youth.

When the above characteristics are accepted by both students and faculty, they are reflected in the interpersonal environment of the educational institution. Faculty members and students acknowledge and value each other as adults. They are respectful of each other's capabilities and experience. In such a setting, faculty members recognize and support individual differences. The student is perceived as competent to identify learning goals and to select learning experiences to achieve stated goals. Faculty recognize that learning is a continuous process and that the student learns in both formal and informal situations. The student learns from faculty and from other students and, likewise, faculty learn from students. While it is the responsibility of the faculty to offer learning experiences, the ultimate responsibility for learning belongs to the student.

Independent learning skills are expected of the student enrolled in higher education. One of the most important skills necessary to success as a nursing student is mastery of the use of a health science library. Current nursing literature is extensive and has its own system of

Table 5–2. **Indexes to Nursing Literature**

CINAHL	*Cumulative Index to Nursing and Allied Health Literature*	Published every two months	Index to periodical articles; listing of book reviews, audiovisuals, pamphlets
INI	*International Nursing Index*	Published quarterly	Includes foreign-language nursing journals; periodical index; listing of doctoral dissertations by nurses; lists publications of organizations and agencies interested in nursing
NSI	*Nursing Studies Index*	Covers 1900–1959 Four volumes complete	Annotated entries. Guide to studies and research in nursing
IM	*Index Medicus*	Published monthly	Literature of biomedicine. Nursing subjects not in nursing journals
MEDLARS	*Medical Literature Analysis and Retrieval System*	Computer-based search	600,000 journal articles. Citations from 1977 are available immediately; from 1966 are available within two weeks

indexes. (See Table 5–2.) Nursing periodicals are often the best source of information since they are more likely to be current than books, hence, the necessity for the nursing student to utilize periodical guides skillfully.

Moreover, because the body of knowledge that comprises nursing is changing so rapidly, the nursing student realizes that a continual educational process is necessary to maintain competence and safe nursing practice. Some of the content the first-year nursing student learns will be out of date by the student's graduation. Use of the hospital library and nursing literature is one way to keep current in both general and specialty areas of nursing. Many states have formally recognized the need for continued learning and have mandated continued education as a requirement for renewal of registered nurse licensure.

Because it is impractical for each nurse to remain in school indefinitely in the traditional student-nurse role, it is essential that each individual develop some skills in the independent learning process. This process consists of:

1. Assessing one's own best learning style
2. Identifying learning needs
3. Selecting ways to gain the knowledge and skills identified as learning needs
4. Implementing selected learning methods
5. Evaluating the learning that has occurred.

Self-Assessment of Learning Style

There are three main learning styles: auditory, visual, and kinesthetic. The *auditory learner* is one who acquires meaning through what is heard; the *visual learner* is one who acquires meaning through what is seen; the *kinesthetic learner* is one who acquires meaning through doing or some form of muscle movement. Table 5–3 provides descriptive characteristics of the major learning modes. It is important to understand that all types of content are not equally appropriate to each learning style. For example, the content related to values and value clarification is difficult to relate to a kinesthetic learning style, while some of the nursing skills, such as giving a back massage, are easily related to a kinesthetic style.

One cursory method of assessing learning style is to imagine that you have just asked directions to City Hospital. How do you prefer to receive the directions? If you listen carefully and understand, you are probably an auditory learner. If you prefer that someone draw you a map to follow, you are probably a visual learner.

Table 5-3. **Characteristics of Learning Styles**

Auditory Learning Style

Acquires meaning through what is heard. "Just explain the directions carefully to me and I will understand."
Prefers lecture and group discussion courses
Prefers verbal directions
Prefers giving oral presentations as a report method
Collects data by interview method when possible
Easily recalls words to songs, poems, famous quotes
Enjoys audiotapes and records

Visual Learning Style

Acquires meaning through what is seen. "Just draw me a map and I can find it."
Prefers written or pictorial instructions
Prefers courses that make extensive use of visual aids: film strips, video cassettes, demonstrations, overhead projectors, slides
Learns new terms by writing them repeatedly
Prefers to study by highlighting, underlining books, outlining content, reviewing notes
Sensitive to and accurately interprets nonverbal communication

Kinesthetic Learning Style

Acquires meaning through muscle movement. "Just let me show you how I do it and you correct me if I make a mistake."
Prefers to learn from "hands on" experience
Prefers demonstration and return demonstration method of learning skills
Utilizes objects within environment to explain statements
Enjoys hobbies that involve use of hands: sewing, carving, woodworking
Enjoys physical activity: biking, walking, skating

Source: From unpublished work of Helen Jones, Ph.D., Consultant, H. B. Jones & Associates, Cincinnati, Ohio. Used with permission.

Finally, if you repeat the instructions back to another person, perhaps using a desk top to represent the freeway, erasers to represent various exits, and coins to represent other buildings, and then do a symbolic trip to the hospital, you probably prefer the kinesthetic mode of learning. Each mode is equally effective for the individual learner; it merely reflects an individual preference.

The student who is aware of personal learning style is able to select learning materials and strategies that maximize potential for success. Conversely, when the student is aware that new essential content is being presented in a mode that is personally difficult, identifying a mode that better suits individual style may facilitate learning. For example, the student who has concluded that the visual mode makes learning easier may be enrolled in a nursing course taught primarily by the lecture method. This student may choose to make extensive use of the nursing library's collection of film strips and video cassettes to supplement auditory learning.

Self-Assessment of Feelings

People have feelings! Although this may seem obvious, it is a fact that is often forgotten or seriously neglected in nursing practice. The feelings of a nurse can directly affect the care given to a patent. For example, consider the student who is angry at a nursing instructor for a reprimand related to reporting late for clinical experience. The student nurse may be unable to talk to an assigned patient and may not be gentle while doing an assigned dressing change. The student does not intentionally hurt the patient, but the stress caused by the anger has affected nursing care.

Feelings are unique reactions that a person has to a situation, event, or another person and can be either pleasant or unpleasant. Feelings are usually described as being of an emotional nature rather than a rational or thinking nature. In addition, feelings have both a physiological and a psychological component. The angry student nurse mentioned above may not be aware of the patient's movements that indicate that the dressing change is causing pain. The nurse may not be able to listen and recall the symptoms the patient is reporting. Depending on the degree of anger the student experienced, it is also possible to assess physiological manifestations of the anger. The nurse may have experienced an increased heart rate, increased respiratory rate, tense rigid muscles, flushed face, and perhaps nausea.

There are many reasons an individual is not aware of personal feelings. Perhaps the most common reason is the lack of teaching to do so or even the admonition not to do so! As children, many people were taught, for example, "You should not feel like that. After all, I was only trying to help you," or "You should not be angry at me. I am your mother." Other individuals may have learned not to share their feelings with peers or authority figures because they fear the judgments that others may make. Although this may be a well-founded fear, it denies the help that others may be able to provide if they were aware of the individual's feelings. Although it is not essential for the individual to share feelings, it is essential for the individual to be consciously aware of personal feelings as they affect interactions with patients.

A nurse might use the following questions to assist in identifying personal feelings:

1. How am I feeling right now?
2. Can I identify, specifically, what I am feeling?
3. What or who caused this feeling?
4. How is this feeling affecting my behavior?

Self-Assessment of Attitudes

Although feelings discussed above may be thought of as temporary subjective states, *attitudes* are feelings that have persisted over time. They are biases or predispositions to act in certain ways. Attitudes are thus strongly held and more resistant to change than are feelings. Attitudes may be formed as a result of interaction with persons, situations, or events. They may have a rational component or be lacking that element. Racial prejudice and sexism are examples of frequently held attitudes. Attitudes can be changed with conscious effort. Consider the student who arrives at college with the attitude that "This will be easy. I always get all As." Following the first series of midterm examinations, the student may revise this attitude to, "This is tough going.

I'd better get some help if I'm going to make it here." The exercise in Table 5–4 will help the student to assess some personal attitudes.

Attitudes may have a very direct influence on nursing care. The nurse who is racially prejudiced may be unable to perceive the needs of a patient who belongs to another group. The nurse may have difficulty touching or providing physical care to this patient. In this case, it is essential that the nurse be aware of personal attitudes and how they affect nursing care. The nurse is bound by professional rules of conduct to provide nursing care without regard to race, color, sex, or creed. Nurses are obligated to practice within the rules of the profession.

Table 5–4. **Self-Assessment of Attitudes**

This exercise provides an opportunity to examine your attitudes toward various topics. First, read each of the following statements and try to identify where you stand on each of the issues. Any of these issues may be selected for discussion in a group setting. In the group, state your attitude as clearly and concisely as possible. Listen to the statement of other persons in the group. Do not attempt to judge, argue, or persuade.

My attitude toward . . . is . . .

1. My attitude toward abortion is . . .
2. My attitude toward euthanasia is . . .
3. My attitude toward professional competition is . . .
4. My attitude toward exercise is . . .
5. My attitude toward divorce is . . .

6. My attitude toward dieting is . . .
7. My attitude toward sexism is . . .
8. My attitude toward homosexuality is . . .
9. My attitude toward smoking is . . .
10. My attitude toward child abuse is . . .
11. My attitude toward spouse abuse is . . .
12. My attitude toward drug abuse is . . .

Rank your three strongest attitudes.
How did you acquire these attitudes?
Do you wish to change any of these attitudes?
Have any of these attitudes changed in the past five years?
How did the attitude change?
If none of the attitudes has changed, how were they reinforced?

Source: Adapted from Thomas W. Muldary: *Interpersonal Relations for Health Professionals.* Macmillan, New York, 1983. Used with permission.

Self-Assessment of Values

Value, in the broadest sense of the word, refers to the worth or the esteem that is accorded to an individual or object by a society. Values (the plural form) take on additional meaning. *Values* refer to the principles or standards considered significant and important to either an individual or a group of persons. A value system is an organized and interrelated group of principles that serve to guide behavior. A value system is highly personal and probably not exactly duplicated by another human being. It is beneficial if individuals are aware of their own value system in order to bring actions and values into agreement. When one's actions and behavior accurately reflect one's values, stress is reduced, with the result of maximizing a health state. In addition, it is important for the nurse to be aware of the fact that personal values may differ significantly from those of the patient and that it is patient values that are most important in the health care system. The patient will ultimately make health care decisions.

Values, like attitudes, are formed as a result of education, experience, culture, and interpersonal relationships. Values are not formed spontaneously but rather evolve over time as a result of much thought and deliberation. This investment of time and energy on the part of the individual makes the value more resistant to change, although a value system must be flexible enough to incorporate the growth of the individual. Uustal (1978), a nurse educator writing about values, summarized the steps in the valuing process as choosing, prizing, acting. The individual is first free to select values after considering the alternatives and the effects of the alternatives. Next, the individual is proud of the choice and is willing to affirm the choice publicly. This is called prizing the values. Finally the individual incorporates the value into action repeatedly and consistently.

As unique as the value system is to the individual, groups of human beings hold values in common, and these are called shared values. Similarly, nurses hold a group of common values which we call professional values. The nursing student brings personal values to the academic setting, but is called upon to incorporate nursing's professional values. Some of the values that members of the nursing profession share are the value of human life, the value of honesty, the value of the individual's right to make decisions about health care, the value of health.

The individual nursing student brings a personal value system to the academic setting. The student is then asked to merge the professional value system with the personal value system. Similarly, the patient brings a unique value system into the health care setting, and a potential for conflict and stress exists between the two systems. For example, if health care personnel place a high value on patient compliance with a prescribed medical regimen and the patient places a high value on individual decision making, a conflict may result. In another example, the nurse who places a high value on accepting the decisions made by patients may experience conflict with a head nurse who does not accept the refusal of a patient to take a prescribed medication. In each example, the individual who is clearly aware of a personal value system is able to identify the source of the stress and to plan coping behavior. This awareness may help to bring values and behavior into agreement.

Within the health care setting, it is also important that the values of the patient take precedence over the values of the nurse, unless harm to others may result. In the latter example above, the nurse may gather more data as to why the patient is refusing the medication or offer more information as to the purpose of the medication, but, ultimately, the patient's decision must be respected. There are legal implications of such nursing actions, and these are discussed in Chapter 3. Table 5–5 provides one tool to assist in value assessment.

Table 5–5. **Values Assessment**

1. You have recently applied to a nursing school. You have been asked to provide three character references from individuals who have known you five or more years.
    a. What things do you wish your references would say about you?
    b. Identify some values indicated by the things you desire included in your reference.
2. Rank the following characteristics in order of decreasing importance to professional nursing. Discuss your reasons for your ranking.
    Attractive physical appearance
    Cleanliness
    Competent
    Cooperative
    Creative
    Legible handwriting
    Punctual
    Religious
    Skilled communicator
    Speed in performing nursing skills
    20/20 vision

Self-Assessment of Transcultural Knowledge

Culture refers to all those human-made aspects, both material and nonmaterial, of a civilization. The material culture consists of such concrete things as art, machines, books, and buildings. The nonmaterial cul-

Table 5-6. Dominant Contrasts: Folk and Professional Comparative Cultural Health Care Systems as Perceived by Clients

FOLK HEALTH CARE EMPHASES	PROFESSIONAL HEALTH CARE EMPHASES
1. Primarily a humanistic focus	1. Primarily a scientific focus
2. Emphases on familiar, practical, and concrete facts	2. Emphases on unfamiliar, less practical, and abstract facts
3. Uses a wholistic, integrated health-illness focus (i.e., culture, religion, kinship, economics, social aspects) with people	3. Uses a fragmented and nonintegrated approach (largely medicine) with people, except for nursing's partially holistic approach
4. Focus is primarily a caring attitude	4. Focus is primarily on a curing attitude with some caring
5. Primarily nontechnological in services, and more sociocultural relationships are stressed	5. Primarily technological treatments and diagnostic services
6. Prevention of illness and disabilities by cultural taboos	6. Diagnostic and treatment regimes of diseases emphasized
7. Modest cost for care or cure services (home-based)	7. High costs for physician and hospital services
8. Health assessment done in relation to cultural, social, political, and economic conditions	8. Illness assessment done mainly on physical and psychological problems of needs of clients
9. Uses familiar local care and cure helpers	9. Uses unfamiliar nonlocal care-givers and curers
10. Uses diverse cultural and community resources to help client in home and community environments	10. Uses limited resources (largely medical and hospital) to help client
11. Uses a wide cultural support system made to help clients	11. Uses professional persons with limited sociocultural supports to help clients
12. Emphases on ways to stay well through local health ways	12. Emphases on ways to be cured according to professional values and beliefs
13. Folk practitioners continue to be the primary care or first-line care-givers	13. Professional practitioners perform mainly secondary and tertiary care services
14. Care and cure occur in familiar home setting	14. Care and cure occur primarily in hospital
15. Participant involvement brings client back to health with instructions on how to keep well	15. Physician, nurse, and others use scientific procedures and ideas to get cured
16. Emphases on group (family and community) in healing process	16. Emphases on individual in curative practices
17. Uses diverse explanations to interpret wellness and illness	17. Uses a focused cause(s) to explain illness and problems

These contrasts of emphases were developed by Leininger through direct participant-observation experiences with approximately 20 cultures.

Source: Madeleine M. Leininger: Transcultural Nursing: Its progress and its Future. *Nurs. Health Care,* 2:365–71, Sept., 1981. Reproduced with permission.

ture consists of abstractions such as family traditions, customs, beliefs, and languages. Thus, culture is highly unique to a specific group of people. It is transmitted largely by life in the culture. It is possible to gain some understanding of life in another culture through academic study, but study will never create as complete an appreciation as that of the individual who has the opportunity to experience another culture by living among its people.

Within the main or dominant culture of a society are small groups of persons (subcultures) who do not participate fully in the life-style of the larger group and who share a common culture different from the dominant culture. Examples of subcultures may include a family, a minority group, drug addicts, and college students. The dominant culture and the subculture may clash when values, life-styles, and norms are different.

In the past, nursing education and nursing practice have been based on Anglo-Saxon and Caucasian culture. This has resulted in *ethnocentrism* in nursing, that is, the tendency to judge other people by the standards of one's own culture. At other points in the history of the United States, this country was seen as a "melting pot," which meant that immigrants assumed the dominant culture of the country, and their own unique culture was blended in and frequently lost. Today, cultural minority groups are seeking to preserve and continue their cultural heritage. The health care system is now challenged to provide services from a multicultural approach.

Madeleine Leininger has been referred to as the founder of *transcultural nursing*. This nursing specialty analyzes cultures and subcultures for their health-illness beliefs, values, and practices. From this type of study, nursing practices can be developed that are unique to a culture (culture specific) or the same between many cultures (culture universal). Leininger (1981) believes that since cultural factors are the major forces that influence the quality of health and nursing care, the omission of cultural factors is a major obstacle in providing quality care. In addition, Leininger states her belief that nursing has an ethical and professional obligation to prepare practitioners to work effectively with people of diverse backgrounds. One of Leininger's major contributions to transcultural nursing has been the study of folk health care compared to professional health care systems. Although most nursing students are aware of the *professional health care system*, few are aware of the *folk health care system*. And, lacking understanding, professionals often refer to folk health care as superstitious, useless, without efficacy. Leininger's research yielded data to describe and contrast professional and folk health care systems. (See Table 5–6.) The professional health care system is learning to exist in harmony and respect with the folk health care system.

Largely due to the work of Leininger, most nursing educational programs now include content related to transcultural nursing. Exhibit 5–1 provides a beginning measurement of transcultural knowledge.

Exhibit 5–1. Transcultural Assessment

Answer the following questions to begin an assessment of your transcultural knowledge.

1. In some American Indian tribes to cut the hair of a child
   a. Is a ceremonial ritual
   b. Is a violation of a taboo
   c. Has no particular significance
2. It is common among young married couples of some American Indian tribes to entrust the care and rearing of children to
   a. Grandmothers
   b. Maternal aunts
   c. Maternal grandfathers
3. Which of the following is not usually seen within the black culture?
   a. Chickenpox
   b. Child abuse
   c. Extended family relationships
4. Who, among the following is seen as a strong, stable figure among the black community?
   a. An elementary teacher
   b. A local YMCA worker
   c. A black minister
5. Within Mexican-American folk medicine, who among the following is seen if one wishes to communicate with a dead relative?
   a. Curandero
   b. Curandera
   c. Espiritista
6. *Mal de ojo* may be prevented in Mexican-American babies by the nurse
   a. Careful handwashing
   b. Encouraging the mother to breastfeed the infant
   c. Touching the baby while admiring it
7. The Puerto Rican culture shares many beliefs with
   a. The American Indian culture
   b. The Mexican-American culture
   c. The black American culture

8. Seventy-two percent of teenage suicide victims less than 15 years of age are
   a. American Indians
   b. Puerto Ricans
   c. Black Americans

9. Illness in the American Indian culture is defined in terms of
   a. One's ability to function properly
   b. The needs of one's family
   c. The inner cycle of birth, life, death

10. Which of the following cultures defines health as an energy flow, a balance between positive and negative?
    a. Traditional Indian medicine
    b. Traditional Chinese medicine
    c. Traditional Puerto Rican medicine

11. The person who is a member of the Church of Christ Scientist
    a. Believes that sickness is cured by mental processes, primarily prayer and counsel
    b. Believes that illness results as a punishment for sin and evil
    c. May request that a clergyman be summoned to practice healing by laying on of hands

12. A Chinese person from a traditional culture may seek health care from
    a. A nurse-midwife
    b. An herb pharmacist
    c. A hypnotist

13. When taking prescribed medications a Chinese person may
    a. Take only one dose of the medicine
    b. Refuse all liquid medications
    c. Require injectable medications

14. Some Chinese patients may prefer
    a. Ice water
    b. Carbonated beverages only
    c. Hot drinking water

15. Afro speech is different from Anglo speech in that
    a. The Afro dialect uses multiple negatives for emphasis
    b. The Afro dialect is a result of the lack of educational opportunities
    c. It is intelligible only to other black Americans

16. Strong kinship bonds among black American families
    a. Serve as a support system against racism and discrimination
    b. Are strongest among low-income blacks
    c. Are a required practice of religious affiliation

17. "Mongolian spots" refer to
    a. A rash related to impetigo common in nonwhite persons
    b. An area of hyperpigmentation primarily on buttocks and thighs common in nonwhite infants
    c. A childhood illness most common among nonwhite preschoolers

18. A Hispanic person is likely to prefer
    a. Rice
    b. Pasta
    c. Potatoes

19. Hispanic clients may refuse to use a psychiatrist because
    a. Of the cultural value against revealing personal or family information
    b. Translators are not available to assist in the treatment process
    c. Mental illness is extremely rare among Hispanic families

20. Within the Vietnamese culture, the authority of the father is absolute, and the role of women is
    a. Related primarily to childrearing
    b. To be the moral authority and financial manager of the family
    c. To assure the continuance of the family by producing male descendants

Answers

1. b
2. a
3. b
4. c
5. c
6. c
7. b
8. a
9. c
10. b
11. a
12. a
13. a
14. c
15. a
16. a
17. b
18. a
19. a
20. b

Scores

18–20. Go to the head of the class!
15–17. There's hope, but start studying!
12–14. Enroll in a transcultural nursing course now.
11 or less. Which half of your own culture do you mind if your nurse does not understand?

Philosophy of Nursing

Each institution in which nursing is taught or practiced, as well as each individual nurse, has a philosophy of nursing. A *philosophy* is a statement of beliefs that guide one's behavior and, in this case, influence the practice of nursing. An understanding of one's own beliefs, feelings, values, attitudes, and culture precedes the development of a philosophy of nursing. Until the nurse has knowledge of self, it is difficult to state beliefs to guide nursing practice. Several concepts must be discussed in any nursing philosophy. These include human beings, health, illness, and nursing. Writing a personal philosophy of nursing is a task that requires a great deal of thought and self-knowledge. Each of the previous self-assessments related to values, attitudes, feelings, and culture provides data that will help the nurse to express personal beliefs. The nurse makes a statement of personal beliefs related to each of the identified concepts. This is a deliberative, rational process that involves a great deal of introspection. For example, the nurse who believes in the Christian religion may express a belief that the human being possesses a life after death and that one function of nursing is to assist the individual to attain this life. These beliefs may influence the care the nurse gives to a dying patient.

Institutions also develop their own philosophy of nursing. The nursing philosophy of a hospice (a place of care for dying patients) and that of a large research center may be very different. Health care institutions developed with strong organizational affiliations may reflect these in their philosophy. Consider a Shriner's hospital, a Jewish community hospital, and a large county hospital in a big city. Exhibits 5–2 and 5–3 are examples of statements of philosophy of organizations. Prior to enrolling in a school of nursing, the prospective student may read the school philosophy in order to consider the level of agreement with personal belief systems. Similarly, the registered nurse who is seeking employment is wise to read the philosophy of the institution and to compare it to a personal philosophy of nursing.

Exhibit 5–2. Example of a Philosophy of Nursing

University of Cincinnati Hospital Nursing Service

The practice of nursing is the care of patients through a professional interpersonal relationship. Nurses apply behavioral scientific principles, biologic scientific principles, and principles of humanism in a skillful, concerted, and compassionate manner to bring patients and their families optimal health status, personal growth, dignity, and peace. Nurses demonstrate the professional use of self and the collaborative involvement of families and related health care providers in bringing about desired change, as established in the patient-nurse contract. Nurses advocate, teach, conduct clinical inquiry, institute planned change, make critical decisions, coordinate and synthesize the efforts of other disciplines, create therapeutic interpersonal contact, perform therapeutic procedures, and establish a therapeutic milieu. The process of nursing causes learning, growth, maturity, and acceptance of responsibility by both the patient and nurse.

The primary function of the Nursing Department is to provide patient services in a manner conducive to the education of health professionals and supportive of appropriate research activities. The Department affirms its commitment to optimal patient outcomes and the highest standards of care possible in the face of increasing technical patient care requirements and the need to make intelligent decisions about the use of resources. Given finite resources, nurses exercise conscious decision making and problem solving, managing environmental and support structures for positive patient care outcomes, thereby realizing a satisfying level of nursing practice.

All patients at the University of Cincinnati Hospital are entitled to excellence in the nursing care they receive. The quality of care given is without regard to race, sex, religious or political belief, socioeconomic status, or ethnic background.

Nursing is the primary professional service received during hospitalization. Posthospitalization, nurses provide continuity of care and contribute to effective interface between hospital and community, emphasizing preventive, health maintenance, and rehabilitative service.

The Department commits to the development of professional nursing through modeling the nursing role in caring for patients, developing new health care providers, and expanding nursing knowledge. Nursing will demonstrate a leadership role in this environment by promoting improved models of organizing and delivering patient care, such as Primary Nursing, in order to increase and clarify our responsibility and accountability for practice.

Source: University of Cincinnati Hospital, Cincinnati, Ohio. Reproduced with permission.

Exhibit 5–3. **Example of a Philosophy of Nursing**

Children's Hospital Medical Center Philosophy of Nursing

We believe that Man is a holistic (bio-psycho-social spiritual) being capable of adapting to many adverse conditions depending upon his stage of development, family dynamics, environment, and cultural influences. We believe that children are individuals as well as members of a family and that they have a right to

a. Be treated as an individual
b. Health care to achieve a better quality of life or dignity in death
c. Be informed
d. Privacy and confidentiality
e. Emotional support
f. A safe environment
g. Maintain family ties in times of disequilibrium
h. An environment where the child experiences a continued sense of parenting

We believe that family-centered patient care requires a collaborative interdependence with other disciplines within CHMC as well as within the community. This is dependent upon a work environment that promotes critical inquiry, free exchange of ideas, and humanistic treatment of personnel. We further believe that decision making must take place at the most effective level of the organization.

We believe that a professional nurse is a skilled, educated provider of patient care with a clear definition of purpose and standards of practice. The nurse is accountable to the child and his family, him/herself, the institution, and society for integrating quality patient care.

We believe that nurses within the department have the responsibility of developing, implementing, coordinating, and evaluating patient care services to insure that the child receives optimal health care. The professional nurse diagnoses and treats human responses to facilitate effective living by the child and his family as they experience actual or potential health problems.

We believe that the professional nurse

a. Is able to use the process of assessment, planning, implementation, and evaluation as a base for practice.
b. Is able to use organizational skills to efficiently direct and implement the appropriate components of a patient care delivery system.
c. Participates in formal and informal learning opportunities to increase skill and knowledge, and communicates new knowledge to other personnel.
d. Performs, analyzes, implements, and communicates nursing research to modify nursing practices for more effective patient care.
e. Has the responsibility to adhere to policies and procedures and assume initiative for improving personal and institutional practices.
f. Fosters open lines of communication with all health team members to assure the best possible care for the client.
g. Conducts formal and informal sessions to facilitate the child's and family's knowledge of his condition and environment.
h. Provides for continuity of the child's care.

Source: Children's Hospital Medical Center, Cincinnati, Ohio. Reproduced with permission.

Summary

Self-assessment is the process of developing an awareness of self. This is essential to the personal growth of a human being, to academic success as a student in nursing, and to professional competence as a nurse. Self-assessment yields an understanding of feelings, attitudes, values, and culture which helps the nursing student begin to formulate a personal philosophy to guide nursing practice.

Terms for Review

attitudes	folk health care system	philosophy	subjective data
auditory learner	kinesthetic learner	professional health care system	transcultural nursing
culture	nonjudgmental	self-assessment	values
ethnocentrism	objective data	self-concept	visual learner
feelings			

Self-Assessment

I. My family as a subculture: Write a description about each of the following statements using your own family as the subject for assessment. If you desire, discuss these with faculty and classmates for similarities and differences.

  1. Religion is defined within my family as . . . and is demonstrated by . . .
  2. Roles within my family.
     Mother is expected to . . .
     Father is expected to . . .
     A male child is expected to . . .
     A female child is expected to . . .
  3. Decisions are made by whom, about what, by what method?
  4. My family spends leisure time doing what, with whom?
  5. Relationships with relatives are . . .
  6. My family celebrates major holidays by . . .
  7. Children would be punished in my family for . . . (offense) by . . . (method).
  8. Education in my family is considered . . .
  9. Political beliefs in my family are . . .
  10. Human sexuality and reproduction was explained to me by . . . at age . . . as meaning . . .
  11. Death in my family means . . .
  12. When a member of my family dies . . .
  13. Disagreements are resolved by . . .

II. Values: For each of the above statements 1 through 13, study your answers and list the values that were transmitted to you by your family subculture.

Learning Activities

1. Values. In a small notebook, list those things you gave up in order to enter a nursing program. Try to include as many things as possible, for example, income, job, family time, leisure activities.
   a. Next, list the values that prompted you to seek a nursing education.
   b. List the benefits or "payoffs," current or future, of your choice.
   c. Review monthly and add or delete from the list.
2. Read several articles about the culture of a minority group living in your community and discuss how health care needs might differ for members of that culture.

Review Questions

1. The most important reason for a nurse to have self-knowledge is
   a. So personal unmet needs do not block awareness of patient needs

   b. To facilitate personal growth
   c. To understand what motivates behavior
2. Which of the following is most likely to be temporary?
   a. Value
   b. Feeling
   c. Culture
3. According to the characteristics of adult learners described by Rosendahl, adult learners
   a. Are likely to use their life experiences as a foundation for building new knowledge
   b. Are likely to have difficulty accepting criticism from younger faculty members
   c. Will experience resistance to change in accepting current educational methods and practices
4. The nursing student requests of an instructor, "Could you please roughly sketch the circulation of the heart to help me understand it?" This is a request to help the student learn in which mode?
   a. Visual
   b. Auditory
   c. Kinesthetic
5. An ethical dilemma
   a. Has the same moral meaning for each and every nurse
   b. Is resolved by consultation with lawyers and clergy
   c. Occurs when a nurse is forced to make a choice between two equally unfavorable alternatives
6. The study of other cultures is important to nursing
   a. In order to provide nursing care that is valued and accepted by patients of other cultures
   b. To avoid ethnocentrism
   c. To expand the body of nursing knowledge

Answers

1. a
2. b
3. a
4. a
5. c
6. a

Suggested Readings

Primeaux, M.: American Indian health practices. A cross cultural perspective. *Nurs. Clin. North Am.,* **12:**55–65, 1977. The author describes characteristics of American Indians and some common health care practices. A case history is presented to demonstrate some conflicts which occurred as a result of cross-cultural misunderstandings.

White, E.: Giving health care to minority patients. *Nurs. Clin. North Am.,* **12:**27–40, 1977. Author discusses health beliefs and health practices of five client groups in the United States: black Americans, Mexican Americans, Puerto Rican Americans, Native Americans, and Asian Americans.

References and Bibliography

Carlin, D.: How to assess your wellness and become a model for your patients. *Nurs. Life*, **2**:48–49, 1982.

DeYoung, L.: *Dynamics of Nursing*, 4th ed. Mosby, St. Louis, 1981.

Leininger, M.: Transcultural nursing: Its progress and its future. *Nurs. Health Care,* **2**:365–71, 1981.

Luft, J.: *Group Processes: An Introduction to Group Dynamics*, 2nd ed., National Press Books, Palo Alto, Calif., 1970.

Roberto, L.: Selected beliefs of Vietnamese refugees. *J. Sch. Health*, **51**: 63–64, 1981.

Rosendahl, P.: Self-direction for learners: An andrological approach to nursing education. *Nurs. Forum,* **13**:136–46, 1974.

Uustal, D.: Values clarification in nursing: Application to practice. *Am. J. Nurs.,* **78**:2058–63, 1978.

THE PROCESS OF INTERPERSONAL COMMUNICATION

Objectives

1. Explain why it is necessary for nurses to study communication.

2. Describe what is meant by the physiological, psychological, and contextual aspects of communication.

3. Describe the purpose served by each of several types of communication.

4. Define what is meant by therapeutic communication.

5. Discuss several factors that influence the communication process.

6. Contrast attitudes that hinder communication to those that enhance communication.

7. Discuss the effect of illness on communication.

8. Give an example of each of the following communication skills: reflection, open-ended questions, clarification, summarizing, silence.

9. State two principles that guide the nurse in dealing with inappropriate communication.

Why Study Communication?

Frequently, beginning nursing students question the need to study communication because, after all, they have been talking, listening, and writing for a minimum of 18 years and some for 50 years or more! Moreover, they complain that practiced communication seems so artificial, so manipulative, so unlike the real "me." It is

Table 6–1. **General Interpretations of Nonverbal Messages**

	INTERPRETATION		INTERPRETATION
Posture		*Eye Contact*	
Erect, relaxed	Confident, interested	Direct	Interest, confidence, honesty
Slouched	Disinterested, depressed, submissive, or hostile	Eyes open unusually wide	Attentive
		Eyelids drooping	Listless, depressed
Stiff	Insecure	Averted gaze	Submissive, untruthful, lacking confidence
Space		*Facial Expression*	
Crouched, body drawn close	Submissive	Pursed lips	Anger
Stretched out, legs and arms apart	Dominant, confident	Relaxed mouth	Calm
		Broad smile	Happy
		Faked smile	Manipulative, placating
		Furrowed brow	Concern, tension, disbelief, lack of comprehension
Gestures			
No gesturing	Disinterest, depression	Flared nostrils	Anger
Excessive gesturing	Anxiety	*Physical Appearance*	
		Well-groomed	Thoughtful, socialized
Touch		Disheveled	Poor socialization, poor mental health
Reciprocal and nonharmful	Caring, intimacy	*Smell*	
Asymmetrical	Dominance, when the toucher is in a higher status position	Bad odors	Poor grooming, poor health

Source: Linda De Villers: What to do when you just can't communicate. *Nurs. Life*, 2:36–39, 1982. Reprinted with permission. Copyright © 1983, Springhouse Corporation. All rights reserved.

important that these feelings be recognized by faculty members and students as a very realistic starting point for the study of communication in nursing.

Communication, as a part of the nursing role, is a skill just as giving injections or changing surgical dressings. Just like other skills, the student must understand the principles that provide the basis for action. Then the student must undertake to practice the skill until it is done easily and well. For example, the first time the nursing student is assigned to complete an admission interview for a hospitalized patient, the student may have difficulty completing the form as required. Later, with additional practice and some knowledge of interviewing skills, the student is able to solicit and clarify important data within the patient's health history which helps to identify problems requiring nursing care.

Relationships are formed through communication. This is true of both the social relationships one has with friends and also of the helping relationship the nurse has with patients. If communication is the means of relating to people, it follows that the nurse must be proficient in this skill. As a nursing skill, communication involves more than the verbal or spoken mode of relating. *Nonverbal communication* is an equally important way to establish relationships. Some modes of nonverbal communication are touching, writing, reading, gesturing, physical movement, and gift giving. The manner in which individuals carry their bodies also conveys nonverbal messages which can be voluntary or involuntary. Table 6–1 includes some nonverbal body messages and possible interpretations.

Touch is a form of nonverbal communication which nurses use daily in providing care. Giving baths and back rubs, moving and positioning patients in bed, and changing surgical dressings all involve touching patients as a part of physical care. At other times, the nurse may touch the patient as a part of psychological care, such as holding the hand of an anxious patient before surgery, or putting an arm around the spouse of a dying patient to offer comfort. Because a nurse needs to be able to both interpret and send messages in verbal and nonverbal modes, communication skills are very important.

Communication Defined

Communication has been very simply defined as "shared meaning." When two people agree on the message that has been sent between them, communication has occurred. Frequently, and for an almost infinite number of reasons, this shared meaning does not result. This is called miscommunication or misunderstanding. For example, consider the nursing student whose instructor told the students to meet for a discussion class when they had finished their patient care assignments at 11:00 A.M. The student who arrived tardy at 11:20 A.M. was surprised to find the instructor irritated. "I told you to be here at 11:00 A.M.," said the instructor. "I thought you said to come when we were finished," said the student. Obviously, a miscommunication has occurred for both persons. The intended message was, "Have your assignment complete shortly before 11:00 A.M. and be ready to start class promptly at 11:00 A.M."

One wise communicator was known to remark, "Understand what I mean and not what I say!" The comment, only partly in jest, illustrates the important fact that speech is highly individualized. Although each person may share the dictionary definition of words, the particular way in which the individual uses the words to convey meaning is unique. Along with the verbal message, the individual adds a personal nonverbal component to the message. The irritated nursing instructor may stand up with crossed arms, tap one foot, and stare directly at the student who is late. All of these nonverbal additions to the verbal words give a very clear message to the student that the instructor is irritated. When shared meaning results, it is because individuals have similar interpretations of verbal and nonverbal messages.

The Individual Communication Process

Three activities or subprocesses make up the complex process of communication. These consist of receiving information, processing information, and transmitting information. In order for communication to occur, the unit or the system producing it must be functional, that is to say, "in working order." When the human being is the communication system, physiological, psychological, and contextual (environmental) aspects of the system must be considered.

The human being receives communication input primarily through three senses: sight, hearing, touch. In order for these sensations to be perceived by the individual, the sensory receptors and the afferent nerves to the nervous system must be intact. If these receptors are damaged, the particular sensation may be impaired or totally lacking. When one of the senses is impaired as a receiver, frequently another sense becomes more acute in an attempt to compensate. The person who is blind may have developed a very acute sense of hearing. The person who is deaf may have a fine visual acuity which enables lipreading.

The activity of processing the information received depends on a physiological component. Processing of information takes place in the central nervous system, that part of the brain and spinal cord that integrates sensory data and initiates a response. This is the part of the brain that can reason, think, understand, and make a response. The speech center is located on the opposite side of the dominant hand in the cerebral cortex. In a right-handed person, the speech center is usually in the left half of the brain. Thus, damage to the left half of the brain is likely to result in impaired ability to communicate.

The activity of transmission within the communication system also depends on some physiological components. The central nervous system directs the body to make a response. The motor nerves, those producing movement, must be intact. In the case of a verbal transmission, the speech apparatus of the body must be functional. This includes both the motor speech center in the brain, which is responsible for controlling the muscles of the face, jaw, and larynx, and a second speech center in the brain which controls comprehension of speech. The primary organs of speech must also be intact: the lips, tongue, larynx. These are the physiological structures that are necessary to verbal communication. Sound is produced when nerve impulses leave the speech center of the brain and innervate the muscles of the larynx, tongue, lower jaw, and lips. When the muscles of the larynx contract, the vocal folds are pulled tight. Exhaled air is passed over the vocal folds, and sound results from the vibration of the folds. The greater the amount and force of exhaled air, the louder is the sound produced. Muscles of the face, tongue, and lips then shape the sound into speech.

Psychological aspects of the communication system

include all the feelings, values, attitudes, and life experiences of the individual. The messages that one receives from a second individual are filtered through this personal backlog, and the response is affected. Consider a nursing student who has a close relationship with a younger brother who is severely mentally retarded. This student is likely to approach a mentally retarded patient with gentleness and understanding based on past experience. A second student, lacking a similar experience, may be very fearful when caring for the same patient.

Finally, the contextual aspect of the communication must be considered. Context refers to the environment, including the people present and the physical setting, in which the system functions. A criticism offered by a classmate during a practice session on hospital bedmaking may be easily accepted by another student. The student-student relationship in a practice setting permits this easy exchange. The same criticism given by a head nurse during a hospital experience may feel quite different to the student. In the latter case, the context has changed. Both the physical environment (the hospital) and the relationship (head nurse–student) have changed to affect the interpretation of the communication.

Functions of Communication

Communication has purpose. It has been said, "You cannot not communicate." Think about it! Even the most withdrawn mentally ill patient who curls up in a ball refusing human contact is communicating a great deal through behavior. The patient's actions tell the nurse that the individual is very ill, in need of help, perhaps fearful, and distrustful of human contact. Understanding the intended purpose of communication helps the nurse to interpret correctly both verbal and nonverbal behavior.

Condon (1966) discusses eight types of communication that serve very distinct purposes:

1. Phatic communication. The purpose of this conversation is not to convey a message but to indicate that the sender is open to further communication, that the presence of another person is recognized. Typical examples of this might include the casual greetings to which no one really expects an answer, "How's it going?" "How are you doing?"

2. Preventive communication. This verbal or nonverbal exchange is designed to discourage any further attempt at communication. The teacher who responds to a question by saying, "That was discussed in yesterday's lecture" and continues the presentation or the student who yawns noticeably during a small group discussion give clear signals about their willingness to continue the communication.

3. Information sending/recording function. This is a purely pragmatic form of communication. Some examples are stock market reports, school absentee lists, charting patients' temperatures and blood pressures.

4. Instrumental function. This type of communication is intended to produce an action or a desired effect. The student may request, "Please demonstrate taking a blood pressure again." The instructor then repeats the demonstration.

5. Affective communication. This form is intended to convey the feelings of the speaker for the listener. These messages can be either positive, as in the case of praise or congratulations, or negative, as in the case of personal criticism or sharp, hostile comments. Some examples are: "Congratulations, you made a fine presentation," or "How could you make such a dumb mistake?"

6. Catharsis. This function of communication permits one to "let off steam," to give vent to emotions. These expressions vary in intensity from the mild "drat it" to the strong expressions that warrant an "expletive deleted" when in print.

7. Magic. In this function, words are thought to have a power, to be able to cause an effect. The expression "knock on wood" is an example of the person believing words have the power to prevent an unpleasant consequence. In another example, a pessimistic individual who says, "I just know it will rain the day of the picnic," is quickly silenced by other members of the group, as if that individual could cause the rain by saying the words. Being afraid to mention the word "cancer" before a biopsy is another example.

8. Ritual. This function of communication relates to the language used in the performance of certain rites or ceremonies which involve other persons on specific occasions with very prescribed detail. Students of nursing often participate in a capping or dedication ceremony which may include taking the Nightingale pledge and having a lamp lit from a ceremonial Nightingale lamp. The sense of solemnity is part of the ritual function of communication.

Intrapersonal Communication

Intrapersonal communication, also called internal communication, refers to the messages the individual gives to self. The messages usually include an evaluative component: positive, negative, or neutral. It is the person thinking about self, putting feelings or reflections into words that may remain unspoken but are brought to a level of awareness. This type of communication contributes to the self-concept of the individual. For example, an individual may critically examine a woodworking project just completed and think: "This isn't much. Even with a lot of help I produced a sloppy project." Depending on how much the individual values woodworking ability, the internal negative message contributes to a low self-concept.

Interpersonal Communication

In order to form a relationship with another human being, the individual engages in interpersonal communication, that is, communication between two people. Some communication between patient and nurse is called *therapeutic communication.* This is defined as planned, deliberate communication the nurse uses in order to help identify and meet the health care needs of the patient. It is therapeutic communication that forms the basis of the nurse-patient relationship. In contrast is social communication which forms the basis of social or friendship relationships. Several characteristics that distinguish therapeutic from social communication are summarized in Table 6–2.

Therapeutic communication is a very complex nursing skill. It is a skill that is taught and then must be practiced if the nurse is to use it to benefit patients. For beginning students, it can be particularly difficult to engage in therapeutic communication while simultaneously giving physical care to a patient. Frequently, patients choose to talk about health-related problems while the nurse is giving a bed bath. This is usually a private, uninterrupted time conducive to conversation. The student gradually learns to give the bath, make observations of the patient's condition, and simultaneously focus on communication. At other times, the nurse will plan a period of time to use only for the purpose of therapeutic conversation. This is a legitimate and valuable use of the nurse's time. Occasionally, nurses have stated that they felt that "sitting with the patient just talking" is shirking responsibility and reflects that they are not "busy." Certainly, "just talking" to the patient is of questionable value to the patient's health care, but therapeutic communication is indisputably beneficial. There are times when therapeutic communication may be the only skill the nurse can offer. Situations might involve being with a client who has been told of a life-threatening diagnosis, caring for the spouse of a dying patient, or helping a patient make a difficult decision regarding treatment alternatives. In each of the above situations, the nurse does not offer advice, give solutions, or tell the patient what to do. The nurse assists the patient to problem solve, to seek personal solutions. To the griev-

Table 6–2. **Comparison of Social and Therapeutic Communication**

SOCIAL COMMUNICATION	THERAPEUTIC COMMUNICATION
Initiation	
By either person	By care-giver: nurse
Purpose	
Not clearly stated: recreation, friendship, relaxation	Goal clearly stated: improve or maintain health. Resolve or alleviate specific health problem
Obligations	
Reciprocal	Unilateral Care-giver accepts responsibility for planning and implementation
Focus	
Any topic mutually agreed upon	Health care and related topics
Termination	
May be ongoing, gradually drifting apart, or abruptly ended. May be decided by one person or mutual agreement	It is the decision of patient or client whether to accept or discontinue health care service

ing spouse, the nurse offers empathy and support through verbal and nonverbal communication.

Beginning students also indicate that they feel a sense of prying into the patient's personal life, or that "It is none of my business," when they first attempt to use therapeutic communication. But be assured that at all times the patient has the right to decline the questions of the nurse, the right to refuse to reveal any information. This right must be respected by the nurse. More frequently, however, the patient is worried and anxious, and welcomes the opportunity to express these feelings to the nurse. Often just the verbal expression of fears and problems to a concerned nurse gives relief to the patient and clarifies problems and possible solutions.

Factors Influencing the Communication Process

Several factors operate to influence either the message sent or the message received in the communication process. These factors apply to either the speaker or the receiver.

Age. The toddler has a very limited vocabulary, while the adult has many more words for expression.

Role. The expectations of each person within a relationship are set to some degree by the roles they assume. Patients are "supposed" to be in pajamas, usually in bed, and to follow the directions of the care-givers. Nurses are "supposed" to be caring, competent, kind, neat, dedicated (Lee, 1979).

Timing. The wise nursing instructor has learned not to present complex or essential information during the last class before holiday vacations. The timing is inappropriate because the students are thinking about the holiday and vacation plans with the result that the teacher's message receives little of their attention. The message of communication should relate to the the primary concern of the person at the time for maximum shared meaning to occur. If a patient is waiting to hear the report of a test result which will confirm or deny the presence of cancer, the nurse does not begin teaching a weight-reduction diet. The weight reduction is not a primary concern for this patient at this time.

Territoriality. This factor considers the questions, "On whose turf is the communication taking place?" and "Which person holds the power and makes the rules in the present situation?" The nurse who is very assertive in communication at work may be timid and reserved in a social situation. A student nurse who is the class president may speak to the class with authority, but when representing the class at a faculty meeting may choose to be more restrained in voicing opinions. Control and power frequently belong to the person operating in the familiar situation or territory.

Distance. Within each culture there are appropriate distances for various types of communication. The distance between sender-receiver reflects the type of relationship that exists between the two people. Persons involved in an intimate relationship are physically very close to each other, such as the newly engaged couple at a candlelight dinner. Business conversation is conducted at a greater distance, approximately three to four feet. A violation of these unwritten rules usually makes people uncomfortable although they would probably find it difficult to identify the source of their discomfort.

Sex. Communication can be influenced by the sex of the speaker and sender, either because they are the same sex or because they are of the opposite sex. Two women may choose to speak of very intimate topics that each woman would decline to discuss with a man. The influence of sex is changing rapidly within the culture of the United States, making it difficult to define in general terms.

Culture. Within each culture are some broad, though unspoken, directives that relate to communication. Frequently, a culture may prohibit members from discussing family problems with strangers. Another culture may prescribe that children are not to participate in the mealtime conversations of adults. Most cultures have a language of their own. The language may be English, but it may contain variations of the language or idioms that are understood only by members of the culture.

Credibility. This factor refers to the believability or reliability of the speaker or sender as evaluated by the other person. An apprehensive patient about to receive an injection from a student nurse, observing the student's obvious stress, asked, "Is this the first time you've done this?" To which the student smoothly replied, "Oh my, no." The patient visibly relaxed, probably because the credibility of the student had increased for the patient. (The student neglected to say that the only other injection she had given was to a mannequin in the nursing laboratory.)

Defensiveness. In an attempt to deal with fear, anxiety, or another unpleasant aspect of a situation, the individual may assume a role of justifying personal beliefs or behavior. This stance effectively cuts off interpersonal communication. A nursing instructor may be very disappointed in the class results of a nursing examination. "I lectured on that topic for three hours; I gave very clear examples; I helped the students to see it in the hospital; the students really didn't study or read the references." This defensive stance cuts off further discussion and problem solving which might lead to identification of the problems related to inadequate learning.

Affect. The mood or general feeling tone that one individual conveys to another influences communication. This is communicated primarily through nonverbal means. Flowers delivered on a birthday may demonstrate affection and promote tender, intimate communication. Yawning and frequent shifting in a chair may indicate boredom and an attempt to "turn off" the speaker.

Attitudes. The tendency to respond in a certain way is the influence of attitudes. They are demonstrated most clearly in our nonverbal behavior. They indicate our acceptance or rejection of others. Attitudes can either hinder or enhance communication. Often we hear a person described as having a negative attitude. This tends to inhibit communication because that individual is not willing to listen and attempt carefully to understand some messages.

Attitudes that Enhance Communication

Caring

Caring is the attitude that tells the patient, "It matters to me what happens to you!" Often patients are well satisfied with the technical aspects of their care, for most patients do not understand machines, surgical procedures, or complex treatments. Nurses are more likely to hear complaints based on interpersonal skills: "Nobody seemed to care that my breakfast was late and I was hungry," or "They were all too busy to listen," or "Nobody had time to answer my questions." The nurse who projects an attitude of caring is not likely to receive these evaluations. However, genuinely caring about patients carries a certain amount of risk for the nurse. This nurse will also grieve when a patient dies or is told of a life-threatening diagnosis. The nurse who is consistently willing to empathize with patients and accept the possibility of this pain risks burnout. The ability to care and to give may be exhausted. But the nurse also may achieve great personal growth and satisfaction from such experiences.

Acceptance

Acceptance has been referred to as a type of discerning, pardoning process. The nurse recognizes undesirable characteristics of the patient but bases a relationship with the patient on the positive characteristics. A neutral tolerance toward the negative aspects is displayed by the nurse. The first stage of acceptance is intellectual. The nurse acknowledges the humanity of the patient and accepts the individual because of a commitment to the code of ethics of the nursing profession. In the second stage, the nurse deliberately and willingly makes the commitment to care for the patient while being fully aware of the negative aspects of that individual's personality. Practicing this attitude is demanding of nurses. It requires that nurses avoid moralizing and that they suspend judgments about the patient's behavior.

Objectivity

Objectivity is the use of the scientific problem-solving process in nursing: collect information, identify the problem, define solutions, implement solutions, evaluate results. The demonstration of this attitude does not imply that the nurse is cold or unfeeling. It does say that the nurse proceeds methodically and knowledgeably.

Commitment

Commitment is the act of solemnly promising to do something to the best of one's ability. In this case, the nurse has pledged to the patient the provision of the best nursing care possible. This attitude is demonstrated by the skill with which the nurse cares for the patient.

Attitudes that Hinder Communication

Superiority

Superiority conveys to the patient that the nurse is more knowlegeable, more competent to judge what is best, and thus is in a position of power. Loosely translated this means, ''And you'd better do what I say without question.'' This attitude does not encourage the patient to ask questions, to participate in the planning of care, or to make decisions.

Extreme Rigidity

Extreme rigidity refers to an excessive degree of regimentation and precision in adhering to hospital routine. The nurse who admits the patient following an inflexible steps 1 through 7 sequence, ignoring the fact that the patient is in obvious pain, is being unnecessarily rigid. The patient in pain is neither willing nor able to communicate effectively. The admission procedure could be completed more effectively after the patient is made more comfortable. The extremely rigid attitude is most often found in inexperienced nurses who have difficulty setting priorities and acting on their own best judgments.

Flexibility requires modification to meet the needs of a particular situation.

Inattention

The nurse who does not focus on what the patient is saying may forget important information which should be added to the patient's record. This attitude clearly conveys to the patient that other more significant things are on the nurse's mind.

Stereotyping

Stereotyping sets expectations for all members of a group to act in a certain way. Difficulty results when an individual does not act in the anticipated manner. When a nurse is admitted to the hospital as a patient, other nurses often feel there is no need to explain tests or procedures because the nurse-patient ''knows it all anyway.'' This nurse-patient is not free to ask questions or express the fears experienced by other patients. Similar situations happen whenever a person is treated as a member of a group rather than as a unique individual.

Effect of Illness on Communication

When a person becomes ill, many additional factors operate that influence the ability to communicate. Anxiety is probably the most common experience of hospitalized patients, yet it is the feeling most individualized when demonstrated in behavior. Some individuals become very irritable when they are anxious. They are critical of the nursing staff, the food isn't right, and the room is not satisfactory. Another individual who is experiencing anxiety may be very jovial, telling many jokes and laughing frequently in an unsuccessful attempt to deal with the anxiety and avoid the real problem. Other persons may be unable to make any decisions, such as coffee or tea for a beverage at mealtime, which nightgown to wear, or whether they would like to order a television set. Most anxious people also show a decreased ability to concentrate and comprehend instructions.

Pain also affects one's ability to communicate, both as a sender and as a receiver. The person who is in pain may not perceive auditory input, perhaps because the pain is occupying conscious perception or because of an attempt to block all sensory input. The medications a

patient in pain receives may also depress sensory awareness and cognitive function. Medication may enable the patient to sleep or rest, eliminating effective communication.

Illness may produce *egocentrism*, that is, a self-centered individual. While in the patient role, the person may be able to think only about personal concerns and needs. Communication focuses almost entirely on self. This self-indulgence has the effect of discouraging relationships and communication with other people. The person is not pleasant to be with and people may choose to ignore such an individual. Egocentrism in a person who has not shown the trait before illness is usually a temporary situation which is resolved when anxiety is lessened.

Illness may also produce depression which causes the patient to withdraw from human contact. Because this patient makes almost no demands on the staff, the depressed individual is more likely to be ignored or neglected when, in fact, a very acute need for human contact exists.

Another response to illness is anger. The patient is

angry at having life interrupted and often wants to know "Why me?" The person who has always enjoyed good health and has an image of self as strong and physically fit may see illness as an intolerable threat to self-concept. This patient may be extremely demanding and may even verbally abuse the nursing staff with comments like, "I bet you're out having coffee while I'm lying here and can't even go to the bathroom alone. Just like a baby!" This patient is lashing out and expressing anger in communication. Certainly this behavior does not endear the patient to the nursing staff, and there is a tendency to avoid this patient who, again, really needs nursing care to deal with problems.

One approach that has helped nurses to empathize, that is, to share the other's feelings, is to consider the usual sequence of events when a "person" becomes a "patient" in a hospital. If the admission has been scheduled and is not an emergency, the would-be patient is told what time to report to the hospital. This is likely the same time that all other persons scheduled for admission that day are to report. This results in the "hurry up and wait game" common to hospitals. After filling out several forms and completing financial arrangements in an often less-than-private semipartitioned cubicle, the patient is tagged with an identification wrist bracelet and given directions to x-ray for the mandatory and unsolicited chest x-ray. When and if the patient finds the location of x-ray, instructions are given on how much to disrobe and where to report. These instructions usually consist of four sentences devoid of commas, periods, expression, or eye contact! "Please take off all clothing above the waist . . . put on this gown . . . tie it in back and sit down on the brown chair when you are ready someone will call for you." (The brown chair is cold plastic.) After the x-ray is completed, the patient is told to wait to be sure that it is not necessary to repeat the x-ray. The patient is given similar instructions to get to the laboratory for a blood test, where the wait is amidst the display of urine, stool, and blood samples. After the blood is taken, the patient is given directions to an assigned room (not of the type requested) or alternately told to wait until a volunteer escort comes to show the way. Once at the hospital room, the patient is greeted by the head nurse who explains that after the change of shift someone will be in to complete the admission procedure but to go ahead and get into pajamas and get into bed. (Why?) By the time the nurse has completed the admission interview and physical examination, it is too late to order a regular supper menu, and the patient is given a light snack from the floor kitchen: Jell-O (what else?), chicken broth, crackers, canned fruit, and semimelted ice cream. After visiting hours end at 8 P.M., there begins a procession of medical students, interns, and residents, all asking approximately the same questions, poking, probing, and telling the patient that "Your own doctor will have to answer that question." The student nurse who will care for the patient the following day also stops by to meet the patient and "gather data." The patient angrily asks the student to leave. Those who have experienced "patienthood" readily understand the above sequence of events and the resulting feelings. Nurses who are skilled communicators can assist the patient to identify the cause of these feelings and perhaps lessen the effects.

Therapeutic Communication

More than 70 percent of the working day of the professional nurse is spent in communication-related activities which include teaching, interviewing, charting, writing referrals, taking nursing histories, group problem solving, and individual or family health counseling. Although most adults communicate effectively enough to satisfy their needs, the professional nurse can gain added skill in communications in order to provide nursing services to patients as effectively as possible. There are techniques the nurse can use to promote therapeutic communication. Conversely, there are common, readily identifiable responses that have the effect of cutting off nurse-patient communication. The nurse can learn both the positive and the negative techniques in order to maximize personal skill.

When beginning to study and practice communica-tion techniques, students frequently complain that their conversation becomes unnatural and stilted, that they feel they are being artificial with patients. These are the honest feelings of students and must be recognized and accepted as a starting point. It may be helpful for the student to remember other skills that were difficult when learned and now seem effortless. These might include cursive handwriting, counting by threes or fives, driving a car, or using a computer. With sufficient practice, the nursing skills of communication, changing a surgical dressing, or giving an injection will seem just as effortless. Moreover, the student who initially loudly doubts the necessity or value of communication techniques frequently reports to the instructor, "It works!" The student has experienced the satisfaction of participating in effective therapeutic communication.

Skills that Facilitate Communication

The following behaviors and responses are communication skills that the nurse uses in therapeutic communication.

Active Listening

To hear is only one part of listening. Hearing is the sensory process of sound waves reaching the ears and being transmitted to the brain. To listen is to attach meaning and interpretation to the perception of sound. *Active listening* is a high-level skill whereby the nurse consciously focuses on the patient whose interests and needs are primary. Active listening demands time and attention. The nurse may be unable to sit and talk to the patient during the middle of administering medications to several patients, but may say, "I'd like to be able to understand this problem better. As soon as I finish passing medications, I will return and have time to talk uninterrupted." The nurse has indicated an interest in what the patient has said, as well as conveyed the idea that the patient is important. When the nurse returns to the patient, it is helpful to structure both the physical and interpersonal environment so it is conducive to active listening. The nurse provides for privacy, perhaps by shutting the door to the room, by walking with the patient to a vacant lounge area, or at least by pulling the curtains between roommates. The nurse may pull a chair up to the bedside of the patient, thus making it easier to maintain eye contact with the patient or making it possible to touch the patient.

The nurse also provides for the comfort of the patient. Offering a cup of coffee or a glass of juice or repositioning the patient more comfortably may increase the patient's comfort and confidence in the nurse as a caring person. If the nurse is taking notes for the medical record, this must be explained to the patient. "This is important information for your record, and I want the dates to be accurate. Do you mind if I take a few notes?" is one approach the nurse may use. Patients are not offended by this approach but seem to feel that the nurse is taking seriously what they have to say. The nurse who takes notes must do so in such a way that it is not a major distraction from the patient's communication. It is helpful if the nurse reviews the notes with the patient at the end of the session as another means of showing attention. Saying something like, "Now to review, in January you had the pain on your left side, but it subsided when you menstruated. By the first week of February, it started again and remained constant until you saw your doctor in March. The pain was first relieved by rest and two aspirin tablets, but that no longer works. Is that accurate?"

Active listening takes energy! It is not a relaxing time or a break for the nurse. It is a demanding process that requires the nurse utilize an extensive knowledge base. Early in their education, nursing students frequently have difficulty "just talking" to patients. They report to faculty that they "feel useless" because they aren't "doing anything" for the patient. Therapeutic communication, of which active listening is a major part, is a most important aspect of nursing. Through communication the nurse establishes the therapeutic relationship, relieves stress, does patient teaching, and identifies health care needs. It may be initially more satisfying for the student to take blood pressures and temperatures for these are skills easily mastered and the nurse feels competent. Active listening is more difficult to master but is a prerequisite to learning all the other communication skills. One must first listen before one can respond appropriately and safely.

Reflection

When using reflection, the nurse attempts to mirror back the patient's feelings, thoughts, or statements. The nurse uses the patient's exact words. The purpose of this technique is to assist patients to view their own statements and then to proceed with further exploration and development of those statements. For example,

Patient: I wonder how long it will be before the doctor will permit me to return to work?
Nurse: You're wondering about returning to work?
Patient: Yes, there are lots of bills and I'm not sure how long my insurance will last. I can't afford much more of this.

In this case the patient has expressed some fears in response to the use of reflection by the nurse. The nurse may now be able to identify some resources that might be helpful to the patient.

Another example:

Patient: It took you fifteen minutes to get here with my medicine. I can't understand why a simple request takes so long! It makes me angry to have to wait.
Nurse: You're feeling angry? [while approaching the bed and maintaining eye contact].

Patient: Oh, I guess I'm more scared of this surgery than I like to admit, and it comes out sounding angry.

Again the nurse in this situation has identified a patient problem that requires nursing intervention. It is important that the nurse's nonverbal behavior enhance the verbal reflection made to the patient. By maintaining eye contact, touching the patient, by sitting down, by approaching the patient, the nurse enhances the verbal response.

There is a danger of overuse of this technique, at which point the patient is likely to shout, "That's what I said! Can't you hear?" But skillfully and compassionately used, the technique aids communication.

Open-Ended Questions

Open-ended questions are used by the nurse to enable the patient to have the freedom of response, or to gather additional data. They are questions that are not answered by a yes-no response. The patient may choose to respond at length, selecting the direction of conversation without leads from the nurse. Some examples of this response are:

Nurse: What brought you to the hospital?
What questions do you have?
Can you tell me more about your illness?
How has this affected your life?

This type of response clearly conveys the willingness of the nurse to listen. It is often used to help establish a therapeutic focus early in the nurse-patient relationship.

Clarification

By using clarification, the nurse seeks to clear up any statements or facts from the patient that are not fully understood. Often clarification techniques are helpful when there is a conflict between the verbal and nonverbal messages sent by the patient. In such a case, the nurse might say, "You said you were not in pain, but I noticed that you grimaced when I asked you to turn over." These techniques have the additional benefit of clearly demonstrating to the patient that the nurse is really listening and cares enough to seek an accurate interpretation. The nurse makes no assumptions but makes the maximum effort to understand the patient's point of view. The nurse may make such statements as:

I'm not sure that I understand . . .
I'm unclear about . . .
Could you tell me that again please?

Other specific examples of clarifying responses are:

1. *Sequencing.* The nurse asks the patient to put the events in the order in which they occurred.

Nurse: I'm confused as to the order in which these symptoms occurred. Can you tell me what happened first . . . and what happened next?

2. *Repeating.* The nurse asks the patient to repeat a statement that was unclear.

Nurse: I'm not sure I understand how you manage to do this treatment at home. Can you tell me that again? ·

3. *Comparing.* The nurse asks the patient to compare a symptom or feeling to something previously experienced or generally known.

Nurse: Was this the same pain you experienced when you had your first heart attack?

Can you compare how this medication makes you feel to how you felt when you took the codeine?

Does this brace give you more or less support than the other model?

4. *Using Examples.* The nurse asks the patient to describe something using specific illustrations.

Nurse: Mrs. Jones, you said that activity seemed to make the pain worse. Can you give me a couple of specific things you do that you notice make the pain worse?

Can you tell me what foods seem to relieve the burning in your stomach?

5. *Estimating Measurement.* The nurse asks the patient to approximate amounts in order to avoid general terms such as "a lot," "a great deal," or "very little."

Nurse: Mrs. Jones, you said you have had vaginal spotting for three days. Was this the size of a quarter, did it stain a small sanitary napkin?

Jennifer, you said you feel thirsty all the time and are drinking a lot of water. Does this mean a glass of water twice a day or about how much?

6. *Paraphrasing.* The nurse restates the meaning of the patient's statement.

Nurse: You say that when he has a temper tantrum, he lies down, kicks the floor, and screams?

When you have severe pain, you are flat in bed and unable to move?

7. *Validating.* The nurse asks the patient to approve the accuracy of an interpretation.

Nurse: Do I understand the situation correctly when I say that you find it easier to breathe while sitting up in a straight-back chair but have extreme difficulty if you lie down in bed?

Is this right? You've been unable to work for the past six months, but for a year before that you had a very difficult time working eight hours without tiring?

Summarizing

The nurse may briefly restate the feelings and content of a particular conversation with the patient. While this may be used as another tool to clarify content, it is also used to conclude an interaction or as a progress review. The nurse might summarize an admission interview as follows: "Thank you, Mrs. Jones, for answering all my questions. Now to review briefly, I understand that you are here for a series of x-rays to determine if you need gallbladder surgery. You are in no pain now, but you do understand that I can give you a medication if the pain recurs. The blood test and urine samples have gone to the lab already. Your doctor will see you yet this evening. You understand about no food or water after midnight. Your test is scheduled for 8 A.M. in the morning. I will be here until 11 P.M. May I get you anything or answer any other questions now?" The nurse has concluded the summary with a final opportunity for the patient to ask questions or make requests.

Silence

The use of silence as a communication tool can either enhance or hinder the interaction. Certainly, there must be enough silence in the conversation for the patient to speak and formulate thoughts and questions. The nurse who is ill at ease may attempt to fill every void in the conversation with "small talk," often to the irritation of the patient. At other times, silence can be extremely comfortable and comforting. If the patient has just been told of the death of her infant child, the nurse may say, "I'll stay with you awhile"' and sit in silence with the patient holding her hand. This silence is probably more appropriate than words. At still another time, there may be long, awkward silences in the conversation. The patient may not wish to talk with the nurse and may wish to be left alone. This is the patient's right and must be respected. The nurse may ask the patient, "Would you like to be alone for awhile?" The nurse

may then determine what to do from the patient's response.

Responding to Inappropriate Communication

Occasionally, the nurse will need to deal with inappropriate conversation. What constitutes "inappropriate" is highly individualized. What is acceptable to one person may be highly offensive to another individual. The following statements are examples of inappropriate communication:

Patient to Nurse: That nurse I had yesterday did a rotten job, just didn't seem to care if anything hurt me. That nurse was actually mean. You seem to really care about the patient.

Nurse to Co-worker: That man is impossible. He complains about everything I do for him and even talks about the other nurses. Do you know what he said about Mrs. Jackson?

Male Patient to Female Nurse: You really are good-looking. I'd sure like to get to know you a lot better.

Female Patient to Male Nurse: So what is a bright, handsome young man like you doing in nursing?

Two general principles can be used in dealing with inappropriate conversation:

1. Politely decline to participate
2. Accompany the verbal response with appropriate nonverbal behavior (Gazda, 1982)

Although declining to participate is difficult, it does prevent hurting innocent parties. It also models appropriate communication behavior. Gazda suggests that, in declining, the nurse be brief and direct. Eye contact is maintained, and a calm tone of voice is used. Neither smiles nor punitive facial expressions accompany a declining statement. After the statement is made, the individual shifts the conversation to an appropriate topic. This is another opportunity to model appropriate communication behavior. Examples of declining responses to the previous statements are:

Nurse: I'm glad if I can make you comfortable. Are you having any pain now?

Nurse to Co-worker: I'm not really concerned with what was said about Mrs. Jackson. By the way, will you be free for coffee in a half hour? I'd really like to hear about the workshop you went to yesterday.

Female Nurse to Male Patient: Thank you for the compliment, Mr. Jones but I am not interested. Now, would you like to shower before your physical therapy appointment at 9:30?

Male Nurse to Female Patient: I've chosen nursing because it is a challenging career. Now, Mrs. Smith, I'd like to check your surgical dressings. Have you had any pain today?

In each of these situations, the nurse responds to the communication without participating in it and without assuming a punitive attitude.

Responses that Hinder Communication

The nurse can make verbal as well as nonverbal responses that discourage communication. Nonverbal responses include a lack of eye contact, very hurried gestures, arms folded or hands placed on hips, standing with back to patient, and foot tapping. Any one of the above gestures would probably discourage a patient from talking to the nurse. The nurse sent a very clear message that now is not the time for talking. Verbal responses that affect communication include false reassurance, judgmental responses, changing the subject, negating or belittling feelings, "a la moding," closed questions, and leading questions.

False Reassurance

False reassurance is a statement of comfort, encouragement, or placation given by the nurse in an attempt to help the patient in a stressful or anxiety-producing situation. The nurse, in many cases, does not know if the statement is true or not. Frequently, the patient responds with silence or an angry retort to such comments. Some examples are the following nurse responses:

I know just how you feel.

I'm sure that everything will be all right.

Dr. Smith is an excellent doctor. Everything will be just fine.

Judgmental Responses

The nurse also hinders communication when offering a judgment or evaluation of the patient or the patient's communication. Examples of such nurse responses are:

I don't think that's a very wise decision. You really ought to give it more thought.

Taking that much medication was really a bad mistake. How could you make that big an error?

Your mother really needs you to take care of her now. She's such a lovely person, I can't understand why you don't want her in your home.

Changing the Subject

Nurses may change the subject when the patient initiates a legitimate topic that the nurse is uncomfortable discussing, does not know the answer, or that may be emotionally charged. This response tells the patient very clearly that the nurse is unwilling to discuss this topic and "don't ask again." It has the effect of treating the patient as a punished child. Some examples of this are:

Patient: I'm getting worse every day. I think that I will die soon.

Nurse: Now don't talk like that. Would you like your bath now? And then I'll get you up in the chair.

Patient: I have been having lots of pain lately during intercourse. I wonder if that's normal after a hysterectomy?

Nurse: You'll have to talk to your physician about that. How did you sleep last night?

Negating Feelings

The nurse may belittle or negate the patient's feelings, however unintentionally, in an attempt to give the patient hope or to help a depressed patient. Unfortunately, the most frequent result is that the patient no longer attempts to express feelings and does not receive the needed help. Some examples of this are:

Patient: I'm so discouraged. I don't think I'll ever be able to walk again.

Nurse: You shouldn't feel like that, Mrs. Jones. You are improving a bit each day.

Patient: If only I wouldn't have insisted on going to the party, the accident would never have happened. I feel so guilty.

Nurse: It was an accident. You have nothing to feel guilty about.

A la Moding

When the nurse asks several questions in a sequence without waiting for a response, the communication is called "a la moding." The nurse is topping question with question, not unlike topping pie with ice cream. The patient is confused and, not knowing which question to answer first, frequently does not respond or does so only in a token manner. Some examples of this are:

Nurse: Mr. Jones, are you having any pain now? Are you able to walk to the bathroom, or would you like some assistance? Have you completed your breakfast menu yet?

Nurse: Mr. Smith, I don't understand what kind of foods seem to help or hurt your stomach? Does fruit help? What about foods like ice cream or milk? Do cooked or raw vegetables seem to make a difference?

Closed Questions

Closed questions require only a "yes" or "no" answer or some similar brief response. They may be useful at times but usually require additional clarification and elaboration. Some examples of this are:

Nurse: Do you have pain? [Requires clarification. What kind of pain? Where? For how long?]

Nurse: Do you understand what will happen in surgery tomorrow? [A better question is "What do you understand about your surgery tomorrow?"]

Leading Questions

Leading questions tend to direct the patient's response and put the patient's response into the words of the nurse. The nurse may ask questions that lead to a particular diagnosis. Consider the following:

Nurse: When your chest started hurting, did the pain radiate into your shoulder and down your left arm? [This question could better be asked, "Can you describe all the places where the pain was felt?"]

Nurse: Have you noticed that you're always hungry and thirsty? [The nurse could better ask the question, "Have you noticed any change in your eating or drinking habits?"]

Summary

Communication is another nursing skill that must be studied and practiced if the nurse is to become proficient. It is essential because therapeutic conversation is the basis of the nurse–patient relationship. Therapeutic communication is the deliberate communication the nurse uses to identify and meet health care problems.

Skills that enhance communication are active listening, reflection, open-ended questions, clarification, summary, and silence. Responses that hinder communication are false reassurance, judgmental responses, changing the subject, negating feelings, a la moding, closed questions, and leading questions.

Terms for Review

active listening
affect
a la moding
clarification
closed questions
communication
credibility

defensiveness
egocentrism
interpersonal communication
intrapersonal communication
leading question
negating feelings
nonverbal communication

open ended question
paraphrasing
reflection
territoriality
therapeutic communication
validating

Self-Assessment

Write a brief response to each of the following statements. Identify the communication skill you used.

1. Friend: So what's it like being a nurse? I bet you really know some juicy stories.
2. Friend: You never have time for me since you started nursing. You're always studying.
3. Friend: You're a nurse so maybe you can help me. I think I'm pregnant and . . .
4. Patient: This is really hard. I don't think I can stand another day here.
5. Patient: Dr. Jones doesn't listen to me. I'm really getting angry. What would you do if you were in my shoes?
6. Patient: I'm so scared. So what if the biopsy report is cancer?
7. Patient: I really feel fine. I don't know why I'm here.
8. Patient: I have to follow the diabetic diet while I'm in the hospital, it's all I get to eat. But when I get home, it's back to normal.
9. Patient: My hot food is cold and my ice cream is melted before I even begin. Then you wonder why patients don't eat.
10. Patient: I had my light on for ten minutes to ask for a pain medication and no one answered it. Nurses here just don't care at all.

Learning Activities

In the nursing laboratory, videotape the following role play. The first student assumes the role of a patient admitted to the hospital for observation and possible gallbladder surgery. The second student is to role play the nurse assigned to care for the patient. The nurse is meeting the patient for the first time and will spend five to ten minutes talking with the patient in order to gather information which will help to plan nursing care. View the videotape and answer the following questions:

1. Identify verbal communication skills that the nurse used to facilitate communication.
2. Identify verbal responses that hindered communication.
3. Identify nonverbal behavior that facilitated communication.
4. Identify nonverbal behavior that hindered communication.
5. Ask the nurse about the feelings experienced during the interview.
6. Ask the patient what things the nurse did that felt helpful or comfortable. What things did the patient wish the nurse had done?

Review Questions

1. Which of the following describe therapeutic communication?
   a. Mutuality, trust, confidentiality, privacy
   b. Patient initiated, problem solving, evaluation
   c. Nurse initiated, goal centered, patient focused, deliberate
2. Which of the following are all examples of nonverbal communication?
   a. Singing, dancing, playing guitar
   b. Shaking hands, eye contact, smiling
   c. Complaining, whispering, grimacing
3. Patient: I'm afraid of having surgery in the morning. Which response of the nurse uses reflection?
   a. You have an excellent doctor.
   b. Are you afraid of dying?
   c. You're afraid of surgery?
4. Patient: I'm not sure how I'll handle all this. Which response of the nurse uses a clarification technique?
   a. Handle all this?
   b. I don't understand what it is you're concerned about being able to handle.
   c. Well, can you ask your sister to help out?
5. You are meeting a patient for the first time. You introduce yourself and state that your purpose is to complete the admission procedure. Which of the following is the most appropriate beginning statement?
   a. Can you tell me what brought you to the hospital?
   b. Are you in pain now?
   c. Do you know if you are having tests in the morning?
6. The primary communication skill is
   a. Clarification
   b. Active listening
   c. Summarizing
   d. Reflection

Answers

1. c
2. b
3. c
4. b
5. a
6. b

Suggested Readings

Diaz-Duque, O.: Overcoming the language barrier: Advice from an interpreter." *Am. J. Nurs.* **82:**1380–82, 1982. A medical interpreter discusses some problems related to interpreting. He offers suggestions how nurses can successfully work with interpreters.

Goodykoontz, Lynne: Touch: Attitudes and practice. *Nurs. Forum,* **18**:4–17, 1979. A nurse discusses procedural and nonprocedural touch, the human being's need for touch, touch throughout the life cycle, including death.

Grasska, M. and **McFarland, Teresa:** Overcoming the language barrier: Problems and solutions. *Am. J. Nurs.* **82**:1376–79, 1982. Two English-speaking nurses who work with many patients who do not speak English describe communication problems and solutions.

Waddell, E.: Quality touching to communicate caring. *Nurs. Forum,* **18**:288–92, 1979. A student describes the use of touch with three patients.

References and Bibliography

Borden, G.; Gregg, R.; and Grove, T.: *Speech Behavior and Human Interaction.* Prentice-Hall, Englewood Cliffs, N.J. 1969.

Condon, J.: *Semantics and Communication.* Macmillan, New York, 1966.

DeVillers, L.: What to do when you just can't communicate. *Nurs. Life,* **2**:36–39, 1982.

Edwards, B. and Brilhart, J.: *Communication in Nursing Practice.* Mosby, St. Louis, 1981.

Gazda, G.; Childers, W.; and Walters, W.: *Interpersonal Communication. A Handbook for Health Professionals.* Aspen Systems, Rockville, Md., 1982.

Hein, E. C.: *Communication in Nursing Practice,* 2nd ed. Little, Brown, Boston, 1980.

Lee, A.: How nurses rate with the public. *RN,* **42**:25–39, 1979.

Muldary, T.: *Interpersonal Relations for Health Professionals.* Macmillan, New York, 1983.

Travelbee, J.: *Interpersonal Aspects of Nursing.* Davis, Philadelphia, 1966.

GROUP COMMUNICATION

Objectives

1. Discuss the importance of group communication skills for nurses.
2. Define what is meant by a group and describe several types of groups.
3. List several advantages of the use of groups that are not found in a two-person relationship.
4. Contrast content and process issues within a group.
5. Describe group tasks during each phase of group development: initiation phase, working phase, termination phase.
6. Describe roles group members may assume related to each of the following: task functions, group maintenance functions, self-interest.
7. Define each of the four major leadership styles and give an example of when its use is appropriate.
8. Describe three methods of decision making and give an example of when the use of each is appropriate.
9. Describe what is meant by "groupthink" as an effect of high cohesiveness in groups.
10. Explain two approaches to group assessment.

Importance of Group Communication Skills

The noted statement of John Donne, "No man is an island entire of itself," is especially appropriate when applied to nursing. No single nurse can provide everything that the patient in a health care setting needs. Nurses work with other professionals and auxiliary workers on the health team to provide the best care possible for each patient. The nurse also works with a group of nurse colleagues. The ability to communicate effectively as a group member or a group leader not only directly affects patient care but probably is related to the job satisfaction of the individual nurse and to the morale of the group. In addition, the nurse communicates with groups of patients. The patient group may be the four to six patients the nurse is assigned that day, or it may be a more formal group, such as a diet therapy group, which the nurse is teaching. In each of these situations, the nurse is more effective if specialized group communication skills can be used.

What Is a Group?

Most authors agree that a *group* is any three or more interdependent persons who share a common goal of which they are all aware. The level of interdependence varies from a high to a minimal amount. A highly dependent group is the operating room team of surgeons, nurses, anesthetists, and technicians who each depend on one another to provide necessary and complementary skills. In contrast is a group of nursing students who are only minimally dependent on each other for successful goal achievement.

Reviewing this definition, one sees that human beings have multiple group memberships. A student nurse may belong to the PTA, the National Student Nurses' Association, Civic Music, a political caucus, a study group of classmates, and a local soccer team. Membership in a group may be achieved, that is, one may work to meet membership requirements, as in the case of a sport team. Membership may be ascribed or assigned, as in the case of a required membership as a condition of employment. Membership may also be voluntary, as in a social group.

Group dynamics is the term given to the study of group function—the way human beings live, work, and play in groups. This includes both content and process issues. Content refers to "what" group members say, while process refers to "how" group members say it. A study of group process focuses on the relationships between the members and how they affect the work of the group.

The main function of any group is to achieve the goal or the purposes for which it was formed. In order to meet this objective, the group must also develop relationships and structures that support goal accomplishment. If member relationships are characterized by a high degree of trust and support, members are free to be creative and take risks without fear of put-downs and personal attack. The group must also agree upon structures that facilitate group work. These may include such things as recording minutes, establishing vote-taking procedures, setting an agenda, and setting policy. All of these structural tasks are not required by every type of group. A nursing staff problem-solving group has a different structure than a patient support group. Each group develops a unique structure to meet its own needs.

Why Use Groups?

There are advantages to using groups that cannot be achieved in a two-person relationship. Perhaps the most obvious advantage is economy. One nurse can teach a group of children about nutrition for the same cost as teaching a single child. It has also been said that groups are a microcosm of human interaction. By studying the individual's behavior within a small group, one can observe how the individual typically relates to persons outside the group experience. Another advantage of groups is the sheer number of persons in the group. If brainstorming or creativity is a value of the group, the varied contributions of several persons are assets. Another advantage is that group members can give peer support such as in weight-reduction groups or study groups. Another potential benefit of group work is the possible cooperation, as opposed to competition, that may be achieved. If the feeling of "we did it" as opposed to "I did it" is present within a group, significantly greater achievement may be accomplished. Consider the soccer team with a star player who refuses to pass the ball but seeks to retain all scoring power. This "one-person team" is rarely as successful as a true team where each player focuses on team play regardless of who scores the goals. The principle of cooperation is equally appropriate to health team members who value achievement of group goals more than personal recognition.

Types of Groups

Most groups are classified by the function they serve for their members. Support groups within the hospital setting provide understanding and hope to patients. An example of such a group is the "I Can Cope" program for cancer patients and their families. Social groups focus on recreational interests, like horseback riding or music, and offer companionship to members. Task groups are organized to carry out a particular function and usually disband once the function is completed. A committee assigned to plan a class party for graduation is a task group. A committee is a specific kind of task group in that it has been given an assignment by a larger organization. Therapeutic groups are organized around a problem common to the members with the goal of group treatment. Examples of therapeutic groups are psychotherapy groups and Alcoholics Anonymous. Personal growth groups offer members the opportunity to expand their human potential through relationships with and feedback from other group members. Consciousness-raising groups, encounter groups, and sensitivity groups are examples of this type. Learning groups are formed around a very specific need. Student nurses may form a group to provide tutoring and joint study for biochemistry. When the need is met, in this case when the biochemistry course is completed, the group may disband. Finally, another large classification of groups is called *primary groups*. These are the basic, face-to-face, small groups in which people transmit and receive values, form and develop self-concepts, and meet needs for love and security. For most individuals, the traditional nuclear family consisting of one generation of parents and children is the most significant primary group. The definition of family currently is being expanded to include many alternatives. The residents of a nursing home, a small group in a college dormitory, several individuals who have worked closely together for a number of years are all possible definitions of alternative families who make up primary groups. When providing care, nurses plan to include members of alternative families, just as they include members of traditional families.

Stages in Group Formation

When several individuals come together with the intent of becoming a group for a specific purpose, there are predictable phases with predictable tasks through which the group progresses. These are similar to the phases and tasks encountered in a relationship with an individual.

The Initiation Phase

The first stage is called initiation. During the initiation phase, both the physical and the psychosocial climates are established for the group. The *physical climate* refers to the meeting place of the group with the chairs, tables, couches, seating arrangements, heat, and light. These factors directly affect the ability of the group to function. For example, if ten chairs are arranged in two lines of five, communication is hindered, whereas, a circular arrangement of ten chairs facilitates communication. An extremely warm room is likely to put group members to sleep, while an extremely cool room may make for a very short meeting.

Next, the group focuses on establishing the *psychosocial climate* which consists of the relationships, feelings, and interaction styles among members. The establishment of social relationships in this culture begins with introductions and frequently some comment on how the individual wishes to be addressed. At the first meeting of a nursing seminar, the faculty member may request that first names be used. Frequently, this formal introduction is followed by "social chitchat," which might include such things as questions related to family, personal life, social, or recreational interests. This communication is an attempt, usually unconscious, to discover similarities and begin to build a group acceptance or cohesiveness. People usually feel more comfortable and more willing to share when they perceive that they have some things in common with other group members. Thus, this task is important to the future functioning of the group.

During this first phase of group formation, a leader emerges, is recognized, or is selected. If the nurse is teaching a group of diabetic patients, the nurse is recognized as the leader of the group. When several students are assigned to complete a group project, one student usually begins the task with a comment like, "All right, how should we begin this project?" and the leadership begins. Finally, another group of students may begin by nominating an individual for the leadership function, thus, a leader is selected. Frequently, a group may attempt to be a "leaderless group," preferring more of a peer group style. This is rarely possible. Close observation would reveal that, although an individual lacks the title, someone has assumed the leadership function. Another alternative is that the leadership function may rotate within the group from meeting to meeting or task to task, depending on the skills of the individual. By whatever method the leadership function is delegated, the leader has an important role during group formation.

During this phase, the group is working on establishing *norms*, which are the rules or standards of behavior for the group. These norms may include such things as not monopolizing the conversation, respecting confidentiality, building trust, attendance at meetings, and handling irrelevant conversation. Some of these norms will be defined in very clear, overt language: "OK. Are we agreed that if anyone misses two meetings without a serious reason, we will select another member as a replacement?" At other times, the norming is more subtle, although equally binding. The leader may respond to a member who, during a support group, has revealed very personal information, "I'm glad that you feel you could tell us something that means so much to you." The leader is setting a norm that gives approval and permission to share personal information. The leader may also set norms against behavior that hinders group work. The leader may say to the person who is using group time for concerns that are irrelevant to the group, "Those are interesting comments, but can we stick to the topic at hand today? Our time together is very limited." Not only does the leader establish norms, but all the group members participate in the process, either by expressing approval or disapproval or by proposing additional or alternative norms. The leader needs to anticipate the effect that such norms will have on group members as well as on the group goal. If, for example, group norms are so rigid as to remove fun and spontaneity from a volunteer committee, the group is likely to disband and the group goal will not be achieved.

The Working Phase

This is the period of time during which the members work on group goals. Members are now clear about the expectations of the group and are willing to cooperate with other members in anticipation of achieving a goal that could not be accomplished individually. Members are either assigned various tasks or volunteer for them. During this phase, subgroups may form that have the potential to facilitate or hinder the group effort. If, for example, a subgroup is especially dissatisfied with the progress of the group, with relationships within the group, or with the leadership style, the efforts of the group can be seriously hampered. Subgroups can also have the effect of facilitating the work of the group. One subgroup may have been very successful in the assigned task and may be able to use this success to motivate a faltering group.

Depending on the type of group, the members will divide their time between content and process topics. *Content* topics deal with the substance or the subject matter of what is said. *Process* topics deal with the manner in which things are discussed, on the relationships between members. Task groups, such as the example of a committee planning a class graduation party, are likely to spend most of their time on content issues. This might include where the party will be held, refreshments, cost, and clean-up. A psychotherapy group would spend the majority of its time on process issues, such as how a member felt when trying out a new assertive behavior, or how did another member feel after a second member had monopolized the entire meeting with a long irrelevant monologue. Each group will have some discussion of both kinds of issues, but either content or process will dominate the allotted time of the group meeting. The group leader during this phase is aware of the two types of issues and may use this knowledge to assist the group toward a goal. If the members of the committee planning the class party are not getting along together, being late for meetings, and not progressing toward the goal, the leader may choose to focus on process issues in an attempt to facilitate task completion. Similarly, if the psychotherapy group spends the majority of its time discussing a sports event, the leader therapist may need to focus the group on process, perhaps by saying, "We have spent nearly half our time together discussing a baseball game. I wonder if we are avoiding another topic that people feel uncomfortable discussing."

Conflict may also occur during the working phase of the group. Examples of issues that may raise hostilities and side-taking are: "Why do we always have to do things your way?" "I'm only one person but I can't go along with this!" or "We're spending the time of this whole group on your one problem!" The conflict issue must be resolved for the group to continue. Successful conflict resolution contributes to group development and cohesion.

The working phase of the group is also characterized by power struggles. Individual members may seek recognition of contributions, may oppose the direction taken by the leader or the group, or may attempt to subvert and take over the leadership role. The leader may retain power, yield it with or without resistance, or become a leader in name only with the opposition wielding the real power. The latter is demonstrated by the example of a head nurse who retains the title of authority, but, in fact, the real power among the staff nurses is wielded by a nurse whose expert clinical skills give power and influence both within the nursing group and from the medical staff. Power struggles occur not only between leader and group members but also among group members. Members may be seeking the attention, rank, or privileges that often coincide with power. Ideally, the group can resolve this issue with cooperation replacing competition.

During the working phase, members may choose to leave the group for a variety of reasons. Some individuals may never have developed a sense of belonging or attachment to the group and during this phase will drop attendance. For others, there is no "payoff" to continued membership, and the demands are too great to continue. This is especially true in volunteer service organizations. The rewards of membership are weighed against the time, energy, and financial costs of membership, and a decision to continue or resign is made. For example, a group of student nurses is attending faculty meetings with the goal of adding student input to the decision-making process. If the students are never asked

for their opinions, they are likely to stop attending these meetings which do not meet their expectations and which cost them time and energy.

The Termination Phase

The final stage of group development is termination. The time of termination may be determined by goal achievement as in a task group, by a certain number of meetings as in a learning group, or by a prearranged schedule as in a psychotherapy group. Prior to the final session of the group, the leader has reminded members of the approaching completion of the group. Thus, not all the work of termination is accomplished during the final meeting of the group.

During termination, there are two main group tasks to be accomplished: summarization and evaluation. The leader frequently begins by condensing and verbalizing the accomplishments of the group. Both content and process achievements are noted. At this time, certain social amenities are also observed. When appropriate, the leader recognizes the accomplishments of individuals and thanks them for their contributions. The group

Table 7–1. **Summary of Group Work During Each Phase of Group Development**

Group Phase	Member Task	Leader Task
Initiation	Participate in establishing climate: physical and psychosocial Seek commonalities with other members Select leader Participate in establishing group norms	Set up physical climate as determined by group choices Begin to build cohesion Identify effect of group climate on members and on goal achievement Identify effect of norms on members and on goal achievement
Working	Formation of subgroups Complete assigned tasks May engage in conflict May engage in power struggles Participates in decision making	Balance time spent on content/process topics Conflict resolution Power resolution Selection of leadership and decision-making style Identify group task, select strategies to accomplish it, delegate to subgroups as appropriate
Termination	Acknowledgment of leader contributions Personal evaluation of group experience Coping with feelings of loss Completion of closure tasks	Summarize accomplishments of group Acknowledge contributions of members Complete or delegate closure tasks Evaluate group process Evaluate goal achievement

Source: Adapted from Benne and Sheats (1948).

members usually respond with similar remarks directed toward the leader. For some groups, termination can be an emotionally wrenching experience which is accompanied by a great deal of stress. This may be the case in a psychotherapy group or patient support group whose members have developed intimate, dependent relationships. These persons may experience a significant loss reaction with accompanying grief that is not unlike the feelings experienced at the death of a loved one. The leader may then focus on summarizing some of the process accomplishments the group has achieved during its life span and bringing feelings into awareness so the group may better deal with them. The leader may comment, "You have helped me to begin to understand how it feels to be facing cancer. We have grown very close over the past few weeks, and I feel sad at the thought of not meeting with you any more." Acknowledging feelings of loss, as well as reviewing progress and accomplishments, will assist members to leave the group with a feeling of well-being. Frequently, group members plan social events or reunions following termination of group membership, or they may even flatly refuse the termination process, saying perhaps, "We don't need to say good-by. We'll get together now that we know each other." Although social relationships are occasionally the outcome of group membership, such behaviors are often a refusal to deal with the pain and loss of an experience that has come to mean a great deal to an individual. Conversely, termination of some groups is accompanied by celebration of goal accomplishment, although even this may not be without a sense of loss.

Termination also involves an evaluative component that can be as formal as completing questionnaires and compiling statistics or as casual as discussing "How did it go?" over coffee. Here, members may acknowledge personal gains such as, "I'm glad I had the opportunity to get to know you," or "I really learned to use a computer by working on this project." If learning to function effectively within groups is a goal of the members, then evaluation is an essential task. Within evaluation, it is also important to seek closure of the group. Closure is roughly defined as tying up loose ends, finishing the group in a satisfying manner. For some groups, this may include creating a file of evaluative comments with suggestions for future use. For another group, such as a diabetic teaching group, closure may mean providing sources of help and information members may use once the group has terminated. The completion of the tasks involved in the termination phase enhances the satisfaction of group participation.

Tasks to be completed during each phase of group development are summarized in Table 7–1.

Roles Within the Group

People assume three main types of roles or customary ways of behaving in group interactions: roles related to task functions, roles related to maintenance functions, and roles related to self-needs. The assumption of a role increases the comfort of the individual and reflects the way the member typically responds in other situations. The following group roles are based on the work of Benne and Sheats (1948).

Roles Related to Task Function

In roles related to task functions, members' communication focuses on helping to achieve the goals of the group. These roles include:

- Information giver—one who provides relevant necessary data to the group
- Initiator—one who proposes new ideas, problems, solutions, or strategies
- Recorder—one who documents the business of the group
- Information seeker—one who asks questions which demonstrate the need for the group to obtain additional data, background information, statistics, etc.
- Evaluator—one who helps the group to judge, assess, or estimate the strategies or proposals of the group
- Timekeeper—keeps the group aware of the time limits.

Roles Related to Group Maintenance

Group maintenance roles refer to those activities of group members that relate to the group process or to the relationships among members. Roles that focus on group maintenance are:

- Gatekeeper—strategic person within the group who can grant an outsider entry into the group. If, for example, the class president welcomes a transferring nursing student and introduces the new student as a friend to a social group, it is likely that the new student will be accepted by the group. The class president is assuming a gatekeeper role.
- Compromiser—one who prevails upon group

members to resolve their differences and to work together to achieve group goals.

- Coordinator—one who brings order, harmony or cooperation to various factions of the group or to diverse ideas
- Tension reliever—uses humor, rest breaks, or other methods to deal with stress and strain among members of the group.
- Communication encourager—recognizes the contributions of each member, tries to give an opening to less assertive members, and limit members who monopolize. Fosters the development of trust by verbally or nonverbally supporting other members.
- Goaltender—appraises group progress toward the goal and brings it to the attention of the group.

Roles Related to Self-Interest

Finally, there is a group of behaviors that serve the individual needs of group members at a negative cost to the group process. In an optimally functioning group, members subordinate their own needs and desires to the group needs and desires. This is not to say that there is no payoff or membership reward to the individual member. But in successful groups, individual rewards are usually closely tied to the achievement of the group goal or some secondary rewards of membership. If this were not the case, individuals would not seek group membership. For example, the students planning a graduation party have the reward of enjoying a good time if they accomplish their goal. There is also the secondary reward of enjoying each other's company as they work in the group. Some groups have individual members who attempt, for various reasons, to meet individual needs

through the group. These individuals may be expressing a low self-esteem, a need for belonging, or a need for psychological security. The satisfaction of these individual needs interferes with the accomplishment of the group goals. The following roles may be assumed by members who seek to meet individual needs through group membership.

- Attacker—this individual verbally assaults the ideas, values, or opinions of other members or of the group. This communication focuses on lowering the esteem or worth of the person being attacked.
- Champion of the underdog—seeks to protect a minority view or personal special interest.
- Sympathy seeker—attempts to solicit understanding and compassion from the group by giving the appearance of not understanding the proceedings, by being incapable, or bewildered.
- Therapy seeker—uses the group to reveal personal matters and intimate problems which are not appropriate to the group goal. While these may be appropriate in a psychotherapy group, they are not suitable topics in other groups.
- Resister—retains original view or proposal and continues to use group time to deal with it even after the group has rejected or voted upon it and proceeded with other business.
- Esteem seeker—seeks recognition and attention by bragging of personal accomplishments, by "blowing one's own horn".
- Joiner—person who enjoys being with the group for the pleasure and companionship of membership but contributes little to the group work, often assuming a witty, joke-telling, and generally distracting role.

Factors Influencing Group Communication

Many factors operate at either a conscious or unconscious level to affect group communication. Some can be easily changed, while others are highly resistant to change.

Number of Participants

The "magic" number of seven to eight members has evolved as the optimal number for small group discussion or participation. If the group greatly exceeds this number, members have little opportunity to state their views and respond to questions.

Physical Climate Considerations

Physical climate refers to all those collective factors that contribute to the well-being and comfort of group members. It includes such things as temperature, beverages, comfortable seating, space, provision for note taking, availability of rest rooms, and rest breaks. At a recent three-day nursing conference, an evening banquet speaker commented on the long day the group had had, which began with a breakfast meeting, followed by continuous meetings, and was only then concluding at 9:00 P.M. After ascertaining that most of the nurses had attended all the scheduled meetings, he questioned the productivity of the group at the late hour and wondered aloud about the abusive physical climate that health care providers had structured for themselves. "Do you also do this to your patients?" he questioned, "And if not, why do you do it to yourselves?"

Territoriality

Territoriality refers to the concept of ownership as it applies to the group. Consider the difference in a group that meets in a public meeting room at a university compared to the group that meets at a member's home. The group at a university would be more likely to disagree freely since territoriality rights are equally distributed. In a home meeting, members feel some constraints on their freedom to aggressively disagree with the member in whose home the meeting is being held. In fact, it is considered a good strategy in group process to have the opposition meet away from its home territory in order to lessen resistance to new proposals.

Cohesiveness

Cohesiveness refers to the closeness or the "we-ness" of the group. One author has described this as the "glue" that holds the group together (Loomis, 1979). Cohesiveness is usually perceived as a positive characteristic of a group which facilitates progress toward a goal. A class of nursing students beginning a program of study is a random group of individuals. Several months into the nursing program, the students have become a group with a high degree of cohesiveness. Loomis says the attraction that the group has for the individual depends on:

The needs of the person that can be met in the group
The goals of the group that relate to the individual's needs
The person's expectation that the group will have beneficial consequences
The person's perception of the effectiveness of the group in providing valuable outcomes

In the case of the nursing students, cohesiveness grows as the class begins to pull together, helping one another study for difficult courses and giving support through emotionally difficult experiences.

Cohesiveness can also have the negative effect of diminishing critical thinking and the healthy discussion of opposing points of view. Irving Janis (1971) made up the word "*groupthink*" to describe a style of thinking in which "group members are amiable and seek concur-

rence on every important issue with no bickering or conflict to spoil the cozy we-feeling atmosphere." Janis further points out that "groupthink" refers to a deterioration in mental efficiency, reality testing, and moral judgments as a result of group pressures.

Type of Membership

Membership in a group may be required or voluntary, by invitation, or open to all interested persons. If, for example, membership is required in order to maintain one's job, the individual may be only a dues-paying member with token participation. This is frequently the case in organizations where a union requires all employees to be members for collective bargaining purposes. Conversely, if membership is perceived as highly desirable with a great many benefits, members are more likely to be active and put energy into developing a group structure that helps to achieve group goals.

Leadership

Group leadership is described as a role exercised by an individual which facilitates the achievement of group goals. Leadership may be assumed by a person who has the most knowledge about the group purpose or by the person who called the first meeting. In a more formal setting, the leader may be elected. Several leadership styles can be identified.

Autocratic Leadership.   An autocratic leader is humorously defined as a "benevolent dictator." This leader has the group goals clearly in mind, delegates tasks to members, supervises performance, and determines policies and procedures for the group with minimal member participation or consultation. This group tends to achieve goals, but low morale and minimal satisfaction may result over time. This leadership style may be most effective in time of crisis when there is not time for group decision making.

Directive Leadership.   Kron (1981) describes directive leadership as a modified form of autocratic leadership. The leader listens to input and gathers data from subordinates but retains decision-making power. This leader retains all responsibility and authority. This style does not enhance cooperation of group members or encourage personal growth. Communication is decreased because it is perceived as not making a difference.

Laissez-Faire Leadership.   Laissez faire is, in reality, an abdication of the leadership responsibility. No leadership exists, perhaps because no one is designated leader, perhaps because the leader is ineffective and has neither the skills nor the influence to move the group toward goal achievement, or perhaps the group works effectively with minimal leadership. Morale may be low, and disinterest and drop-out rate high. This style of leadership may be a direct response of the group to a previous autocratic leader, but little satisfaction is usually found with this solution.

Democratic Leadership Democratic leadership is based on the consent of the governed. Power and authority are delegated by the group members to the leader, usually for a limited time period or until the group members are so dissatisfied that they remove the leader from office. Under this leader, communication is free and open without fear of reprisal because a high degree of trust exists within the group. Satisfaction and morale are high within the group as long as the group continues to be effective in meeting group goals.

No one style of leadership can be determined to be best or most effective. Individuals may use a combination of all types depending on a specific situation. One author (Borden, 1969) suggests that it is more valuable to study "leadership acts" which he defines as any behavior within the group that makes a difference in the group's activity and thinking to the extent that it affects the group goal. Borden argues that this approach helps the student to study leadership where it occurs rather than only from one designated leader. It is also helpful in evaluating which leadership acts enhance or hinder group goals.

Group Norms

Group norms are the rules for behavior that the members have established formally or informally. Examples of group norms might include: meetings are to begin promptly at 2 P.M., no nonmember guests are permitted to attend meetings, or discussion of absent members is not permitted. Each of the norms developed by the group has a direct effect on communication.

Conflict Resolution

How members resolve disputes and differences of opinion is governed both by leadership style and by the norms the group has established. Conflict is inevitable and potentially valuable within the group. Any time people attempt to merge ideas and interests within a group, conflict results because no two people act or believe in the same manner. This can have the result of en-

couraging change, stimulating member interest and cooperation, and clarifying the purpose of the group. Alternatively, it can weaken or destroy a group by personal attacks on members, by generating anger, or by increasing competition between members.

Effective groups welcome disagreements as a way of generating new ideas and alternatives. Members examine reasons for opposing points of view and do problem solving in order to find a solution that incorporates the views of both factions. Groups may strengthen their effectiveness through conflict. In less effective groups, conflict becomes a win-lose divisive situation or may be ignored by members.

Trust

Trust is the confidence that other group members will consistently act with integrity, honesty, and justice for the well-being of the group and individual members. When the trust level in the group is high, members are free to respond openly, and communication is fostered.

Cultural Influence

In some cultures, illness is considered extremely private and not to be discussed outside the family. In another culture, it may be unacceptable to express one's feelings, thus, group psychotherapy designed to foster the expression of feelings may not be helpful. Cultural influences are deeply ingrained, pervasive in their effects, and highly resistant to change. It is in keeping with the ethics of nursing to accept the culture of the patient as a valuable and significant part of the human being, not to be altered to fit the health care organization. Cultural practices that jeopardize the health of an individual are identified, but change is the choice of the individual.

Power

Power is the influence an individual exerts within the group. Power can be either formal or informal. Formal power is that given to the individual by virtue of an elected office within the group, by an appointment from a higher authority, or by virtue of holding a position requiring knowledge and expertise, such as the nurse who is teaching a group of patients about nutrition. Informal power lacks the official recognition of a vote but is equally or even more influential than formal power. It may be demonstrated by a member with seniority who "knows the ropes" of an organization and is repeatedly called upon by group members for advice and information. It may be the nursing student who has a high academic average who is called upon by a study group to settle a disputed question. Frequently, both types of power are found as attributes of the same person.

Decision Making

Decision making within the group can be done by majority vote, by consensus, by an authority figure with or without group input, or by a small subgroup of the total group. A majority vote is frequently the most expedient way to reach a decision but has the effect of negating the views of the members who are in the minority. This may so alienate the minority members that they refuse to participate in future group work. Decision making by consensus means that discussion continues until a decision or a compromise is reached that is satisfactory to all members. The obvious limitation to this method is the time involved in reaching this understanding. It may result in an excellent decision which incorporates the best of the majority and minority points of view, but it may also result in a diluted or second-rate decision from excessive compromise. Frequently, out of sheer frustration or exhaustion, members agree to what they feel is less than the best decision. Another method empowers a small subgroup of the total group to make a decision. This is efficient but may cause disagreement if the total group is dissatisfied with the decision. If, for example, the committee planning the class graduation party schedules a place and time that many students dislike, the event will be less than successful unless a compromise is reached. In this type of decision making, it is important that the subgroup is representative of the larger group. Finally, in some instances, the designated leader of the group may make a decision, with or without group input. Frequently, the leader has this power under the rules of the organization, and no difficulty results. Occasionally, a leader may overstep the boundaries of authority, and group members may refuse to abide by the leader's decision. This may result in a confrontation between the leader and group members.

Each method of decision making affects communication among the members of the group. The leader anticipates and evaluates the effects of various styles of

Table 7–2. **Characteristics of a Good Group Decision**

1. The group demonstrates efficiency in the utilization of time, money, energy, skills, and talents.
2. The views of the minority are considered and, if possible, incorporated into the decision.
3. The decision is accepted and implemented by group members.
4. The group has gained decision-making skill from the experience.

decision making before entering into the process. The leader considers the time available to make the decision, the nature of the decision, and the acceptance on the part of group members needed to implement the decision. If the time available to make the decision is brief, the leader may choose to make the decision alone or by the decision of a majority vote. If the decision is relatively insignificant, such as holding a meeting at 2 P.M. or 3 P.M., the leader may choose merely to announce a decision. If the decision has widespread implications, for example, costing a large amount of money and altering the schedules of individuals, the leader may seek extensive member input. Finally, the leader considers who is to implement the decision. It is generally accepted that the more an individual is affected by a decision, the more the individual should participate in making the decision. This enhances the possibility of the individual accepting the decision and being committed to its operation. Consider the patient who must adhere to a strict therapeutic diet. If the health team presents the patient with a typed diet and instructions to "Do it," the chances for adherence to the diet are very low. In contrast, consider the health team that meets with the patient, explains the nature of the disease process, the reasons the therapeutic diet is necessary, and includes foods that are acceptable to the patient. The team then begins to work with the patient to plan a diet that is agreeable to the patient but still meets the desired therapeutic goals. The chances are very high the patient is going to adhere to this diet because the person has participated in the decision-making process. Like many other processes in nursing, there is no one best method of decision making. The variables in each instance must be considered, and a professional judgment made. (See Table 7–2.)

Assessing Group Communication

In addition to reviewing each of the factors that influence group communication, it may be helpful to assess who talks to whom in the group, how often, and for how long. One way to do this is to draw diagrams de-

picting the direction and frequency of communication. (See Figure 7–1.) The observer first draws a circle to indicate each of the group members and their position within the group. Then, while observing the group in

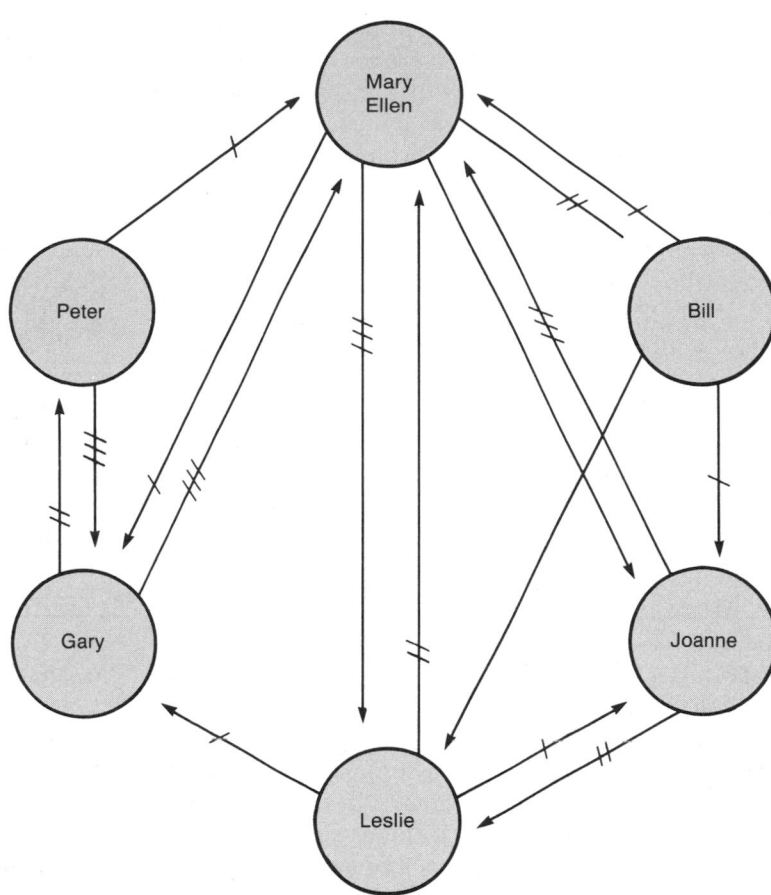

Figure 7–1. Example of group communication diagram.

process, the observer draws arrows to indicate the direction of conversation and the responses. Slash marks may be used on an arrow to indicate frequency. An analysis of the frequency marks will indicate levels of participation, as well as giving some indication of leadership—formal or informal. The observer may also note how much of the group time each member uses. A group leader might use this technique to identify members who monopolize group time or members who need support in order to enter the group communication. It may also be used to identify conflict and strengthen the group process.

Another method of assessing group communication is the analysis of the communication network, that is, the pattern of communication that exists within the group. (See Figure 7–2.) The diagram of the open network is ideal for most groups since the diagram indicates that everyone speaks to and responds to everyone in this group. A second type of network is the wheel which indicates that group communication, at least for

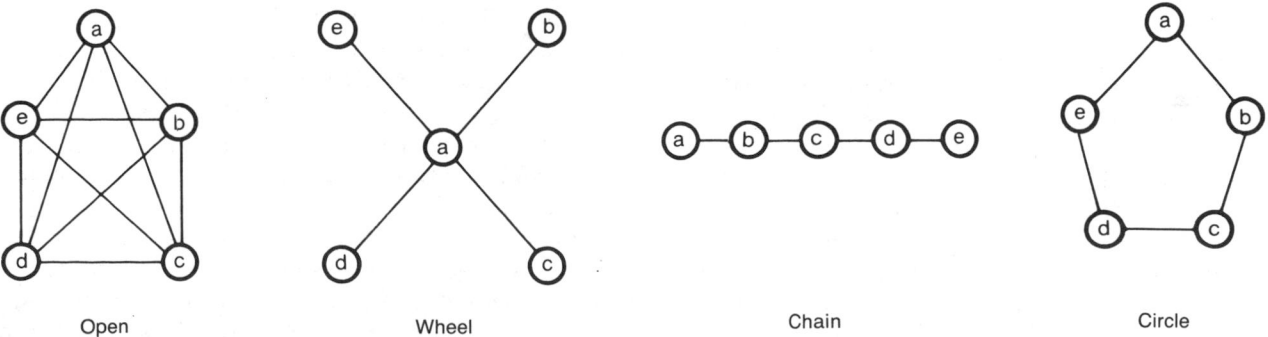

Figure 7–2. Communication networks.

a time, centers around one person, perhaps a leader, an information giver, a recognized expert. A chain network implies a hierarchy, such as nurse aid, staff nurse, team leader, assistant head nurse, head nurse, supervisor. In a chain, communication flows both up and down, but not across. If, for example, the staff nurse had an idea for how to improve patient care in this organization, the nurse would most likely present the idea to the team leader who would, in turn, communicate the idea to the next level. The circle network indicates communication between superiors and subordinates and cross-communication at the lowest level, but not at higher levels.

Researchers have studied how the circle, chain, and wheel affect communication. They discovered that the circle is the slowest network for transmitting information and the poorest in accuracy, but it produced the highest morale in the participants. When groups were working on very complex problems, however, the circle network was found to be faster and more effective than other networks.

Another assessment variable is called "triggering" (Johnson and Johnson, 1975). This pattern of communication has several forms. In one type, person A speaks and is always responded to by person B. Johnson and Johnson state that the second remark may be an attempt to give support ("Atta boy") or dilute the first remark ("Yea but"). Observations of triggering give clues as to how members see their own power and roles within the group. Members who perceive themselves as occupying high-power positions within the group are more likely to give support and to feel free to interrupt.

Effect of Illness and Hospitalization of Group Member on the Group

How a group responds to the crisis of illness and hospitalization will depend to a great extent on the way the group has handled stress in the past. If the usual group response to stress is to assume a "grin and bear it" stoic stance, that is the response the group will most likely assume toward illness. If the usual response is to approach stress in an intellectual manner, the group will most likely use that approach. This might include reading extensively, consulting experts, reviewing recent statistics on the problem, and finally making a decision. In general, past experience determines present response. The strategies that have been successful in the past will be among the first utilized in the new situation.

The group that is better organized with clearly defined roles may give better support to the hospitalized member and may also exert more control. For example, in the work group of an organization, who does what is clearly defined. When one worker becomes ill, the tasks of the ill member are redistributed to other members. Co-workers generally visit the hospital and send some gift to the person. All these activities are clearly defined and expected.

Hospitalization interrupts established group relationships. During illness, it is important to maintain communication between the patient and the primary group so the patient retains a feeling of membership and group support. The communication network between the patient and the group is kept open and functioning in order that the patient can easily rejoin the group after recovery. If this is not done, the group may close ranks, and the ill member may no longer have a place in the group. A head nurse who has been away for a lengthy illness may return to find that an assistant has directed the operation of the unit equally well. The nurse may question personal need and role within the group.

Summary

Group communication skills are essential for nurses to develop since nurses work with groups of patients, groups of nurse colleagues, and groups of health team members. There are three stages in the development of a group: initiation phase, working phase, and termination phase. During each phase, there are predictable content and process tasks that each group completes.

Group members assume roles within the group both to facilitate goal achievement and to increase the comfort of personal functioning. These roles are related to task functions, group maintenance functions, or self-interest.

Some major factors that influence group communication are number of participants, cohesiveness, leadership style, decision making, group norms, conflict resolution, and trust. Group communication is assessed by studying the frequency and direction of individual communication, as well as the patterns of group communication as a whole.

The illness of a member affects other group members. The way the group responds is determined largely by past experiences in handling stress. Communication between the ill member and the group is maintained to provide continued group support to the patient.

Terms for Review

climate	group development phases	group roles	leadership style	norm
physical	initiation phase	maintenance roles	autocratic	primary group
psychosocial	work phase	self-serving roles	democratic	process
content	termination phase	task roles	directive	
group	group dynamics	groupthink	laissez faire	

Self-Assessment

Briefly describe one group to which you belong: name, goal, number of members. Ask permission of the group to tape record one meeting for the purpose of looking only at your own participation, after which the tape will be discarded. Use the following tool (Exhibit 7-1) to assess your own roles as a group member as you listen to the tape of the meeting. Each time you participate in the group make either a check mark or a brief note in the appropriate column. Try to make a note of the group response to your comment. Then, using your completed tool to provide the data, respond to the following questions:

1. The role I assumed most often was . . . .
2. Conflicts arose which were about . . . .
3. During conflict I (assumed what role) . . . .
4. Decisions that were made were about . . . .
5. During decision making, I (assumed what role) . . . .
6. I performed a leadership act when I . . . .
7. My contributions that facilitated the group goals were . . . .
8. I hindered group goals when I . . . .
9. When I work in groups, the thing I do best is . . . .
10. When I work in groups, the thing I would most like to change about myself is . . . .

Exhibit 7-1. Tool for Assessing Role as a Group Member

MY PARTICIPATION

Task Roles

Information giver
Initiator
Recorder
Information seeker
Coordinator
Evaluator

Maintenance Roles

Gatekeeper
Compromiser
Tension reliever
Communication encourager
Goaltender

Self-Serving Roles

Attacker
Champion of underdog
Sympathy seeker
Therapy seeker
Resister
Esteem seeker
Joiner

Learning Activity

Attend any public meeting as an observer. This might be a political meeting, a school board meeting, or a nurses' association meeting. During the meeting, function only as an observer of group content and process. Answer the following questions and cite the data upon which you based your answers.

1. Identify the leader of the group and state how the leader obtained the office.
2. What was the leadership style of the individual?
3. Describe the type of power used by the leader.
4. Were there any other individuals present who demonstrated informal power?
5. Identify the major content issue of the group.
6. Identify the major process issue of the group.
7. Identify one decision made by the group and evaluate it using the characteristics of a good decision listed in Table 7-2.
8. Describe the phase of development of the group.
9. Evaluate the effectiveness of the group related to goal accomplishment.

Review Questions

1. The best reason for a nurse to be knowledgeable about group behavior is
   a. Nursing care that uses groups is most cost effective.
   b. All human beings live in groups.
   c. No single nurse can provide all the care a patient in the health care setting needs.
2. An example of a primary group is
   a. A family
   b. The National Organization of Women
   c. The American Nurses' Association
   d. The Democratic Party
3. Which of the following is a function of the leader during the initiation phase of the group?
   a. Directing energies to the group goal
   b. Commenting on group process issues
   c. Summarizing group accomplishments
   d. Establishing rules of group behavior
4. Ms. Jones, the local tennis club president, introduces new member Smith to the members of her tennis club and schedules a doubles match as Smith's partner. This is an example of which of the following group roles?
   a. Tension reliever
   b. Initiator
   c. Joiner
   d. Gatekeeper
5. Which of the following characteristics predispose a group to make the errors described as ''groupthink''?
   a. Low cohesion, frequent membership turnover, decision by majority vote
   b. High cohesion, stable membership, decision by consensus
   c. Autocratic leadership, high creativity, decision by authority
6. In which of the following decisions would a nursing leader be most likely to involve staff nurses?
   a. Patient menus and diet-selection procedures
   b. Purchasing of paper office supplies
   c. Uniform code requirements
   d. Housekeeping and maintenance scheduling
7. The response of a group to illness of a member is largely determined by
   a. The degree of cohesion among members
   b. The way the group handled stress in the past
   c. Number of members
   d. The length of time the group has been together

Answers

1. c
2. a
3. d
4. d
5. b
6. c
7. b

Suggested Readings

Janis, I.: Groupthink. *Psychology Today*, pp. 43–46, 74–76, Nov., 1971.

A psychologist describes the effect of high group cohesion on the decision-making process of the group.

References and Bibliography

Benne, K. B., and Sheats, P.: Functional roles of group members. *J. Soc. Issues,* **4:** 41–49, Spring 1948.

Borden, G. and Gregg, R. and Grove, T.: *Speech Behavior and Human Interaction.* Prentice-Hall, Englewood Cliffs, N.J., 1969.

Bradley, J. and Edinberg, M.: *Communication in the Nursing Context.* Appleton-Century Crofts, Norwalk, Ct. 1982.

Edwards, B., and Brillhart, J.: *Communication in Nursing Practice.* Mosby, St. Louis, 1981.

Janis, I: Groupthink. *Psychology Today* pp. 43–46, 74–76, Nov. 1971.

Johnson, D., and Johnson, F.: *Joining Together.* Prentice-Hall, Englewood Cliffs, N.J., 1975.

Kron, T.: *The Management of Patient Care.* Sanders, Philadelphia, 1981.

Loomis, M.: *Group Process for Nurses.* Mosby, St. Louis, 1979.

Sampson E., and Marthas, M.: *Group Process for the Health Professions,* 2nd ed. Wiley, New York, 1981.

CHAPTER 8

COMMUNICATION AMONG THE HEALTH TEAM

Importance of Communication Among Health
   Team Members
Purpose of Professional Communication
Ethical Considerations Related to Professional
   Communication
Legal Considerations of Professional
   Communication
Assertiveness in Communication
Written Communication
      Contents of the Patient's Chart
      Documentation of Health Care
      Legal Responsibilities in Charting
      Nurses' Notes

Verbal Communication
      Change-of-Shift Report
      Giving a Verbal Report
      Receiving a Verbal Report
      Physicians' Telephone Orders
      Physicians' Verbal Orders
Patient Care Conferences
Staff Conferences

Objectives

1. Discuss why communication among health team members is important.
2. Describe the use of documentation as part of a nursing audit.
3. Discuss the requirements related to communication of one ethical code for nurses.
4. Describe how the ethical requirements of the nursing code related to communication apply to nursing students.
5. State a major advantage and disadvantage of consumer access to medical records.

6. Differentiate between assertive and aggressive communication.
7. Differentiate between problem-oriented medical records and source-oriented medical records.
8. State six times or events that require written documentation in the patient's record.
9. Discuss the legal requirements of documentation.
10. State the sequence of one format a nurse may use to organize a verbal report.

Importance of Communication Among Health Team Members

The single most important reason to strive for clear, open communication among the members of the health team is that it contributes to the quality of patient care. Stated more emphatically, if health team members are not communicating with each other, they are probably not working together and may even be working against each other. This may be overdramatic, but the frag-mented health care that results when team members do not communicate is a serious disservice and breach of responsibility to the patient. Maintaining quality communication is not easy. It is another professional skill that requires both study and practice to attain a high level of proficiency.

Purpose of Professional Communication

Communication among members of the health team includes verbal and written messages. Within the practice of nursing, verbal communication focuses on reporting functions; written communication focuses on *documentation* or recording functions.

The patient's chart is a health record which details the patient's condition, all treatments received, and the response to them, as well as recommendations and plans for future care. Each member of the health team contributes to the record and uses the notations of other team members to provide care. Charting that is well done contributes to improved patient care because it informs nurses and other health team members of the patient's condition and any changes that have occurred. A nurse may review the charted notes of a particular patient, for example, and decide that, although a nursing treatment has been completed four times a day for the past three days, there is no improvement in the patient's condition, and a change in plan is necessary.

Another way in which quality charting contributes to improved patient care is in the nursing *audit*. This is a peer evaluation system in which a second nurse (or a committee of nurses) examines the record of nursing care and compares it to standards. *Standards of care* are written by nurses to describe what would be considered safe, competent, reasonable care for a patient having a certain condition. These standards are a listing of the observations that the nurse must make and care that should be given to the patient. Using these standards, a nurse conducting an audit will select a patient chart, usually at random, and make a determination about the quality of nursing care the patient received based on the recorded data. Table 8–1 is an example of a patient care standard for rest and sleep. The audit method of nursing care evaluation has been criticized because many nurses feel that much nursing care is given that is not recorded. Because the chart is also a legal document, these nurses are reminded of the legal maxim: if it is not recorded, it is not done. In other words, if a nurse forgets to record on the patient's chart that a medication was given, then another nurse has no indication that the medication was actually given. A serious mistake may be made if the second nurse gives another dose of the medication while attempting to correct the apparent omission.

Not only does documentation serve as a record of care, but in some cases it may serve to protect the nurse. If a patient refuses to take a prescribed medication, for example, the nurse must document the fact, along with the explanation given to the patient, if the physician was notified, and any other action taken. If a lawsuit arises at a later date, the facts of the situation are well docu-

mented, and the nurse has a dated record of the events. The legal aspects of communication are more fully discussed in Chapter 3 of this text.

Patient records may also be used as a source of data for research. At times only grouped data (data that combine the statistics from many patients without individual identification) are used; for some research purposes, the individual data with a long-term history are more beneficial. The more specific the charted data about the patient and the nursing care received, the more useful are the records for research purposes.

Records may be used in cost analyses within the hos-

Table 8–1. **Example of Patient Care Standard**

REST AND SLEEP

Observations

Inappropriate fatigue
Lassitude
Loss of muscle tone
Incoordination
Restlessness
Irritability
Muscle tension
Interrupted sleep
Dreams

Assessment

Patient's normal sleep patterns
Aids used for sleep
Alterations in sleep needs due to illness
Level of anxiety
Extent of daytime activity and its compatibility with degree of convalescence

Ongoing Care

Maintain patient's normal sleep pattern whenever possible
Utilize patient's normal sleep aids—reading, warm drink, etc.
Arrange appropriate plan for daytime activity
Provide planned rest periods as needed
Provide appropriate environment
Provide physical comfort
 Warmth
 Positioning for body parts
 Pillows
 Back rub
 Administer sedation as ordered
Provide psychological comfort

Source: Susan Martin Tucker, Mary Anne Breeding, Mary M. Canobio, Eleanor Vargo Paquette, Majorie Fyfe Wells, and Mary E. Willman: *Patient Care Standards*, 3rd ed. Mosby, St. Louis, 1984.

pital. If a review of records reveals that certain brands of medical care products are found to last longer, this may affect both the purchasing of equipment and the cost the patient is charged.

In addition, records may be used to determine third-party payment (usually insurance coverage) for hospitalization and related fees. Because an expensive diagnostic procedure might accidentally be charged to the wrong patient, it is important that records be complete and accurate.

Ethical Considerations Related to Professional Communication

Because nursing provides a very intimate, personal service to other human beings, nurses are exposed to a great deal of confidential information. The "International Code for Nurses" (ICN), the "Code of Ethics" of the Canadian Nurses' Association (CNA) and the American Nurses' Association's (ANA) "Code for Nurses" require that the nurse respect the client's right to privacy by using professional judgment in revealing confidential information to other persons. The ANA Code requires that confidential information be shared only when it is necessary in planning and implementing that patient's care. The nurse consciously decides if others need to know personal information about a patient. Casual conversation about a patient or family for purposes other than improving nursing care is unethical. The Code also states that it is permitted to reveal patient information for purposes of documenting care as required by third-party payment, or perhaps for use in nursing audits. Even in these situations, the Code requires that the data be disclosed only in accordance with established, written policies that assure that confidentiality is maintained.

Student nurses using patient data for learning purposes are bound by the same rules of ethics related to confidentiality. Discussions about patient situations are conducted in a private setting with other nursing students and are supervised by a nursing instructor. Patients are identified by pseudonyms such as Ms. X. Pseudonyms are also used on written learning assignments related to the care of a particular patient.

The Code points out that the nurse-patient relationship is built on trust, and any violation of patient's confidentiality could destroy this relationship. A violation of the Code may result in censure of the nurse by the professional organization or reconsideration by the licensing agency of the individual nurse's right to practice nursing.

Legal Considerations of Professional Communication

A violation of the confidentiality of the nurse-patient relationship could also have legal implications for the nurse. These are based on a breach of the patient's right to privacy. For example, the nurse may be required to give testimony in a court of law about a patient. The nurse may claim that the information is privileged communication, protected under law, and the court cannot force the nurse to reveal it. The nurse would be well advised to seek legal counsel in this case since the law regarding privileged communication varies both from state to state and to whom it applies. The law frequently includes the physician-patient, attorney-client, priest-confessor relationships but does not usually extend to the nurse-patient relationship.

In recent years the ownership and right to access of the patient's chart have become controversial issues. Although it is generally agreed that the chart is the property of the institution collecting the data, there is less agreement over the control of the information. The ANA "Code for Nurses" states that the individual has the right to control the information provided by self, family, and environment. Professionals may exercise the right of control over the information generated by them. Many patients and professionals currently believe that patients are entitled to a full disclosure of their health records to them. The question has been raised as to why health professionals, review committees, insurers, government agencies, and researchers should all have access to the patient's records and not the patient? Stating that there are important advantages to the patient to be gained by having patient access to medical records, one consumer research group has published a step-by-step guide for the individual to use in obtaining medical records (Sarath, Auerbach, and Bogue, 1980).

Some of the advantages of consumer access to records cited by this group are:

1. Protection of privacy. Only the patient who knows what is in the record can make an informed decision as to whether or not to grant authorization for disclosure

2. Improved understanding of the medical condition
3. Open patient-physician relationships
4. Continuity of health care in a mobile society

Conversely, one concern that some health professionals have when patients have full access to medical records is that they may make inaccurate conclusions about their diagnoses and prognoses.

Computer access to patient information is a final legal issue involving communication. The topic is extremely timely since computer terminals are currently installed on many hospital stations, with many more predicted for the future. With the massive data storage and retrieval capabilities of computers, the issues become those of who has access to the data, for what purposes, with whose consent. This will be discussed in Chapter 10.

Assertiveness in Communication

Communication skills that reflect the individual's rights and power are called *assertiveness skills*. These result in communication in which there is an honest and direct verbalization of feelings, wants, needs, or opinions. This communication respects both the sender and the receiver. It is not done at the expense, punishment, or threat of either party. Assertive communication is accompanied by appropriate nonverbal behavior. The nurse maintains eye contact and assumes good posture. Hands are in a position that is neither threatening nor timid. Muldary lists four reasons for assertive behavior:

1. It tends to increase one's self-respect.
2. It enables the individual to meet needs and wants.
3. It promotes open, honest relationships characterized by mutuality or give and take.
4. It has a higher probability of effecting better relationships than either aggression or nonassertion. Successful aggressive behavior puts the person in a dominant position; nonassertive behavior places the person in a subservient position. Assertion promotes equality (Muldary, 1983).

In contrast, *nonassertive communication* is indirect, hesitant, apologetic, a failure to express oneself. It is not respectful of the self.

Aggressive communication conveys disrespect for the other person. It places the other person on the defensive and sets up a win/lose situation. The aggressive person attempts to secure rights at the expense of the rights of others.

The following statements clarify the differences among assertive, nonassertive, and aggressive communication.

1. Nursing student to instructor:

I do not understand the skill. I need another demonstration. Could you please repeat it for me? [assertive]

I'm so slow and uncoordinated that I just can't catch

on in one demonstration. Please, repeat it for me. [nonassertive]

If you'd give just one, good, clear demonstration I could learn this. [aggressive]

2. Staff nurse to head nurse:

I have a family emergency and need a personal leave day tomorrow in order to settle the problem. [assertive]

I'm sorry to have to ask for this but I really need to have tomorrow off to handle a family emergency. Do you think maybe it could be arranged? [nonassertive]

You'll just have to do without me. I won't be in tomorrow because my family needs me and that is most important. I'm taking a personal leave day. Just this once someone else will have to cover for me. [aggressive]

3. Nursing student to friend who has just asked to borrow notes the night before an examination:

No, I will be using my notes tonight. [assertive]

Oh, I need my notes, too, but maybe we could study together or maybe we could each use them half of the evening? [nonassertive]

Why don't you learn to take good notes and you wouldn't have this problem. My notes are for my use and you're on your own! [aggressive]

Some assertive verbal communication skills the nurse may use are:

1. Positive self-statements. The more the nurse respects self, the greater will be the respect given by others. The nurse gives messages to the self like, "I really did a fine job today. Mrs. Jones was very uncomfortable, and I was able to help her using those alternative methods of pain relief that I just learned."

2. Owning personal behavior. One way this is done is by using "I" statements. For example. "I need to stay home and study tonight and cannot go out."

3. Confrontation. This is a statement about confu-

sion in a verbal message, nonverbal behavior, or both. This is not angry or attacking behavior. It is a statement of fact delivered in a calm, firm voice. Example:

Nurse A to Nurse B: I needed you to help me walk Mrs. M. I thought you were coming but you went on a break. Now Mrs. M. has visitors and refuses to walk.

Nurse A to Nurse B: I had to stay over because you were late for work again today. Now you are smiling and I do not feel this is funny.

There are many other assertive communication skills the nurse may use. The nurse practicing assertive communication maintains self-respect and grants respect to others.

Written Communication

Contents of the Patient's Chart

The chart is a record of the health care the patient has received, as well as the response to treatment and future health plans. It has space for each member of the health team to make contributions. Each hospital or health care institution develops various record-keeping forms to meet its own needs. Some variation of the following forms are usually found within each chart.

Face Sheet. Identifies the patient and includes data such as complaint that necessitated hospitalization, attending physician, nearest relatives, food or drug allergies, current medications, ambulatory status.

Medical History and Physical Examination Form. Should be completed by a physician or nurse practitioner.

Nursing History. Documents past health care experiences, and the patient's physical and psychological response to illness. The purpose of the nursing history is to identify problems that require nursing intervention. It also helps to make the patient's adjustment to the health care setting as easy as possible (See Figure 8–1.)

Graphic Sheet. A graph page that permits the nurse to document temperature, pulse, respirations, blood pressure, intake, output, and weight.

Flow Sheet. A page usually divided into columns which the nurse may date and then check or initial to indicate such activities as bathing, ambulation, and treatments completed. This sheet is intended to save time by reducing repetitive handwritten notes, but the nurse is still obligated to make and record observations. A check mark in the column for ambulation would indicate that the patient walked, but in the nurses' notes the response of the patient would be documented. (See Figure 8–2.)

Medication Record. It may be in the patient's chart or in a separate chart with the medication cart, depending on the system of medication administration used. There is space to record the medication, dose, route, date, time, and signature of the person administering the medication.

Nursing Notes. They are used to record nursing treatments, patient response to treatments, and observations of the patient. Nurses may include documentation of activities of other health team members such as, "Consultation and exam completed by Dr. J. Smith."

Physicians' Progress Notes. They are the documentation of observation, progress, treatments, and visits by the physician written by the physician.

Laboratory and X-ray Sheets. They are frequently attached to a special section in the patient's chart by self-adhesive or three-ring binder paper.

Problem List. If the institution is using the problem-oriented charting approach, a separate sheet for numbered patient problems is included. Under this system, some of the above forms will be altered since all health team members chart on the same form.

Health Team Notes. Physical therapy, inhalation therapy, or other departments will have designated forms within the chart for the purpose of recording patient problems, treatments, and progress.

Discharge Plan. The health team's plan for ongoing health care after the patient is discharged from the hospital or facility. This may include such things as diet instructions, activity restrictions, scheduling a follow-up examination, and further outpatient treatment.

Although some variation of each of these forms is being used in most hospitals, the trend is toward using the computer to complete many charting functions. Nurses enter the data into the computer, either by typ-

UNIVERSITY OF MINNESOTA HOSPITALS

NURSING DATA BASE (General Adult)

All questions must have an answer. Patient has the right to refuse to answer. "NA" indicates "Not Applicable".

DATE 12-1-84	TIME 2 pm	INFORMANT (IF OTHER THAN PATIENT) N.A.		PATIENT IDENTIFICATION PLATE

| NAME OF RELATIVE IN CITY MRS. J. BERSIN | PHONE 659-8310 | PATIENT ADMITTED FROM Home | PATIENT ADMITTED PER ☑WALKING ☐WHEELCHAIR ☐LITTER ☐OTHER: |

| AGE 59 | HEIGHT 5'6" ☐IN. ☐CM. | ☐LITTER ☑STANDING | WEIGHT 135 ☑LB. ☐KG. | TEMPERATURE 99° | ☐A ☑O R |

| PULSE 84 ☐A ☑R | REGULARITY/QUALITY Regular, full | RESPIRATIONS 26 | QUALITY & POSITION PATIENT IS IN Sitting on chair |

| BLOOD PRESSURE 142/76 ☐R. ARM ☑L. ARM | NOTE IF HX OF HYPER/HYPOTENSION none | DOES PATIENT KNOW HIS REGULAR B.P.? 140/80 |

GENERAL APPEARANCE (BODY SIZE, SKIN CONDITION, CLEANLINESS, LEVEL OF CONSCIOUSNESS, LEVEL OF COMFORT, PHYSICAL HANDICAP, ETC.) Well groomed, oriented female admitted ambulatory accompanied by daughter. No complaints of pain, nausea or dizziness at present. Pale skin color, warm to touch.

PATIENT'S STATEMENT AS TO REASON FOR ADMISSION (PATIENT'S OWN WORDS) "I got dizzy & flushed last night after getting up from a chair. The dr. wants to run some tests."

PROBLEMS—PAST & PRESENT

DATE OF ONSET	PROBLEM TITLE	DESCRIPTION OF PROBLEM (INCLUDE PATIENT'S UNDERSTANDING)
12/84	#1 Possible bleeding ulcer	Pt. describes episode of dizziness previous evening which subsided c̄ rest. States, "I feel OK now but Dr. Losby wants to do some tests because my blood was low & she suspects I have a bleeding ulcer."
	#2 Knowledge deficit related to diagnostic tests	"I've never been in a hospital since I had my babies. These tests really scare me. What are they like?"

CURRENT MEDICATIONS (Rx and/or self-prescribed)

NAME	DOSE, FREQUENCY	REASON FOR TAKING & HOW LONG	TIME OF LAST DOSE

MEDICATIONS BROUGHT WITH PATIENT WERE REMOVED FROM PATIENT'S BEDSIDE   ☐ YES   ☐ NO   ☑ NOT APPLICABLE

17038, FEB 78

Figure 8–1. Example of nursing data base form. (Courtesy of the University of Minnesota Hospitals, Minneapolis, MN.)

ALLERGIES/ SENSITIVITIES	MEDICATION/FOOD/MATERIALS	TYPE OF REACTION
	PENICILLIN	Hives, rash, "wheezing breathing"
	no food allergies	

DOES PATIENT UNDERSTAND HIS/HER RESPONSIBILITY FOR PERSONAL BELONGINGS?	[X] YES [ ] NO →	IF "NO", TO WHOM EXPLAINED?	HAS PATIENT BEEN ORIENTED TO ROOM? [X] YES [ ] NO
DOES PATIENT HAVE IDENTIFICATION BAND ON WRIST?	[X] YES [ ] NO →	IF "NO", WHERE?	HAVE CALL LIGHTS BEEN EXPLAINED TO PATIENT? [X] YES [ ] NO
DOES PATIENT HAVE A COPY OF PATIENT'S BILL OF RIGHTS?	[X] YES [ ] NO →	IF "NO", TO WHOM GIVEN?	HAVE SMOKING REGULATIONS BEEN EXPLAINED TO PATIENT? [X] YES [ ] NO

CHECK ANY OF THE FOLLOWING BELONGINGS OF THE PATIENT'S THAT HAVE BEEN BROUGHT TO THE HOSPITAL AND IDENTIFY LOCATION OF EACH ITEM IF NOT IN PATIENT'S ROOM:

LOCATION, IF NOT PATIENT'S ROOM		LOCATION, IF NOT PATIENT'S ROOM
[X] GLASSES	[X] WATCH	
[ ] CONTACT LENSES	[X] RING	
[ ] DENTURES	[ ] OTHER (LIST BELOW):	
[ ] HEARING AID		
[ ] PROSTHESIS		
[ ] CRUTCHES		
[ ] WALKER		
[ ] CANE		
[ ] BRACE		
[ ] WHEELCHAIR		

	PROBLEM	DESIRED OUTCOME	I IMMEDIATE D DISCHARGE	NURSING INTERVENTION
INITIAL PLANS	1 Possible injury related to "dizzy spells"	1. Physical safety maintained until discharge.	I	1. a. Side rails up b. Instructed to ring for nurse to assist when up c. √ vital signs q.2h.
	2 Knowledge deficit related to G-I tests	2. Pt. will give accurate description of GI x-rays prior to test.	I	2. Explain upper G-I x-ray a. NPO b. Barium c. no pain d. expelling barium

SIGNATURE OF ADMITTING NURSE/TITLE   X _S. Riley, R.N._

Figure 8–1. (*Continued*)

137

137

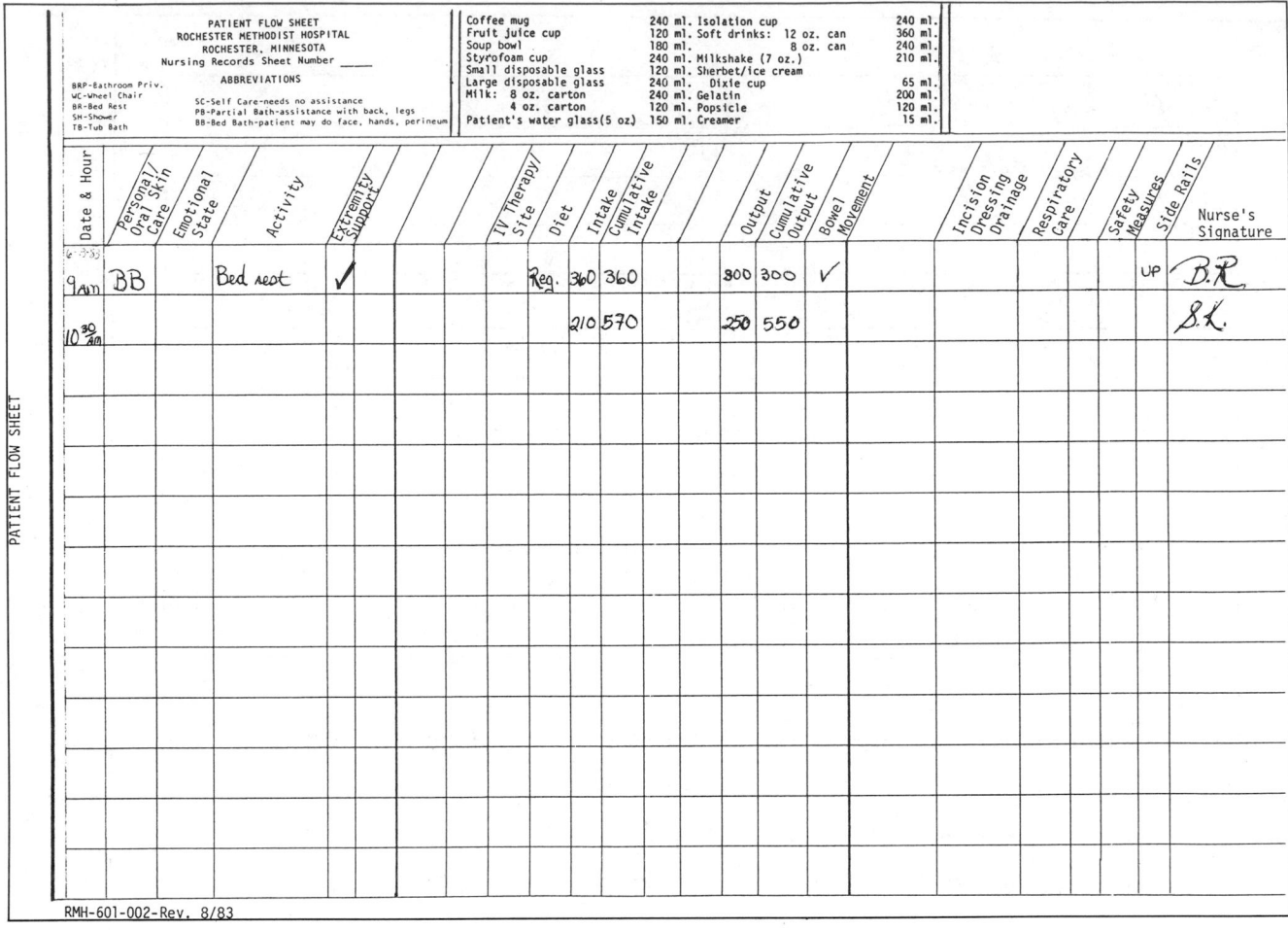

Figure 8–2. Example of a flow sheet. (Courtesy of Rochester Methodist Hospital, Rochester, MN.)

ing it in or by using a sensing device to select printed data from a screen. Under such a system, data are immediately available to the entire health care system. The potential time and energy savings of such a system are great. However, it does present a new set of skills for health professionals to learn. (See Chapter 10.)

Documentation of Health Care

In order to make written communication effective, there are several guidelines the nurse can use to improve clarity.

1. Writing must be legible. First, and most essential, write legibly in black ink. If your writing is not easily read, print the notation and sign your name in cursive style. If you cannot read another notation in the chart, ask for clarification from the writer. Guessing at the words of another person's handwriting may result in harmful errors and is indefensible in a court of law. This applies to physicians as well as nurses. Do not guess at the content of a physician's order. Black ink is usually preferable because it reproduces when photocopied. Many institutions will have policies requiring specific ink color for certain time periods.

2. Nurses notes are to be factual observations without unsupported judgments or conclusions. For example, consider the following examples of the same notation.

Smoking aggravates condition.
Smoking (two cigarettes) followed by three minutes of hacking cough. States, "Smoking really makes it harder to breathe, but I haven't been able to stop."

The first observation is an unsupported conclusion while the second is a statement of facts including the patient's own words.

3. Include the date and time of all entries in the patient's chart. Some institutions are now using military time to avoid confusion. In this 24-hour system, no A.M.

or P.M. is used: 0100 hours is 1 A.M., 0200 hours is 2 A.M., 1200 hours is noon, 1300 hours is 1 P.M., and so forth to 2400 hours at midnight. Minutes are designated by the last two numbers in the sequence: 1230 is 12:30 P.M., 1515 is 3:15 P.M. This system eliminates confusion between A.M. and P.M. times. Institutions not using military time may require that all evening and/or night charting be done in red ink to distinguish it from the daytime hours.

4. Include all necessary information but still be as

Table 8–2. **Medical Abbreviations**

a	before	N & V	nausea and vomiting
abd	abdomen	NPO	nothing by mouth
ac	before meals	N/S	normal saline
ad lib	as desired	ō	nothing, none
ADL	activities of daily living	O & P	ova and parasites
AP	apical pulse	OD	right eye
AROM	active range of motion	OOB	out of bed
bid	twice a day	OR	operating room
BM	bowel movement	OS	left eye
BMR	basal metabolic rate	os	mouth
BP	blood pressure	OU	both eyes
BR	bathroom	p̄	after
BRP	bathroom privileges	pc	after meals
c̄	with	PE	physical examination
CBC	complete blood count	per	by, through
CC	chief complaint	po	by mouth
cc	cubic centimeter	prn	as needed
C/O	complains of	PROM	passive range of motion
C & S	culture and sensitivity	PT	physical therapy
CSF	cerebrospinal fluid	q	every
CTDB	cough, turn, deep breathe	qd	every day
dc	discontinue	qh	every hour
DOA	dead on arrival	qid	four times a day
DOE	dyspnea on exertion	qod	every other day
Dx	diagnosis	q4h	every four hours
ECG (EKG)	electrocardiogram	R	rectally
EEG	electroencephalogram	RBC	red blood cells
EENT	eye, ear, nose, throat	RLQ	right lower quadrant
FF	force fluids	R/O	rule out
FUO	fever of unknown origin	ROM	range of motion
Fx	fracture	RUQ	right upper quadrant
GI	gastrointestinal	Rx	treatment
gm	gram	s̄	without
gr	grain	sc	subcutaneous
gt/gtt	drop/drops	SG	specific gravity
h	hour	SOB	shortness of breath
Hct	hematocrit	stat	immediately
Hgb	hemoglobin	subq	subcutaneous
HS	hour of sleep	s̄s̄	one-half
H & P	history and physical	tab	tablet
I & O	intake and output	TCH	turn, cough
IM	intramuscular	tid	three times a day
IV	intravenous	TKO	to keep open
lb	pound	TPR	temperature, pulse, respiration
LLQ	left lower quadrant	UA	urinalysis
LP	lumbar puncture	URI	upper respiratory infection
LUQ	left upper quadrant	VS	vital signs
mg (mgm)	milligram	w/c	wheel chair
ml	milliliter	wt	weight

↑	Increase		∴	Therefore
↓	Decrease		♂	Male
>	Greater than		♀	Female
<	Less than		°	Degree
×	Times		#	Number
=	Equal to		ʒ	Dram
≠	Not equal to, unequal		℥	Ounce
1°	Primary		@	At
2°	Secondary			

Figure 8–3. Symbols used in health care records.

brief as possible. Although no one is suggesting that the nurse write pages, it is important that significant data not be excluded to achieve brevity. For example, if a patient is complaining of pain, the nurse notes the time, describes the pain, and actions taken to relieve the pain. Later, the nurse makes a notation regarding the effectiveness of the pain-relief measures. This documentation does take more time than merely documenting that a pain medication was given on the medication record,

Table 8–3. **Common Prefixes and Suffixes Used in Medical Terminology**

Prefixes

a-, an-	not or without		hypo-	deficiency
ab-	away from		inter-	between
ad-	toward		intra-	within
adeno-	gland		kines-	movement
ambi-	both		leuko-	white
ante-	before		macro-	large
anti-	against		mal-	bad
bi-	double		mega-	large
brady-	slow		melano-	black
cardio-	heart		micro-	small
cephal-	head		myo-	muscle
circum-	around		neo-	new
contra-	against		nephro-	kidney
dent-	teeth		ped-	foot
derma-	skin		per-	through
dis-	apart		peri-	around
dorso-	back		phlebo-	vein
dys-	difficult		photo-	light
en-	within		post-	after
ex-	outside		pre-	before
eryth-	red		pseudo-	false
ferro-	iron		pyo-	pus
gastro-	stomach		pyro-	fever
glyco-	sugar		reno-	kidney
hemi-	half		steno-	narrow
hepato-	liver		sub-	under
hydro-	water		tachy-	fast
hyper-	excess		trans-	across

Suffixes

-algia	pain		-oma	tumor
-ase	enzyme		-ostomy	opening
-cele	tumor/swelling		-otomy	incision
-ectomy	surgical removal		-penia	lack of
-emesis	vomit		-phobia	fear
-emia	blood		-phylaxis	prevention
-esthesia	sensation		-plasty	repair
-itis	inflammation		-rhea	flow
-lith	stone		-scopy	examine visually
-lysis	destroy		-uria	urine
-megaly	enlargement			

Table 8-4. **Guides for Determining When Written Documentation Is Required**

1. Chart any time the patient's condition warrants it.
2. Admission data must be recorded as soon as possible after the patient is admitted.
3. Record medication administration as soon as possible.
4. If the patient leaves the nursing unit for surgery, diagnostic studies, specialist consultation or examination, make a notation in the chart before the patient leaves and upon the patient's return. Relevant observations might include method of transportation, fatigue or pain assessment, blood pressure, pulse, and temperature readings, or expressed concerns of the patient.
5. Record any unusual or untoward incident, the resultant nurse actions, and patient responses promptly and completely. This might include such examples as a patient fall in the bathroom, an incident of vomiting, a drop in blood pressure that is greatly different from the previous recording, or an episode of blood in the urine.
6. Document anytime the nurse gives care, treatments, or makes an assessment of the patient. The nurse may occasionally feel that it is a waste of time to chart when nothing noteworthy was observed. Often nurses check a patient who had surgery during the day hourly or more frequently in the first few hours postoperatively. Although charting these observations may seem repetitious, if the patient should suddenly start bleeding or have difficulty breathing, the status of the patient preceding the hemorrhage is well documented. This frequent documentation also would establish that the nurse had not neglected the patient.

but it is much more useful in assessing the patient's condition. It may be that the patient requires a different medication if the first was found ineffective in relieving the pain, or that a different method of pain relief is needed. Thorough documentation provides the data to support that decision.

5. Document events chronologically: what happened first, next, and last. This is especially important if changes are occurring rapidly in the patient's condition or treatments.

6. Sign each recording and include the first initial, last name, and the title of the person making the notation. Such signatures might read, "J. Smith, R.N." or S. Jones, S.N." The "S.N." designates student nurse.

7. Use only approved abbreviations. There are many abbreviations used within the medical professions to shorten written communications. Convenient as these abbreviations are, they can be equally confusing. Table 8-2 lists common medical abbreviations. Figure 8-3 lists symbols commonly used in health care records. Each institution and clinical area will have a list of acceptable abbreviations for use within the facility. Abbreviations may be easily confused. Consider the abbreviation "po." This may be interpreted as *per os*, meaning by mouth, as phone order, or as post operative (Robinson, 1978). Seek clarification when in doubt about the meaning of an abbreviation or symbol.

Table 8-3 is a list of common prefixes and suffixes used in medical terminolgy.

Where to document within the chart is determined by the kinds of chart forms available and the system of charting used within the institution. When to chart also reflects institutional policies but includes some profes-

sional judgments by the nurse. The usual rule is to chart anytime the condition of the patient warrants it. This may include times when the nurse observes progress or deterioration in the patient's condition. It may include observations recorded as subjective data about the patient's feelings, worries, or mental health. It is important to include both the presence and absence of signs. An example of this is the charting done on a patient in a leg cast. It is important to record whether the patient is able to move toes on request or is unable to do so. The presence or the absence of these signs is an indication of the quality of blood circulation in the leg. Absence of sensation or unusual sensations are also recorded.

When to chart is usually covered by institutional policy. This specifies the minimum amount that must be done in order to document adequately patient care and serve as a legal safeguard for the nurse. Table 8-4 contains guides that may be used by the nurse in deciding when written documentation is necessary.

Legal Responsibilities in Charting

The most important purpose of documentation is to provide communication that improves patient care. But additionally, there are several guidelines the nurse can follow to assure that charting meets legal requirements.

1. *Never erase* on a chart. To do so could result in an accusation of altering medical records. If an error is made, either circle the mistake or draw a line though the mistake, and write "error," adding the date and your signature.

2. *Never alter* charting once it has been written in

the chart. Occasionally a nurse may be asked by a supervisor to remove charting that may reflect poorly on the hospital or that may be felt to be improper. Once documentation is in the chart, it is permanent. To alter the chart is to make oneself vulnerable to charges of fraud, misrepresentation, or possibly the criminal charge of obstruction of justice (Hemelt and Mackert, 1978). The nurse may use only the method of correcting errors described above. This method does not obliterate the charting but still leaves it readable. It has happened that a nurse will chart an entry on one patient in another patient's chart. In this case, the whole section is crossed out, leaving it legible, "error wrong patient" written, and signed.

3. *Do not leave blanks* in the record. A nurse entering a note in the record begins immediately following the last entry. When completed, the nurse draws a line to the right to fill in any blank space, leaving enough room for a legal signature. This format also assures that no one else may alter a record at a later date.

4. *Understand what is meant by countersigning.* To countersign means to "place one's signature to a writing already signed by another to attest to the authenticity of that writing" (Hemelt and Mackert, 1978). In some institutions, nurse aides are not permitted to chart, although they perform many tasks that require documentation. The registered nurse is required to chart these activities, often without any personal knowledge of them. Legal experts recommend that those who give the service should initial or sign for the service. If this is not possible, the nurse might consider adding a note to the chart which more accurately reflects the situation such as, "Care given by S. Smith, N.A. Recorded by J. Jones, R.N." Nursing instructors or other registered nurses may be required to countersign charting done by student nurses. When this is the policy, the chart must be countersigned by the responsible nurse before the student leaves the clinical area.

5. *Record only data.* Unsupported judgments and conclusions do not contribute to the quality of patient care. Statements that include "appears" or "seems" are not factual and weaken the legal value of the document. Describe the situation in clear, precise language.

6. *Avoid the use of general terms.* Be specific. Statements like "Had a good night" or "No complaints" provide no helpful information and say nothing about the nursing care that was given, or not given! Chart instead, "Slept for six hours without need of medication for sleep or pain."

7. *Chart frequently!* If several hours pass without some notation on the chart, it can legally be assumed that no one has seen the patient or provided care. Although this may not be true, it would be difficult to prove otherwise in the absence of documentation.

8. *Document the safety precautions* taken to protect the patient. This may include side rails, restraints, allergy identification bands, seizure precautions, or care of valuables the patient has brought to the hospital.

9. *Document the observations taken to prevent complications.* This indicates competent assessment of patient problems. For example, in a patient who has had abdominal surgery, the nurse notes repeatedly that the surgical dressing was clean and dry, that the blood pressure has been checked repeatedly. Both of these observations indicate that the nurse is aware of the possibility of postoperative bleeding.

Nurses' Notes

Nurses' charting, if done well, is one of the most valuable contributions to the patient's care. This record includes a statement of patient problems, often in the patient's own words, or as nursing diagnoses, as well as treatments and the response to them. There are two general forms that the nurses' notes may take: source-oriented notes (also called traditional or narrative) and problem-oriented notes (also called POMR, SOAP notes, or SOAPIER notes). Regardless of the method used, learning the skill of charting is usually an anxiety-producing task for beginning nursing students because they are unsure of what to document and the correct words to use. It may be helpful for students to write their notes on a piece of paper and have them checked by an instructor before transferring them into the permanent record. This avoids the need to correct the actual charting if the instructor feels that some of the student's charting is inappropriate.

Source-Oriented Documentation. The source-oriented record separates the professions of the health team members making the entry into the record. There are separate sheets for nurses, one for physicians, one for physical therapy, and so forth. In addition, there are separate sheets for graphing vital signs, for laboratory data, and for x-ray reports. Thus, it is necessary that a nurse collect data from several areas in the chart in order to review a patient's problem. Many nurses using this system feel that the separation of different professional notes detracts from their value as a communication tool for health team members.

Problem-Oriented Documentation. Problem-oriented documentation, developed by Weed (1968), is organized around identified patient problems. In this system, all health team members may chart on the same sheet. Although the perspective and contribution of each health care professional are different, each team member uses the same numbered problem list as a starting point. Because problem number 1 entries are labeled throughout the chart, the notes provide a complete record and plan of care for that problem. The POMR (problem-oriented medical record) has four main parts:

Data Base. Data base consists of all the information about a patient, including physical examination, nursing history, medical history, diagnostic test results, consultation reports.

Problem List. Problem list is a series, in chronological order, of identified patient problems. Any member of the health team may add a problem to the list. Space is included on this form to indicate the date of onset of the problem, as well as the date of resolution. Some agencies draw a single line through a problem to indicate that it has been resolved.

Initial Plan. Initial plan is completed as soon as possible after admission and is the beginning working plan of the health team. Each person entering a problem into the record has the responsibility of completing a plan related to it.

Progress Notes. Progress notes include both a narrative sheet and a flow sheet. The flow sheet is designed to facilitate the recording of recurring treatments or observations in a graphic form. Data are recorded in numbered sequence corresponding to the problem-list numbering. For example, if problem #1 was recorded as muscle weakness associated with insufficient exercise, there may be spaces on the flow sheet for the nurse to indicate that the patient has completed certain exercises four times each day. Another type of flow sheet might provide space for the recording of temperature, pulse, respiration, and blood pressure readings. The health team member can fill in the flow sheets to meet the specific needs of patients. Flow sheets also serve an important legal function in the absence of a progress note. An entry on the flow sheet indicates that the patient was seen and observed by a member of the staff, a fact that might be difficult to prove in the absence of documentation. (See Figure 8–4.)

Progress or narrative notes are added by the various health team members as required by the patient's condition. All members of the health team add progress notes on the same type of sheet. Progress notes are numbered to correspond to the problems in the problem list and are written in a specific format designated by the acronym: SOAP or SOAPIER.

S = subjective data. These include any statements made by the patient pertaining to an identified problem on the problem list.

O = objective data. These include the data observed by the health team member related to the same problem.

A = assessment or analysis of the data. This is usually a brief statement of interpretation of data. This may change as the patient's condition changes.

P = plan for action based on the above data. The original plan is written by the person entering the problem into the record. All subsequent plans are revisions entered into the progress notes. The plan includes the activities being done to resolve a particular problem. The plan may be to terminate certain activities if the problem is resolved, or to begin new activities if the problem is not improving.

I = implementation or intervention. This records activites in the plan that were actually done for the patient. This must be extremely specific.

E = evaluation. This is the documentation of the patient's response to the plan. This should be stated in behavioral terms. What did the patient see, do, or say as a response to the plan? Based on patient behavior, was the plan successful in lessening or alleviating the problem identified in the assessment?

R = revision or reassessment. Based on the notation and decisions in the evaluation, this note will include any changes in the original plan that must be made. There may be additional data that are now available, or the condition of the patient may have either improved or deteriorated. All the letters of the SOAPIER format will not be included in each recording. At times, it will be helpful to make a notation as to why a portion is missing. Many institutions use only the SOAP format, omitting the last three entries I, E, and R.

There are several advantages to the use of the POMR. In this approach, the patient's problems are the focus of the team which includes many health disciplines. Because problems are not eliminated from the problem list until resolved, this approach assures that problems will not be inadvertently forgotten or omitted. In addition, this approach makes certain that the patient's view is solicited as the S, the first step in the process. Evaluation of patient care is also easier in this system when problems and interventions are so clearly identified. Each professional has access to the assessments and plans of the rest of the team and may contribute to identified problems, thus ensuring a comprehensive approach. Communication among team members is facilitated since all members use the same record. The problem-oriented record is being rapidly adopted by health care institutions and being modified to meet the unique needs of each setting.

Other Written Documentation. While providing care for a patient, the nurse may find it necessary to complete other documents. These might include:

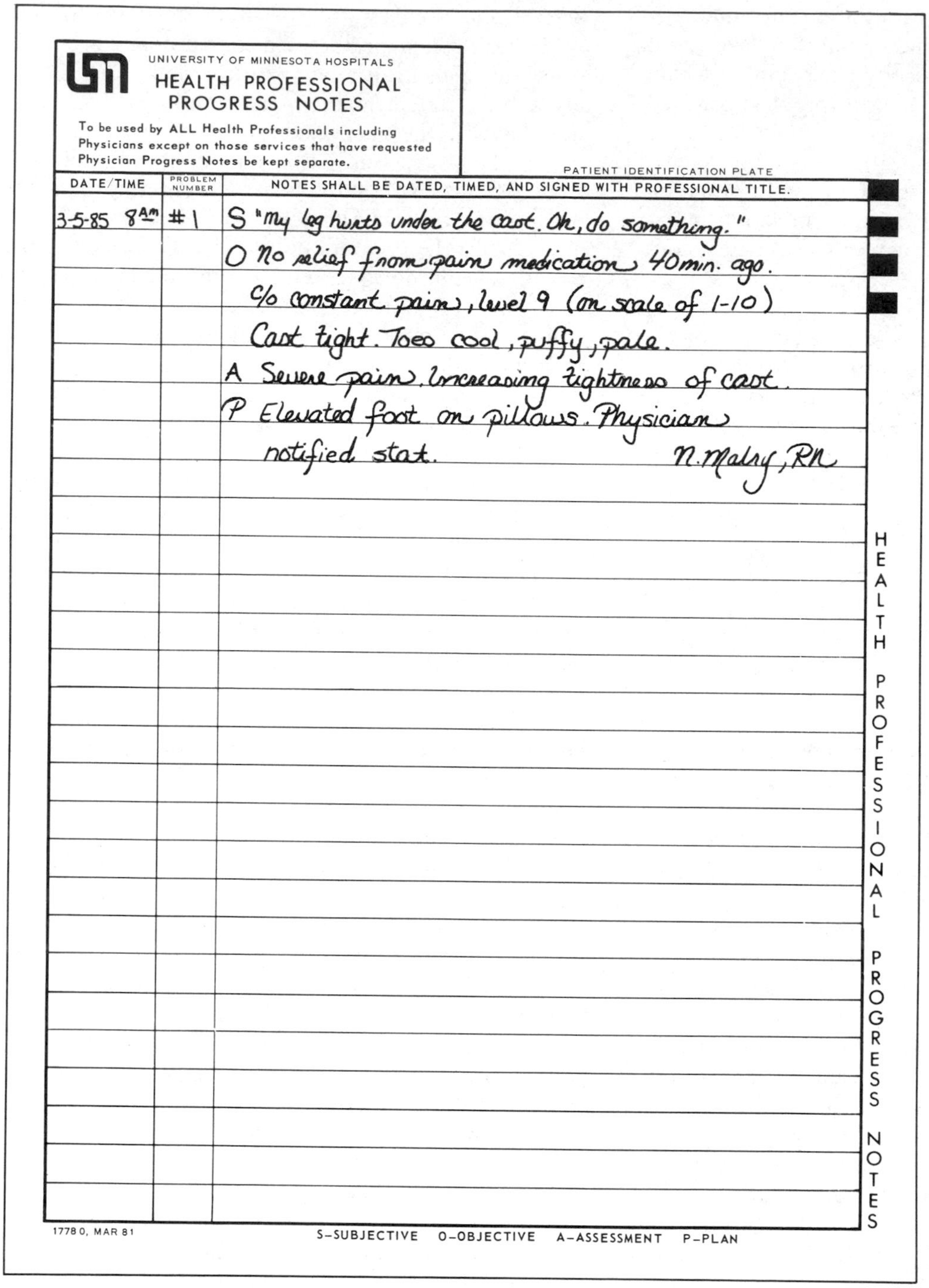

UNIVERSITY OF MINNESOTA HOSPITALS
HEALTH PROFESSIONAL PROGRESS NOTES
To be used by ALL Health Professionals including Physicians except on those services that have requested Physician Progress Notes be kept separate.

PATIENT IDENTIFICATION PLATE

DATE/TIME	PROBLEM NUMBER	NOTES SHALL BE DATED, TIMED, AND SIGNED WITH PROFESSIONAL TITLE.
3-5-85 8AM	#1	S "My leg hurts under the cast. Oh, do something."
		O No relief from pain medication 40 min. ago.
		c/o constant pain, level 9 (on scale of 1-10)
		Cast tight. Toes cool, puffy, pale.
		A Severe pain. Increasing tightness of cast.
		P Elevated foot on pillows. Physician
		notified stat. N. Malry, RN

HEALTH PROFESSIONAL PROGRESS NOTES

17780, MAR 81

S–SUBJECTIVE O–OBJECTIVE A–ASSESSMENT P–PLAN

Figure 8-4. Example of nurses' notes in the SOAP format. (Courtesy of the University of Minnesota Hospitals, Minneapolis, MN.)

NURSING KARDEX. This is an abbreviated written plan of care which contains all the nursing care for a particular patient. Whatever the format of the Kardex, it serves as a quick reference point for the nurse at times when using the patient chart would be inconvenient or cumbersome, such as at a change-of-shift report. At some institutions, the Kardex is written in ink, signed with the name and title of the person making the entry, and retained as part of the permanent record. In other agencies, the Kardex is written in pencil, viewed as a worksheet, and not saved as part of the patient's record.

MEDICATION KARDEX. Although not used in all agencies, this Kardex contains the current listing of all the medications the patient is receiving. This may be kept in the medication preparation area so nurses pre-

UNIVERSITY OF MINNESOTA HOSPITALS & CLINICS
INCIDENT REPORT

NAME OF PERSON INVOLVED (LAST / FIRST / M.I.)	AGE	SEX	INCIDENT DATE	INCIDENT TIME	INCIDENT LOCATION (AREA AND ROOM#)
MARINS SUSAN L.	46	F	1/3/85	10:30 [X] AM [ ] PM	UTILITY ROOM 3-SOUTH

CATEGORY OF PERSON INVOLVED: [ ] PATIENT → UH# — CONDITION [ ] AMBULATORY [ ] UP WITH HELP [ ] BEDREST [ ] SEDATED; [ ] EMPLOYEE → JOB TITLE — DEPARTMENT; [X] OTHER → SPECIFY (E.G., VISITOR, VOLUNTEER, ETC.) VOLUNTEER — HOME PHONE (AREA CODE) (638) 249-7013

GENERAL TYPE OF INCIDENT: [X] INJURY / FATALITY; [ ] THEFT (CALL SECURITY IMMEDIATELY); [ ] PROPERTY / FACILITY DAMAGE; [ ] PATIENT PROPERTY OR VALUABLES; [ ] MEDICATION ERROR; [ ] DEFECTIVE PRODUCT; [ ] POTENTIAL HAZARD; [ ] ADVERSE DRUG REACTION; [ ] OTHER (SPECIFY) ______

DESCRIPTION OF INCIDENT - PLEASE OBJECTIVELY DESCRIBE ALL INCIDENTS IN THIS SPACE. IN ADDITION, A CHECKLIST HAS BEEN PROVIDED FOR MEDICATIONS, FALLS AND LABORATORY-RELATED INCIDENTS FOR YOUR CONVENIENCE. CONTINUE ON REVERSE IF NECESSARY.

Ms. Marins was removing flowers from a container at the request of a patient. She cut her hand (R) on the wire inside the container when attempting to remove it. Seen by Dr Jones in the employee health service. Received four stitches on (R) index finger and a tetanus booster. Ms. Marins states, "This was my own fault. I really was careless."

CHECK HERE IF CONTINUED ON BACK [ ]

MEDICATION RELATED INCIDENTS

TYPE (CHECK ALL THAT APPLY): [ ] DIFFERENT MED/DOSE/SOLUTION ARRIVED ON STATION; [ ] DIFFERENT MEDICATION GIVEN; [ ] DIFFERENT DOSAGE GIVEN; [ ] MED. GIVEN TO DIFFERENT PATIENT; [ ] MED. GIVEN AT DIFFERENT TIME; [ ] MED. GIVEN BY DIFFERENT ROUTE; [ ] MEDICATION OMITTED; [ ] OTHER ______

STEPS WHICH MAY HAVE CONTRIBUTED TO INCIDENT (CHECK ALL THAT APPLY): [ ] ORDERING MEDICATION; [ ] TRANSCRIBING ORDER; [ ] LABELING MEDICATION; [ ] READING MEDICATION LABEL; [ ] COMPARING LABEL W/MED KARDEX; [ ] CHECKING PATIENT I.D. BAND; [ ] GIVING MEDICATION; [ ] PATIENT DISREGARDED INSTRUCTIONS; [ ] OTHER ______

INTRAVENOUS FLUIDS (CHECK ALL THAT APPLY): [ ] TOO FAST; [ ] TOO SLOW; [ ] DIFFERENT SOLUTION; [ ] DIFFERENT ADDITIVE; [ ] DIFF. ADMINISTRATIVE APPARATUS; [ ] I.V. INFILTRATED; [ ] OTHER ______

INCIDENTS INVOLVING FALLS

TYPE OF FALL: [ ] FROM COMMODE; [ ] FROM WHEELCHAIR; [ ] FROM CHAIR; [ ] FROM BED; [ ] OTHER ______

ACTIVITY AT TIME OF INCIDENT: [ ] WALKING ALONE; [ ] WALKING ASSISTED; [ ] TRANSFER ALONE; [ ] TRANSFER ASSISTED; [ ] SITTING UP; [ ] LYING DOWN; [ ] OTHER ______

CIRCUMSTANCES (CHECK ALL THAT APPLY): [ ] SLIPPERY WALKING SURFACE; [ ] TRIPPED; [ ] FAINTED; [ ] LOSS OF BALANCE; [ ] SEIZURE; [ ] DISREGARDED INSTRUCTIONS; [ ] OTHER ______

LABORATORY RELATED INCIDENTS

TYPE OF INCIDENTS: [ ] RESULTS REPORTED INCORRECTLY; [ ] SPECIMEN HANDLED IMPROPERLY; [ ] RESPONSE TIME; [ ] MISLABELED SPECIMEN →; [ ] UNLABELED SPECIMEN →; [ ] OTHER ______; STATION/CLINIC SENDING SPECIMEN WAS; PHLEBOTOMIST WAS

PHYSICIAN NOTIFIED? [X] YES [ ] NO — IF YES, NAME: J.E. Jones, M.D. — SIGNATURE: X J.E. Jones
PHYSICIAN'S FINDINGS: Laceration (R) index finger. Cleansed, sutured. Tetanus Toxoid 0.5 ml. IM — CHECK HERE IF CONTINUED ON BACK [ ]

PERSON COMPLETING — SIGNATURE: X M. L. Fransen, R.N. — TITLE: H.N. 3-South — DATE: 1/3/85 — PHONE: 289-1604

UH 1038, APR 81

Please forward to Box 708 Mayo within 24 hours.

Figure 8–5. Example of incident report. (Courtesy of the University of Minnesota Hospitals, Minneapolis, MN.)

paring medications may use it as a safeguard to check medications prior to administration to patients.

Incident Reports. This document is used when an unusual event, action, or situation occurs within the agency setting. The most frequent events requiring such documentation are medication errors and patient falls. Events involving possible injury to a patient's relatives or visitors also require this documentation. This might include the spouse of the patient who slipped and fell on a wet floor, or who entangled an arm in an electric bed. This report includes a brief, clear, concise statement of what happened, observations of the results to the parties involved, any subjective statements of the involved parties, who was notified, actions taken by the nurse, and perhaps how the incident might have been prevented. It is not appropriate to assess blame or make accusations in these reports, only the facts are necessary. Nurses do make mistakes and accidents do happen. This record provides documentation of incidents for insurance purposes and for identification of repeatedly unsafe settings, activities, or personnel. The worst mistake, legally and ethically, is to attempt to cover up a mistake. This may cause additional harm to the patient and more severe legal implications for the nurse. (See Figure 8–5.)

INFORMED CONSENT. This document is a written acknowledgment that the patient has been informed, in language that the individual can understand, of the procedure to be performed, the risks and consequences of the procedure, and the alternatives to the procedure. This explanation is to be done by the physician. The nurse does not have the authority or knowledge to interpret medical findings and discuss alternatives. The nurse may witness a consent form, but this only means that the nurse is witnessing the patient's signature, something anyone may do. The patient does have the right, however, to withdraw consent up to the time of the procedure. In this case, the nurse is obligated to inform the physician of the patient's changed decision.

RELEASE OF INFORMATION. This document is frequently used for the purpose of providing information to insurance companies which require the information prior to payment. This may also be used for press releases. A variation of this form may be used to grant permission for patient data to be used in research.

REFERRAL SUMMARY. The nurse may complete a referral summary when the patient is being discharged and transferred to another institution. This is frequently the case when patients are to be discharged from the hospital to a nursing home setting or when a public health nurse may visit the patient at home. This summary may include such things as eating and sleep habits, method of ambulation, current medications and treatments that are to be continued, family support, religious preferences, and life-style choices. Any active health care problems are documented and the current plan recorded. This exchange of information between agencies helps to provide better care for patients.

Verbal Communication

Verbal communication among health care professionals is another method of contributing to patient care. Like written documentation, verbal communication must be factual, concise, and descriptive. Formal verbal communication among professionals includes the change-of-shift report, physicians' telephone orders, physicians' verbal orders, patient care conferences, and nursing staff conferences.

Change-of-Shift Report

At the end of each duty period, usually every 8, 10, or 12 hours, the nurse who is leaving is responsible for reviewing the events of the shift with the oncoming nurse. This may be done in a variety of ways. Some agencies require that each nurse tape-record the patient report. This tape is then played for the oncoming staff. Although this method has the advantage that the tape can be repeated for clarity or latecomers, it has the disadvantage of not permitting questioning of the reporting nurse. Because the reporting nurse can edit the report or retape any part that was unclear, this method usually results in an efficient report. A more traditional method involves the responsible nurse giving a report on all the patients cared for by the team members. This necessitates that previously all team members have reported to the team leader. The obvious disadvantage to this method is that the information given to the oncoming shift is already second hand. In still another method, one nurse reports directly to a second nurse who will be responsible for the patient care during the next duty period. This ensures the maximum opportunity to ask questions and plan for the nursing care to continue. Other agencies prefer to use "walking rounds." In this method, the nurse who has cared for the patient during the day is accompanied by the oncoming nurse, and the report is given at the patient's bedside. The nurse is introduced to the patient, and the brief report is given. A patient may add something the nurse has omitted or may ask a question that suggests some teaching or additional information is indicated. Some nurses express concern over talking about the patient in front of the patient. Most patients are fully informed about their conditions and treatments, and usually nothing is said in report that patients do not already know, and some things can be clarified by the patient. Moreover, this open discussion serves to enhance the trust between the nurse and the patient.

Giving a Verbal Report

Whatever method of reporting is used, the nurse develops the skill of both giving and receiving a verbal report. A verbal report is concise and to the point. It is brief but still contains all the necessary information. The report is presented in a clear voice, loud enough to be easily understood, and slow enough to permit necessary note taking. The following suggestions may serve as a guide for oral reporting.

1. Establish a format so listeners are ready for what they will hear. This may include name of patient, admitting medical diagnosis or chief complaint, attending physician, diagnostic procedures completed that day, condition of the patient, and responses to treatments and medications. Some nurses may include reminders to the next nurse regarding observations or specific treatments to be completed during the next shift.

2. Use a logical order or sequence for the report of several patients. Some nurses follow the order of the patient rooms, others follow the practice of reporting on the most seriously ill patient first.

3. Use the SOAP format to organize the report on a particular patient. For example:

S = Susie Jones complains of a sore throat, no appetite
O = Red throat, enlarged tonsils, temperature 103.2 F (39.8 C)
A = Possible streptococcal infection
P = Treat as contagious until culture is back
TYLENOL is to be given for fever
I = TYLENOL elixir 2 tsp at 1200
Sleeping for past two hours
Culture sent to lab

4. Respect patient confidentiality. Be guided by the criterion: do team members need this data in order to give care to the patient? If the answer is yes, the data are to be included in the report. If the answer is no, the data are best omitted.

5. Be specific, exact, and brief! Although brevity is admirable, the report is as long as necessary to include the essential data.

Receiving a Verbal Report

Nurses beginning a shift or duty period receive a report on the patients for whom they will be providing care. In addition, they have a general awareness of the condition of all the patients in the immediate area in order that they will be able to assist both other patients and staff as necessary. Prior to beginning report, the patients the nurse will be caring for are identified. This information is recorded on a worksheet that hospitals usually provide for this purpose. If no worksheet is available, the nurse uses any blank paper with lines or boxes drawn as needed. While listening to the report,

the nurse takes notes about assigned patients. This might include such things as ability to ambulate, time of last pain medication, preparation or follow-through needed for diagnostic procedures or test results. In addition, the nurse may jot down relevant information about other patients in the area that may be helpful. This information will help the nurse who is not the primary care-giver to give safe assistance to patients. After the completion of the oral report, the nurse will check the Kardex of each of the assigned patients in order to complete the worksheet. The Kardex will provide medication schedules, nursing and medical treatments, and the care plan for the patient. The nurse uses the combination verbal report and the Kardex to organize and plan the care of the patients.

Physicians' Telephone Orders

Frequently the physician is not able to be present to write orders in the patient record and will request that a nurse accept an order over the telephone. If such a request is made of a student nurse, the correct response is, "I am a nursing student and am not authorized to accept a telephone order. Please wait and I will find a registered nurse to help you." The registered nurse will then record the physician's order on the order sheet of the chart with the additional notation, "Telephone order of Dr. Smith recorded by J. Jones, R.N." The nurse then reads the order back to the physician for verification. The nurse may then carry out the order. The physician is required to sign the order at the earliest time possible, usually within 24 hours.

Physicians' Verbal Orders

During the course of working with physicians to provide patient care, the nurse is frequently asked to accept their verbal orders. This might be the case when the nurse is making rounds with a physician who asks, while at the patient's bedside, "Would you discontinue the IV, start a low-sodium, clear-liquid diet, and give a daily multivitamin." This may or may not be interpreted by the nurse as an order and is generally confusing. The nurse requests that the physician write the order. This avoids confusion and assures that the patient receives the necessary care.

In the case of an emergency situation where speed is crucial, common sense must prevail. If, for example, a patient has a cardiac arrest, the physician may give fast and frequent verbal orders. The nurse responds to the orders as rapidly as possible. When preparing medications, the nurse repeats out loud the medicine and the dose before giving it or before passing it to the physician for administration. The nurse notes the time and amount of the medications given on a note pad. (In some institutions, the second or third nurse to arrive at the scene of the emergency routinely assumes the re-cording function.) This information is necessary to remind everyone of the time and the amount of specific medications so an overdose or an inadequate dose does not occur. When the emergency treatment is completed, the nurse and the physician must document the events and the medications on the chart.

Patient Care Conferences

Members of the health team may meet either on a regularly scheduled basis or as a patient situation requires to discuss and plan the care of a patient. The skills studied in the group communication chapter are helpful to the nurse in working within this group. (See Chapter 7.) Often this group functions as a problem-solving group, working together to discover solutions to complex problems in patient care. Such a conference may be requested by any member of the health team. Frequently, a group of nurses may meet to discuss only the nursing care needs of a particular patient. Either of these meetings, of the nursing staff or of the health team, is usually begun with a brief summary of the patient's history. Current problems are then identified. The majority of the time is spent producing alternative approaches and deciding which to implement. The pa-

tient may be asked to be present and contribute to the plan of care. The patient care conference usually results in a written plan of care for the patient.

Although student nurses frequently attend these conferences as part of their learning experiences, they may be reluctant to make their opinions or contributions known in these groups. There is a great deal of perceived risk involved in speaking in such a group. However, student nurses often have more time to spend with a single patient than does a staff nurse. Students are likely to know the patient well and are able to make an excellent contribution. At first, students may be comfortable contributing only data rather than problem identification and solutions. However, this is a first step, and the student may be able to make additional contributions in the next conference.

Staff Conferences

Nurses working together often choose, or are required by administration, to meet on a regular basis to discuss work-related matters, changes being considered, or other things that affect the work environment. This is another form of verbal communication within the health team. The same group skills learned in Chapter 7 are used here to facilitate communication.

Summary

Communication among members of the health team is important because it contributes to the quality of patient care. This communication includes both written documentation and verbal reporting functions. Both aspects have ethical and legal implications. Documentation of health care can take the form of either traditional source-oriented records or problem-oriented medical records. Verbal reporting functions include both receiving and giving a verbal report as well as taking verbal physicians' orders. Patient care conferences and staff conferences are additional forms of professional verbal communication.

Assertive communication skills are presented as a means of maintaining self-respect and conveying respect for others.

Terms for Review

aggressive communication	countersign	POMR	SOAPIER
assertiveness skills	documentation	problem-oriented record	source-oriented record
audit	nonassertive communication	SOAP	standards of care

Self-Assessment

1. The following samples of charting are taken from the case of an 11-year-old boy admitted after surgical reduction of a fractured radius. Read the charting and identify each error. Explain what is wrong with the documentation. (The lines have been numbered on the left for the purpose of identification.)

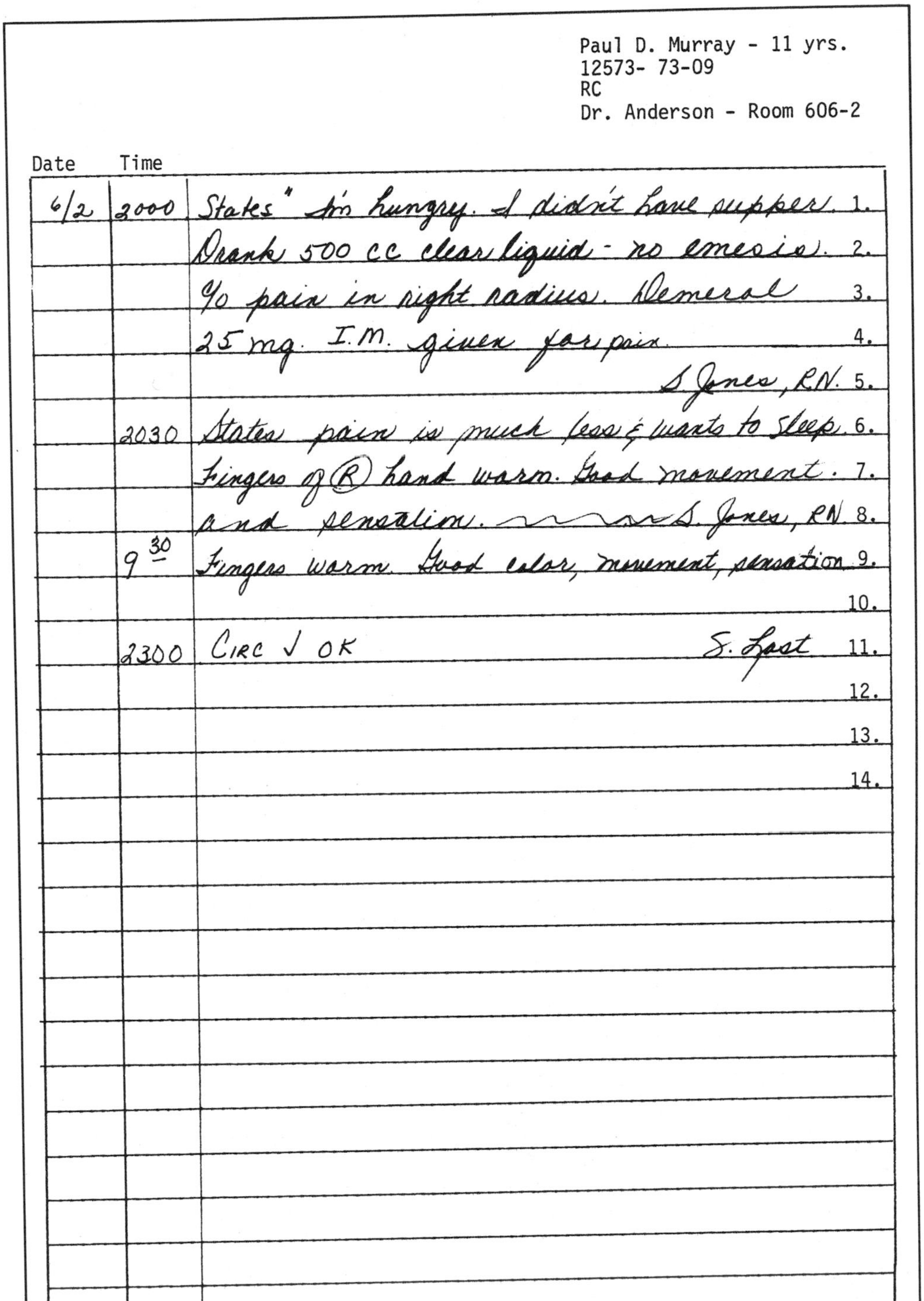

```
                                    Paul D. Murray - 11 yrs.
                                    12573- 73-09
                                    RC
                                    Dr. Anderson - Room 606-2
```

Date	Time		
6/2	2000	States "I'm hungry. I didn't have supper.	1.
		Drank 500 cc clear liquid - no emesis.	2.
		No pain in right radius. Demerol	3.
		25 mg. I.M. given for pain.	4.
		S. Jones, RN.	5.
	2030	States pain is much less & wants to sleep.	6.
		Fingers of (R) hand warm. Good movement.	7.
		and sensation. S. Jones, RN	8.
	9³⁰	Fingers warm. Good color, movement, sensation	9.
			10.
	2300	Circ ✓ OK S. Last	11.
			12.
			13.
			14.

Figure 8-6. Sample charting #1. (Courtesy of Rochester Methodist Hospital, Rochester, MN.)

PATIENT PROGRESS NOTES
ROCHESTER METHODIST HOSPITAL
ROCHESTER, MINNESOTA

SHEET NO.

Paul D. Murray - 11yrs.
12573-73-09
RC
Dr. Anderson - Room 606-2

ROOM 606=2   NAME Paul D. Murray   CLINIC NO. 12573-73-09   DR. Anderson

DATE	TIME	PROBLEM/NEED		
6/2	2000	#1 Fracture ℝ arm	S = fracture ℝ radius c̄ surgical reduction.	1.
			O = "my arm hurts"	2.
			A = Pain related to fracture and immobility	3.
			P = Follow nursing care plan.	4.
			I = Demerol given for pain.	5.
			S. Jones, RN.	6.
	2030		O = Fingers warm, pink, good sensation and movement. S. Jones RN.	7.
				8.
				9.

S—SUBJECTIVE
O—OBJECTIVE
A—ASSESSMENT
P—PLAN
NURSING RECORD

Figure 8–7. Sample charting #2. (Courtesy of Rochester Methodist Hospital, Rochester, MN.)

Answers

Sample #1
1. Correct
2. Correct
3. Correct
4. Blank space
5. Blank space
6. Correct
7. Correct
8. Correct
9. Wrong use of time
10. Blank space
11. Very general
    Blank space
    No title on signature

Sample # 2
1. Objective data
2. Subjective data
3. Correct
4. Correct
5. Not specific
6. E is missing
7. Belongs in flow sheet

Learning Activities

After reading each of the following summaries, document the situations as you judge necessary, indicating which forms you would use and writing out the necessary information.

Situation 1. Mrs. Jones is a 70-year-old retired postal worker. She lives at home with her husband and is independent in all activities of daily living. Dr. J. Hurst admitted Mrs. Jones after she complained of rectal bleeding, weight loss, and feeling "bloated." Although you had instructed Mrs. Jones to call a nurse if she wished assistance to the bathroom in the night, she stated, "I am very capable of caring for myself." At 2 A.M. the signal lighter from Mrs. Jones's bathroom is on, and you enter to find that she has tripped and fallen, hitting her head on the sink. She states, "No harm done. I'm going to have a real egg on my head. I guess I should have called you."

Situation 2. You, the registered nurse, are returning to duty after two weeks' vacation. The evening is very busy with several new patients to be admitted and other seriously ill patients. After administering medications at 8 P.M. (2000 hours), you realize that there are two Mr. Smiths on the unit: Joseph Smith, a patient of Dr. Meast admitted with diabetes, and John Smith, a patient of Dr. Ward admitted with a peptic ulcer. You mistakenly gave Joseph Smith the medication that should have been given to John Smith: methantheline bromide 75 mg (BANTHINE).

Situation 3. Mrs. Smith's relatives have visited her and are leaving at 3 P.M. There is a delay in the arrival of the elevator and they decide to walk down the steps. From the hallway you hear a scream and you hurry to investigate. Joan Henly, Mrs. Smith's 45-year-old daughter, has slipped on a candy wrapper which was on the step and fallen 15 steps to a landing. She states, "I didn't see the paper until it was too late. It was just like wax—zoom! I can't move my leg. It hurts too much."

Review Questions

1. Standards of nursing care are
   a. An individualized nursing care plan
   b. Required by law for each patient in an acute care facility
   c. A description of what would be safe, competent, reasonable care for a patient with a certain condition
   d. Part of a performance review of an individual nurse
2. The most important reason for clear documentation and reporting is
   a. Legal protection of the nurse
   b. Providing data for cost analyses of health care
   c. Providing important data for medical research
   d. Providing quality patient care
3. A nurse is required to give testimony in a court of law. The nurse refuses to discuss certain matters claiming that to do so would violate the nurse-patient relationship. Which statement best describes the stance of the nurse?
   a. The nurse is an uncooperative witness and may face contempt charges.
   b. The nurse claims that the matter involves a privileged communication that the court cannot require be breached.
   c. The nurse may be guilty of slander or libel if the information is revealed.
   d. The nurse is under oath to reveal the whole truth.
4. A nursing student answers the telephone during a busy time on a medical unit. Dr. I. Markeln requests that the student take a telephone order since he is in an extreme rush. He states that he will accept responsibility for her action. The student
   a. States, "I will find an R.N. to take the order immediately."
   b. Writes the order and reads it back to the physician for verification.
   c. "I'm sure my instructor will approve just this once."
   d. Hangs up and breaks the connection.
5. When using the POMR method of documentation, where would the following be placed: "My mother died of cancer and now I think that I have it too."
   a. S
   b. O
   c. A
   d. P

Answers

1. c
2. d
3. b
4. a
5. a

Suggested Readings

Begerson, S.: Charting with a jury in mind. *Nurs. Life*, **2:**30–33, Aug., 1983.

An attorney describes how a jury interprets a chart.

Eilers, K.: How to stand up for yourself and get away with it. *Nurs. Life*, **3:**46–49, July/Aug., 1983.

A nurse describes verbal and non-verbal assertiveness techniques. A self-assessment quiz is included.

Kunkel, J.: Charting: Some pointers for doing it better. *Nurs. Life*, **3:**57–64, Mar./Apr. 1983.

A nurse identifies common charting mistakes and offers suggestions for how to avoid them.

References and Bibliography

American Nurses' Association: *Perspectives On the Code for Nurses.* ANA Publication Code G-132, Kansas City, Mo., 1978.

Hemelt, M., and Mackert, M.: *Dynamics of Law in Nursing and Health Care.* Reston Publishing Co., Reston, Va., 1978.

Herman, S.: *Becoming Assertive.* Van Nostrand, New York, 1978.

Muldary, T.: *Interpersonal Relations for Health Professionals.* Macmillan, New York, 1983.

Murchison, I; Nichols, T.; and Hanson, R.: *Legal Accountability in the Nursing Process.* Mosby, St. Louis, 1978.

Robinson, J. (ed.): *Documenting Patient Care Responsibly.* Nursing Skillbook Series. Springhouse Corporation, Springhouse, Pa., 1978.

Sarath, M.; Auerbach, M.; and Bogue, T.: *Medical Records: Getting Yours.* Public Citizen's Health Research Group, Washington, D.C., 1980.

Tucker, S.; Breeding, M.; Canobbio, M.; Paquette, E.; Wells, M.; and Willmann, M. E.: *Patient Care Standards.* Mosby, St. Louis, 1980.

Weed, L.: Medical records that guide and teach. *New Engl. J. Med.*, **278:** 593–600, 1968.

CHAPTER 9

THE TEACHING-LEARNING PROCESS

The Nurse and the Teaching Role

Teaching and Learning Defined

Student/Teacher Ratios in Teaching
  Individual Teaching
  Small Group Teaching
  Large Group Teaching
  Teaching Through the Media

Benefits of Patient Teaching
  Independence
  Maintenance of Optimum Health Status
  Cost Reduction
  Decreased Severity of Illness
  Decreased Anxiety

Inadequate Teaching—Legal and Ethical Aspects

Developing Teaching Skills

Flexibility and Rigidity

Motivation for Learning

Types of Learning—Cognitive, Affective, Psychomotor

Principles Related to Learning

The Process of Teaching
  Identifying Problems Related to Unmet Learning Needs
  Assessment of the Learner
  Developing Learning Goals
  Selecting Teaching Methods
  Implementing the Teaching Plan
  Evaluation

Objectives

1. Identify competencies related to patient teaching appropriate to your own level of nursing education upon entrance into nursing practice.

2. Describe three characteristics of learning.

3. Contrast the concepts of teaching and learning.

4. Describe situations in which learning might best occur in the following student/teacher ratios:
   Individual patient teaching
   Small group teaching
   Large group teaching

5. Identify benefits of effective health teachings: for the patient, for the family, for the nurse, for the larger community.

6. Describe situations in which health education by the nurse may present ethical/legal concerns.

7. Discuss motivation for learning and relate it to learning needs.

8. Identify the learning principles guiding your patient teaching.

9. Identify activities of the teacher that facilitate learning.

10. Identify activities or situations that often interfere with learning.

11. Identify nursing diagnosis related to patients' learning needs.

12. Describe nursing assessment of learners that will facilitate development of a teaching plan to meet individual patients' learning needs.

13. Identify learning goals for patients with diagnosed learning needs.

14. Describe various teaching methods and the teacher preparation and responsibilities of the learner appropriate to each.

15. Describe the relationship between evaluation of learning and the learning goals.

The Nurse and the Teaching Role

Teaching is an integral part of nursing. The five roles of practice for the associate degree nurse include the role of client teacher. Roles and competencies of nursing graduates from diploma and baccalaureate degree programs contain statements regarding patient and family teaching. Competencies are descriptions of behavior expected of the individual nurse. (See Chapter 2.) There is also an expectation that the nurse will function as a teacher for various other health care personnel and assume responsibility for continued personal learning. Almost all situations involving patient care have teaching potentials. The nurse is most often concerned with helping patients and their families learn how to maintain health, restore health, or adjust, with maximum independence, to altered levels of health. Patient teaching, rather than performing treatments, is a major role for some nurses, such as in the public health field. Other areas may involve lesser amounts of teaching due to the critical status of patients' health and the priority of other needs such as oxygen, elimination, or nutrition. Teaching in these acute settings often involves simplified explanations to patients and their families. Students in nursing may find some of their earliest patient care experiences involve some form of patient teaching. The skills and confidence necessary to be a good teacher come with knowledge, experience, and the ability to take risks and try new things. This chapter will provide the student with some basic knowledge related to teaching and learning, but it is up to each individual to develop skill in teaching.

Teaching and Learning Defined

A very wise man, named Robert Mager (1968), once wrote, "If telling were teaching, we'd all be so smart we could hardly stand it." In fact, some nurses are quite surprised to discover that just telling a patient something in no way guarantees that learning will occur. Nurse faculty members have been known to comment after low examination scores, "I've taught it. Why haven't you learned it?" Students in nursing have experienced various types of teaching, some good and some not so good. But what exactly is teaching? There are many different definitions, but there seem to be several common elements. Teaching is a deliberate activity. Teaching should be purposeful and not accidental. Teaching involves developing learning goals, which are specific outcomes of learning. Planning is also part of teaching as activities and content are chosen to help learners achieve these identified goals. Teaching involves anticipating and creating a predetermined change in the learner. It may be an observable change, as when a skill such as deep breathing is taught to a patient. The change in the learner may not be observable, as when the teaching involves altering feelings or ways of thinking. *Teaching*, then, may be defined as the process of assisting the learner to change behavior in a predetermined direction.

The definition of learning often reflects the theoretical framework of the person defining it. Some people view learning in terms of a stimulus and a response. The development of the desired response is based on reinforcement (rewards.) Much of this work comes from animal studies. From this orientation, learning may be defined as an increase in the probability that a particular response will be made to a given stimulus. This concept of learning is exemplified in many preparation-for-childbirth classes, as the woman learns to begin a particular breathing pattern in response to the stimulation of the contracting uterus. There does not seem to be a lot of credit given to an individual's ability to think and reason in this type of definition.

A completely different orientation defines learning in terms of nerve cells and chemicals. For the physiologist, learning may be defined as the alterations occurring in the neurons of the brain. For a nurse working with a patient-learner, the goal of changing the structure of macromolecules within the neurons of the patient's brain is interesting but impersonal.

In a more personal definition, three elements are identified as involved in learning. First, learning is a process involving some type of change in the learner. For example, an individual may learn a completely new activity such as typing, writing, or giving an injection. The individual may learn to change a previously learned behavior, as when a student in nursing learns to make a bed using hospital corners. Learning to use good body mechanics in moving and lifting patients often involves changing previous learning. A new response to a situation is another type of change that may be the result of learning. Learning to substitute new activity for an old habit may be the goal of learning, as when people try not to overeat by going for a walk or doing some other activity.

The second element in defining learning is that the

change is a result of practice or experience and not due to a temporary physical/mental state or normal growth and maturation. Pulling your hand away from a hot object is not learning; it is a natural reflexive response. The ability to retain urine in the bladder over time is not learned but is a result of normal growth and maturation. Learning occurs when the person avoids touching the hot object or empties the bladder (voids) only in an appropriate recepticle.

The third element of learning is that its occurrence is inferred from behavioral changes in the learner. Teachers consider that learning has occurred when a student is able to answer test questions correctly. But what does that student actually understand about the material that was taught? As nurses teach patients and their families to change behavior, some of the learning that occurs is hidden. Some people feel that there is a different type of learning taking place within each student, even though all students are hearing the same material. The type and amount of learning that occurs depend on how the individual student interprets what is being taught in relation to individual needs at the time.

To summarize, *learning* is not observable but is inferred from a change in the learner's behavior which is not the result of a temporarily altered state or normal growth and maturation.

Student/Teacher Ratios in Teaching

The first clinical experience a nursing student has with a patient may involve some form of teaching. In the simplest form, the student will be answering direct patient questions. If the student is unable to answer the patient's question, the patient should be told that the student will come back later with the requested information. The student would find out the answer to the patient's question, using any of several resources available, and return to the patient with the requested information as soon as possible. An example of a more complex form of teaching involving nursing is the development and implementation of health education programs such as community classes on cardiopulmonary resuscitation. Three broad categories of teaching done by nurses are described below. These categories are based on the ratio of learners to teacher.

Individual Teaching

In this type of teaching, the nurse is involved with one person at a time. This form of teaching can be extremely individualized to a particular patient's learning needs. Individual teaching may involve simple questions and answers, or development, implementation, and evaluation of entire teaching plans. Complex skills that require a great deal of patient learning may best be taught on an individual basis. An example of this type of teaching would be helping an individual patient learn self colostomy care or home care of an intravenous infusion (IV). One-to-one teaching can be very time consuming and difficult to work into an eight-hour schedule, especially if a nurse has several patients, all requiring large amounts of care. Individual teaching may be most appropriate, in the sense of efficiency, when a patient has unique needs from other patients or has a learning disability that requires different teaching methods in comparison to most patients. One-to-one teaching is usually less threatening to a new nursing student than teaching a group. This is also true for many experienced nurses who continue to find they are uncomfortable or anxious when asked to teach groups of patients or nursing students.

Small Group Teaching

In a small group of several learners, there continues to be a good opportunity for individualizing the teaching to patients' needs, especially if the nurse is familiar with all patients in the group. The session can be quite structured or more free flowing, with patients sharing feelings, concerns, and questions. This form of teaching usually requires more planning than may occur in a spontaneous one-to-one teaching session, simply because several people and their schedules are involved. To conserve time, the meeting is set up when it is convenient for all members of the group to attend. Small group teaching allows individual patients to hear the concerns of others and perhaps the answers to questions they are afraid to ask. There is some comfort gained when people share feelings with others experiencing similar problems. Knowing they are not alone and that others share their fears may make people more willing to talk honestly about their concerns. This does not happen in individual teaching and is something to consider in planning to teach. Small group teaching can be very effective for patients and others who are trying to learn new skills such as injections or newborn bathing. Even complex skills, such as cardiopulmonary resuscitation, may be taught in small groups. The nurse is able to demonstrate and explain the skill with everyone close enough to hear and see the details. With only three or four people practicing a skill, the nurse can give enough feedback to each individual to ensure safe, effective performance with a minimum of learner and teacher frustration. A class in which inadequate guidance is provided because there are too many learners and too few teachers is a potentially negative situation. As you may remember from your first clinical experience, there just did not seem to be enough instructor time to go around, and that can be upsetting and frightening.

Large Group Teaching

Large groups are usually composed of ten or more people who feel that the nurse-teacher will be able to help meet their individual learning needs. Often, the nurse does not know the individuals. The large class has a tendency to be more formal, in the sense of more listening and less responding by the learners. A nurse may be presenting information on a very specific topic, such as nutrition, in which the patient contact is brief and limited to one session. Other large groups may meet for several weeks and cover a wider range of information and activities, as is the case in education-for-childbirth classes or diabetic teaching. Patients may not be willing to share their feelings and experiences in a large group because they are afraid of how others, unknown to them, may react. Large groups may be the most efficient way of communicating information, if this is the goal of the teaching session. Demonstration of anything but very large-scale activities is often inappropriate since many people may not be able to see what the nurse is doing. Details can be shown in a large group with films, but practice sessions require a smaller teacher-learner ratio.

Teaching Through the Media

Nurses in the future will be doing more health teaching through devices such as cable television, videotapes, visual telephone communication, and computers. This type of teaching has the potential advantage of reaching large numbers of people through repeated use. The learner can select the time for viewing the teaching media to meet personal schedules. The learner may also view media repeatedly to improve understanding of the content. The disadvantage of this type of teaching is the lack of personal contact. Individualization and learner involvement is enhanced when the learner interacts with the nurse and reacts to the material as it is presented. Through the media, skills requiring close observation by the learner can be demonstrated through camera close-ups. Media teaching is enhanced by personal follow-up by the nurse for maximum learning. The nurse's time is then occupied less by initial teaching and more with helping patients practice the skills they have seen through the media. Individualization of teaching will have to occur in the follow-up visits, as will evaluation of learning.

Benefits of Patient Teaching

There are many benefits of patient teaching for the individual patient and family, the community, and the health care facilities. In the long run, each of us is both healthier and wealthier as a result of health education. The cost of health care is shared by all of us in the form of insurance premiums, benefits to employees, and that great certainty of life—taxes! Every time health teaching is effective, one less person is using the resources of the system and relies instead on independent management or outpatient care for health problems. Listed below are several general benefits of health teaching.

Independence

Health teaching helps people learn the information and necessary skills to manage their own health care during illness and recovery. Patients are being discharged from hospitals earlier than in past years. Much of the impetus for this comes from various forms of health insurance that will only pay hospital costs for a specified time with common uncomplicated procedures and surgeries. A relaxing recuperation in the hospital is a thing of the past. Many patients are leaving the hospital while they are still quite ill. They must learn how to meet their health needs at home for optimum recovery. Individuals and their families are usually highly motivated and capable of learning what is needed to manage these health problems at home safely.

Maintenance of Optimum Health Status

Health teaching may help people understand and reach their personal peak level of health. A terminal cancer patient can learn to maintain the self at an optimum level of wellness for as long as life continues. People who are presently free of health problems can be taught how to decrease their risks of developing problems in the future through healthy living practices. People can be taught how to live with chronic illness and remain as healthy and active as possible.

Cost Reduction

When people live longer, life insurance premiums cost less. When families stay healthy and require less medical care, health insurance costs go down. When people are able to manage their care at home and are quickly discharged from the hospital because of this, hospital costs per admission go down. When people are able to maintain their health and earn a living despite physical problems, taxes should go down. When individuals stay healthy and are able to maintain productive lives, family finances are less drained. Health costs are increasing at an alarming rate. In a year, when inflation was close to 4 percent, health costs increased by 11 percent. Health education is one way of slowing this rise.

Decreased Severity of Illness

Teaching people the signs and symptoms of various common health problems allows them to identify problems early while treatment is often less drastic and outcomes are more positive. Individuals, families, and whole communities are being trained in cardiopulmonary resuscitation (CPR). Imagine how this could affect the outcome of a heart attack (MI or myocardial infarction) for any given individual. Another example is the reduction in deaths and complications associated with choking when people are taught how to dislodge objects in the throat obstructing air flow.

Decreased Anxiety

Anxiety is a common reaction when people encounter new problems and they do not know what to expect. The unknown is usually worse then the known. Minimally, people can begin to work through their fears when they know what is wrong and know what options they have for correcting or improving the problem. Knowing what will be experienced in any selected treatment is very effective in decreasing anxiety. Teaching about what will be experienced before, during, and after surgery does reduce patients' anxiety, as well as the anxiety of affected family members. Patients gain reassurance from sharing their feelings with other patients experiencing similar health problems.

Inadequate Teaching—Legal and Ethical Aspects

Failing to teach can be an act of negligence, and the nurse may be held legally liable for resulting problems that patients experience. Patients' lack of knowledge or incorrect knowledge can result in critical illness and death. Inadequate teaching usually means inadequate learning. Consequences of inadequate teaching and learning may result in an individual being unnecessarily admitted to the hospital for the same or a related health problem. It is difficult to work with patients who are frequently admitted for the same problems; there often is a sense of failure and futility experienced by both the patient and the staff. Appropriate health teaching at the right time may reduce or eliminate these readmissions.

Patients experience anxiety and a feeling of loss of control over the environment when health teaching is neglected. For people to take responsibility for their own health problems and manage safely at home, they must understand how all the elements of treatment fit together. How do diet, exercise, rest, medications, stress, follow-up health examinations, and smoking all fit together to affect a patient's risk of another heart attack? If teaching is poorly done, a patient may not put the new information or skills to use because they are associated with a negative teaching experience. Patients may even avoid future health care following negative teaching experiences in a health care facility.

Ethical issues can arise in several ways. When a nurse realizes a patient has been given inaccurate or incomplete information, the nurse is expected to contact the patient directly or through another health professional and correct the mistake. Both ethical and legal issues are involved. Not only can the patient experience problems because of the inaccurate information provided by the nurse, but the nurse may be sued for malpractice. Another example with ethical and legal considerations is teaching a minor about health-related concerns when parents or guardians feel the material is inappropriate. Teaching the young teenage couple about birth-control measures may be offensive to their parents for various reasons. Does the child have the right to accurate information about preventing conception when parents have refused to consider the sexual functioning of a son or daughter? Does the pregnant, 14-year-old girl have a right to ask for and obtain information about the actual procedure of abortion when her parent's religious or personal values are opposed to artificial termination of pregnancy? The nurse should know the policy of any institution in which employed when these ethical issues associated with patient education arise. The decision to honor institutional policy, patient requests, or individual conscience is an ethical question each nurse must answer at the time.

Developing Teaching Skills

Wilbert McKeachie (1969) wrote, "The instructor can occasionally be wrong. If he is wrong too often, he should not be teaching. If he is never wrong, he belongs in heaven . . . ." As a student begins to develop skills as a patient teacher, the discovery is quickly made that all the answers are not known. In fact, as an experienced patient-teacher, the nurse will probably still find that all the answers are not known. Medical and nursing knowledge and treatment are constantly changing, and specialization is one way of knowing most of the answers in a confined area. Initially, patient teaching will involve responding to direct patient questions. Later, patient teaching may involve entire communities. Table 9–1 shows a possible progression in the development of teaching skills during the course of formal nursing education and beyond graduation. At first, a primary concern may relate to personal feelings of adequacy, rather than the patient's needs. This is very typical. No one wants to appear ignorant or incompetent. People think of their own needs when self-esteem is threatened. As confidence develops in teaching, the nurse is able to focus less on self and more on the patient. Eventually, as concern about personal competence decreases, the nurse devotes maximum attention to how the patient is responding to the learning experience. Watching patients gain knowledge and skill in handling their own health needs is rewarding for the nurse.

Narrowing the scope of early teaching may increase personal feelings of competence. This enables the nurse to obtain all the needed information ahead of time and feel well informed on a topic. Short-term teaching goals usually have a narrow focus of content. Usually only one thing is being taught, and it is to be evaluated in the near future prior to a patient's discharge. Short-term teaching goals are often part of comprehensive teaching plans involving multiple learning needs of patients, families, and even communities. The evaluation of these comprehensive teaching plans may be done through long-term, follow-up visits. As students gain experience

Table 9–1. **Development of Teaching Skills for Patient Care**

(Listing is in order of increasing difficulty)

Responding to patients' questions

Seeking more information to better answer patients' questions on a given subject

Volunteering explanations to patients on what is being done and why it is being done

Offering health-related information to patients (beginning with normal body functions and measurements, such as patient's normal BP, and progressing to more complex problems involving altered body functions)

Providing information to family (teaching several people concerned about one individual)

Teaching a skill or behavior upon request of patient or another more experienced nurse

Anticipating learning needs based on patients' health status and medical treatment

Initiating common forms of patient teaching, independently, based on assessed patient need

Evaluating learning

Teaching family members specific skills they will need to perform for the patient after hospital discharge

Developing a teaching plan on a specific subject for a group of patients

Developing a comprehensive teaching plan for individual patients with multiple learning needs. Identifying needs, developing and implementing teaching, evaluating learning

Teaching other nursing personnel, identifying learning needs, developing and implementing teaching, evaluating learning

Developing family teaching plans, coordinating teaching efforts of various health care providers and the family in planning, implementing, and evaluating a variety of short-term teaching goals, they will begin to understand what is involved in organizing the personnel, time, and materials to meet multiple learning needs in patients experiencing complex health problems. Patients and families learning how to cope with chronic illness or dramatic changes in physical or mental abilities require comprehensive teaching plans to organize the teaching efforts of various health care personnel. (See Figure 9–1).

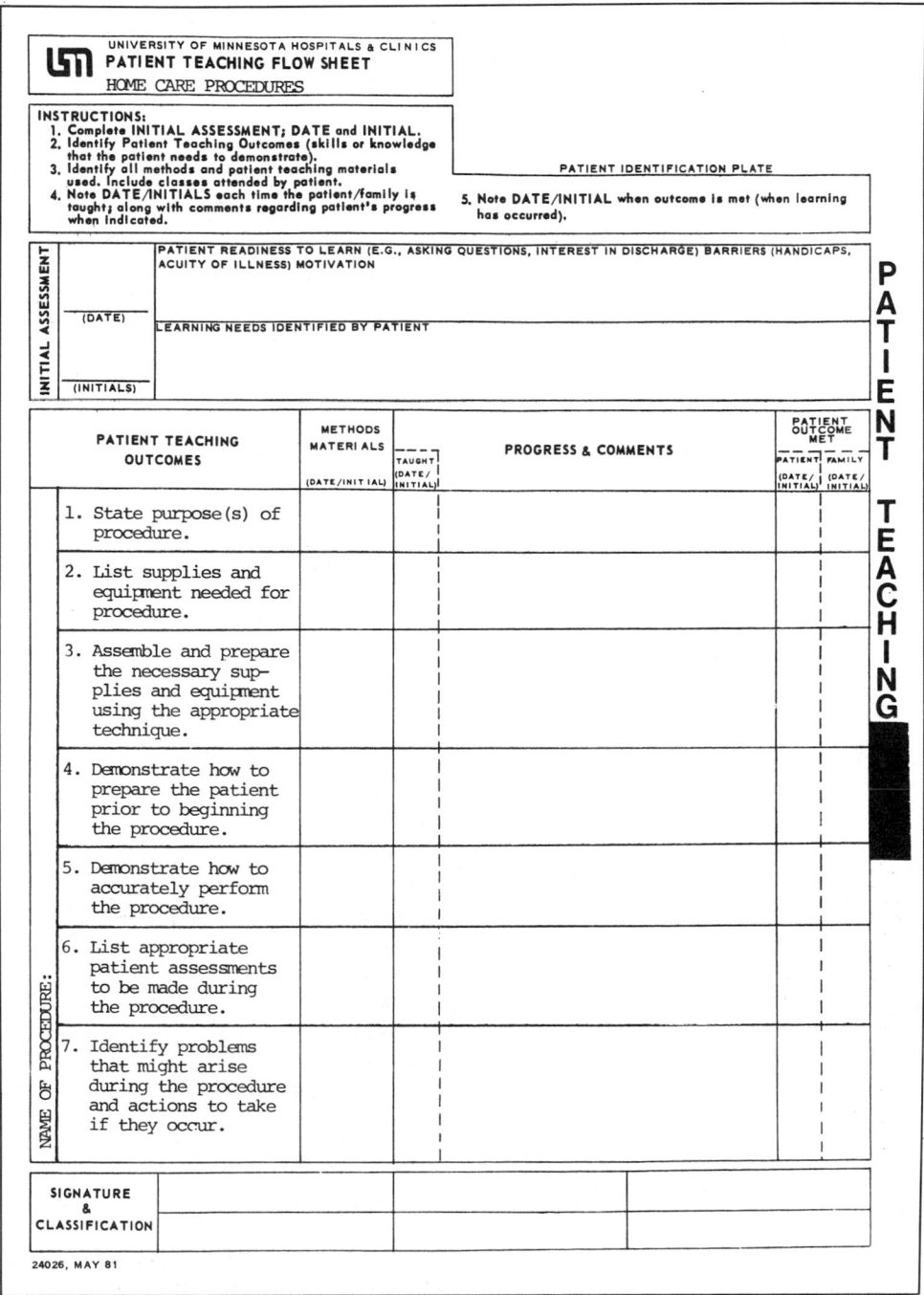

Figure 9–1.   A patient teaching form. This particular form from the patient's chart identifies teaching outcomes (goals) for home care procedures being taught by the nurse. (Courtesy of the University of Minnesota Hospitals and Clinics, Minneapolis, MN.)

PATIENT TEACHING OUTCOMES	METHODS MATERIALS (DATE/INITIAL)	TAUGHT (DATE/INITIAL)	PROGRESS & COMMENTS	PATIENT OUTCOME MET	
				PATIENT (DATE/INITIAL)	FAMILY (DATE/INITIAL)
8. Explain how to care for the supplies and equipment following their use.					
9. State how new supplies and equipment can be obtained when needed.					
10. Name resources to contact if questions about the procedure arise after discharge.					
SIGNATURE & CLASSIFICATION					

Figure 9–1. (*Continued*)

Flexibility and Rigidity

It is 7 P.M. and you are walking down the hall to your patient's room. Your nursing instructor has made the assignments, and yours is preoperative teaching for Mr. Klein in Room 210. His wife is also in the room with him. Just what you need! Now two people will know how unprepared you feel! You are going over your notes on preoperative teaching as you enter the room. You are feeling anxious and have an uneasy feeling in your stomach. Why you ever entered nursing school escapes you at this moment. You hope no one asks any questions. You begin your presentation and follow your outline from beginning to end, with occasional pauses to catch your breath. As you finish, you wish your patient well for tomorrow's surgery and head for the door, escaping as quickly as possible. You survived your first teaching assignment!

The example above may seem exaggerated, but some students find patient-teaching assignments very stressful. When people are stressed, their perception of external events tends to narrow. The result of this in the teaching role is rigidity. Outlines for content presentation are closely followed as a lifeline to pull the student through the experience. It is often difficult for students to explore the patients' reactions to the teaching as it progresses because of their own inner focus. Questions are usually not encouraged and are seen as a source of possible embarrassment if answers are not known. Teaching tends to be a presentation of information about do's and don'ts, rather than an exploration of patients' options and their consequences. This rigidity eases with experience. As students feel more confident in the clinical area and with the material to be taught, they can begin to talk *with* patients rather than *at* them. Questions will be welcomed because they help the nurse-teacher evaluate the patient's understanding. When ap-

propriate, family members are encouraged to participate in learning experiences with patients. They will help reinforce the teaching in the nurse's absence. Often, the family is better able to learn than the patient, depending on the patient's physical needs and discomforts at the time the teaching was done.

Teaching that has meaning for the learner increases the chances that the information and skills taught will be utilized and remembered. Teaching is a process to be adapted for each individual if it is to meet unique learning needs. The teacher who adheres to a prepared teaching plan may appear very competent to the learner. Sometimes, though, the teacher who is more flexible and seeks reactions to the teaching as it occurs and adjusts, repeats, or modifies the material is more effective, even though the presentation does not seem as polished. Patients will ask some very creative questions as they apply knowledge or adapt skills to their home environments or personal preferences. Consider patients' questions carefully before telling them they cannot do something in a manner they devise. Is it safe? Does it accomplish the goal? It may not be the way the nurse would do it, but that does not matter. If it works for the patient, it should be supported if it is safe and results in similar outcomes.

Motivation for Learning

What motivates people to learn? Some theorists believe people do not require external motivation to learn, but rather a natural curiosity and willingness to learn are inherent. They believe in the appropriate environment where freedom to explore and make mistakes is acceptable, people will be naturally motivated to learn. Other theorists believe people are motivated to learn by being rewarded or by avoiding punishment, and that it is often up to the teacher to motivate individuals to learn. A third point of view gives the credit for motivation to the learner, who identifies personal learning needs. A *learning need* is recognized when the person perceives a difference between the real situation and the desired situation. Learning is viewed as a means of reducing the difference between the two. As the time for skills testing approaches, many nursing students are able to identify personal learning needs by contrasting current abilities with performance levels expected by nursing instructors. Practicing the skills the student performs incorrectly leads to improved dexterity and reduction in the difference between actual and desired performance. Nurses are frequently able to identify learning needs of patients after assessing current knowledge and skill levels. Identification of a patient learning

need is a nursing diagnosis. These diagnoses are often stated in the form: Inadequate information (or skill) related to . . . or knowledge (skill) deficit associated with . . . .

People in the hospital are often highly motivated to learn health-related practices compared to people who are not currently experiencing problems severe enough to require hospitalization. There are several reasons for the increased willingness to learn in the hospitalized patient. These are discussed below:

1. Captive audience. The person in the hospital does not have to exert much energy to come in contact with people qualified to help meet personal learning needs. If questions are asked, people in the immediate environment will be able to respond. The patient has the professional nurse and, intermittently, the physician as a captive audience. The reverse is also true. Patients are readily available to nurses, no trip to a private home nor waiting for an appointment. When patients are hospitalized, nurses can schedule teaching time into their patient assignments just as they schedule medication administration or x-ray procedure preparations. Teaching can also be incorporated into many of the repeated nurse-patient contacts throughout the eight-hour shift.

2. Seriousness of the health problem recognized. By the time most patients are admitted to the hospital, they are willing to accept the fact that they have unmet health needs. They realize they can no longer manage their health problems independently and that professional help is needed. Recognition of the problem is a strong motivator for learning. If new learning is presented as a way of lessening the problem to allow independence from the hospital, patients are usually eager to learn. Families are also made aware of the serious nature of a member's health status. Hospitalization is disruptive to family functioning. Most families want to learn information and skills that will allow the hospitalized member to return home and remain healthy.

3. Increased anxiety. Many people experience some degree of anxiety when moved from the familiar to the unfamiliar. For most people, the hospital is an unfamiliar environment, and anxiety, in varying degrees, is common. If anxiety is mildly to moderately increased, a patient is more alert and ready to learn. Extreme anxiety narrows perception and tends to interfere with learning.

4. Time out from usual responsibilities. When people are hospitalized, they are not expected to continue to meet their outside responsibilities. Others usually take over work and home activities, while the hospitalized person is free to focus on health-related problems. This allows the patient time and energy to devote to learning about the health problems which resulted in this hospitalization. It also provides time to learn new skills or ways of behaving to minimize chances of future hospitalization. There is time in the hospital to think about the future and consider the alternatives to personal behavior which may result in improved health and longer life. Hospitalization sometimes helps people realize what their real priorities are.

Types of Learning—Cognitive, Affective, Psychomotor

Goals of learning and teaching will generally fall into three areas. Cognitive learning, affective learning, and psychomotor learning are common terms used to describe these areas. *Cognitive learning* deals with information and mental processes such as remembering signs and symptoms of a disease. Solving a problem such as the correct number of 0.125-mg tablets to give a patient who is ordered to receive 0.25 mg is a cognitive learning skill. *Affective learning* emphasizes feelings, emotions, or some degree of acceptance or rejection. Affective learning goals can range from simply getting a person to pay attention to internalizing values such as accountability and professionalism. The third area, *psychomotor learning*, involves some form of physical activity and coordination between the brain and the muscles at a voluntary level. Learning to drive a car, give an injection, and perform cardiopulmonary resuscitation are all examples of psychomotor learning. Learning often has components of all three forms. All learning has motivation, emotion, and cognition present to some degree. The lowest level of affective learning, the attention of the learner, is needed for all other types of learning.

Principles Related to Learning

Principles related to learning provide some of the rationale for what to teach, when to teach, and how to teach. Learning is an extremely complex phenomenon which is not completely understood. The principles, described below and listed in Table 9–2 are statements which have been shown to hold true for most people in a teaching-learning experience. Suggestions for applying the principles to promote learning are listed in Table 9–3. Table 9–4 identifies some factors which may interfere with learning.

Learning is more likely to occur when the learner perceives a need to learn.

Patients and families do not always recognize their learning needs. One of the early activities in effective teaching is to help the patient recognize the difference between the current, real situation and the desired situation for improved health status. When the patient realizes that a problem exists, motivation for learning is increased. If the patient does not agree with the nurses's diagnosed learning need and goals of teaching, the patient may respond with lack of attention, making learning impossible.

Learning is more likely to occur when the learner believes the subject matter is helpful in meeting personal needs.

Many of us have had the experience of thinking, "Why in the world is this being taught? It doesn't relate to anything." Many people file this unrelated teaching

Table 9–2. **Principles Related to Learning**

Learning is more likely to occur when the learner perceives a need to learn.

Learning is more likely to occur when the learner believes the subject matter is helpful in meeting personal needs.

Learning occurs more rapidly when the learner perceives both a learning need and a way to meet that need.

The learner's active participation in the learning experience increases the chances that learning will occur.

The learner's physical, emotional, and mental status can have a positive or negative effect on amount, type, and rate of learning.

Retention of learning is increased when learning occurs over time rather than in one massed exposure.

Retention of learning is increased when the new learning is used and applied immediately and frequently.

Retention of learning and repetition of learned behavior is more likely when the learner receives positive reinforcement for the learned activity.

Learning, which involves changes in the learner's self-concept, may be perceived as threatening and, as a result, learning may be resisted.

Learning involving accepting changes in the learner's self-concept is more likely to occur when external threats are perceived to be at a minimum.

Material that is integrated into the learner's prior knowledge/behavior is more likely to be learned.

Learning experiences that are rewarding for the learner serve to motivate further learning.

Practice with corrective, positive feedback to the learner leads to improved performance.

in the useless category and do not bother to learn it or quickly forget the material. Later, the learner may realize that this seemingly useless information was an essential part of the overall learning to meet personal needs safely. This relationship should be made clear to the learner from the beginning to promote learning. At this point, the patient not only recognizes that a learning need exists, but also that what the nurse is teaching is going to help lessen or alleviate the health-related problem. A patient who has a weakened heart muscle following a myocardial infarction may view teaching related to avoiding the Valsalva maneuver (breath-holding while bearing down) during defecation unrelated to either the heart problem or the constipation problem. The relationship between what is being taught, in this case, the Valsalva maneuver and the weakened heart muscle, must be understood by the patient if the teaching is to have meaning for the patient. It should be clearly explained that holding the breath while bearing down to pass a stool and then suddenly releasing the air and taking a breath creates dramatic changes in the blood pressure which can cause excessive strain on the heart as a sudden surge of blood returns to the weakened heart. This explanation of the relationship between the Valsalva maneuver and the heart will help motivate most patients to learn alternatives to current behavior.

Learning occurs more rapidly when the learner perceives both a need and a way to meet that need.

When the learner recognizes the unresolved problem and has learning materials available, learning occurs rapidly. Compare this situation to one in which the learner is unsure of what is expected and how to learn. When patients want to learn something and are given the material and help they need to learn, skills or information can be learned quickly. When the test is tomorrow, a student can learn material rapidly, if a passing grade is important. For example, a patient knows she is going to be discharged from the hospital as soon as she can demonstrate safe administration of her insulin. If personnel and supplies are readily available for practice and encouragement, the skill will be learned rapidly if the patient is eager to go home. If learning materials are not available, difficult to obtain, or sources for the learning are unknown, learning will occur more slowly owing to less practice time and expenditure of energy on finding information. Time may also be wasted on inappropriate learning materials if patients are not guided in their choices of learning strategies.

Active participation in the learning experience increases the chances that learning will occur.

Learning is an active process. The more routes of communication that can be used, the clearer the mes-

Table 9–3. **Suggestions to Promote Learning**

As the Teacher

Be well informed on the subject.

Assist people to recognize personal learning needs.

Respect the learner as a capable individual.

Believe in yourself as a capable teacher.

Organize the presentation of material in some logical form; organize resources and references for learners; organize teaching aids such as charts, transparencies, slides.

Develop the goals of teaching with the individual learner whenever possible.

Clarify purposes of teaching and expectations of learners.

Recognize and admit personal limitations; seek help as needed to meet learner's needs.

Consider learning-style preferences of individuals: visual, auditory, or kinesthetic (see Chapter 5 on Learning Styles).

Involve learners as much as possible.

Take some risks; try new methods of teaching.

Be available to the learner; let learners know where and how to reach you with questions; allow time during and after teaching to have contact with individual learners; limit number of learners based on amount of individual help needed from teacher.

Create a relaxed, accepting environment: relaxed posture, quiet environment, unhurried pace of presentation, smile, allow time for questions, consider all questions, good eye contact.

Create a challenging environment where learners feel capable of achieving learning goals; break down complex learning into small steps.

Encourage expression of feelings and reactions to teaching.

Evaluate learning and discuss with the learner.

Solicit and consider suggestions from learners on helpful changes in teaching plan.

Develop adequate communication: speak slowly, clearly, and as loudly as necessary or get a microphone; make sure learner can read and understand printed material; make sure seating allows clear view for learners; use terms and words familiar to learners; vary voice tones to avoid a constant monotone; clarify verbal content with writing and diagrams.

Do not assume anyone else has done patient teaching—ask the patient.

Sit in with the patient when others explain or teach; reinforce what others have taught; bring up prior patient questions and concerns with other health personnel during teaching.

Discuss your desire to teach each patient with the head nurse/team leader—does the patient know medical diagnosis? What does the family know about the patient's problems? Clarify conflicting information on treatment, prognosis, discharge plans before teaching.

Do not assume patients managing chronic illnesses have current, accurate information or adequate skills, assess for learning needs.

sage is for the learner. If a patient can hear about a skill, see it demonstrated, and have practice doing it, the level of involvement is much greater than when only reading about the skill. Kron (1982) points out from a study some years back by the Socony-Mobil Company that people remember:

10 percent of what is read
20 percent of what is heard
30 percent of what is seen
50 percent of what is seen and heard
80 percent of what is said and done

The more active the learner in hearing, seeing, discussing, and performing activities to be learned, the greater the learning. The nurse also recognizes that the more ac-

tive the patient is in learning, the more energy is required from the patient. The physical status of each patient should be considered in devising a teaching plan. Does the patient have the strength and ability at this point in recovery to participate in the learning experiences chosen? Will fatigue, pain, and medications limit this patient's ability to participate in some methods of learning?

The learner's physical, emotional, and mental status can have a positive or negative effect on amount, type, and rate of learning.

The patient's physical status will affect ability to perform skills and activities requiring coordination, muscle strength, endurance, hearing, seeing, and speaking. Can the patient see well enough to read or observe a demonstration? Can the patient hear the nurse's expla-

Table 9-4. **Factors/Activities that May Interfere with Learning**

Overwhelming the learner—presenting too much material too quickly

Environmental distractions—noise, interruptions, uncomfortable temperature, telephones, televisions

Inadequate communication—inability to hear, see, understand, read

Internal distractions—pain, fatigue, medications, nausea, gastrointestinal distress, hunger, thirst, fear, anxiety, anger, apathy, grief

Rigidity of learner—learners wanting right/wrong answers to complex problems; unable or unwilling to consider alternatives; rejection of unfamiliar; unwilling to take risks

Lack of resources/learning experiences

Inadequate feedback on learning progress

Negative feedback or repeated failure associated with attempted learning

Lack of confidence or trust in the teacher

Fear of negative reactions of others—embarrassment, ridicule, dislike

Inadequate motivation to learn

Learner perceiving self as unable to learn—learner feels threatened or learning experiences too advanced for learner's current capabilities

Decreased level of consciousness related to illness, medications, anesthesia

Beginning to teach before the learner is ready to learn

---

nations and information either in person or through the media? Is there damage to a patient's communication skills that will interfere with learning? Is the patient too tired to learn or in too much discomfort to concentrate? The patient's emotional status may block learning if anxiety levels are too high. Fear may interfere with learning. Refusing to accept a problem will definitely block any learning related to lessening it. Some anxiety may stimulate learning. Positive feeling about learning and enthusiasm about the topic are attitudes that encourage learning. The patient's mental status can be affected by pain, medications, or oxygen supply to the brain. Are the patient's thinking processes functioning at an adequate level for learning? Greatly decreased mental functioning makes all but the most basic learning very difficult. The nurse considers the current and future status of the patient in planning learning experiences.

Retention of learning is increased when the learning occurs over time rather than in one mass exposure.

The student who crams for a test the night before the examination usually retains less of the learning over time than the student who studies material each day. Patients learning a cluster of related skills retain the information and skills longer if they are given the opportunity to practice frequently for shorter periods of time. Skills can be broken down into simple steps, and learning can build over time. One long teaching episode tends to tire people, and they often feel overwhelmed and incapable of learning so much material.

Retention of learning is increased when the new

learning is used and applied immediately and frequently.

If there is a considerable gap in time between learning and application, some of the learning is forgotten. After a patient is taught a skill, the more frequently the skill is performed during the remainder of the hospital stay, the more likely the patient will perform the skill safely at home. If the nurse is teaching patients how to take their own medications after discharge from the hospital, letting them practice by giving themselves their own medications under supervision while in the hospital improves retention. If the patient is learning how to do dressing changes, encourage performance of as many dressing changes as possible so the patient has a regular routine established before discharge. This may take more of the nurse's time to observe the patient apply the learning. The nurse has already established and perfected a routine for doing dressing changes and can do it more rapidly than the patient. But if the goal of teaching is to have the patient do safe dressing changes at home, the patient should be active, not the nurse.

Retention of learning and repetition of learned behavior is more likely when the learner receives positive reinforcement for the learned activity.

When people receive positive outcomes from learning, the learned activity tends to be repeated and remembered as a means of receiving the initial reward. Positive rewards can come in the form of praise from the nurse, from the family, from the patient, and from outside sources, such as employers. When patients reward themselves for learning through sense of pride in what has been accomplished or pleasure from the increased independence gained, no external source of reward is necessary. In the early stages of learning, many people want the positive reinforcement from someone they identify as an authority in the form of praise and encouragement.

Learning that involves accepting changes in the learner's self-concept may be perceived as threatening and tends to be resisted.

A dramatic example of this is the healthy young teenager with a high spinal cord injury. Teaching this patient the skills and information needed to function as a quadriplegic will be resisted until this patient begins to have a concept of self as a quadriplegic. Give patients time and support in accepting themselves in their new status before teaching skills and information they will need in the future. A newly diagnosed diabetic will need time to incorporate the new body image into self-concept. Teaching done before this process begins is not very effective and often angers the patient.

Learning involving changes in the self-concept is more likely to occur when external threats are perceived to be at a minimum.

When a patient perceives too many threats in the environment, the reaction tends to be defensive rather than open exploration and risk-taking. Defensive behavior is designed to protect the self-concept of the individual and maintain it in its present form. A more open examination of potential new aspects of oneself is difficult to risk if the person is worried about negative reactions from other people. If an environment can be created between the nurse and the patient that is accepting and open, the patient may feel secure enough to begin to learn about the changes an altered health status may impose on personal life-style. An environment in which the patient is valued as an individual and viewed as a competent participant in health care contributes to giving patients security and confidence to learn new behaviors.

A safe environment does not allow patients to harm themselves when they attempt new skills. There is enough help in the form of personnel and equipment to assist patients if they should run into problems. A safe environment is also free of interruptions that could distract or embarrass a patient or family, such as the interruptions during visiting hours as the nurse is teaching the patient how to do self-catheterization of the bladder.

Material that is integrated into the learner's prior knowledge/behavior is more likely to be learned.

This principle suggests that teaching should begin at the learner's level of understanding or skill. What may seem simple to the nurse may seem very difficult to the patient. Assess a patient's level of understanding before beginning to teach. Begin with what is familiar to the patient. Use examples that are common in the patient's experience. Use words that are familiar to the patient. Common words may not sound as professional as the nurse would like, but unfamiliar medical terminology will make teaching unclear. Information that is incorporated into prior learning and experience will also be remembered longer than unrelated information. Teaching that begins at a level below the patient's level of understanding or performance can be equally offensive. It seems as though the nurse is talking down to the patient. No one likes to be taught information or skills they already know. Reading an information pamphlet to a patient who is capable of reading it alone is an example of this. It is a waste of the teacher's time and learner's time. Find out what patients and their families already know. Give the individual credit for prior learning by beginning to teach at the appropriate level for each patient.

Learning experiences that are rewarding for the learner serve to motivate further learning.

People who experience rewards from learning tend to be lifelong learners. If people meet frustration and failure in their learning attempts, they will tend to avoid similar learning situations. Choosing learning experiences to match patients' abilities will help to ensure patients' success in their learning attempts. Offering sincere praise for learning efforts is appreciated and encourages patients to keep trying. Helping patients to see the progress they have made over time is also helpful in encouraging further learning. Rewards may be very different from one patient to another. For a small child, favorite foods and drinks can make learning a positive experience. For other children, added playtime earned through learning efforts is effective. Praise from health personnel and family is important for all ages and is a very effective reward for learning. If learning can be fun, even better. Can learning be incorporated into a social event? Can a learning contest be created where everyone is a winner? Can a fresh new environment be selected for learning so patients can get out of their rooms and enjoy stimulating scenery?

Practice with corrective, positive feedback to the learner leads to improved performance.

The art of correcting without discouraging a patient is a vital skill for the teacher. People have the right to be wrong in a learning situation. Do not take patients' errors or confusion personally as a reflection that you are a poor teacher. Correct the mistakes or misinterpretation. Avoid comments that may be taken as a negative evaluation of the person. Try to incorporate what the patient is doing correctly and make suggestions for improving the inappropriate behavior.

The Process of Teaching

Teaching, like the nursing process discussed in Chapter 17, has several separate activities. Assessment, planning, implementation, and evaluation are also applicable to patient teaching. As the nurse does an initial *assessment* of a patient, learning needs may become apparent. The learning need can then be explored with the patient and clearly identified to the satisfaction of both the nurse and the patient. Occasionally, there may be disagreement when the nurse thinks the patient should learn one thing and the patient, either because of a lack of understanding of a health problem or because of information unknown to the nurse, thinks learning is unnecessary or inappropriate. Through discussion and further assessment, the nurse and the patient can usually identify mutually acceptable learning needs and goals. Some general examples of nursing diagnoses related to learning needs are listed below:

Knowledge deficit related to . . . (some specific area)
Inadequate skills related to . . . (some specific area)
Incorrect information or understanding related to . . . (specific area)

Some specific nursing diagnoses related to learning needs are listed below:

Knowledge deficit in all aspects of diabetes
Knowledge deficit related to process of normal labor and delivery
Unfamiliarity with skills related to infant care
Unfamiliarity with cast care
Incorrect information related to self medications
Inadequate skills related to care of pressure sore

Identifying Problems Related to Unmet Learning Needs

Patients need accurate, current information to make choices about health care and treatments. Any patient admitted to the hospital is a potential learner. Find out what a patient knows about personal health problems. "Can you tell me what problems resulted in your being admitted to the hospital?" "What has your physician told you about your health problems?" "What do you know about . . . [particular illness/problem]?" These are all possible questions to pose as the nurse begins to assess patients' learning needs. Asking patients to demonstrate how they have been performing a skill at home is another way to assess learning needs. Asking patients

if they understand their diagnosis, treatments, and medications is another place to begin.

Assessment of the Learner

After the nurse has identified a learning need based on data from the patient, family, or other health care personnel, a more thorough assessment of the learner is helpful to individualize the eventual teaching. What are this patient's strengths and weaknesses? Where should teaching begin? At what level? What exactly does the patient know compared to what is necessary to know? Listed below are areas to consider in patient assessment related to learning.

Readiness to Learn

1. Is the patient motivated to learn? Does the patient recognize personal learning needs? Does the patient feel the potential learning will be valuable in meeting personal needs? If the answer to these and similar questions is no, then the nurse can assist the patient to understand these things before beginning to teach.

2. Consider a patient's developmental level and age. Is the patient capable of learning the needed information at this time, or is it more appropriate to teach family members? Are there adequate motor and sensory skills for learning?

3. Consider the illness/medical problem of the patient. Are other needs of greater importance at this time? If so, it would be better to delay teaching. If a patient is in an acute stage of illness, anything other than simple explanations may be inappropriate. Delay teaching until the patient is more stable. The family of the patient may be ready to learn before the patient is. Teaching the family while giving care to the acutely ill member is usually much appreciated. Illness will also affect the patient's level of consciousness. Patients who are not alert, oriented, nor relatively comfortable will have a hard time concentrating on any teaching. Waiting until the patient feels better makes teaching more effective. Medications for pain may also affect ability to learn. Patients receiving large doses of analgesics do not usually comprehend and retain information as they normally would. Wait until medication is reduced and the patient is more alert.

4. Consider the level of anxiety in the patient. If the patient is quite anxious, teaching can be delayed. Help the patient talk through the feeling and concerns causing the anxiety. Try to identify specific fears and deal

with these before beginning to teach. Highly anxious patients often do not even hear teaching, or they hear it incorrectly, and retention is very poor.

Learning Strengths and Deficits

1. Find out what the patient already knows or is able to do. This will help the nurse plan what to teach, the type of language to use, and what other health professionals might be needed, such as a dietary referral or a referral to pastoral services. Find out what the patient wants to know or be able to do and incorporate this into the teaching.

2. The patient's attitude toward learning may be positive or negative as a result of past experiences. If it is negative, find out what went wrong in the past and try to avoid a repetition of the problem. If it is positive, find out what went right for the patient and consider building this approach into the teaching.

3. Discuss the patient's resources in terms of time, energy, money, and help or support from others. Including other people in the teaching may be important, especially if these individuals will be active in helping the patient at home. Will special equipment be needed at home? Is a referral to social service for financial assistance going to be necessary?

4. Consider whether to include or exclude the family in the teaching. For some patients, including other family members may be very helpful. For other patients, it may be an added threat. They may not want family members with them as new skills are learned. Some family members may not be ready to accept the medical diagnosis of the ill member and may interfere with the patient's learning.

5. Ask patients how they like to learn; this preference can then be incorporated into your teaching plan. Give them examples, such as, "When you have learned to do something in the past, what seems to be the easiest way for you to learn? Do you prefer to read about something first, for example, or do you prefer to watch someone else perform the activity?" Consider whether the patient is an auditory, visual, or kinesthetic learner and adapt teaching strategies accordingly.

Developing Learning Goals

What is it specifically that the nurse wants a patient to learn? Write these things down as a teaching plan is developed. Learning goals are the desired outcomes of learning which correspond to the identified learning need. What should the patient be able to do as a result of learning? Is knowledge enough, or will the patient

---

Table 9–5. **Nursing Diagnoses and Goals Related to Patient Learning Needs**

Nursing diagnosis: Anxiety related to lack of information about cardiac stress test.

Learning goal: Patient will understand activities involved in a stress test and the safeguards for decreasing risks during test.

Teaching method: One-to-one discussion with patient and family, if family available.

Evaluation: Asking patient to describe what will be happening during the stress test several hours prior to the test.

Nursing diagnosis: Unfamiliarity with relaxation and breathing techniques for labor.

Learning goals: Patient will use slow chest breathing in early labor. Patient will use rapid-rate chest breathing in active labor. Patient will relax between contractions.

Teaching methods: Explanations of learning need. Demonstration of breathing techniques. Practice with reinforcement for breathing and relaxation.

Evaluation: Patient demonstration of breathing techniques and relaxation during course of labor.

Nursing diagnosis: Lack of knowledge about taking own medications.

Learning goal: Patient will describe correct dose and administration time for each medication prior to hospital discharge.

Teaching methods: Discussion with patient and spouse about medication; reason for taking medication, dose, time; number of days to take medication; any side effects; reasons to discontinue medication and notify M.D.; take home instruction card.

Evaluation: At time of discharge, ask patient to explain medications, when to take them, and the dose of each.

have to apply the knowledge in solving problems. Is understanding how and why an activity is done adequate, or is it necessary for the patient to be able safely to perform an activity independently? As the nurse considers patient outcomes as a result of teaching, the content and teaching methods become easier to select. The methods for evaluation of learning are also made clear when learning goals are identified. If the patient is to be able to perform an activity as a result of learning, then evaluation would involve the patient demonstrating that activity to the nurse. If the patient is to be able to identify the signs of low blood sugar (hypoglycemia), then evaluation involves asking the patient to write or describe these signs and symptoms. Some examples of learning goals are listed in Table 9–5. The learning goals are related to the diagnosed patient learning needs in the sense that they are a means of helping the patient meet the identified need.

Selecting Teaching Methods

When beginning to teach patients, consider the variety of teaching methods available. Lectures, demonstrations, discussions, printed material, role-playing and audiovisual material are some common methods most students have encountered during the course of their own education. Try not to let one bad experience with a particular method prevent use of that method again. Table 9–6 describes various teaching methods and when they may be most effective. Each method has certain expectations of the learners and the teacher, and these can be compared to personal and patient capabilities at the time teaching is planned. Consider individual strengths, familiarity with a method, and the perferred type of interaction with patients. Choose the teaching method that gives the patient practice in the activity to be evaluated as evidence of learning. If a patient is to learn how

Table 9–6. **Teaching Methods**

Demonstration

Performance of an activity for other people to watch for the purpose of learning about an activity or how to perform it.

Useful in teaching skills

Useful in helping learner visualize application of information or principles

Preparation and responsibility: practice ahead of time; assemble all equipment; arrange environment so everyone can see and hear; if practice session is to follow demonstration, have enough equipment and help to assist learners; inform learners what is expected of them before, during, and after demonstration

Lecture

A verbal presentation of information by one individual to a group of learners; communication is one way from teacher to learner.

Useful in presenting information to large group of learners

Method allows an "expert" to share information/experience with large group

Useful when learners have common informational needs and backgrounds

Preparation and responsibility: organization of content in logical form prior to lecture; arrange for a microphone if there is a need; break up information presented with personal experiences, slides, transparencies, and other things to provide variety and reinforce important points; provide breaks at least every hour

Role-Play

Creation of an imaginary situation in which individuals take on the roles and behaviors of others.

Useful in rehearsing communication and behavior for real situation

Useful in developing communication skills

Useful in anticipatory problem solving

Useful in dealing with feelings, expressing feelings, and trying out response alternatives

Useful combined with videotaping to allow people to see and hear themselves as others do for increased self-awareness

Helpful in discovering how an individual views other people and experiences

Preparation and responsibility: creation of a "safe" environment so people will be willing to participate; creation of the role-play situation and characters; describing to the learners the purpose of the role-play and their responsibility; deciding when to stop each role-play situation; helping the learners to identify and discuss what occurred and why; be prepared to encounter and work through strong emotions of participants; be willing to participate in the first role-play; use volunteers rather than recruits for the role-play situations

Table 9–6. **Teaching Methods** (*Cont.*)

Discussion

A group, interacting primarily verbally, which investigates various aspects of a topic by sharing information, experiences and feelings.

Useful in discovering different viewpoints on a topic

Useful way of sharing experiences and information so each individual understands the topic from a broader perspective

Useful in involving several people in identifying and resolving problems

Useful in clarifying questions arising from other learning experiences

Preparation and responsibility: identify for the learners what is expected of them in preparation for the discussion; suggest appropriate resources; study the topic and bring questions or situations to stimulate the discussion; plan what the topic for discussion will be; take notes as necessary to make occasional summaries of ideas as discussion progresses; bring group back to topic as necessary during discussion: plan how to deal with impatience, frustration, nonparticipation of learners who want quick, right/wrong answers from an ''expert''

Site Visit

This is a tour of an environment unfamiliar to the learner for the purpose of becoming acquainted with a physical environment and with equipment, personnel, and functions.

Useful when verbal descriptions are difficult to visualize

Useful in reducing anxiety related to the unknown, as when a child tours the hospital prior to admission

Useful in showing real situations and individuals' behavior/skills

Useful in exposing people to new ideas, equipment, procedures, and ways of thinking; creates interest in further study

Preparation and responsibility: arranging time for visit; preparing learners for what they will see; have someone at the site who can describe what is seen and answer questions (or be prepared to do this yourself); prepare people at the site for the visit; get permission from all necessary people prior to the visit; arrange for transportation if needed; select a meeting place at the site; plan time for discussion or questions following site visit

Audiovisual Material

This is a method of teaching using the learner's senses of hearing and/or seeing through the use of media such as slides, audiotapes, films, videotapes.

Useful for showing activities in the real world

Useful in demonstrating skills

Useful in creating moods and showing emotional situations

Useful in orienting people to new places, equipment, procedures

Useful when learners have busy schedules; each learner can view media at own convenience

Useful as a common stimulus for discussion

Useful in exposing the learner to unusual situations that they may not encounter in other learning experiences

Preparation and responsibility: select the film or media only after personal preview; make sure all needed equipment is available and functioning; prepare learners for what they will see and why they are seeing it; provide a handout, if necessary, so learner does not have to take many notes since this interferes with the learner keeping pace with the media (unless rate is regulated by learner); show learner how to operate equipment if appropriate

to apply warm moist heat to a leg, a combination of demonstration and practice would be more effective than printed material on this activity as the sole teaching method.

Exhibit 9–1 is an example of a preoperative teaching plan based on a patient's diagnosed learning needs.

Implementing the Teaching Plan

Selecting the Learning Environment. When the nurse is ready to begin teaching, an environment that meets the needs of the patient and the teaching method can be chosen. Assess the patient's current physical status first.

Exhibit 9–1. **Sample Teaching Plan—
Preoperative Teaching**

Assessment Data

A 28-year-old man is admitted to the hospital for removal of torn cartilage from the right knee. He has never been a patient in a hospital before. He is married and has one child, aged three years. He is in good health in other respects. He smokes one pack of cigarettes a day. He takes no medication other than several EMPIRIN #3 prescribed for the knee pain several days ago. He is questioning how long he will be unable to work after the surgery but is receiving workmen's compensation since the injury to the knee was work related. He says his physician briefly described the surgery to him several days ago. Surgery is scheduled at 8 A.M. Patient does not enjoy group teaching, prefers reading material privately and talking with health personnel directly. Has a real fear of general anesthesia and is unsure what will be used for surgery. States, "This whole thing scares me to death—not knowing what they are going to do and how I'll feel. I don't even know when I might walk again let alone go back to work. I really hate pain. This knee has bothered me for six years, but right now I'm not so sure the cure isn't going to be worse than the problem." He feels his wife would like to hear about the surgery, and she will be in to visit after 6 P.M.

Nursing Diagnoses

1. Inadequate information related to surgical experience
2. Inadequate information related to activities in the postoperative period
3 Inadequate information about recovery from surgery and return to work

Learning Goals

1. Patient will understand the normal preoperative routines and the things he will experience during surgery by this evening.
2. Patient will understand common activities and sensation of the early postoperative period by this evening. (See Figure 9–2.)
3. Patient will be knowledgeable about normal course and length of recovery from knee surgery prior to discharge.

Planning the Teaching Methods

1. Discussion with patient and wife at 7 P.M.
2. Printed information on operative experience for patient's reference
3. Referral to anesthesia department for someone to talk with patient about type of anesthesia to be used
4. Return later in evening to answer any further questions

Content and Organization

1. Night before surgery
   a. Lab work; diagnostic tests—chest x-ray, blood tests, urine specimen
   b. Signed consent form for surgery
   c. Restrictions on food and fluid after midnight
2. Events immediately preceding surgery
   a. Application of elastic stocking on left leg
   b. Preoperative medication
   c. Voiding on call to OR
   d. Transfer to OR holding room
   e. Starting IV
   f. Skin preparation of right knee area
3. Events during surgery
   a. Level of consciousness with anesthesia
   b. Approximate time in OR
   c. Type of incision and dressing
4. Events in recovery room
   a. Level of consciousness
   b. Probable feelings, amount of discomfort to expect
   c. Nursing interventions such as frequent assessment of pulse in left foot, blood pressure, dressings
5. Postoperative events
   a. Feelings in leg
   b. Availability of pain medication
   c. Positioning and ambulation restrictions
   d. Use of urinal or bedpan if needed
   e. Diet and removal of IV
   f. Deep-breathing activities to prevent respiratory complications
   g. Nursing interventions—frequent assessment of pulse and sensation in right leg and foot, frequent pulse and blood pressure check, auscultation of chest for any problems with secretions
   h. Discharge approximation

Is the patient able to leave the room or has a recent treatment such as bed rest or traction made it difficult to move to another area? Is the patient waiting for the physician, important phone calls, or visitors which results in a reluctance to leave the room at this time? If some of these factors are occurring, patient teaching at the bedside may be the best environment for learning. If it is possible to change the patient's environment, select a room with adequate light, temperature, seating, and privacy. Make sure the person in charge of the hospital

UNIVERSITY OF MINNESOTA HOSPITALS & CLINICS
OPERATIVE CHECKLIST

STATION

PATIENT IDENTIFICATION PLATE

DESCRIPTION BY PATIENT OF WHAT WILL HAPPEN TO HIM IN SURGERY: (E.G. NAME OF SURGERY, WHAT WILL BE DONE)

_____

WHAT PATIENT EXPECTS AS RESULT OF SURGERY: (E.G. CHANGES IN APPEARANCE, FUNCTION OR PAIN)

_____

INSTRUCTIONS GIVEN TO
☐ PATIENT ☐ FAMILY ☐ BOTH

TITLES OF WRITTEN OR AUDIOVISUAL MATERIALS USED:

_____

PATIENT TEACHING

INITIAL AND DATE AREAS LISTED BELOW WHICH HAVE BEEN REVIEWED. IF NOT APPLICABLE, CHECK N/A BOX.

PREOPERATIVE	√ N/A	INFORMED INIT.	DATE	POSTOPERATIVE	√ N/A	INFORMED INIT	DATE
1. TIME OF SURGERY/POSSIBLE CHANGE/OPERATIVE PERMIT				15. SENSATIONS AS RESULT OF SURGERY OR POSITIONING			
2. DIET/NOTHING BY MOUTH, IV, PRE AND POSTOPERATIVELY				16. POSTOPERATIVE ACTIVITY/ RESTRICTION			
3. SMOKING REGULATION				17. POSTOPERATIVE UNIT/POSSIBLE SURGICAL INTENSIVE CARE			
4. PREP/SHAVE/ENEMA				18. MONITORING TO EXPECT OF NURSE			
5. REMOVAL OF DENTURES/JEWELRY/ WIGS/MAKEUP/GLASSES/ CLOTHES				19. MONITORING TO EXPECT OF PATIENT			
6. PREOPERATIVE & SLEEP MEDICATION/ EFFECTS				20. WHY PULMONARY EXERCISES ARE NECESSARY			
7. VOIDING/POSSIBLE CATHETER				21. SAFETY PRECAUTIONS			
8. ELASTIC STOCKINGS				22. POSSIBLE ADVERSE EFFECTS FOR PATIENT TO WATCH FOR			
9. VISITORS PRE AND POSTOPERATIVE/ HOW MANY/WAITING ROOM/ CAFETERIA/SMOKING				23. RESPIRATORY EQUIPMENT			
POSTOPERATIVE				**DEMONSTRATION/PRACTICE**			
10. POST ANESTHESIA RECOVERY				24. TURNING			
11. VITAL SIGNS FREQUENCY				25. LEG EXERCISES			
12. EQUIPMENT SPECIFIC TO SURGERY/ DRAINS/MONITOR/SUCTION				26. COUGHING			
				27. DEEP BREATHING			
13. DRESSINGS				28. OTHER			
14. PAIN MEDICATION							

COMMENTS (PATIENT'S & FAMILY'S UNDERSTANDING & REACTION TO INFORMATION & SURGERY)

_____

AREAS TO REINFORCE

_____

SIGNATURE/CLASSIFICATION
X

SIGNATURE/CLASSIFICATION
X

22012, AUG 80

Figure 9–2. A preoperative teaching form. This form indicates possible content areas for the nurse to consider when teaching patients and their families about their surgical experience and serves to document any teaching the nurse did. (Courtesy of the University of Minnesota Hospitals and Clinics, Minneapolis, MN.)

station knows where you and the patient are in case something unexpected develops. Get all needed equipment into the room before bringing in the patients.

Adjusting Teaching During Implementation. Try to be flexible when implementing a teaching plan. If the learners start to look confused, slow down or go back and clarify the confusion. Ask the patients for feedback. "You look confused. Is something unclear?" Ask for questions and allow time for learners to formulate them before moving on to the next topic. Try to involve the learners in decisions about starting and stopping times, breaks, need for additional practice, and the amount of information they can handle at one time. If the learners are having trouble with a skill, consider a demonstration where the skill is broken down into smaller steps and have the learners practice these more simple activities. Later, learners can put the smaller skills together to perform the original complex skill. New teachers frequently underestimate the amount of time it will take to teach a certain amount of information or skill. A seasoned teacher once said, "Figure out how much time you will need to cover each topic and then multiply by four."

Hints to Implementation. When beginning to teach, the more flexible the nurse can be in adapting the plan, the more effective the nurse will be in meeting the needs of the patient. Remember:

- Large chunks of time are not essential to effective teaching; teach a little during each contact with the patient; combine physical care and treatments with teaching (this becomes easier as proficiency in physical care skills improve).
- Provide written materials to complement teaching.
- When teaching one patient, find out if another nurse has a patient with similar needs and teach them together; this is more efficient, and patients often have reduced anxiety levels if they can share concerns with others experiencing similar problems.
- Face the learners; use frequent eye contact; speak slowly, clearly, and loudly enough to be heard.
- Try to solicit the patient's feeling and reactions to the material as it is being taught.
- Encourage patients' learning efforts by praising their abilities and understanding; correct erroneous information or skill performance by explaining why it is incorrect and helping them learn the preferred information or activity.
- Schedule teaching time just as other treatments; include the patient in planning the time.

Evaluation

Evaluation involves deciding whether or not the desired learning actually occurred. It also involves analyzing the effectiveness of the teaching method, the teaching plan, and the skills of the teacher. When evaluating whether learning actually occurred, review the goals of learning and choose a form of evaluation to match the behavior identified in the goal. Evaluation may take the form of a talk between the nurse and patient in which the patient reviews the information learned. The nurse can evaluate a skill taught to patients by having them demonstrate the skill back to the nurse. A public health referral may be needed to have a nurse visit the patient at home to evaluate learning that occurred in the hospital. Follow-up phone calls to patients after discharge are another way of evaluating learning.

Asking the patient to fill out an evaluation form is one way of gathering data about the teaching which was done. Asking another nurse or student to sit in on your teaching session is called peer review, and this is another way of getting feedback on your strengths and weaknesses in the teacher role. Tape recording teaching sessions will give the nurse valuable information on personal communication skills. Self-evaluation of teaching will lead to improved skills because it helps the nurse-teacher identify personal learning needs for improved performance.

Summary

The nursing competencies related to patient teaching that are associated with various nursing education levels for entry into practice are discussed in the early part of the chapter. They include the assessment of patients' learning needs, development of short-range to comprehensive teaching plans, implementation of teaching plans, and evaluation of learning. The nurse is expected to work with individual patients or groups of patients and to incorporate learning needs into the individual's total plan of care. The nurse is further expected to be a lifelong learner, keeping current with new medical and nursing procedures. In addition, the role of educating other health personnel on new techniques for patient care is presented.

Teaching is defined as the process of assisting the learner to change behavior in a predetermined direction. Learning is not observable but is inferred from a change in the learner's behavior which is not the result of a temporarily altered state or normal growth and maturation.

Teaching on an individual basis, in a small group, or in a large group is based on the particular type of learning desired and other needs of the patients. One-to-one patient teaching sessions may be most amenable to individualization but are also less efficient. Large groups tend to be the least individualized but may be very efficient if patients' learning needs are quite similar.

Benefits to the patient of effective teaching include independence, maintenance of optimum health status, lowered costs, decreased severity of illness, and decreased anxiety. Inadequate or inaccurate patient teaching may cause unnecessary harm to the patient if not corrected and presents the nurse with the ethical choice of admitting an error and taking corrective action. Giving health information to minors that conflicts with parental values is presented as another example of an ethical conflict in the teaching role.

Motivation for learning may be inherent in the human race or may be caused by anticipating rewards or avoiding negative outcomes. When the learner recognizes a difference between the real situation and a desired situation, and new learning is viewed as a means of reducing the difference, a learning need is present. Recognition of learning needs facilitates learning. Assessment by nurses of a learning need in a patient is a form of nursing diagnosis.

Types of learning include cognitive, affective, and psychomotor areas. Most learning incorporates aspects of all three types while focusing on one.

Principles of learning are presented as a guide to personal learning and patient teaching. Planning and implementation of teaching plans are based on these principles as they apply to each patient's needs and situation. Activities and situations that can facilitate learning or interfere with learning are discussed. Assessment of a patient's readiness to learn, learning style, strengths, and deficits is important prior to the planning phase to facilitate an individual's learning.

Learning goals are specific patient outcomes which correspond to the diagnosed learning needs. Evaluation is guided by the type of behavior selected in the learning goal. Learning is viewed as having occurred if the patient can perform the specific behaviors identified in the learning goals.

Various teaching methods are discussed: demonstration, lecture, role-play, discussion, site visit, and audiovisual teaching. Effective use of each method is based on the goals for learning and adequate preparation and guidance of learners before, during, and after use of each method.

Terms for Review

competencies	learning	learning need	role-play
demonstration	learning goals	lecture	teaching
discussion			

Self Assessment

A student in nursing is a learner. The personal feelings associated with particular learning experiences are unique to each student. Nursing students are often under a great deal of stress. Their learning needs are many and not always easily met. Students may find some comfort in the following table, which demonstrates feelings and concerns of other students in nursing. (See Table 9–7.)

Learning Activities

1. Observe other nurses involved in teaching patients and their families. What techniques do they use to involve the learners? Are the learners motivated to learn? Is the environment appropriate? Is the pace slow enough to allow questions and practice time as needed by the patients?

2. Plan to identify one learning need for your next patient and do some simple teaching. Does the patient understand why each medication has been prescribed? Does the patient understand the reason for all treatments? Are the reasons for restrictions on such things as activity, diet, or smoking understood?

3. Evaluate the teaching you are receiving in your nursing program in terms of your felt needs and the learning goals identified by your nursing instructor. How are you affected when your personal goals are similar to those of the instructors? When they are different? Do the learning experiences match your preferred learning style? How do you feel using new learning methods? Is practice with positive reinforcement part of skills learning? How do you feel when your instructor compliments your efforts and developing skill? How do you feel when you receive too little practice and no feedback or only negative feedback in your learning efforts? Remember these feelings and try to take the best from your education and incorporate it into the patient-educator role as a nurse.

4. Talk with nurses who have primary responsibilities in the area of patient education. Plan an independent laboratory time with one nurse as patient teaching is done. How does the nurse evaluate learning? How does the nurse evaluate teaching? How long did it take before confidence was gained in the nurse-educator role? What additional type of education, either formal or informal, was helpful to the teacher role?

Table 9–7. **Feelings and Concerns of Nursing Students**

Fears of Nursing Students During Their First Week of School

	PERCENT
1. Failure in school	46
2. Taking responsibility	19
3. Making a dangerous mistake	13
4. Not liking the profession	6
5. Dealing with death	4.4
6. Dealing with sick people	3
7. Relating to people	2.2
8. Financial worries	1.5
9. Family problems	.7

Negative Experiences of Nursing Students After Eight Months in School

1. Overall pressure and stress	30
2. Fear of failing out of school	13
3. Relating to certain people	13
4. Anxiety about clinical work	6.5
5. Lack of confidence	4.3

Positive Experiences of Nursing Students After Eight Months in School

1. The instructors	19.5
2. Being competent	14.4
3. Helping patients	13.6
4. Working with people	12.7
5. Clinical work	11.9
6. Getting a good education	9.3
7. Personal growth	6.8
8. Positive self-image	5.9
9. Professionalism	5.9

Reprinted from the *Journal of Nursing Education*, June 1981, Vol. 20, no. 6, pp. 12–13. Published by Charles B. Slack Inc., Medical Publishers, copyright 1981.

Review Questions

1. All of the following are elements common to teaching *except*
   a. Teaching is a purposeful activity.
   b. Teaching involves identifying learning goals.
   c. Teaching involves changing the learner in some predetermined direction.
   d. Teaching creates identical changes in all learners in a group.
2. Which of the following activities is a result of learning?
   a. The newborn who sucks and swallows
   b. Withdrawing your hand quickly when something hot is touched
   c. Blinking of the eyes
   d. A feeling of probable failure when attempting to learn a new skill

3. Benefits of patient education include all of the following *except*
   a. Reduced health costs
   b. Increased number of hospital admissions for any given individual
   c. Feelings of independence for the patient
   d. Decreased patient/family anxiety related to health care
4. Which of the following statements is true about individual patient teaching?
   a. This form of teaching has the potential for being the most individualized to a patient's learning needs.
   b. This is one of the most time-efficient forms of teaching.
   c. Patients' ability to share feelings with other patients experiencing similar problems is an advantage of this form of teaching.
   d. This form of teaching is indicated when similar learning needs are shared by several other patients.
5. Which of the following activities tends to promote learning?
   a. Rigidity of learner
   b. Repeated failures associated with prior learning experiences
   c. Creating a situation where learner feels threatened
   d. Active involvement of learners
   e. Discussing all aspects of a complex problem in one extended teaching session
6. True or False
   _____ a. Students who are more anxious about their own behavior than the learning needs of the patient when they begin to do patient teaching should get out of nursing.
   _____ b. Flexibility is more common than rigidity in the teaching style of nursing students in their early patient teaching experiences.
   _____ c. The ability to develop comprehensive, long-term teaching plans for patients with complex medical problems is appropriate for the licensed practical or vocational nurse.
   _____ d. Hospitalized patients are usually inadequately motivated to learn about personal health needs.

Answers

1. d
2. d
3. b
4. a
5. d
6. a. F
   b. F
   c. F
   d. F

References and Bibliography

Adams, D., and Wright, A.: Dissonance in nurse and patient evaluations of the effectiveness of a patient-teacher program. *Nurs. Outlook,* **30**:132–36, Feb., 1982.

Busl, L.: The teacher as manager of the learning environment. *J. Nurs. Educ.,* **20**:42–47, May, 1981.

Combs, A.; Blume, R.; Newman, A.; and Wass, H.: *The Professional Education of Teachers,* 2nd ed. Allyn & Bacon, Boston, 1974.

Commission on Nursing Education: *Educational Preparation for Nursing—A Source Book 1980.* Pub. #NE-105M4/81, American Nurses' Association, Kansas City, Mo., 1981.

Commission on Nursing Education: *Standards for Nursing Education.* Pub. #NE-1 10M6/75, American Nurses' Association, Kansas City, Mo., 1975.

Elhart, D.; Firsich, S.; Gragg, S.; and Rees, O.: *Scientific Principles in Nursing* Mosby, St. Louis, 1978.

George, G.: If patient teaching tries your patience, try this plan. *Nursing 82,* **12**:50–55, May, 1982.

Hassid, P.: My way—teaching couples to be flexible. *Childbirth Educator* **1**:15–18, Summer, 1982.

Jacobs, A.; Fivars, G.; Edwards, D.; and Fitzpatrick, R.: Critical requirements for safe/effective nursing practice. Pub. #B41, Council of State Boards of Nursing, American Nurses' Association, Kansas City, Mo. 1978.

Krathwohl, D.; Bloom, B.; and Masia, B.: *Taxonomy of Educational Objectives.* McKay, New York, 1964.

Kron, T.: *The Management of Patient Care,* 5th ed. Saunders, Philadelphia, 1981.

MacMillan, P.: Teaching and learning, insight and growth. *Nurs. Times,* **77**:1513–14, Aug. 26, 1981.

Mager, R.: *Developing Attitudes Toward Learning.* Lear Siegler/Fearson, Belmont, Calif., 1968.

McKeachie, W.: *Teaching Tips—A Guidebook for the Beginning College Teacher* Heath, Lexington, Mass., 1969.

Mitchell, P., and Loustau, A.: *Concepts Basic to Nursing,* 3rd ed. McGraw-Hill, New York, 1981.

Redman, B.: *Patterns for Distribution of Patient Education.* Appleton-Century-Crofts, New York, 1981.

Rogers, C.: *Freedom to Learn.* Merrill, Columbus, Ohio, 1969.

Snelbecker, G.: *Learning Theory, Instructional Theory, and Psychoeducational Design.* McGraw-Hill, New York, 1974.

Standards of Nursing Practice. American Nurses' Association, Kansas City, Mo., 1973.

Tyler, R.: *Basic Principles of Curriculum and Instruction.* University of Chicago Press, Chicago, 1974.

Vander, A.; Sherman, J.; and Luciano, D.: *Human Physiology—The Mechanisms of Body Function.* McGraw-Hill, New York, 1980.

CHAPTER 10

COMPUTERIZED INFORMATION SYSTEMS
COMMUNICATION TOOLS FOR NURSING*

Objectives

1. Discuss why it is important for nurses to have an understanding of what a computer system can do.
2. Describe several features of computers that are designed to make them user friendly.
3. Explain how a computer is used to facilitate admission procedures to the hospital.
4. Describe the process used to prevent unauthorized access to confidential data stored in the computer.
5. Describe the use of a light pen with a menu screen.
6. Explain how the computer may help eliminate some types of medication errors.

7. Discuss how computers may be used to help the nurse to write patient care plans.
8. Discuss potential advantages and disadvantages of computer-assisted charting.
9. Describe the use of computers for physiological monitoring.
10. Explain why physiological monitoring systems will not replace a skilled intensive care nurse.
11. Discuss how the computer may be used to assist in discharge planning.
12. List some actions the nurse may take during downtime.

*Written by Linda Edmunds the Practice Editor of *Computers in Nursing*. She is nursing systems consultant, with Travenol Laboratories, Inc., and was formerly Systems Nurse and Clinical Assistant Professor in Adult Health Nursing at State University of New York at Stony Brook, New York.

Introduction

Computer systems installed in health care facilities are usually called information systems. They are called information systems because their function is to assist in the communication of patient-related information. Computerized information systems are used to collect, organize, and transmit patient data between departments, among health care providers, and to patients. Because nurses play a central role in the patient-related communication process, these systems offer nursing an unusual tool for assisting with the efficient delivery of high-quality patient care.

For nurses, understanding what a computer system can do is more useful than understanding the technical complexities of how a computer works. Most of this chapter, therefore, will center on what computers can do for nurses. It will explain the types of applications that have been developed to assist nurses to take care of patients.

But because we live in a society where computers are being used in all spheres of activity, it is helpful to be familiar with some of the terminology and some of the technical concepts associated with how computers work. This will keep us from feeling left out when friends and colleagues, even our children, discuss what they are doing with their computers. More important, it may help us to communicate more effectively with the data-processing people who design computer systems.

Why do nurses need to be able to communicate with programmers, systems analysts, data-base administrators, hardware engineers, and other types of data-processing professionals? The reason is that despite all the ways computers are currently used in nursing practice, we are still only at the edge of exploring what these machines can do to assist with health care delivery. The more nurses understand about the technology, the more successful they will be in working with data-processing staff to develop systems that will help nurses plan, implement, and evaluate care.

Computer Terminology and Concepts

Computers come in three basic sizes: small, medium, and large. The smallest computers are called *microcomputers*; medium-size computers are called *minicomputers*, and the largest computers are called *mainframes*. The important difference between micros, minis, and mainframes is not really size, but their relative capacity to store data and the speed with which they manipulate it.

Hardware

Computer systems are described in terms of their hardware and their software. Computer *hardware* refers to the devices or equipment that make up the computer system. A home computer, which is an example of a microcomputer, may consist of just two pieces of hardware: a typewriterlike keyboard connected by wires to a television set. In a basic home computer, the two most essential hardware components—memory and central processing unit (CPU)—are contained within the keyboard. *Memory* is the place where data entered into the computer are stored, either temporarily or permanently. The *CPU* is the part of the computer that manipulates data to produce requested results. For example, suppose a user wants to add two numbers: 375 and 459.3. Using the keyboard, the numbers are typed on the TV screen and *inputted* (entered) into the computer's memory. The addition is done by the central processing unit and the result, 834.3, is *outputted* (displayed) on the TV screen.

A more complex microcomputer used in a home or office would have two additional pieces of hardware: a printer and a disk drive. Data are outputted to a printer which provides the user with a permanent copy of the requested information. A paper printout of computer data is termed *hardcopy*. Disk drives are devices that read floppy disks. Floppy disks look like flexible plastic records. They are used to store data, just as cassette tapes are used to store sound. The disk drive reads the data stored on the disk and transmits it to the CPU just as a cassette recorder reads a tape and sends it to an amplifier. Disks are used to expand the memory of a computer system. Two floppy disks store twice as much data as one disk.

Software

If it's part of a computer system and you can touch it, it's hardware. If you can't touch it, it's *software*. Software is another name for computer programs. *Programs* are sets of instructions, written in a language understandable to the computer, that tell the central processing unit what to do with the data that are inputted to it. In the example used above, two numbers, 375 and 459.3, are entered temporarily into the computer's memory. How does the central processing unit know whether to add, multiply, divide, subtract, or just permanently store the two numbers? It knows because it follows the instructions in a program, designated by the user, which has also been stored in memory. Before the user enters the numbers, the name of the program that is to be used by the CPU is typed on the TV screen and entered. Most home and office computers are programmed in a language called BASIC. Other more complex programming languages are COBOL, PASCAL, FORTRAN, and ASSEMBLER. There is even a language called MUMPS which is used to write software for some health care facilities that use minicomputers.

Data Base

A data base is a collection of related information organized into discrete units called records. A user who owns two floppy disks might decide to store a different data base on each disk. On the first disk, one might store the names, addresses, phone numbers, and birthdays of acquaintances. The name, address, phone number, and birth date of one acquaintance would be considered a record. If the user had 400 friends, the data base would have 400 records, each including the four pieces of data indicated. The second disk might be used to store a data base made up of all the items in the user's house along with their cost, location, and date of purchase. Of course, if the user had a lot of valuables (or a lot of junk), the data base might be very large and two or more disks required to store it.

Suppose the user had written a program that could alphabetize any list of words or phrases inputted to it. The user could use the program to alphabetize either possessions or friends by loading the data from one of the two disks into the computer. In a microcomputer system, a user can move disks into or out of the machine as needed. In mainframe computer systems, where many users share the same data base, the disks on which the data are stored cannot be moved. A hospital with a computer system would be in quite a fix if one of its employees could take a disk filled with patient data home for the weekend.

Hospital Information Systems

As you might expect, the hardware, the software, and the data base of a computer system used in a hospital are more complex, and there is more of it. The central processing unit is more powerful, there are a variety of devices to store data, hundreds of programs are used, and the data bases may be numerous with each one complexly organized and including thousands, even millions, of records. But happily, the hardware that the nurse uses on the patient care unit is very simple to operate. And the nursing software is designed to be user friendly. *User friendly* means that programs are written so that entering data into the computer and retrieving information from it are as simple as possible.

If you walk into a 30-bed nursing unit in a hospital with an information system, you will probably see one, two, or three computer terminals at the nursing station. These terminals, sometimes called CRTs, look like small television sets with keyboards attached to them. A terminal keyboard looks like a standard typewriter keyboard with the keys for the letters and numbers in the same places. The only difference between the two keyboards is that the computer keyboard may have some additional keys not found on a typewriter. For example, there may be an "Enter" key. After the user types some information on the video screen, the Enter key is pressed. This sends the information to the CPU which processes it.

The Enter Key is a nice feature because it helps to prevent errors. If you make a mistake when you are typing on the computer screen, you have the chance to correct the mistake before the information is entered for processing. This is one example of how systems installed in hospitals are made to be user friendly. They are designed so that a user has multiple opportunities to correct errors. Understanding how to correct their errors usually stops nurses from being afraid to use the terminals.

Nurses may also fear that when they use a computer they will somehow cause the system to malfunction, either by breaking a piece of hardware or by entering some data that are so bad they will mix up or destroy the programs that run the computer. Causing a system to break down by entering bad data is almost impossible. Information systems are designed so that only highly trained programmers can alter the system sufficiently so that it crashes (breaks down). The hardware on the patient care units is also pretty sturdy. If reasonable care is taken to prevent food, or drink, or heavy objects from falling on the terminals, they won't break.

Data can be entered into the system by using the keyboard attached to the terminal. For example, if a nurse is using the system to enter an order for a patient, instructions might appear on the screen that state, "Key in the name of the ordering physician." The nurse would use the keyboard to type "Dr. Spock," for example. On most terminals used in hospitals, there is another device for entering data which is called a *light pen* (Figure 10–1). The light pen is about the size and shape of a pen

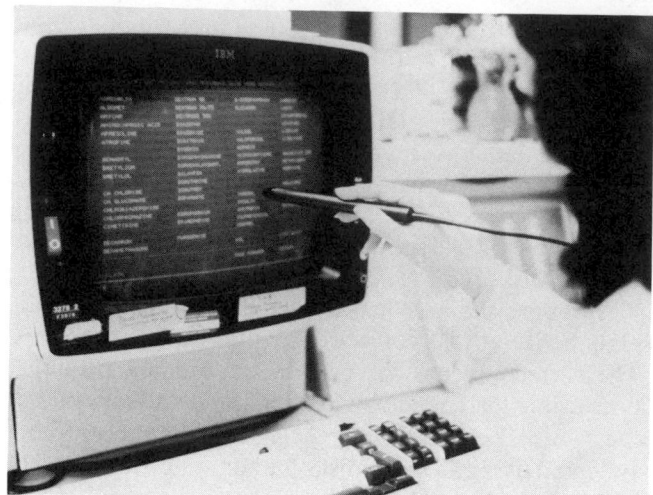

Figure 10–1. Videodisplay terminal. A computer terminal used on a nursing unit resembles a small television set with a typewriter keyboard attached to it. The penlike device in the user's hand is called a light pen and is used for entering and retrieving data.

light and is attached to the terminal by a wire. The light pen speeds up the process of data entry by allowing users to enter data by selecting what they want from screens with menu lists. If a nurse were going to enter an order for a patient, the computer would display a list of all patients on the unit, and the nurse would select the appropriate patient by touching the computer screen with the light pen at the place where the patient's name was displayed. Similarly, if the nurse were going to enter an order for a clear-liquid diet, the computer might display a list of 20 diets. When the nurse touches the phrase "clear-liquid diet," the diet order is sent into the computer. Most information systems are designed so that the light pen is used more frequently than the keyboard for data entry. This is because most clinical staff do not like to type or do not type quickly. Designing systems around light-pen entry is another example of how computer designers try to make systems user friendly.

The other piece of computer hardware that is usually found on a nursing unit is a printer. Many types of printers are relatively noisy and have to be kept away from patient rooms. Other printers are quiet and can be positioned closer to patients. Since patient test results, as well as other confidential information comes across the printer, it is important in all cases to keep these devices away from public areas of the hospital.

Some printers have a great many buttons and look complicated. Generally, however, the nurse only needs to know how to use a few of the buttons to remove the printouts that are needed. Keeping the machine supplied with paper and ribbons may be more difficult and time consuming. Clerks or unit managers, therefore, should be assigned these routine maintenance responsibilities. If nurses work on shifts where these support personnel are not available, or in areas of the hospital that are isolated by dress codes such as the OR, it may be useful for them to know how to change a printer ribbon or add paper.

All the terminals and printers are connected by means of cables to a large mainframe computer. A cable is simply a group of wires enclosed within a layer of rubber insulation. Sometimes the mainframe computer is not located in the same building as the hospital. It may even be in another city. In this case, the information is transmitted between the terminals and the computer via telephone lines.

Wherever the mainframe is located, it looks like a large box the size of several refrigerators standing next to each other. Connected to the mainframe are at least two types of memory devices: disk drives and tape drives. The disks used with mainframes are hard, not floppy, and are about the size of 33-rpm records. A number of them are stacked in a protective box. Data stored on these disks, immediately accessible to users, are considered *online data*. When the disks get full, some of the data stored in them may be off loaded onto magnetic tape. *Off loaded* means that a copy of the data stored on the disk is transferred to tape. Then the disk is erased so that it can be reused. Data stored on tape are not available unless the user is willing to wait.

Because the hardware used in a large information system is complex and there is so much of it, there is usually a person called an operator who sits at a console in the main computer room and makes certain that the system is operating properly. If nurses have problems with hardware on the nursing units, they will call the console operator for assistance. If they have problems with software, they would call the programming department or the nurse who acts as liaison with the programming department.

Communicating with Hospital Departments

A variety of companies market information systems for hospitals. Although each of these systems may have some unique capabilities, almost all of them are designed to assist with the communication of patient data, orders, and results between the nursing units and the main ancillary departments such as admitting, laboratory, radiology, pharmacy, dietary, and medical records. If a system is really broad based, communication with other departments such as ECG, EEG, respiratory and physical therapy, cental supply, biomedical engineering, housekeeping, and transport will also go through the computer system. Computerization assists nurses with interdepartmental communication by making the clerical procedures more efficient. Patients benefit because supplies, services, and, most important, test results are available sooner to the medical and nursing staff.

Admitting

It is important to understand how the admitting office uses the computer because it is in this department that the patient first enters the computer system. A patient entering the hospital stops at the admitting department. The admitting officer collects basic information, including the patient's name, address, phone number, age, sex, religion, and social security number. The name, address, and phone number of the patient's nearest relative and employer are also requested. Next, the admitting officer asks if the patient has health insurance. If the patient does, the insurance carrier and policy number are noted. The admitting diagnosis, which is also required, is obtained from the admitting physician prior to the patient's arrival. Hospitals without computer systems type this information on special forms. One of these forms becomes the face sheet (first page) of the patient's chart.

In a hospital with a computer system, the first thing the admitting officer does after greeting the patient is to type the patient's name onto the terminal screen. When the Enter key is pressed, the computer does a search of its memory to see if the patient has been in the hospital previously. If the patient has had a previous admission, all the admission information collected at that time—age, sex, next of kin, insurance carrier, and so forth—is displayed on the computer screen. If there are changes, these are entered into the terminal, as are the name of the admitting physician and the admitting diagnosis. A great deal of clerical time is saved because information that is unchanged does not have to be retyped.

The next step in the admitting process is to find a bed for the patient. When computers are not available, records of occupied and unoccupied beds are kept in a notebook or on a large blackboard. When a computer is available, manual records are unnecessary. The admitting officer can request a list of beds for any unit to be displayed on terminal. This list, called a bed census, shows which beds are empty and which are filled. A bed is selected for the patient by touching the light pen to a bed listed as unoccupied (Figure 10–2). As soon as this is done, the unit to which the patient has been admitted gets a notice on its printer stating that the patient has arrived in the hospital. Other departments, such as dietary and pharmacy, are also notified. In admitting, a face sheet for the chart with all the admission information prints out. If plastic addressograph cards are used, the computer may activate the machine that makes the card.

Communication over the information system between nursing and admitting does not end with the patient's admission. Anytime the patient is transferred to another unit, the admitting office is notified via computer. When the patient is discharged, the nurse will again use the computer to notify admitting.

```
@@@@@@@@@@@@@@@@@@@@@@@@@@@@@@@@@@@@@@@@@@@@@@@@@@@@@@@@@@@@@@@@@@@@@@TOP
         B E D   C E N S U S   F O R   S U R G E R Y   N O R T H
         TO ADMIT PATIENT TO UNIT SELECT AN UNOCCUPIED BED WITH LIGHT PEN
-------------------------------------------------------------------------------
ROOM   BED   NAME                     SEX   AGE   SMOKER?   VACATED        CLEANED
1501   D     FREZNER, MAXINE          F     56    Y         . . . . . . . . . .     .
1501   W     ..  UNOCCUPIED ........   .     . .   .         042284 0600            Y
1502   D     COHEN, JOSEPH            M     23    N         . . . . . . . . . .     .
1502   W     DANDENELO, MARTIN        M     34    N         . . . . . . . . . .     .
1503   S     BRETZ, JANINE            F     45    Y         . . . . . . . . . .     .
1504   S     MALONEY, JOSEPH J.       M     78    N         . . . . . . . . . .     .
1505   1     BACCORDIALI, MICHAEL     M     34    N         . . . . . . . . . .     .
1005   2     HOLLINGTON, FRANK        M     44    N         . . . . . . . . . .     .
1505   3     DETINGER, ERNEST P.      M     21    N         . . . . . . . . . .     .
1505   4     PEOONI, ANTHONY          M     54    N         . . . . . . . . . .     .
1506   D     REUBEN, ALICIA           F     38    Y         . . . . . . . . . .     .
1506   W     ..  UNOCCUPIED ........   .     . .   .         042384 1000            N
1507   D     MONTOFORO, SAMUEL        M     65    Y         . . . . . . . . . .     .
1507   W     RIZZO, MARIO             M     43    Y         . . . . . . . . . .     .
1509   S     MASON, NELLIE            F     43    N         . . . . . . . . . .     .
1511   1     VASSER, LESLIE           F     31    N         . . . . . . . . . .     .
1511   2     REIESNOR, KATHERINE      F     67    N         . . . . . . . . . .     .
-------------------------------------------------------------------------------
                              MASTER

@@@@@@@@@@@@@@@@@@@@@@@@@@@@@@@@@@@@@@@@@@@@@@@@@@@@@@@@@@@@@@@@@@@@@@BOT
```

Figure 10–2. Bed census. An admitting officer can display a bed census for any unit in the hospital. The bed census shows which beds are filled and which are unoccupied. To admit a patient to the unit, the admission officer touches the light pen to one of the unoccupied beds listed on the screen.

Transmitting Physicians' Orders

One of the major uses of information systems in hospitals is for the communication of physicians' orders to the clinical ancillaries such as laboratory and radiology. In some hospitals, physicians sit at a terminal and enter their orders directly into the computer themselves. In other hospitals, physicians handwrite their orders, and nurses or clerks transcribe them into the computer system. Each approach has its advantages and disadvantages, but the order entry process is basically the same. For the purpose of this discussion, we will assume that nurses are responsible for order entry. The reader should be aware of one other thing. It would be unlikely for two hospitals using paper laboratory requisitions to have exactly the same forms. It is just as unlikely that any hospital would use a computerized order entry sequence exactly the same as the one that will be described here. Nonetheless, order entry sequences, if not identical, do resemble one another. Understanding the details of the order entry process to be described here should be of help in grasping any other sequence encountered.

Signing On.   The first step in using a computer system for entering physicians' orders, or for any other reason, is to *sign on*. An information system in a hospital has a great deal of confidential data stored in it. To protect these data from being displayed by nonauthorized staff and to prevent untrained persons from entering incorrect data into the computer's memory, access to the system is limited by secret code. Personnel who are authorized to use the computer, and who have completed a computer training course, are assigned their own personal identification number and password. Before they can use the computer system, they type this code onto a special computer screen (Figure 10–3A). This is called "signing on." If the computer recognizes the code, the user is allowed to proceed. If the computer does not recognize the code, it will display a message to the person at the terminal. The message will say something like, "You have keyed in an invalid code." If the user has just made a typing mistake, the code can be retyped.

In some institutions, the code not only allows the individual to use the computer system, but defines the access level of the user. What this means is that not all staff in an institution need to use the computer for the same functions. A housekeeper does not need to display a patient's laboratory results on a terminal, and a pharmacist should have no reason to enter a radiology report into the system. A nurse taking care of babies in the nursery may have reason to look at clinical data for mothers in obstetrics, but there is no reason for this nurse to display data for patients in psychiatry. When a valid code is correctly keyed into the computer, the computer only allows the user to display and update data appropriate for the job. An alternative way of limiting access to patient data is by terminal. This means that to get information about a patient in the emergency room, the user must sign on to a terminal in the emergency room. To get information about a patient in the labor and delivery suite, the nurse must be there.

Entering a Laboratory Order.   Regardless of the specific procedures for securing patient data, to enter an

```
@@@@@@@@@@@@@@@@@@@@@@@@@@@@@@@@@@@@@@@@@@@@@@@@@@@@@@@@@@@@@@@@@@@@@TOP

        HOSPITAL    INFORMATION    SYSTEM
................................................................................



          TO SIGN ON TO THE SYSTEM KEY IN YOUR
              ID NUMBER AND PASSWORD


          ID NUMBER:*            *

          PASSWORD:*            *


      THEN PRESS THE ENTER KEY ON YOUR KEYBOARD


................................................................................

@@@@@@@@@@@@@@@@@@@@@@@@@@@@@@@@@@@@@@@@@@@@@@@@@@@@@@@@@@@@@@@@@@@@@BOT
```

Figure 10–3 (A).   This sequence of screens illustrates a typical computerized order entry sequence. ID/ password sign-on screen. To use an information system, the nurse must type in an ID number and a password that the computer recognizes.

```
@@@@@@@@@@@@@@@@@@@@@@@@@@@@@@@@@@@@@@@@@@@@@@@@@@@@@@@@@@@@@@@@@@@TOP
            S U R G E R Y    M A S T E R    S C R E E N
         SELECT THE APPROPRIATE APPLICIATION WITH YOUR LIGHT PEN
               TO SIGN OFF THE SYSTEM SELECT ' SIGN OFF'.
-----------------------------------------------------------------------

  *** CENSUS FUNCTIONS ***              *** REFERENCE DATA ***
  PT CENSUS: SURG NORTH                 HELP SCREEN INDEX
  PT CENSUS: SURG SOUTH                 MATH CALCULATORS
  BED CENSUS: OCCUPIED/EMPTY            QUALITY ASSURANCE STANDARDS
  PTS WITH ADMITTING DX                 VISITOR GUIDE

                                        *** MESSAGE FUNCTIONS ***
                                        SEND MESSAGE
  *** PATIENT DATA ***                  INFECTION CONTROL MESSAGE
  PT LOCATION INQUIRY                   SYSTEMS SUGGESTION BOX
  PT MEDICAL RECORD# INQUIRY            TRANSPORT/MESSENGER REQUEST
  PREADMISSION LAB RESULTS              EXCHANGE CART ITEM REQUEST
  LAST E.R. VISIT DATA                  IMED PUMP REPLY
                                        DIETARY REQUEST MESSAGE
                                        BIOMEDICAL ENGINEERING REQUEST

-----------------------------------------------------------------------
                                                         SIGN OFF

@@@@@@@@@@@@@@@@@@@@@@@@@@@@@@@@@@@@@@@@@@@@@@@@@@@@@@@@@@@@@@@@@@@BOT
```

Figure 10–3 (B). Surgery master menu screen. The surgery master screen lists the functions assigned to nurses who work on the surgical units of the hospital. To enter an order for a patient on Surg North, the nurse probes "Patient Census: Surg North." (Note the sign-off command on the bottom of the screen. When a user leaves a terminal, this command is probed so that access from the terminal is ended.)

order the nurse must first sign on to the system. If the password is keyed in correctly, the nurse's master menu screen appears (Figure 10–3B). The screen is called a master because it lists only those applications appropriate for the nurse. It is called a menu screen because the nurse chooses one application from the list with the light pen, just as a diner might choose an item from a restaurant menu by pointing to it.

The nurse works on a unit called Surg North. One of the functions listed on this master screen, which is assigned to all nurses on the surg north unit, is "Patient Census:Surg North." When the nurse touches any part of the phrase "Patient Census: Surg North" with the light pen, a list of all patients on this unit appears on the video screen (Figure 10–3C). Another function on the nurse's master menu screen is "Patient Census: Surg South." If this function is selected with the light pen, the patients on Surg South are listed on the terminal. Most likely, the nurse has access to patients on both Surg North and Surg South because staff float between the two units.

The physician, Dr. Spock, has written orders for a

```
@@@@@@@@@@@@@@@@@@@@@@@@@@@@@@@@@@@@@@@@@@@@@@@@@@@@@@@@@@@@@@@@@@@TOP
      P A T I E N T   C E N S U S   F O R   S U R G E R Y   N O R T H
            SELECT THE APPROPRIATE PATIENT WITH YOUR LIGHT PEN
-----------------------------------------------------------------------
ROOM BED NAME                   PT NUMBER  SEX AGE ATTENDING MD
1501 D   FREZNER,MAXINE         I0088004    F   56  GOAL,NEIL
1501 W   METRAS,CATHERINE       I0087065    F   65  SPOCK,JONAS
1502 D   COHEN,JOSEPH           I0087089    M   23  NELSON,GREGORY
1502 W   DANDENELO,MARTIN       I0087034    M   34  SESKA,JOSEPH
1503 S   BRETZ,JANINE           I0087047    F   45  GOAL,NEIL
1504 S   MALONEY,JOSEPH J.      I0087121    M   78  GOAL,NEIL
1505 1   BACCORDIALI,MICHEAL    I0086999    M   34  VARET,THEODORE
1505 2   HOLLINGTON,FRANK       I0087089    M   44  NELSON,GREGORY
1505 3   DETINGER,ERNEST P.     I0087125    M   21  BERNSTEIN,HOWARD
1505 4   PEOONI,ANTHONY D.      I0087134    M   54  SESKA,JOSEPH
1506 D   REUBEN,ALICIA          I0087111    F   38  BERNSTEIN,HOWARD
1507 D   MONTOFORO,SAMUEL       I0087167    M   65  DIANOPALI,JAY
1507 W   RIZZO,MARIO            I0087194    M   43  GOAL,NEIL
1509 S   MASON,NELLIE P.        I0087134    F   43  HOROWITZ,MILTON
1511 1   VASSER,LESLIE NEAL     I0087115    F   31  HOROWITZ,MILTON
1511 2   CAPELLUTE,THERESA      I0087155    F   67  WEEK,HOWARD M.
1511 3   REIESNOR,KATHERINE     I0087256    F   23  VARET,THEODORE
-----------------------------------------------------------------------
                    PAGE  FORWARD              MASTER

@@@@@@@@@@@@@@@@@@@@@@@@@@@@@@@@@@@@@@@@@@@@@@@@@@@@@@@@@@@@@@@@@@@BOT
```

Figure 10–3 (C). Census screen. The census lists all the patients on Surg North. To enter an order for the patient Catherine Metras, the user touches that name with the light pen.

```
@@@@@@@@@@@@@@@@@@@@@@@@@@@@@@@@@@@@@@@@@@@@@@@@@@@@@@@@@@@@@@@@@@@@@TOP
          P A T I E N T   F U N C T I O N   S C R E E N
       CHECK THAT YOU HAVE ACCESSED THE APPROPRIATE PATIENT, THEN PROBE
              APPROPRIATE FUNCTION WITH YOUR LIGHT PEN
     -----------------------------------------------------------------
              PATIENT SELECTED IS   <   METRAS, CATHERINE   >
     . . . . . . . . . . . . . . . . . . . . . . . . . . . . . . . . .
        *** ENTRY FUNCTIONS ***              *** DISPLAY FUNCTIONS ***

        ENTER ORDERS BY DEPT                 DISPLAY ORDERS
        HIGH FREQUENCY ORDER ENTRY           DISPLAY REQUISITION STATUS
        ADMISSION ORDERS                     DISPLAY RESULTS
        PHYSICIAN ORDER SETS                 DISPLAY MEDICATION PROFILE
        UPDATE ORDERS                        DISPLAY INTRAOPERATIVE RECORD
        CANCEL ORDERS

                                             PRINT PATIENT ORDERS
        PATIENT CARE PLAN                    PRINT MEDICATION WORKLIST
        DISCHARGE PLANNING GUIDE
        PATIENT PROFILE DATA
        PATIENT ACUITY DATA

        MEDICATION CHARTING

     -----------------------------------------------------------------
                                  MASTER          CENSUS
@@@@@@@@@@@@@@@@@@@@@@@@@@@@@@@@@@@@@@@@@@@@@@@@@@@@@@@@@@@@@@@@@@@@@BOT
```

Figure 10-3 (D). Patient function screen. The patient function screen lists functions that allow data to be inputted or retrieved for the patient whose name is displayed on top. The nurse checks that the correct patient has been selected and then probes "Enter Orders."

CBC and a barium enema for Catherine Metras who is a patient on Surg North. To enter the order, the nurse first probes "Patient Census: Surg North" with the light pen. When the list of patients appears, the nurse touches the light pen to Catherine Metras' name. The next screen that is displayed has the name "Catherine Metras" displayed on top and a menu of functions listed below. It is called the patient function screen (Figure 10-3D) because whatever function is selected by the nurse will be done for the patient Catherine Metras. For example, if the nurse probed "Display Orders" with the light pen, it would be Catherine Metras' orders that would be displayed.

In this case, the nurse wants to enter orders for Catherine Metras, so the function "Enter Orders" is probed with the light pen. A screen listing the clinical ancillary departments appears (Figure 10-3E). The nurse is going to enter the laboratory order first, so "Laboratory" is selected and the laboratory index is displayed (Figure 10-3F). The nurse has two options for ordering a CBC. If the nurse knows that a CBC means a complete blood count and is done by the hematology laboratory, the nurse can probe "Hematology." If the nurse is uncertain as to which section of the laboratory performs a CBC, the nurse can request a list of all laboratory tests beginning with the letter C. When the letter

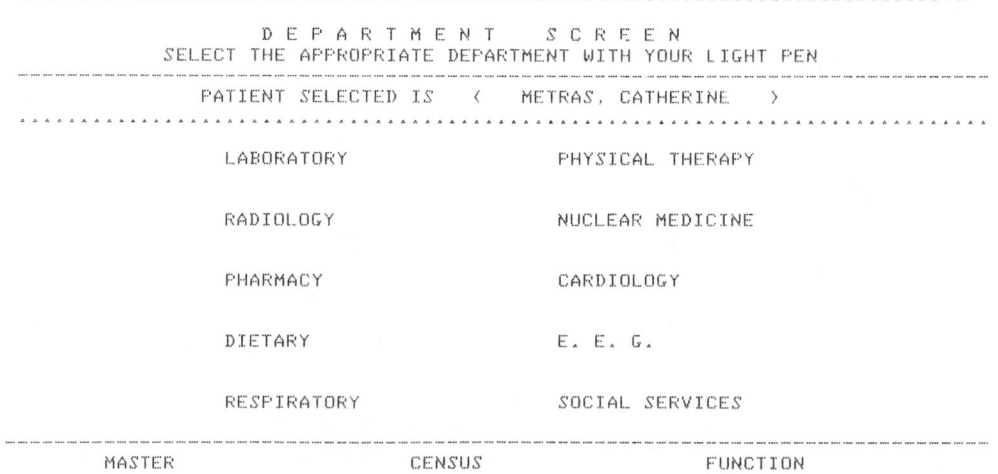

```
@@@@@@@@@@@@@@@@@@@@@@@@@@@@@@@@@@@@@@@@@@@@@@@@@@@@@@@@@@@@@@@@@@@@@TOP
          D E P A R T M E N T   S C R E E N
       SELECT THE APPROPRIATE DEPARTMENT WITH YOUR LIGHT PEN
     -----------------------------------------------------------------
              PATIENT SELECTED IS   <   METRAS, CATHERINE   >
     . . . . . . . . . . . . . . . . . . . . . . . . . . . . . . . . .

          LABORATORY              PHYSICAL THERAPY

          RADIOLOGY               NUCLEAR MEDICINE

          PHARMACY                CARDIOLOGY

          DIETARY                 E. E. G.

          RESPIRATORY             SOCIAL SERVICES

     -----------------------------------------------------------------
        MASTER            CENSUS            FUNCTION
@@@@@@@@@@@@@@@@@@@@@@@@@@@@@@@@@@@@@@@@@@@@@@@@@@@@@@@@@@@@@@@@@@@@@BOT
```

Figure 10-3 (E). Department screen. The department screen lists the clinical ancillaries that are connected to the computer. To enter an order for a CBC (complete blood count), the nurse probes "Laboratory."

```
@@@@@@@@@@@@@@@@@@@@@@@@@@@@@@@@@@@@@@@@@@@@@@@@@@@@@@@@@@@@@@@@@@@@@@@@TOP
              L A B O R A T O R Y     I N D E X
       SELECT APPROPRIATE LAB OR APPROPRIATE LETTER OF THE ALPHABET.
-----------------------------------------------------------------------
          PATIENT SELECTED IS   <   METRAS, CATHERINE   >
. . . . . . . . . . . . . . . . . . . . . . . . . . . . . . . . . . . .

        ** LABS **                  A      I      Q

        CHEMISTRY                   B      J      R

        HEMATOLOGY                  C      K      S

        IMMUNOLOGY                  D      L      T

        MICROBIOLOGY                E      M      U

        PATHOLOGY                   F      N      V

        TISSUE TYPING               G      O      W

        BLOOD BANK                  H      P      XYZ

-----------------------------------------------------------------------
     MASTER          CENSUS          FUNCTION         DEPARTMENT
@@@@@@@@@@@@@@@@@@@@@@@@@@@@@@@@@@@@@@@@@@@@@@@@@@@@@@@@@@@@@@@@@@@@@@@@BOT
```

Figure 10-3 (F). Laboratory index screen. The nurse can order a CBC by probing the letter *C*. If the letter *C* is selected, a list of laboratory tests beginning with that letter is displayed. If "Hematology Lab" is probed, all tests done by that laboratory are listed. In this case, the nurse probes the letter *C* with the light pen.

C is probed with the light pen, tests beginning with this letter are listed (Figure 10-3G). If all the tests beginning with the letter *C* do not fit on one screen, there will be a probe point on the bottom of the screen which says "Page Forward." Probe points such as "Page Forward" and "Page Backward" allow the user to page back and forth through a series of screens in the same way a reader would page back and forth through a book. The nurse uses the light pen to select the CBC. The next screen that appears has the instructions "Key in the name of the ordering person," and there is a place designated on the screen to type in these data (Figure 10-3H). The keyboard is used to type in Dr. Spock's name.

Typing on a computer is even simpler than using a typewriter because it is so easy to correct errors. On the screen there is a small movable marker. It looks like a dash and is called a *cursor*. If the letter A is pressed on the keyboard, the letter A will print on the screen over where the cursor is located. When the letter A is typed, the cursor moves one position to the right. The cursor can also be moved backward and forward by special

```
@@@@@@@@@@@@@@@@@@@@@@@@@@@@@@@@@@@@@@@@@@@@@@@@@@@@@@@@@@@@@@@@@@@@@@@@TOP
              L A B O R A T O R Y     T E S T S
          SELECT THE APPRORIATE TEST WITH YOUR LIGHT PEN.
-----------------------------------------------------------------------
          PATIENT SELECTED IS   <   METRAS, CATHERINE   >
. . . . . . . . . . . . . . . . . . . . . . . . . . . . . . . . . . . .
CADMIUM, BLOOD                    CATECHOLAMINES, URINE
CADMIUM, URINE                    CATHETER TIP, CULTURE
CAFFEINE                          CBC WITH DIFFERENTIAL
CALCITONIN                        CBC NO DIFFERENTIAL
CALCIUM, SERUM                    CEA
CALCIUM, 24HR URINE               CELL COUNT, CSF
CALCIUM, SPOT URINE               CELL COUNT, BODY FLUID
CALCIUM, TOTAL SERUM              CELONTIN
CALCULI                           CEREBRALSPINAL FLUID, CULTURE
CANDIDA ANTIBODIES                CERULOPLASMIN, SERUM
CARBAMAZEPINE, SERUM              CHEM 6 PROFILE
CARCINIOEMBRYONIC ANTIGEN         CHEM 12 PROFILE
CARISOPRODOL                      CHLORAL HYDRATE, BLOOD
CAROTENE                          CHLORAMPHENICOL
CATECHOLAMINES, PLASMA            CHLORIDE, 24 HR URINE
-----------------------------------------------------------------------
     PAGE BACKWARD                             PAGE FORWARD
@@@@@@@@@@@@@@@@@@@@@@@@@@@@@@@@@@@@@@@@@@@@@@@@@@@@@@@@@@@@@@@@@@@@@@@@BOT
```

Figure 10-3 (G). Laboratory tests—*C* screen. There are more tests beginning with the letter *C* than can be listed on one screen. The "Page Forward" and "Page Backward" commands listed on the bottom of the screen allow the user to page back and forth through the tests as necessary. To order the CBC, the nurse selects "CBC No differential" with the light pen.

```
@@@@@@@@@@@@@@@@@@@@@@@@@@@@@@@@@@@@@@@@@@@@@@@@@@@@@@@@@@@@@@@@@@@@@@@@@@@TOP
                     O R D E R I N G     P H Y S I C I A N


         ----------------------------------------------------------------
              PATIENT SELECTED IS   <    METRAS, CATHERINE    >
              TEST   ORDERED IS     <  CBC WITH DIFFERENTIAL  >
         ................................................................/


                       KEY IN THE NAME OF THE PHYSICIAN
                            WHO WROTE THIS ORDER


                    *      DR. SPOCK               *



                      THEN PRESS THE ENTER KEY OR
                   PROBE 'ENTER' WITH YOUR LIGHT PEN




         ----------------------------------------------------------------
                                                       ENTER
@@@@@@@@@@@@@@@@@@@@@@@@@@@@@@@@@@@@@@@@@@@@@@@@@@@@@@@@@@@@@@@@@@@@@@@@@@@BOT
```

Figure 10–3 (H).   Enter ordering physician. The screen requests the nurse to type in the name of the ordering physician. The name is typed in the designated field. Then the Enter key is pressed to send the information into the computer's temporary memory.

keys on the keyboard. To correct a typing error, all the user has to do is move the cursor under the character that is incorrect and type over the incorrect character with the correct key. This is certainly faster and less messy than using liquid whiteout.

Once the doctor's name is keyed into the computer, the last screen in the order entry sequence appears. This screen is a review screen (Figure 10–3I). It is called a review screen because the nurse has the opportunity to review the information that has been entered and to make any corrections or modifications. For example, if the physician has ordered the CBC stat, the frequency of the test would be changed from routine to stat at this time. On the other hand, if the nurse had selected the wrong test or the wrong patient, the entire order could be deleted by probing ''Delete'' on the bottom left-hand corner of the screen. This is another example of how systems are designed to be user friendly. If a user knows

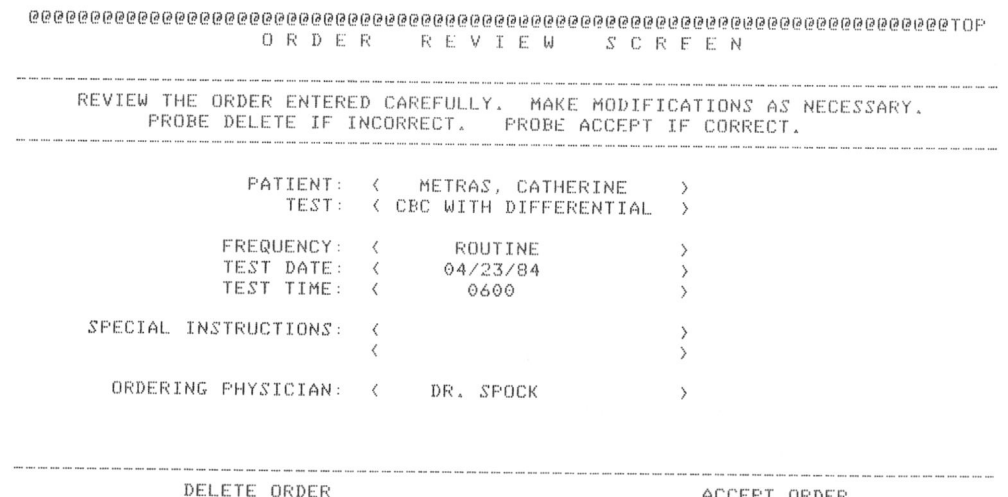

```
@@@@@@@@@@@@@@@@@@@@@@@@@@@@@@@@@@@@@@@@@@@@@@@@@@@@@@@@@@@@@@@@@@@@@@@@@TOP
                  O R D E R    R E V I E W    S C R E E N

         ------------------------------------------------------------------
           REVIEW THE ORDER ENTERED CAREFULLY.   MAKE MODIFICATIONS AS NECESSARY.
              PROBE DELETE IF INCORRECT.    PROBE ACCEPT IF CORRECT.
         ------------------------------------------------------------------

                      PATIENT:  <    METRAS, CATHERINE    >
                         TEST:  < CBC WITH DIFFERENTIAL   >

                    FREQUENCY:  <        ROUTINE          >
                    TEST DATE:  <       04/23/84          >
                    TEST TIME:  <         0600            >

          SPECIAL INSTRUCTIONS:  <                         >
                                 <                         >

          ORDERING PHYSICIAN:   <     DR. SPOCK           >


         ------------------------------------------------------------------
              DELETE ORDER                              ACCEPT ORDER
@@@@@@@@@@@@@@@@@@@@@@@@@@@@@@@@@@@@@@@@@@@@@@@@@@@@@@@@@@@@@@@@@@@@@@@@@BOT
```

Figure 10–3 (I).   Order review screen. The nurse has completed entering all the required data for ordering the laboratory test. The review screen displays all the data that have been entered so that the nurse can check it for accuracy. If the wrong test or the wrong patient has been selected, the order would be deleted by probing ''Delete'' on the bottom of the screen. If order has been correctly entered, the nurse probes ''Accept'' on the review screen. This sends the data into the computer's permanent memory. It also initiates the printing of a requisition which will accompany the specimen to the laboratory.

that the opportunity exists to correct errors made in entering an order, then the computer will seem less intimidating, especially when the user is new.

If the order is correct, the nurse probes "Accept" on the review screen (bottom right, Figure 10–3I). The computer then automatically prints out a laboratory requisition for the CBC. The requisition is like a manual paper laboratory slip, except that it does not have to be stamped with the patient's nameplate. One of the first things the nurse did on entering the order was to indicate to the comptuer who the tests were for. When the computer prints out the laboratory requisition, it prints the patient's name on it. It also searches through the computer's memory for information about the patient's age, medical record number, sex, admitting diagnosis, and admitting physician, and prints this information on the requisition. If you recall, these data were entered by the admitting officer on the patient's arrival. This sharing of a centralized data base illustrates one of the most significant advantages of a large mainframe computer used by the entire hospital over minicomputers with separate data bases in individual departments. When a housewide mainframe computer system is available, data entered by one department are available to be used as necessary (and as appropriate) by other departments. The requisition may also have information about the minimum volume of blood needed for the test and the type of container to be used. Storing this information in the computer's memory and printing it out on the requisition facilitate appropriate specimen collection. This is especially useful when unusual laboratory tests are ordered or in areas of the hospital, like the intensive care units, where nurses rather than laboratory technicians draw most of the blood specimens.

Transporting the Specimen. After the blood is drawn from the patient, it must be transported with the requisition to the laboratory. Most hospitals have messengers who make hourly rounds picking up specimens, delivering medications, and transporting supplies and equipment from place to place. At times, it is not possible to wait for the routine messenger service, and the nurse will require a special messenger. In a hospital without a computer system, the telephone is used to notify the messenger service. If the line is busy or the dispatcher has stepped away from the desk, the nurse may waste several minutes waiting for the phone to be answered. An information system saves a nurse time. The nurse can select a function from the master screen, "Transport/Messenger" request. On the screen that appears, the nurse types in what the messenger is needed for, e.g., "Transport specimen from Surg North to Hematology Lab." The message prints out immediately in the transport office, and the nurse can continue with other patient care activities.

The Laboratory. When the blood for the CBC is received in the laboratory, it is accessioned. This means that the specimen type, patient name, and date and time of receipt are recorded. In a manual system, accessioning is done in a logbook. When a computer system is available, accessioning is done on the terminal. This provides certain benefits to the laboratory, but it is also useful because the nurse can determine, from the terminal on the unit if the specimen was received in the laboratory.

Much of the equipment in modern laboratories is automated. For routine hematology tests like a CBC, a sample of blood is put into a special machine, and the machine does the tests and prints out the results on a laboratory slip. When a hospitalwide system is available, instead of printing out the results in the laboratory, the results are transferred electronically to the main computer system. As soon as a laboratory technician verifies that the results are valid, they print out on the patient unit. Instead of having to wait an hour or so until a messenger transports the laboratory results up to the unit, the nurse can immediately pull the CBC results off of the unit's printer.

There are other advantages to computerizing results reporting beside the speed with which the results reach the unit. In addition to printing at the nursing station, the results are stored in the computer's memory. If a physician is in another area of the hospital and wants to check a patient's test data, the physician can sit at a terminal anywhere and review these data. This saves the nursing staff from having to stop what they are doing to answer the phone, find the chart, and look up the results for the doctor. It also means that if the nurse on the unit is writing in a chart, the physician can look up the same patient's laboratory results on the terminal without interrupting the nurse. The computer can also summarize data and produce reports that show the trend of a patient's laboratory results over time. For example, if a patient has had seven CBCs since admission, the results would print on a single page. Trends, such as a falling hematocrit or an increasing white cell count, are more quickly apparent when data are presented tabularly than when they are available only on multiple laboratory slips.

Automation of laboratory order entry and results reporting helps the hospital to maintain financial solvency. When the laboratory results for the CBC are entered into the computer, a charge is automatically put on the patient's bill for the test. Because this is done automatically, fewer charges are lost. A lost charge is one that is not entered on a patient's bill because of clerical error. Communicating charges by computer from ancillary areas to the business office where bills are prepared saves the hospital the expense of hiring staff to do these tasks manually. Of course, the hospital still needs to pay for the computer hardware and personnel, so the issue of cost-effectiveness becomes a complex one.

Entering a Radiology Order.   We have looked in some detail at how a nursing unit communicates with a laboratory using a housewide information system. Similar communication procedures are used between nursing and other clinical departments. If a physician orders a radiology test such as a barium enema, the nurse would go through the same steps that were necessary to enter the laboratory test. (It might be helpful to return to Figure 10–3 at this point and make believe you are sitting at a terminal getting ready to enter a barium enema order for Catherine Metras.)

The nurse sits at the terminal and types in the secret password. The nurses' master menu screen appears. The patient is on Surgery North so the nurse probes "Patient Census: Surg North" with the light pen. When the list of patients on the unit is displayed, Catherine Metras is selected. The next screen is the patient function screen and the nurse checks to see that Catherine Metras' name is on top. The nurse probes "Enter Orders" and a list of the ancillary departments is displayed. This time the nurse picks radiology, and from here on you will need to use your imagination and perhaps sketch what you would expect the nurse to see on the terminal.

When the nurse selects "Radiology," the radiology index screen presents itself. This screen has an alphabetic index to tests just as the laboratory index did. The nurse probes the letter B and radiology procedures that begin with the letter B are listed. "Barium enema" is on the list, and the nurse selects this test. The next screen instructs the nurse to key in the physician's name. When

this information is entered into the system, the final screen in the order entry sequence appears. It is the review screen and looks like the laboratory review screen. The nurse carefully checks that all the information is correct and probes "Accept" on the bottom of the review screen. When the radiology order is accepted by the nurse, it prints out in the radiology department. The secretary or technician in the radiology department removes the requisition from the printer and schedules the procedure for the following day. In some hospitals, the computer itself will check the patient's other appointments, schedule the radiology examination, and notify the nursing unit. After the patient has had the barium enema, the radiologist reads the x-ray film and dictates the results of the analysis. Clerks in the radiology department type the dictation into the computer. When the radiology report has been entered into the computer, it prints on the patient unit. It is also stored in the computer memory like the laboratory results.

Cardiograms, EEGs, blood gases, physical therapy, diets, medications, pulmonary function tests, and any other procedures are ordered in the same way. Of course, the nurse does not have to sign on to the computer each time a test is ordered. If Dr. Spock had written ten orders for Catherine Matras, the nurse would not sign off the computer until the orders for each department had been entered into the system. Computer systems are designed to be as efficient as possible. If, for example, the nurse had typed in Dr. Spock's name as the ordering physician for the CBC, it would not request the ordering physician again. The computer would assume that the same doctor had written all ten orders and would enter that information by itself. If this were not

```
@@@@@@@@@@@@@@@@@@@@@@@@@@@@@@@@@@@@@@@@@@@@@@@@@@@@@@@@@@@@@TOP
     S U R G E R Y   H I G H   F R E Q U E N C Y   O R D E R   E N T R Y
          SELECT ALL APPROPRIATE ORDERS.  THEN PRESS ENTER KEY.
--------------------------------------------------------------------------------
          PATIENT SELECTED IS   <    METRAS, CATHERINE    >
--------------------------------------------------------------------------------
** LAB **              ** LAB **            ** RADIOLOGY **       ** DIETARY **
?TYPE & CROSS          ?C/S SPUTUM          ?ROUTINE CHEST        ?REGULAR HOUSE
?FF PLASMA             ?C/S WOUND           ?ABDOMEN              ?SOFT
?PACKED CELLS          ?C/S SPUTUM          ?BARIUM ENEMA         ?FULL LIQUID
?CHEM 6                ?C/S BLOOD           ?CHOLECYSTOGRAM       ?CLEAR LIQUID
?CHEM 12                                    ?UPPER GI SERIES      ?NPO
?CBC WITH DIFF        ** PHARMACY **        ?IVP                  ?LOW NA
?CBC NO DIFF           ?PREOP MEDS          ?BONE SCAN            ?LOW CHOLESTEROL
?PLATELET COUNT        ?PAIN MEDS           ?LUNG SCAN
?PRO TIME              ?ANTIBIOTICS         ?LIVER SCAN          ** PT CARE **
?PTT                   ?MULTIVITS           ?CAT SCAN: HEAD       ?I&O
?URINALYSIS            ?DUCOLAX             ?PORTABLE CHEST       ?GUIAC
?VDRL                  ?DALMANE             ?PORTABLE HIP         ?S&A
?T3,T4                                      ?UPPER EXTREMITIES    ?DAILY WTS
?HEP B SUR ANTI       ** MISC **            ?LOWER EXTREMITIES    ?NEURO CHECK
?SERUM DIGOXIN         ?ECG                 ?OTHER PORTABLES      ?SPIROMETRY
?SERUM AMYLASE         ?ABG                                       ?ROUTINE VITALS

       MASTER                   CENSUS                  FUNCTION
@@@@@@@@@@@@@@@@@@@@@@@@@@@@@@@@@@@@@@@@@@@@@@@@@@@@@@@@@@@@@BOT
```

Figure 10–4.   High-frequency order entry screen. High-frequency order entry screens list the most common orders for patients in a specific clinical area. The nurse can select as many orders as necessary from the screen. This type of screen speeds up the order entry process.

the case, the nurse could change the doctor's name on the review screen.

High-Frequency Order Entry. To speed up the process of order entry, some hospitals have developed high-frequency order entry screens and standard order screens. A high-frequency screen is developed for a specific nursing area such as pediatrics. It lists on it the 70 to 80 most common laboratory, radiology, dietary, and other medical orders for that clinical area (Figure 10–4). Instead of going from the laboratory index to the radiology index or to the dietary index and ordering one test at a time, the nurse can enter most or all of a patient's orders from a single screen.

A standard order screen is similar to a printed physicians' order sheet. An obstetrician, for example, may use a standard set of orders for women in normal labor. Instead of handwriting the orders for each new admission, the doctor has a preprinted sheet with the orders listed on it. When the patient is admitted, the doctor makes any necessary modifications and signs the printed sheet. The orders listed on a standard order screen are the same as the orders listed on the physician's printed order sheet. This speeds up the process of transcribing the orders to the computer. In hospitals where physicians enter orders into the computer themselves, this type of screen is essential.

In the emergency room when speed is sometimes critical, block ordering can be done on the computer. If the patient has had a cardiac arrest or infarction, the nurse makes a single selection with the light pen ''Cardiac Orders'' without going through any other screens. Requisitions for predetermined laboratory, radiology, blood gas, and cardiogram procedures print out in the appropriate areas of the hospital. This can save critical minutes in life-threatening situations.

Other Hospital Departments

Because computerization can decrease the amount of clerical time involved in interdepartmental communication, many of the smaller departments in the hospital come online (are connected to the computer) once software development for the clinical ancillaries is complete. Central supply, for example, may store its inventory catalogue in the computer's memory, so that nursing units can order equipment and disposables using the system. When a nurse orders additional suction tubes, for example, a notice may automatically go to the transport office so that a messenger can be sent to pick up the item and bring it to the unit.

Both the information desk and the hospital switchboard are usually connected to the mainframe computer. The information desk uses the system to locate patient rooms for visitors. If a nursing unit enters a patient's condition into the system, (for example, critical, fair, satisfactory), the operators on the switchboard can retrieve these data on their terminals to respond to inquiries from callers.

One of the most important departments connected to the computer, in terms of direct benefit to nursing staff, is medical records. When a patient is discharged from the hospital, the physician writes one or more diagnoses. Medical records staff assign each discharge diagnosis a numeric code according to ICD (International Classification of Disease) protocols. The number and diagnosis are stored in the computer's memory. If the patient should suddenly come back to the emergency room, the nursing staff there can look up the patient on the computer and find out the discharge diagnosis for previous admissions, as well as orders, information about test results, allergies, and so forth. In any hospital, it usually takes at least 15 to 30 minutes to retrieve a paper chart from the medical records department. A housewide information system with terminals in the ER provides critical clinical data instantaneously.

The other benefit of storing discharge diagnoses in the computer's memory is that patients can be quickly identified for research, evaluation, and planning studies. Suppose your nursing research class were doing a project on female adolescents between the ages 12 and 18 with a diagnosis of scoliosis. Once the ICD codes had been identified for the different types of scoliosis, a program could be written that would provide a list of patients fitting the indicated criteria.

Communication on the Nursing Care Unit

Computer systems can facilitate communication on the nursing care unit by assisting nurses with patient care planning and by providing nurses with up-to-date worklists of a patient's medical orders. In some hospitals, nurses use the computer for all or part of their charting. Information that is charted on the computer is legible, available to more than one practitioner at a time, and can be retrieved in a variety of formats depending on what the user's interest is. Bedside computer systems that monitor a patient's vital signs extend the nurse's ability to accurately assess the status of unstable patients.

Computerized Care Planning

Developing a care plan for a patient helps nurses organize their thoughts about a patient's problems, the goals they want the patient to achieve, and the nursing care necessary to assist the patient to meet those goals. When a nursing care plan is available, it serves as a focal point for coordinating patient care across all shifts and for assessing, from a nursing perspective, how well the patient is doing.

Writing a good care plan generally requires a substantial knowledge base, the ability to clearly formulate nursing diagnoses, patient outcomes, and appropriate interventions. This is, even for an experienced nurse, a process that takes time—time to think and time to write. When a nurse is inexperienced or unfamiliar with the actual or potential problems a patient faces, the process may be difficult and even more time consuming. Unfortunately, what often happens in real-life nursing is that the care plan is not written. Faced with uncertainty about what to include, the nurse may opt to spend all available time doing bedside care. On a busy unit, there is certainly almost never enough time to provide every patient with all the physical care and emotional support that are necessary. But something is lost when the care plan is not formulated. Without a set of nursing orders to guide staff, the patient loses because there is no agreed-upon direction for nursing care. And without defined goals against which to compare patient progress, nurses lose the opportunity to objectively assess what their nursing skills have accomplished.

Computerization of the care planning process can provide valuable assistance to busy nursing staff by prompting them to include appropriate diagnoses, goals, and orders in the care plan. Not only can computerized care planning help the nurse formulate a comprehensive care plan, but the clerical time necessary to actually write the care plan is decreased.

Computerized care planning applications can be separated into two categories: standardized care planning and care planning by nursing diagnoses. In the first type of application, a series of standard care plans are stored in the computer's memory. Standard care plans are care plans written for a particular condition by nurses expert in caring for patients with it. The patient condition can be a medical diagnosis, a surgical procedure, or a nursing problem. For example, standard care plans might be available for the patient with congestive heart failure, the preoperative patient for a Harrington rod insertion, or the patient who, for any reason, is immobilized in bed for a long period of time.

How each standard care plan is organized will depend to some extent on the policy of a hospital's nursing service. But, generally, standard care plans list the actual or potential problems a patient with the condition is expected to face. For example, the care plan for the patient with congestive heart failure might list the following associated problems: "Respiratory distress related to increased fluid level in the lungs," "Dependent edema in lower extremities and potential renal failure," "Fatigue due to decreased cardiac output," "Anxiety related to physical condition," "Potential skin breakdown due to immobility," "Potential mismanagement at home due to lack of understanding or acceptance of diet and medication regimen."*

For each actual or potential problem stated in the standard care plan, expected outcomes and related nursing orders are stored. For the problem of "dependent edema and potential renal failure," the expected outcomes that might be stated would be: (1)no edema, (2) return to normal body weight, (3) urinary output of 240 ml per shift. The nursing orders written to assist the patient in achieving the expected outcome would include: weigh patient daily, elevate legs, record urinary output and specific gravity, and measure ankle circumference at bath time. Some standard care plans include a deadline for when the patient is to meet the outcome and the frequency with which the nurse is to assess the patient. For this potential problem, the standard care plan directs the nurse to assess the patient q8h and indicates that the outcome is to be met prior to discharge.

If a nurse works in a hospital that has standard care plans stored in the computer's memory, the patient's care plan is formulated by sitting at a terminal. The first thing the nurse does, after signing on to the system and selecting the patient from the census, is to call up a list of all the available standard care plans. If the patient has a diagnosis of congestive heart failure (CHF), the nurse would use the light pen to select "Congestive Heart Failure" from the care plans noted. The first screen in the care planning sequence for CHF would list the common, actual, or potential problems described above. At this point, the nurse would decide which of the problems listed were applicable to the individual patient. The nurse might select all of the problems or only some of them. In addition, the nurse might use the terminal keyboard to type in additional problems unique to the patient. For example, if the patient were concerned about financial problems related to the disabling effects of illness, the nurse might add a problem "Anxiety related to family welfare."

For each problem selected, the related outcomes and

---

*The content for this care plan on congestive heart failure is from Marlene Mayers and El Camino Hospital: *Standard Nursing Care Plans*. K/P Medical Systems, Stockton, Calif., 1974. El Camino Hospital in Mountain View, California, was one of the first hospitals to make computerized care planning available for its nursing staff.

nursing orders stored in the computer's memory would display sequentially. For each problem, the nurse selects the appropriate goals and interventions, deletes the inappropriate, and makes necessary modifications and additions so that the care plan conforms to the individual patient's needs. Once the nurse is satisfied with the care plan, a copy might be printed for the chart. The modified care plan would also be stored in the computer's memory under the patient's name. If additional problems become apparent and further nursing orders are required, these are added to the care plan. As each problem is resolved by the patient's meeting the stated outcome, the date and time are recorded in the computer.

Standardized care plans help a nurse to plan care by reviewing common problems and usual care associated with a particular condition. The nurse still has to assess the individual patient and think carefully about which parts of the standard care plan are applicable and what needs should be added. But a lot of the time that is usually involved in deciding on appropriate phrasing is eliminated, and the likelihood that some important part of the care process will be overlooked is reduced. Also, the time spent in writing the care plan by hand is saved. This is particularly true in instances such as care planning for the normal newborn where the same initial care plan is used for all babies. Instead of nursing staff copying by hand the care plan for each infant, it can be called up on the computer system, stored under the infant's name, and printed for the chart. Later on, if problems develop, additions can be made.

Using standard care plans as the basis of computerized care planning is one of two approaches that have been developed to utilize the computer in the care planning process. The other approach is based on nursing diagnosis, with the patient's care plan built in modular fashion. The nurse assesses the patient and formulates the nursing diagnosis, for example, anorexia, altered sleep pattern, or potential for skin breakdown. The exact form that the nursing diagnosis takes will depend on the policy of the nursing service, although many are deciding to adopt diagnoses accepted by the National Group for the Classification of Nursing Diagnosis. (See Chapter 17.) Once the nursing diagnoses are formulated, the nurse sits at the terminal and selects from an alphabetic list of diagnoses stored in the computer memory one of those applicable to the patient. For example, when the nurse selects anorexia, the computer may request that the nurse indicate what the anorexia is related to. The nurse, for example, may key in "Anorexia related to depression," "Anorexia related to chemotherapy," or "Anorexia related to difficulty in swallowing." The next screen in the care planning sequence would display expected outcomes (goals) and nursing

actions (orders) for anorexia. For anorexia, general goals for the patient might be stable weight and intake of priority nutrients. The related orders might include "Offer preferred food and small frequent feedings." But probably these orders would have to be modified orders depending on the cause of anorexia. Company during mealtime might be helpful to the depressed patient who is anorexic but not to the patient with dysphagia. As with standardized care planning, the nurse uses the light pen to select applicable goals and orders and uses the keyboard to modify or add to what has been suggested on the screen. After outcomes and nursing actions have been inputted for each nursing diagnosis, the care plan is stored for the patient in the computer's memory and updated as necessary.

Whether computerized care planning is done using standard care plans or by nursing diagnoses, or using a combination of the two approaches, the advantages are the same. Less clerical time is spent in developing the care plan. Nurses who have difficulty phrasing nursing diagnoses, outcomes, or orders are assisted with the writing process. Students or inexperienced nurses who may not know what actual or potential problems are associated with a patient's condition, or what constitutes an appropriate outcome or time frame, can learn a great deal about good nursing care as they review what has been stored in the computer's memory by their more experienced peers. Also, the result of making the care planning process easier and more efficient for staff is that more patients have good care plans developed for them.

Computerized Worklisting

Most nursing units maintain some form of Kardex. A Kardex, whatever its format or configuration, summarizes briefly and by category, a patient's current active orders. In addition to the patient's name, age, sex, religion, doctor, and diagnosis, there may be space for the patient's diets, medications, laboratory tests, radiology procedures, physical therapy appointments, activity level, and any treatments or procedures. Nursing orders may be included also.

When a computer system is available, it may be possible to eliminate the manual Kardex. Many systems produce reports, either once a shift or on a demand basis, that list all of the patient's active orders. Of course, this report is only as accurate as the patient's data base. If a new diet order is entered without existing diet orders being cancelled, the report will be cluttered with outdated data. If house staff or attending physicians don't read a patient's orders before writing new ones, duplicate orders are a likelihood. If the order transcribed into the computer is not verified against the written order, errors will creep into the computer data base, and staff will not trust the printed output. If nursing orders are not written in the nursing care plan, they will not be included in the worklist. The computer can save the nurse a lot of time by making available a legible, well-organized document summarizing current health care orders. Multiple copies can be printed without additional work so that the nurse, the aide, the clerk, and the physician can each have a copy. But there is a saying among computer people: "Garbage in, garbage out." If nurses want a manual Kardex to be useful, it has to be updated on a constant basis. Similarly, a computerized worklist will only be as useful as the care taken to maintain an accurate data base in the computer.

Charting

Some facilities with information systems have nursing staff do some of their charting on the computer. Information charted may include the admission history, progress notes, medications administered, vital signs, or even the intraoperative record. One advantage of charting online is that what is written is clearly legible. Another is that the charted data can be recalled in multiple formats. For example, if problem-oriented charting is computerized, the user can display all progress notes in chronological order or just call up notes related to a single problem. When charting is done manually, only the person in physical possession of the chart can write it in or review what has been written. On a busy unit when there are residents, social workers, dietitians, and other health care providers all using the chart, just finding it can be problematic. With a computer system available, several people can chart at the same time, and others can look at data previously entered. All that is needed is a free terminal.

Therein lies one of the problems with computerized charting. If a hospital has a limited number of terminals, say two for each 30-bed unit, and a lot of data must be charted for each patient, queuing problems can result, particularly at the end of the shift. What this means is that nurses may have to wait in line to use a terminal to complete their charting, in the same way that they would have to wait to write their notes if the unit had only two pens which had to be shared.

Another problem with computerized charting, particularly of progress notes, is that notes often lose a degree of sensitivity. Most nurses don't like to type. Therefore, when hospitals put up charting applications, an attempt is usually made to develop screens with phrases on it that the nurse can select to build a progress note. One screen might have phrases related to appetite, with options such as "appetite excellent," "appetite good," "appetite fair," "appetite poor," "refuses food." What if the patient could be described by none of these categories? Suppose the patient indicates he is hungry but doesn't like the salt-free diet that has been ordered for him and so refuses to eat. If the nurse picks "appetite excellent," the reader might assume that the patient ate well. If the nurse selects "refuses food," the assumption might be that the patient has a poor appetite. Even if the nurse selects both "appetite excellent" and "refuses food," the specific nature of the patient's eating problems would not be identified. Usually, to overcome this problem, charting systems allow nurses to type in notes as well as to select phrases for inclusion. The advantage of computerized charting is that it can be quicker and more complete because the system can remind the nurse to chart in all areas of patient care. The danger of computerized charting is that nursing notes begin to sound canned. The phraseology is so similar between notes that they can be boring to read and thus ignored by other disciplines.

One of the areas in which computerized charting has proved quite effective is in the recording of medications administered to patients. Medication administration charting is tied in closely with pharmacy order entry. Depending on the institution, the physician, the nurse, the clerk or the pharmacist enters a patient's drug orders into the computer. For example, suppose the physician has ordered timolol eyedrops, 1 gtt, bid in both eyes; clonidine, 0.1 mg, po qid; amikacin, stat, IV push q6h; and meperidine q4h prn for pain. Each of these orders is entered into the computer system. The orders print out in the pharmacy, with labels that the pharmacist will use when sending up the medications to the unit. The amikacin order might trigger a bell on the pharmacy printer to alert the pharmacist because it is to be filled stat.

Each of the patient's medications is to be given at a different frequency. The eyedrops will be given once a day; the antihypertensive clonidine twice a day, the antibiotic amikacin q6h, and the merperidine as necessary. For each frequency, a time schedule is stored in the computer memory. For example, when a physician orders a medication to be given bid in this hospital, the nurse knows that the time schedule it is to be given at is 8 A.M. and 8 P.M. All qd orders will be given at 9 A.M. The times for a q6h order are 6 A.M., 12 noon, 6 P.M., and 12 midnight. The computer has the same schedules programmed into it.

Every hour the computer goes through all the medication orders for the patients on Surg North. If it is 10 A.M. in the morning, it checks to see which patients have 10 A.M. medications ordered. The computer then prints out a list of all the patients in the unit who are due for a medication. Under each patient's name is listed the complete medication order.

The nurse may use this computer-generated list as a

worksheet as medications are distributed. After completing medication rounds, the nurse returns to the terminal and enters into the system which medications have been given. If a medication was not given, the computer will request that a reason be inputted. If an injection was administered, the nurse may note the location. Information about IV or IV piggybacks, including starting time, volume, drip rate, and so forth, will also be entered. The computer will automatically record the initials of the nurse charting the medications.

In addition to providing a list of medications to be given each hour, some systems will even print out a reminder notice if no one has charted that the medication has been administered. Another way the computer helps the nurse to save time and decrease errors is by eliminating the transcription of medication orders to medication tickets or from page to page in a medication book. Once the order is entered into the computer, there is no discrepancy between the order in the pharmacy, the order on the nursing unit and the order on the medication label. With manual systems discrepancies of this type may cause medication errors.

When charting is done on the computer, a nurse can look up the last time a prn medication for pain was administered. The nurse with the keys to the medication room, or the nurse with the medications cart, does not need to be bothered, unless it is actually time for the patient's next dose. A physician or pharmacist can quickly scan a patient's drug profile without looking for the chart. Furthermore, some systems generate a cumulative report each day that lists all the medications given to a patient during the past seven days. Missed doses are also listed on this printout.

One of the gravest of the potential pitfalls of using computers for patient care becomes apparent when considering medication charting. Computerized printouts can be somewhat intimidating. The reports look so official a nurse may be less likely to review or check critically information displayed on the printout than when the data is handwritten. Now, computers, left to themselves, really don't make errors. But computers are rarely, if ever, left to themselves. People enter the data which the machine manipulates. If incorrect data are inputted, the computer will also output incorrect data. If an order is entered into the computer as a q4h order, it will reliably appear on the medication lists for 6 A.M., 10 A.M., 2 P.M., 6 P.M., 10 P.M., and 2 A.M. But suppose the order originally written by the physician was a q4h prn order, and it was transcribed into the system incorrectly. Or suppose the physician typed in clonidine 1 mg qd, instead of correctly writing the dosage 0.1 mg qd *by error*. In either case, the patient might be seriously overmedicated. The point is that orders for patients or other data outputted by a computer must be reviewed as carefully and with the same amount of clinical expertise as any other data the nurse uses. The content of computer-printed orders must be examined. Errors in transcription must also be looked for. The nurse needs to check that there are no duplicate orders and that outdated orders are cancelled. The computer is a tool of great value, but it is still just that—a tool. Used competently, it can help nurses provide better patient care more efficiently. Used sloppily, or relied on uncritically, it can be dangerous.

Physiological Monitoring

In the critical care areas of a hospital where patients are actually or potentially unstable, minicomputers, independent of the hospital's mainframe, may be used to support bedside physiological monitoring. Physiological monitoring is, in a sense, an extension of cardiac monitoring which most nurses are familiar with. Cardiac monitors measure two parameters: heart rate and heart rhythm. Physiological monitoring systems track these two parameters, but, in addition, they can also measure respiratory rate, temperature, EEG, and arterial, venous, and intracranial pressures.

The equipment used for physiological monitoring parallels that used for cardiac monitoring. For cardiac monitoring, sensors are attached to specific areas of a patient's chest. Wires from these sensors are attached to a bedside terminal which has a video display screen. The terminal electronically converts the incoming data into a numeric display of heart rate and a graphic display of the cardiac rhythm. If the patient's heart rate falls outside of set limits, or the rhythm shows an atypical or life-threatening pattern, an alarm sounds to alert the nursing staff. The nurse at the bedside will check to see if the patient is truly in danger or if the alarm is caused by an equipment-related problem. Many times a sensor on a patient's chest will become loose or detached. This interferes with accurate sensing of the heart rate. If the monitor picks up a heart rate of 0, it interprets this to mean cardiac arrest, and the alarm is sounded. At the central nursing station where screens display the heart rates and rhythm of all patients being monitored, a rhythm strip prints out. This documents for the nurse and the physician the cardiac events occurring at the time of the alarm.

Basically, the same equipment configuration is used for physiological monitoring. Electronic sensors are connected to the patient. Some of these may be attached to the surface of the patient's body like the ECG or EEG leads. Others, used to measure central venous or arterial pressures, are connected to invasive lines inserted into a patient's vein or heart. The sensors are wired to a bedside video display terminal. Like the cardiac monitor, this terminal converts incoming data into numeric displays of all monitored parameters as well as graphic displays of selected variables.

A bedside monitor might indicate a heart rate of 100, a systolic blood pressure of 125, a diastolic of 56, mean arterial pressures equal to 75, a central venous pressure of 6, a mean pulmonary arterial pressure of 15, a temperature of 100, and a respiratory rate of 18. In addition, the screen might show a graphic display of the values for the systolic, diastolic, and mean blood pressures for the past hour (Figure 10–5). A momentary pressure of 100 is meaningless without knowing what the patient's systolic pressure has been in the past. A graphic display of an hour's worth of data gives the clinician some assistance in determining if the systolic pressure is stable within a range of 105 to 115 or if the pressure is dropping or spiking precepitously. In a computerized physiological monitoring system, if an hour's worth of systolic pressure measurements is not sufficient, the clinician can request a graphic display of the data for the past eight hours or the past day or the past week. Physiological monitoring systems have monitors that display data for all patients at the nurse's station. Like the cardiac monitors, alarms are sounded when incoming data are beyond preset limits.

The advantages of these computerized monitoring systems for the care of critical patients should be obvious. Most important, electronic monitoring is continuous. No nurse takes a patient's blood pressure or other vital sign every few seconds. A machine can and does. The chances, therefore, of missing a life-threatening event are decreased; and the opportunity to pick up in the early stages of a gradual decline or improvement in a particular parameter is increased. The ability to store incoming data and present them as required in graphic form helps the nurse document events and trends for physician review.

Fully computerized physiological monitoring systems may also integrate laboratory results, medications administered, input and output data, and nurses' notes with the monitored data. For example, if medications administered are entered into the physiological monitoring terminal, the nurse and physician may be able to request a graphic display of mean arterial pressure over time, showing when each dose of antihypertensive (medication to lower blood pressure) was administered. Graphics of this type can help the clinician conceptually correlate therapeutic interventions with outcomes. Physiological monitoring systems can also take laboratory data and monitored data and do the necessary mathematics to calculate acid-base balance, cardiac output and stroke volume, or mean intracranial pressure. Calculations which are arithmetically complex can be done more accurately and more quickly by the computer than by the nurse.

If the physiological monitoring system is connected into a hospitalwide network, all of a trauma patient's data can be transferred with the patient from, for example, the emergency room to the operating room, into the recovery area, and, finally, to the surgical intensive care unit. The physician who ultimately is responsible for postoperative care in the intensive care area can review in detail all of the patient's monitored data since admission, not just what busy nursing staff have had time to record in an emergency situation.

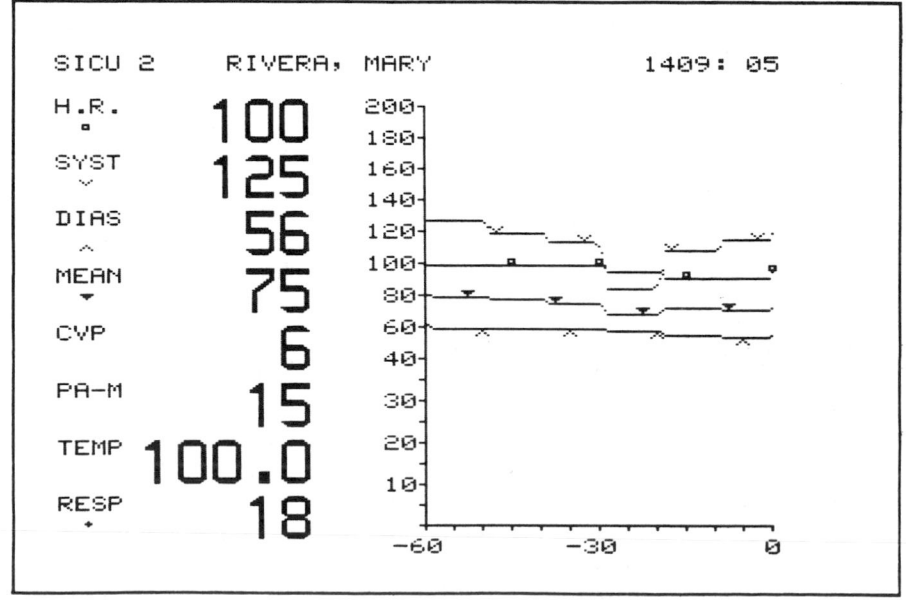

Figure 10–5. Physiological monitoring. The physiological monitoring terminal at the patient bedside displays numeric values of selected physiological variables. In addition, four of these variables—systolic BP, heart rate, mean BP, and diastolic BP—are trended graphically over the past 60 minutes. In many physiological monitoring systems, the variables monitored can be changed, depending on the patient's medical condition. (Reproduced with permission courtesy of the Hewlett-Packard Company, Waltham, MA.)

Can physiological monitoring systems replace the skilled intensive care nurse? The answer to this question is such an emphatic negative that the page is not big enough for the appropriate "No." First, physiological monitoring systems run into the same problems as the cardiac monitoring systems in terms of artifactual data. When a patient is on a cardiac monitor and loses a chest lead, it may look like a cardiac arrest. Obviously, the nurse who observes the patient moving in bed will not begin rescuscitation procedures. The more sophisticated sensors used in physiological monitoring also malfunction. A catheter inserted into a vein may block and provide invalid data. The ICU nurse has to be able to interpret and continuously validate monitored data. When data are really in question, manual readings must be taken to determine whether the electronic data are correct. With all the information the physiological monitoring system can collect, it can never replace the subtlety of an evaluation made by an observant nurse experienced in assessing the physical and mental status of a patient.

Currently, most physiological monitoring systems are not connected to hospital information systems. This can be a problem because it means that nurses must manually enter laboratory results, blood gas values, medications administered, in addition to nursing notes and basic admission data. Manual entry can be time consuming, transcription may be delayed, and errors can occur as results are copied from one computer system to another. For this reason, some facilities are working toward connecting the physiological monitoring systems into hospitalwide systems so that data can be automatically and quickly transferred between the two networks.

Communication Within the Nursing Service

Most of the direct communication about an individual patient's care occurs among clinical personnel on the nursing unit or between the nursing unit and the ancillary departments. But there is a great deal of general communication related to nursing care that goes on within a hospital nursing service. A computerized information system with printers and terminals on all nursing units can make the process of distributing up-to-date information about hospital policies, nursing procedures, new computer applications, inservice programs, operating problems, and other departmental issues very simple. A computer can also assist with a nursing department's quality assurance program and assure that the amount of nursing staff assigned to a unit is based not just on the number of patients on a unit, but on how sick those patients really are. Also, an information system can supplement a hospital's continuing education program by maintaining large amounts of reference material in its memory. This reference data can be accessed by nursing staff when it is needed during the course of patient care.

Message Applications

One of the simplest functions to use in most hospitalwide computer systems is the message function. This type of application lets a user send a message from one area of the hospital to another. The user types the message on a specially formatted screen and picks a destination for the message from another screen that has a menu list of areas in the hospital with printers. When the user finishes typing the message, the computer sends it to the selected destination, and it is outputted on their printer.

Suppose a nurse coming on night duty at 11 P.M. notices that a car with license plate ATG-074 has its lights on. To find the staff member who owns the car, the nurse might sit down at a terminal, sign on, select the "Send Message" application, and type in "To all staff, from Nurse Rosemans, Surg North: Lights left on yellow Dodge with license plate ATG-074." Since the nurse wants to get the message to as many staff as possible, all destinations listed would be selected. As soon as the "send" command is given to the computer, the message begins printing all over the hospital.

In order to organize the distribution of hospital-related announcements, a nursing service may develop a computerized newsletter by modifying the message function. All notices are copied to one secretary who types them onto special newsletter screens once a day. When the day's issue is entered into the computer, it prints at all nursing stations. A typical newsletter (Figure 10–6) might include a schedule of basic cardiac life support classes available for nurses needing recertification, an announcement of meeting times between night staff nurses and the Director of Nursing, a notice from a local motel indicating an offer of free Christmas holiday housing to families of hospital patients living more than 50 miles away from the institution, a description of a new drug added to the formulary, and a posting of available positions for nursing staff. Nursing staff, as well as staff from other departments, use the computerized newsletter to disseminate information because their

```
@@@@@@@@@@@@@@@@@@@@@@@@@@@@@@@@@@@@@@@@@@@@@@@@@@@@@@@@@@@@@@@@@@@@@@@@@@
@ * * * * * * * * * * * * * * * * * * * * * * * * * * * * * * * * * * * @
@ *                                                                   * @
@ *    Q Q Q         DD D  D        AAA      YYYY YYYY      DAILY      * @
@ *   Q     Q        D      D      A    A     YY YY         NEWS       * @
@ *   Q     Q        D      D     AAAAAAA      YY           NOTES      * @
@ *   Q    QQ        D      D     AA    AA     YY           NOTICES    * @
@ *    Q Q QQQ       DD D  D     AAAA  AAAA   YYYY          FOR THE    * @
@ *                                                        NURSING     * @
@ *    THURSDAY         APRIL 10, 1984                     DIVISION    * @
@ *                                                                   * @
@ *  * * * * * * * * * * * * * * * * * * * * * * * * * * * * * * * *   * @
@@@@@@@@@@@@@@@@@@@@@@@@@@@@@@@@@@@@@@@@@@@@@@@@@@@@@@@@@@@@@@@@@@@@@@@@@@
*                                                                       *
*   BASIC CARDIAC LIFE SUPPORT RECERTIFICATION CLASSES FOR APRIL        *
*      APRIL 12    THURSDAY        9-12 NOON                             *
*      APRIL 17    TUESDAY      1-4 PM                                   *
*      APRIL 19    THURSDAY        7-10 AM                               *
*      APRIL 23    TUESDAY         3:30-6:00 PM                          *
*                                                                       *
*      CALL JOANNE SLATER TO REGISTER.                                  *
*                                                                       *
* * * * * * * * * * * * * * * * * * * * * * * * * * * * * * * * * * *   *
*                                                                       *
*   * NEW ON THE HOSPITAL INFORMATION SYSTEM: ATTENTION E.R. NURSES     *
*                                                                       *
*     LABELS ARE NOW AVAILABLE AS A FUNCTION OFF THE PATIENT FUNCTION   *
* SCREEN.  YOU CAN PRINT SINGLE LABELS OR 5, 10 OR 15 LABELS AT A TIME. *
* RECOMMENDED USE: LABORATORY SPECIMENS                                 *
*                                                                       *
* * * * * * * * * * * * * * * * * * * * * * * * * * * * * * * * * * *   *
*                                                                       *
* MEETING CANCELLATION:      O.R. STAFF MEETING SCHEDULED FOR 4/24 HAS  *
*                            BEEN CANCELLED.  RESCHEDULED FOR 4/25      *
*                            AT 0700. MS. LATOUR WILL MEET WITH OR NURSES*
*                            IN THE OR LOUNGE                           *
*                                                                       *
*    MEETING SCHEDULED:      QUALITY ASSURANCE                          *
*                            APRIL 26                                   *
*                            1:30 PM  SURG NORTH CONFERENCE ROOM        *
*                            IF UNABLE TO ATTEND PLEASE CALL LEE DORSET.*
*                                                                       *
* * * * * * * * * * * * * * * * * * * * * * * * * * * * * * * * * * *   *
*   LECTURE: DR JACK PEDMONE, MEDICAL SCHOOL LECURE HALL 7  - 4/26  3PM *
*            DIC: DISSEMINATED INTRAVASCULAR COAGULATION                *
* * * * * * * * * * * * * * * * * * * * * * * * * * * * * * * * * * *   *
*   DAY CARE CENTER                                                     *
*      THE DAY CARE CENTER WILL OPEN AT 6:45 AM INSTEAD OF 7:45 AM      *
*      BEGINNING NEXT MONDAY.                                           *
*                                                                       *
*   OFFICE SUPPLIES/FORMS:  ATTENTION NURSING STATION CLERKS           *
*      DIRECT PICKUP FOR OFFICE SUPPLIES WILL BE 8:00-11:00 AM          *
*      AND 1-300 PM ON TUESDAYS AND THURSDAYS. ORDERS MAILED OR DROPPED *
*      OFF WILL BE FILLED AS SOON AS POSSIBLE.                          *
*                                                                       *
* * * * * * * * * * * * * * * * * * * * * * * * * * * * * * * * * * *   *
*            P O S I T I O N S     A V A I L A B L E                    *
*   STAFF NURSE - PEDIATRICS - EVENINGS.  CALL PAT SURMAN IF INTERESTED.*
*          - MEDICAL INTENSIVE CARE - DAYS.  CALL MARY GARNER.          *
*   CLINICIAN - SURG NORTH  - EVENINGS.  CALL NANCY PENNY IF INTERESTED.*
*                                                                       *
*                                                                       *
*************************************************************************
```

Figure 10-6. Nursing newsletter. A computerized nursing newsletter transmits daily announcements to staff all over the hospital quickly and efficiently. All announcements are telephoned to one secretary who types them onto specially formatted computer screens. When the data have been entered, a print command sends it to all nursing units. (Reprinted with permission courtesy of University Hospital, Health Center, SUNY at Stony Brook, NY.)

notices go out the same day they are delivered to the secretary. Staff read the newsletter because it relieves them of searching for multiple notices posted on bulletin boards all over the unit.

The computer is unusually helpful when there is a need to notify staff of a temporary or critical problem in the hospital. Suppose, for example, there is a personnel shortage in the transport service on a particular shift. The supervisor of this department can use the computer to notify all nursing staff that transport service will be limited to stat calls and routine runs. Instead of multiple nurses calling the transport office or one person in the transport office calling each nursing unit, everyone in the hospital can be notified immediately of the temporary cutback in services.

Equipment shortages are another type of problem that is critical and common to many facilities. A patient may be admitted with a critical need for an IMED Pump. An IMED Pump is a special device used to regulate infusion rates of IV medications. If central supply has no more of these pumps in stock, it is essential that a pump be located that is either not in use or being used for a patient who can be managed without it. Without a housewide computer system, the nursing supervisor has to go through the time-consuming process of telephoning each unit to relay the problem and determine if any pumps are available. With a computer system, the supervisor can sign on to a terminal anywhere in the hospital and send out a preformatted message requesting nurses to report any pumps not in use or not critically needed. The nurse on the unit can use the computerized message function to reply to the supervisor. The time necessary to locate a pump is reduced and the patient gets the care that is needed sooner.

The computer can even be used to improve itself. One of the functions that can be put on each nurse's master screen is a systems suggestion box. If a nurse has an idea for a new application that would assist with patient care or for a modification to an existing application that would make it work more efficiently, the idea can be sent to the data-processing department using the suggestion box. Many hospitals have a nurse working as a liaison between the nursing service and data processing. In this case, the suggestion would go to the nursing liaison. It would be the responsibility of the nursing liaison, often called a user coordinator or systems nurse, to work with the nurse and with the programmers to develop the application.

The most effective way to design a computer system that nursing staff find useful is to listen to and implement their suggestions. A system designed purely by data-processing people would work wonderfully if programmers and engineers were on the patient units giving bedside care. But if nurses are going to be the primary users of the computer on the nursing units, they must be integrally involved in guiding application development.

Patient Classification/Staff Scheduling

No matter what hospital or health care facility a nurse works in, one of the problems that invariably comes up is staffing. Nurses often complain that there are not enough staff on the unit to provide the care that the patients need. Hospital administrators, on the other hand, who see a large proportion of their operating budget going to pay nursing salaries, may decide there are too many nurses.

To support the need for an adequate nursing staff and to allocate nursing personnel according to actual nursing care needs, some hospitals have developed criteria for classifying patients and assigning staff. Sometimes the criteria are simple. The head nurse or the primary nurse might rate each patient according to whether

the patient requires intensive care, full care, partial care, or is a self-care patient. Because the categories in this example are not specifically defined, some subjectivity is involved in this type of rating system. To eliminate much of the subjective component, other rating systems provide the nurse with a long list of criteria, and the nurse checks off the ones that are appropriate for each patient. Criteria are usually grouped into categories. Under the category of elimination, for example, the nurse might check one or more of the following: "Incontinent of urine or feces," "OOB (out of bed) to bathroom with assistance," "OOB to bathroom, no assistance," "requires bedpan, urinal, or diaper changes," "monitor output," "bowel or bladder training."

Each criterion has a point value assigned to it. This is based on studies that have been done to determine how much nursing time is required to provide care for each criteria: the more nursing time required, the higher the point value. A patient who can go to the bathroom with no assistance may get one point, whereas the patient who is incontinent will acquire five points.

After the nurse finishes checking all the criteria which fit the patient, the points for the selected criteria are summed. The more nursing care a patient requires, the higher this total score will be. Each patient is then placed in a category based on the score. Patients might be placed in one of four categories: 0–25 points, 26–50 points, 51–75 points, and 76–100 points. If a patient accumulated 60 points, the patient would be a category-3 patient in the 51–75-point range.

Each patient on the unit is placed in a category, and then a nurse or clerk figures out the number of patients in each category. The purpose of all this is to determine how many nursing care hours are needed, thus, how many nurses are needed for all patients on the unit for the shift. For example, the hospital may have decided that each category-1 patient needs a total of one hour of nursing care on the day shift. If there were 16 category-1 patients, they would need 16 hours of nursing care. Since one nurse can only do eight hours of work on the day shift, the unit would need at least two nurses for these 16 patients. But now the nursing care hours needed for the other 14 patients (this is a 30-bed unit) must be calculated to determine the total staff needed for the day shift. Then all the calculations would have to be done for the evening and night shift because patients who are not critically ill generally need less care, thus, fewer nurses during the evening and at night.

There are two things to remember about these types of detailed procedures for classifying patients and ascertaining the number of nursing care hours and staff needed. The first is that the procedures are very cumbersome to do manually. In addition to checking the appropriate criteria for each patient, there is a lot of detailed arithmetic involved in classifying all patients and summarizing the needs for all patients on the unit. Often the calculations are more complex than those discussed here because staff requirements are broken down in terms of RNs, LPNs, and nursing aides.

But the second thing to remember is that the figures are very useful. If a 30-bed unit is only 75 percent filled, it may be hard for head nurse to justify a request for two additional staff members for the day shift. But if the nurse can show that the majority of the patients are category-3 and category-4 patients requiring more nursing care hours than is usual for that unit, the request for additional staff may be met. In many hospitals, patients are classified every shift, and float nurses are assigned based on the results. Using a patient classification/staff scheduling system helps the staff nurse because there is greater congruence between patient care needs and nursing hours available.

In addition to daily adjustments to staffing levels, these systems are very useful for justifying the need for more permanent staff. If a nursing director can document for a six-month period that the average number of nurses needed on Surg North for the day shift was five, but only an average of 3.5 nurses could be assigned, hospital administration may approve the hiring of two more staff nurses for that unit.

Where do computers fit in? Basically, they make implementation of very useful, but cumbersome, procedures practical. The computer takes over the job of adding up the scores of individual patients, determining the number of patients in each category, calculating the number of staff needed for each shift, and providing post hoc graphic comparisons of needed staff against actual staff.

When a computerized classification system is available as part of a hospitalwide system, the nurse may sit at a terminal and use the light pen to select those criteria appropriate to each patient. The computer takes all the available input, does the number crunching (this is what computerniks call calculations), and sends the results to the nursing office.

More commonly, patient classification systems are run on microcomputers located in nursing administration offices. Nurses on the units use paper forms to rate their patients. For each patient, the nurse marks the appropriate criteria using a lead pencil in the same way answer sheets are marked when taking **SAT** examinations or Nursing Boards. The completed sheets are collected and sent to the nursing office. Here each sheet is placed in a machine which electronically scans the items marked for each patient and inputs the data into the microcomputer. The microcomputer does the calculations and provides the tallies of nurses needed for each unit (see Figure 10–7).

Reference Data

There are many times during the course of taking care of patients that nurses need information about a medication, a diet, a laboratory test, a nursing procedure, or a hospital policy. Nursing units may have textbooks or manuals with the needed information, but in many cases these volumes move from place to place, and just finding the appropriate information is time consuming.

One of the ways a hospitalwide information system can be of real use to nursing staff on a daily basis is to make reference data quickly available. Pages and pages of information can be stored in a very small amount of space in a computer's memory, and the information can be accessed from any terminal on any nursing unit. Also, computer terminals don't get moved, misplaced, lost, or worn like a book.

Keeping reference information updated is also easier when it is stored in a computer's memory. Consider, for

```
**  SURG NORTH - DAY SHIFT - STAFFING REQUIREMENTS  **

                                APPROVED           TOTAL
                NUMBER PTS     NURSING HRS       NURSING HRS
                IN CATEGORY      PER PT         PER CATEGORY

CATEGORY 1          16             1                 16

CATEGORY 2           7            1.7               11.9

CATEGORY 3           4            2.3                9.2

CATEGORY 4           3            3.5               10.5


              TOTAL NURSING CARE HOURS      47.6
                   DIVIDED BY 8 HOURS        5.95
                      NURSES NEEDED          6
```

Figure 10–7. Patient acuity. Classifying patients into categories and calculating the number of nursing care hours required, based on accepted standards, helps allocate nursing staff according to actual patient care needs.

example, what happens when a policy changes in a hospital without a computer system. First, the policy has to be typed over by a secretary. Then, copies have to be xeroxed and distributed to every nursing unit and department in the hospital. When the new policy is received, a person in each of these areas has to locate the policy manual, find the old policy, remove it, and replace it with the revised copy.

When policies or other reference data are stored in a computer, the only place the data have to be changed is in the computer's memory. In most systems, this is a relatively simple procedure which does not require a trained programmer. Once the changes are made in the computer's memory, the process is complete. Anyone who calls up the policy on any terminal obtains a corrected version.

What types of reference data can be stored in a computer's memory? The answer is any type, but unless a hospital has unlimited hardware and personnel resources, it will probably set some priorities based on what is used most often by the nursing and other clinical staffs. The best way a hospital can determine what is needed is to ask. This can be done formally through user evaluations or informally. An easy way of gathering informal suggestions from nurses about useful reference data is to encourage them to use the computerized system's suggestion box described previously.

Telephone numbers are easily stored in the computer's memory and useful to staff throughout the hospital. The phone numbers of ancillary departments and the nursing units can be listed on one screen. Another screen can show maintenance phone numbers, so it is

clear who to call if there is a problem with plumbing, heating, and elevators, wall suction, call bells, or the computer system itself. This is particularly useful on weekends and off shifts when inhouse maintenance crews are scarce.

Some hospitals even store phone numbers of staff members willing to serve as foreign language translators. If a patient comes into the hospital who speaks a little English but is fluent in Italian, a nurse can look on the computer and find the names and phone numbers of those staff who have volunteered to do English-Italian translation (Figure 10–8).

Suppose nurses on the night shift are finding that translators are not available for their patients. This can be a real problem in the emergency department where it is critical to find out quickly what the patient's complaint is and something about the medical history. An ER nurse might suggest that the computer store in its memory common phrases translated into several languages which can be used to assist with patient communication (Figure 10–9). If an Italian translator could not be found, the ER nurse could print out Italian translations of phrases such as "How old are you?" "How long have you had this problem?" "Where is the pain?" "Are you allergic to any medications?" A sheet with a variety of responses, also with Italian-English translations, could be given to the patient. This obviously is not an optimal solution but in the absence of a family or staff member who can serve as a translator, the availability of this information on the computer can help.

Nurses need information about drugs and laboratory tests frequently. If a nurse has to draw blood speci-

```
@@@@@@@@@@@@@@@@@@@@@@@@@@@@@@@@@@@@@@@@@@@@@@@@@@@@@@@@@@@@@@@@@@@TOP
                  H E L P    S C R E E N
                FOREIGN LANGUAGE TRANSLATORS
       PAGE FORWARD FOR ADDITIONAL FOREIGN LANGUAGE TRANSLATORS
-----------------------------------------------------------------------

AFRIKAANS .............. JASON POPLER, MD ....... ANESTHESIOLOGY ....... 4732

CHINESE ................ MARY SOO ............... HEMATOLOGY LAB ....... 4657
                        SARA WANG .............. EMPLOYEE HEALTH ...... 4322
                        CHARLES TSO ............ MEDICAL RECORDS ...... 4667
                        MAY LIU, RN ............ SURG NORTH ........... 4896

CZECHOSLOVAKIAN ........ VASILY JIREKEK ......... PHYSICAL THERAPY ..... 4436

DUTCH .................. JASON POPLER, MD ....... ANESTHESIOLOGY ....... 4732
                        ANDRE MEDILE ........... BIOMEDICAL ENGIN ..... 4555

FILIPINO ............... LYDIA TEDASCO, RN ..... PEDIATRICS ........... 4317

FLEMISH ...............JASON POPLER, MD ....... ANESTHESIOLOGY ....... 4732
-----------------------------------------------------------------------
     MASTER                                 PAGE FORWARD

@@@@@@@@@@@@@@@@@@@@@@@@@@@@@@@@@@@@@@@@@@@@@@@@@@@@@@@@@@@@@@@@@@@BOT
```

Figure 10–8. Foreign language translators. Storing the names and phone numbers of staff willing to serve as foreign language translators assists nursing staff in caring for non-English-speaking patients. A paper memo with the same information is easily misplaced. The same data stored in the computer's memory are always accessible.

mens for TSH (thyroid-stimulating hormone) or urine for a 24-hour urea nitrogen, it may be necessary to check the type of tube necessary for the first test and the preservative necessary for the second. If the nurse has trouble drawing blood from the patient, or if the patient is a child, it may be useful to know the minimum volume needed. The nurse may be unfamiliar with the purpose of a test that is ordered, or wonder why the results are not back after three days. All this information might be available if the nurse telephoned the laboratory and convinced the laboratory secretary to interrupt a techni-cian who could answer the question. On the other hand, if the laboratory manual on the unit was up to date and could be found, the information might be there. But if the same data are stored in the computer's memory, it is always available as long as the nurse has access to a ter-minal.

Information about patient medications also can be stored on a computer. A sheet with information about a drug's actions, side effects, dosage ranges, contraindi-cations, and the nursing implications can be printed out on demand (Figure 10-10). The nurse may also be able

```
UU    UU   HH   HH   IIII   SSSSS
UU    UU   HHHHHHH   II     SS
UU    UU   HH   HH   II     SSSSS
UU U  UU   HH   HH   II        SS
UU U  UU   HH   HH   IIII   SSSSS        S U G G E S T I O N    B O X

                                                    01/28/84

TO:      LINDA EDMUNDS, SYSTEMS NURSE
FROM: KAREN LOHANDI          UNIT: E.R.        SHIFT: NITES    EXT: 4432
SUBJECT:  U.H.I.S

================================================================

   HOW ABOUT HAVING A LIST OF BASIC TERMS IN SPANISH-ENGLISH, FRENCH, GERMAN,
   CHINESE, ETC AVAILABLE ON THE COMPUTER IN CASE TRANSLATORS ARE NOT AVAIL-
   ABLE. THIS WAY ASSESSMENT OF NON ENGLISH SPEAKING PATIENTS CAN BE DONE WITH
   OUT WAITING. TERMS THAT MIGHT BE USEFUL ARE: PAIN, BATHROOM, HUNGRY, NURSE,
   DOCTOR, ETC. THANK YOU.




*************************************************************************
            PLEASE DELIVER TO THE SYSTEMS NURSE ON T-14
*************************************************************************




-------------------------------------------------------------------
FROM T14A TO NADM                     SENT ON 01/28/84  AT 11:30:39
```

Figure 10-9. Systems nurse sug-gestion box. A computerized sug-gestion box is useful in collecting ideas from staff about needed ap-plications. Nurses can sit at a ter-minal and type their suggestions on a screen. The suggestions are automatically printed out for the systems nurse or data-processing department. (Reprinted with per-mission courtesy of University Hospital, Health Sciences Center, SUNY at Stony Brook, NY.)

to look up which intramuscular or intravenous drugs can be mixed together. Some hospitalwide information systems and physiological monitoring systems do dosage calculations. For example, if a physician orders an IV to run at 250 ml per shift, the computer will calculate the number of drops or microdrops to be administered each minute (Figure 10–11). In some pediatric units, a list of drugs to be used in emergency situations with the correct dosages is posted near each child's bedside. Since a pediatric unit has newborns as well as adolescents, these dosages are always calculated according to patient weight. If a computerized calculator is available, the nurse can type in the child's weight and all the calculations will be done. Once a calculator like this is thoroughly tested, it is much more accurate than when the nurses do the calculations manually. It may also save a nurse 10 to 15 minutes, which is the time it takes to do and check the arithmetic involved in calculating dosages for 15 to 20 emergency medications.

In addition to information about phone numbers,

```
*********************************************************************
*           UNIVERSITY HOSPITAL: DRUG REFERENCE GUIDES FOR NURSING STAFF        *
*********************************************************************
*                                                                   *
*   DRUG:   TENSILON (EDROPHONIUM)                                  *
*                                                                   *
*   USED FOR:                                                       *
*       1. USED FOR THE DIFFERENTIAL DIAGNOSIS OF MYASTHENIA GRAVIS. *
*       2. USED IN THE EMERGENCY TREATMENT IN MYASTHENIA CRISIS.    *
*       3. USED TO REVERSE THE NEUROMUSCULAR BLOCK PRODUCED BY CURARE. *
*       4. USED INVESTIGATIONALLY TO CONVERT SVT AND PAT TO NSR, ONLY WHEN *
*          SIMPLER PROCEDURES SUCH AS REST, SEDATION AND CAROTID SINUS MASSAGE *
*          ARE INEFFECTIVE.                                         *
*                                                                   *
*   DOSAGE AND METHOD OF ADMIN:                                     *
*       1. MOST COMMON TOTAL DOSE IS 10MG GIVEN IV VERY SLOWLY, AS FOLLOWS: *
*          FIRST, 2MG IS GIVEN OVER 15-30 SECONDS. THE NEEDLE IS LEFT IN *
*          SITE FOR 45 SECONDS, IF NO COMPLICATION OCCURS, THE OTHER 8MG *
*          IS GIVEN.                                                *
*       2. GIVEN IM IN PATIENTS WITH INACCESSIBLE VEINS.            *
*                                                                   *
*   DESIRED EFFECTS:                                                *
*       ANTICHOLINESTERASE AGENT PRODUCES CHOLINERGIC RESPONSES OF SHORT *
*       DURATION.                                                   *
*                                                                   *
*   ACTION:                                                         *
*       TENSILON INHIBITS THE ACTION OF ACETYL-CHOLINESTERASE. ITS EFFECT IS *
*       MANIFESTED WITHIN 30-60 SECONDS AFTER INJECTION AND LASTS AN AVERAGE *
*       OF 10 MINUTES.                                              *
*                                                                   *
*   SIDE EFFECTS:                                                   *
*       1. BRADYCARDIA, CARDIAC STANDSTILL.                         *
*       2. INCREASED LACRIMATION, PUPILLARY CONSTRICTION, DIPLOPIA, CONVULSION, *
*          DYSPHAGIA, INCREASED TRACHEOBRONCHIAL SECRETIONS, LARYNGOSPASM, *
*          BRONCHIOLAR CONSTRICTION, PARALYSIS OF MUSCLES OF RESPIRATION, *
*          ARRHYTHMIAS, HYPOTENSION. INCREASED SALIVARY, GASTRIC AND INTESTI- *
*          NAL SECRETION, NAUSEA, VOMITING, INCREASED PERISTALSIS, ABDOMINAL *
*          CRAMPS. INCREASED URINARY FREQUENCY, INCONTINENCE, DIAPHORESIS AND *
*          WEAKNESS.                                                *
*                                                                   *
*   NURSING IMPLICATIONS:                                           *
*       1. SHOULD NOT BE ADMINISTERED IN URINARY AND INTESTINAL OBSTRUCTIONS. *
*       2. SHOULD NOT BE GIVEN TO PATIENTS WHO ARE KNOWN TO BE HYPERSENSITIVE *
*          TO ANTICHOLINESTERASE AGENTS.                           *
*       3. USED WITH CAUTION IN PATIENTS WITH BRONCHIAL ASTHMA AND THOSE *
*          RECEIVING DIGITALIS AND CARDIAC ARRHYTHMIAS.             *
*                                                                   *
*                                                                   *
*--------------------------------------------------------------------*
*   NREFP41      REFERENCE DATA PRINTED FOR  EDMUNDS,LINDA           6/81   *
*********************************************************************
```

Figure 10–10. Medication guide. If a nurse wants information about a medication, the name of the medication is selected from a list, and a guide prints out. (Reprinted with permission courtesy of University Hospital, Health Sciences Center, SUNY at Stony Brook, NY.)

```
@@@@@@@@@@@@@@@@@@@@@@@@@@@@@@@@@@@@@@@@@@@@@@@@@@@@@@@@@@@@@@@@@@@@@@@@TOP
                                                         01/21/84  1517
        KEY IN ONE OF THE FOLLOWING FIELDS. PRESS ENTER TO CALCULATE OTHERS.
                          KEY IN ONE FIELD ONLY
-----------------------------------------------------------------------------


            MICROGTTS/MIN:  *          *

               GTTS/MIN:  *          *

                ML/MIN:  *          *

               ML/HOUR:  *          *

               ML/4 HR:  *          *

               ML/8 HR:  * 250       *

               ML/24HR:  *          *



   ^ ^ ^ ^ ^ ^ ^ ^ ^ ^ ^ ^ ^ ^ ^ ^ ^ ^ ^ ^ ^ ^ ^ ^ ^ ^ ^ ^ ^ ^
        RETURN                     PRESS ENTER TO CALCULATE

NWANKIV1
@@@@@@@@@@@@@@@@@@@@@@@@@@@@@@@@@@@@@@@@@@@@@@@@@@@@@@@@@@@@@@@@@@@@@@@@BOT
```

A

```
@@@@@@@@@@@@@@@@@@@@@@@@@@@@@@@@@@@@@@@@@@@@@@@@@@@@@@@@@@@@@@@@@@@@@@@@TOP
                                                         01/21/84  1517
                        IV DRIP RATE DISPLAY.
-----------------------------------------------------------------------------


          MICRO GTTS/MIN:  31.25

               GTTS/MIN:  5.2083           FOR 10 GTTS/ML ONLY

                ML/MIN:  0.5208

               ML/HOUR:  31.25

               ML/4 HR:  125

               ML/8 HR:  250

               ML/24HR:  750


   ^ ^ ^ ^ ^ ^ ^ ^ ^ ^ ^ ^ ^ ^ ^ ^ ^ ^ ^ ^ ^ ^ ^ ^ ^ ^ ^ ^ ^ ^
                                            RETURN

NWANKIV2
@@@@@@@@@@@@@@@@@@@@@@@@@@@@@@@@@@@@@@@@@@@@@@@@@@@@@@@@@@@@@@@@@@@@@@@@BOT
```

B

Figure 10-11. IV drip calculator. Computerized calculators assist nurses with routine medication calculations. On the first screen of this calculator, the nurse types in that the IV is to run at a rate of 250 ml per shift (**A**). The answer screen (**B**) provides the appropriate drip rate per minute and the volume to be administered over 1, 4, and 24 hours. (Reprinted with permission courtesy of University Hospital, Health Sciences Center, SUNY at Stony Brook, NY.)

medications, and laboratory tests, the computer can be used to store patient care protocols, quality assurance standards, dietary information, and patient preparation procedures and policies. To obtain any of this reference data, the nurse signs on to the computer system. When the master menu screen appears, the nurse may use the light pen to select a function called the help screen index (Figure 10-12). The screen that appears lists all the reference data stored in the computer. If the nurse wants information about a diet, the light pen is used to probe "Dietary Information." A list of diets, such as "low cholesterol," "high fiber," "lactation," appears. The nurse selects the diet of interest with the light pen and goes to the unit printer to obtain the stored information. The printout might include a list of foods allowed and foods to be avoided, as well as a sample menu. If the information is not lengthy, it will display on the terminal screen instead of printing out.

```
@@@@@@@@@@@@@@@@@@@@@@@@@@@@@@@@@@@@@@@@@@@@@@@@@@@@@@@@@@@@@@@@@@@@@@@@TOP

            H E L P    S C R E E N    I N D E X
       SELECT THE APPROPRIATE REFERENCE MATERIAL WITH YOUR LIGHT PEN
-----------------------------------------------------------------------------

** PHONE NUMBERS **        ** MEDICATION INFO **      ** PROCEDURES **
NURSING STATION            ADULT MED PRINTOUTS        HELICOPTER TRANSPORT
OUTPATIENT CLINICS         PEDIATRIC MED PRINTOUTS    VAN TRANSPORT
HOSPITAL DEPTS             PATIENT MED GUIDES         PEDIATRIC TRANSPORT
MAINTENANCE                IV MISCIBILITY             NEWBORN TRANSPORT
SYSTEM PROBLEMS            IM MISCIBILITY             PSYCH ADMISSION
STAFF DEVELOPMENT
FOREIGN LANGUAGE
    TRANSLATORS            ** HOME CARE **            ** OTHER **
                           ER INSTRUCTION SHEETS      LAB TEST INFORMATION
** CALCULATORS **          OSTOMY CARE GUIDES         RADIOLOGY PREPS
IV DRIP                    DIET PRINTOUTS             STANDARDS OF CARE
LB/KG CONVERSION           COMMUNITY AGENCIES         FOREIGN LANGUAGE
EMERGENCY PEDIATRIC                                       PHRASES
IN/CM CONVERSION                                      VISITOR INFORMATION
MCG/KG/MIN DOSE                                       PEDIATRIC GRAPHICS
HEPARIN DOSE

@@@@@@@@@@@@@@@@@@@@@@@@@@@@@@@@@@@@@@@@@@@@@@@@@@@@@@@@@@@@@@@@@@@@@@@@BOT
```

Figure 10-12. Help screen index. When the help screen index is selected from the master screen, the index to reference data stored in the system is displayed. The nurse uses the light pen to select the information category of interest.

Communicating with Patients

Although computer technology is of little use in most of the communication that goes on between patient and nurse, there is one area of interaction in which the computer can provide the nurse some assistance. The area is patient education. The computer can help the nurse by providing the patient with easily readable materials which supplement and reinforce the nurse's verbal explanations.

Discharge Planning

When patients leave the hospital or other health care facilities, it is essential that they go with a clear understanding of the care they will need at home. A clear understanding of needed home care may not ensure a patient's compliance with a regimen, but when a patient is confused about diet, medications, treatments, or follow-up appointments, the chances that medical and nursing instructions will be followed are reduced even further.

Writing a discharge plan on the computer helps the nurse clearly organize instructions for the patient. To prepare a discharge plan, the nurse signs on to the computer system and asks for the patient census. When the patient is selected with the light pen from the census, the patient function screen appears. If you remember the beginning of this chapter, you will recall that the screen sequence for discharge planning is, up to this point,

identical with the one described for order entry. This is why learning to use a computer system is not very difficult. The screens used in many different applications usually follow similar patterns. Once you grasp the basic pattern, it is easy to master its variations.

Suppose the nurse is preparing a discharge plan for a baby named Jeffrey Lang. On the patient function screen, the nurse checks that Jeffrey has been selected from the census by reviewing the name displayed on top (review Figure 10-3**D**). The application "Discharge Planning Guide" is selected with the light pen. The nurse progresses through three screens, each of which is formatted to prompt the nurse to type in specific information for the baby. The first screen has four sections (Figure 10-13**A**). One section is headed "Activity," the other headings are "Diet," "Medications," and "Referrals." There is space under each heading for the nurse to key in the appropriate instructions. For this newborn baby, the nurse might type in the following activity instructions, "Keep away from large crowds or people that are sick for the first few weeks." Under diet, the nurse might write "ENFAMIL, 20 calories with iron, 2-4 oz every 4-6 hours." Since most newborns are not sent home from the hospital on medications, the medication section would be left blank. If a referral were made to public health nursing or the mother were breastfeeding and might want to call the LaLeche League, information about these referral agencies—phone number, contact person, an explanation of services—could be included. The nurse might also want to include the phone number of the nearest poison control center on the discharge plan.

The second screen has a heading "Special Instructions." If, for example, the baby has had a circumcision, specific instructions for circumcision care could be written here. Instructions about bathing the baby, cord care, and safety precautions, such as using a car seat, might also be typed in under the special instruction section. On the last screen of the discharge planning sequence there are only two headings "Notify MD If" and "Follow-up Appointment." Under "Notify MD If" the nurse states the conditions that require physician consultation such as "Rectal temperature is 100.4 F or above" or "Baby refuses to eat three times in a row." The plan is completed by the nurse making an appointment for the baby in the pediatrics clinic and typing in the date, time, place, doctor's name, and phone number on the screen.

After the nurse writes the discharge plan on the terminal, a copy is printed out for the child's mother (Figure 10-13B). Another copy is printed for inclusion in the patient's manual chart. Because the outpatient clinics and inpatient modules are connected to the same computer system, a copy of the discharge plan can be sent to the pediatric clinic. A final copy is printed in the office of the discharge planning coordinator.

The patient or, in this case, the parent benefits because it is easier to read a computer-printed discharge plan than one that is handwritten. Sending a copy of the discharge plan to the outpatient clinic encourages continuity of care between the two areas. The outpatient nurses have specific information about the instructions given to the patient and can determine whether these instructions have been followed. The risk that they will confuse the patient by giving conflicting instructions is minimized. Because the discharge planning coordinator receives a copy of the home care instructions, any serious deficiencies in the plan can be corrected. If patients on a particular unit are not being given discharge plans on a consistent basis, this becomes quickly obvious to the discharge coordinator, and intervention in the form of staff education can be started quickly. Although nursing staff without a computer might use carbon paper so that copies of discharge instructions could be distributed as indicated, this is in reality rather cumbersome and is not usually done.

Often many patients on specialty units will be treated for the same condition and discharged with very similar home care instructions. In these cases the computer can save the nurse time in the preparation of the discharge plan. Prewritten instructions can be stored in the computer's memory and incorporated into the instructions given to the patient. For example, instructions related to the care of a circumcision can be added to a newborn's discharge plan by a single probe of the light pen. The mother gets a clearly written list of what to do for the baby without the nurse's having to com-

```
@@@@@@@@@@@@@@@@@@@@@@@@@@@@@@@@@@@@@@@@@@@@@@@@@@@@@@@@@@@@@@@@@@@@@@@@@TOP

           D I S C H A R G E    P L A N N I N G    G U I D E
          THIS IS THE FIRST OF THREE DISCHARGE PLANNING SCREENS
           TYPE IN THE REQUESTED DATA THEN PRESS YOUR ENTER KEY
       -------------------------------------------------------------
                 PATIENT: <    LANG, JEFFREY          >
       -------------------------------------------------------------
ACTIVITY:
   *  KEEP BABY AWAY FROM LARGE CROWDS OR PEOPLE THAT ARE SICK FOR THE   *
   *  FIRST FEW WEEKS.                                                   *
   *                                                                     *
DIET:
   *  FORMULA, 20 CAL WITH IRON Q4-6HRS.                                 *
   *                                                                     *
   *                                                                     *
MEDICATIONS:
   *                                                                     *
   *                                                                     *
   *                                                                     *
COMMUNITY RESOURCES REFERRALS:
   *  PUBLIC HEALTH NURSING, CALL MRS VICKERS AT 555-4466 FOR APPOINTMENT. *
   *                                                                     *
   *  POISON CONTROL CENTER:    542-2323                                 *

@@@@@@@@@@@@@@@@@@@@@@@@@@@@@@@@@@@@@@@@@@@@@@@@@@@@@@@@@@@@@@@@@@@@@@@@@BOT
```

A

Figure 10-13. Discharge planning guide. The discharge planning guide is a three-screen sequence that prompts the nurse to include instructions for patients in several categories. On the first screen (**A**), the nurse types in information about activity, diet, medications, and community resources. The discharge guide that prints out for the patient and/or family (**B**) is legible, organized, and comprehensive, and copies can be sent to the pediatric outpatient clinic as well as to the discharge planning coordinator. (Reprinted with permission courtesy of University Hospital, Health Sciences Center, SUNY at Stony Brook, NY.)

```
**************** DISCHARGE PLANNING COORDINATOR COPY *********************
*  09N2                                                                  *
* DISCHARGE PLAN FOR: 09N2 09012- 3 LANG,JEFFERY        00000029         *
*           MRN: 000070           PREPARED BY: LINDA EDMUNDS             *
*  NEWBORN NURSERY * 516-444      SIGNED: L   Ed      DATE: 0128         *
*************************************************************************
* ACTIVITY:                                                             *
*   KEEP BABY AWAY FROM LARGE CROWDS OR PEOPLE THAT ARE SICK FOR THE FIRST *
*   FEW WEEKS.                                                          *
* DIET:                                                                 *
*   ENFAMIL. 20 CALORIES WITH IRON Q4-6H.                               *
*                                                                       *
* MEDICATIONS:                                                          *
*   NONE                                                                *
*                                                                       *
*                                                                       *
* SPECIAL INSTRUCTIONS:                                                 *
*                                                                       *
*                                                                       *
*                                                                       *
*                                                                       *
*                                                                       *
*   CIRCUMCISION CARE FOR YOUR NEWBORN:                                 *
*                                                                       *
*   1. MAKE SURE YOU HAVE WASHED YOUR HANDS CAREFULLY.                  *
*                                                                       *
*   2. LEAVE THE VASELINE GAUZE ON THE TIP OF THE PENIS UNTIL YOUR BABY *
*   URINATES FOR THE FIRST TIME. AFTER FIRST URINATION TAKE A GAUZE     *
*   PAD. OPEN IT UP AND APPLY VASELINE IN THE CENTER BEING CARE-        *
*   FUL NOT TO TOUCH THE GAUZE. PLACE THE GAUZE OVER THE TIP OF THE     *
*   PENIS AND DIAPER LOOSELY. CONTINUE DOING THIS AT EACH DIAPER CHANGE *
*   FOR ABOUT 24 HOURS. MAKE SURE THAT THE DIAPER AREA IS KEPT VERY     *
*   CLEAN.AFTER ABOUT 24 HOURS APPLY VASELINE WITHOUT GAUZE TO THE PENIS. *
*   CONTINUE TO DO THIS UNTIL THE PENIS LOOKS HEALED.                   *
*                                                                       *
*   3. AFTER 24 HRS YOU MAY NOTICE A YELLOWISH WHITE MEMBRANE ON THE HEAD *
*   OF THE PENIS. THIS IS NORMAL AND NOT A SIGN OF INFECTION. YOU MAY   *
*   ALSO NOTE THAT THE PENIS BLEEDS SLIGHTLY OVER THE FIRST DAY. THIS   *
*   BLEEDING SHOULD DECREASE GRADUALLY. CONTINUE TO OBSERVE THE CIRCUM- *
*   CISION SITE FOR FOUL ODOR, SWELLING OR EXCESSIVE DISCHARGE. REPORT  *
*   ANY ABNORMAL FINDINGS TO YOUR PHYSICIAN.                            *
* NOTIFY MD IF:                                                         *
*   CALL MD IF YOU NOTE FOUL ODOR, SWELLING OR EXCESSIVE DRAINAGE AT THE *
*   SITE OF THE CIRCUMCISION.                                           *
*   RECTAL TEMPERATURE IS 100.4 DEGREES OR ABOVE.                       *
*   THERE IS A FOUL SMELL FROM THE CORD.                                *
*   BABY HAS 3 WATERY STOOLS OR REFUSES TO EAT 3 TIMES IN A ROW.        *
*   INFANT IS EXCESSIVELY IRRITABLE OR SLEEPS MORE THAN USUAL.          *
* REFERRALS/ COMMUNITY  RESOURCES:                                      *
*   PUBLIC HEALTH NURSING. CALL MRS VICKERS AT 555-4466 FOR APPOINTMENT. *
*                                                                       *
*   POISON CONTROL CENTER:      542-2323.                               *
* FOLLOW UP APPOINTMENT:                                                *
* DAY: MONDAY   DATE: FEBRUARY 1, 1984  TIME: 0900     TELE: 555-5444   *
* DR: JOAN SELLAB             PLACE: PEDIATRICS CLINIC                   *
* APPT INSTRUCTIONS:                                                    *
*                                                                       *
*************************************************************************
*   IF YOU OR YOUR FAMILY HAVE ANY QUESTIONS CONCERNING YOUR HOME CARE  *
*     FEEL FREE TO CALL THE  NEWBORN NURSERY * 516-444-.                *
*************************************************************************
```

B

Figure 10-13 (B).

pose and type the information for each male child who is circumcised.

Patient Instruction

Computer-stored preformatted discharge instructions can be used efficiently in the emergency room. Most ERs do keep mimeographed instruction sheets for common conditions such as head injury, diarrhea, or cast care. But there is a limit to the number of piles of instruction sheets that can be stored in a busy ER. Re-

stocking also takes time. When the same instruction sets are stored in the computer's memory, stocking and filing problems are ended. If a nurse needs to give a patient instructions about poison ivy care, the light pen is used to select "Poison Ivy" from a list on the computer screen, and the poison ivy guide prints out. A large variety of instruction sets are available, the supply never runs out, and clutter in the ER is diminished.

Other types of reference material written especially for patients can also be stored on the computer. If physicians in the outpatient area are receiving many questions about AIDS, or genital herpes, a three- or four-page informational guide that interested patients can read at home is useful. Information about drugs, written in language that is clear, can help the patient understand what each medication does, the expected side effects, and adverse reactions requiring physician notification. Guides of this type reinforce a nurse's verbal instructions. This is particularly important when patients go home on multiple medications with complicated dosage schedules.

Learning to Use an Information System

Learning to use a computerized information system is somewhat like learning to drive a car. The first time at a terminal is like the first time behind the wheel. There is a tendency to feel out of control and afraid that one wrong move may damage the machine irreparably.

The first thing to remember about learning to use a system is that it takes a tremendous amount of programming background to understand enough about a computer system to make it stop working. Unless a user spills hot coffee over the keyboard or takes a sledgehammer to the video screen there is little chance of making the computer break.

The second thing to remember is that system analysts design hospital information systems so that clinical users—nurses, doctors, technicians—will find them easy to use. They do this by working in collaboration with nurses, doctors, or technicians when developing screens and printouts that will be used by these professional groups. As a result, most nurses do not find learning to use a system too difficult. It takes some time, some concentration, and some practice. To master a system, nurses must become accustomed to using a light pen and become familiar with the extra keys that are found on a computer keyboard. After that, the two most important things to learn are pattern recognition and error correction.

Pattern recognition is important in helping nurses understand what to expect as they progress through the screens and screen sequences that make up to an application flow. As an analogy, consider a seven-story hospital. If nurses know how the patients rooms are laid out on the third floor of the building, the chances are they will be able to find their way around the fifth-floor patients' rooms with ease. Computer sequences are similar. Screens follow each other in predictable patterns and, once the patterns are learned, the nurse will be able to figure out how to use applications that are being viewed for the first time.

Error correction is critical because, no matter how proficient nurses become in working with the computer, they are bound to make some errors in entering or retrieving data. Knowing how to correct these errors not only protects the integrity of the data stored in the system, but also gives the user a better sense of control over the system. Because the user knows how to correct mistakes, anxiety about making them is decreased. This is particularly comforting to the nurse who is just beginning to use the computer.

To ask a nurse to learn to use a computer system on the nursing unit would be like asking a person to take a first driving lesson in midtown Manhattan traffic. So most hospitals provide nurses and other users with a special computer training course. For new nursing staff, the course will be incorporated into the orientation schedule. If the hospital is in the initial process of installing a system, nurses should be given time off from their regular duties to attend classes.

Computer training may begin with a general lecture about the system. The most important part of the training program, however, is hands-on training. Hands-on training refers to the time the nurse sits at a terminal and actually practices using the applications that will be needed on the unit. An effective training program provides the nurse with between 6 and 20 hours of hands-on practice time, depending on the number of nursing applications available. Generally, there is a training room with five or six terminals in it. An instructor helps users as they proceed through detailed training guides (see Exhibit 10–1). These guides are written to assist each person learn and practice every application that will be used on their nursing unit. There is also a printer in the training room so that the students can become familiar with the various printouts and learn to remove them from the printer correctly.

Downtime Procedures

Any system that goes up in a hospital will come down. *Down* means that the computer is not working. Data cannot be entered or retrieved because of a hardware malfunction, a software problem, or scheduled maintenance procedures. But a hospital cannot stop functioning because its computer system is temporarily unavailable. For this reason, hospitals that use computers develop special downtime procedures. A computer training program should include an introduction to these procedures for the nursing staff.

During downtime, a hospital reverts to using paper requisitions similar to the ones that are used in hospitals without computers. Nurses need to know how to use

Exhibit 10–1. **Training Guide**

Step-by-step training materials assist nurses who are learning to use an information system. The training materials
explain each application and guide the nurse through its
use.

Figure 1
University Hospital Information System
Nurse Training Course

Training Guide

Note: As you proceed through the Training Guide, be sure
to read the comments in the right-hand column, as well as
the instructions on the left-hand side.

INSTRUCTIONS

I. Sign On
1. Press clear key.
2. Key in UHIS. Press En-
   ter key.
3. Key in ID and
   Password. Press Enter
   key.
4. Observe Master Screen.
5. Sign off.
6. Sign on again (follow
   steps 1–5).
7. Sign off.

EXPLANATION

I. Sign On
Keying in the hospital
code (UHIS) notifies the
computer that you are at
the terminal and wish to
access or input data. The
ID and Password cue the
computer to display the
appropriate Master
Screen. In training, we
all use the same Master.
On the patient units, you
will have a special Mas-
ter designed for that
unit.
The Master Screen lists
12 of the functions that
can be done at the nurs-
ing station. The other
functions are listed on
the Function Screen
which you will see later
in this training course.

II. Help Screen Index
1. Sign on.
2. Probe "Help Screen In-
   dex."
3. Note the different types
   of reference data that
   are currently available.
4. Probe "Hosp/Ancil-
   lary Phone Numbers."
   "What is the phone
   number of pharmacy
   dispensing area?"
5. Probe return.
6. Probe "Foreign Lan-
   guage Translators."
7. Who would you call to
   translate for a patient
   who speaks Greek?
8. Probe return.
9. Return to Master
   Screen.
10. Sign off.

II. Help Screen Index
Help screens are de-
signed to provide you
with easy access to reference data that are de-
fined as critical, fre-
quently needed, unique
to this hospital, or difficult to locate manually.
We are in the beginning
stages of developing help
screens and prints. Addi-
tions, as they occur, will
be announced in the Up-
Date.

Note: Figure 1 shows page 1 of the Training Guide. After
initially "Signing On," the learner repeats this function
once for practice. The next step in the learning process is
introduction of another simple application, the "Help
Screen Index."

Source: Linda Edmunds: Teaching nurses to use computers. *Nurse
Educator*, Autumn, 1982. Reprinted with permission.

each form, where the forms are located on the unit, and
how to obtain more forms if the supply runs out. There
are usually some general criteria set for instituting
downtime procedures which nurses need to be familiar
with. If a system is down for 15 to 30 minutes, most
noncritical care units can wait until the computer is
working again. If the computer engineers are uncertain
as to how long it will take to fix the system, an announcement may be made over the loudspeaker that
downtime procedures are to be instituted until further
notice. The overhead page system has to be used because when the system is down, there is no way to send a
hospitalwide message to all units.

When a system comes back up, after downtime, all
the orders and results that have been transmitted on paper forms have to be entered into the computer. If this is
not done, the patient's computer record will have big
gaps in it, making it essentially unusable to clinicians.
The process of entering downtime data into the computer's memory is called *recovery*. Downtime recovery
may be done from the nursing care units by nursing station clerks, or it may be completed in the clinical ancillaries. In any event, recovering from an extended downtime efficiently takes some coordination between
departments, and it is essential that nursing staff be
clear about their roles in this process.

Information Systems: Questions, Issues, Problems

This chapter has detailed many of the ways computerized information systems are currently used to assist nursing staff. It has been argued that the technology benefits patient care by making communication among nurses, between departments, and with patients more efficient and more effective. But this does not mean that there are no actual or potential problems associated with computer technology in a health care environment. It is realistic for concerned nurses to have questions about issues such as the privacy of patient information, the introduction of error into data transmission, the effect of automation on the patient-nurse relationship, and the cost-effectiveness of the technology.

Privacy

Because online computerized information systems can store a great deal of patient data and make that data accessible almost instantaneously, the potential for the abuse of patient privacy is great. It is much easier to sit at a terminal on a nursing unit and look up your neighbor's pregnancy test results than it is to go into the medical records department and sign out that person's chart. This is exactly what can happen in a hospital where policies and procedures are not established and enforced to protect the patient. Since most nurses use the health care facilities of their own institution, protecting patient privacy means protecting themselves as well.

Although the software design of a system is extremely important in tailoring a system so that users get the amount of information they need to practice but no more, the single most important factor in maintaining system security is the users themselves. Systems are almost always password-protected, with each staff member having a secret access code. If staff do not respect the secrecy of these codes, or if they share them with colleagues on other units or departments of the hospital, the probability for the violation of patient privacy escalates. This is also true if a staff member leaves a terminal without signing off from the computer because any other individual can continue working under that ID on that terminal.

If nurses do not respect the precautions set up to protect the patient data base, they are not only violating professional ethics but may be putting themselves in a serious legal situation. Although many legal issues surrounding computer-based documentation are unsettled, nurses may be considered responsible by the hospital and, perhaps some day, by the courts for data entered into a system under their ID codes, in the same way that they are responsible for the accuracy of information written in a chart under their signatures.

Errors

Nurses often worry that computers, or nurses who use computers, will make errors in the transmission of patient data. Every time data are transcribed from one place to another, the potential for transcription error exists. When data are transcribed into a computer, usually some translation is involved which may increase the possibility of error. In this case, translation means that the person entering the information into the system may need to interpret what is written manually and convert it to one of the choices listed on a menu screen. For example, if the physician handwrites an order for a "CXR," the appropiate x-ray for the nurse to select from a list of chest x-rays might be "Chest PA and lateral." On a manual requisition, whatever had been written in the order sheet could be copied directly, whether or not the person picking up the order recognized the test requested.

On the other hand, unless a programming error has been made and has remained undetected, computers do not usually make transcription errors. If a medication order is entered into a computer system and it is entered correctly, it will show up correctly on every label that is printed, on the medication administration record, in the computerized Kardex, and on the renewal notice. The chance for transcription errors in this case is less than it would be if the order was hand copied to all these places.

Many examples could be advanced to demonstrate that computerization either increases or decreases errors in data communication. But the bottom line is that, whatever the method of documentation, errors are minimized if a nurse has a good understanding of the patient's treatment plan, if the physician's orders and notes are reviewed carefully, and if the work done by nursing station clerks and hospital aides is well supervised.

Patient-Nurse Relationship

Will a computer take a nurse away from the patient's bedside or, in the case of physiological monitoring systems, will the presence of the computer at the bedside isolate the patient from the nurse? Many nurses are concerned that if machines are used in the care of patients, the nurse will become so involved in the care of the machine, that the personal relationship between patient and nurse will suffer. Suppose a nurse sits down at a terminal and, prompted by the screens displayed, writes a comprehensive set of individualized discharge instructions. In addition, the nurse prints out detailed diet and medication guides for the patient. If these computer printouts are handed to the patient, without the nurse sitting down and explaining the material, answering the patient's questions, and assessing whether potential problems with noncompliance exist, the computer is certainly interfering with the appropriate patient-nurse relationship. But a skilled nurse would not use any type of educational material in this fashion, whether or not it comes from a computer. A computer is simply a tool which, if used wisely, can extend a nurse's ability to provide good patient care.

Cost

One of the most important questions that needs to be addressed in relation to the use of computer technology in health care is cost versus benefit. Does the introduction of computerization into health care facilities increase the cost of medical care for patients or does it decrease costs? The question is a very complicated one because of the multiplicity of economic factors that must be considered. The issue is made even more complex if the quality of care is considered at the same time. If costs per patient increase, but so does the quality of care, is the cost justified? But the measurement of quality is at least as difficult, if not more, than the measurement of cost. There are probably lots of opinions about the cost/benefit ratio of computerization on health care, but professional nurses must be critical in their evaluation of the data and arguments.

In short, computers have the potential for assisting nurses in many aspects of patient care. But the potential will be realized only if nurses become actively involved in the design and implementation of hospital information systems. Furthermore, unless nurses respect and pay close attention to the inherent problems of computerization, the benefits of the technology will be undermined.

Summary

Computerized information systems are made up of a network of video display terminals and printers located in all areas of a hospital and cabled to a large computer. Information systems are used to facilitate communication between departments, among clinical staff, and with patients.

A patient's computerized record begins with the entry of demographic and insurance data in the admitting department. Physicians' orders are communicated to ancillaries, such as the laboratory, radiology department, and pharmacy, over the system, and test results are sent back the same way. When the patient is discharged, the medical records department inputs the discharge diagnoses and other abstract information into the patient's data base.

Computer systems are used to help nurses develop care plans and for charting medications administered and other clinical data. Bedside physiological monitoring systems, which may or may not be connected into the hospital information system, monitor and trend physiological variables such as blood pressure, respiratory rate, and temperature.

Reference data about laboratory tests, medications, protocols, or diets can be stored in a computer's memory and displayed on a terminal or printed out for use by nurses as they care for patients. Similar reference data, written at a layman's level, can supplement patient teaching and discharge planning.

Computers are useful tools for nursing services. They can improve the efficiency with which clerical tasks are performed. They make clinical data legible and instantaneously accessible to multiple users at the same time. They can help guide and structure nursing practice. But all powerful tools require critical evaluation. Nurses who use computer systems are concerned about issues such as the privacy of information, the introduction of error, and the effect of the technology on the cost as well as the quality of patient care.

Terms for Review

CPU	downtime recovery	light pen	minicomputer	programs
cursor	hardcopy	mainframes	off loaded	sign on
data base	hardware	memory	online data	software
downtime	inputted	microcomputer	outputted	user friendly

Self-Assessment

1. You are going for a job interview in a hospital with a computerized information system. Make a list of five questions that you want to ask the person interviewing you about the system.
2. The interviewer asks you how you feel about the prospect of working with computers on the nursing units. Truthfully, you feel somewhat excited about the possibility but also a little nervous. You want to be honest about your concerns but also let the interviewer know that you are knowledgeable about the benefits of computerization. What would you say?
3. You have passed your computer training course. The hospital has assigned you the following ID number: 765991. You are allowed to select your own password. It can be 5, 6, or 7 letters long and can be any word except your first, middle, last or maiden name. What word would you select?

Learning Activities

1. This learning activity may at first seem more appropriate to the cut-and-paste activities of the kindergarten set. But it is probably the best way to give yourself an idea of what it feels like to sit in front of a terminal and use a computer system.

    First, xerox or copy out Figures 10–3A through 10–3I. Cut each figure out so that you have nine separate paper screens and put them in order. Take a piece of cardboard and cut out an opening the size of the paper screens. Tie a piece of string about 1½ ft long to a pencil. Attach the other end of the string to the cardboard. Prop the whole thing up on a typewriter keyboard.

    Find a partner. The partner will sit behind the typewriter and hold up the first of the screens (Figure 10–3A). You will sit in front and use the typewriter key board as your computer keyboard and the pencil as your light pen. Go through the order entry sequence as described in the chapter. Each time you enter data on the keyboard or make a selection with the light pen, your partner will display the next appropriate screen.

2. This chapter has described some of the types of reference data that can be stored in a computer's memory. There are many other possibilities. Use your imagination to think of another category of reference data that could be valuable to you or your patients on a computer. Describe in detail what would be stored in the computer's memory, how nurses would access the information, and what a typical screen or printout would look like.

3. One of the applications that can be designed for children who are inpatients on the pediatric unit or outpatients in the emergency room is a medal. The nurse types in the child's name on the computer screen, the reason for the award, and a graphic in the form of a medal prints out with the child's name on it as well as the reason. Applications like this are fun for children and can also be used therapeutically. Try to think of another application you might design for pediatric patients (Figure 10–14).

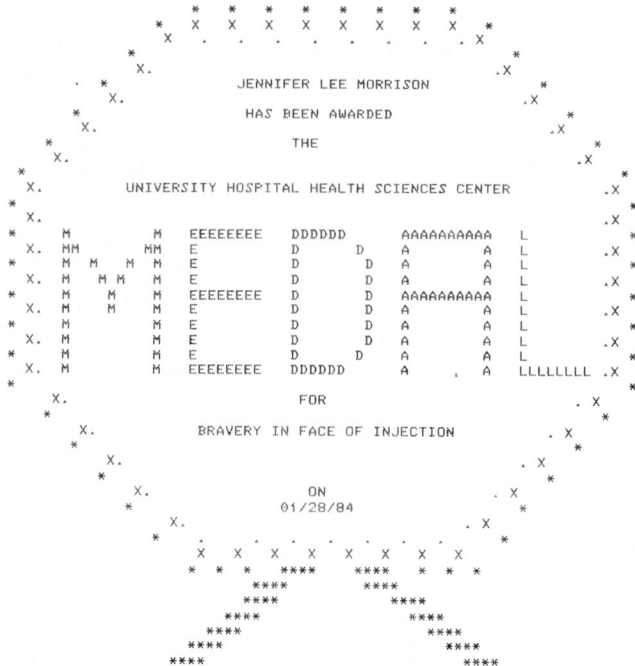

Figure 10–14. Pediatric medal. A medal with the child's name on it is both fun for the child and useful therapeutically.

Review Questions

1. Would a light pen be classified as hardware or software?
2. Explain what user friendly means.
3. What prevents visitors to a hospital from using the hospital's computerized information system?
4. What is a high-frequency order entry screen?
5. What is a standard care plan?
6. What are some advantages of standardized care plans?
7. List five variables that a physiological monitoring system can track.
8. Give one example of how a computerized message function can assist a nursing department.
9. Who would you expect to need more nursing care—a patient with an acuity score of 39 or one with a score of 57? Explain.
10. The computer system in your hospital is going to be down for one to two hours. How will you order tests from the laboratory and radiology during this time?

Answers

1. Hardware.
2. Programs are written so that entering and retrieving data are as easy as possible.
3. Access to the computer is limited by secret code.
4. A high-frequency order screen is developed for a specific clinical area. It lists 70 to 80 common laboratory, radiol-

ogy, dietary, and other medical orders often used in that clinical area. The nurse can enter most or all of a patient's orders from a single screen.

5. A standard care plan lists the usual actual or potential problems of a patient with a certain condition. For each problem, goals and nursing orders are stored. The nurse can select those appropriate to a specific patient or add alternatives.

6. Standardized care plans prevent errors of omission, save time of handwriting a plan, and make multiple copies readily available.

7. Heart rate, heart rhythm, respiratory rate, temperature, EEG, arterial, venous, and intracranial pressures.

8. The computer can be used to send a message to all destinations in the hospital.

9. A patient with a score of 57 would require more nursing care. The higher the score of the patient, the more nursing time required.

10. Tests must be ordered manually, using paper requisitions, during the downtime period. During recovery, downtime data are entered into the computer's memory.

References and Bibliography

Barnett, G. Octo, and Zielstorff, Rita D.: Data Systems can enhance or hinder medical, nursing activities. *Hospitals,* **51**: 157–61, 1977.

Baron, Judith A., and Brown, Janet: Nurse in computerland, A practical guide for the professional interested in working with computers. *Comput. In Health Care,* **4**(11): 4–27, 1983.

Cook, Margo, and McDowell, Wanda: Changing to an automated information system. *Am. J. Nurs.,* **75**:46–51, 1975.

Edmunds, Linda: Computer assisted nursing care. *Am. J. Nurs.,* **82**:1070–79, 1982.

Edmunds, Linda: Teaching nurses to use computers. *Nurse Educator*, pp. 32–38, Autumn, 1982.

Edmunds, Linda: Making the most of a message function for nursing services." In Ruth E. Dayhoff (ed.): *Proceedings of the Seventh Annual Symposium on Computer Applications in Medical Care.* Computer Society Press, Silver Springs, Md., 1983.

Fishman, Rosalie, and Dusbabek, Sister Charlotte: An information system for managing nursing productivity and quality of patient care NPAQ. *Comput. Nurs.,* **1**(5): 1–3, 1983.

Kelly, Janet: Computers in hospitals, nursing practice defined and validated. In Ruth E. Dayhoff (ed.): *Proceedings of the Seventh Annual Symposium of Computer Applications in Medical Care.* Computer Society Press, Silver Springs, Md., 1983.

Light, Nancy: On line nursing care plans. *Comput. Nurs.* **1**(3):4, 1983.

Lombard, Nick and Light, Nancy: On line nursing care plans by nursing diagnosis. *Comput. In Health Care,* **4**(11): 22–23, Nov., 1983.

Mayers, Marlene, and El Camino Hospital: *Standard Nursing Care Plans*, Vols. I, II, III, K/P Medical Systems, Stockton, Calif. 1974.

McNeill, Donna Jane: Developing the complete computer based information system. *J. Nurs. Admin.* pp. 34–46, Nov., 1979.

Milholland, Delores Kathleen: Computers at the bedside. *Am. J. Nurs.* **83**:1304–07, 1983.

Norwood, Donald; Hawkings, R. Edwin; and, Gall, John, Jr.: Information system benefits hospital, improves patient care. *Hospitals,* **50**:79–83, 1976.

Zielstorff, Rita (ed.): *Computers in Nursing.* Nursing Resources, Wakefield, Mass., 1980.

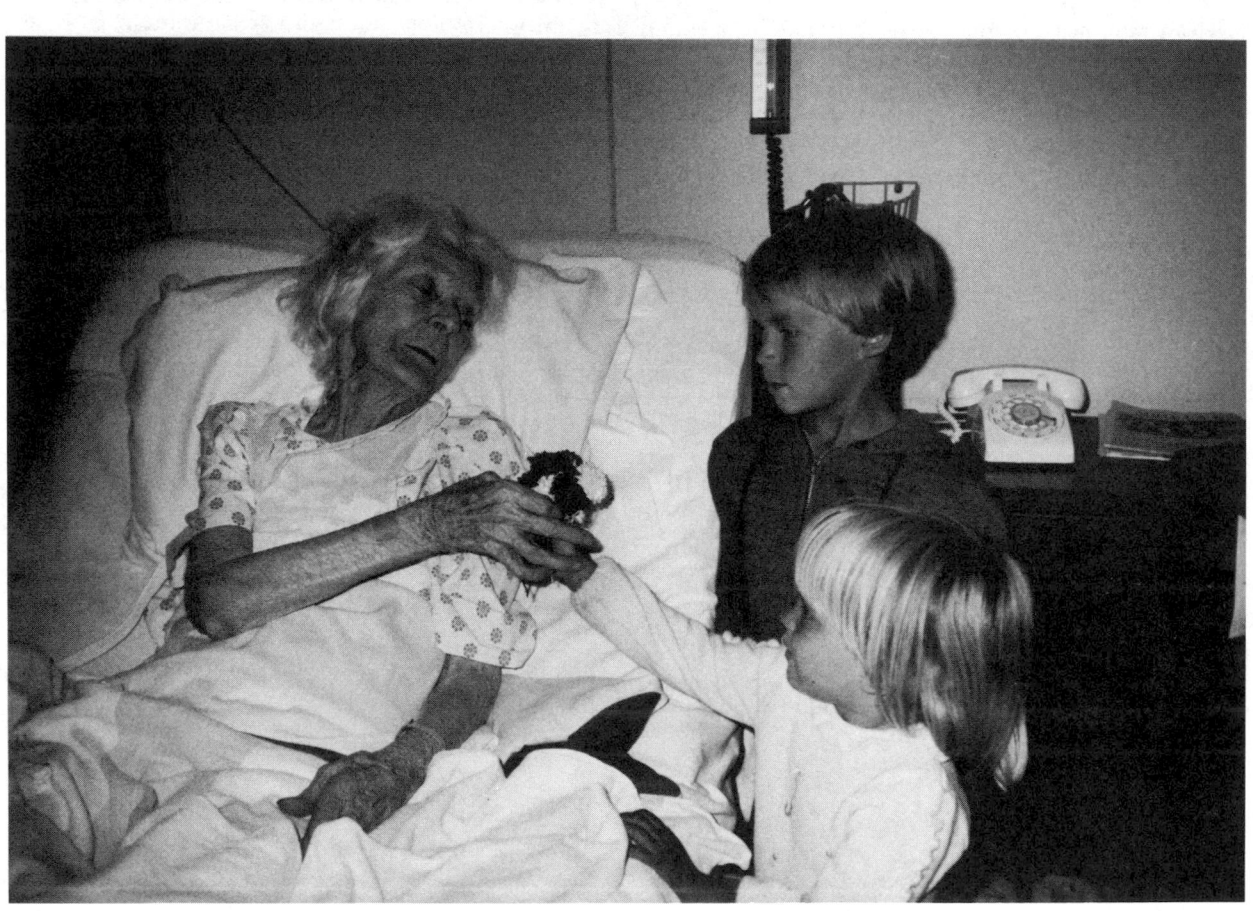

UNIT III
THE DEVELOPMENTAL PROCESS

Introduction

Your personal level of growth and development will affect your nursing education and your nursing practice. It will affect the way you relate to people, your knowledge, and your personal goals. Each of you is facing the challenge of developing your own potential as you progress through your nursing education. For some students still in the adolescent stage, financial support in the form of tuition, food, shelter, and clothing may be provided by parents. For others, the responsibility for providing financial and emotional support for your own children may be added to the goal of obtaining an education. Men or women who have children of their own may be better able to relate to the parents of a sick child because of the experience they have had from their own life, added to their nursing education. Caring for dying patients and grieving families may be very difficult for nurses who have not dealt with their own mortality or with death on a personal level, which is often the case for people in the adolescent and young adult years.

How you feel about different ages of people and the stereotypes you hold about them may interfere with your ability to see each of your patients as individuals. What many of us believed about middle-aged people when we were 18 years old is often very different from our beliefs about middle age when we are 40 years old.

Your patients also will have preconceived ideas about you, based on your stage of growth and development. They may feel you are too young to be competent or too old to understand their problems. With advancing age comes the expectation for increased skills and knowledge based on education and life experiences. A nursing student in the middle-age years may feel more pressure to be competent quickly compared to an 18-year-old student who is often viewed as less competent solely because of age. Patients may be willing to give the older nursing student more credibility and value the guidance offered based on nothing other than age. The responsibility to admit a lack of knowledge and experience to the patient is the same for all students when confronted with problems beyond their capabilities.

Knowledge of normal growth and development is helpful to the nurse giving care to individuals and families of various ages and stages of development. Intellectual ability, motor function, coordination, body structure and function, and social and emotional behavior of patients will be affected by their level of maturation and development. The needs of a healthy newborn are very different from the needs of an active teenager. An understanding of the different ways people meet their needs for optimum health based on their stage of development will serve as a resource to nurses providing care to individuals with health problems. Chapters 11 through 14 on individual growth and development are organized around the concept of basic needs, introduced by psychologist Abraham Maslow. Death and dying are discussed in Chapter 15, and Chapter 16 presents the family as an evolving unit from conception to separation, involving various numbers of people and various relationships.

Since the subject matter presented in Chapters 11 through 15 is so closely related the chapter sections on Self-Assessment and References and Bibliography have been consolidated and appear at the end of Chapter 15. *These basic needs are summarized as follows:*

1. Physiological Needs. These are needs that must be met to some degree in order for the individual to survive. They include the need for oxygen, nutrition, fluid, temperature maintenance, elimination, pain avoidance, sex (reproduction and sexuality are included here), and stimulation (sensory and muscular functioning).

2. Safety and Security Needs. These needs are satisfied by conditions that make the person feel safe and comfortable. They also include things that protect the physical safety of the individual.

3. Love and Belonging Needs. These represent the human need to give and receive love and affection. They also are fulfilled by feelings of belonging to a group in the sense of companionship, mutual enjoyment, shared concerns and goals.

4. Self-Esteem Need. This is the need individuals have to feel positive about themselves. For optimum health, people need to feel they are important and valuable; they have a need to love themselves.

5. Self-Actualization. This is the human need to continue to expand and develop throughout one's life. Striving to achieve identified goals and develop one's potentials are goals related to self-actualization.

These needs are believed to be in a hierarchy with the individual focusing on meeting survival needs such as oxygen and elimination before higher needs, such as developing a positive self-concept. The physiological needs of the individual will take priority over other needs, such as concern for family members.

Concepts Related to Growth and Development

Presented below are several basic concepts related to human growth and development. *Growth* involves increases in size or structure by addition of materials through assimilation into living cells. *Development* involves movement from an undifferentiated state to a unique, organized state of functioning.

1. The rate of maturation is unique to each individual and is based on a combination of genetic and environmental factors. An environment that is less than optimal will compromise the individual's genetic potential. On the other hand, an enriched environment can do a great deal to overcome an abnormal genetic trait or genetic predisposition. Even though these chapters refer to various stages and corresponding age groups, the reader should remember the enormous differences within and between normal individuals.

2. Stages of development are not absolute divisions. An individual does not completely leave a previous stage of development with maturation, but occasionally goes backward and forward in response to needs felt at the time.

3. Development proceeds in a head-to-toe (*cephalocaudal*) pattern in all people. The head develops before the limbs in embryonic life. In infancy and preschool years, development and coordination of the arms occur before those of the legs.

4. Growth and development follow a near-to-far (*proximodistal*) pattern in human maturation. This means that maturation proceeds from the center of the body outward to the arms and legs and then to the hands and feet. Movement of the arms and legs is possible before the infant can coordinate movement in the hands and feet.

5. Development tends to move from gross to specific. The gross, awkward attempts of the child to hold a crayon and draw are replaced by the specific ability for increased detail work with maturation of the neuromuscular system.

Understanding the physical abilities of patients based on knowledge of normal growth and development helps nurses approach patients with more realistic expectations of behavior. Age-related concerns and interests are still important to the patient with health problems, and nursing care should help each patient maintain optimum progress in personal development at all stages of life. Illness and hospitalization create physical and psychological stress and tend to delay or stop the normal progress of development. Regression to earlier stages of development is also common with this type of stress. Knowing how to minimize this stress for each patient will be based partly on the nurse's knowledge of growth and development and partly on information obtained from talking with and caring for the individual.

CHAPTER 11

GROWTH AND DEVELOPMENT: CONCEPTION THROUGH INFANCY

Conception to Birth—Thirty-eight to Forty-two Weeks
> Physiological Needs
> Higher Level Needs

The Newborn (Neonate)—Birth to Twenty-eight Days of Age
> Physiological Needs
> Higher Level Needs
> Common Problems of the Neonate and Nursing Implications

Infancy—One Month to One Year of Age
> Physiological Needs
> Higher Level Needs
> Common Problems During Infancy and Nursing Implications

Objectives

1. Describe changes occurring in the pregnant woman leading to satisfaction of oxygen needs in the fetus.
2. Identify the function of the placenta.
3. Identify the function of testosterone in the fetus during the first trimester of pregnancy.
4. Describe maternal activities that may be harmful to the developing embryo or fetus.
5. Identify changes occurring following clamping of the umbilical cord that stimulate neonatal respirations.
6. Identify alterations in blood flow in the neonate compared to that in the newborn.
7. Identify nursing activities designed to protect the neonate from health problems in the future.
8. Explain why the neonate and infant are at risk for problems with temperature maintenance.
9. Discuss the importance of a constant, attentive care-giver for the neonate and infant.
10. Describe the abilities of the neonate and infant to initiate and maintain social interaction.
11. State the range of normal vital signs (temperature, pulse, and respirations) for the neonate and the infant; state pulse range for fetus.

Conception to Birth—Thirty-eight to Forty-two Weeks

The period of time from conception until birth, usually 40 weeks, is a time of such rapid growth that the rate will never again be repeated in a human life span. Changing from a single cell to an 8-lb, alert, responsive newborn involves very rapid cell division and differenti-ation of tissues and organs. Abnormal cell growth and function often result in spontaneous abortion before 13 weeks of age. Abortion after 13 weeks is usually related to maternal problems in maintaining an adequate environment for the developing fetus. An *embryo* is the fertilized egg from the time of implantation in the uterus until eight weeks of life. The *fetus* is the developing baby from eight weeks until birth.

Physiological Needs

Oxygen Needs. The placenta, attached to the wall of the uterus within the pregnant woman, serves as the exchange station for all fetal wastes and supplies the oxygen and nutrition needs of the growing fetus. Maternal blood flow through the uterus is crucial for adequate oxygen levels in fetal blood. The pregnant woman develops an increased blood volume (hypervolemia of pregnancy), about one-third greater than her normal blood volume, to supply fetal needs. This slow increase in blood volume peaks by 32 to 34 weeks into the pregnancy. Respiratory rate increases in the mother by 40 percent over the course of the pregnancy, and the amount of blood pumped out of the heart each minute (cardiac output) is significantly increased to meet fetal needs. Maternal blood and fetal blood never mix during a normal pregnancy. Exchange of fetal wastes and needed oxygen and nutrients occurs as a result of differing concentrations of these substances in the mother's blood and in fetal blood. This results in movement of these substances from an area of higher concentration to the area of lesser concentration (diffusion). The fetus makes respiratory movements during gestation which can be seen on sound-wave pictures called ultrasound. Fetal circulation bypasses the fetal lung for the most part, traveling to the placenta through the two umbilical arteries carrying oxygen-depleted blood away from the fetus and from the placenta through the one umbilical vein carrying oxygen-rich blood back to the fetus. The embryo grows with its heart on the outside of its body for several weeks. This organ is repositioned within the chest by the end of the first trimester (13 to 14 weeks). The fetal heartbeat is audible by 12 to 14 weeks of age, with a device called a doptone, which uses sound waves reflected from the beating fetal heart for amplification. The heart rate ranges from 120 to 160 beats each minute and is fairly regular. By 20 weeks, the heartbeat can be heard with a specially adapted stethoscope. The heart rate remains constant during the pregnancy and is one of the best indicators of adequate oxygenation in the fetus.

Temperature Maintenance. The amniotic fluid surrounds the fetus and provides a constant temperature. Changes in maternal temperature may affect fetal temperature. A rise in the mother's temperature caused by hot baths, saunas, or illness may result in problems with fetal development, such as birth defects. Most health clubs and hotels have warnings about using saunas and hot whirlpool baths during pregnancy.

Elimination. The fetus does not normally pass any stool during the course of the pregnancy, but stool (*meconium*) is formed in the fetal intestines from swallowing amniotic fluid. The fetus does urinate into the amni-

Table 11–1. **Milestones in Fetal Development**

Week 1	Fertilization
	Cell mass enters uterine cavity
Week 2	Implantation
Week 3	Head and tail areas present
	Heart tube
	Primitive vascular system
Week 4	Limb buds appear
	Placenta begins to form
	Enlarged and beating heart
	Blood formation in yolk sac
	All major systems and structures beginning to take shape
Week 6	External genitalia developing
	Blood formation in liver
	Fingers and toes developing—still webbed
Week 8	Neck develops
	Separation of fingers/toes
	Tail disappearing
	Chambers of heart separate
	Rapid growth of central nervous system
	Fetal muscular movement begins
Week 12	Rapid increase in length
	External ears have moved up to position on side of head
	Eyelids fused
	Fingernails and toenails developed
	External genitalia recognizable as male or female
	Blood formation in liver and spleen
	Kidneys start secreting urine
	Tooth buds present
Week 16	Blood formation in bone marrow begins
	Joints develop
	Eyes, ears, and nose in final position on face
	Meconium starts to accumulate in the gut
	Fetus swallowing amniotic fluid
Week 20	Mother feels fetal movement
	Heartbeat heard with stethoscope
	Hair present on head
Week 24	Eyelids open
Week 32	Subcutaneous fat being laid down
	Nail growth to end of fingers
Week 36	Fetus gaining weight rapidly
	All structures nearly mature
Week 40	Maturity—labor and delivery

otic fluid as kidney function matures. The stress caused by inadequate oxygen levels in the fetus during the third trimester (last 13 weeks of pregnancy) may cause relaxation of the anal sphincter with meconium passing into the amniotic fluid.

Nutrition and Fluid Needs.   Nutrition is provided to the fetus through the placenta and by the amniotic fluid being swallowed. If the pregnant woman is inadequately nourished or dehydrated, the fetus will grow more slowly and be born at a lower than normal birth weight. A well-balanced diet, approximately 300 calories above the woman's optimum normal intake, is required to meet the nutritional needs of the fetus.

Rest and Sleep.   The fetus spends much of its time in some form of sleep or inactivity. A normal wake and sleep pattern develops in the fetus and may persist after birth.

Pain Avoidance.   It is uncertain at what stage of development the fetus becomes capable of perceiving pain. Immediately after birth, the newborn is capable of perceiving pain and responding in a withdrawal behavior.

Sexual Needs and Sexuality.   The male and female sexual organs, the testes and ovaries, develop from the same place within the body of the embryo. During the seventh week of life, male physical structures or female physical structures develop. The male testes develop first, and several weeks later the ovaries in the female develop. The developing testes in the male produce the male hormone, testosterone, necessary for the normal development of a male. Without the production of testosterone, the fetus will develop female genital structures, even though the chromosome pattern of an X and Y sex chromosome indicates a male. This is true for both external and internal structures. The uterus, oviducts, clitoris, vagina, and labia will develop unless tes-

tosterone is present to cause male structures to form. The female hormone, estrogen, seems to take little part in the development of female structures. The absence of testosterone is the critical factor. By the 12th week of life, the external genital structures are developed to the point that the sex can be determined by visualization.

Stimulation Needs.   By eight weeks, fetal muscular movement begins and continues until birth. By 20 weeks, the pregnant woman is able to feel the fetus moving within the uterus. By 16 weeks, the eyes, ears, and nose are in their final position on the head. By 24 weeks, the fetal eyelids open. The fetus is able to hear and taste in the uterus at some time during development since these senses are functioning at birth. The darkness within the uterus prevents vision. The sense of touch develops, and some fetuses are able to coordinate the activity of thumb-sucking while still in the uterus. Stimulation in the fetal environment is created by such events as the maternal heartbeat, external noises, and maternal activity. Most external stimulation reaching the fetus is vague and muffled by the protection of the uterus and amniotic fluid. Table 11–1 shows milestones in fetal development.

Higher Level Needs

Safety and Security Needs.   The safety of the fetus is dependent on the provision of a safe environment within the mother. Alcohol, medications, illness, and maternal disease, such as diabetes or hypertensive disorders, may put the fetus in physical jeopardy for retarded growth, birth defects, and death. Maintaining optimum maternal health by prenatal education and medical care is the best way available to protect the fetus during gestation. Careful nursing assessment of the mother and fetus during labor and delivery is essential to provide data indicating possible fetal or maternal problems.

The Newborn (Neonate)—Birth to Twenty-eight Days of Age

The neonatal period is a time of transition from intrauterine life to extrauterine life. The newborn can no longer rely on maternal blood flow through the placenta to meet its basic survival needs. The changes discussed in this section relate to the normal full-term neonate.

Physiological Needs

Oxygen Needs.   At birth, the umbilical cord is clamped, and the newborn must immediately begin to

meet its own oxygen needs. Within one minute, most newborns have established adequate respirations to meet their oxygen needs. When the umbilical cord is clamped, the blood level of carbon dioxide (PCO_2) begins to rise in the newborn's blood. At the same time, the oxygen concentration in the blood begins to drop as does the pH of the blood (the blood becomes more acidic). These three events provide strong stimulation to the respiratory center in the medulla of the brain to initiate and maintain respirations. At birth, the head is born before the chest in most instances, and the nose and

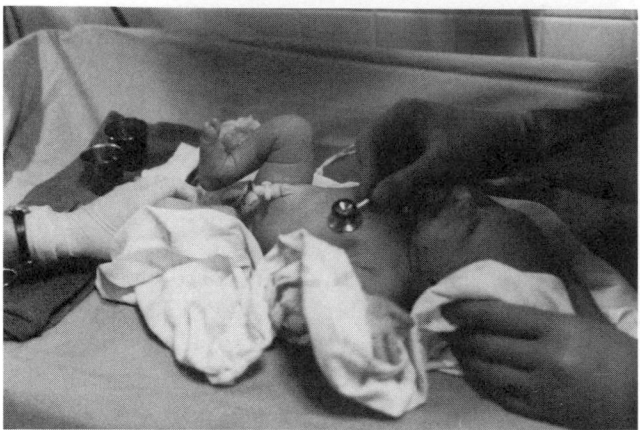

Figure 11–1. This nurse is assessing the apical heart rate and respiratory rate within several minutes of delivery.

mouth of the newborn are suctioned to clear the air passages before the first breath. With the birth of the chest, there is a sudden release of external pressure which had been provided by the vaginal canal around the chest. This decrease in pressure on the chest is another stimulus for inspiration and the first breath.

Changes in the circulatory system are essential to move blood through the lungs after birth instead of bypassing them as was the case for the major blood flow in the fetus. Figure 11–2 illustrates these changes. As the

umbilical cord is clamped, the blood flow to the placenta from the newborn is terminated and aortic blood pressure rises in the newborn. At the same time, blood flow returning to the newborn from the placenta is terminated, and venous blood pressure decreases. With expansion of the lungs, after the first breath, pulmonary blood pressure decreases, becoming lower than the now elevated aortic pressure. This causes blood to move into the newborn's pulmonary system rather than into the foramen ovale. The foramen ovale is an opening in the wall of the heart between the right and left atrium present during fetal life. This allows blood to move from the right atrium to the left atrium, bypassing the fetal lungs. The changing pressure between the right and left atria of the heart, which results from clamping the cord and expansion of the lungs, reverses the pressure differences present *in utero*. After birth, the right atrium pressure becomes lower than that of the left atrium which closes the foramen ovale, preventing unoxygenated blood from being circulated throughout the newborn's body. The ductus arteriosus also closes within approximately 15 hours after birth and becomes fibrosed within about three weeks. This closure prevents blood from bypassing the lungs and moving directly from the pulmonary artery into the aorta prior to receiving oxygen in the lungs as it did during the fetal stage. The ductus venosus also closes at birth and becomes fibrosed within the first week of life. The ductus venosus

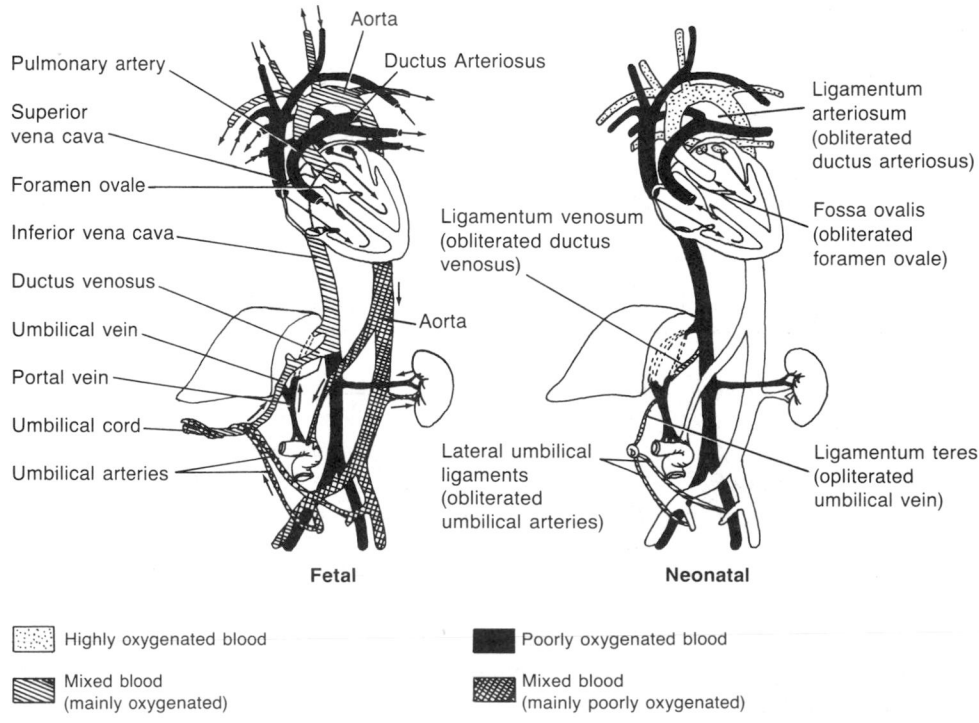

Figure 11–2. A comparison of fetal and neonatal circulation. The largest and most critical circulatory changes involve routing blood to the lungs for oxygenation after delivery. (Adapted from M. Miller *et al.*: *Kimber-Gray-Stackpole's Anatomy and Physiology*, 17th ed. Macmillan, New York, 1977.)

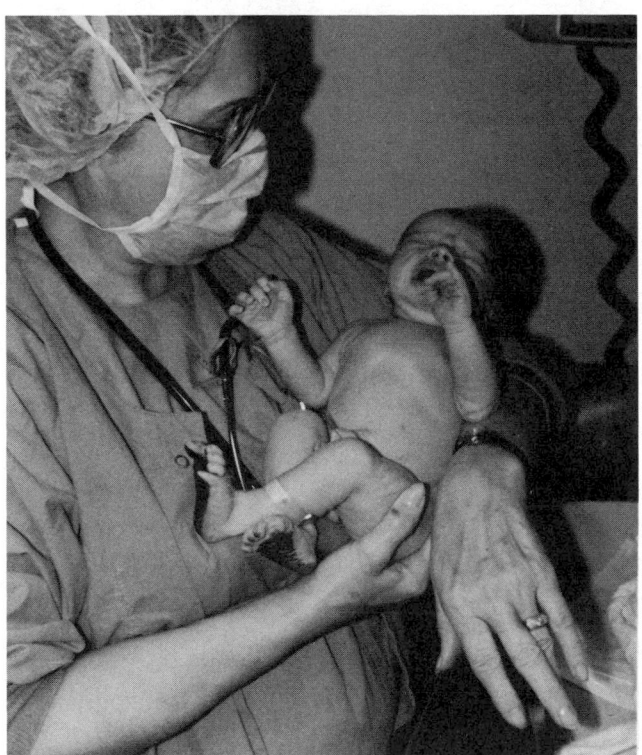

Figure 11–3. A nurse assessing a newborn's respiratory rate.

was the route the blood took from the umbilical cord into the fetal venous circulatory system.

Newborn respirations are often irregular with a rate between 30 and 60 breaths per minute. Newborns are *obligate nose-breathers* and will open their mouth to breathe only as a last resort, so nasal passages should be kept clear to prevent respiratory distress. Neonates have an inborn response, called the defense reaction, to any-

thing obstructing their nasal opening. They bring their arms and hands up to their face and claw at the area around the nose in an attempt to remove the obstruction. Normal pulse rates range from 120 to 160 beats per minute, and blood pressure at birth is in the area of 70/30 to 80/40 mm Hg. By about one week of age, this has increased to approximately 90/50 to 100/60 mm Hg. Blood volume in a seven- or eight-lb neonate is between 200 and 300 ml, which is approximately the amount of blood an adult donates at one time to a blood bank. Table 11-2 shows blood values and vital signs for the neonate.

Temperature Maintenance.   Newborns are at risk for reduced body temperature (hypothermia). The thermal regulating mechanism within the hypothalamus of the brain is not fully mature, and neonates are unable to shiver to increase body temperature as the child or adult does. In addition, they have a larger body surface in comparison to their weight, and heat loss through evaporation can be excessive, especially if they are not dryed immediately after birth. They have less fat between muscles and skin (subcutaneous fat) than older children and adults, so heat is lost more rapidly due to decreased insulation. Newborns cannot put on warmer clothing or take off coverings when they are too warm and must rely on the attention of others in their environment.

Newborns may respond to infection with a drop of several degrees in body temperature below the normal 99°F measured by the rectal route. A continual dropping or low temperature not caused by external chilling is a sign of possible infection and should be reported to the physician or nurse in charge. The only way a newborn can increase body temperature is through increasing the metabolic rate to produce heat through acceler-

Table 11–2. **Blood Values and Vital Signs in the Neonate**

	PULSE	RESPIRATIONS	BP
Birth	120–160	30–60	80/46
2 weeks	120–150	25–55	100/50
1 month	110–150	25–45	90/60

	HEMOGLOBIN* (GM)	HEMATOCRIT† (PERCENT)	WHITE BLOOD CELLS‡ (WBC)
Birth	14–24	44–64	15,000–45,000
2 weeks	15–20	35–49	5,000–20,000
1 month	11–17	30–40	5,000–19,500

*Hemoblobin (Hgb): Oxygen-carrying molecule in the red blood cell measured in grams per 100 ml of blood; normal adult values, 12–18 gm/100 ml.

†Hematocrit (Hct): Number of red blood cells in 100 ml of blood; measured as a percentage of the total blood volume; normal adult range is 37 to 52 percent.

‡White Blood Cells Count (WBC): Number of white blood cells in a cubic millimeter of blood; normal adult range, 4,500 to 11,000; increases in response to infection.

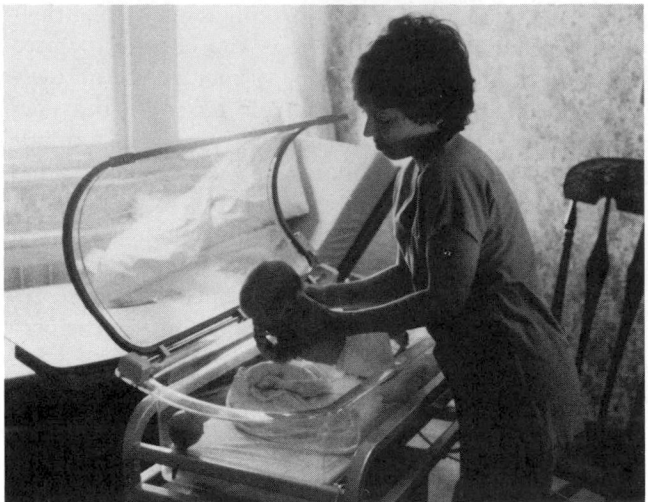

Figure 11-4. A newborn being placed into a cradle warmer for the first few hours after delivery to assist with thermal regulation.

ated chemical reactions within the body's cells (*nonshivering thermogenesis*). A cold newborn will have increased oxygen needs until the body temperature returns to normal. Oxygen needs are increased because oxygen and glucose are needed for nonshivering thermogenesis. If increased oxygen is not available, the newborn will begin to use methods of heat production without oxygen (anaerobic metabolism) to raise the temperature. This will cause the baby gradually to de-

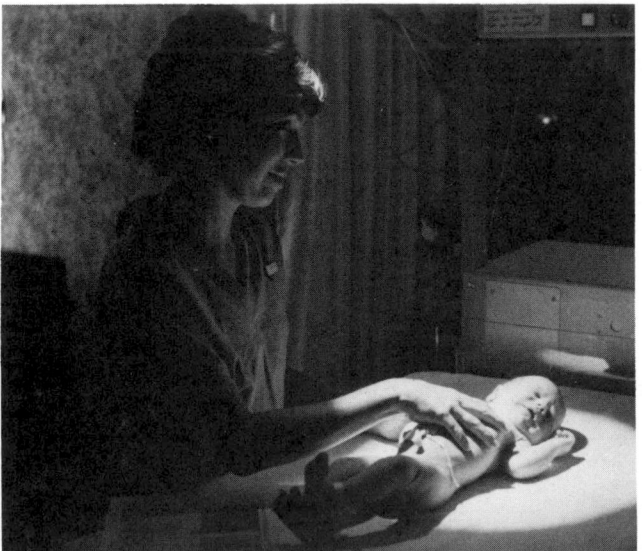

Figure 11-5. During examination of a newborn, a radiant heat source is needed to help maintain the baby's temperature. In this examination area, the heat source is focused on the newborn from above, providing the nurse with more access to the baby compared to a cradle warmer.

velop respiratory distress. Keeping the newborn warm is a critical responsibility of the nurse and the parents.

Elimination. Within 24 hours, most newborns have urinated and passed their first stool, known as *meconium*. The dark, tarlike meconium stool changes during the first few days of life until it is more yellow in appearance. Some newborns have several loose or soft stools in one day, while others may have only one. The number of voidings is a reflection of the degree of hydration in the newborn, so a vigorous eater will have more output than an uninterested eater. Urine output is 16 to 60 ml in 24 hours shortly after birth, and this increases to volumes of 250 to 400 ml by one month of age.

Nutritional/Fluid Needs. The newborn's intake is all fluid, in the form of formula or breast milk. No further supplement is usually recommended for several months. Additional fluid, in the form of water, is generally unnecessary unless the environment is very warm and water is lost through increased perspiration. Most mothers will have breast milk within several days of delivery. During the interval when the mother's milk supply is developing, small amounts of sterile water or 5 percent dextrose water may be used if the newborn seems hungry after breastfeeding. After the milk comes in, the healthy, breastfeeding newborn will establish its own milk supply based on individual need. The more the newborn takes, the more milk the breast will make, given a little time. Neonates usually need 117 calories for every kilogram of body weight to be adequately nourished. Breast milk and most formulas provide 20 calories per ounce. The average-size neonate will usually be eating between 16 and 23 oz of formula or breast milk each day. All newborns lose weight after birth. An average weight loss is between 5 and 10 percent of their body weight at birth. This birth weight is usually regained by one to two weeks after birth. The neonate moves from an early feeding pattern of seven to eight feedings to five to six feedings in a 24-hour period by the end of the first month. Night feedings are common at this age. The newborn has a rooting reflex for feeding. When the lips or cheeks are stroked, the baby turns toward the nipple and opens its mouth. The suck, swallow, and gag reflexes are also mature and functioning in the full-term newborn. Inadequate nutrition in the neonatal and infancy periods can result in fewer numbers of brain cells, decreased mental abilities, and retarded growth.

Rest and Sleep. The newborn is alert approximately 3 percent of daylight hours, and most of the neonate's time is spent in some form of drowsiness or sleep. At birth, the newborn sleeps approximately 22 hours out of

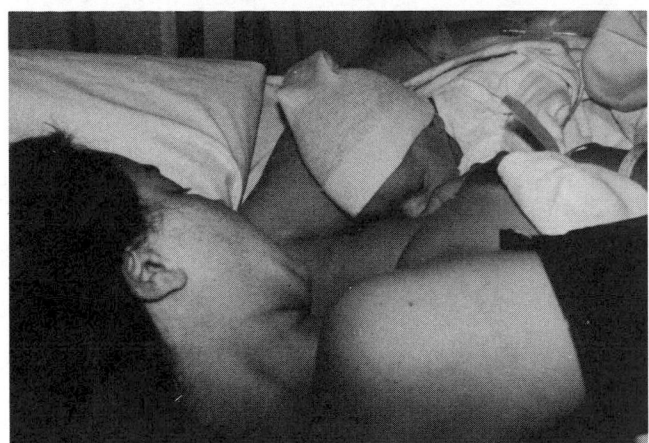

Figure 11-6. A newborn breastfeeding shortly after birth. The cap on the baby's head is to reduce heat loss.

24 hours. By one month, this is down to 15 to 18 hours. The newborn usually has seven to eight periods of sleep in every 24-hour period, and, by one month, this may have changed to three to four naps during the day with a longer stretch of five to six hours at night. Neonates are mostly light sleepers. Only 20 to 30 percent of their sleep is deep sleep; the remaining sleep is similar to adult dream sleep (see Chapter 25).

Pain Avoidance.   There are individual differences in newborn's response to pain. A newborn cannot provide subjective data about pain, but the perception of pain can be inferred from neonatal behavior. Generally, the perception of pain is decreased at birth and increases during the first few weeks of life. The newborn will try to avoid pain by withdrawing the body part receiving the painful stimulus. A newborn having blood drawn from a foot will pull the foot away or, if that action is prevented, the other foot may come over to push the painful stimulus away. Circumcision for male infants is initially painful as indicated by the loud crying which accompanies part of the surgery. This period of crying is usually fairly brief.

Sexual Needs and Sexuality.   At birth, the parents and others begin to relate to the newborn as male or female. Newborn male infants frequently have penile erections, and parents should be aware that this is normal. Pediatricians usually do not recommend routine circumcision of male newborns and believe this is a religious or cultural concern but not a medical one. Breast enlargement may be noticeable in the newborn. This is related to maternal hormone levels, and the newborn's breast size decreases to normal within several days after birth. Newborn females have thick vaginal secretions that gradually decrease during the first week of life, again re-

lated to hormone levels in the mother during gestation. Parents who planned on one sex and delivered the opposite-sexed baby may initially have difficulty forming a close attachment to the newborn when compared to parents who had no preference or delivered the desired-sexed baby. Although this delay is usually brief, it may affect the way the child is raised.

Stimulation Needs.   The neonate's senses of touch, hearing, smell, and vision are functioning at birth. Neonates begin to learn through interaction with an interesting, varied environment. The newborn prefers the human face and spends much time looking at mother's and father's faces. The brain is still growing, especially during the first six months. Environmental stimulation and handling are needed for optimum development. Muscle movements of arms and legs are mainly reflexive at this age. Table 11-3 describes reflexes in the neonate. The neonate can hold its head up for brief periods and may be able to roll slightly toward the side. The neonate does not have the coordination to reach for objects. Holding or swaddling the newborn usually quiets any crying.

A cultural difference is noted in the muscle tone and coordination among Caucasian, Negro, and Oriental newborns. The black newborns, especially African blacks, have advanced motor development compared to the other two groups. The Oriental and American Indian newborns show the least motor development and muscle tone at birth of the three groups. The African black infants remain advanced in their motor development until close to the second year of life, when the other two cultural groups catch up. This may be partly due to environmental childrearing practices, but the differences are apparent within the first few days of life and seem to imply a strong genetic component (Papalia, 1975; Cultural Differences in Newborn Behaviors, 1974).

Higher Level Needs

Safety and Security Needs.   The safety and security needs of the neonate are related to having basic physical needs met by constant, attentive care-givers. The neonate may start to recognize the mother's and father's voices and respond by quieting. The greatest safety needs of the newborn are associated with preventing accidents. One example of this is the ride home from the hospital in an approved infant car seat. The nurse should be familiar with state laws affecting children under four years of age and the use of car seats and discuss the law with new parents.

Within the hospital, the nurse performs many activities to protect the newborn from potential problems. If

Table 11–3. **Reflexes in the Newborn**

REFLEX	DESCRIPTION	DISAPPEARANCE OF REFLEX
Rooting reflex	The newborn will turn and open its mouth toward the cheek being stroked. Mother strokes the cheek closest to the breast and the infant turns toward mother's nipple	3–4 months (while awake)
Sucking	Stimulation of upper palate will stimulate sucking. Anything touching the lips or mouth may induce sucking	Persists during first year, especially during sleep
Grasp reflex	The newborn will grasp and hold a narrow object, such as a pencil, when it is placed in the palm	5–6 months
Moro reflex	Same as startle response; elicited by quickly lowering the infant's head while in a supine position (on the back). Extension and flexion of arms and legs; may end in crying	4–7 months
Babinski	Fanning of the toes in response to stroking up from the heel along the outside edge of the foot	Disappears when child begins walking and changes to an incurving of the toes
Tonic neck	Newborn extends the arm and leg on the same side to which the head is turned, and flexes the extremities on the other side. Elicited by turning the head to one side. The side to which the head is turned will then extend	6 months
Stepping	The newborn picks up its feet, alternating right and left, as if taking steps. Elicited by holding newborn upright with feet touching a firm surface and then leaning infant forward	3–4 months

the mother has gonorrhea, the newborn is exposed to it during the process of birth. The eyes of all newborns are protected from possible infection from this organism by the application of erythromycin ophthalmic ointment to both eyes or by the instillation of a 1 percent solution of silver nitrate. Gonorrheal infection in the eyes of the newborn can cause permanent blindness. Prophylactic treatment is given to all newborns unless parents specifically refuse treatment.

Another prophylactic treatment the newborn frequently receives is an injection of vitamin K (AQUAMEPHYTON) to prevent any problems with inadequate blood clotting. Vitamin K, needed for clotting, is not produced in the intestines until several days after birth when bacteria begin to colonize the area. It is the bacteria in the gut that produce the body's supply of vitamin K.

Another safety consideration in the care of the newborn is the umbilical cord stump which could serve as an entrance for bacteria into the circulation. Careful handwashing and application of an alcohol solution to promote drying and a BETADINE solution to reduce bac-

terial growth are common nursing interventions. The umbilical cord is usually dried to the point that the cord clamp can be removed 24 hours after birth. The remaining stump falls off within the next week or two.

Neonates have immature immune systems and have a decreased ability to produce effective antibodies until about two months of age. A virus, such as herpes simplex, can be fatal to the newborn if it enters the circulation. Nursing and other medical personnel are unsafe in the nursery if they have active cold sores, a form of herpes simplex. This immature immune system is the reason immunization against diphtheria, tetanus, pertussis, and polio is delayed until the infant is several months old.

Neonates are also screened for inborn metabolic disorders. Examples of these include phenylketonuria, galactosemia, and hypothyroidism. Most states require by law that the nurse take a blood sample for these tests before the newborn is discharged from the hospital. Specific diets or medication will prevent permanent damage from these problems when started in the neonatal period.

Common Problems of the Neonate and Nursing Implications

The problems discussed here relate to the full-term newborn in no apparent physical distress. The emphasis of nursing care for the newborn is on helping the new parents develop the skills and confidence they will need to care for the baby independently. Many parents have inadequate skills and knowledge related to infant care so the major part of nursing care has an educational-supportive focus on the parents. Breastfeeding is a new skill for many women and a critical one for the newborn. With a majority of women selecting this feeding method, nurses are spending much of their time teaching this activity. Teaching other skills, such as diapering, bathing, and use of car safety restraints, is also part of nursing care for families of newborns.

One problem common to many newborns in the first week of life is elevated bilirubin levels in the blood, causing the baby to appear jaundiced. For the full-term newborn this problem is usually most apparent on the third or fourth day of life. If the level of bilirubin in the blood becomes excessively elevated, there is a risk of a condition in which the bilirubin is deposited in the cells of the brain, *kernicterus*. This can result in varying degrees of mental retardation. Most healthy newborns never get close to this dangerous level, but some have elevations of bilirubin which are treated with phototherapy to prevent any further rises. During phototherapy, fluorescent lights, especially those with a predominance in the blue light spectrum, are used to lower the bilirubin levels. The newborn's skin is exposed to the lights over a period of time, usually about 24 hours, and the lights break the bilirubin down into a form that can be excreted through the intestines. This is a temporary problem and usually relates to immature liver function at birth. Nursing responsibility involves explanation to the parents and providing adequate heat, fluids, and hygiene care. The eyes of the newborn are covered to protect them from possible damage. Keeping the eye covers in place is a nursing responsibility.

Infancy—One Month to One Year of Age

Infancy is the period of time from the end of the neonatal period until one year of age. Some differences of opinion exist about the length of this period, with an upper age limit of two or three years. The changes and growth occurring in the first year of life are so remarkable and rapid that they are second only to the time from conception to birth. It is for this reason that the one-year length was chosen in describing the rapidly changing infant. Mobility, language, and a sense of self will be achieved to some degree by the end of the first year, as the infant grows to nearly three times its birth weight. During the first six months, the infant is growing in length at a rate of 1 inch a month and ½ inch the remaining six months. If that rate continued until people were 15 years old, the average height would be 9½ ft. Different areas of the cortex of the brain mature at different rates within any one infant. This progressive maturation of the brain's cortex makes it possible for the infant to develop new motor and intellectual abilities over time. The brain continues to grow and develop very rapidly during the first six months of life, and by approximately 18 months to two years, brain growth is slowed and the fontanels become closed over by bone growth (ossified). Differences among infants in their levels of development result from a combination of environmental factors, genetics, and individual differences in their timetables for brain cortex maturation.

Physiological Needs

Oxygen Needs. Infants remain obligate nose-breathers until sometime toward the end of infancy, when they become comfortable with mouth-breathing. Until this time, any obstruction in the nasal passages may give the infant varying amounts of respiratory distress, and it is important to keep these passages clear. A bulb syringe is a convenient tool for the parents, babysitters, and nurses to use in keeping the airway open through the nose. Compressing the bulb syringe, inserting it into one nostril, and then releasing it will usually clear any obstructing material. Both nostrils should be cleared for optimum respiratory ease in the infant. The infant is predominantly an abdominal breather, using the muscles of the abdomen rather than those of the chest. Respiratory rates in infancy usually range from 20 to 40 breaths per minute.

For some infants, the foramen ovale and the ductus arteriosus do not close completely until several months after birth. The resulting heart murmur will be present in varying degrees until complete termination of fetal circulation patterns. There is no accompanying cyanosis or other clinical signs or symptoms of distress with either of these openings unless there are other defects in the heart. Most murmurs will disappear during the neonatal period, but some may take several additional

Table 11–4. **Blood Values and Vital Signs in the Infant**

AGE	HEMOGLOBIN (GM)	HEMATOCRIT (PERCENT)	WBC
Blood Values in the Infant			
3 months	10–13	37	11,000
6 months	10.5–14.5	37	11,900
12 months	11–15	37	11,400

AGE	PULSE (PER MINUTE)	RESPIRATIONS (PER MINUTE)	BP
Vital Signs in the Infant			
3 months	110–150	25–45	90/60
6 months	100–140	22–40	90/60
12 months	95–135	20–40	96/66

months to achieve complete closure. The heart rate in the infant is in the range of 100 to 120 beats per minute in normal health. The blood pressure of the infant averages 90/60 mm. Hg. Some infants exhibit a slightly irregular heartbeat associated with changes in respiratory rates. Table 11–4 shows normal ranges for blood values and vital signs in the infant.

Temperature Regulation.   Infants, like neonates, continue to be at risk for problems with temperature maintenance. Infants sweat very little because they have an immature system and are, therefore, susceptible to increased temperatures from environmental heat. They must depend on those caring for them to remove clothing when external temperatures rise and add additional clothing as the external temperature cools. The infant gradually develops the ability to shiver to raise body temperature. During the first year of life, shivering begins at lower temperatures than in the adult so the infant has already lost considerable heat by the time shivering begins. The story is told by Pozos and Born (1982) of a couple who went cross-country skiing with their one-year-old son who was warmly dressed in a backpack on the father's back. The temperature was 20°F and fairly calm. The parents were quite warm from the exercise of cross-country skiing, but the father's heat was not reaching the infant because of all the layers of insulation. The infant's body temperature continued to drop, and he died of hypothermia. Education of parents by nurses regarding the risks of temperature extremes on the infant can be lifesaving in some climates. Infants have difficulty maintaining their temperature when stressed by infection and often show rapid rises in their temperature of 104°F or higher. Temperature elevation from infection is so common that many physicians recommend not treating with antipyretics such as aspirin or

acetaminophen (TYLENOL) until the infant's fever is above 102°F. The normal temperature in the infant is 99°F taken rectally or 97 to 98°F taken axillary.

Elimination.   The majority of infants remain incontinent of both urine and stool during the first year of life. Many parents do not begin toilet training until close to the second year of life, when bladder capacity is greater and sphincter control and mobility are at more mature levels. Infants tend to have six to eight wet diapers a day when adequately hydrated, equaling approximately 400 to 500 ml of urine in 24 hours by late infancy. Bowel movements may be as frequent as four to five times in a 24-hour period, or the infant may only have a stool once a day or every other day. The infant is not constipated as long as the stool continues to have a soft-formed consistency. Hard, pellet-type stools usually indicate a need for additional fluid.

Nutrition and Fluid Needs.   Because of the rapid growth rate in the infant, nutrition and fluid needs are extremely important. Brain cells are forming and developing during infancy, and malnutrition, especially during the first six months of life, may reduce the total number of brain cells. Reduction in number of brain cells is a permanent consequence of inadequate nutrition during this period of rapid brain growth and may affect future mental potential. Adequate nutritional intake for the infant is calculated by body weight in kilograms. During the first six months of life, the infant needs 115 kilocalories for every kilogram of body weight and 2.2 gm of protein for every kilogram of body weight. In the second six months, the nutritional needs decrease slightly with 105 kilocalories and 2.0 gm of protein needed for every kilogram of body weight. For example, an infant weighing 8 lb at one month of age would need approximately 21 oz of formula or breast milk in a 24-hour period.

Calculations

3.6 kg = 8 lb   20 cal = 1 oz
(20 calories are present in 1 oz of breast milk or standard formula)
115 cal × 3.6 kg = 414.0 total calories needed in 24 hours
414 cal ÷ 20 cal/oz = 20.7 oz/24 hr

By 12 months, the infant usually weighs 19 to 25 lb and is 27½ to 30½ inches in length. Breastfed children, who nurse every two to five hours for ten minutes or more on each breast and seem content after eating for several hours, are usually meeting their nutritional needs for the first half of infancy. After six months, the gradual addition of foods is begun by most parents, and breastfeeding may continue or be eliminated and replaced with formula feedings. Many women breastfeed their children for a full year or longer. Formula or breast milk is recommended by the American Academy of Pediatrics for the first year of life. After that time, cow's milk may be used instead of formula or breast milk.

Fluid needs in the infant require 100 to 165 ml of water per kilogram of body weight to be met adequately. This usually amounts to 1,100 to 1,300 ml of fluid in 24 hours by the time the infant is 12 months old. This is the equivalent of 36 to 43 oz of fluid. There is an increased fluid need in infancy compared to older children because the infant has an increased water loss through evaporation of fluid from the epidermal skin layers. Added fluid seeps into the epidermal skin layer during early infancy, increasing the fluid content of this tissue. Added fluid is also lost through respirations.

With maturation in the infant, changes occur that affect nutritional intake and digestion. The volume of the stomach gradually increases, with accompanying delayed emptying of a full stomach. This allows the older infant to wait for a longer time between feedings. Hydrochloric acid production in the stomach reaches adult levels by about four months of age, and this is important for digestion of more complex foods. Amylase, which is needed for digestion of complex carbohydrates, is not present until three months of age, and after that it gradually reaches adult levels in the older child. By the end of the first year, most other enzymes needed for digestion are present in sufficient amounts to digest most foods. As the infant matures, a more active role in feeding becomes characteristic. Holding and drinking from a cup, self-feeding, and expressing food preferences are common activities of the older infant. Teeth begin to erupt through the gums at about six months of age, and by one year, most infants have six teeth and can eat finger foods.

Overfeeding in infancy resulting in a plump baby is

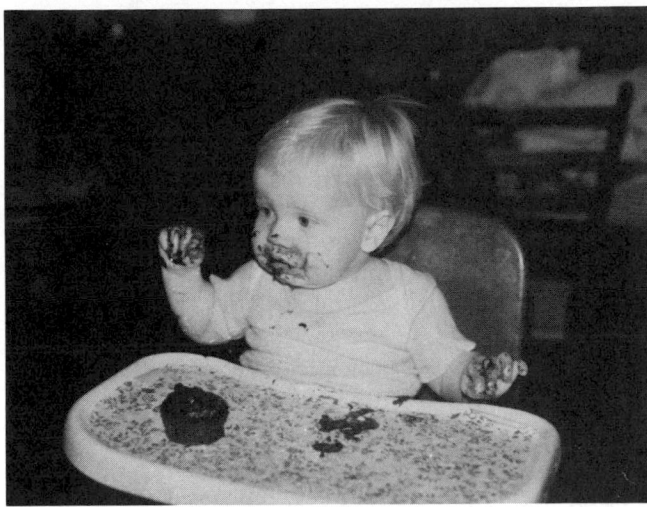

Figure 11-7. An infant involved in self-feeding. Some children this age may refuse to eat if others attempt to feed them, but will eat soft finger foods themselves.

no longer considered optimum nutritional status. Trimmer infants are believed to run less of a risk for obesity in later life because they will actually have fewer fat cells than overweight infants. These fat cells, which are formed during infancy, remain with the individual throughout life and predispose the individual to excessive weight gains.

Rest and Sleep.   Approximately 14 hours of the infant's day are spent in sleep. They are awake about as much as they are asleep by the end of the first year. Many infants begin to sleep through the night around three to four months, and others may continue to waken for a night feeding until later infancy. Some infants will take a morning and an afternoon nap, while others prefer one long nap during the day.

Pain Avoidance.   The infant will communicate pain through crying. Crying due to pain has a different sound than does crying for other reasons. By the end of the neonatal period, pain perception in the full-term newborn is mature. The source may be unrecognized by the infant, but the pain is perceived, and affected parts will be withdrawn whenever possible.

Sexual Needs and Sexuality.   The time of infancy is a time of exploration, and the infant's body is one more fascinating thing to examine. Pleasurable sexual sensations are associated with genital manipulation and exploration in the infant. During diapering and cleaning, the infant's genital area is stimulated by the parents and other care-givers. Infant boys have penile erections, and when infants gain hand control, both sexes explore the genital area with the hands on frequent occasions.

Early responses from the parents begin to affect the child's self-image as male or female. The infant may learn that touching and exposing the genital area are unacceptable and may even be related to some form of punishment. A very negative parental attitude toward the normal sexual exploration of self that occurs in infancy may have damaging effects on future sexual functioning, especially if parental attitudes continue during childhood. Sigmund Freud viewed the infant as operating on the pleasure principle with oral gratification through sucking and mouthing objects as a form of sexual pleasure. The sexuality of a woman breastfeeding an infant and the close tactile contact make the time of feeding a very intimate time between mother and infant.

The way the infant is treated is often affected by the sex of the newborn. The infant may be handled and talked to differently depending on its sex. Infant boys may be handled more roughly and played with in a more physical manner than infant girls. Infant girls may be talked to more than infant boys and cuddled and held more than their male counterparts. Clothes, toys, and the appearance of the infant's bedroom may all be affected by the infant's sex, so that the environment the infant boy explores may be quite different from the environment of the infant girl. These factors will help form the concepts of maleness and femaleness as the child grows and learns from the environment.

Stimulation Needs.   As the infant grows and matures, the reflexive movements of the newborn are gradually replaced by purposeful activities in the one-year-old. The infant learns to roll over, sit, crawl, stand, and walk, all in the course of 12 months. Table 11–5 shows the age at which some of these behaviors develop. The ability to use the hands to manipulate the environment is comprised of many separate parts which depend on neuromuscular maturation, intact and functioning senses, and a responsive, stimulating environment. The one-year-old infant with a capacity to understand much of what is said and a beginning ability to respond with several words is progressing well. The senses develop during infancy, with vision and hearing at mature levels by 12 months. The ability of the infant to focus on objects (accommodation) is at an adult level by approximately four months. Binocular vision is well developed by 11 to 12 months, and depth perception seems to be present at an age as young as experimenters are able to measure. The six-month-old will not move beyond a visual illusion of a drop-off, and younger infants show an increase in pulse and respiratory rates when placed near such a drop-off. Coordinated movement of both eyes occurs around two to three months.

Table 11–5. Behavioral Developments in Infants

	APPROXIMATE AGE (MONTHS)
Smiles in response to people, events	1
Laughs, squeals	2
Rolls over	2–3
Sits when held with head steady	3
Reaches for objects	3–4
Bears some weight on legs while being held	4–5
Turns to voice	5–6
Passes block from one hand to the other	5–6
Sits without support	5–6
Stands holding on to furniture	6
Plays peek-a-boo (cultural)	6
Imitates speech sounds; mama/dada	7
Able to get into a sitting position	7–8
Shy of strangers	9–10
Stands and walks holding on to furniture	9–10
Pincer grasp of small objects	10–11
Drinks from cup	11–12
Stands unassisted	11–12

Source: Adapted from Denver Developmental Screening Test. Frankenburg, W., Dodds, J., Univ. of Colorado Medical Center, 1969.

Some cultural differences are present in the rate of growth and the acquisition of motor abilities. The African black infant when compared to other infants is precocious in both growth and motor activity. These differences are noted in the neonatal period and seem to persist until close to the second year of life when other racial groups catch up.

A varied, stimulating environment, with different sights, sounds, tastes, and textures for the infant to explore, tends to stimulate the infant's development. A severely deprived environment, in which the child is restrained because of illness or lack of attention by care-givers, tends to retard the development of motor and cognitive skills in the infant.

Higher Level Needs

Safety and Security Needs.   Providing physical safety for the exploring infant is no easy task, and accidents are a constant problem. Everything goes in the mouth, and objects that can be accidentally swallowed are a danger. Anything less than about 2 inches in diameter should be considered dangerous for infants. Infants are crawling and walking, so poisons are a real danger. Using safety latches on cupboards containing anything at all dangerous if swallowed is one way of protecting infants not confined to a playpen or play area. Falling off changing tables, beds, and down stairs is another danger

Table 11–6. **Recommended Schedule for Active Immunizations of Normal Infants and Children**

AGE	IMMUNIZATION
2 months	DTP (diphtheria and tetanus toxoids plus pertussis vaccine) TOPV (trivalent oral poliovirus vaccine)
4 months	DTP, TOPV
6 months	DTP (optional TOPV for areas with high incidence of poliomyelitis)
1 year	Tuberculin test (not an immunization—diagnostic)
15 months	Measles, rubella, mumps combined vaccines (MMR)
18 months	DTP, TOPV
4–6 years	DTP, TOPV
14–16 years	Tetanus and diphtheria toxoids (to be repeated every 10 years)

Source: Recommendations of the Immunization Practices Advisory Committee (ACIP), a branch of Center of Disease Control (CDC), Atlanta, Ga. 1983.

for the infants whose motor skills may be underestimated by caretakers and parents. Infant walkers pose a particular danger of falls when stairs are in the area. Infants can move around very rapidly in walkers and may fall down open stairwells.

Immunizations are begun during this period and Table 11–6 shows a common sequence. Table 11–7 shows past incidence of diseases now preventable by immunizations.

Many infants begin to show fear of new places and people around seven to nine months. Separation from one or both parents often results in anxiety, and the infant will try to bring the parent back through crying and motor activity. Many infants learn to comfort themselves with thumb- or finger-sucking. A favorite toy or blanket may become very important to the infant in the absence of the parent and during sleep times. The infant gradually gains a sense of security about the environment when parents respond consistently to the infant's needs. The infant learns that efforts to communicate needs will result in attention from parents. This is the beginning of trust in interpersonal relationships, and people like Erik Erikson see this development of trust and security as a basic developmental task upon which all other tasks in future stages are built. The important factor seems to be that the care-givers are constant in the infant's environment and that they respond to the infant's needs as those needs arise, rather than on the set schedule of a busy caretaker. If the infant feels all efforts to communicate personal needs have no relationship to the appearance of the caretaker and need satisfaction, then the infant may feel powerless to control the environment and withdraw, becoming very passive, verbally and physically.

Love and Belonging Needs.   Good parenting provides the close, affectionate bond that infants need for nor-

Table 11–7. **Current and Past Incidence of Preventable Diseases in the United States**

	MEASLES	RUBELLA	MUMPS	DIPHTHERIA	PERTUSSIS	TETANUS	POLIO
1920	465,048 cases 7,600 deaths	*	*	147,991 cases 13,211 deaths		*	2,338 cases
1930	419,465 cases 3,783 deaths	*	*	66,576 cases 5,741 deaths	166,914 cases 5,671 deaths	*	9,220 cases 1,364 deaths
1940	291,162 cases 706 deaths	*	*	15,536 cases 1,457 deaths	183,866 cases 2,926 deaths	*	9,894 cases 1,026 deaths
1950	319,124 cases 468 deaths	*	*	5,796 cases 410 deaths	120,718 cases 1,118 deaths	486 cases 336 deaths	33,300 cases 1,904 deaths
1960	441,703 cases 380 deaths	*	*	918 cases 69 deaths	14,809 cases 118 deaths	368 cases 231 deaths	3,190 cases 230 deaths
1970	47,351 cases 89 deaths	56,552 cases 31 deaths	104,953 cases 16 deaths	435 cases 30 deaths	4,249 cases 12 deaths	148 cases 79 deaths	33 cases 7 deaths
1980	13,506 cases no deaths	3,904 cases no deaths	8,576 cases no deaths	3 cases no deaths	1,730 cases no deaths	95 cases no deaths	9 cases no deaths
1982	1,697 cases no deaths	2,283 cases no deaths	5,196 cases no deaths	3 cases no deaths	1,784 cases no deaths	81 cases no deaths	7 cases no deaths

Source: Division of Disease Control, Immunization Unit, Center for Disease Control, Atlanta, Ga., 1983.
*No National Data Available

Table 11–8. **Theories Related to Infant Growth and Development**

SENSORIMOTOR STAGE—BIRTH TO 24 MONTHS

Piaget—Four-Stage Theory of Cognition

Substage I—birth to 1 month	Reflexive stage. Through use of inborn reflexes, the neonate begins to adapt and organize experiences. Sucking, rooting, crying, smiling, and grasping are a few of these early reflexes
Substage II—1–4 months	Primary circular reaction. Beginning to recognize objects. Tries to repeat behaviors in body movement. Thumb-sucking
Substage III—4–8 months	Secondary circular reactions. Tries to duplicate events discovered by accident. Learns that objects have permanence outside of infant's perception. Reaches out to touch a mobile and make it move
Substage IV—8–12 months	Coordination of secondary schemata. Concerned with manipulating environment. Early beginning of problem solving

Freud—Oral Stage (up to 1½ years)
Primary pleasure through sucking and oral stimulation

Havinghurst/Hurlock—Developmental tasks of infancy and early childhood

Learning to walk, talk, take solid foods, and control the elimination of body wastes
Learning sex differences and sexual modesty
Achieving physiological stability
Forming simple concepts of social and physical reality
Learning to relate emotionally to parents, siblings, and other people
Developing a conscience, a sense of right and wrong

Erikson—Stage of development for the infant

Infancy (birth to 1 year)   development of trust versus mistrust

mal growth and development. By the end of the third month, most parents are closely attached to their new infant. By the end of the first year, the infant has completed attachment to the parents. This process of attachment is dependent on a reciprocal interaction between the parent and the infant. The infant stares at the parent's face, smiles, quiets when spoken to, and laughs with approval. All the varied activities the infant displays which please the parent will help solidify the loving bond between them. A fussy, unresponsive child may discourage parent's efforts to interact with their infant, and attachment may be delayed or incomplete. Autistic children often appear unresponsive during infancy and seem to give the parents little positive feedback in the form of socialization. Infants who fail to develop an affectionate bond with a caring, attentive adult, because of being institutionalized in a nonresponsive environment, may fail to grow and develop normally. This syndrome is called "failure to thrive," and the infant is severely retarded in growth and development in the absence of any known pathology. The element that is missing is a relationship with a loving, responsive adult who attends to the child's needs, especially nutritional needs.

Self-Esteem Needs. By the end of the first year, infants have begun to develop a sense of self. They recognize that they are separate from other people and things in their environment. They have also discovered that they can manipulate the environment through verbal and motor activities. The infant expresses a definite need to do things independently. The infant is learning to master body movements and begins to show a sense of pride and pleasure in achievements. Infants have learned that the adult can be very helpful in satisfying their needs and that language is one way to make needs known. A sense of conscience is beginning to develop. Temper tantrums begin to appear in some infants as they demand their own way. Table 11–8 describes several different theories related to infant development and developmental tasks.

Common Problems During Infancy and Nursing Implications

1. Accidents are among the leading causes of death in infants. The most common accidents are from falls, poisoning, burns, and auto accidents. Providing safety

information to new parents in the early postpartum period may help them look at their home for safety hazards before their infant begins to crawl. Many states require infants and children to be restrained in federally approved car seats when being transported in an automobile or truck. The first ride the infant ever takes, which is often home from the hospital, should be in a car seat. It is the nurse's responsibility to inform new parents about motor vehicle laws in their state relating to infant restraints and to assist them in obtaining and using car seats from the beginning of their child's life.

2. Infections are a common problem in infants. Respiratory tract infections are the most common. Infants are more susceptible than older children and adults because of the small size of the respiratory tract. Bacteria have a much shorter distance to travel from a contaminated source in the air or skin surface to the inner lung. Ear infections are another problem encountered by many infants. The eustachian tube is shorter and straighter in the infant, forming a direct opening for bacteria located in the pharynx. Feeding infants flat on their backs increases the risk of bacteria moving from the throat to the inner ear. Nurses and parents should hold infants upright during feedings to reduce this risk.

3. Intestinal problems are frequently seen in the form of diarrhea and colic. Infants are more susceptible to diarrhea because of the immature immunological response of the intestinal mucosa. Usually the problem bacteria is *E. coli*. The infant's endocrine system is also immature, and production of antidiuretic hormone, important for reabsorption of water by the kidney, is limited. This means that diarrhea can rapidly dehydrate the infant, compared to an older child. Colic is experienced by some infants in the first part of infancy, but the cause remains unclear. The infant experiences abdominal pain as evidenced by constant crying, a rigid abdomen, and legs flexed up onto the abdomen. Parental efforts are often unsuccessful in quieting the infant, and the periodic episodes seem to resolve on their own. By three months of age, most infants have stopped having colic.

4. Anemia is a problem common to the infant at approximately two to three months. Many physicians recommend iron-fortified formula until the infant is a year old. Iron supplements may be recommended in breastfed infants, since iron is available in only small amounts in human milk.

5. The infant is sensitive to sunlight and easily burned because the melanin in the epidermal layers of the skin is only slowly being laid down. The infant's and child's skin color darkens with age from melanin.

6. Sudden infant death syndrome (SIDS) is probably the most frightening and puzzling problem of all. SIDS claims up to 10,000 infants a year in the United States and is the leading cause of death in this age group (Whaley and Wong, 1982). Most infants die from SIDS after the neonatal period. Deaths from SIDS drop off dramatically after the fourth month of life and rarely occur after six months. Beckwith (1970) defined this syndrome as: "The sudden and unexpected death of an infant who was either well or almost well prior to death and whose death remains unexplained after an autopsy." There are many theories on what causes these deaths. This usually indicates that no one really knows. The infant at greatest risk has the following traits: male, born prematurely, mother smoked during pregnancy, and family belongs to the lower socioeconomic class. However, this tragedy strikes healthy, full-term infants from all family backgrounds, and these infants are never viewed as high risk so no special precautions are taken. With infants known to be high risk, apnea monitors may be sent home from the hospital with the parents and used whenever the infant sleeps. If the infant fails to take a breath after a set period of time has elapsed, the monitor sets off an alarm which startles the infant to stimulate respiration and alerts the parents to check on the infant. These monitors are used until the infant is approximately six months old. Support groups are available for parents who lose a child to SIDS.

7. Child abuse does occur during infancy and may be second only to SIDS as a cause of death in this age group. It is defined by the 1974 Child Abuse Prevention and Treatment Act as: "The physical or mental injury, sexual abuse, malignant treatment or maltreatment of a child under 18 years of age, by a person who is responsible for the child's welfare, under circumstances which indicate that the child's health or welfare is harmed or threatened." Adults who abuse infants and children have totally varied backgrounds, but some things are characteristic. Many abusive parents were abused by their parents when they were young. Parents seem to have failed to develop a sense of trust with their own parents. The marriage is more often unstable in abusive families. The parents often have unrealistic expectations for the infant and child compared to normal patterns of growth and development. For example, the parent may expect the child to be toilet trained by 12 months, which is highly unlikely for most infants. The child seems to be unable to meet the parent's expectations and often is viewed as different, in a negative way, from other children. Usually a crisis or disruption of some sort is necessary to trigger the episode of abuse. It is the nurse's legal responsibility to report any suspected abuse to the police, social services, or the district attorney's office. There are also various support and help groups available to parents who react to stress with abuse to their children. Parents Anonymous may be the most widely known support grop for abusive parents.

In providing nursing care to infants, the following suggestions may be helpful:

1. Be as attentive as possible in responding to the distress expressed by the infant. Demand-feeding schedules are important when possible.

2. Encourage parental participation in the infant's care. Make sure the parents can meet their own needs for food and rest, especially if the mother is breastfeeding.

3. Provide close physical contact and stimulation through holding, rocking, singing, and talking. Bring the infant out into the hall to view the activity. Provide toys, wall decorations, and mobiles to stimulate the senses.

4. Provide consistent nursing care by the same individuals whenever possible.

5. Encourage the parents to bring familiar objects from home to make the infant feel more secure in the absence of the parents.

6. Recognize that an infant who crys and becomes extremely upset is showing a positive sign of attachment to the parents. The infant who withdraws from the environment and offers no resistance when the parent leaves may have lost the sense of trust for the parent and feel helpless to control the environment. This is a dangerous sign for future interpersonal and social development.

Summary

The length of time it takes for the single fertilized egg cell to become a fully developed fetus is between 38 and 42 weeks. This rate of growth will never again be equaled. All major body systems and structures are formed and beginning to mature and function at the end of 13 weeks of gestation. Development of male internal and external structures is dependent on the production of testosterone during the first 13 weeks of life, or the embryo will develop female physical structures. The placenta is the site for exchange of substances between mother and fetus, but their blood does not mix. Transfer of substances, such as oxygen, nutrients, and carbon dioxide occurs as a result of diffusion from a higher to a lower area of concentration. During pregnancy, drinking alcoholic beverages and inadequate nutritional intake are known to risk fetal health and development.

The fetal heart rate, in the range of 120 to 160 beats each minute, is one of the best indicators of fetal health and satisfaction of oxygen needs. Inadequate oxygen to the fetus in the last trimester may cause a reflex defecation, and the first stool, meconium, is passed into the amniotic fluid. The healthy fetus is active from the end of the first trimester until birth, swallowing amniotic fluid and passing urine. The neonatal period is a time of transition from fetal life to independent life. Major changes in the heart and the circulatory system must occur with clamping of the umbilical cord if the neonate is to survive. The lungs must expand with the first few breaths and receive a major supply of blood if the newborn's oxygen needs are to be met.

The newborn is especially prone to problems with temperature regulation because of the immaturity of the system regulating body temperature. The large body surface area, combined with an inability to sweat or shiver and total lack of control over environmental temperature, makes the newborn a high risk for hypothermia or low body temperature.

The newborn sleeps most of the time, waking to eat five to eight times in a 24-hour period. The newborn is basically reflexive in movement with little purposeful activity. Some newborns are able to coordinate the movement of fingers to mouth and suck their thumb hours after birth. They are able to see and prefer to focus on the human face.

Assessments of blood are made to determine the presence of any metabolic disorders, such as phenylketonuria so they can be corrected before permanent damage occurs. Protection of the eyes from possible gonorrheal infection is also done by the nurse shortly after birth.

The period of infancy spans the age from one month to one year. Rapid growth continues, especially during the first six months. Adequate nutrition is essential during this rapid growth for maximum development. Malnourished infants will be smaller, with a reduced number of brain cells which cannot be corrected later in life.

By infancy, the pulse has decreased slightly to 100 to 120 beats per minute. Temperature regulation gradually improves, but shivering and sweating remain ineffective.

The purposeful movements of the infant gradually replace the reflexive movements of the newborn, and most early reflexes disappear. Fine hand coordination begins to develop, and objects can be picked up, held, and released at will by the end of this period.

The infant is constantly exploring everything in the

environment, and accident prevention is a primary health concern. Falls are especially common.

The attention and responsiveness of a few constant care-givers is needed by the infant for normal development. Responding to the infant's needs, when expressed, leads to security and a trusting relationship with parents.

Terms for Review

cephalocaudal	fetus	meconium	proximodistal
development	growth	nonshivering thermogenesis	sudden infant death syndrome
embryo	kernicterus	obligate nose-breather	

Learning Activities

1. Talk with friends and family who have recently been pregnant or are now pregnant. What information or warnings were they given to help ensure satisfaction of fetal physiological needs? What kinds of advertisements or public statements have you seen designed to protect the fetus?

2. Attend a prenatal or parenting class in the community for information on normal growth and development. What kind of help do the parents receive for meeting the needs of the newborn and growing infant? What kinds of concerns are parents expressing related to pregnancy, labor and delivery, and infant care?

3. Attend a day care center or watch infants with their parents. To what types of stimuli are infants of various ages responding? How does the infant make needs known? How do the care-givers know which of the infants needs are unmet? What behavior of the infant gives a clue?

Review Questions

1. The development of normal internal and external reproductive structures in the male fetus is dependent on which of the following hormones?
   a. Estrogen
   b. Testosterone
   c. Progesterone
   d. Growth hormone

2. Which of the following fetal activities is abnormal and a sign of possible problems?
   a. Fetal respiratory movements
   b. Swallowing amniotic fluid
   c. Voiding into the amniotic fluid
   d. Passing meconium into the amniotic fluid

3. Which of the following activities should the nurse caution a pregnant woman to avoid in order to protect the developing fetus?
   a. Dancing
   b. Soaking in a hot whirlpool bath
   c. Increasing her prepregnant caloric intake by approximately 300 calories
   d. Working full time

4. All of the following changes occurring at birth stimulate the newborn to breathe *except*
   a. Rising level of carbon dioxide in the newborn's blood
   b. Dropping level of oxygen in the newborn's blood
   c. Dropping blood pH
   d. Rising body temperature within the newborn

5. Neonates are at risk for problems with temperature maintenance. Which of the following factors is a reason for this problem?
   a. Immature thermal regulating center within the medulla
   b. Excessive subcutaneous fat
   c. Shivering in the neonate is not quite as effective as in the adult
   d. Neonates have a small body surface area in relation to their weight

6. True or False
   _____ a. At birth, a newborn's hemoglobin is higher than that of most adults.
   _____ b. Respirations in the newborn are often irregular.
   _____ c. The heart rate in the neonate is significantly slower than that of the fetus.

7. Which of the following descriptions most accurately describes the infant's activities for meeting oxygen needs?
   a. Uses chest muscles and diaphragm to breathe at a rate of 60 to 80 breaths each minute.
   b. Maintains a patent foramen ovale and ductus arteriosus in the circulatory system
   c. Maintains a heart rate of 100 to 120 beats per minute and a respiratory rate of 20 to 40 breaths per minute.
   d. Breathes mostly through the mouth at a rate of 40 to 60 breaths per minute.

8. Which of the following data indicate adequate hydration and elimination in the infant?
   a. Intake of 20 oz per day at 12 months; output of 400 ml of urine in 24 hours.
   b. Intake of 80 oz per day at 12 months; output of 200 ml of urine in 24 hours.
   c. Hard, pellet-type stools every third day.
   d. Three soft stools each day, six to eight wet diapers each day, nursing well at breast, ten minutes each side.
9. An infant who is fed, kept clean and warm, but rarely talked to, held, and responded to is likely to show which of the following behavior patterns?
   a. Aggressive behavior, throwing temper tantrums, crying
   b. Withdrawn behavior, unresponsive, quiet, and inactive
   c. Accelerated physical and mental growth; talking to self
   d. Vigorous crying and activity when separated from parents due to hospitalization

Answers

1. b
2. d
3. b
4. d
5. a
6. a. T
   b. T
   c. F
7. c
8. d
9. b

CHAPTER 12

GROWTH AND DEVELOPMENT: CHILDHOOD AND ADOLESCENCE

Objectives

1. Identify trends in pulse rate, respiratory rate, and blood pressure as a child ages from one year to 18 or 20 years.
2. Describe trends in nutritional and fluid needs for the child from one year through adolescence.
3. Identify developmental tasks at the different stages of development during childhood and adolescence.
4. Describe major health concerns for children at various stages of development and possible nurs-

ing interventions to reduce the risks of these problems occurring.
5. Trace the role of the family and peer group in helping the individual meet love/belonging and self-esteem needs from the toddler to the adolescent.
6. Describe how hospitalization might interfere with need satisfaction in the various age groupings of childhood.

Early Childhood—One to Six Years of Age

The years from one to six cover a time of remarkable cognitive, physical, and social growth in children. The toddler, aged one to three years, and the preschooler, aged three to six years, are common age divisions within the early childhood category. The toddler experiences the most rapid changes, with a slowing toward the end of the preschool years. Genetically determined traits become more apparent toward the end of the preschool years, and more individual differences develop among children from three to six years.

Physiological Needs

Oxygen Needs. By two years of age, the heart has doubled its weight. The child at this age has approximately 40 ml of blood for each pound of weight. A 20-lb child, two years old, would have a blood volume of 800 ml, compared to the newborn who may have a normal blood volume of 200 to 300 ml. There is a steady growth in the capillary beds throughout the body during early childhood, and the vessel walls of arteries and veins be-

Table 12–1. **Blood Values and Vital Signs in the Early Childhood Years**

Common Blood Values

	HEMOGLOBIN (GM)	HEMATOCRIT (PERCENT)	WBCs (PER CU MM)
Toddler (1–3 yr)	11.8–13	36–38	9,000–10,500
Preschooler (3–6 yr)	12.5–15	38–40	8,500–9,000

Vital Signs

	PULSE (PER MIN)	RESPIRATIONS (PER MIN)	BP (MM HG)
2 yr	90–130	20–30	98/64
3 yr	90–120	20–30	100/60
4 yr	90–110	20–28	100/60
5 yr	80–110	19–25	100/60
6 yr	75–105	18–24	100/60

come thicker and more sturdy, compared to those of the infant. Some arrhythmias (irregularities in the heartbeat rhythm) may still be present in toddlers. Heart murmurs may continue to be present during early childhood as the child experiences rapid growth of the chest, lungs, and muscles used in breathing. The tracheobronchial tree, which conducts outer air into and out of the exchange areas deep within the lung, grows rapidly in the toddler and then grows more slowly until adolescence. The lung has tripled its weight by two years of age, and breathing changes from mainly abdominal to diaphragmatic with chest muscle involvement. The pulse and respiratory rate remain rapid by adult standards, with toddlers having pulses from 90 to 120 beats per minute and preschoolers having slightly slower ranges from 80 to 100 beats per minute. Respirations in early childhood are in the 20 to 30 range at rest. Blood pressure in the toddler averages 100/60–70, and in the preschooler 90/60 mm Hg. Table 12–1 shows common blood values and vital signs for this age group.

Temperature Maintenance. With maturation and growth of the capillary beds, the child in this age group becomes better able to respond to temperature extremes. The body becomes equipped to conserve or release heat into the environment by regulating the amount of blood flowing through the capillary beds near the surface of the body. The hypothalamus within the brain also matures, and since it is the primary regulator of heat production and heat loss, temperature maintenance becomes more stable. During early childhood, the body's ability to sweat and thus lose heat through evaporation is still limited, so very little body heat is lost through this mechanism until later childhood

and adolescence. High fevers continue to be associated with infections in this age group, and fevers of 104°F are not uncommon and often develop very rapidly.

Elimination. During the toddler years, peristalsis in the bowel (muscle activity which moves food through the intestines) begins to slow. This allows more water to be absorbed from the stool, resulting in darker, more formed bowel movements. The toddler and preschooler also have a more varied diet with more roughage. This results in bowel patterns more like those in the adult with one stool a day at a more consistent time each day. Control of the bowels is usually achieved by the toddler who is around two to three years old.

The kidneys are mature and producing approximately 500 to 600 ml of urine in the well-hydrated toddler and 600 to 750 ml of urine in the preschooler. The child's kidneys take longer to return to normal levels of functioning following severe physical stress when compared to those of adults. Kidney dialysis may be needed on a temporary basis in the critically ill child until the return of adequate function. Bladder function usually is controlled in the toddler for daytime wetting, but complete nighttime control may not be achieved until the preschool years. Involvement in play activities can easily distract the child from internal signals of voiding needs, and periodic reminders are useful in maintaining bladder control. Stress, which occurs with illness and hospitalization, may cause the child to regress to an earlier stage of development, and loss of bowel and bladder control is common in the hospitalized toddler. Inability to meet elimination needs in the normal way established at home can cause the toddler and preschooler much distress and may be responsible for incontinence. The nurse can help the child maintain control by duplicating patterns developed at home as much as possible. A familiar potty chair, a stool to reach the toilet, loose-fitting clothing, and offers for help may be needed by the child if wetting is to be avoided. A child who has just recently gained bowel and bladder control may be so inflexible about behavior that an unfamiliar potty chair may be refused.

Nutrition and Fluid Needs. The functioning of the gastrointestinal tract matures in toddlers, and they are capable of digesting most foods. Peristalsis in the intestinal tract slows, and this results in delayed emptying of the stomach. The stomach is also enlarging during this time, and the combination of the greater stomach capacity and delayed emptying makes it easier for the child to adjust to three meals a day. By two years of age, the stomach capacity is approximately 500 ml, and this increases gradually as the child matures. The teeth continue to erupt and, by the age of three, the 20 primary teeth have appeared. Calcification of the permanent teeth is also occuring during early childhood.

The toddler is learning to eat, using utensils common to the family and its cultural background. Drinking from a cup and giving up the bottle or breast are dealt with during the ages of one to three years. Until the age of 16 or 17 months, most toddlers lack sufficient wrist control to manage cups and glasses, and many spills should be expected. The child is often very insistent on self-feeding and may refuse to eat if fed by others. Many children in the years from one to three go through episodes of poor eating. They may want to eat only certain foods and refuse all others for a brief time. They may then switch to another favorite food. Over time, when offered a variety of nutritious foods, they seem to meet their nutritional needs. Ritualism with food and drink is common, and unless home patterns and activities related to eating are followed, the child in this age group may refuse to eat. Food may have to be cut in a certain way, served on a certain plate, or topped with a particular food product before the child will eat. Hospitalization may create many problems related to nutrition for this age child. If the nurse can plan with the parents how to adapt hospital food services to the individual child's routines, life will be easier for all involved. The toddler and preschooler are less susceptible to fluid and electrolyte imbalances compared to the infant. This is due to more maturity of the gastrointestinal system, decreased peristalsis, and a lesser percentage of total body weight composed of water. Table 12–2 shows average gains in weight and length and nutritional needs.

The toddler tends to gain 5 to 6 lb each year, and the preschooler averages 4 to 5 lb per year. The potbellied look of the toddler slims down during the preschool years.

Rest and Sleep Needs. The toddler usually sleeps 12 to 14 hours in every 24 hours. The preschool child sleeps 11 to 12 hours each day on the average. The toddler begins to have nightmares and may awaken very upset and unable to differentiate between dreams and reality. Children in this age group have bedtime routines which become very important and, when not followed, may interfere with ability to sleep. Quiet activities before bedtime also help children to gear down from activity so

Table 12–2. **Growth and Nutritional Needs of the Young Child (1–6 Years)**

	AVERAGE WEIGHTS (LB)	AVERAGE LENGTHS (INCHES)
2 yr	20	32–36
3 yr	30	36–40
4 yr	36	38–43
5 yr	40	41½–45½
6 yr	47	43½–48½

	CALORIES	WATER	PROTEIN
Age 1–3 yr	100 cal/kg (45 cal/lb) Total: 1,200–1,300 cal/24 hr	125 ml/kg (20 oz/lb) Total: 1,300–1,500 ml/24 hr	1.8 gm/kg (23 gm/24 hr)
Age 3–6 yr	90 cal/kg (41 cal/lb) Total: 1,400–1,600 cal/24 hr	100 ml/kg (1½ oz/lb) Total: 1,600–2,000 ml/24 hr	1.5 gm/kg (30 gm/24 hr)

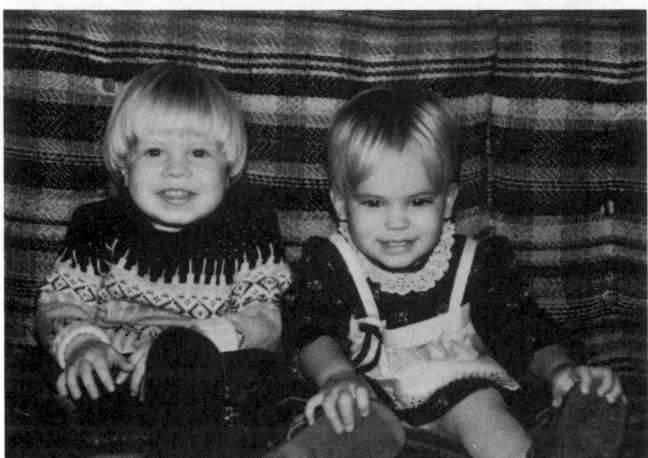

Figure 12–1. Toddlers of the same age learning differences in dress between males and females on some occasions.

and nipples; father does not. Men have a penis; women do not. Preschoolers know which sex they are and vigorously assert this when teased about being the opposite. There are normal manipulation of the genitals and exploration of the genitals of others in peer play. Masturbation is common. There is an attraction to the opposite-sexed parent, and the child may become jealous when that parent shows attention to others in the family. Play may involve imitation of the parents in playing "Mommy" and "Daddy." Diapering each other, mimicking parents diapering the baby, is another form of toddler play involving genital exploration. By about four years of age, the child recognizes that overt exploration and manipulation of the genitals are unacceptable in some cultures, and such activities among children may become more secretive and private.

they are more likely to fall asleep. Favorite security items such as stuffed animals or a blanket may be very important to give children when putting them to bed.

Sexual Needs and Sexuality. Children in this age group have an increased interest in the body and differences between men and women. They may want to watch others when they dress, toilet, and bathe. The toddler is aware of the differences between men and women in general physical traits. Fathers have whiskers; mothers and other women do not. Mother has breasts

Stimulation Needs. Development of the brain and nerve tissue is not complete until sometime during the fourth year of life. Fine motor coordination is not possible until this development is complete. As the toddler matures into a preschooler, the ability to coordinate muscles improves. Fine motor activities, such as cutting with scissors, drawing, and catching a ball, become possible. Tables 12–3 and 12–4 give examples of various motor and cognitive skills and the ages during which they commonly develop.

Most muscle growth and strength come from enlargement of muscle fibers already present during infancy. The toddler exhibits a swayed back with a convex

Table 12–3. **Behavioral Developments in the Toddler**

	APPROXIMATE AGES
Walks unassisted	12 mon
Says three words besides "Mama" or "Daddy"	12–13 mon
Imitates activities in the home	13–14 mon
Scribbles with crayon, pencil	13–14 mon
Uses spoon fairly well	14–15 mon
Builds tower of two blocks	14–15 mon
Walks backward	14–15 mon
Walks up steps; backs down steps	17 mon
Follows simple directions	19–21 mon
Throws a ball overhand	19–21 mon
Kicks a ball	20–21 mon
Jumps in place	22–23 mon
Begins to dress self	22–23 mon
Pedals tricycle	2 yr
Plays games involving other children	2–2½ yr
Balances on one foot	2½–3 yr
Builds tower of eight blocks	3 yr
Gives first and last name	3 yr
Walks down steps, alternating feet	3 yr

Source: Adapted from Denver Developmental Screening Test. Frankenburg, W., Dodds, J., Univ. of Colorado Medical Center, 1969.

Table 12–4. **Behavioral Developments in the Preschooler**

	APPROXIMATE AGES
Able to button clothing	3–3½ yr
Separates from mother easily	3–3½ yr
Recognizes colors	3–3½ yr
Describes objects, concepts such as tired, hungry	3–3½ yr
Hops on one foot	3½ yr
Dresses without supervision	3½–4 yr
Catches bounced ball	4 yr
Draws person with three parts	4–4½ yr
Balances on one foot	4½ yr
Copies shapes in drawing	4½–5½ yr
Draws person with six parts	6 yr

Source: Adapted from Denver Developmental Screening Test. Frankenburg, W., Dodds, J., Univ. of Colorado Medical Center, 1969.

lumbar curve (lordosis). This, along with the classic pot-belly, gives the toddler a definite posture unique to this age group. As the child grows into the preschool years, this lordosis decreases, and the muscles of the abdomen strengthen to pull in the stomach, giving the child a much leaner look.

Play becomes an important form of stimulation during early childhood. Play provides an avenue for social, emotional, and physical development, and friends become very important by the end of this age group. Children in the toddler age group often exhibit a parallel form of play where they play alongside each other in small groups, but each child plays independently of the others. In the preschool years, cooperative play develops where children play with each other in some form of imaginative play. A nurse may use play therapy to help children act out fears and aggression they are unable or unwilling to express verbally. Play therapy also gives the nurse an opportunity to better understand the child's perception of events and people in the new environment. Unfounded fears or unrealistic events can be corrected for the child as play progresses. Most hospitals offer a variety of props for play therapy in the toy room, such as doll nurses and doctors, stethoscopes, beds, and injured dolls with casts or bandages.

Stimulation of the senses remains critical for normal growth and development. The developing language abilities of the child are affected by the quality of the child's hearing. Poor vision may affect the child's motor development if he or she is unable to judge distance or objects are too blurred to recognize. The child's safety needs are also greatly affected if the senses of hearing and vision are inadequate. Children who cannot see or hear as others do will need additional supervision as they interact with an enlarging environment through the preschool years.

By four years of age, the child's auditory system is completely developed, and hearing has reached adult levels. By five years of age, the child's vision is reaching adult acuity levels, and most children will have 20/20 vision. There is a slight decrease in visual acuity during the early preschool years because of more rapid growth of several parts of the eye. By five years, this growth is usually complete, and the child will exhibit optimum vision. The senses of taste, smell, and touch continue to develop during early childhood. The tear ducts are mature by age four.

A common problem related to vision, called *strabismus*, occurs in early childhood. With this problem, the eye deviates to some degree toward the inner or outer corner of the eye. The eyes do not focus on a point of light equally, but rather the child tends to use one eye or the other but not both as in normal binocular vision. The treatment involves patching the nondeviated eye to stimulate usage of the other weaker eye so the vision center within the brain develops. The deviated eye often has decreased visual acuity which will deteriorate further over time if no treatment is initiated. The visual acuity problem may be unrelated to the structure of the eye itself, and therefore, be uncorrectable with glasses. The problem in this case is in the brain, and patching is the only method currently available to stimulate development of the visual area of the brain responsible for vision in the affected eye.

Higher Level Needs

Safety and Security Needs. The immune system continues to develop during early childhood, and by the age of five it is functioning at an adult level. The need for immunizations continues, with most children receiving their last injections just prior to entering school.

Accidents are the leading cause of death in this age group with automobile-related accidents at the top of the list, followed by drowning, and by burns in third place. Specially designed and federally approved car seats for children under 40 lb continue to be the best way of protecting the child and reducing injury and death. Poisonings have decreased over the years as a major cause of death in this age group. Part of this may be the "Mr. Yuk" campaign for warning stickers on all poisonous products. (See figure 12–2). Other factors involve childproof safety caps on medicines, better-educated parents on child safety, and poison control centers where information and appropriate treatment can be initiated very rapidly. Poison ingestion still remains a significant problem. Illness and injury (*morbidity*), as a result are more commonly seen today, with *mortality* (death) at much lower rates of about 6 percent of all poisonings.

Regular visits to the dentist should begin in the toddler between the ages of two to three years. Children who are allowed to fall asleep drinking a bottle often have many dental caries, and the practice should be discouraged for this reason. Regular brushing of the teeth is important in the toddler group to protect the primary teeth and teach the child healthy dental habits.

Children have an active imagination in this age group and may become very fearful. They may want to sleep with their parents because of a fear of the dark. Night-lights become important for psychological safety and physical safety as children often get up in the night

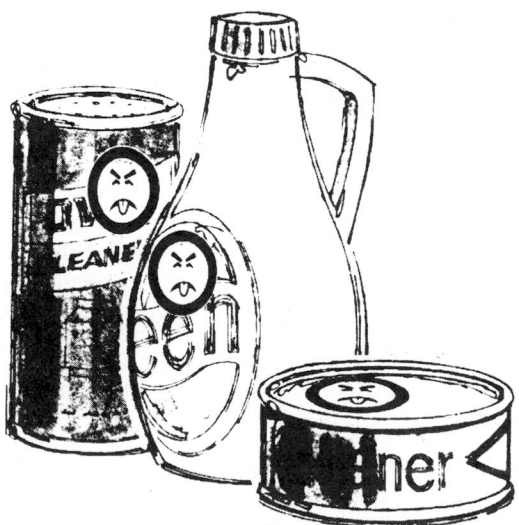

Figure 12–2. The "Mr. Yuk" emblem, designed to be placed on containers of substances that are harmful if ingested, which is part of a national poison prevention program.

to empty their bladder and should be able to see where they are going. Children in this age group are commonly fearful of the following problems:

1. Being physically hurt
2. Rapid changes in environmental factors, such as sudden noises, new places, and new people
3. Experiencing differences between what the child expects to happen and what actually happens
4. Actual or anticipated separation from parents and other security objects, such as a favorite stuffed toy or blanket.

Rituals are important in maintaining a sense of security in children this age. They give the child a sense of predictability and control in an often confusing environment. Children may create imaginary playmates to do things they are fearful of doing or saying. The imagined playmate may provide the child with a sense of security and usually disappears during the schoolage years when it is no longer needed.

Love and Belonging Needs.   Toddlers continue to need the love and attention of caring parents as they explore the environment. As children move through the years from one to six, they begin to venture further and further from the parent. Peer friendships become important during the preschool years. Sibling rivalry may also appear with the birth of another child. For the safety of the new infant, toddlers and preschoolers should not be left alone with their new sibling. They may try to hurt the baby, or they may overestimate their ability to handle the baby as they have seen adults do. Regressive behavior may develop as the child tries to compete with the new baby for parents' attention. Providing additional attention whenever possible during this adjustment time may minimize undesirable behavior in the child.

Self-Esteem Needs.   The child usually receives much attention for efforts to master new motor skills and language skills. As the child gains a sense of control over body and environment, a positive self-image begins to develop. Children in this age group have a drive to do things for themselves and then show their success to their parents or other interested adults. The child feels pride over accomplishments when adults in the environment respond with positive attention. Limits are important in children of this age, not only to ensure their physical safety but to help the child develop a sense of self-control. Temper tantrums occur as children pit their wills against the desires of others. The child's ability to communicate gives more control over other people and helps the child understand events. At two years of age,

Table 12–5. **Theories Related to Development in Early Childhood**

Piaget

Substage V (12–18 months)	The child seeks out new experiences, repeats a series of actions just seen. Develops new ways of reaching goals; begins to view objects and people as permanent when out of view.
Substage VI (18–24 months)	Beginning of true thought and problem solving. Imagination and memory develop. Imitates events from past. Begins to understand causality. Completes concept of object permanence.
Preoperational stage, 2–7 years	Able to create mental images to represent objects and events. Active, concrete thought rather than abstract. Thinks about only one aspect of a thing at a time. Unable to identify patterns or similarities among things. Confuses imagined events with reality. Cannot reverse sequence of events. Begins to be capable of concept of "God" at 4 years. Poor understanding of time, quantity.

Erikson

Autonomy versus shame and doubt (1–4 yr)	At this age the child struggles with demanding increased independence from parents and the fear of loss of self-control, which results in guilt and shame. Loss of self-control is associated with a decreased self-esteem and a feeling of unworthiness.
Initiative versus guilt (3–6 yr)	The child develops an ability to plan and engage in activities which are new and interesting. Creativity, sexual exploration, increased mobility, and language are used to initiate exploration of the environment. The developing sense of conscience and parental reactions to the child's initiative may result in guilt and fear leading to the child's overcontrolling behavior.

Freud

Anal stage (1–3 yr)	Primary pleasure through developing control of bowel and bladder function.
Phallic stage (3–7 yr)	Increased interest in genitals and body function; may want exclusive love of opposite-sexed parent.

Havinghurst/Hurlock—Developmental Tasks of Early Childhood

Developing skill in walking, eating, and controlling elimination by socially accepted methods.
Developing communication skills.
Recognizing differences between the sexes.
Developing sexual modesty appropriate to culture.
Recognizing which behavior is culturally right or wrong; conscience develops.
Developing emotional relationships with family and other people.
Understands social and physical concepts and uses them in thought and language.

the vocabulary averages around 300 words. By five years, this has increased to 2,000 to 2,500 words.

Illness and hospitalization may threaten the child's self-esteem by forcing the child to relinquish some of the mastered, self-care activities. The child may feel illness or hospitalization is a punishment for bad behavior. Children may also fear body mutilation, and this would be an additional threat to self-esteem. Encouraging children to do as much for themselves as possible and giving them praise are ways the nurse has of helping them maintain positive feelings about themselves. Explanations and honesty about procedures and treatments are also helpful to the child in a new environment, such as a clinic or hospital.

Table 12–5 presents theories related to development in early childhood.

Common Problems in Early Childhood and Nursing Implications

Infections are still a very common problem among toddlers and preschool children. Toddlers are most likely to develop middle ear infections (otitis media), and preschoolers are more likely to have respiratory infections. A narrowing of the trachea in response to a viral infection (croup) is common in the toddler. In very severe cases, the trachea may be blocked off (occluded), and an emergency situation would exist. Most cases are relieved by comforting and holding the child while in a steam-filled room. Cool, moist, outside air also helps to relieve the swelling in the trachea, and symptoms often improve on the ride to the hospital. Hospitalization and use of a croup tent providing cool, moist vapor may be needed for a brief time.

When working with young children, the following suggestions may be helpful:

1. Use simple language to communicate. Use short sentences and simple words. Do not give the child a choice unless the child can really choose. Asking if the child is ready to take the medicine now may be met with a definite "no." Telling the child, "It is now time to take your medicine. Would you like to take it with water or apple juice," sets a limit for the child, yet gives a real choice, so the child retains some sense of control.

2. Try to maintain consistency in the child's environment by following home routines and preferences as much as possible. Consistent nursing personnel for each child provides the child with more of a sense of security.

3. Be truthful with the child. Compare feelings to be experienced during procedures with those familiar to the child. Lying to the child destroys the child's ability to trust that person in the near future.

4. Use distraction and relaxation with children to reduce fear and pain.

5. Involve the parents in the child's care and encourage them to remain with the child as much as possible.

Middle Childhood—Six to Twelve Years of Age

The middle childhood years are when the child moves away from the family's constant support and enters school. For many children, this separation begins at a much earlier age with approximately 50 percent of preschoolers in the United States in day care or nursery school facilities for up to nine hours each day. Traditionally, the break with the family begins with mandatory school enrollment at age five or six. Most of the child's physical systems are mature, with continuing development in neuromuscular areas.

Physiological Needs

Oxygen Needs. By the end of middle childhood, the circulatory and respiratory systems are reaching adult levels of functioning. The vital capacity of the lungs, which is the amount of air that can be exhaled after a full breath, doubles from age six to age twelve. The heart rate is slightly slower with each passing year during middle childhood. Heart murmurs may still be present even through the heart is functioning normally and has no damaged areas or defects. The blood pressure slowly rises during middle childhood, and respirations remain fairly constant in the range of 19 to 21 breaths per minute. Table 12–6 shows normal ranges in the vital signs and blood values for children from six to twelve years.

Temperature Maintenance. Temperature maintenance has become well established by the middle years of childhood. The ability to perspire and thus lose heat is more mature but far from adult levels. Very high fevers in response to infection are less likely to occur in the older child with maturity of the immune system and improved thermal regulation. This age child will express thermal discomfort and put on or take off clothes independently. These children are more likely to stay under the blankets during the night than younger ones.

Elimination. The kidneys continue to grow with the rest of the child's body and are better able to concentrate urine. The amount of blood purified by the kidney's each minute (glomerular filtration rate) decreases during middle childhood because of more efficient kidney function. The six- to eight-year-old child produces about 650 to 1,000 ml of urine in 24 hours, when well hydrated. The ten- to twelve-year-old produces slightly more urine, in the range of 700 to 1,500 ml per 24 hours.

Nutrition and Fluid Needs. Children's bodies in the middle years continue to grow. Table 12–7 shows a range in heights and weights for six- to twelve-year-olds. The range goes from the third percentile to the 97 percentile, so only extremely small or large children were excluded. The schoolage child appears thinner than the preschool child. Boys are slightly heavier and taller than

Table 12–6. **Vital Signs and Blood Values in Middle Childhood**

Vital Signs

AGE (YR)	PULSE RATE (PER MIN)	BLOOD PRESSURE (MM HG)	RESPIRATIONS (PER MIN)
6	75–105 (ave. = 90)	100/60	18–24
8	75–95 (ave. = 85)	102/60	17–23
10	70–90 (ave. = 80)	106/60	16–22

Blood Values

AGE (YR)	HEMOGLOBIN (GM)	HEMATOCRIT (PERCENT)	WBCs (CU MM)
6	13–15.5	40	8,500
8	13–15.5	40	8,000
10	13–15.5	42	8,000

girls until sexual maturity begins with the accompanying accelerated rate of growth. Since girls mature before boys, they tend to be taller, starting at about age ten. The average weight gain each year in the child from six to twelve years is 6.5 lb and growth is approximately 2.5 inches each year. Adequate nutrition will allow the child to reach maximum growth, while inadequate or inappropriate nutrition may slow the child's growth rate and decrease adult height. Obesity may develop during middle childhood as during any other age. Humphrey (1979) found that 27 percent of schoolage children were overweight. Eating patterns established during this time of growth and development will affect future health. Being overweight may affect the child's self-esteem, motor development, and social development. The child requires 35 to 36 calories for each pound of body weight to grow optimally. This amounts to 2,000 to 2,400 calories each day for most children. Protein needs are approximately 36 gm in a 24-hour period, which is an increase over early childhood needs of 23 to 30 gm. Fluid needs for the six-year-old are 1½ oz of water per 24 hours for each pound of body weight, and for the older

child this drops to 1 oz. Total fluid intake is in the range of 2,000 to 2,500 ml in 24 hours. When the child begins more rapid growth between age ten and twelve years, total caloric needs are increased to 2,200 to 2,700 in 24 hours.

The permanent teeth begin to erupt around the age of seven years. By twelve years, the permanent teeth are all in place except for the third molars (wisdom teeth), which erupt in late adolescence or early adulthood. Prior to eruption, the teeth become calcified in the gums, and inadequate nutrition can interfere with this process.

Children in this age group are often in a hurry to eat and get back to playing with friends. They are free to select what they will eat during lunch at school, with no parental encouragement to eat certain foods. Frequent requests for in-between feedings are common, and fruits and vegetables offered at this time, along with juices and milk, will help balance the child's diet. In the hospital, in-between snacks are very important, especially when normal appetite may be decreased or procedures may require food restrictions.

Table 12–7. **Normal Growth Patterns in Middle Childhood**

AGE (YR)	HEIGHT (IN.)	WEIGHT (LB)
6	42–51	34–67 (ave. = 47–48)
7	43–54	37–86 (ave. = 52–53)
8	45–57	42–89 (ave. = 57–61)
9	47–59	46–104 (ave. = 63–66)
10	49–62	51–131 (ave. = 70–78)
11	51–66	57–134 (ave. = 81–87)
12	54–68	64–144 (ave. = 91–95)

Rest and Sleep Needs   The child will usually sleep nine to eleven hours during these years. The naps of the toddler and preschool child have been eliminated. Getting the schoolage child to bed at an appropriate time, as identified by the parents, can be a challenge. Interest in favorite television programs, playing with friends, projects, and reading usually take priority for the child. Nighttime bed-wetting may still continue for some children and is often related to very deep sleep. Often this deep sleeping is a genetic trait from a parent who was also a nighttime bed-wetter at this age.

Sexual Needs and Sexuality.   The schoolage child is interested in the anatomy and functioning of the male and female body. Children become interested in conception and birth, and slightly later their focus moves to changes that are occurring, or anticipated, within their own bodies and those of the opposite sex. Conception and pregnancy in schoolage children are rare, but they do occasionally occur in a child who has matured at an earlier age than the majority. Fertility control, sex education, and sexual exploration are areas to which most schoolage children are exposed. Masturbation is not usually associated with sexual drives in the childhood years but with pleasurable sensations. Children are taking on the sex-related roles in their culture, and children usually prefer same-sex playmates. The child develops a sense of modesty and may get angry or embarrassed when anyone interrupts privacy during bathing, dressing, or toileting. The hospitalized child may be very upset about the lack of privacy and the need for assistance with intimate activities such as bathing and using the bathroom, urinal, or bedpan. Providing privacy while ensuring the child's safety is important in providing nursing care to schoolage children.

Stimulation Needs.   The child's environment enlarges with entry into school. New places, people, and information provide the child with a wide range of stimulation. Manual dexterity, muscle strength, and endurance for physical activity increase in schoolage children as they play and learn with enthusiasm. Play with other children continues to be a needed activity for adequate muscular and social development. Boys develop an increased muscle mass compared to girls and tend to be better performers at big muscle activities such as running, jumping, and throwing a ball. Fine muscle coordination develops around age seven to eight years to allow the child to write cursively instead of printing. The senses of taste and smell develop increased discrimination, and food preferences may continue to change. The child's visual acuity and hearing are at adult levels. Myopia (inability to see clearly into the distance), often called nearsightedness, may develop during the school-

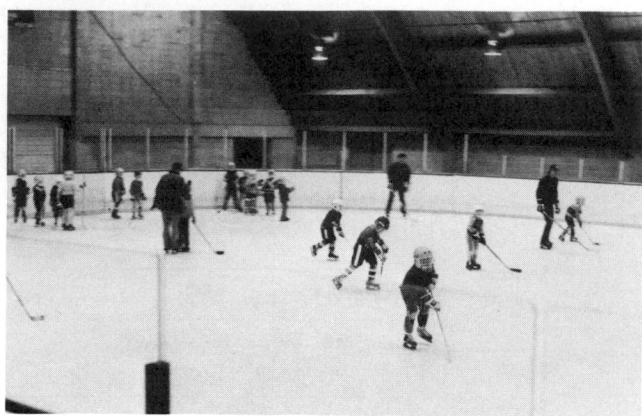

Figure 12–3.   Schoolage children (six to seven years) developing the motor coordination and strength for the team sport of hockey.

age years, and it tends to worsen with age. Frequent vision checks (yearly) are done to identify children whose vision is less than optimal.

Higher Level Needs

Safety and Security Needs.   Accidents continue to be the leading cause of death in children from six to twelve years of age. Estimates are that 40,000 to 50,000 children are permanently injured from accidents each year in the United States. Automobile accidents, drownings, and firearms accidents are leading causes. Teaching the child about water safety and how to swim is helpful in reducing water-related accidents. Anticipating emergencies and planning actions ahead of time are family practices that can reduce mortality and morbidity for the entire family. Smoke alarms and practice fire drills should be encouraged. Emergency phone numbers should be on or near the phone so the child can call for help if the need arises.

Dental care and health care are usually viewed as family responsibilities. The school nurse may be the first to identify possible problems during routine health screening of schoolage children. Teachers also may refer possible health problems to the school nurse for further assessment. Conferences between the parents and the school nurse may be appropriate when health problems are identified in school. Dental examinations are recommended every six months. Children often lack the muscle coordination to floss their teeth until approximately age ten, so parents will need to assist the child with dental hygiene, as will the nurse when the child is hospitalized.

Love and Belonging Needs.   During the middle childhood years, parents lose their omnipotence in their child's eyes. The child starts to enjoy relationships with

Table 12–8. **Theories Related to Growth and Development During Middle Childhood**

Piaget

Ages 5–7 years
Operational stage of development. The child begins to use abstract symbols in thinking. Ability to understand another's differing viewpoint develops. The child is less self-centered (egocentric) and thinks and acts more independently from parents. The child is able to consider various aspects of a situation, making thinking more realistic and logical.
Ages 7–11 years
Concrete operations. This stage is characterized by more logical thinking. The child understands how to categorize things by noting similarities and differences. Children understand that specific things may belong to broader groups, such as trout and fish. The child is now capable of reversing a sequence of events in the mind and knows what is real and what is imagined.

Freud

Ages 6–12 years
Latency period. The focus during this time is seen as acquiring skills, knowledge, and attitudes appropriate for sex roles in the child's culture. Sexual interest was viewed as dormant or minimal.

Erikson

Age 6–12 years
Industry versus inferiority. This developmental task involves the child's developing a sense of competence in projects undertaken. Children are seen as involved in goal-related activities such as building, writing, drawing, and playing. If the children feel good about the work they are doing because of favorable reaction from others, a positive self-image develops. If children feel incompetent or inadequate in the activities of middle childhood, they may develop a sense of inferiority and be afraid to try new skills or be involved in new situations. The fear of failing may be related to unrealistic expectations for children, by parents, or by the children themselves.

Havinghurst/Hurlock—Developmental Tasks of Middle Childhood

Learning physical skills necessary for games common to the child's culture.
Developing positive feelings about oneself as a growing and maturing person.
Learning to play and work cooperatively with peers.
Learning sex roles appropriate to child's culture (masculine/feminine).
Developing fundamental skills in reading, writing, and calculating (cultural).
Developing conscience, morality, and a set of personal values.
Developing an understanding and attitudes about concepts, such as democracy, freedom, occupation, and religion.
Development of personal independence from parents.
Developing attitudes fostered by the culture and governmental groups in the society in which the child lives.

other adults such as teachers and coaches. Children strive to receive approval, not only from their parents, but also from the other adults important in their expanded lives. The family still is the primary force influencing the child, but parents may feel children do not love and need them the way they did in earlier years. Sibling rivalry is less acute since the schoolage child has many outside interests. Peer groups are important to the child and give a sense of belonging to something apart from the family. The peer group helps the child deal with the new situations encountered in and out of school. These groups are often comprised of children of similar ages, backgrounds, and sex. Around the age of ten years, the child will often develop a very close relationship with another child of the same sex. This "best friend" stage is viewed as a child's first love relationship outside the family and is seen as important for future heterosexual relationships.

Self-Esteem Needs. During the middle childhood years, the self-concept continues to mature. Children recognize differences between themselves and other children. The child feels competent if others recognize and praise efforts to make or build things. Competition and winning are important to this age group as proof of physical or mental abilities. A sense of control over the environment and others comes with logical thought and understanding of reasons behind other's behavior. Acceptance by peers is especially important during middle childhood and further reinforces the child's positive self-concept. Rejection by peers and unrealistic expectations by parents, or the child, can lead to unmet self-esteem needs where the child feels inferior and incapable. Table 12–8 presents several theories on development during middle childhood and the associated developmental tasks.

Common Problems In Middle Childhood and Nursing Implications

1. The schoolage child is more mobile and daring than younger children. Most children are riding bicycles in the street, often more concerned with their ability to do tricks than with safety. Fractures and lacerations are the most common result of accidents in the child. The child usually heals rapidly compared to the adult. Children in casts will need help in many of their normal activities, but the nurse should encourage as much independent activity as possible to preserve the child's self-esteem.

2. Muscle aches are a problem for some children when bone growth is more rapid than muscle and ligament growth. The increased stretch put on these structures may cause aches and pains.

3. Respiratory infections are the most common problem in the schoolage child who experiences three to four colds each year on the average. Ear infections still occur but are much less common than in preschoolers. Sore throats and streptococcal infections (strep throat) occur among schoolage children, and throat cultures are frequently done to determine if antibiotic drug therapy is needed. Urinary tract infections occur in 5 percent of the girls in this age group but rarely in boys.

4. Chronic problems such as allergies, asthma, scoliosis (abnormal curving of the spine), and juvenile-onset diabetes may develop during middle childhood.

When working with schoolage children, the following may be helpful:

1. The schoolage child is less fearful of medical treatment and personnel compared to the younger child. Schoolage children have a better ability to understand their health problems and treatments, without feeling they are being punished. Explanations and answers to questions at the child's level of understanding are important in nursing care of children. Talking below children's level may insult their self-esteem. Talking above their level may confuse them. Asking children what they understand about health problems is one way of discovering their level of understanding.

2. As with younger children, consistent nursing personnel are helpful in reducing anxiety in this age group.

3. Children in this age group enjoy and need peer relationships, and providing an opportunity for interaction with other patients of the same age, or with the same problem, can be helpful to the child. Encouraging conversations and visits by friends is another way of easing the stress of hospitalization for the schoolage child.

4. The hospitalized child may need help keeping up with classmates in school and provisions for tutoring may be necessary.

Adolescence—Twelve to Twenty Years of Age

Adolescence is the time of life between childhood and adulthood. It begins with puberty and ends with psychological, physiological, and sexual maturity. *Puberty* or pubescence is the beginning stage of adolescence, as rapid growth and development of the reproductive structures and secondary sexual characteristics begin. Girls tend to enter puberty at about age 10 to 11 years and boys slightly later, around age 11 to 12 years. Adolescence can be divided into three stages of development:

1. *Early adolescence—ages 12 to 13 years.* During this time, the growth in height is most remarkable. Girls begin to develop breast tissue, and their internal reproductive organs begin to mature. *Menarche* (onset of menstruation), begins in girls at the age of 12 years, on the average, with a range from 10 to 15 years. Pubic hair appears in both sexes during these years. Menstrual periods are often irregular, and no egg is released from the ovary during the monthly cycle (anovulatory). Boys begin to have growth of the testes around age 11 years. Growth of the penis begins slightly later between 12 and 13 years. This is a very unstable emotional time, partly due to fluctuating hormone levels and partly due to a changing body image and less self-control. The rapid growth in height may leave the teenager uncoordinated and unsure of physical abilities. Conformity to peer-

group standards becomes more important. The individual begins to develop a personal value system and often has problems relating to parents as separation from the family begins. Close, same-sexed friends are characteristic.

2. *Middle adolescence—ages 14 to 16 years.* Physical growth continues, especially in boys. Boys begin to develop facial hair, and shortly later their voices change. Growth of the penis continues and will double in length by age 17 years. Girls continue to have breast development and growth of pubic hair. The female hips begin to widen as pelvic bone structure changes to facilitate childbearing. Increased vaginal secretions may also be experienced in response to the hormone estrogen released from the ovary. The ovary begins to ovulate (release an egg) more consistently in most girls. Adolescents develop relationships with the opposite sex, but peer groups still remain very important. Dating is often in groups for specific activities. Problems relating to parents may continue as the teenager develops personal values which may be different from those of the family. Experimentation with personal appearance may be supported by the peer group and discouraged by the family. Parents may have difficulty relating to their child's developing sexuality.

3. *Late adolescence—ages 17 to 20 years.* This time is a more calm, stable stage for most adolescents. Body growth has slowed or stopped, and secondary sexual characteristics are well established; there are no major physical changes left to anticipate. Teens continue to adapt to the new body image and feel more self-control over their body and emotions. They become more secure in relationships with both sexes. Relationships with parents often improve, as teens become better able to understand their parent's views. Most teens, during this stage, are involved with planning their future and eventual economic independence from their family.

Physiological Needs

Oxygen needs. The heart continues to enlarge until about age 17 to 18 years. The adult lung weight is also reached at this age. The vital capacity of the lungs con-tinues to increase during adolescence but is greater in males, even when body size is adjusted to that of the female. The pulse continues to slow during adolescence until adult rates are reached. Teens may have slower pulse rates than the average adult rates, with those of males tending to be slightly slower than those of females. Respiratory rates also decrease during adolescence. Blood pressure increases gradually during this time. Girls tend to show an earlier rise in blood pressure in comparison to boys. A blood pressure above 130/90 mm Hg during adolescence should receive further evaluation and may be related to some underlying disease process. Table 12–9 gives the vital signs in adolescence. Table 12–10 shows normal blood values for this age group. Females experience blood loss through menstruation, which is why their hemoglobin tends to be lower than that of males. Testosterone, which is predominant in males, also stimulates red blood cell production.

Elimination. Kidney function and gastrointestinal functioning are mature. The kidney produces approximately 700 to 1,500 ml of urine on the average in a 24-hour period. Fluid is also lost through increased perspiration related to emotional stress. Unusual eating patterns, because of involvement in activities, skipping meals, and eating "fast food" may affect bowel movement patterns.

Nutrition. The accelerated growth rate occurs during adolescence. Adequate nutrition will allow the adolescent to reach maximum height potential without undue fatigue and other nutrition-related problems. Calcium is essential in the diet for optimum bone growth. Protein needs are between 50 and 60 gm in 24 hours, which is a considerable increase from middle childhood needs of 36 gm. Protein needs are higher in males because of the greater growth of muscle tissue, compared to females. Total caloric needs in males range from 2,400 to 3,200 calories, and in females the range is 2,300 to 2,400 calories in 24 hours. A teen's activity level and rate of growth will affect the individual's nutritional needs. Fluid needs decrease to ¾ oz for each pound of body weight, which is the same as in the adult. The volume of fluid taken in to meet this need ranges from 2,200 to

Table 12–9. **Vital Signs in the Adolescent**

AGE (YR)	PULSE (PER MIN) (MALES)	(FEMALES)	RESPIRATIONS (PER MIN) (MALES)	(FEMALES)	BLOOD PRESSURE (MM HG)
12	69	71	19	19	110/64
14	65	68	19	19	112/66
16	63	66	17	18	114/70
18	61	65	16	17	120/70

Table 12-10. **Normal Blood Values in Adolescence**

AGE (YR)	HEMOGLOBIN (GM)		HEMATOCRIT (PERCENT)		WBC (CU MM)	
	(MALES)	(FEMALES)	(MALES)	(FEMALES)	(MALES)	(FEMALES)
12	13	13	38	38	8,000	8,000
14	14	13	41	39	8,000	7,800
16	15.5	13.5	45	40	7,800	7,800
18	16	13.5	47	40	7,800	7,800

2,700 ml for most teens. The basal metabolic rate decreases in adolescence, with the greater decrease in BMR occurring in females. This will add to the tendency to gain weight when growth stops if eating patterns remain the same as in early adolescence. Most teens do not begin to fill out and gain weight until after most growth is completed. Table 12–11 shows average weights and heights and caloric needs for adolescents.

The adolescent has more control over eating than at any other stage of growth and development in the past. Most teens have some money and will buy foods that they enjoy and that others in their peer group enjoy. Activities and social plans begin to interfere with family mealtimes, and the adolescent may skip some meals completely, especially if the teen views gained weight as a problem. Snacking between meals often supplies as much as one-third of the daily calories for teenagers. Teenagers with braces on their teeth may experience periodic discomfort when eating after orthodontic visits and may eat only soft foods or drink only fluids. The third molars usually erupt sometime during late adolescence.

Rest and Sleep. Adolescents need slightly less sleep than the schoolage child. Most teens require eight to ten hours of sleep to avoid feeling tired or fatigued. Boys begin to experience sleep orgasms, known as wet dreams (*nocturnal emissions*) during adolescence, often before they become sexually active with girls. Nocturnal emissions of semen may occur several times each month. Confusion with bed-wetting by an uninformed boy, or

by his parents, can cause embarrassment and fears of being abnormal. These feelings can be reduced by providing information to teens on this normal body response to sexual development.

Sexual Needs and Sexuality. Changes related to developing reproductive functioning are the driving force behind almost all physical changes occurring during adolescence. Testosterone is the primary male hormone, and estrogen is the primary female hormone associated with developing sexual function and secondary sexual characteristics. Progesterone is the female hormone associated with the cyclical maturing of the lining of the uterus for implantation of a fertilized ovum (egg). Premature or postmature development of body changes during adolescence can be a cause for concern in the affected teen. The teen uses the support of the peer group to adjust to body changes in structure and function. Modesty and embarrassment of being seen by others are common in early adolescence when the individual is still uncomfortable with personal physical development. Sexual identity becomes firmly established by the end of adolescence following much experimentation with appearance, relationships, and values. The time teenagers spend in front of the mirror may help them integrate their changing body image with their self-concept. Intimacy with the opposite sex may begin through verbal or written exchanges, which the uncertain adolescent views as safer compared to face-to-face communication. The telephone is well used by most adolescents, and the majority of the teen's communication is with peers of both

Table 12-11. **Heights, Weights, and Caloric Needs in Adolescence**

AGE (YR)	WEIGHT (LB)		HEIGHT (INCHES)		CALORIC NEEDS (CAL/LB)	
	(MALES)	(FEMALES)	(MALES)	(FEMALES)	(MALES)	(FEMALES)
12	85	88	59	60	30	30
14	108	110	64	63	31	24
16	130	117	68	63.5	31	21
18	140	120	68.5	64	25	19

sexes rather than with family members. Teenagers in the hospital may feel less isolated if telephone communications are maintained with members of their peer group.

Masturbation is related to sexual urges during the period of adolescence. Approximately one-half of teenagers are sexually active (Tyler and Josimovich, 1977), and there is experimentation with both heterosexual and homosexual relationships by some individuals. Peers may put pressure on individual members to be sexually active before he or she feels ready. Initial experience with intimate sexual relations may not meet expectations. Approximately 20 percent of males are unsuccessful at their first attempt with intercourse because of inadequate erections or premature ejaculations (Siemons and Brandzel, 1982). One-fourth of women, in one study, remembered their first intercourse as a positive, happy experience (Siemons and Brandzel, 1982). The rest of the women had more negative memories of initial attempts at intercourse. Adolescents may be uneasy discussing sexual concerns with their parents and may turn to their peer group for information. Health promotion among teens is aimed at providing them with accurate information about sexual changes and function. Providing adolescents with choices for safeguarding sexual contact in regard to sexually transmitted diseases and fertility control is important in health education.

Stimulation Needs. Adolescents need physical, mental, and social forms of stimulation to promote optimum development. Physical activity is important to improve muscle strength and coordination and to regain a sense of body control. An individual who begins a sedentary life in adolescence is more likely to be a sedentary adult with the added risks to health that this life-style creates. Team and individual sports, social activities, and continued learning in school provide the teen with opportunities to learn new skills and test out personal limits. The teen begins to recognize personal strengths and weaknesses by participation in a wide variety of activities. Future life choices about occupation and lifestyle will be affected by the variety of experiences during adolescence.

Higher Level Needs

Safety and Security Needs. Teenagers often seem to be full of daring to the adult and to take unnecessary risks with themselves and others. Teens are striving to be recognized as separate and mature individuals and to demonstrate those characteristics they associate with their adult role models. They may be more willing to take risks because of a sense of being infallible. They may lack personal experience with the negative or dangerous

consequences of their actions. Their coordination may be temporarily impaired, as rapid bone growth exceeds muscle and ligament growth. The teen also begins driving motor vehicles, and these increase the risk to physical safety. Safety devices such as helmets, flotation devices, and automobile seat belts should be encouraged to reduce the injuries from related accidents. The nurse's role in educating the teen may include work with parents. Providing the family with an opportunity to discuss fertility control issues with a health professional in their home or at a clinic may be needed to protect the teen from unwanted pregnancy.

Dental care and health care continue to be needs for the adolescent to safeguard physical health. Teaching teens about the need for self-breast examination may be frightening and embarrassing for the teenage girl. Pro-

---

I'm writing this letter in memory of my very special daughter Tracy who was killed last March 27th in an automobile accident.

She was much loved by us all. Her mother, sister, brothers, grandparents, friends and her cat.

Her zest and excitement energized everyone. She loved dramatics, music, her guitar, warm weather, the ocean, family vacations, pasta, late nights and sleeping in.

If she'd worn her seat belt she'd be here with us now. We miss her and love her so. Just like your family and friends love you.

So on this first anniversary of her death I wanted to take this opportunity to remind you to please wear seat belts when you drive or ride in any car, with anyone. No matter how good the driver.

I don't want to have happen to you what happened to Tracy. She wouldn't either. Because people who love you will miss you more than words like these can ever say.

With love,

Her Dad

Figure 12–4. "A Love Letter to the Children of Minnesota." This letter appeared in a Minneapolis newspaper emphasizing the importance of seat belts for all children, including teenagers. (Reprinted with permission from the *Minneapolis Star and Tribune*.) March 26, 1982

viding information about what will be done and support during the procedure are nursing responsibilities. Teens may feel uncomfortable with the opposite-sexed nurse or physician, and offering the patient a choice, whenever possible, may relieve some fear of embarrassment. Immunizations are also completed during the teen years with the booster injection of tetanus and diphtheria toxoids. Education about the need for repeated immunizations every ten years or following penetrating wounds will help protect the teen's future health.

Love and Belonging Needs. A feeling of belonging and being accepted is very important during the teenage years. The family continues to provide love and support for the teen, but the process of separating from the family and examining its values often causes disharmony. The teen may feel the parents don't understand, and turn away from them as a primary support. The peer group gives the teen the support needed to separate

from the family. Close relationships with both sexes begin to replace part of the role previously filled only by the family. The family continues to provide stability to the adolescent's life and is critically needed during these years when the teen is facing so many changes. Teens who cannot form close, loving relationships with other individuals may have a difficult time breaking away from their family since the need for love and belonging will be unmet.

Self-Esteem Needs. The adolescent is faced with major changes in body structure and function. The range of behavior acceptable for this age group is very different than activities acceptable in middle childhood. New skills are learned to move the teen into the adult world with assumption of added privileges and responsibilities. All these new skills and changes begin to be incorporated into a new self-image. Teens who are accepted and valued by their peers and family tend to develop

---

Table 12–12. **Theories Related to Development During Adolescence**

Piaget

Formal operations stage	Adolescents move into the stage of formal operations and use abstract thinking and are able to conceptualize. They are able to use inductive and deductive reasoning to think logically. They are able to understand and work with things and ideas without prior direct experience. They can think in hypothetical terms. Personal morality is based on individual's judgments and beliefs rather than being externally determined by laws, rules, or beliefs of others. Teens are able to consider intentions and consequences of various actions. They may question and reevaluate religious beliefs.

Erikson

Identity formation versus identity diffusion	The adolescent establishes personal identity as separate from family. In an optimum situation, the peer group, family, and other adults support and contribute to the individual's attempt to clarify identity. Confusion over roles and identity leads to feelings of inadequacy and self-consciousness. The individual is confused about adult roles and feels incapable of taking on role-related responsibility.

Havinghurst/Hurlock—Developmental Tasks of Adolescence

Achieving new, more mature relationships with peers of both sexes.
Achieving a masculine or feminine social role.
Accepting physical changes in the body.
Becoming emotionally independent from parents and other adults.
Assuring future economic independence from family, preparing for a career.
Preparing for marriage and family.
Developing personal values and a code of ethics.
Developing socially responsible behavior.
Developing skills needed for competent behavior in civic affairs.
Building conscious values in harmony with a realistic view of the current world situation.

positive self-images and feel good about themselves. They gain confidence in themselves and their ability to become adults.

Teens who are unable to form relationships or who are rejected by peers because they are different, or perceived as too different to fit in, may develop more unfavorable images of themselves and feel unsure of their ability. Teenagers with illnesses, physical defects, or handicaps may have a more difficult time in adolescence if they feel rejected by their peers or unable to participate in activities. Educating the peer group, so they understand the individual's problems and are less uncomfortable with the physical differences between them, may help to foster acceptance of the affected teen. Peer groups of adolescents with similar problems may also give the teen a chance to develop close relationships with others and feel accepted and valued. Providing opportunities for teens to meet each other in the hospital, especially during long-term illness, is important in promoting the teen's social development, and positive self-image.

Table 12–12 presents several theories on adolescent development and associated developmental tasks.

Common Problems in Adolescence and Nursing Implications

Teenagers are the only age group in the United States with an increasing death rate. The death rate among teens is up 9 percent from 1960 and totals approximately 50,000 annually.

1. Automobile accidents are the leading cause of mortality and morbidity among teens with almost four times as many males affected compared to females.

2. Suicide is the second leading cause of death among adolescents. Most of those attempting suicide tell someone about their plans a few hours to a few weeks before attempting to kill themselves. Health education for this age group should include some type of discussion with teens about suicide, alternatives, and what to do if they think one of their peers might be suicidal.

3. Drug abuse, including alcohol, affects over one million teenagers each year. Automobile accidents and drug abuse are often related. It is estimated that one out of four adolescents is a moderate to heavy user of alcohol (Rachal *et al.*, 1975), and approximately one million teens are dependent on alcohol. Danger signs that a teen may be abusing drugs include lost interest in school, lower grades, personality changes, trouble with peer relationships, deterioration in personal grooming habits, and decreased coordination. Pupils may appear dilated,

constricted, or normal, depending on what substance is being abused.

4. Sexually transmitted diseases include gonorrhea, syphilis, herpes type 2, moniliasis, trichomonal vaginitis, and chlamydia. In the past, these were referred to as venereal diseases, but the preferred term is now sexually transmitted diseases (STD). It is estimated that one out of eight teens acquires one of these infections each year, adding up to some 2.5 million cases each year. Education about these diseases, their treatment, and methods of prevention is an important aspect of health care during adolescence. Health information related to STD and treatment, along with information on fertility control, should be readily available to the teen in places that guarantee privacy and anonymity. Literature available inside bathroom stalls in the school reaches a wide audience and ensures privacy.

5. Fertility control and pregnancy become a problem for sexually active teenagers. An estimated one million births occur each year to teens between the ages of 15 and 19 years and some 30,000 to younger girls (Lincoln *et al.*, 1976). One-fifth of all births in the United States are to teenagers. Teenage girls are at high risk for developing physical complications related to pregnancy because of the immaturity of the reproductive system, poor diets, and emotional stress when support systems are lacking. Some teens view pregnancy as a positive indicator of their sexual maturity and a way of establishing independence from their family. Others may not even be able to accept the idea that they are pregnant, and energy is directed toward concealing the physical signs. Failing to seek prenatal medical care until very late in the pregnancy may also occur. Many unwanted pregnancies result in abortion, with one-third of all abortions in the United States being done on women in their teens. Girls under 15 years of age have an induced abortion (AB) rate of 45 percent, with older teens running an AB rate of 27 percent, (Lincoln *et al.*, 1976). During the early adolescent years or before, discussions and information on fertility control should be part of every teen's preparation for adulthood and optimum health. Family, church, schools, and health care providers are sources teens should be able to consult for this health need.

6. Sexual abuse affects some 100,000 children each year, and this is believed to be a conservative figure, since many cases go unrecognized and unreported. Sexual abuse is a reportable crime, and people who work with teens should be alert to possible cases. The average age for sexual abuse is nine to ten years but occurs at almost all ages. Sexual abusers of children can be parents, grandparents, adult friends of the family, older children, adolescents, and babysitters. Pregnancy occurs in approximately 12 to 24 percent of the victims who are

female, but both sexes can be victims. Father-daughter incest is the most common form and can leave the child with feelings of guilt, fear, and permanent problems relating to others in a mature sexual relationship.

7. Acne and pimples are problems to some extent for most adolescents. The problem seems to peak in later adolescence and then decreases, affecting males more severely than females. Pustular lesions often require antibiotic therapy and should be referred by the nurse to a physician for evaluation. The diet does not seem to be the causative agent but rather the fluctuating hormones and physical changes affecting the skin and secretory cells.

8. Menstrual irregularities are common among teenage girls. *Amenorrhea* (absence of menstruation) and *dysmenorrhea* (painful menstruation) may have both physical and psychological causes. Pregnancy, rapid weight loss, strenuous exercise, illness, and stress can all cause amenorrhea. Most pain from menstruation is caused by the hormone prostaglandin, which constricts smooth muscle in the uterus causing cramping. Aspirin and a drug called ibuprofen are prostaglandin inhibitors and are effective in reducing pain by reducing the cause of the pain. Hospitalization for health problems can be very stressful, both physically and emotionally. Amenorrhea or irregular menstrual periods may be a related problem in long-term care. Talking with the teen about how stress can affect normal cycling within the woman's body may be important in reassuring her that nothing further is wrong.

Summary

The early childhood years span the time of life from one to six years and are divided into the toddler group (ages one to three) and the preschooler (ages three to six). Dramatic changes in intellectual and behavioral abilities occur as the child moves from dependence to independence with entrance into school. Maturation of all body systems continues as the nervous system develops, and finer muscle control is gained. The child becomes "a real person" with a unique personality and way of behaving. The child is gradually able to achieve independence in performing all activities of daily living such as dressing and washing. Body control is achieved. Peers begin to play an increasingly important role in play for the child from the age of two years on. Investigation of sexual differences among peers is common in the preschooler, and modesty begins to develop at the end of early childhood.

The middle childhood years (ages 6 to 12) are often considered a quiet time with fewer changes occurring compared to early childhood or adolescence. Children in this age are busy doing or making things. Peers are very important and same-sexed friendships develop. School and group activities with peers are two major areas of focus for the child. Curiosity and interest in learning about changes that will occur in boys and girls in adolescence are areas for health education.

The adolescent (ages 12 to 20) experiences many physical and social changes as the reproductive system matures. Rapid growth in height, growth of reproductive structures, elevated hormone levels, and increasing social responsibility are changes teenagers encounter. The adolescent often feels a loss of control over the body because of rapid changes. This loss of control and conflict between increasing pressure to be independent from family restrictions and fear of doing so may jeopardize the person's self-esteem. The peer group serves as a buffer for the individual's self-esteem by providing positive feedback on dress, behavior, and similar problems. Early, middle, and late phases of adolescence show a progression from maximum change to stabilization, reaching adult maturity levels both physically and emotionally. Satisfaction of needs is transferred from the family to the individual and a few close peer relationships. The individual becomes responsible for earning an income from which to provide food, clothing, housing, and transportation.

Accidents are a major health problem during all ages of childhood. Auto accidents, fractures, drownings, poisoning, and burns affect all three age groups. Suicides and drug abuse begin in the middle childhood years and peak in adolescence. Fertility control and sexually transmitted diseases are health issues of adolescence.

The pulse and respirations gradually decrease as the child ages, from rates of 20 to 30 breaths per minute in the toddler, slowing to 16 to 17 breaths per minute in late adolescence. Heart rates decrease from 90 to 120 beats per minute in the toddler to 62 to 66 in late adolescence. Blood pressure gradually rises from 100/60 mm Hg in the toddler to 120/70 mm Hg in late adolescence. Total fluid intake and nutritional intake gradually increase, as does total urine output. Nutritional and fluid needs per kilogram of body weight actually decrease as body growth rate slows. These needs increase slightly during adolescence.

Terms for Review

amenorrhea	morbidity	myopia	puberty
dysmenorrhea	mortality	nocturnal emissions	sexually transmitted diseases
menarche			

Learning Activities

1. Visit a busy park and observe toddlers and preschoolers, schoolage children, and adolescents. In what kind of activities is each group engaged? Compare coordination between toddlers and preschoolers. Attempt to correctly guess a child's age by physical abilities, types of play, and general appearance, and then ask the child's age to check your assessment. Do different age groups of children dominate the park at different times of the day? If so, what might be some reasons for this?
2. Visit a center for children with physical disabilities. How are these children different and how are they similar to the same age group you observed in the park? Are activities involving the physically disabled geared to helping them with age-related developmental tasks, or is the focus on physical functioning only?
3. Talk with nurses who specialize in caring for children, such as a school nurse, pediatric nurse practitioner, or a pediatric staff nurse. Do they have any suggestions for working with children and teenagers? What types of health problems are commonly seen by these nurses, and could health teaching have prevented the problem in that nurse's opinion?

Review Questions

1. Children in early childhood develop an increased ability to maintain a stable temperature. Which of the following explanations most accurately presents one reason for this ability?
   a. The thermal regulating center in the medulla of the brain reaches maturity.
   b. Capillary growth in the skin allows the individual to lose and conserve heat by increasing or decreasing blood flow through the skin.
   c. The child is now capable of losing a great deal of heat through heavy perspiration.
   d. The surface area of the child is now greater in relationship to weight than in the infant.
2. True or False
   _____ a. As the child ages, respirations gradually decrease in rate.
   _____ b. As the child ages, pulse gradually decreases in rate.
   _____ c. As the child ages, temperature gradually decreases.
   _____ d. As the child ages, BP gradually decreases.
3. Which of the following statements describes nutritional needs during early childhood?
   a. Breastfeeding during the toddler years is unsafe, and the child should be switched to cow's milk.
   b. The toddler is growing at a more rapid rate than the preschool child and has greater caloric needs for each pound of body weight.
   c. Total caloric and fluid intake over a 24-hour period should be greater in the toddler than in the preschooler.
   d. The child in the toddler and preschool years needs more fluid for each pound of body weight than the infant to meet fluid needs.
4. Which of the following data indicate normal behavior in meeting oxygen needs for a schoolage child?
   a. Respirations at rest of 40 to 50 breaths per minute.
   b. Heart rate of 90 beats per minute at rest
   c. Heart rate of 65 during activity
   d. Respirations at rest of 12 to 14 breaths per minute
5. Which of the following data indicate normal amounts of urine output in a schoolage child?
   a. 2,000 ml/24 hr
   b. 1,000 ml/24 hr
   c. 500 ml/24 hr
   d. 300 ml/24 hr
6. Which of the following activities, occurring during middle childhood, is related to sexuality needs?
   a. Development of modesty
   b. Increased ability to perspire
   c. Nighttime bed-wetting
   d. Play involving building or making things
7. Which of the following statements best describes physical changes occurring to the boy during puberty?
   a. Rapid physical growth in height beginning around age 10 years
   b. Growth of the testes and penis beginning at age 17 years, on the average
   c. Development of facial hair between 14 and 16 years
   d. Change in voice occurring around ages 10 to 12 years
8. Which of the following data is a normal finding in the healthy teen?
   a. Pulse of 65 beats per minute in the male
   b. Pulse of 54 beats per minute in the female
   c. A higher hemoglobin value in most teenage girls compared to teenage boys
   d. A blood pressure of 140/96 mm Hg

9. True or False
   _____ a. Testosterone in the male stimulates red blood cell production.
   _____ b. Protein needs for adequate nutrition are greater during middle childhood than during the teenage years.
   _____ c. Nocturnal emissions of semen in teenage boys occur only in sexually active individuals.
   _____ d. The 18-year-old generally needs more calories for each pound of body weight than the 12-year-old for optimal nutrition.

10. Mr. Anderson is 19 years old, financially independent, and the father of a three-month-old child. He and his family live in a trailor home of their own, and he is attending college on a part-time basis. What stage of growth and development is most appropriate for Mr. Anderson?
    a. Adolescence
    b. Young adult
    c. Middle adult

Answers

1. b
2. a. T
   b. T
   c. F
   d. F
3. b
4. b
5. b
6. a
7. c
8. a
9. a. T
   b. F
   c. F
   d. F
10. b

CHAPTER 13

GROWTH AND DEVELOPMENT: ADULTHOOD

Young Adult—Eighteen to Forty Years of Age
  Physiological Needs
  Higher Level Needs
  Common Problems During Young Adulthood and
    Nursing Implications

Middle Adult—Forty to Sixty-five Years of
  Age
  Physiological Needs
  Higher Level Needs
  Common Problems During the Middle Adult Years
    and Nursing Implications

Objectives

1. Identify criteria used for separating adolescence and young adults.
2. Describe physical changes beginning to occur in young adulthood which are progressive and have a potential for interfering with satisfaction of physiological needs.
3. Discuss differences in fertility between men and women during the early and middle adult years.

4. Discuss the effects of exercise on changes associated with aging.
5. Describe nursing interventions designed to reduce people's risk of developing serious health problems during adulthood and in later years.
6. Identify developmental tasks of early and middle adults.

Young Adult—Eighteen to Forty Years of Age

The division between adolescence and adulthood occurs at various ages within different societies. Some individuals remain emotionally and financially dependent on their family for many years after age 18. Other people are very independent at an early age because of choices they have made, social expectations in their culture, or circumstances beyond their control. Death or illness of family members may force an adolescent to take on an adult role and responsibilities at an earlier age than individuals whose families are supporting them through college and postgraduate study.

Legally, an 18-year-old has the right to vote and participate in civic activities and even hold some offices within the government structure. The choice of participation in the military is open to the 18-year-old without parental approval. The legal age for alcohol consump-

tion outside the home varies from 18 to 21 years, depending on the laws in different states.

Financial independence is another criterion applied to determining adult status. Adults are viewed as individuals who have achieved financial independence from the family.

Others use maturity to take on and successfully deal with the developmental tasks of adulthood as evidence of adult status. Personality traits may also be used to clarify the difference between the adolescent and the young adult. Traits such as self-control, responsible behavior, ability to tolerate frustration, ability to plan realistically for the future and implement those plans, acceptance of differences in others, formation of prolonged intimate relationships, and development of one's potentials are characteristics associated with the maturity level of adult status. For most young adults, this is a time of minimal physical problems and changes. It is more a time for expanding socially and emotionally in coping with work, community, and close personal relationships.

Physiological Needs

Oxygen Needs. Young adulthood is a time of peak functioning of the cardiovascular and respiratory systems. The heart muscle (myocardium) begins a very slow, imperceptible loss in strength during the young adult years. This loss in strength is estimated to be about 1 percent each year in the average person. Changes in the coronary arteries (arteries supplying the heart's oxygen needs) are known to begin during young adulthood, and people in their twenties may have fat deposits (*plaque*) and narrowing of the lumen (opening) in these vessels. Autopsies done on Korean War casualties found at least one artery narrowed by 50 percent in 15 percent of the victims examined. Diets high in cholesterol are believed to play a significant role in the formation of plaque which causes this narrowing. The pulse in young adults averages 72 beats each minute. Blood pressure remains stable and 140/90 mm Hg is considered an upper normal limit. Table 13–1 shows vital signs and blood values in the young adult.

Elimination. Kidney function is mature, producing approximately 1,000 to 2,000 ml of urine each 24 hours.

Nutrition. Full growth is reached during adolescence or during the twenties. With no further growth, except during pregnancy, caloric needs decrease. Fluid needs remain fairly constant at ¾ oz for each pound, as during adolescence. Caloric needs in women are between 15 and 20 calories per pound, and in men needs are slightly higher, running 18 to 25 calories per pound. Total caloric intake in men averages 2,700 to 3,000 calories and in women 2,000 calories in 24 hours. Protein needs in men are 56 to 60 gm per 24 hours and in women 46 to 50 gm per 24 hours.

The third molars erupt during the twenties if that has not occurred earlier. Some people will have third molars

that fail to erupt and should be evaluated by their dentist for any problems. Some people will not have any molars at all; others will have these teeth grow inappropriately within the gums, and this may affect the health of other nearby teeth.

Food selection and preparation are now the responsibility of the individual. Work environments and schedules will affect the types of foods consumed. Foods from the basic four food groups continue to be important in meeting the nutritional needs of adults. Frozen dinners, fast foods, and an inability or unwillingness to prepare meals at home can contribute to an unbalanced diet, often lacking in fruits and vegetables and overly high in carbohydrates.

Rest and Sleep. The amount of sleep required by most individuals decreases slightly during adulthood. The young adult requires seven to nine hours of sleep, on the average, each night. This decreases further in later adulthood to five to seven hours for people in their fifties and beyond.

Sexual Needs and Sexuality. The sexual identity of most young adults is well established by the time they reach their twenties. The ability to enter into a prolonged intimate relationship with someone of the opposite sex is a characteristic of an adult. Sexual intercourse is no longer needed as a way for clarifying sexual identity and role as in earlier years. It becomes less self-centered and more of an intimate, shared experience with a loved partner. Giving pleasure becomes as important as receiving pleasure from sexual encounters in the mature individual. Fertility control is a basic need related to sexual function, whether a couple is trying to have children or trying to prevent pregnancy. There is a trend toward delaying pregnancy until later in life. Many women are having their first baby in their thirties rather than in their late teens and early twenties as was common in years past. With increasing age of a woman comes a gradual loss in fertility over time. Many couples in the years from 20 to 40 find infertility a very real problem, with the incidence estimated to be 15 to 20 percent of all married couples. Stress in other areas of life, with new responsibilities and challenges, can affect sexual function in a negative way. Exhaustion, alcohol con-

Table 13–1. **Blood Values and Vital Signs in the Adult**

	PULSE (PER MIN)	RESPIRATIONS (PER MIN)	BP (MM HG)	HEMOGLOBIN (GM)	HEMATOCRIT (%)	WBC (CU MM)
Men	60–80	18	126/74	16	47	7,500
Women	60–80	17	126/74	14	42	7,500

sumption, job anxiety, and depression are a few of the things that can interfere with normal sexual function. The ages of 24 to 25 years are considered to be the peak of a woman's fertility.

Women experience regular ovulatory menstrual periods during young adulthood. Men may begin to experience baldness and increased growth of facial hair.

Stimulation Needs.   The creative and productive peak for many individuals is reached during the young adult years. The brain is completely developed by age 25 years, and sensory acuity and cognitive functioning are at optimal levels. Adults require some type of meaningful purpose for their lives, usually gained through work, family, and participation in other activities viewed as important by the individual. A stimulating work environment provides opportunities to learn new skills and maintain the individual's interest. Boredom and stagnation may be the result of a life situation with little variety and change. Use of leisure time to stimulate the senses, exercise the muscles, and entertain the mind, is increasingly important for people working indoors at repetitive tasks or high-stress jobs. After several years at a job, nothing may seem new, and leisure activities can provide the stimulation needed to maintain enthusiasm for life and promote health. Challenging activities and stimulation to the senses and muscles are even more important to the adult in a compromised state of health. Pain, worry, and depression can be reduced or prevented when people become involved in an enjoyable or valued activity. Reading or being read to, participation in creative activities, listening to music, writing, participation in patient discussion groups, and religious activities are a few of the things that may be stimulating to the hospitalized adult without being overtiring.

Higher Level Needs

Safety and Security Needs.   The individual during the young adult years experiences many life changes, depending on the kind of choices made regarding career, marriage, family, and living environment. Patterns are developed that can have a positive or negative effect on current and future health. The level of activity and exercise chosen at this time may continue into later life and minimize many of the problems related to aging. Physical activity is an excellent way of maintaining an optimum weight and avoiding weight-related health problems. Dealing with stress, learning what to expect, and how to cope with changes, such as pregnancy, birth, and childrearing, make the young adult a prime target for health education. Developmental changes are experienced by most individuals and families moving through

different age stages. These changes can be anticipated and planned for ahead of time with the help of health educators and care-givers, making changes less stressful when they occur. Adequate finances are necessary for individuals and families to meet their needs for food, shelter, clothing, and to have a sense of security and independence. Illness can interfere with an individual's ability to earn an income, either temporarily or permanently. Young adults faced with new responsibilities and financial commitments may need help with financial matters during illness. Nursing care for individuals in their adult years involves discussing these potential problems with the patient and making necessary referrals to social services if necessary. A patient worried about being unable to pay bills and provide for personal and family needs is using a lot of energy which might better be used for physical recovery. Stress over such concerns can interfere with optimum recovery and comfort.

Love and Belonging Needs.   The majority of people will marry at some time during their life. The choices made during young adulthood will be affected by the individual's need to be loved and to feel a sense of belonging. This may come from a family, a group of friends with similar interests, a church group, or the sense of companionship many people receive from their jobs and the people with whom they work. Work, school, and church are a few of the places in which most people find a chance for social interaction. Some couples marry and begin new families to fulfill their need to be loved by others. People choosing to live alone and remain single may have to depend more heavily on work and other social activities outside the home to meet love and belonging needs. Separation from family and friends during hospitalization and illness may interfere with a young adult's ability to meet these personal needs. Providing opportunities for children to visit hospitalized parents is important for both the child and the parent. Giving couples some private time in the hospital, free of disturbances, may give them an opportunity to have physical contact and feel loved and needed by each other.

Self-Esteem Needs and Self-Actualization.   Work provides the adult with a source for recognition and prestige. Many people feel a sense of pride and importance from their work, and this leads to a positive self-concept. Some careers are assigned prestige by the society, such as physicians, attorneys, and professional athletes. The person in this type of career is given recognition from others by the title of the profession. This tends to enhance the individuals' feelings about themselves and helps them meet their self-esteem needs. Other people are unemployed or have jobs that carry little or negative recognition, such as sanitary engineer

Table 13–2. **Theories Related to Development During Young Adulthood**

Erikson

Intimacy versus isolation	Young adults are viewed as developing close physical and emotional relationships with a partner and making a lasting commitment to maintain the relationship "even though they may call for significant sacrifice and compromises." The young adult is less self-centered and able to risk the sharing of self with another individual in an ongoing, intimate relationship. Avoidance of close intimate relationships because of fear of a loss of self-esteem can lead to a sense of isolation and a self-centered focus.
Generativity versus stagnation	The young adult becomes concerned and active in establishing (through reproduction) and guiding (through childrearing) the next generation. The concepts of individual productivity and creativity are encompassed in generativity. Stagnation can result when the individual no longer plans for the future and is afraid or unwilling to change and learn new things.

Hurlock/Havinghurst—Developmental Tasks During Young Adulthood

Selecting a mate
Learning to live with a marriage partner
Starting a family
Rearing children
Managing a home
Getting started in an occupation
Taking on civic responsibility
Finding a congenial social group

Hill/Humphrey—Alternate Developmental Tasks

Breaking away from the family
Establishing intimate relationships
Making commitments to a career
Establishing a personal set of values
Forming an adult life of one's own
Establishing a social network

(garbage collector) or assembly-line worker. These people will get personal recognition and pride from others based on their performance. People who feel they are good at their job or are using their time productively, no matter what they do, have a sense of pride in their work and themselves. Working in isolation from one's peers is perhaps the most difficult job for receiving positive feelings of pride and accomplishment. Individuals must be able to tell themselves they are good at what they do with little or no confirmation from others. Adults who choose roles having little contact with other adults may have trouble feeling good about how they spend their time. Staying home to raise children can be very rewarding but also very hard on an individual's self-esteem. Children are not known for telling parents what a good job they are doing, and frequently neither is the working spouse.

The young adult sets life goals and plans for a positive future. Individuals begin to recognize and develop their potentials. There is a striving to experience life to the fullest measure of one's abilities.

Table 13–2 presents theories related to development during young adulthood and associated developmental tasks.

Common Problems During Young Adulthood and Nursing Implications

Most people enjoy optimum levels of health during the years between 20 and 40. Many of the problems encountered are social and economic in nature but may have a bearing on individual and family health.

1. Alcohol abuse seems to be an increasing problem as people encounter added stress in their lives. The National Institute on Alcohol Abuse and Alcoholism (1975) estimates that there are nine million alcohol abusers in the United States. Statistics show men have peak abuse time from 18 to 20 years and again at 37 to 40 years. Women have a peak abuse time in the late thirties. Automobile accidents and alcohol abuse are clearly related, as are other health problems such as inadequate

nutrition, tissue damage to vital organs, and birth defects. Regardless of the health setting in which nurses are employed, education and assessment for potential problems related to alcohol abuse are part of health care.

2. Abuse within families affects several million men, women, and children each year. Two million couples are reported for spouse beating. Abuse of elderly parents within the home is also a newly recognized problem involving young and middle adults. Wife abuse is most common in the young-adult years, with related factors being young children in the home, no outside employment or income for the wife, and an unwillingness on the part of the wife to leave the home for self-protection. The wife and the husband may view abuse as part of their role if their parents were abusive to each other. Abuse of women during pregnancy is not uncommon, possibly related to her increasing dependence on the man, altered sexuality, and the stress related to the added future responsibilities of a new baby. Nurses should be aware that the problem exists and that community and legal resources are available for the abused individual. Alcohol is sometimes involved and often blamed for loss of self-control.

3. Sexually transmitted diseases continue to be health problem among young adults.

4. Cancers, such as Hodgkin's disease, typically affect young adults. Breast cancer, which is currently affecting 1 out of 13 women, strikes most commonly in the ages of 35 to 55 years. Teaching women the need and technique for self-breast examination is often a nursing responsibility. Testicular cancer accounts for 12 percent of all deaths from cancer in the young adult, yet it is one of the most curable if detected early. Men are often uninformed about testicular cancer and how to do a self-examination. Health teaching by the nurse and physician may prevent needless deaths from this form of cancer. Figures 13–1 and 13–2 describes self examinations for men and women.

5. Stress-related illness is a problem at many ages, but the young adult may be especially vulnerable because of high personal aspirations, lack of experience,

How to examine your breasts

In the shower:

Examine your breasts during bath or shower; hands glide easier over wet skin. Fingers flat, move gently over every part of each breast. Use right hand to examine left breast, left hand for right breast. Check for any lump, hard knot or thickening.

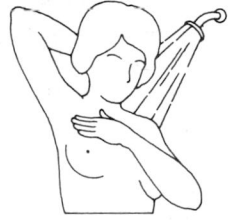

Before a mirror:

Inspect your breasts with arms at your sides. Next, raise your arms high overhead. Look for any changes in contour of each breast, a swelling, dimpling of skin or changes in the nipple.

Then, rest palms on hips and press down firmly to flex your chest muscles. Left and right breast will not exactly match—few women's breasts do.

Regular inspection shows what is normal for you and will give you confidence in your examination.

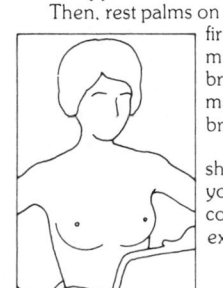

Lying down:

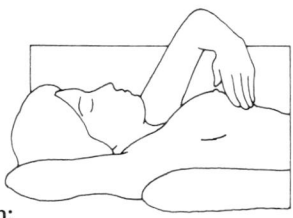

To examine your right breast, put a pillow or folded towel under your right shoulder. Place right hand behind your head—this distributes breast tissue more evenly on the chest. With left hand, fingers flat, press gently in small circular motions around an imaginary clock face. Begin at outermost top of your right breast for 12 o'clock, then move to 1 o'clock, and so on around the circle back to 12. A ridge of firm tissue in the lower curve of each breast is normal. Then move in an inch, toward the nipple, keep circling to examine *every part of your breast*, including nipple. This requires at least three more circles. Now slowly repeat procedure on your left breast with a pillow under your left shoulder and left hand behind head. Notice how your breast structure feels.

Finally, squeeze the nipple of each breast gently between thumb and index finger. Any discharge, clear or bloody, should be reported to your doctor immediately.

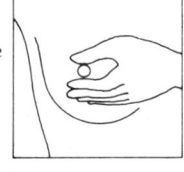

Figure 13–1. Technique for self-breast examination (courtesy of the American Cancer Society).

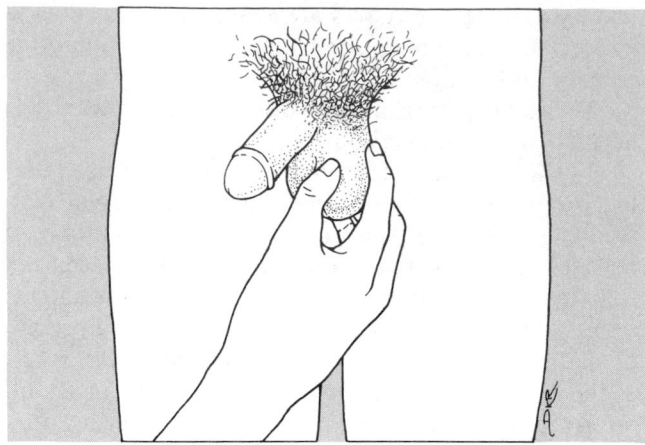

When:
Every month—after warm shower or bath (relaxes scrotal skin).
How:
Roll each testicle between fingers and thumb checking for any hard lumps between fingers. Testicular Cancer is one of most common forms of cancer in men age 15–34 and accounts for 12% of all cancer deaths in this age group.*
Seminoma (most common form) has almost 100% survival rate if detected and treated early.
(*American Cancer Society)

Figure 13–2.   Technique for self-testicular examination (as recommended by the American Cancer Society).

and major life changes with family and work responsibilities. Helping people deal with stress becomes part of the nurse's role during a patient's hospitalization and recovery. Relaxation techniques may be helpful to some individuals, and expressing feelings and frustrations may be helpful to others. Back rubs, warm baths, limiting stimulation, and talking with clergy are additional ways to help people relieve some of their stress and become more relaxed.

6. Pregnancy is most commonly achieved during the young adult years. The need for early prenatal care is important to reduce the risk of serious complications for the mother and fetus. Practices known to be dangerous during pregnancy should be discussed with the pregnant woman so she can make an informed decision on whether to reduce activities such as drug and alcohol consumption, smoking, and exposure to such things as x-rays, or medications related to birth defects.

Middle Adult—Forty to Sixty-five Years of Age

The middle years of a person's life generally involve a slow, often unrecognized, decline in the functioning of the body systems. These changes are a continuation of the imperceptible decline which began in the young adult years. The changes occurring in body systems do not usually affect normal functioning but rather the reserve capacity of most organs and systems. Gradually, changes in appearance, strength, coordination, and sensations are recognized by the middle adult who begins to see life as finite. Overall intelligence tends to increase, for most people, with the accumulation of knowledge and life experiences. The skills needed for an individual's occupation or profession are often at their peak during middle adulthood, and this is commonly a time of financial security and optimum status. Appropriate nutrition, exercise, rest, and management of stress will help to maintain optimum health and vigor during this time of life and may delay or prevent changes often associated with aging.

Physiological Needs

Oxygen Needs.   Cardiac muscle strength continues to decrease at an average rate of 1 percent each year, especially in people with sedentary life-styles. This gradual decline does not affect the cardiac output during middle age. The blood vessels, especially the arteries, become less elastic because of the gradual deposition of *lipids* (fats) within the lining of the vessels (*atherosclerosis*). This also causes narrowing of the vessel and a decreased ability to transport the same volume of blood to the tissues, compared to earlier years. Calcification may occur within the blood vessels, causing an actual hardening of the arteries with loss of elasticity. With loss of elasticity in the arteries, the blood pressure will begin to rise, and hypertension may develop with blood pressures above 140/90 mm Hg. The vital signs during middle age are expected to run in the same range as those during young adulthood in the absence of known disease. Pulse is in the range of 60 to 80 beats per minute, respirations range from 14 to 20 breaths per minute, and blood pressure fluctuates around 126/74 mm Hg. The lungs are also gradually losing their elasticity and permeability, which affects the ability to exchange waste products for oxygen. Most people experience no problems related to this minimal loss in function during middle age, and shortness of breath and fatigue are more likely related to an underlying disease process or inactivity.

Elimination.   During middle age, there is a gradual loss of the small functioning units within the kidney, called nephrons. Because of the abundance of these nephrons, this gradual loss is not reflected in kidney function. Urine output continues to be the same as during earlier years, approximately 1,000 to 2,000 ml in 24 hours. Enlargement of the prostate gland in men will sometimes occur during this time of life and may obstruct urine flow by compressing the ureters which lead from the bladder to the penis. The man may experience a decreased urine output, difficulty voiding (dysuria), or small amounts of urine voided more frequently (oliguria). Medical or surgical treatment may be needed to restore normal elimination patterns. Peristalsis also tends to decrease because of lessening muscle tone in the gut and general inactivity. This may cause problems with constipation unless exercise and a diet high in bulk-producing foods are used to counteract this decreased peristalsis. People should be cautioned against using mineral oil as a laxative for extended periods of time, since it will prevent absorption of vitamins A, D, E, and K which are fat-soluble and excreted with the mineral oil.

Nutrition.   Most adults experience little change in their nutritional needs during middle age.

The basal metabolic rate gradually decreases during middle age and will result in weight gain unless food consumption is decreased or exercise is increased. Caloric needs gradually decline so that after age 50 most people need 200 to 300 calories less each day to maintain their weight, compared to earlier adult years. The woman in her fifties consumes approximately 1,800 calories to maintain normal weight, and the man consumes approximately 2,400 calories each day to maintain weight. These figures will vary for each individual, based on body size and activity level. The larger, more active individual will have increased caloric needs compared to the smaller person with a sedentary life-style. Fluid needs remain the same as during early adulthood, which is approximately ¾ oz for each pound of body weight, or 2,000 to 3,000 ml in 24 hours.

Many people begin to loose their teeth during middle age but good dental hygiene and care will prolong the health of the gums and teeth. By age 65 years, 50 percent of middle-age adults have lost half of their permanent teeth. This will affect chewing ability and food choices if false teeth are not being used. There is also a progressive loss of taste buds on the tongue, leading to a decreased sense of taste. Bland foods may have very little taste by later middle age because of lost taste buds, and people may refuse to eat these foods or fail to adhere to a bland diet prescribed by their physician.

People often have more money to spend on food and entertainment at this age, and activities such as dining at restaurants, business luncheons, and consumption of richer foods and alcohol may increase. This will lead to a tendency to gain excess weight unless exercise is increased proportionately.

Rest and Sleep.   The need for rest and sleep remains fairly constant for any given individual during adult life. As people approach the later middle-age years, the amount of sleep required tends to decrease. People over 50 need approximately two hours less sleep each night. The comment, ''I'm just not able to sleep anymore,'' is common, and older individuals may be very early risers.

Sexual Needs and Sexuality.   During the middle adult years, men and women experience a decreasing production of sex hormones, testosterone and estrogen/progesterone, respectively. For women, there is a very definite physical sign of aging with cessation of ovarian function and menopause. *Menopause* refers to the cessation of menstruation and occurs in women from 35 to 60 years of age. The most common ages for menopause are during the mid-forties. *Climacteric* refers to a period of time during which reproductive function is gradually lost and usually spans several years prior to actual menopause. The woman loses the ability to produce estrogen and progesterone in quantities sufficient to maintain tissues dependent on these hormones for structure and optimal functioning. The ovary and the woman's eggs are as old as she is, and eventually the aging eggs are no longer able to respond to follicle-stimulating hormone (FSH) from the anterior pituitary gland within the brain. The eggs no longer mature, and ovulation ceases. Before total loss of reproductive ability, most women experience a gradually decreasing fertility. Eventually, irregular menstrual periods occur with decreased bleeding or breakthrough bleeding at abnormal times during the monthly cycles and, finally, menopause. Atrophy (tissue degeneration) occurs in the internal and external sexual tissues of the breasts, vagina, ovary, fallopian tubes, and uterus. Pubic hair tends to become more sparse, and there is an increased alkaline pH in the reduced vaginal secretions which is related to an increased risk for vaginal infections. The classic "hot flashes" are a result of inadequate amounts of estrogen, causing dilation of the arteries in the skin, flushing, and perspiration. Estrogen replacement therapy will alleviate many of these symptoms, but supplemental estrogen is related to increased incidence of cancer in women and is being used with much caution. Women with a family history of breast or cervical cancer would probably not be candidates for this treatment. The female sexual drive during climacteric and postmenopause is frequently reported to be unaltered or increased, now that the worry of fertility control is in the past.

Men experience a slow decrease in testosterone production from the testes. The declining production of testosterone levels off during the years between 40 and 60, but for most men it never decreases to the point that spermatogenesis (production of sperm) ceases. Some men in their eighties are capable of fathering children, as case-history evidence shows. Changes the man may experience related to aging and decreased testosterone include increased time required to achieve an erection, decreased force of ejaculation, and decreased number of sperm within the ejaculated fluid (semen). Men have also reported experiencing "hot flashes," nightmares, and emotional instability with further decreased testosterone production.

Intimate sexual relations with one's partner may be altered somewhat as the effects of aging are felt. The woman may need a water-soluble lubricating jelly to replace the normal vaginal secretions lost from inadequate amounts of estrogen. More time may be necessary during sexual foreplay to give the man time to achieve an erection and to provide the woman with the added time needed to achieve optimum levels of normal vaginal lubrication. As with any activity, the people involved with sexual counseling tell us that use improves and maintains function.

Stimulation Needs.   Changes are occurring in the acuity of the senses during middle age. Already mentioned is the decreasing sense of taste. The senses of smell, vision, and hearing are also losing function. The eye loses some of its ability to focus on near objects because of decreasing elasticity in the lens. This loss of clear vision at close distances is called *presbyopia* and affects approximately 50 percent of people by the age of 65 years. Color discrimination in the blue-green part of the spectrum is also lessened because of the yellowing of the lens with increasing age. The need for more light in order to see clearly begins in the thirties and increases with age, giving the individual reduced vision in dim light. Brighter lighting becomes important for many activities such as reading and detailed handwork. Dim lighting

also may become a safety hazard, especially if the individual is in an unfamiliar setting, such as the hospital.

Muscle mass declines with aging, and there is a loss in strength of 10 to 20 percent from the beginning to the end of middle age, and jobs requiring heavy physical labor may be more tiring as the individual ages. Regular physical stimulation of the body's muscles also helps to maintain weight levels and gives the individual a more positive outlook, a sense of "feeling good."

Higher Level Needs

Safety and Security Needs.   For most individuals, middle age is a time of financial and job security. Good health and vigor for life are common. The gradual physical changes make some safety considerations important for this age group. Dental care is extremely important to maintain healthy gums and teeth. Booster shots of tetanus and diphtheria toxoids remain important every ten years or following injuries causing deep skin breaks. Increased lighting will help prevent falls and accidents. Railings, nonskid shoes, and complete ice and snow removal on walks and steps will help prevent falls and bone fractures. Fractures have become more likely by late middle age due to loss of calcium from the bones (*demineralization*), decreasing their strength.

Love and Belonging Needs.   The individual between 40 and 65 years will usually experience many events that affect satisfaction of love and belonging needs. If the individual married, the death of the spouse may be a crisis to face, leaving a very large gap in the individual's life. If the couple had children, the children may be leaving the home and becoming independent adults. The physical and emotional separations of the children can leave parents feeling unneeded and unloved, especially if the child is not recognized as an independent adult with an independent life to lead. The individual's parents are reaching advanced years, and the loss of one or both parents through death will decrease the number of close, loving relationships for the middle-aged individual. This is also a time for marriage of one's children, birth of grandchildren, and even remarriage for the individual who has lost a spouse through death or divorce. All these new relationships give the individual the opportunity to feel loved and needed.

Self-Esteem and Self-Actualization.   An individual's self-esteem can be affected in a positive and a negative manner during the middle adult years, as is the case in most of life's stages. The physical changes related to aging, such as graying hair, appearance of skin wrinkles, baldness, thinning hair, and menopause are often seen as negative traits in a youth-oriented society. Possession of these traits indicating aging may make the individual feel less valued and unattractive. There may be a grieving or depression over lost youth and failure to accomplish the goals set in younger years. A person who is able to maintain a positive self-concept is more able to adapt to changes during middle age and continue to be flexible and optimistic about the present and the future. Many people reach the peak of their career during middle age and are respected and valued by their fellow employees. Skills and knowledge have increased over time for many individuals, and they know they are good at what they do. This sense of pride and respect from others increases a person's self-esteem.

The parent who chose to stay at home and raise the children may find middle age a very difficult time as the children become adults and strive for independence. The feeling of no longer being needed is common, and the question of what to do with the rest of one's life often causes major changes. Many people choose to re-

enter the work force or return to school. Some people become active in civic, social, or charitable organizations. Middle age is often a time for personal assessment of how one has measured up in occupational and interpersonal performances. Time is viewed as running out for accomplishing those goals that were important in the individual's life plan. Some people choose to make drastic changes in their life, trying to reach those goals before they are too old. Other people may feel that life has passed them by and treated them unfairly. This will lead to a loss of self-esteem and possibly stagnation in future development. Depression and suicide occur in the middle-aged woman at a higher rate than at any other age. The ability to develop and enjoy life and its many changes is partly dependent on a positive feeling about one's self and partly dependent on the human need to continue to learn and expand one's abilities.

Table 13-3 describes several theories related to development during the middle adult years and associated developmental tasks.

Table 13-3. **Theories Related to Development During the Middle Years**

Erikson

Generativity versus stagnation continues from young adult years.

Peck

Valuing wisdom versus valuing power	With decreasing muscle strength and stamina, the adult needs to place more emphasis on experience, knowledge, and skills gained during life to maintain self-esteem.
Socializing versus sexualizing	Interpersonal relationships should focus more on sharing and understanding and less on intimate sexual behavior.
Cathectic flexibility versus cathectic impoverishment	The person's successful adjustment to middle age and the future depends partly on replacing lost relationships with new ones. Extended family relationships and new peer relationships fill the gap left from death, divorce, and relocation of friends and children.
Mental flexibility versus mental rigidity	Remaining open to new experiences and ideas is important for the individual's continued development.

Havinghurst/Hurlock—Developmental Tasks of the Middle Adult

Reaching and maintaining satisfaction in a job that interests them
Establishing and maintaining a satisfactory standard of living
Achieving social and civic responsibility
Acceptance and adjustment to physiological changes of middle age
Relating to one's spouse as a person
Developing adult leisure activities
Adjusting to aging parents
Helping teenage children to become responsible and happy adults

Common Problems During the Middle Adult Years and Nursing Implications

1. In the United States, 1.5 million adults have heart attacks each year, with death the outcome in one-third of the victims (Trafford, 1982). It is the leading cause of death in the middle adult years. Cancer, the second leading cause of death, occurs most frequently in the breasts and cervix of women and in the lung and prostate gland of men. The seven warning signs of cancer should be familiar to all adults and are part of the nurse's responsibility in health education. See Table 13–4 for these warning signs.

2. *Glaucoma* affects 2 percent of the population over 40 and commonly develops between 40 and 65 years of age. The increased intraocular pressure occurring in glaucoma damages the optic nerve and may eventually result in blindness. Gradual loss of peripheral vision, halos around lights, headaches, and blurred vision are warning signs.

3. The incidence of diabetes mellitus increases after age 40 years and is seen most often in people who are overweight and have a family history of diabetes.

4. Degenerative changes cause many problems for some adults in the form of *osteoarthritis*. This is a degenerative change in joints affecting most people over 45 years of age to some degree. The incidence is slightly higher in men under 55 years compared to women. Af-

Table 13–4. Seven Warning Signs of Cancer

1. Persistent cough or hoarseness
2. Change in wart or mole
3. Abnormal bleeding or discharge
4. Thickening or lump in breast or other body sites
5. Change in bowel or bladder functioning
6. A sore that heals very slowly
7. Indigestion or difficulty in swallowing

Source: American Cancer Society, Pamphlet #2066, 1979.

ter age 55 years, the incidence is remarkably higher in women.

5. Hypertension is related to loss of elasticity in the arteries and occurrs in 18 to 24 percent of individuals during their middle adult years. It is more common in black people, but the reason is unknown. Yearly blood pressure checks offered through places of employment, during physical examinations, and at any location where large numbers of people congregate, such as shopping malls, will help to alert an individual to possible problems. Hypertension can be a symptom of underlying disease in the body, and it can cause damage to the heart and other organs. People should be aware of their normal blood pressure and the need for yearly checks.

6. Drug abuse and alcohol consumption continue to be problems during the middle-age years, as do family abuse and violence. Widowed women are a group known to be at risk for drug and alcohol abuse.

Summary

The division between the adolescent and the young adult may be based on several criteria including age, financial or emotional independence from family, and characteristics of maturity indicating ability to deal with the developmental tasks of young adults. The developmental tasks of the young adult focus on independence, intimacy, career, establishing personal values, and a social network.

For most people, the early adult years are a time of optimum health and functioning. Choices of life-styles, which are active and not overly stressful, will help to reduce the deterioration and changes in body structures leading to aging and health problems.

There is a trend toward delayed pregnancy in young adult families with parenthood beginning in the mid-to-late twenties or early thirties. Peak fertility occurs in women during the early twenties and decreases progressively until menopause. Infertility problems are related to this trend and affect approximately 15 to 20 percent of married couples.

Sexually transmitted diseases, alcohol abuse, abuse of children, spouse, or aging parents, and cancer are problems common to both young and middle adults. Some young adults are also affected by pregnancy-related health concerns.

Middle adults are viewed as having fairly good health but recognize that age-related changes are occurring. Cardiac muscle strength and general physical strength decline gradually as aging progresses. Atherosclerotic changes in the blood vessels begin and progress during the adult years. Loss of bone mass gradually occurs in men and is delayed somewhat in women until after menopause. Women lose their fertility during the middle adult years, while men often retain fertility throughout their lives.

Choices regarding marriage and children are often made during the early adult years. Childbearing and childrearing activities then occupy a large portion of adult life. Helping children become independent and leave home occurs in middle adulthood. The need for self-esteem and self-actualization may take on new meaning when children no longer occupy the adults' en-

ergy, time, and financial resources. Depression and suicide are not uncommon problems during middle adult life when people, traditionally women, are uncertain what to do with the rest of their life once the children have left home.

Encouraging regular exercise, maintenance of optimum weight, self-examinations for cancer, and routine health examinations are some ways in which nurses are effective in reducing health problems in adults.

Terms for Review

atherosclerosis	glaucoma	menopause	plaque
climacteric	lipids	osteoarthritis	presbyopia
demineralization			

Learning Activities

1. Talk with a nurse clinician about problems commonly encountered in young and middle adults. Consider your own and your family's health problems. Are they related to changes or conditions associated with normal aging?
2. Ask various adults if they have received any health teaching to help them maintain optimum health and identify any serious problems early when treatment is more successful. Do you know where in your community adults can receive information or screening for hypertension, fertility control, warning signs of cancer and self-breast or testicular examination, vision and hearing testing, or counseling on drug/alcohol abuse?
3. In a public area, such as an airport or shopping center, observe various aged adults. Do you see physical changes associated with aging in these adults? What is the incidence of obesity in young and middle-aged adults you observe?

Review Questions

1. Nutritional needs in the young adult are different from needs during adolescence. Which statement describes one of these differences?
   a. Males generally have higher caloric needs than women during young adult years and similar needs during adolescence.
   b. Fluid needs are less in the young adult than in the adolescent.
   c. Caloric needs are generally less in both sexes in the young adult years compared to adolescence.
   d. Protein needs are higher in the teenage female and lower in the young adult female compared to the needs of same aged males.
2. True or False
   _____ a. Female fertility peaks around 25 years of age and then begins to decline.
   _____ b. Young adults begin to have a very small loss in muscle strength of the heart as they age.
   _____ c. Urine output is commonly between 500 and 1,000 ml in 24 hours for most young adults.
   _____ d. Peak abuse times for alcohol are during the young adult years.
3. As changes occur related to normal aging, the person in the middle adult years may have which of the following signs and symptoms?
   a. Elevated respiratory rates in the range of 40 to 50 breaths per minute
   b. Lowered pulse rates in the range of 50 to 60 beats per minute because of reduced strength of the heart muscles by age 55 years
   c. Difficulty or inability to void
   d. Difficulty sleeping more than six hours each night at age 58 years
4. Lessening muscle tone in the gut may cause which of the following problems for the middle and elderly adult?
   a. Constipation
   b. Incontinence of stool
   c. Difficult urination
   d. Poor absorption of fluid from the digested food in the gut

5. Changes occur in the senses during middle age and beyond. Which of the following relates to changed needs because of altered sensory perception?
   a. The sense of taste becomes more discriminating and highly seasoned foods are often dislike because of this.
   b. People commonly need glasses to help them focus on far objects as the lens of the eye loses its elasticity.
   c. Brighter lighting is needed for clear vision as a person ages.
   d. Color vision is almost completely lost by the end of the middle-age years because of yellowing of the lens of the eye.

Answers

1. c
2. a. T
   b. T
   c. F
   d. F
3. d
4. a
5. c

CHAPTER 14

GROWTH AND DEVELOPMENT OF THE OLDER ADULT

Theories Related to Aging
Physiological Needs and Nursing Implications
Higher Level Needs

Objectives

1. Describe several biological theories related to aging.
2. Describe several psychosocial theories related to aging.
3. Identify developmental tasks of the older adult.
4. Describe physical changes of aging that may interfere with satisfaction of physiological needs.

5. Describe physical and psychosocial changes affecting the elderly that may interfere with satisfaction of higher level needs.

6. Identify nursing interventions helpful in reducing health risks in the elderly.

Theories Related to Aging

The number of people living to the age of 65 years and beyond is increasing more rapidly than the number of people in any other age group. In 1982, the estimated life expectancy for newborns was 74 years of age. For people who live well into their nineties, this is the longest phase in their lives. The census bureau has estimated that there will be close to thirty million older adults by 1990 and 55.5 million by 2050. The percentage of people over 65 years of age in the total population is expected to increase from 4 percent in 1900 to an estimated 17 percent by 2030. Nursing care for patients in their later years will become an increasingly important issue in the future. Table 14–1 describes some biological and psychosocial theories related to aging. Aging is a complex process which is not well understood at this time, as evidenced by the many different theories on the topic. Some factors such as stress, obesity, smoking, and sedentary life-styles seem to accelerate the aging process. Many older people remain actively involved in life for as long as they live. Others seem to gradually withdraw from the active life and choose a quiet, slower paced life-style with advancing years. Some elderly are relatively free of active, obvious disease or illness until they die suddenly. Others are bothered by some of the chronic health problems associated with old age such as osteoporosis, hearing and vision losses, and arteriosclerosis, to name only a few. Most people over 80 years of age (80 percent) continue to live in their own homes with friends or relatives. Only a small portion of the elderly require nursing home care.

Physiological Needs and Nursing Implications

Oxygen Needs. The need for oxygen is decreased in the elderly for two main reasons. The basal metabolic rate (BMR) decreases with age. People's activity levels also tend to decrease with age. As muscle activity and the BMR decrease, less oxygen is needed because there are fewer chemical reactions occurring at the cellular

Table 14–1. **Theories Related to Aging**

Biological Theories of Aging

Genetic theory	Aging is a result of biochemical changes programmed into the DNA molecule within each cell.
Mutation theory	Aging is a result of errors in cell division occurring over time, which alter the effectiveness and function of the mutated cells.
Cross-linkage theory	As cells age over the life span of the organism, there is increased cross-linkage of collagen molecules within the connective tissues of the body. This cross-linkage forms stable clusters of molecules and results in a loss of elasticity and a hardening of the tissue, with loss of function progressing over time.
Free-radical theory	Over the course of time, groups of atoms, called free radicals, are formed through oxidative (oxygen-using) chemical reactions within the cell. These free radicals are highly reactive and cause altered biochemical reactions in the cell. The cell membrane is highly susceptible to damage from these reactions. The free radical, *lipofuscin*, accumulates in the cells, especially nerve tissue, with aging and alters cell function. (Vitamin E binds free radicals and may extend the life of the aging cells.)
Autoimmune theory	Production of autoantibodies (antibodies against self) increases with age. The effectiveness of the immune system is altered with age, and people become more susceptible to infections, tumor growth, and autoimmune diseases such as rheumatoid arthritis.
Stress theory	The changes associated with aging are a result of the body's failing ability to maintain a stable internal environment. The accumulated wear and tear on the body eventually exceeds the ability to rebuild and repair. Stressors in the environment increase the rate of aging.
Nutrition theory	Diet can affect rate of aging and length of life. Lean, trim individuals experience fewer health problems and tend to live longer than overweight individuals.
Cell replacement	As people age, cell destruction gradually exceeds cell production. The result is a decreasing number of functioning cells over time. Tissues and organs atrophy and shrink with advancing age.

Psychosocial Theories of Aging

Disengagement theory	As people age, they gradually withdraw from society. Society simultaneously withdraws from people as they age. There is a decreased number of relationships among individuals over time.
Activity theory	Healthy aging involves maintaining an active involvement in life. Physical, intellectual, and social activity is important to the elderly to preserve a healthy quality of life.
Continuity theory	As people age, they attempt to maintain values, habits, and ways of behaving. The focus gradually is to preserve a past way of life rather than incorporate the new and change with the times.

level. Since the human organism utilizes primarily aerobic (with oxygen) metabolism at the cellular level, decreases in metabolism result in decreased utilization of oxygen.

Changes gradually occurring with age affect the ability to satisfy individual oxygen needs. Lung capacity decreases with age. There is a loss of elasticity within the lung over time. Elderly individuals often experience a reduced capacity to cough and remove secretions from the lungs due to decreased strength of the expiratory muscles and an increased rigidity of the chest.

Some changes in the vascular system may affect an individual's ability to meet oxygenation needs. There is a gradual increase in the rigidity of the arterial system which creates increased resistance to blood flow and elevated blood pressure in some individuals. If the resistance to blood flow is great enough, it will overcome the pumping force of the heart, the amount of blood reaching certain tissues and organs is decreased, and blood tends to pool in the venous system. If the blood flow is decreased to a point where oxygen needs are unmet at the cellular level, there will be altered function and possible cellular death.

Atherosclerosis, which is a form of arteriosclerosis, is associated with aging. In this disease, plaques of lipid and cholesterol material are deposited in the walls of the arteries and can obstruct blood flow. Cardiac output, which is the heart rate per minute multiplied by the stroke volume (volume of blood ejected into the aorta with each ventricular contraction), is decreased. This reduction is caused mainly by a reduced stroke volume, with the heart rate remaining fairly similar to middle adult rates. By age 80 years, cardiac output may have decreased 50 percent from output in earlier years. There is a reduced ability to increase the heart rate in relationship to stress, and a longer period of time is required to return to normal heart rates after the stress is removed. Infrequent activities, such as shoveling snow and carrying heavy loads, may demand more oxygen than the elderly individual's body is able to supply, and cellular damage to vital organs, such as the heart, may result. A progressive fibrosis of the heart valves is associated with aging, which decreases the efficiency of the heart. Vital signs remain about the same as during middle adulthood.

Most older adults meet their oxygen needs with little difficulty. The body adapts to the individual's life-style over time to meet differing needs. Many runners are over 65 years of age and are able to maintain satisfaction of oxygen needs during this physical stress. Many older adults maintain an active life, beginning each day with jogging or brisk walking for several miles. This activity helps to establish new collateral circulation (new blood vessels grow in) to vital organs such as the heart. This helps counteract the tendency toward atherosclerosis and narrowing or obstruction of arteries from the build-up of plaque. Daily physical activity also maintains healthy lung function well into the older adult years. The older person who smokes, eats fatty foods, is overweight, and has little or no daily physical activity is the person who will have the most difficulty meeting oxygen needs when stressed by illness or rare strenuous activity.

Nursing intervention should focus on both prevention and ways of assisting patients who are having difficulty in meeting oxygen needs. Health education begun in the young adult years, which discourages smoking and encourages people to maintain a physically active life, and an optimum weight, along with regular self- and medical examinations to detect problems early, is the best way nurses can help people reduce their health risks. Chapter 20 discusses nursing interventions for patients unable to meet their oxygen needs.

Temperature Maintenance. The elderly, as a group, are at high risk for developing problems with maintaining their body temperatures. "Hypothermia is a continuing and all-pervasive threat to the elderly" (Pozoz and Born, 1982). There are several reasons for this, which are listed below:

1. There are decreased sensory perception to cold and slowing of neural function with advancing age. The result of this is that the elderly may not detect cold as soon as when they were younger. The physiological response to cold for maintaining temperature (vasoconstriction of vessels in the skin) is delayed. Cold may be sensed but not perceived or recognized, and no protective action is taken, such as adding clothing.

2. For many elderly people, there is a reduction in overall activity levels which decreases heat production.

3. The metabolic rate is decreased in the elderly, which also means less heat production from chemical reactions at the cellular level.

4. Vascular changes with aging tend to decrease the individual's ability to respond to cold with vasoconstriction to conserve heat. The vessels are less elastic and more rigid, making them less able to contract or dilate maximally from nervous signals originating in the brain.

5. Medications such as those for sleep, blood pressure control, sedation, and mood elevation have the potential for causing hypothermia.

6. Elderly people who experience a stroke affecting the hypothalamus, which regulates body temperature, are at risk for hypothermia and hyperthermia (elevated body temperature).

7. Elderly people on a fixed income may not be able to afford to maintain comfortable temperatures in the home due to rising heating costs. Failing to pay bills may result in heating service being discontinued. Drafty, poorly insulated housing is also a cause of hypothermia in the elderly.

8. The elderly are in danger of hyperthermia when environmental temperatures are excessive. Their less elastic blood vessels cannot dilate to lose heat. The elderly also have a decrease in sweat gland activity, which is usually the most effective means of losing heat for younger adults. Purchasing and running air conditioners are added expenses beyond some people's financial resources. The people most at risk for these temperature problems are those who are relatively inactive and on barely adequate, fixed incomes or in a facility where they cannot regulate heating and cooling for personal comfort. The active older adult maintains muscle mass longer and retains a good shivering response to cold.

Activity, also, increases heat production. Many people choose to remove themselves from excessively cold or hot temperatures by vacationing in warm areas during the winter months and cooler, northern areas in the summer. Many older people maintain their homes at a temperature for their comfort, often in the high 70s or 80s. This may be uncomfortable for others who visit the older couple or individual, but the elderly are meeting their needs for additional external heat to maintain a normal body temperature.

Nurses working with the elderly should be alert to signs of hypothermia (see Chapter 21). Thermometers, which are designed to measure body temperatures below 96°F should be used with elderly patients to detect low body temperatures. Some patient's mental confusion has been attributed to long-term hypothermia, which improves as body temperature is brought into the normal range. A comfortable working environment for staff in a hospital or nursing care facility is usually not warm enough for inactive patients. Add insulation for patients in the form of clothing and blankets, and position wheelchairs and beds away from drafts. If the patient's hands and skin feel cool, the body is probably trying to conserve heat. This means the person is experiencing some degree of cold stress, and warming measures or added insulation is needed.

Nutrition and Fluid Needs. The elderly are at risk for inadequate nutritional intake for several reasons. Some of these factors relate to physical changes experienced by many people with advancing age. Other factors relate to socioeconomic aspects of life. Some factors related to the altered ability of the elderly to meet nutritional needs are listed below:

1. A decreased sensitivity to taste affects the flavor of foods and may decrease consumption. Along with this, the sense of smell may be decreased, which may make foods less appealing. There is an actual reduction in the number of taste buds with a resulting decreased sensitivity to sweet and salty. To compensate for this reduced taste, people may increase the amount of added salt and sweets in the diet. For some medical conditions, this can be a problem. It may also lead to weight gains.

2. Tooth loss is increased over time due to decreasing bone density and gum disease. This may alter the ability to chew certain foods, and they may be omitted from the diet. Poorly fitting dentures or failing to wear dentures will also affect the type of food consumed. A sore mouth or loose teeth will affect ingestion by limiting the types of foods that can be comfortably eaten.

3. Secretion of gastric enzymes is decreased with age, and this can lead to problems with digestion.

4. There is an increased tendency toward problems with glucose metabolism related to advanced age.

Adult-onset diabetes occurs with more frequency in the elderly than in middle age.

5. Gastrointestinal motility (peristalsis), is decreased frequently related to decreased activity levels. This may lead to constipation problems.

6. The ability to obtain quality food may be affected by inadequate finances, generalized weakness, and feeling too tired to grocery shop and prepare meals. In many cultures, eating is a social activity. Eating alone can be a negative experience. Often, people lose interest in cooking and eating when they are alone. However, poverty may be one of the biggest obstacles to optimum nutrition in the elderly.

7. Inappropriate nutrition leading to obesity is a common problem in the elderly when previous intake patterns are maintained while the BMR decreases and life becomes more sedentary.

8. The elderly who are institutionalized may not have foods and fluids of their choice readily available to them. Rather then requesting special things to eat or drink, they may choose to eat or drink only small quantities of what is available. On the other hand, in retirement many people have time and money available to experiment with cooking, and this becomes a new, shared interest. Different spices can do much to compensate for loss of some of the taste for sweet and salty. Salt and sugar substitutes may be used if weight control or medical conditions contraindicate increased use of sugar and salt. Many people maintain an active life through work, exercise, or both, well into their eighties and nineties. This increases their caloric needs over those of a more sedentary individual and counteracts the tendency to gain weight. Many older people working on farms continue to eat three big meals each day and remain trim and fit. Good dental care and a healthy diet during younger years does much to prevent tooth loss. Many adults maintain their natural teeth in good health their entire life. People in their young adult and middle adult years are wearing braces to straighten their teeth, reduce future cavities, and have healthier gums and teeth in their older years.

Nurses are active in educating older adults about changes affecting nutrition and ways to meet the body's nutritional needs. Referrals are made to dietitians for patients needing help with meal planning. Social service referrals are necessary if the patient's finances are interfering with adequate nutrition. Educating older people about community resources for food and meal service is another area of responsibility for nurses in the public health area. See Chapter 22 for suggestions on feeding patients and improving their ability to feed themselves.

Elimination Needs. The elderly may experience several different types of problems with solid and liquid elimination. The elderly have a tendency toward constipation, resulting from a lack of bulk in the diet, poor fluid intake, decreased activity, poor muscle tone, and possibly from abusive use of laxatives. Some problems are a result of infections such as of the bladder. Impaired thinking ability will also affect the ability to control bladder and bowel function. The immune system of the elderly person is not as effective in combating infection when compared to that of a younger person, so the risks of infection from catheterization for lost bladder function can be great. Prostatic hypertrophy (enlargement of the prostate gland) may make urination difficult in men, while older women may be troubled with the problem of stress incontinence due to relaxed muscle control of the bladder. Any forceful activity such as laughing, coughing, or running may result in the uncontrolled passage of urine in people with stress incontinence. Incontinence is a problem seen in residents of nursing homes and other facilities for elderly adults needing nursing care. This problem can be related to lack of help in getting to the toilet, medications such as sedatives or diuretics, bed rest, disease, and confusion.

Drinking alcohol, coffee, or tea in the evening may lead to nighttime incontinence in the elderly since these beverages tend to increase urine production (diuretic effect). Also, the capacity of the bladder is decreased with age. This leads to the need for frequent voiding. Elderly people may decrease their intake of fluid to reduce the number of times they must empty their bladder. This reduced fluid consumption may lead to constipation and bladder infections. Total urine output should be similar to that during middle adult years—1,000 to 2,000 ml of urine in 24 hours. Again, regular physical exercise, foods high in bulk, such as fruits, grain foods, and vegetables, and adequate fluid intake can counteract most of the problems involving elimination related to age. Not using bubble bath or nylon underpants and drinking cranberry juice are also helpful in preventing bladder infections in women. During illness, activity is reduced, and normal intake of foods and fluids is altered. This is when older people are most likely to experience problems with normal elimination.

Nursing interventions can focus on adequate fluid intake to reduce urine concentration and bowel constipation. Caution with using nighttime sleep medications will help patients maintain better nighttime elimination control. The attitude of health personnel will also affect the patient's willingness to seek assistance with elimination needs early before incontinence occurs because of overfilling. Negative remarks and nonverbal communication, which tells the patient the staff is too busy to be bothered, will make a patient reluctant to request help in the future. In fact, urinating in the bed may cause less distress than exerting the energy to get to the bathroom with help, only to receive negative comments from the staff, such as, "Not again. I just took you to the bathroom one hour ago. This is ridiculous." As the nurse in charge of patient care, education of health staff may be part of your role when working with elderly patients. See Chapter 24 on assisting patients to meet their elimination needs.

Rest and Sleep.   The amount and type of sleep needed change with age. Women seem to be able to maintain previous sleep patterns longer than men.

1. The total amount of sleep in a 24-hour period is decreased to five to seven hours.
2. The elderly are more easily awakened from sleep.
3. It often takes longer for people to fall asleep.
4. Stage-4 sleep (deep sleep) is decreased by 50 percent compared to young adults.
5. Medications for sedation may alter sleep. Usually there is a decrease in dreaming sleep after taking these medications. See Chapter 25 for nursing interventions to promote rest and sleep.

Pain Avoidance.   Sensitivity to pain seems to decrease with advancing age, but at the same time there are often more causes of pain. The chronic nature of pain related to bone and joint problems and frequent falls and injuries because of decreased muscle strength is often difficult to tolerate and can be physically and emotionally exhausting. See Chapter 26 for nursing interventions to reduce pain and promote the patient's comfort.

Sensory Stimulation Needs.   The changes related to sensory stimulation and physical mobility are described below. These changes, which occur to varying degrees with aging, make some people in this group at risk for sensory deficits. Mobility, agility, and balance can also be compromised. See Chapter 28 for nursing interventions to help patients meet their needs for stimulation.

Sensory Stimulation.

1. Taste. Sensitivity decreases with age with the loss of taste buds. There are increased perception of bitterness and decreased perception of sweet and salty. Artificial sweeteners may taste more bitter.

2. Tactile sensation. Sensitivity to touch decreases with age; this may create problems with manipulating small objects and performing activities such as reading braille printing. There may be a delayed reaction time in withdrawing from hot or cold objects and less awareness of irritations to skin areas which may cause damage, such as when poorly fitting shoes create blisters.

3. Smell. This sense seems to remain fairly stable with age. Some women note a decrease in smell after

menopause. Estrogen may be related to increased olfactory acuity.

4. Sense of balance. Sudden movement of the head may lead to dizziness in some elderly individuals due to changes in the inner ear.

5. Vision. There is a slow, gradual decrease in the ability to focus on close objects (*presbyopia*) and a gradual decrease in overall acuity. Contact lenses or glasses with bifocal visual areas are effective in correcting both problems. The ability to adapt to the dark decreases with age. Moving from bright light to a poorly lit room will result in a longer period of darkness for the elderly as their eyes slowly adjust. The pupil becomes smaller in diameter with age, so less light is admitted to the retina. Lumination requirements increase with age since the retina of people in their sixties only receives about one-third the light it received when they were twenty. There is also a loss of color discrimination, especially in the blue areas of the spectrum. The elderly often experience more problems with glare and will be more comfortable with sunglasses when in bright light. The elderly have a decrease in tear production and may become more sensitive to irritants in the air. Wearing contact lenses may be uncomfortable without artificial tear eyedrops. The most common eye disease in the elderly is *cataracts* where the lens of the eye becomes opaque and vision is gradually lost. Eye surgery to remove the lens is common. Thick glasses, contact lenses, or implanted replacement lenses are used to restore vision. Glaucoma is also common in the elderly and can be effectively treated when recognized early. Peripheral vision is lost first and should serve as a warning sign of this problem.

6. Hearing. There is a slow, gradual hearing loss beginning in the late thirties affecting both sexes. High-pitched sounds are lost sooner. With advancing age, ability to understand the spoken word is decreased, especially if other sounds are in competition. The female voice seems to remain easier to understand than a deeper male voice. Hearing aids will amplify the sound for the individual experiencing problems with diminished hearing. Devices on telephones and television sets can amplify sound so the individual can continue to use and enjoy them.

Physical Mobility Stimulation Needs

1. Nerve conduction velocity is decreased with age, which leads to slower reaction times. This results in a slower rate of performing motor activities.

2. The muscle mass of the body is decreased over time. This results in a gradual loss of strength, endurance, and agility. These changes may be minimal in a physically active person but quite noticeable in someone who is inactive.

3. *Osteoporosis* (loss of bone) is related to the aging process. The gradual loss of bone leads to increased risk of fractures since the bone is more fragile. Immobility increases the rate of bone loss, while weight-bearing activity, such as walking, decreases bone loss. The elderly person confined to a bed or wheelchair for any length of time will be especially likely to experience osteoporosis and related fractures with falls or trauma.

4. Inflammation or deterioration of the cartilage in the joints makes movement painful and increases the chance for fractures and deformities in the joint for some older people.

5. Older people may begin to have changes in their posture. *Kyphosis* is a gradual collapsing of the vertebrae in the spinal column. This slowly leads to a stooped posture with the head and neck forward, and the individual may appear to develop a humped back. Some people lean backward, especially when there is a fear of falling. This has been observed in people who spend much time in bed or slumped in a wheelchair. Other people may notice a slight decrease in height of about ½ inch with no other noticeable problems.

Sexual Needs and Sexuality. The elderly person's need to continue sexual activity and feel sexually attractive is often ignored. The thinking of many professionals specializing in human sexual needs is that people are sexual beings from the moment of conception until the moment of death. Both sexes continue to enjoy and need close physical relationships, long after reproductive ability is lost. "The most sexually disenfranchised members of our society are the permanent residents of nursing homes" (Siemans and Brandzel, 1982). Part of the problem relates to the attitudes of the staff who view sexual activity in the elderly as unnatural or inappropriate. They may fear reactions from family members of the residents if they discover "grandma" is sleeping with another resident. When an elderly married couple enters a nursing home, it is not uncommon to separate them and give them same-sex roommates. The problems of providing privacy are a major obstacle to close intimate relationships in any institutional setting. Some medications may decrease sexual ability and interest. Physical handicaps and discomforts may make sexual activity difficult without support and help from the nursing staff. A confused patient in a nursing home cannot be permitted to repeatedly upset or embarrass other residents. But the alert resident has a right to expect a professional attitude from the staff in regard to sexual needs and the need for close physical contact with another human being. Loss of one's sexual partner due to death is something most elderly people must face. The majority of elderly people (80 percent) remain independent and continue to enjoy close physical contact with a loved partner into their seventies, eighties, and nineties. See Chapter 27 for nursing interventions to assist patients with sexual need satisfaction.

Higher Level Needs

Safety and Security Needs. The physical safety needs of the elderly are associated with the individual's alterations in sensory and physical abilities. Accidents, especially falls, are among the top ten causes of death in the elderly. Periodic examinations for vision and hearing may lessen or correct problems before they become dangerous. When working with elderly patients, make sure glasses, hearing aids, walkers, and other aids are in good repair and are being used by the patient if they are needed. Make sure lighting is adequate, especially at night. Keep bathrooms well lit at all times, and make sure hand rails are safe and installed where necessary. When elderly people are taking medication, make sure they can follow the directions, open the cap, read the label, and understand any special precautions or potential side effects. If the nurse finds that an individual patient has several different medications with different physicians' names on the label, a check with the pharmacy is in order to find out if there are any potentially dangerous drug interactions.

Psychological security in the elderly can be severely jeopardized. People who are forced to move in with relatives or into a nursing home because of failing health face the loss of many of their possessions. They lose their home which is often full of memories and a place where they have felt safe and comfortable. They lose their privacy and quiet when institutional living becomes necessary. Loss of a marital partner through death can be a terribly frightening event. Now one person must perform all the activities associated with maintaining a home, instead of two. The elderly in a nursing home, hospital, or at home may be unable to meet their religious and spiritual needs, and this can affect their feelings of well-being. Depression and suicide are not uncommon in the elderly when living becomes too painful, too frightening, or too lonely. Maintaining social contact with friends, relatives, and religious leaders can do a great deal to promote a feeling of security in older adults.

Love and Belonging Needs. The elderly are at risk for unmet needs related to feeling loved and belonging to a group or family of people who care about them. Loss of spouse and friends over time may leave the person of advanced years feeling very alone. If these lost relation-

ships are not replaced by new friends and by contact with children and new grandchildren, the problem of social isolation grows. Family get-togethers, senior social activities, babysitting for grandchildren, and communicating with friends or relatives on the telephone—all help the older person feel loved and needed.

Hearing and vision losses, if uncorrected, can also make the elderly at risk for social isolation. Physical handicaps that limit mobility will add to feelings of isolation unless these people receive help in getting to social and family functions. See Chapter 29 for nursing interventions to assist patients in meeting their needs for love and belonging.

Self-Esteem Needs. As people age, their physical characteristics change. In a youth-oriented society, it is often difficult for people to accept these physical changes and still feel attractive. People continue to need to feel good about themselves as they are and not feel bitter or grieve lost physical attributes. An individual's self-esteem may interfere with obtaining bifocal glasses or hearing aids because they are related to aging. The elderly often feel young inside and have a hard time accepting the aging exterior. American society, as a whole, tends to devalue old age. People are retiring at earlier ages and may find they no longer feel useful or important. Decreasing strength may also conflict with the individual's self-image as a strong, robust person.

The elderly are often faced with increasing dependency on family and friends. This is a role reversal for most adults who are accustomed to caring for others. The grown child may become the "parent" by providing a home, food, transportation, and financial support to aging parents. This can have a negative effect on the value older people see in their lives if they do not feel they are contributing to the family. Sharing family costs, babysitting, and helping with household chores can make the older person feel needed and useful. The impact of institutionalization can be very difficult for

Table 14–2. **Common Stressors in Aging Adults**

Decreased physical attractiveness and ability
Fear of growing old
Retirement
Fear of helplessness or actual increasing dependency on others
Decreased sexual abilities or activity
Reduced financial resources
Giving up a long-time residence
Belief in negative stereotypes about aging and the elderly
Death of loved ones and close friends
Illness and debilitating disease
Becoming a grandparent for the first time

Table 14–3. Theories Related to Development During Older Adult Years

Erikson

Ego integrity versus despair	This relates to accepting one's life as valuable and appropriate. Despair is associated with dissatisfaction with one's life and a belief that it is too late to change. There is a greater fear of death among people who remain dissatisfied with the course of their life throughout their older adult years.

R. C. Peck

Ego differentiation versus work role preoccupation	Elderly persons who are retired from the occupation or profession that had occupied the major part of their time for several decades must find new activities for self-expression and continued productivity. New interests are needed to replace the gap left by retirement, if individuals are to feel useful and valued by themselves and by society.
Body transcendence versus body preoccupation	The elderly person is frequently confronted with major and minor physical discomforts and changes as part of the aging process. The task in old age is to focus on the positive aspects of one's life and the abilities one still has rather than the losses. Enjoying life while remaining as active as possible in spite of physical changes is viewed as a healthier approach to aging then dwelling on physical problems and limiting activity and social interaction.
Ego transcendence versus ego preoccupation	The adjustment to this final task involves a recognition and acceptance that life is finite. Rather than dwelling on death, the individual continues to be involved with life and the lives of those who will continue living.

Duvall—Developmental Task Related to Older Adults

Developing a belief system that helps the individual face aging and death with a sense of peace
Maintaining values and beliefs in spite of life's disappointments
Maintaining cognitive abilities
Maintaining an enjoyable relationship with one's spouse
Maintaining relationships with adult children
Developing relationships with grandchildren and new members of the extended family
Maintaining relationships with people outside the family
Remaining socially active
Adjusting to a reduced income in retirement
Adjusting to decreased physical abilities
Adjusting to loss of spouse and finding alternate sources for receiving affection
Accepting help from others, when necessary, with a positive attitude

Hurlock/Havinghurst

Adjusting to decreasing physical strength and health
Adjusting to retirement and reduced income
Adjusting to death of spouse
Establishing satisfactory physical living arrangements
Adopting and adapting social roles in a flexible way

the elderly. Loss of bodily functions and ability to perform even simple tasks unassisted can give the individual a sense of personal failure and worthlessness.

Factors associated with high morale in the elderly include adequate financial resources, high educational level, and involvement in valued groups or organizations. A life of varied activities, in which the individual receives recognition as a valuable member, improves the self-esteem of elderly people and helps to protect them from depression and social isolation.

Self-Actualization Needs. The need to continue to grow intellectually, creatively, and emotionally is apparent in the elderly. In fact, continued striving and interaction with people and the environment seem to keep people healthy. Retirement offers a time to develop talents that may have been dormant during the years when the breadwinner or childrearing roles were most important. The elderly are a great resource for the entire community, and their talents and time can benefit all. The leaders of many countries are well past retirement age, as are many artists, writers, physicians, actors, and reli-gious leaders. These people continue to change and develop as they remain actively involved in various aspects of life. Illness, handicaps, and physical discomforts do not remove the need for self-actualization in the affected elderly population; they only make it more difficult.

Table 14–2 is a summary of common problems encountered by aging adults. Table 14–3 presents some theories on development in the older adult and associated developmental tasks.

Summary

The actual cause of aging remains a mystery, but several theories are discussed. The number of people over age 65 years is increasing and they are predicted to become a larger percentage of the total population in the future, increasing from 4 percent in 1900 to an estimated 17 percent in 2030. This means that nurses will be working with more patients in their later years. An understanding of physical and psychosocial changes encountered by people in this stage of life will help the nurse better meet patients' individual needs.

Many physiological need levels decrease with age, such as caloric needs, total oxygen used, and the amount of sleep needed. Many other needs remain constant, but the ability to meet the need decreases, such as with oxygen, stimulation, and mobility.

Some people are active and vigorous their entire life while others prefer a more sedentary, reflective life-style in retirement. Many people never retire. For most, the changes imposed by retirement in the middle to late sixties require the individual to reassess personal life events and plan activities to occupy the mind and body for the next decade or more. Loss of work-related activities and relationships, declining physical strength and abilities, and death of friends and family can lead to depression and possibly suicide if higher level needs remain acutely unmet.

Involving patients in group activities and enabling them to be as physically active as possible decrease social isolation and often improve patients' self-concept. Nurses play a vital role in helping elderly patients meet physiological and higher level needs and helping family and other health professionals understand the special needs of the elderly.

Terms for Review

| cataracts | kyphosis | osteoporosis |

Learning Activities

1. Visit a nursing home and observe the residents in the lobby. What physical changes do you notice? Are personnel attentive to their patients' needs for temperature maintenance, nutrition, fluids, and elimination? Talk with the patients about their concerns when they entered the nursing home and could no longer manage independently. What possessions could they bring with them? Did they have a loved pet they could not bring with them? What would they change about the care facility? What would they leave the same?
2. Talk with staff in a nursing home about their feelings about caring for older adults and common problems they encounter in the patients. Contrast the attitudes of aides to those of nurses. Contrast the attitudes of young care-givers with middle-aged and older-aged care-givers. What physical safety modifications have been made in bathrooms, on stairs, and in the halls?
3. Talk with an elderly person who is still active and independent. What does that person do to maintain physical health, financial independence, and social interaction? What major stressors has that person encountered with advanced age? Has that person successfully dealt with some of the developmental tasks associated with older adults?

Review Questions

1. Oxygen needs may be decreased in the older adult for which of the following reasons?
   a. Decreased basal metabolic rate
   b. Increased blood volume
   c. Continuation of physical activities on a daily basis
   d. Increased blood pressure

2. The elderly person is at risk for developing hypothermia. All of the following are reasons for this *except*
   a. Decreased sensory perception to cold
   b. Increased ability to respond to cold with vasoconstriction of the blood vessels near the body's surface
   c. Decreased ability to shiver in response to cold
   d. Decreased metabolic rate
3. True or False
   _____ a. The need for close physical contact with another person decreases with age.
   _____ b. The majority of people over 80 years old are residents of nursing homes.
   _____ c. Loss of hearing, if uncorrected, can predispose the individual to feelings of social isolation.
   _____ d. It often takes elderly people longer to fall asleep compared to their younger years.
4. What is the best preventive teaching a nurse can offer a healthy person entering the older adult phase of life?
   a. Activity should be reduced along with decreased caloric and fluid intake.
   b. A gradual daily program of exercise does a great deal to minimize many of the health problems that develop with aging.
   c. Working at a strenuous job such as a construction worker, physician, or nurse can be dangerous after age 65 years and should be discontinued.
   d. Walking five miles each day will prevent changes associated with aging.

Answers

1. a
2. b
3. a. F
   b. F
   c. T
   d. T
4. b

CHAPTER 15
DYING AND DEATH

Dying as the Final Phase of Life
Defining Death
Causes of Cellular Death

Physiological Needs and Nursing Implications
Higher Level Needs and Nursing Implications
Physical Changes with Death

Objectives

1. Describe your feelings about working with a dying patient and the family.
2. Identify several causes of cellular death and compare cellular death to total body death.
3. Describe how various age groups generally conceive of death.
4. Describe changes in physiological need satisfaction as death becomes imminent.
5. Identify nursing activities to assist the dying patient with unmet needs.

6. Describe changes associated with terminal illness and dying that jeopardize higher level need satisfaction.
7. Describe the stages of dying as identified by Kübler-Ross and responsive nursing care.
8. Describe the physical changes just before and after death.
9. Perform postmortem care of the body as guided by the institution in which nursing care is given.

Dying as the Final Phase of Life

Dying is the final phase of life. It is a certainty for every living creature from the moment of conception. The dying individual may not be in familiar surroundings since many people do not die in their homes. However, no person should be allowed to die alone unless it is a personal choice. Most people are not familiar with dying and death. Unfamiliarity with this aspect of life may make caring for the dying patient a frightening experience for the student in nursing. It is sometimes difficult for people to confront their own mortality, and this is what happens when nurses care for dying patients. It can be even more distressing if the patient is close in age to the nursing student. It may be easier for a young person to work with an elderly patient, who is in the process of dying, compared to giving care to a dying young person. This is not to say that one life is more valuable than another but that the closeness in age makes the identification more likely and makes the care-giver more vulnerable to the loss. Nurses who are parents often feel great empathy for the parents of dying children, to the

point that they may be unable to give support to the family. People born in the 1980s have a life expectancy in the middle seventies, and there is a tendency to feel cheated by life if those years are taken away because of illness or accidents. Many people are gamblers and risk-takers and think they can beat the odds and live on into their eighties or nineties. When newborns, infants, and young children die, our grief is not only for the lost loved one but also for what might have been and the loss of the future. Death is usually unexpected in the young. In the elderly, death is expected within some fairly predictable time span and is anticipated by family and by the elderly person as a part of the life cycle.

Table 15-1 describes how various age groups view death. Table 15-2 identifies the leading causes of death in the United States.

Defining Death

Death occurs when the vital organs of the body are no longer able to function to meet our human survival

Table 15–1. **Understanding Death in Different Stages of Growth and Development**

STAGE OF DEVELOPMENT	UNDERSTANDING OF DEATH
Fetus-Infancy	No known understanding of death.
2–3 years old (toddler)	Does not understand the concept of death. Confuses it with sleep. Responds to lack of movement in dead animal rather than death. Does not fear death but reacts to physical discomforts and separation from parent if death occurs.
3–6 years old (preschool)	Beginning to understand the concept of death. Has some trouble accepting the permanence of death which may be related to television shows and cartoons where characters rarely die. The idea of being badly hurt is often associated with death rather than an illness. The child fears separation from parents in own death. The fear of being left alone, especially in a dark place, may be associated with dying. Children may believe that wanting to hurt someone or thinking about bad things happening to another person can cause another's death. As children reach the age of five or six years, they know that they will die some day.
6–12 years old (schoolage)	This age group has many spontaneous questions about death. There is a fear of painful medical procedures related to dying. This age group begins to view death as part of the life cycle and not a punishment or a result of violence.
12–18 years old (adolescent)	Feelings of omnipotence are common in this group. Their own mortality is rarely considered and, in fact, many behaviors seem to invite physical harm. Fear of death is related to fear of not becoming an adult.
20–65 years old (adult)	Death viewed as something in the distant future. People dying in this age group may feel cheated out of their remaining years. Concerns about leaving young families who are dependent on them is a common worry. The feeling of frustration from having succeeded with getting an education and establishing profession or occupation only to be cheated out of the rewards of enjoying success in retirement may also lead to anger.
65 years and beyond (elderly adult)	The elderly recognize that they are in the last phase of the life cycle. Elderly are more conscious of death since the longer one lives, the more friends and relatives one sees die. The elderly may see their coming death as part of an internal process which is natural and appropriate. The elderly often view themselves as having had a full life and recognize it will soon be their time to die.

needs for oxygen, nutrition, fluid, temperature maintenance, and elimination. The cells of the body gradually loose their ability to function and eventually die. When enough cells die within a particular organ or tissue, the function of that tissue or organ is lost. If it is an essential organ or tissue for meeting survival needs, the person will die if function cannot be restored or replaced.

Causes of Cellular Death

There are many specific causes for cellular damage and death, but most will fall into the following eight categories:

1. Hypoxia. Hypoxia is a condition in which there is inadequate oxygen, at the cellular level, to maintain life. Common causes are obstructed blood flow to an area, cardiac arrest, respiratory failure, and carbon monoxide or cyanide poisoning which interfere with the oxygen available to the body cells. Hypoxia is the most common cause of cell damage and death.

2. Physical injury. Physical injuries actually damage the structure of the cell. Examples are excessive heat and cold, mechanical injuries, and electrical injuries.

3. Radiation. Sunlight and x-ray and gamma rays are all forms of radiation capable of causing cellular damage and death. Radiation is used therapeutically to destroy the cells of malignant growths because more

Table 15–2. **Leading Causes of Death in the United States (1982) by Age (Rates per 100,000 population)**

	UNDER 1 YR	1–14	15–24	25–44	45–64	65–84	85 +
All causes	1,143.7	35.8	104.7	334.8	1,848.8	9,254.8	15,228.6
Diseases of the heart	19.8	1.2	2.9	49.4	632.7	3,968.4	7,473.2
Malignant neoplasms	2.2	3.7	6.5	58.5	622.2	2,065.1	1,598
Cerebrovascular diseases	3.8	0.2	1.0	10.2	81.4	873.9	2,056.4
Accidents	28.6	16.2	52.1	73.9	71.2	157.5	278.5
Chronic obstructive pulmonary disease and related conditions	2.2	0.2	0.6	2.1	50.9	367.9	281.4
Pneumonia and influenza	20.3	0.7	0.9	3.9	24.5	242.1	748.5
Diabetes mellitus	0.8	0.1	0.3	4.4	34.2	180.6	194.3
Suicide	--	0.3	12.5	32.0	38.5	36.4	17.2
Chronic liver disease and cirrhosis	1.1	0.1	0.2	14.3	60.8	69.9	14.3
Atherosclerosis	--	--	--	0.3	4.9	124.9	548.5
Homicides	2.7	1.4	13.9	30.3	17.8	9.0	6.1
Conditions originating in the perinatal period	565.9	0.2	--	--	--	0.1	--
Nephritis, nephrotic syndrome, and nephrosis (kidney diseases)	6.3	0.1	0.2	2.0	13.3	93.9	190.6
Congenital anomalies	241.1	2.8	1.4	2.4	2.9	7.6	4.1
Septicemia	7.4	0.2	0.2	1.2	9.3	55.9	104.3

Source: National Center for Health Statistics: *Monthly Vital Statistics Report*, Oct., 1983, Hyattsville, Md.

rapidly growing cells are most susceptible to damage by radiation. This is also why the unborn fetus is so susceptible to damage by x-rays.

4. Chemical injury. Contact with chemicals through direct application to the skin, inhalation, or ingestion can result in cell damage and death.

5. Biological agents. Biological agents are such things as viruses, bacteria, and parasites. These organisms are capable of reproduction and produce material that can cause cellular damage (toxins).

6. Genetic derangements. These are changes in the cell occurring with cell reproduction that are incompatible with life or jeopardize cell function. They are a major cause of spontaneous abortion.

7. Nutritional imbalances. The cellular environment is closely regulated to remain fairly stable during health. With major and minor chemical changes created by inappropriate nutrition, the cells' function is compromised and, if uncorrected, these imbalances can lead to death.

8. Inflammation and immune response. The normal responses designed to protect the body, at times, lead to its death. This is the case in severe allergic reactions to foods, drugs, or insect bites. Individuals' immune systems may develop antibodies to their own tissues and cause cellular death by attacking tissues as if they were invading viruses or bacteria.

The degree of cellular damage is related to the type of injurious agent, the duration of exposure, and the type of cells affected.

Physiological Needs and Nursing Implications

Oxygen Needs

1. Respirations become irregular and may be rapid or slow. The term "Cheyne-Stokes breathing" is used to describe respirations that are irregular with periods of apnea (no breathing). These may develop as a person nears death.

2. Peripheral circulation to the rest of the body gradually decreases and finally fails. Extremities feel cold and are inadequately perfused with blood. The heart and brain receive a blood supply longer than other parts of the body.

3. Mental alertness will be affected by the adequacy of oxygenated blood reaching the brain. Some patients remain completely alert while others are in a coma.

4. With peripheral circulation failure, the extremities appear mottled and lose sensation to all but pressure.

5. Blood pressure decreases as peripheral circulation fails. First systolic pressure drops (the top number), and then diastolic pressure drops (the bottom number).

6. The radial pulse (pulse at wrist) is weak and eventually lost. The apical pulse (over the heart) can usually be heard for a brief time after the radial pulse can no longer be palpated.

7. The patient may be restless due to hypoxia.

8. The pulse becomes weak and rapid; it may become irregular.

9. Secretions may accumulate in the esophagus and

trachea as the swallow and gag reflexes are lost; the patient will require suction to maintain patency of the airway. Elevating the head of the bed may ease respirations.

Elimination

1. Analgesics used to control pain in the dying patient may cause constipation.

2. There is a generalized decrease in muscle tone and peristalsis leading to both urine retention in the bladder and incontinence; incontinence of stool is related to relaxation of the sphincters in the rectum. Indwelling catheters may be necessary if urinary retention is present.

3. Decreased blood flow to the kidneys and eventual kidney failure will result in very low or no urine output.

4. Decreased oral intake contributes to constipation and low urine output.

5. With circulatory failure, there is often a drenching sweat, and the extremities cool.

Nutrition and Fluid Needs

1. There is a generalized decrease in peristalsis with resulting abdominal distention since fluids and food may not be emptying from the stomach.

2. Weight loss and general weakness may make it difficult for patients to keep their dentures in place. If they are loose fitting or beginning to obstruct breathing, they should be removed and kept in a safe place to prevent accidental breakage.

3. The mouth may be open with the patient breathing by mouth; lips may become very dry and need to be lubricated, and the mouth may need cleaning and moistening with wet swabs.

4. As death becomes imminent, the swallow and gag reflexes will be impaired or absent so fluids must be given very cautiously or the patient will choke and inhale the fluids into the lungs (aspirate).

5. An intravenous infusion may be used until death to maintain some degree of hydration and to serve as a route for analgesics.

6. Nausea and vomiting may occur.

7. Some patients experience hiccupping spells.

8. Weight loss is frequently associated with patients dying from terminal illness, since the body's nutritional needs are unmet.

Temperature Maintenance

1. The patient's extremities usually feel cold as peripheral circulation fails and blood flow is reduced to the arms and legs.

2. Patient's internal temperature is frequently elevated. The patient may be restless because of a feeling of excess heat; blankets and heavy covers may increase the patient's restlessness and discomfort, even though the extremities feel cold.

Stimulation Needs (Sensory)

1. Vision is gradually lost; the patient will turn toward light in the room or from the window; the blink reflex may be lost and eyes may appear to stare.

2. Hearing is believed to be the last sense to remain intact during the process of dying; speaking slowly, clearly, and in simple phrases increases the patient's understanding. Assume the patient hears and understands all that is said by people in the room

3. The sense of touch is diminished in the lower extremities first as circulation fails; sensations of the face are probably the longest lasting tactile awareness; lips may lose sensation and be difficult to move; speech may become difficult.

Mobility Needs.   Dying patients are often too weak to move and reposition themselves and will require gentle help in changing position every few hours. Pressure areas on the skin where bony areas of the body come in contact with the mattress are easily damaged because of weight loss and inadequate blood supply of oxygen and nutrients to the cells. An alternating pressure mattress (air mattress) may help relieve pressure areas on the skin to minimize damage.

Pain Avoidance

1. Sensation and perception of pain are gradually lost; patients near death seldom report feeling pain.

2. Pain medications should be given intravenously when peripheral circulation fails because medication will be poorly absorbed by intramuscular or subcutaneous routes.

3. Patients who are alone often experience more pain than when they are with someone. Spending time with the dying patient may reduce the fear of being alone and also provide some temporary diversion from physical discomfort.

Higher Level Needs and Nursing Implications

Safety and Security Needs.   The goal of nursing care for the dying patient is to make the patient as comfortable and alert as possible, while maintaining safety from further injuries as body systems gradually fail. Many patients are afraid of a painful death or of dying alone. Talking with patients about specific fears they have and what might be done to improve the problem can make them less anxious. Maintenance of some degree of hope without giving false reassurance is also important to many patients. Spiritual and religious needs are often of

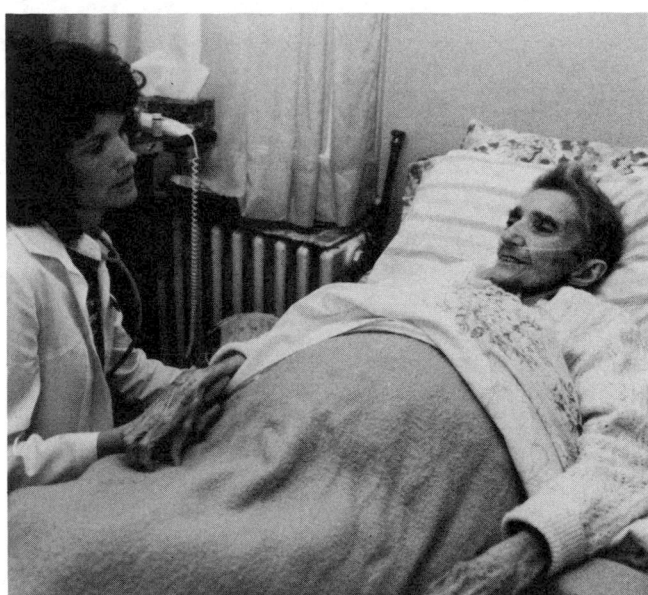

Figure 15-1. A visiting nurse with a patient who is dying in her home. (Courtesy of Fairview Hospitals Home Nursing Service, Minneapolis, MN.)

increasing importance to the dying patient. Continuing religious practices and talking with religious leaders can be very comforting to the patient and family. Most hospitals have ministers, priests, and rabbis available who will come to the patient's room as often as needed to meet religious and spiritual needs. Attending religious services may be important to the patient and the family, and such services are usually available within the hospital. Some people may panic when they are told they have a terminal illness and turn to alternate healing methods or suicide. Many people fear dying in the hospital and prefer the security and closeness with family that a home death offers. If a home death is chosen, families will need help in preparing the home for the dying patient and will usually need continued support and frequent home visits by the nurse during the dying process. (See Figure 15-1.) Planning how to handle problems before they arise can help the patient and family feel more secure in their ability to manage a death at home.

Love and Belonging Needs. Being with loved ones is usually very important to the dying person. People who are dying are facing the loss of all the people they love and will grieve the loss of these loved people and may continue to want close physical contact with another person. The feelings of loneliness and isolation are common to dying patients, and having one or two loved ones with the individual as death approaches is helpful in reducing these feelings of isolation. If family is not

available, it is often the nurse who stays with the patient as death occurs. The dying patient is still a composite of roles maintained during healthier times. Family, coworkers, and friends may all help to make patients feel that people continue to love and care about them. Flexible visiting hours, live-in arrangements for family, and remaining at home for as long as possible may help the patient meet love and belonging needs.

Self-Esteem Needs. The dying person has the same need as other people to maintain self-esteem. The dying person may be grieving the physical changes and losses associated with dying and ineffective medical treatments or surgeries. Patients' feelings of self-worth may come from the way the medical and nursing staff relate to them during the process of dying. It is often difficult to go into a dying patient's room to sit and talk or to give needed physical care. Health professionals may feel helpless to stop death, and this may also leave the health professional with a sense of failure. However, spending time with the patient and giving gentle, complete physical care as it is needed convey to patients that they are still respected and valued as living human beings. The increasing dependency that often accompanies dying can also negatively affect a person's self-esteem. Giving the patient all possible choices and abiding by the decision that each person makes leave the patient with more self-respect as a person still capable of making decisions and having some control of life. Helping the patient maintain optimum physical appearance may be helpful in promoting a patient's self-esteem. People relate to each other differently when they feel uncomfortable about their physical appearance. Assisting the patient with personal hygiene and cosmetic habits can make the dying person feel better about himself. Helping patients wear their own clothes or pajamas as long as possible may make them feel more at ease. Encouraging independence as long as possible gives the patient a further sense of personal control. Some patients may be very angry about their disease and the fact that they are dying. This may conflict with their spiritual beliefs and be difficult for the patient to express. Strong emotions of any kind may be in conflict with some people's self-concept, and expression of these emotions may be upsetting to the patient and the family. Elizabeth Kübler-Ross describes five stages that many people experience with death and dying. Progression through these stages is very individualized. Not all people pass through each stage or follow the same order. It may be comforting for a person to know that many people experience similar feelings when they are confronted with a terminal illness. These are described in Table 15-3.

The process of life review (Ramon, 1983) is offered by some nurses as a means for maintaining a patient's

Table 15–3. **Stages of Dying**

STAGES	NURSING CARE
Stage 1—Denial	
This is a stage of disbelief. Common when people first learn they are dying. May last until death or person may move on to next stage. Patient may talk about future plans, incorrect tests or diagnosis, or denial of symptoms. Patient may use denial in presence of family in an effort to protect them; may only be honest with nurse about seriousness of illness. "No, not me!" reaction.	Try to avoid directly contradicting the patient; find out what the patient and family were told. Maintain an open communication with the patient. Try not to avoid the patient. If the patient begins to talk in realistic terms about an illness, take time to listen. Reassuring the patient that everything will be all right is not helpful.
Stage 2—Anger	
Patients may be angry at God, at physicians, at the nurses and at family, or at themselves. The reaction here is "Why me!" Patient may revert to denial periodically.	Try not to take the patient's outbursts or criticism personally. The patient is angry about dying, not at you as a person or as a nurse. Try to maintain contact with patients rather than avoiding them.
Stage 3—Bargaining	
Patients realize that they are going to die but try to make a bargain for more time. Bargaining often done with God. Usually done privately and not discussed with others. Reaction is "Yes, me but. . . ."	The nurse cannot give the person the promise of extra time no matter how much this is wanted for the person. If the person shares the bargain with the nurse, listen without judging or falsely reassuring.
Stage 4—Depression	
Reaction is "Yes, me." Recognizes and accepts the closeness of own death. Patient often withdrawn and may be grieving the loss of loved ones, and of own existence.	Trying to cheer patients with comments about the good things in their lives or in the environment is usually inappropriate. Let the patient be upset. The dying person is about to lose all that has been important and loved. Try to be there if the patient needs to talk or cry.
Stage 5—Acceptance	
Reaction is "Yes, me and that's OK." Described as neither happy or sad, but separate from feelings. Often wants one other loved person to stay until death occurs—someone who is able to accept death for the other.	The patient has accepted death as inevitable, and the nurse who can do the same will be the one who can comfort the patient during the final moments. The nurse will also be supporting family members who may then be able to sit quietly with the patient and maintain physical contact until death.

Source: Elizabeth Kübler-Ross: *On Death and Dying*. Macmillan, New York, 1969.

self-esteem. *Life review* involves helping people examine the positive aspects of their life, while also identifying any unresolved conflicts that may still be troubling them so that some form of resolution can be achieved before death. It is believed that most people do some form of life review before death. If family is unable or unwilling to do this with the patient, the nurse may be able to help the patient with this activity. Life review is related to self-esteem and a need to feel comfortable with the course and outcome of one's life. Talking with patients during physical care or scheduling time for talking about the patient's life does not require a great deal of time and can be accomplished over several separate sessions. Active listening and good communication skills are important to nurses as they work with the dying patient and the family.

Exhibit 15-1 presents the dying person's bill of rights as a means of maintaining respect for the individual and assisting with meeting needs for self-esteem, safety and security, spirituality, love and belonging, and pain avoidance.

Self-Actualization. Many people are able to view death as a culmination of life and use this time for continued self-growth and maturation. The feelings and reactions of family, friends, and health care providers can facilitate this development or block it. People who die from causes that were sudden or unanticipated, are the least likely to be able to focus on their self-actualizing needs. Other needs are of greater priority and will occupy the patient's attention. The patient who is diagnosed as having a terminal illness has time before death to deal with other needs. The patient may want to accomplish something before death or participate in a valued endeavor such as medical research or doing something to help others with a similar terminal illness. The composer, Wagner, wrote a major composition for a full orchestra while terminally ill with leukemia. Many other people have continued cognitive, creative projects during terminal illness.

Exhibit 15-1. The Dying Person's Bill of Rights

I have the right to be treated as a living human being until death.

I have the right to maintain a sense of hopefulness, however changing its focus may be.

I have the right to be cared for by those who can maintain a sense of hopefulness, however changing this might be.

I have the right to express my feelings and emotions about my approaching death in my own way.

I have the right to participate in decisions concerning my care.

I have the right to expect continuing medical and nursing attention even though "cure" goals must be changed to "comfort" goals.

I have the right not to die alone.

I have the right to be free from pain.

I have the right to have my questions answered honestly.

I have the right not to be deceived.

I have the right to have help from and for my family in accepting my death.

I have the right to die in peace and dignity.

I have the right to retain my individuality and not be judged for my decisions which may be contrary to beliefs of others.

I have the right to discuss and enlarge my religious and/or spiritual experiences, whatever these may mean to others.

I have the right to expect that the sanctity of the human body will be respected after death.

I have the right to be cared for by caring, sensitive, knowledgeable people who will attempt to understand my needs and will be able to gain some satisfaction in helping me face death.

Source: Barbus, A. "The Dying Person's Bill of Rights." In H. Whitman and S. Lukes: Behavior modification for terminally ill patients. *Am. J. Nurs.,* **75**:98–101, 1975.

Physical Changes with Death

Shortly before death, the blood pressure is usually well below normal for the individual, respirations are very irregular, pulse is elevated, and temperature is often elevated. Respirations usually stop before heart contractions, but the heart stops within several minutes of respiration failure. The pupils become fixed and nonreactive to light. After death, the body begins to cool rapidly at first and reaches room temperature within 24 hours. This is called *algor mortis.* Immediately after death, there may be some jerky body muscle movement, but within several hours the muscles of the body go into a contracted state known as *rigor mortis.* This is caused by the lack of fuel (adenosine triphosphate, ATP) within the dead or dying cells of the body. ATP is needed for muscle cell relaxation. After the cells of the body die and decompose, they release enzymes that gradually destroy the fibers of tissue holding the muscles in the contracted state of rigor mortis and the muscles begin to relax. Rigor mortis has usually disappeared within 96 hours after death. After death, blood may settle in the lower (dependent) tissues such as the buttocks and back. A bruised appearance of the skin may result if the head and face are level with the rest of the body.

This is called postmortem hypostasis, and the resulting discoloration is known as *livor mortis*. Normal bacterial action within the body continues after death and gradually begins to soften and liquefy the cells of the body as decomposition occurs. Heat increases this process, and chemicals used in embalming stop it by destroying the bacteria within the body.

A flat (nonreactive) electroencephalogram (brain wave test for electrical activity) for 24 hours is also used as a sign of brain death in patients maintained on artificial life support for organ donor status.

Several nursing activities are based on the changes that occur after death. To prevent unusual muscle con-tractions and positioning after death, the nurse puts the patient in good body alignment, on the back (supine) with the head of the bed slightly elevated. This prevents livor mortis in the face and upper chest. The nurse will close the patient's eyes and mouth after death before rigor mortis sets in. These are done out of respect for the patient and for the culturally accepted appearance of the dead body with eyes and mouth closed. The appearance of the person in a normal, relaxed sleep state seems to be the goal of the mortician in our culture. It is toward this end that some of the immediate care of the body is aimed. (See Nursing Skill 15–1, Postmortem Care of the Body.)

Nursing Skill 15–1.   **Postmortem Care of the Body**

Preparation	Explanation
1. Rearrange work load as needed.	1. The nurse caring for the dead patient will have added time commitments with the patient's family, care of the body, and documentation in the chart, before transporting to the morgue. Other patients under this nurse's care may be neglected unless some of the work assignment is delegated to other capable people.
2. Notify appropriate people: Charge nurse Physician Clergy Morgue Family	2. Notification of the nurse in charge of the medical area, the physician, and the morgue is important so hospital personnel can do their jobs effectively. The charge nurse can help with reassigning the nurse's work load and assuring hospital policy is followed. The physician will pronounce the patient dead and identify whether an autopsy is desired. Care and notification of the family may be shared by the nurse, the physician, and the clergy.
3. Review the institution's policy on postmortem care.	3. Each institution may have slightly different ways of caring for the body; there may be differences within the institution, depending on the age of the patient and cause of death.
4. Talk with the family about their wishes to spend time with the deceased or help in preparing the body. Find out if the family wants any religious activities before transporting the patient to the morgue.	4. Some family may want to see, touch, and help in giving the final physical care. Offering the family some choices may help meet their needs. If the family feels the patient's religious needs were omitted, it can be a further source for distress.
5. Follow institutional policy for handling the patient's possessions. Have relatives sign for any possessions they take with them.	5. Possessions are very important to the family even when actual value may be minimal. Giving the patient's belongings to identified relatives and having them sign for what they received will eliminate confusion and provide documentation for the institution.
6. Consider any necessary precautions because of patient contamination if there was infection or isolation.	6. If the patient was infected, the organisms are still present and could infect other people coming in contact with the body.
7. Assemble equipment: clean gown, envelope for valuables, container for personal possessions, wash basin, towels, body wrap, masking tape, identification tags, and dressings for draining wounds left when and if tubes are removed.	7. Organizing what will be needed ahead of time saves time and energy. Going in and out of the room can be distressing to the family and other patients.
8. If deceased patient had a roommate, move that person to another room if possible.	8. The activities related to caring for the deceased patient may be very upsetting to another patient in the same room. It is also difficult to provide privacy for the family to be with the deceased with another patient in the room.

Procedure	Explanation
1. Provide privacy for the deceased.	1. Care of the body by not exposing the body to others is the last way the nurse can show respect. Other patients may also be upset by seeing a dead patient.
2. Remove any valuables and place in envelope and seal. If the family wants the patient to keep a ring on, secure it with tape or according to institutional policy.	2. Valuables removed by the nurse should be identified on the envelope and sealed so there is no opportunity for theft or loss. Valuables should be locked in a safe place, and this should be documented and signed in the patient's chart to protect the nurse.
3. Position the body in good alignment in the supine position with the head elevated slightly.	3. This will prevent possible problems with rigor mortis and livor mortis of the face and upper chest.
4. Close eyelids if open by placing fingertips over each lid for a few seconds and gradually closing the eyes.	4. When rigor mortis sets in, the eyes will be held open, and this is usually undesirable for an open-casket funeral.
5. Place dentures in patient's mouth if possible. Send with body to mortician if unable to put in the patient's mouth.	5. Without the teeth in place the patient will have a sunken, altered appearance. The teeth are in place for an open-casket funeral. Rigor mortis may make it difficult to position dentures if not done shortly after death.
6. Close patient's mouth if open by placing rolled towel under the chin.	6. The mouth is expected to be closed in death, and rigor mortis may make this difficult later.
7. Remove all tubes and drains as identified in policies for institution. Apply dressings if there is drainage.	7. This equipment is no longer needed and should be removed and disposed of appropriately.
8. Soiled areas of the patient's body are washed, hairpins are removed, and the hair is combed. A clean gown is put on the patient if family is to view body. Some institutions do not use a gown under the morgue wrap.	8. Prevention of contamination and damage to the body by sharp objects. If family views body before it goes to the morgue, a clean gown and combed hair convey respect and optimum care.
9. Place absorbent pad under buttocks.	9. Relaxation of sphincters may cause release of stool or urine.
10. Attach identification tag to body. Leave hospital ID band in place.	10. Loss of outside tag could cause confusion on patient's identity if no identification is on the body.
11. Wrap body as described for particular institution. (See Figure 15–2.)	11. This serves to protect the body and provide privacy.

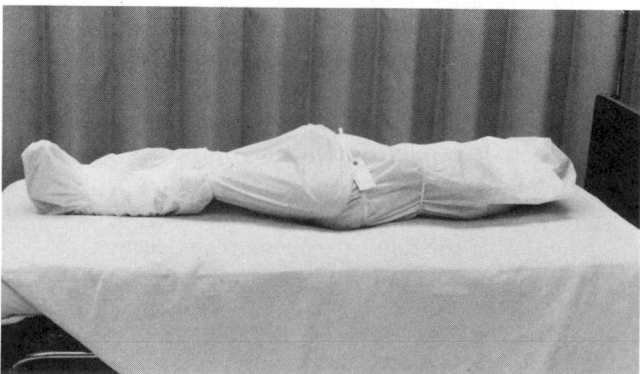

Figure 15–2. A postmortem body wrap with identifying tag.

12. Attach outside ID tag to wrapped body.

12. This is for ease in identification by the morgue and mortuary. Make sure both tags are identical to name on hospital ID band.

13. Pack all remaining personal belongings in a container for the relatives. Label accurately. Wash hands.

13. Patient's belongings can easily be forgotten if upset relatives collect them. Accurate labeling is helpful in getting the belongings to the right family members.

14. Arrange for transportation of the body to morgue or mortuary.

14. This avoids confusion for the relatives and assures that no one arrives to claim the body before the nurse and family are ready for it to be moved.

15. Document care given in the patient's chart.

15. Documentation allows others to know what was done to the body and with patient's possessions.

16. After body is transported, the unit is stripped of linen and utensils. Wash hands. Notify housekeeping or appropriate personnel that the room is ready to be cleaned.

16. This is done to protect other patients and cleaning personnel from possible contamination.

Summary

Dying is presented as the final phase of life in this chapter. The nurse working with the dying patient is confronted with the concept of personal mortality. Some nurses and students may find it very difficult to work with dying patients when "cure" is no longer the goal of medical care.

Until about ages three to six, children have a vague concept of death, often confusing it with sleep. It is difficult for children to understand the permanence of death in this culture. Fears of separation from parents and fear of pain and punishment are often associated with death for children. By age six and above, death is seen as a part of life. The adolescent may fear death because it will prevent attainment of adult status. Many young and middle-aged adults have not considered their own eventual mortality and view death or terminal illness as premature and unfair. Concern for families left behind who are still dependent on them is another problem to work through. The older adult recognizes and is dealing with the concept of death as friends or one's spouse dies.

There are several causes for cellular death, the most common being hypoxia. When enough individual cells die, tissues and organs lose function. When basic physiological needs are acutely unmet, the total body dies.

Physical changes associated with the physiological needs are discussed. Measures to ease discomfort are the primary focus for physical care of the dying. The higher level needs can be met as a patient dies. Attention to spiritual needs by referrals to hospital pastoral services may be helpful. No person should die alone unless it is a specific request. Family, religious counselors, or nurses can help reduce the fear of dying by staying with the patient. Even the patient who seems nonresponsive as death approaches may be aware that others are there, since hearing often remains functioning when other senses fail. Life review is offered as a technique to help patients assess their life and identify any last-minute actions needed to give them personal peace. Denial, anger, bargaining, depression, and acceptance are presented as states related to dying. All people may not pass through all stages but most will experience some of these stages identified by Kübler-Ross.

Postmortem care of the body following death is a skill presented in this chapter.

Terms for Review

algor mortis	death	livor mortis
Cheyne–Stokes respiration	life review	rigor mortis

Learning Activities

1. Visit the hospital morgue and watch an autopsy. Compare the appearance of a dead person in the morgue with the appearance of a dead person at funerals you have attended. Remember your first reactions when you saw a dead person. A negative reaction may have been based on inadequate preparation for what you would see. Prepare the family for what they will see if they view the patient after death has occurred.

2. Discuss with other students the following deaths and how you might react as a nurse caring for the patient and family:
   a. A full-term, physically perfect fetus is stillborn because of a knot in the umbilical cord.
   b. A child, two years old, dies of biliary atresia because a liver donor could not be found.
   c. A teenager dies of injuries received in a motorcycle accident.
   d. A young woman of 30 years dies of cancer, leaving a husband and two schoolage children.
   e. An 82-year-old man dies from injuries suffered in a farming accident, leaving his wife of 60 years alone on their family farm.

3. Discuss the self-assessment exercises related to this chapter with other students. Has experience with death altered people's feelings?

Review Questions

1. Which of the following is the most common cause for cell death?
   a. Radiation
   b. Hypoxia
   c. Physical damage
   d. Bacteria

2. A dying child, four years of age, would most likely have which of the following feelings related to death?
   a. Unable to understand death; no specific feelings
   b. Fear of not becoming an adult
   c. Concerns about how the family will manage after child's death
   d. Fear of being left alone and separated from parents
   e. Confuse death with sleep; no fear of death
3. As a person nears death, all of the following changes can be expected to occur *except*
   a. Decreased peripheral circulation to arms and legs
   b. Irregular respirations
   c. Decreasing blood pressure
   d. Excessive urine production
4. Which of the senses or abilities is believed to remain functioning the longest during the process of dying?
   a. Clear vision
   b. Hearing
   c. Tactile sensations in arms and legs
   d. Perception of pain
5. Which of the following nursing actions is designed to assist the dying patient meet individual needs?
   a. Life review
   b. Turning off all lights in the room
   c. Reducing family visiting times to five minutes each hour
   d. Leaving the patient in one position for six to eight hours to prevent unnecessary discomfort from turning

Answers

1. b
2. d
3. d
4. b
5. a

Individual Growth and Development—Self-Assessment (Chapters 11 through 15)

Presented below is a self-assessment tool based on developmental tasks from adolescence through later maturity. Select the response most representative of you and compare with tasks appropriate to your age grouping; more than one answer may apply.

1. a. I am trying to become more self-reliant and not count on my parents for all my financial needs, but they meet most of them now.
   b. I am beginning to assume almost all of my financial responsibilities and expect to be earning more soon.
   c. I am economically independent from parents, with resources expected to rise in the future.
   d. My financial resources are reduced and fixed, and I am no longer employed as I once was.
2. a. I have a well-established social network of friends.
   b. I am beginning to make intellectual, emotional, and social relationships with peers of both sexes.
   c. My close friends are only of one sex.
   d. I am losing some close relationships as friends die, but am making new ones among younger people and those my age with similar interests.
   e. I do not have time for any relationships.
3. a. I am making commitments to a career by employment in my chosen field.
   b. I am trying to decide what to do with my life.
   c. I am preparing for a career in a specific field.
   d. I am satisfied with my career as it has evolved.
   e. One aspect of my career is over, and I have chosen a new area for commitment.
4. a. I have a close, intimate relationship with a special person.
   b. I have sexual encounters but do not feel I have a close intimate relationship with a partner.
   c. I am adjusting to the death of my loved life partner.
   d. I see my life's partner as a unique person whom I enjoy being with.
5. a. I am actively dating.
   b. I have selected a mate.
   c. I have started a family and plan to add to it.
   d. I am busy rearing children.
   e. I am helping my children make and implement plans for future independence.
   f. All my children have left home and are independent.
6. a. I am adjusting to decreasing physical abilities.
   b. I feel I am just beginning to reach my full physical potential.
   c. I feel I am at my full physical potential.
   d. I have started to notice minor physical changes in my appearance which I associate with aging.
7. a. I have just registered to vote for the first time.
   b. I understand how officials are elected, and I know who my local representatives are.
   c. I vote regularly and am generally informed on major issues.
   d. I am just beginning to become involved in politics and civic issues.

Answers

The answers correspond to the age group for which the developmental task is appropriate. Remember developmental tasks are for people in general but cannot be applied to individuals as "right" or "wrong." It may be interesting to see how your chronological age matches some developmental tasks you identified as representative.

1. a. Adolescence, 12–20 years
   b. Young adult, 18–40 years
   c. Middle adult, 40–65 years
   d. Older adult, 65 and older
2. a. Young or middle adult, younger older adult
   b. Adolescent
   c. Adolescent
   d. Older adult
   e. Failure to attend to developmental task spanning all age groups in some form
3. a. Young adult
   b. Adolescent
   c. Adolescent
   d. Middle adult
   e. Older adult
4. a. Young, middle, and older adult
   b. Adolescent
   c. Older adult
   d. Middle and older adult
5. a. Adolescent
   b. Young adult
   c. Young adult
   d. Young and middle adult
   e. Middle adult
   f. Older adult
6. a. Older adult
   b. Adolescent
   c. Young adult
   d. Middle adult
7. a. Adolescent
   b. Adolescent
   c. Young, middle, and older adult
   d. Young adult

A person who is involved with very different developmental tasks from similar-aged people may feel more stress and find less support from friends and family. The student who is 50 years old and coming back to school may feel isolated from other students and also from long-standing friends who find the tasks of preparing for a career hard to understand at their stage of development. The very young 18-year-old student may also find older students have more life experiences and different outside interests.

The following two exercises deal with death and dying and your personal feelings.* Feelings about one's own mortality and working with dying patients can be

helpful to consider before actually working with patients and their families coping with death and dying. The following exercise may help you consider these issues. Sharing your feelings with other students with different life experiences may also be helpful.

Place a check after each statement that applies to you.

Personal Mortality

1. When I read statistics of traffic deaths, I think it unlikely that such a thing can happen to me. _____
2. I have never had someone close to me, of my own age, die. _____
3. I think that my death will be only a temporary separation from those I love. _____
4. Inside, I really believe that the secret of eternal life will one day be discovered. _____
5. I don't think much about death. _____
6. Of course, I know that all living things die. But if I take care of myself and avoid foolish risks, there's no reason to think about dying for a long, long time. _____
7. I think when a relatively young person gets sick and dies, there must have been something in his (or her) attitude and approach to life that made him (or her) susceptible to the disease. _____
8. It is impossible for anyone to accept the knowledge of his (or her) own death peacefully. _____
9. No one has a right to decide that at some arbitrary point it is useless to continue medical treatment. _____

How Do I Feel About Caring for a Dying Patient?

1. I expect to feel very uncomfortable when I talk to a dying patient. _____
2. I wish I knew what to say to a patient who knows he (or she) is dying. _____
3. I wouldn't want to be the one to tell a patient he (or she) is dying. _____
4. At the point when there's nothing more medical science can do for a patient, then the responsibility of the doctor and nurse is only to make him (or her) as comfortable as possible, physically. _____
5. I am frankly frightened at the thought of caring for a dying patient. I am afraid the patient will ask me if he (or she) is dying—or other questions about his (or her) condition that I am not supposed to answer. _____
6. I think I can help make a patient more comfortable with the fact of his (or her) death. _____
7. I worry that I will get too fond of a dying patient. _____
8. I can't imagine anyone ever being free of the fear of dying. _____

*C. Epstein: *Nursing the Dying Patient*. Reston Publishing Company, a Prentice-Hall Company, Reston, Va, 1975, pp. 13–16. Reprinted with permission.

9. I don't think a person should be told he (or she) is dying. There's no point in adding to his (or her) suffering. _____

10. I think people are most afraid of death when they are about my age than at any other age. _____

11. I don't think death should be discussed in front of children. _____

12. I must admit to a feeling of disgust at the thought of being around a person who is dying. _____

13. Being around a dying person would just keep reminding me that I will also die. _____

14. I think people can wish you dead. _____

15. Being around someone who is sick or dying would make me feel proud of my good physical condition. _____

Discuss your answers with those of another student with whom you feel comfortable. Compare your feelings to the dying patient's bill of rights in Chapter 15.

References and Bibliography (Chapters 11 through 15)

Beckwith, J.: Discussion of terminology and definition of sudden infant death syndrome. In Bergman, A., *et al.* (eds.): *Proceedings of the Second International Conference on Causes of Sudden Death in Infants.* University of Washington Press, Seattle, 1970.

Bodinski, L.: *The Nurse's Guide to Diet Therapy.* Wiley, New York, 1982.

Clemens, S.; Eigsti, D.; and McGuire, S.: *Comprehensive Family and Community Health Nursing.* McGraw-Hill, New York, 1981.

Corbett, J.: *Laboratory Tests in Nursing Practice.* Appleton, Englewood Cliffs, N.J., 1982.

Cultural Differences in Newborn Behavior. (Film) Pennsylvania State University, 1974.

Elhart, D.; Fersich, S.; Gragg, S.; and Rees, O.: *Scientific Principles in Nursing.* Mosby, St. Louis, 1978.

Epstein, C.: *Nursing the Dying Patient.* Reston Publishing Co., Reston, Va., 1975.

Erikson, E.: *Childhood and Society.* McLeod, New York, 1963.

Goffnett, C.: Your patients' dying—Now what? *Nursing 79,* 9(11):27, Nov., 1979.

Guyton, A.: *Textbook of Medical Physiology,* 6th ed. Saunders, Philadelphia, 1981.

Hale, M.: Better care for adolescents. *Contem. OB/GYN,* 21:150–75, 1983.

Havinghurst, R.: *Developmental Tasks and Education,* 3rd ed. Longman, New York, 1972.

Hill, P., and Humphrey, P.: *Human Growth and Development Throughout Life: A Nursing Perspective.* Wiley, New York, 1982.

Humphrey, P.: Weight/height disproportion in elementary school children. *J. School Health,* **49**:25–29, 1979.

Hurlock, E.: *Child Development,* 3rd ed. McGraw-Hill, New York, 1956.

Kandzari, J., and Howard, J.: *The Well Family: A Developmental Approach to Assessment.* Little Brown, Boston, 1981.

Kozier, B., and Erb, G.: *Techniques in Clinical Nursing.* Addison-Wesley, Menlo Park, Ca. 1982.

Kübler-Ross, E.: *On Death and Dying.* Macmillan, New York, 1969.

Lincoln, R.; Jaffee, F.; and Ambrose, L.: *11 Million Teenagers.* Alan Guttmacher Institute, Planned Parenthood of America, New York, 1976.

National Institute on Alcohol Abuse and Alcoholism: *Alcohol and Health.* HEW, Washington, D.C., 1975.

Nursing 77 Skillbook: *Dealing with Death and Dying.* Intermed Communications, Jenkintown, Pa., 1976.

Olds, S.; London, M.; Ladwig, P.; and Davidson, S.: *Obstetric Nursing.* Addison-Wesley, Reading, Mass. 1980.

Papalia, D., Olds, S.: *A Child's World—Infancy Through Adolescence.* McGraw-Hill, New York, 1975.

Peck, R.: Psychological developments in the second half of life. In *Middle Age and Aging.* University of Chicago Press, Chicago, 1968.

Pelliteri, A.: *Maternal-Newborn Nursing.* Little Brown, Boston, 1981.

Pozos, R., and Born, D.: *Hypothermia—Causes, Effects, Prevention.* New Century, Piscataway, N.J., 1982.

Rachal, J. et al.: *A National Survey of Adolescent Drinking Behavior, Attitudes and Correlates.* National Institute of Alcohol Abuse and Alcoholism, HEW, Washington, D.C., April, 1975.

Rambo, B., and Wood, L.: *Nursing Skills for Clinical Practice.* Saunders, Philadelphia, 1982.

Ramon, P.: The final task-life review for the dying. *Nursing 83,* pp. 44–49, Feb., 1983.

Ramsey, J.: *Basic Pathophysiology. Modern Stress and the Disease Process.* Addison-Wesley, Reading, Mass., 1982.

Sanfilippo, J.: Meeting the unique needs of teenage patients. *Contem. OB/GYN.* 21:177–92, 1983.

Siemens, S, and Brandzel, R.: *Sexuality—Nursing Assessment and Intervention.* Lippincott, Philadelphia, 1982.

Tilkian, S.; Conover, M.; and Tilkian, A.: *Clinical Implications of Laboratory Tests,* 2nd ed. Mosby, St. Louis, 1979.

Trafford, A.: America's $39 billion heart business. *U.S. News and World Report,* p. 53, March 15, 1982.

Tyler, L., and Josimovich, J.: Contraception in teenagers, *Clin. Obstet. Gynecol,* 20:651, 1977.

Vander, A.; Sherman, J.; and Luiciano, D.: *Human Physiology—The Mechanisms of Body Function* 3rd ed. McGraw-Hill, New York, 1980

Whaley, L., Wong, D.: *Essentials of Pediatric Nursing.* Mosby, St. Louis, 1982.

Yurick, A.; Robb, S.; Spier, B. and Ebert, N.: *The Aged Person and the Nursing Process.* Norwalk, Ct., 1980.

GROWTH AND DEVELOPMENT OF FAMILIES*

Objectives

1. Define family structure, developmental task, family life cycle, family crisis, developmental crisis, and situational crisis.

2. List the eight stages of the family life cycle.

3. Compare and contrast situational and developmental crises.

4. Use a family diagram as a basis for family assessment.

5. Differentiate family-centered nursing activities from individual-centered nursing activities.

6. Define the purpose of the family conference and when it is most appropriately used.

7. Identify the goals of family-centered nursing care and apply them to a case situation.

8. Explain the interrelationships among crisis events, family resources, and family perception of crisis event(s) and the outcome to the family.

9. Explain why nursing care can be part of the crisis prevention in illness situations.

10. Identify means to develop self-awareness and clarify one's own values about family living and related issues.

Introduction

The family in our society, as in most societies, is the institution responsible for the physical, emotional, and social support of its members—especially the very young. Without basic nurturance by caring adults, the newborn will not thrive. In most Western societies, individuals typically live in two different families during their lives. The first is the family into which they are born, called the *family of orientation*. The second is the one created when they marry or form a significant and lasting bond with another adult, called the *family of*

---

*Written by Barbara J. Leonard a Pediatric Nurse Practitioner with experience in pediatric neurology. She is currently an Assistant Professor in maternal child health in the School of Public Health at the University of Minnesota. She currently heads the childhood chronic illness curriculum within that program.

procreation. Most individuals requiring nursing services will be part of one of these two types of families. An individual's need for family support varies with age and health status. For the very young, very old, and the infirm, family support is critical. Typically, nursing care is approached from the perspective of the individual patient. Although short-term goals may be achieved, long-term goals may fail if the family is not considered the basic unit of nursing care. For example, an otherwise healthy infant who is failing to thrive due to parental neglect will make remarkable progress in the hospital environment. However, the infant will not maintain progress if the family unit is unable to provide care. In other words, the family environment must be made suitable for the care of an infant. This means intense work with the parents. The focus of nursing care in this example is the family which includes the parents as well as the child.

Nurses hold a privileged position in our society in that they have contact with people at critical transition points in their lives—birth, illness, and death. Together with physicians and clergy, nurses share this strategic position. Nurses are in a place to enhance the lives of others. People in transitions and crisis are more vulnerable to education and learning than those who are not. Even in very tragic situations such as the loss of a child, the nurse who takes a family perspective can help the family cope with their loss, grieve, and move on to enriched living (Martinson, 1980).

This chapter will focus on (1) the family as it is defined in our society, (2) the growth and development of families, (3) the effects of illness on family function and structure, (4) family support systems, (5) family-centered nursing care, and (6) self-assessment considerations.

The Family Defined

Culture and Family Structure

The family is defined as two or more persons related by marriage, blood, birth, or adoption (Duvall, 1977). The family form is determined by the culture of a particular society. The culture's values, traditions, and historical perspective prescribe family form. Worldwide, three family forms dominate. These forms follow the pattern of the marital bond. (1) The *nuclear family* is one husband and wife and their children which is based on a monogamous marital union. (2) *Polygamous families* are many husbands and/or wives and their children which derive from one of three types of polygamous marital types—one male and several females, polygyny; one female and several males, polyandry; and many males and many females, group marriage. (3) The *extended family* is either a nuclear or polygamous family extended to include the parental generation and sometimes relatives such as aunts and uncles (Reiss, 1980). Polygyny accounts for about 75 percent of marital unions in the world. About 24 percent are monogamous, and 1 percent is polyandrous (Reiss, 1980).

The monogamous type of family structure is typical in the United States. The extended family structure was characteristic of the rural American family in the last century. Later, the two-generation household with extended family nearby was typical in urban communities. The nuclear family became more prominent when grandparents and other relatives moved away.

According to Dempsey (1981), the following seven family structures appear today in the United States. They are nuclear intact family—husband, wife, and offspring in an intact household (28 percent); nuclear dyad—husband and wife living alone without children (13 percent); single-parent household (18 percent); remarried nuclear family, parents previously married (15 percent); the kin family—unmarried relatives living together or in close proximity to one another (21 percent); and experimental families—group marriage, living together (5 percent). Thus, family form or structure is shaped by the marital bond which, in turn, is determined by the culture, its traditions, values, and moment in history. Great variety in structure is the norm in this society today.

The Family as a Social System

The family, regardless of its form, is conceptualized as a social system. The family as a unit is made up of individuals who play certain roles within the family which contribute to the system's functioning as a whole. These roles, guided by culturally prescribed norms, are made up of specific tasks and responsibilities. In the nuclear family, for example, the husband-father role may be assigned the task of provider. The mother role may be comprised of child and household care tasks. The exact roles with their specific tasks are determined by the family with its unique values and traditions derived from its cultural group. Ten years ago, the wife-mother stayed home and cared for young children, while the husband-father assumed the provider role exclusively. Today, about 50 percent of mothers with children under 18 years of age work, assuming a provider role in their family units (Dempsey, 1981). The provider task is split or shared by the two adult members of the family unit. In past generations, it was not at all uncommon to find the oldest male child assuming a provider role with the father (Bane, 1976). Although the structure of the family unit may vary, as well as the role assignment of members, *family functions* (the expected tasks assigned by the larger society) must be carried out.

Family Functions

Duvall (1977) defines family functions as what a family does to meet the needs of its members, to survive, and to make a contribution to the larger society. There are eight basic tasks of the American family life: (1) providing for the basic necessities of life—food, clothing, and shelter; (2) meeting costs and allocating resources such as time, space, facilities in accordance to each member's needs; (3) determining who does what to support, manage, and care for the home and the members; (4) socializing each member through the internalization of mature roles within the family and beyond; (5) establishing ways of interacting, communicating, giving affection, expressing aggression, and sexuality within limits acceptable to society: (6) bearing and rearing children; (7) cooperating with other institutions such as church, work, and school, and establishing roles for the inclusion of inlaws, relatives, guests, friends, mass media into the family unit; (8) maintaining family morale and motivation, rewarding achievement, meeting personal and family crises, setting attainable goals, and developing family loyalties and values.

The family in American society is charged and expected to transmit the culture from generation to generation. This is an exceedingly complex task in a pluralistic society.

The Growth and Development of Families

Family Life Cycle

The family may be conceived as having a life cycle of its own, analogous to the life cycle of individuals. The family life cycle is a sequence of characteristic stages beginning with the formation of the family and proceeding through the life of the family until it dissolves. Each of these stages is said to have its unique tasks which must be resolved in order for the family unit to move forward successfully. Just as the individual must acquire intellectual and social skills, a family must develop specific skills in order to grow and develop. The family enters a new stage of the family life cycle when the first child enters a new developmental phase. The child's development causes the family to adapt its patterns of living together. Typically, the family with a child entering formal education must learn ways to interact with another highly complex social institution, the educational institution, so that the child acquires the skills necessary for success in our society. Likewise, a family with early adolescents needs to renegotiate family roles and responsibilities. Successive life-cycle stages require family members to acquire new skills and patterns of coping, as well as adapting old patterns of behavior.

The family life cycle typically has eight distinct stages: (1) the married couple without children; (2) childbearing families, the oldest child not older than 30 months; (3) families with preschool children, the oldest child not older than six years; (4) families with schoolchildren, the oldest child not older than 13 years; (5) families with adolescents, the oldest child under 20 years of age; (6) families with young adults; the launching family is one in which the children are young adults, and the family stays in this stage from the time the first child enters it until the last one is launched; (7) the middle-aged parents alone again; and (8) the aging family from the time of retirement to the death of both spouses (Duvall, 1977).

Developmental Tasks. The new skills and patterns of interaction required by each succeeding stage in the family life cycle are called developmental tasks. They are tasks occurring in families as a result of the oldest child's individual development, causing the family to learn new skills. The developmental tasks are expected in the natural order and are, therefore, typical for all families with children. The term *developmental crisis* is often applied to these tasks which underscores the critical nature of the tasks. A developmental crisis implies that a family is at a transition point in its developmental path requiring members to learn new ways of coping. For example, the family with its first infant is and has been described as being in a developmental crisis (LeMaster, 1957). New parents must quickly learn to nurture the newborn, not only acquiring the skills necessary to care for the baby but also adjusting their ways of relating to each other with their work environments and extended family. The new role must be learned and some old tasks discarded, shared, or exchanged. A new mother may have to quit working, leaving the father as sole provider for the family unit. The developmental crisis is the result of the rapid change necessary to meet the urgent needs of the young.

Developmental Crises Versus Situational Crises. Unlike developmental crises, situational crises are not expected events. Examples of situational crises are serious illness in a family member, divorce or separation of marital partners, unemployment of the provider(s), a premature death of a family member, or adding a family member such as an elderly parent to the family unit. As with developmental crises, family members must learn to cope with the problem. Initially, they will use old patterns of coping. When they find these patterns ineffective, it is hoped they will develop new coping strategies.

Crises are either developmental (predictable developmental tasks) or situational (events that are unexpected within the usual course of the family life cycle). The family crisis model was first described by Hill *et al.* (1970). They asserted that a particular event may or may not produce a crisis for a family. Whether it did or did not depended upon the interaction of several factors. For example, unemployment of a provider in one family may be very disruptive, while in another it would be considered a minor inconvenience. This would depend upon the circumstances of the family at the time of the unemployment. Thus, the event interacts with the family's crisis-meeting resources and their ability to perceive the event in a healthy perspective.

Crisis Events

Crisis events can be divided into two types—those that are external to the family and those that are internal. The external events include natural disasters, war, economic recession and so forth. These events, although very difficult for families to withstand, may be less destructive than internal crisis events. Internal family crises include events such as unwanted pregnancy, imprisonment, divorce, separation, desertion, death by suicide, mental illness, alcoholism. These events are not only disruptive, but they carry negative social sanctions as well. Consider, for example, the disruption caused in an Orthodox Jewish family when the father-provider loses his job for sexual harassment. This family must cope not only with loss of the provider but also with the accompanying social disgrace in their community. Thus, some internal family crises are disruptive because of negative social sanctions.

Family Crisis-Meeting Resources

Family crisis-meeting resources are all those things that the family brings to bear on the events that befall them (Duvall, 1977). (1) Past experience with events of a similar nature may provide an "immunity effect" for the family. This can be observed in families who seem to function well in spite of tragedy. Older people who have lost loved ones and have experienced grief develop strength to deal with subsequent losses and eventually their own deaths. (2) Commitment to the family is another crisis-meeting resource. (3) Family togetherness, referred to as family cohesion, is another resource which has been shown to be associated with families that cope well. (4) Flexibility of the family unit is associated with successful resolution of crisis events. The flexible family is a resilient family. An example would be a mother who is able to return to work, assuming the provider role, when her husband is found to have a serious illness. The mother's ability to earn money helps the family avoid further losses. (5) A family's ability to use resources outside the nuclear family and in the community is also adaptive. Thus, past experience and successful coping with crisis events, commitment to the unit, cohesion, role flexibility, and outside resources are some of the factors that enable families to cope successfully with crisis events.

Family Perception of the Problem

The family's crisis-meeting resources interact with their perception of the problem to give definition to the event. Whether or not the event is perceived as a crisis is determined by the family's definition of the event. The ability to reframe an event in a positive perspective is a highly adaptive mechanism. For example, divorce is generally considered a very disruptive event for all family members. However, the parent who sees the divorce as an opportunity for growth will be better able to avoid the negative impact of the situation. Another example is the birth of a child with Down's syndrome, which in some families becomes an opportunity for growth. Thus, for many families the ability to reframe a situation into positive terms will enable them to cope with the problem successfully.

Although the nature of an event is important in producing stress in a family unit, it, alone, is insufficient to produce crisis. Crisis is the result of family resources being overwhelmed, negative perception of the situation, and inadequate outside support. In other words, the crisis event interacts with a family's crisis-meeting resources and its perception of the stressor event. Families particularly vulnerable to crises and subsequent disruption are those families with few or poorly developed crisis-meeting resources, few outside supporters or services, and a negative perception or attitude toward their situation. The family unit may dissolve or continue in a marginally functional manner. In the case of the latter, the families are susceptible to stress and become "crisis-prone."

The Effect of Illness on Family Function

The impact of illness in one family member will affect all other family members to some extent. The specific illness (the nature of the illness itself, whether it is acute or chronic, and the degree to which it disables the ill individual) and the individual who is affected by the illness are factors to consider in predicting the impact of disease on a family unit. Each of these factors is considered separately even though they are interrelated.

The Nature of the Illness

Acute Illness.   The nature of an illness will influence the ill individual's coping behavior as well as that of other family members. An acute illness is usually of short duration, has few, if any, long-term effects, and involves specific treatment of short-term duration. In other words, acute illness, while often serious, is of relatively short duration and leaves little residual disability. The individual is disabled only a brief time, requiring minimal family adjustment. For example, a simple inguinal hernia in the husband-father has a very good prognosis for full recovery. The family is inconvenienced temporarily.

Chronic Illness.   Chronic illness is defined as an illness that lasts over three months (Ireys, 1981). It is usually characterized by permanency and requires long periods of treatment and rehabilitation. Approximately 15 percent of the child population from birth to 18 years of age has some form of chronic illness with a physiological basis (Ireys, 1981). Chronic illness in the adult population increases gradually until after 65 years of age. Almost all adults have at least one chronic health problem (Minnesota Dept. of Health, 1982). The degree of disability varies with the nature and stage of the chronic illness. In children, most (67 percent) will be mildly affected by their diseases. However, even mild disease in a developing child can cause serious academic and psychosocial consequences. Chronic illness requires adjustment in all areas of living. Likewise, family members must adapt to the chronically ill family member as well. The degree of family adjustment will depend upon the type of disease and roles played by the ill individual.

The Ill Individual, Family Roles, and Change

The typical nuclear family, comprised of husband-father, wife-mother, and children is organized to carry out the developmental tasks of that unit dependent on their particular stage of family life cycle. Chronic illness in one of the members has implications for all. Serious chronic illness in a parent may jeopardize a family's integrity as a unit. For example, a father who is seriously injured on the job, but who receives only minimal compensation, may increase the family's risk of being in crisis. If the father's disability is extensive, preventing him from caring for the children while his wife works, the unit may be very stressed. If the father was injured as a result of his own carelessness, family members may blame him; adding even greater stress to the unit. Older children may have to take on child care functions for the absent mother if she assumes the provider role for her husband. The children may receive less emotional support and environmental protection under these circumstances. Thus, it is very important for the nurse to consider the implications of the impact of illness, not only on the individual but on other family members. The nature of the disease is considered, as well as the individual who is ill and how the family compensates for role impairment or absence due to that individual's illness. Illness in an adult person who is also a husband-father or wife-mother has serious implications for the other family members. Chronic impairments in children, however, are not without their long-term implications for the integrity of the family unit. Cairns and Lansky (1980) found that parents of children with cancer had moderately disturbed marital relationships. Although they were not as disturbed as families in counseling for marital problems, they were more disturbed than families in the control group. Thus, illness, particularly chronic illness in one family member, will affect all members to some degree, dependent upon the roles played by the individual.

Family Crisis

Family crisis as the result of illness is dependent upon the above factors, as well as those discussed earlier in this chapter. Family cohesion, commitment to the family unit, flexibility of family members or the unit's adaptability, and their ability to use resources outside the family are all factors that mitigate against a crisis. Even if the family avoids a crisis, it will experience considerable stress as it adapts to illness in one of its members. It is not so much the disease itself (just as it was not the particular event so much) as the family's crisis-meeting resources coupled with their ability to "reframe" the event into manageable terms, if not positive terms, that determine the outcome or the impact of illness on the family unit. Families will need support, varying in kind and degree, which goes beyond caring for the individual during the acute phases of an illness if the unit is to effectively adjust to the illness in one of its members, especially if that illness is long-term or chronic in nature.

Consequently, a serious illness may have positive effects on a family unit also. The author's experience with chronically ill children has shown that many families view their child's disease as a learning experience. Although they will admit to the hardships imposed by the illness, they view the experience as having taught them to live better lives. They said that they were closer, valued each other more, and set better priorities for living (Leonard, 1983). These families were not the exception but the rule in the author's research and clinical practice.

Family-Centered Nursing

Family-centered nursing care is nursing care focused on the patient within the context of the family. The nursing process is based upon an understanding of the patient's family unit. Nursing assessment includes both the patient and the family. This is true of planning, implementing, and evaluating nursing care. In other words, the family is central to the nursing process. For example, a child with diabetes, aged ten years, is instructed in self-care. The child has to have a basic understanding of the disease, its treatment, and personal care. A ten-year-old child is dependent on the family for many aspects of care: diet, receiving medical care, and emotional support. The nurse assesses not only the child's needs but the family's as well. The child's well-being is in no small way determined by how well his parents and siblings adjust to his illness. Nursing care is focused on the family as well as the individual.

Implementation of Family-Centered Nursing Care

To implement family-centered care, the nurse has a working knowledge of family growth and development and is able to apply it to family situations. For example, the nurse anticipates the needs of the family whose oldest child (aged two years) is diagnosed as having acute lymphocytic leukemia. Without knowing the family, the nurse anticipates that they are relatively new parents and may be somewhat inexperienced in their parental roles. They may lack experience with illness of any kind and especially life-threatening illness. When meeting the family, the nurse modifies the anticipated perception with the actual concerns of the family. The nurse needs to be aware of the nature of family developmental crisis and situational crises, realizing that similar events may not produce the same results, dependent upon the unique circumstances of a specific family's resources and coping abilities.

The nurse will bring to nursing care of families a unique set of beliefs about family life based upon life experience. It is important to be aware of one's individual values and attitudes about family life. If, for example, the nurse does not believe that three generations should live in one household it is important that the individual nurse be aware of this and not pass judgment on patients who prefer this life-style. A nurse's values and biases, in other words, must be in awareness and not imposed unconsciously on patients. Because of the rapidly changing values regarding family life, sex roles, and sexuality today, widely divergent beliefs exist. Respect for beliefs and practices different from one's own is essential to family-centered nursing care.

To gain insight into one's beliefs and values, the nurse can participate in values-clarification exercises, discuss issues with colleagues, attend classes and workshops on the subject of values, and read professional literature. It is critical to call into question one's own belief system and be aware of the values held as important. Nurses may choose not to participate in the care of a particular patient if values are in conflict. For example, a nurse may withdraw from caring for a dying patient who is intentionally uninformed about the prognosis. It is preferable to withdraw and to allow someone else to care for a patient and family in such a case. It is unlikely that high-quality nursing care is provided when one's values are severely compromised. Communication with the patient and family is not effective, and emotional support would be difficult at best.

Skills Required for Family-Centered Nursing Care

Nursing care can be divided into three components: psychosocial care, physical care, and the coordination of care on behalf of the patient. All three of these components of nursing care can be further subdivided. For example, psychosocial care includes the education of the patient and family, provision of emotional support, assistance in problem-solving, and counseling. Physical care is subdivided into tasks which are typically carried out for medical professionals on their orders and those physical interventions that comfort the individual and promote health and healing. The third area of care is that based on the concept that nurses coordinate the care of other professionals in order to assist the patient and family. For example, the nurse might arrange to have social service personnel visit the patient and family to facilitate discharge planning. The nurse might also arrange to have the physician meet with the family to explain the implications of a new diagnosis. Nurses are commonly involved in helping to coordinate care for a patient with other institutions such as nursing homes, schools, and other treatment centers.

The degree to which a nurse emphasizes any one of these three components of care in practice is somewhat dependent on the employment setting. The coordination function, although part of all nursing practice regardless of setting, is integral to the practice of public health nurses and nurse practitioners. Physical care and direct psychosocial intervention is typical of nursing practice in the hospital setting. In each of these roles, however, the family is the focus of care. The salient skills required are identified below.

Communication.   The nurse must first identify the family member with whom to communicate. Responsible adults communicate directly with the nurse and family members are involved with the patient's permission. In the case of young children, or dependent adults such as those who are mentally ill or retarded, the nurse should establish an appropriate family member with whom to communicate. Although beyond the scope of this discussion, open communication is preferred in patient-family interactions. The nurse conveys a willingness to listen to patient/family concerns by setting aside time to answer questions and to listen to concerns. The nurse who is dealing with a number of family members must be very careful not to reveal confidences. To illustrate, a child is not told the diagnosis without the parents first being told and allowed time to decide how and when to tell the child. The nurse encourages family members to share their concerns and needs with each other, but they are not forced to do so.

Open communication requires specific skills. Listening is basic to good communication; following through on agreed assignments is also important, as is setting aside time to get to the heart of problems when appropriate.

Family Assessment.   The nurse collects information about the family in four general areas. The first is in the area of *family structure*—the organization of the family. The second is the interaction of the usual way family members exchange information and feelings. Third, the nurse is concerned with the family's relationship to the community, and fourth, the family's health behaviors (Green, 1982).

A convenient as well as nonthreatening way to begin assessment with a family is to use the family tree concept (see Figure 16–1). The family tree is a three-generational family diagram. Often, the family tree will appear in the individual's health (medical) records. When it does, it is used for nursing assessment. If not, the nurse generates a family tree by interviewing the patient, parent, or other responsible adult or family member. The family structure is immediately apparent as well as other health problems, such as diabetes. In Figure 16–1 observe that the parents are married, have the potential support of the father's family, and have experienced two deaths, one of them recently. The cause of death is also part of the tree. The stage in the family life cycle is observable. This family is entering the adolescent stage of the family life cycle, a major transition point. Using the family tree as a springboard for further assessment, the nurse can review the family's reactions to the major events in the family's past history. It is noted in the family in Figure 16–1 that the mother's mother had cancer. It is also noted that the mother is an only child. Perhaps she had difficulty coping with her own developmental needs and the health needs of her mother. It could be a fruitful area for discussion.

Apart from the family tree, the nurse will also note the education and occupation status of the family members, particularly the adult members. The parents depicted in Figure 16–1 are both providers. Thus, how they share household chores and what difference their child's illness will make in their roles, both as providers and as parents, can be discussed.

The nurse will also want to assess the family's ability to communicate. Are members open in sharing thoughts and feelings, or do they tend to withhold sensitive material? As the nurse is interviewing the family, they will give cues as to their usual ways of communicating with each other. For example, does one member do all the talking? How do others react to this person? Do they speak for themselves—express how they feel and what they think—or do they talk for each other without asking how the other person feels or thinks? Do they interrupt each other? Do they express conflict and disagree with each other comfortably or not?

The nurse also needs to assess family support. Does the family have relatives, neighbors, or friends upon whom they depend for emotional and other types of support? Is the family well integrated into their community, or are they relatively isolated? Families who have few support systems and are greatly stressed by an illness situation need professional intervention. The nurse discusses this with other members of the health team so that support can be built into the plan of care. For example, an elderly, frail widow was able to remain in her own home and neighborhood, even though she did not have family to help her, when the nurse was able to find

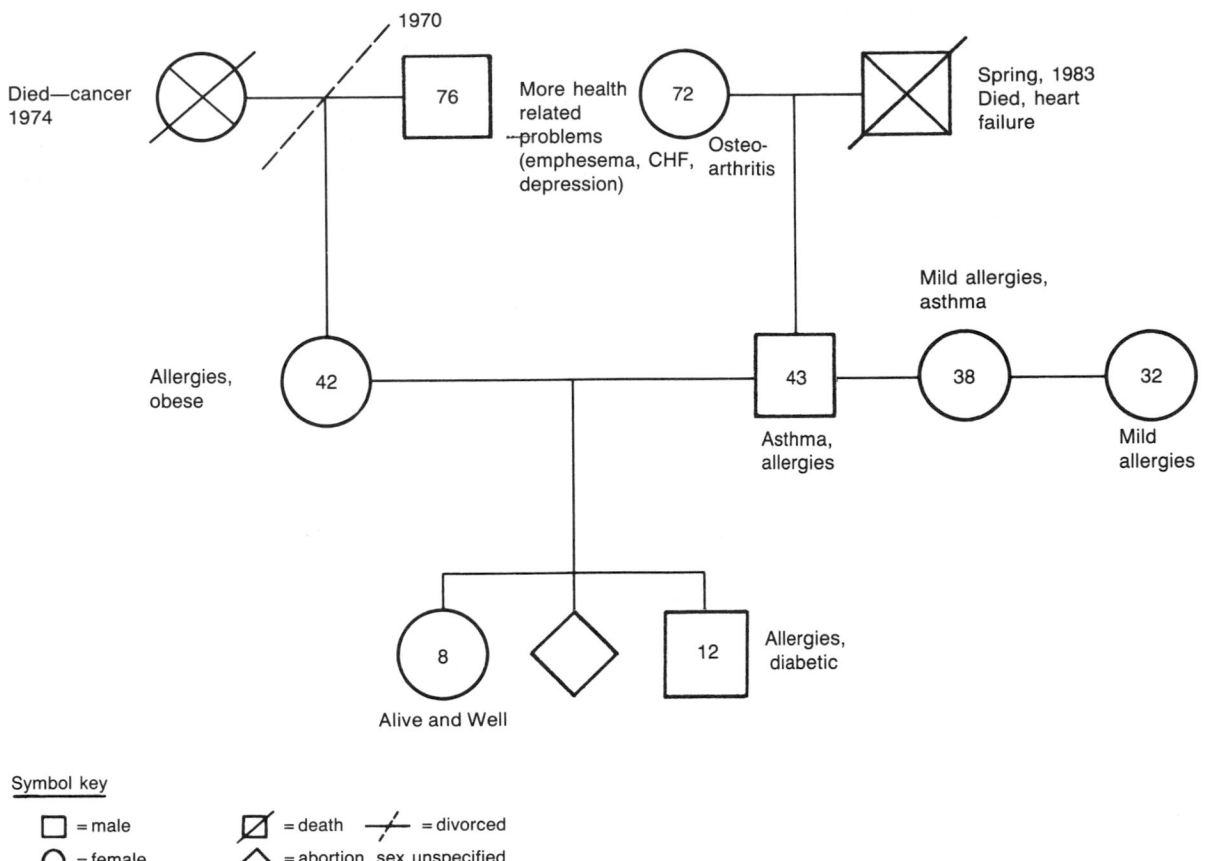

Died—cancer 1974

1970

76   More health related problems (emphesema, CHF, depression)

72   Osteo-arthritis

Spring, 1983 Died, heart failure

Mild allergies, asthma

Allergies, obese

42

43   Asthma, allergies

38

32   Mild allergies

8

12   Allergies, diabetic

Alive and Well

Symbol key

☐ = male   ◻ = death   ╱ = divorced
○ = female   ◇ = abortion, sex unspecified
☐─○ = mated, married   Numerals age in years

Figure 16–1. Family diagram.

neighbors who were willing to provide the care necessary to sustain her at home.

The final area of assessment is the understanding of the family's health beliefs and practices. The nurse needs to be aware of cultural differences with regard to such things as self-medication, perception of illness, diet, and perception of medical and health care providers.

These differences are considered before a plan of care is initiated, or misunderstanding can lead to undesirable results. For example, it is customary for certain Native Americans to assign the parent role to grandparents. If this is not understood by the health care provider, the parents may be perceived as negligent or irresponsible in caring for their children. An example of this occurred when the chief of a medical specialty service told a Native American grandmother the negative psychosocial consequences of her grandson's living with her. In fact, the grandmother was a competent, responsible person who was the child's greatest advocate. The child was thriving in her care. Rightly, the grandmother refused to return to the physician.

Thus, family-centered nursing care begins with as-

sessment of the family as well as the individual. Nursing care is based on the unique structure, communication, support systems, and health beliefs and practices of the individual family.

Nursing Goals and Objectives for Family-Centered Nursing Care of Families with Ill Members

Specific Nursing Goals. Although it is beyond the scope of this chapter to describe nursing interventions in detail, it is important to consider some guides for planning and intervention of family centered-nursing care. First, the nurse provides care that permits *the family to continue to carry out its functions as a unit*—its life cycle stage, appropriate developmental tasks. The nurse supports family members in making their own decisions and doing their own problem solving with regard to the care of the ill member. For example, the nurse supports a family's decision not to extend the life of a child with a fatal illness when further treatment would be painful and ineffective. In addition, the nurse will provide all necessary information and interpretation of nursing care and medical care so that families can make informed decisions about their ill members. Whenever possible, the nurse will inform family members as a group about critical changes in the course of their ill member's disease. Families are informed as units about such things as diagnosis, prognosis, and changes in the disease.

Second, the nurse attempts to *foster communication between and among family members*. Family members are encouraged to talk with each other and to share their feelings, when appropriate. The nurse respects the expression of feelings of family members and encourages appropriate action on the basis of those feelings. Third, the nurse *supports the family's unique cultural values and patterns of living*, except when these would compromise the health of the ill member or others.

Fourth, the nurse *encourages the family's care of the ill member throughout the patient's illness*, except when it would be harmful to the patient or the family member. The nurse not only encourages family members to care for their ill member but teaches them how to do so and supports their efforts. Even in the intensive care unit, new parents can be taught to care for some aspects of their baby's care. The nurses encourage increasing amounts of care until the parents are fully comfortable in caring for their newborn at discharge.

Specific Nursing Interventions. The nurse, as a matter of routine, plans nursing care with the patient and family. This is critical in the area of pediatrics. The parents are the child's source of emotional support and comfort, know the child best, and are able to give the staff suggestions. Nursing care is planned with family members whenever appropriate. This principle holds true for discharge planning as well. Family members are involved in this process, or it may not be successful. Family members who are confident in their abilities to care for the ill member in the home are going to need encouragement, instruction, and support. Martinson (1980) found that with these three ingredients family members were able to care for children dying with cancer. In fact, her research has changed the manner in which terminally ill children are cared for in this country. Instead of the child's dying in the hospital environment, the child is able to spend the last days of life in the care of family and friends. What was thought impossible ten years ago has become the norm for the care of dying children.

Family Conferences. The family conference is a cruicial part of nursing care and is an appropriate method of intervention at any phase of the care of a patient. The nurse or the family may initiate a conference. Generally, the nurse or another member of the health care team initiates the conference for the purpose of sharing new information about the patient's progress, for planning health care interventions or for decision making about a critical issue. Family conferences are appropriate at the beginning and ending of a patient's hospitalization, regardless of the degree of impairment. The members present vary with the family's wishes and the gravity of the situation. However, it is the author's experience and belief that children over six years find family conferences valuable if they are included in the discussion. Recently, children 9 and 12 were present for a family conference called by the family to discuss their grandfather's care. The decision to discontinue treatment was made with the physician's support amid tears. The children shared in an important part of the family's life and participated in his care until his death. They were present at his death which they accepted with amazing strength. No negative consequences of their experience occurred because of the support they received by the entire family. Thus, family conferences are an important means of sharing information with family members, as well as for mutual planning of nursing and medical care. Family members are able to rely upon each other for support when they receive bad news about a family member. The ability to share with one another helps them sustain themselves in times of tragedy.

Summary

This chapter has identified the family as the focus of nursing care. The family was defined, family structure related to the form of the marital bond, family developmental tasks defined and discussed, family functions listed, and situational and developmental crises identified and applied. Illness was viewed as a potential crisis event for a family. Interrelated factors, such as the family's crisis-meeting resources, their perception of the illness, and outside support and service, were discussed and applied to patient/family care situations. The goals of family-centered nursing were elaborated, and a guide for family assessment suggested. This chapter has emphasized the need for family-centered nursing care on the basis that nurses are in a position to enhance family well-being because of their strategic role in the lives of families. They are often present at birth, illness, terminal illness, and death—critical transition points in human lives.

Terms for Review

chronic illness	family-centered nursing care	family of orientation	polygamous family
developmental crisis	family crisis	family of procreation	roles
developmental tasks	family functions	family structure	situational crisis
extended family	family life cycle	nuclear family	

Self-Assessment

The following statements provide an opportunity for students to assess their own values and beliefs regarding family life and care of families. Read each statement and indicate whether you strongly agree, agree, disagree, or strongly disagree with the statement.

	Strongly Agree	Agree	Disagree	Strongly Agree
Women working outside the home has contributed to the breakdown of the family.	1	2	3	4
Physical punishment of children is an effective means of discipline.	1	2	3	4
Children whose parents divorce should go to the parent who is best able to provide financial support.	1	2	3	4
As a rule, grandparents should not live in the same household with their own children and grandchildren.	1	2	3	4
Fathers should not be given custody of children under the age of six years.	1	2	3	4
Teenage girls who bear children should be encouraged to live at home with their parents.	1	2	3	4
Children with terminal illness should be cared for in their own homes rather than in the hospital.	1	2	3	4
Infants with severe irreversible mental retardation and other handicaps should be allowed to die if their parents do not want to continue treatment.	1	2	3	4
Househusbands make inadequate male role models for their young male offspring.	1	2	3	4
Nurses should be able to refuse to care for patients whose families refuse to tell them they are dying.	1	2	3	4
A nurse who learns that a woman is beaten by her husband should keep that information out of the patient's record.	1	2	3	4
A homosexual couple should not be allowed to raise children.	1	2	3	4
Children need two married parents to develop normally.	1	2	3	4

Review Questions

True or False

_____ 1. Irrespective of one's own values, the nurse is obligated to care for a patient and family who unquestionably violate one's values.

_____ 2. The nuclear family, with mother in the home and father working outside the home, is the most common form of the family in the United States.

_____ 3. Crisis events that carry negative social sanctions are often more traumatic for families than those that do not.

Multiple Choice:

4. Family *structure* is determined by which one of the following:
   a. Family size
   b. Roles and tasks
   c. Marital form
   d. Economic status

5. The most common family structure in the United States in the last century (1800s) was which of the following:
   a. Polygamous
   b. Nuclear
   c. Kin
   d. Extended

6. Which of the following *best* describes a *developmental crisis*?
   a. An unexpected event occurring outside the usual time frame of the family life cycle
   b. A highly traumatic but anticipated event within the expected time frame
   c. An expected stressful event occurring within the usual sequence of life-cycle events
   d. A mildly stressful event which was unanticipated

7. Which of the following is a *family developmental task*?
   a. Coping with an unplanned pregnancy in a teenage daughter
   b. Preparing oneself as a parent for the children leaving
   c. Learning to live alone after divorce
   d. Institutionalizing a retarded adult child

8. The *impact* of illness in a family member on the family as a whole is dependent upon several interacting factors. Identify all that apply.
   a. Roles played by the ill member
   b. The flexibility of the family
   c. The nature and impact of the disease
   d. The level of family cohesion

9. The *family tree diagram* is useful for family assessment. The nurse is able to identify all *but one* of the following facts about a family from use of the family tree.
   a. Structure
   b. Occupation and educational status
   c. Illness of family members
   d. Number of family members

10. Family-centered nursing care includes which of the following activities:
    a. Education of new parents to care for a premature infant
    b. Identifying a drug treatment program for a young adult with an addiction problem
    c. Arranging for the public health nurse to care for an aged adult
    d. Meeting with family members to discuss a new diagnosis

Answers

True or False

1. False. If the nurse is not going to be as effective as needed for the welfare of the patient/family, he or she should decline caring for the patient/family unless it is an emergency situation.
2. False. This type of family is a mere 13 percent of families today.
3. True. Negative social sanctions add to the family's burden psychologically.

Multiple Choice

4. c
5. d
6. c
7. b
8. All apply
9. b
10. a, d

References and Bibliography

Bane, M.: *Here to Stay: American Families in the Twentieth Century.* Basic Books, New York, 1976.

Bertman, S.: Lingering terminal illness and the family: Insights from literature. *Fam. Process,* **19**:341–48, 1980.

Boyle, J.: The diminishing family and its impact on health (substitution resolution 55, I–81). A Report to the Board of Trustees of the American Medical Association, Chicago, Ill., 1983.

Cairns, N., and Lansky, S.: MMPI indicators of stress and marital discord among parents of children with chronic illness. *Death Educ.,* **4**:29–42, 1980.

Dempsey, J.: *The Family and Public Policy: The Issue of the 1980's.* Paul H. Brookes, Baltimore, 1981.

DeParra, M. L. V.: Changes in family structure after a renal transplant. *Fam. Process,* **21**:195–201, 1982.

Drotar, D.: Family oriented intervention with the dying adolescent. *J. Pediatr. Psychol.,* **2**:68–71, 1977.

Duvall, E.: *Marriage and Family Development.* Lippincott, Philadelphia, 1977.

Goldson, E.: The family care center. *Child. Today,* **10**:15–20, 1981.

Green, C.: Assessment of family stress. *J. Adv. Nurs.* **7**:11–17, 1982.

Grotberg, E.: Changing family structures and parental responsibility. ACYF, Department of Health and Human Services, Washington, D.C., 1978.

Hill, R., et al.: *Family Development in Three Generations.* Schenkman, Cambridge, Mass., 1970.

Ireys, H. Health care for chronically disabled children and their families. *In Better Health for Our Children: A National Strategy.* U.S. Dept. of Health and Human Services/Public Health Service, Washington, D.C., 1981.

LeMaster, E. E.: Parenthood as crisis. *Marr. Fam. Liv.,* **19**:352–55, 1957.

Leonard, B.: The psychosocial consequences on siblings of chronic illness in a brother or sister. A doctoral dissertation, University of Minnesota, 1983.

Martinson, I.: Impact of childhood cancer on the child and family. Final Report to the St. Paul Foundation, University of Minnesota, School of Nursing, March 1, 1980.

Minnesota Department of Health: *Healthy People: The Minnesota Experience.* Minnesota Center for Health Statistic, Minneapolis, 1982.

Montgomery, R.: Impact of institutional care policies on family integration. *Gerontologist,* **22**:54–58, 1982.

Reiss, I.: *Family Systems in America.* Holt, Rinehart and Winston, New York, 1980.

Selig, A., and Berdie, J.: Assessing families with a developmentally delayed handicapped child. *Dev. Behavior. Pediatr.,* **2**:151–54, 1981.

Spinetta, J.: Impact of cancer on the family. *Front. Radiat. Ther. Oncol.,* **16**:167–76, 1982.

Suelzle, M.: Changes in family support networks over the life cycle of mentally retarded persons. *Am. J. Ment. Defic.,* **86**:267–74, 1981.

White, M., and Dawson, C.: The impact of the at-risk infant on family solidarity. *Birth Defects* **27**:253–84, 1981.

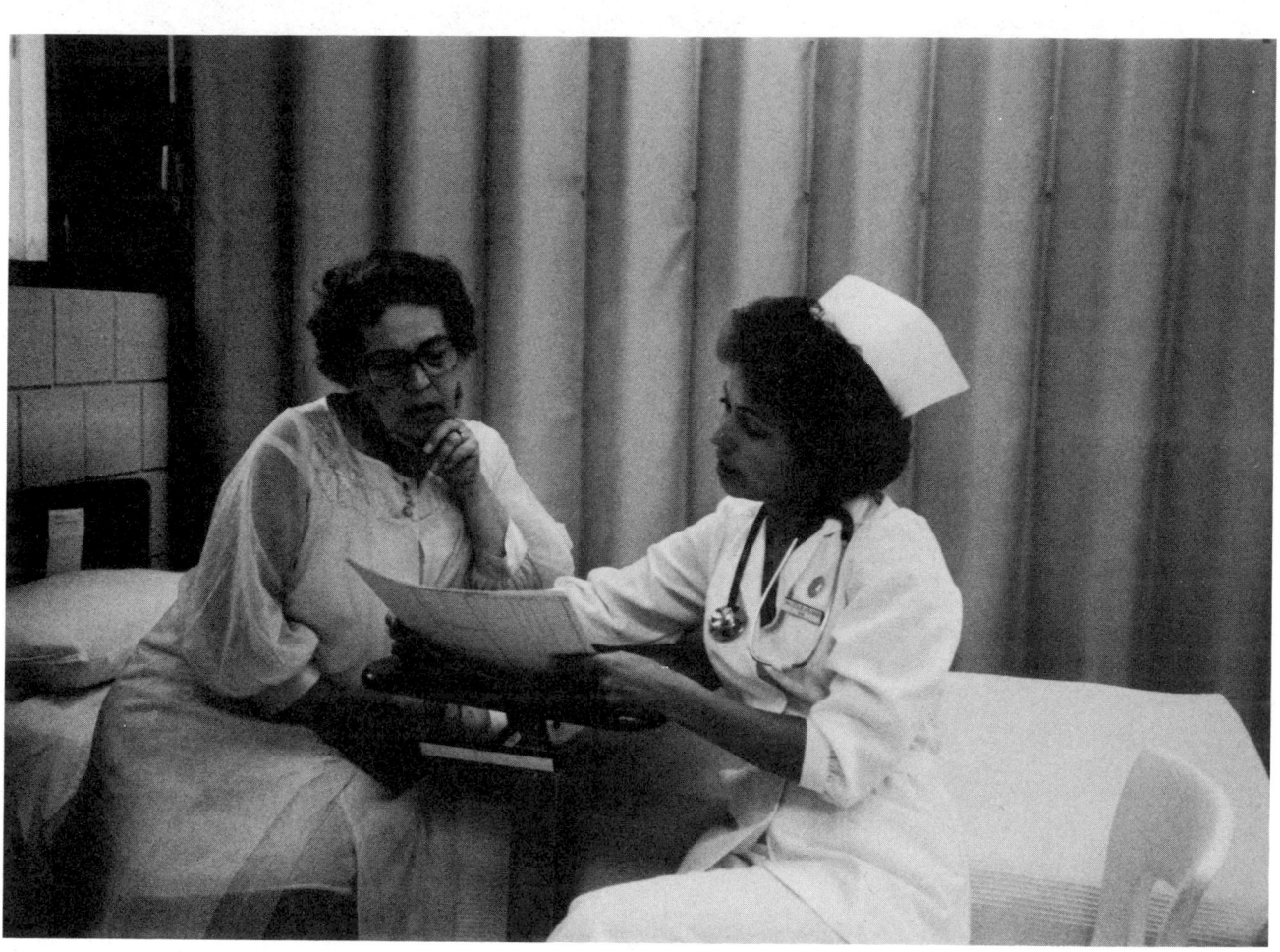

UNIT IV
THE NURSING PROCESS

THE NURSING PROCESS AND PATIENT CARE PLANNING

Objectives

1. Discuss the benefits to the nurse and to the patient of using the nursing process to plan nursing care.

2. Describe the four steps of the nursing process.

3. Describe the activities of the nurse in each of the four steps of the nursing process.

4. Define what is meant by the term "baseline data" and discuss the importance of such a data collection.

5. Contrast nursing diagnosis and medical diagnosis.

6. List guidelines for writing nursing diagnoses.

7. List guidelines for writing nursing goals.

8. Discuss some factors the nurse considers in setting priorities for patient care.

9. Discuss factors the nurse considers in selecting nursing actions for a particular patient.

10. Identify two factors the nurse considers in validating a care plan for a colleague.

Introduction to the Nursing Process

When nurses provide care for patients, they use a systematic, scientific approach. This approach is much like any problem-solving method which all individuals use daily. For example, consider a student nurse who has been ill for several days and has missed important nursing classes. First, the student attempts to figure out how much has been missed, what topics were covered, were there any tests given or announced. Then the student reviews all the information and decides that some of the missed work can be read independently, some notes can be borrowed, but one problem remains. An instructor gave a demonstration of giving insulin injections, and the student will need help learning this skill. The student wants to learn to give insulin injections safely and correctly. The student identifies the alternative methods of learning this skill as requesting a private session with the instructor to learn the skill, using videotapes in the library to learn the skill, or asking another student to teach the skill. The student decides that the first action is more likely to result in learning the skill correctly. The student then contacts the instructor, sets an appointment for the learning session, and later keeps the appointment. At the end of the session, the instructor evaluates the student's ability to do the procedure correctly. The instructor assures the student that the procedure is correct, but that additional practice is needed in order to perform the skill in a reasonable amount of time. In this example, the student is using the problem-solving process: collect information, clearly state the problem, consider alternative ways to solve the problem, choose one solution, try it out, judge its results, and try another alternative solution if the first was not successful.

The nursing process is much the same as the problem-solving process. Using the nursing process, the nurse collects relevant information related to the patient's health care needs, analyzes the data, and identifies problems. This is called the assessment phase. Next, the nurse determines what it is that the nurse hopes to be able to accomplish with the patient (goals). Then the nurse considers many nursing actions to resolve or reduce the problem, and selects those most likely to accomplish the desired results. This step is called planning. Finally, the nurse gives nursing care to the patient directed toward solving the identified problem. This step is called implementation. Last, the nurse makes a decision as to the achievement of the goals set during the planning phase. If the goals have not been accomplished or only minimally accomplished, the process may need to be reviewed and revised.

One outcome of the nursing process is a patient care plan. This is a written plan designed to reduce or eliminate one of several identified problems experienced by a particular patient. Each patient is expected to have a plan of care written by a registered nurse soon after admission to the hospital. All people caring for patients are expected to read and follow the plan of care, updating it as needed.

The Importance of the Nursing Process

The nursing process is an approach that can help ensure quality patient care. The nursing care is planned to meet the unique needs of the patient and is then written so all persons caring for the patient have access to the plan of care. Without this written plan of care, omissions and duplications begin to occur. In the absence of a written care plan, the patient must repeat personal information and preferences for each care-giver. With a written care plan, each nurse is able to provide care that incorporates the patient's individual preferences and needs. This helps to provide for continuity of nursing care. The American Nurses' Association's Standards of Nursing Practice reflect the use of the nursing process. (See Exhibit 17–1.)

Another benefit to the patient is participation in care. If the patient is able to work with the nurse to plan care, the patient gains experience in problem solving related to health care. Moreover, if patients are involved in developing care plans, they are more likely to be committed to the goals in the care plan.

In addition to the benefits for patients, the use of the nursing process has many benefits for the nurse. Perhaps the most important benefit is graduation from a school of nursing. Each type of nursing program has an expectation that the student can, at graduation, write a nursing care plan and think like a nurse, using the steps of the nursing process. In addition, the licensure examination for nurses in the United States is now organized around the activities of the nursing process. Thus, a knowledge of and ability to apply the nursing process are essential to a career as a nurse. Another accrediting agency, the Joint Commission for Accreditation of Hospitals, states:

> Standard IV: Individualized, goal directed nursing care shall be provided to patients through the use of the nursing process. . . . The nursing process (assessment, planning, intervention, evaluation) shall be documented for each hospitalized patient from admission through discharge. (Joint Commission, 1981)

The job satisfaction of the individual nurse is increased because there is no uncoordinated trial-and-error nursing. Well-written care plans also give the nurse confidence that nursing actions are based on correct identification of patient problems. A sense of pride and

Exhibit 17–1. **Standards of Nursing Practice**

Standard I

The collection of data about the health status of the client/patient is systematic and continuous. The data are accessible, communicated, and recorded.

Standard II

Nursing diagnoses are derived from health status data.

Standard III

The plan of nursing care inlcudes goals derived from the nursing diagnoses.

Standard IV

The plan of nursing care includes priorities and the prescribed nursing approaches or measures to achieve the goals derived from nursing diagnoses.

Standard V

Nursing actions provide for client/patient participation in health promotion, maintenance, and restoration.

Standard VI

The nursing actions assist the client/patient to maximize health capabilities.

Standard VII

The client/patient's progress or lack of progress toward goal achievement is determined by the client/patient and the nurse.

Standard VIII

The client/patient's progress or lack of progress toward goal achievement directs reassessment, reordering of priorities, new goal setting, and revision of the plan of nursing care.

Source: The American Nurses' Association, 1973. Reproduced with permission.

accomplishment is felt when the goals in a care plan are reached and the patient's problems are lessened.

The nursing process also contributes to the professional growth of the individual nurse. As the nurse completes the plan and is able to evaluate how effective it was in meeting the needs of an individual patient, the nurse learns additional skills which can be adapted to meet the needs of other patients in the future. As this learning continues from experience with many patients, the nurse gains skill and expertise.

Finally, a review of an existing care plan can also help the nurse in charge determine patient care assignments. Perhaps a nursing assistant is able to give the required care or perhaps the needs of the patient require the skill of the registered nurse. Perhaps a student nurse has the knowledge and experience to provide care for this patient. These decisions are based on the degree of skill required to carry out the activities in the patient's plan of care.

Beginning the Process

While almost all nursing students begin the process of writing care plans with less than rampant enthusiasm, all who become proficient in the skill agree that it was worth the time and effort. Using the nursing process to develop care plans is a skill, just like giving injections and bathing patients in bed. All of these skills take time and practice to develop. Initially, the written care plan will probably be lengthy in order to clarify the thought processes the student is using. The student may become discouraged and respond with some variation of the comment, "I know that staff nurses couldn't possibly use this. They don't have time to write all this." "Why am I learning this? I'll never use it when I get out of school!" Be assured that writing the long care plan

which demonstrates the use of the nursing process is an educational tool used to communicate between student and instructor. When the student is proficient in the use of the process, the lengthy written work is omitted and only a brief form is used. Patients whose conditions require complex nursing care may require long care plans. The point of using the nursing process is to provide the nurse with a pragmatic, practical tool to provide quality care.

Also be assured that no one has yet written the perfect nursing care plan! Although initial efforts may be a bit rough, the experience gained from writing one care plan can be used to improve the next.

Assessment

The assessment phase is the first step in the nursing process. It consists of three activities: data collection, data organization and analysis, and formulating nursing diagnoses. The thoroughness and skill of the nurse in this phase are crucial since they will determine the accuracy of the entire nursing care plan.

Data Collection

The nurse begins data collection at the first meeting with the patient and continues until the patient is discharged from care. All the additional data that the nurse learns about the patient in the course of providing care are incorporated into the care plan. Additions to the data base may necessitate additions or revisions to the care plan.

The nurse uses three methods to collect data: observation, interview, and examination. There are many sources of information available to the nurse. The patient is the primary source even if unable to communicate verbally. Perhaps the patient is able to communicate in writing or in sign language using an interpreter. The nurse collects data from an unconscious patient through the use of observation and physical examination. The nurse may also interview members of the patient's family or another primary group. In addition, the nurse may collect data from other members of the health team who are involved in the patient's care. Many nurses report that the men and women who clean patients' rooms are often very knowledgeable about patients' feelings. Nurse clinical specialists and more experienced staff nurses can often contribute to data collection. Professional journals and reference texts can also add to the data base.

All data collection results in data that are free of the judgments and conclusions of the nurse. This is not to say that nurses do not judge, evaluate, and draw conclusions. Certainly these processes are a part of the professional role of the nurse. However, during data collection, the nurse attempts to remain free of biases, open to all new input. In addition, data recorded as judgments and conclusions are highly individualized. A statement that the patient is "neatly groomed" or "experiencing moderate pain" may mean different things to each nurse. However, if the nurse notes that the patient "has hair combed, makeup applied, and is fully dressed," there is little confusion about the facts. Similarly, the data about pain are very clear when they are noted as, "I can't walk more than twenty feet without stopping because of the pain, but I have no pain when I am flat in bed." In addition, if the nurse has already made a judgment about some aspect of the patient's care during data collection, important data may be disregarded.

Both objective and subjective data are recorded without judgments or conclusions. Objective data (*signs*) are that information observed by the nurse that could be noted by any other observer. Subjective data (*symptoms*) are that information given verbally by the patient and not directly observable by the nurse. Table 17–1 gives examples of both types of data correctly noted without judgments or conclusions.

Finally, data collection is systematic, organized, and methodical. If it proceeds in a random fashion, the nurse may inadvertently omit important areas. The nurse may use a cephalocaudal (head-to-toe) approach or perhaps a body systems (respiratory, digestive, cardiovascular, etc.) approach, or a needs approach (oxygen, food, fluid, etc.). Whatever approach is selected, it is used simultaneously with the other activities of data collection: observation, interview, and examination.

It is important that the initial data collection of the nurse be complete and accurate. The first data collection is known as the baseline data and is the standard against which changes in the patient's condition are measured. For example, if the patient weighed 185 lb at the time of admission and one week later weighed 179 lb, the nurse notes a weight loss of 6 lbs. If this piece of data was omitted from the baseline data, it would not be possible to determine the weight loss for the week.

Observation. The process of observation begins with the first contact between the nurse and the patient and continues throughout the nurse-patient relationship. Observation is a high-level skill which requires a great deal of effort from the nurse. Observation continues throughout every activity the nurse does with the patient. Not only does the nurse observe verbal and nonverbal communication and the physical responses of the patient, but the nurse must be able to recall what has been seen and heard for accurate recordings in the chart. Frequently, beginning nursing students are concentrating so hard on the performance of a skill, such as taking a blood pressure, that they are unable to recall data once they have left the patient's room. For this reason, many nurses carry a small paper to promptly jot down a significant piece of information which they wish to be certain to include.

At other times, the data gathering will be structured by a form which the nurse will fill out in an interview with the patient. If the nurse does write in the presence

Table 17–1. **Examples of Data**

	DATA	JUDGMENTS AND CONCLUSIONS
Subjective	"I'm really feeling crummy. Nothing is going my way."	Patient is depressed
	"I've never had pain like this."	Patient complains of severe pain
	"Please, I'd like to be alone."	Patient angry and withdrawn
Objective	Three-inch diameter circle of red drainage through three 4 × 4 dressings at incision site	Moderate amount of red drainage
	Voided 300 ml light-amber, clear urine	Voiding OK
	Ate 120 ml orange juice, two toast, egg, and coffee	Ate well

of the patient, it should be explained to the patient so it does not become a secretive element that detracts from the nurse-patient relationship. The nurse may explain it by saying something like, "I'll just write down your blood pressure so I don't forget it. That's 176/72" or "Mr. Jones, I'll be filling out this record as we talk. It will help the nursing staff to plan care with you while you are in the hospital." At times, the nurse may either summarize what has been written for the patient or read back the notes for the patient's information or clarification. This open and honest approach enhances the nurse-patient relationship.

Interview. The interviewing process is both formal and informal. When the nurse meets the patient for the first time, the nurse initiates a formal interview during which the nurse seeks information to establish a nursing history. Unlike the medical history which focuses on disease and treatment, the *nursing history* focuses on the patient's perception of illness and the response of the patient to it. Prior to beginning the interview, the nurse provides as much privacy as possible for the patient. This may simply mean closing doors, or it may mean walking to a vacant lounge or office. The nurse selects a time for the interview when other people or duties are not likely to interrupt. An interview is begun with an introduction and a statement of purpose. The nurse may say something like, "Good evening Mrs. Jones. My name is Susan Keyes. I will be your primary nurse during your hospitalization. That means I will be responsible for the nursing care you receive while you are here. I'd like to ask you some questions about your health so I can work with you to plan nursing care. This should take about one-half hour. Are you comfortable? May I get you anything before I begin?"

In the example, the nurse has explained the use of the information, as well as assuring that the patient is comfortable prior to beginning. An opening question that is often helpful in beginning an interview is, "Mrs. Jones, can you tell me what brought you to the hospital?" The patient responds with an understanding of the illness as she defines it. Occasionally, a patient may respond by stating a medical diagnosis like, "I have a stomach ulcer." The nurse may respond to this by saying, "And what was that like for you?" Or "How did you know things were not right?" Or "How did you handle that?" Any of these responses or a similar remark will usually yield the patient's perception of the illness. Many hospitals or other agencies have developed a printed form to be followed for the nursing interview. Specialty areas dealing with particular types of problems such as sleep disorders or infertility problems will usually have their own unique forms. In using such forms, it is important that the nurse adapt it to the individual situation and put it into the nurse's own words. It is also important to maintain eye contact with the patient during the interview process.

When beginning the interview process, nursing students may feel that they are prying into personal matters. The patient has the right to refuse to answer any questions and know that this right will be respected. When patients do discuss personal information with the nurse, they can be assured that this information will be shared only with those in need of the information in order to provide care.

The nursing interview has three parts: beginning, working, termination. During the beginning phase, the nurse gives an introduction of self and a statement of purpose. The nurse also provides for patient comfort. In the second or working part of the interview, the nurse attempts to achieve the purpose of the interview. During termination, the nurse summarizes what was said in the interview. The nurse gives the patient an opportunity to provide clarification and ask questions. The nurse also thanks the patient, tells the patient of any scheduled procedures and assures the patient's comfort before leaving.

The informal interview process continues each time the nurse has contact with the patient. Experienced nurses often state that some of the best therapeutic conversation is conducted during the time the nurse bathes a patient. During this time, the patient is comfortable, relaxed, and has the undivided and uninterrupted attention of the nurse. A skilled nurse is able to give physical care while simultaneously focusing on what the patient is saying.

Examination. The nurse establishes a relationship with the patient whenever possible prior to any physical examination. But, carrying out a physical examination may also enhance a nurse-patient relationship. If the patient complains of abdominal pain and the nurse is able to skillfully palpate the abdomen, listen for bowel sounds, and ask questions seeking further information, the credibility of the nurse is increased in the eyes of the patient. The use of these skills also tells the patient that the nurse is taking the complaint seriously.

When the patient is admitted to the hospital, the nurse routinely performs a limited physical assessment of the patient. Any necessary equipment is brought to the room before the nurse begins. After handwashing, the nurse explains the content and purpose of the examination. Next, the nurse provides for the privacy of the patient. The door to the room is closed, and the curtains around the patient's bed are pulled. Depending on the extent of the examination, the nurse may offer the patient a hospital gown. In a systematic manner, the nurse then completes the examination. This will minimally include height and weight, temperature, pulse and respirations, heart and lung sounds, skin assessment, general appearance, and mobility limitations. Nurses with additional training in physical assessment may perform more extensive examinations. The data the nurse collects are recorded as objective data, clearly and concisely stated.

The data in Table 17–2 have been collected by the

Table 17–2. **Case Study—Mrs. L. Johnson**

DATA COLLECTION	DATA ORGANIZATION
1. 42-year-old female	*Growth and development*
2. Bank officer	1–3
3. Mother of 12-year-old (daughter) and 15-year-old (son)	*Maslow*
4. Married 20 years	Physical needs—6, 8–11, 15
5. Admitted 8/25 for gallbladder removal 8/27	Safety/security needs—12–14, 16
6. Height 5′6″, 140 lb, BP 126/84, T = 99° F, P = 80, R = 22	Love/belonging needs—3, 4, 7, 16
7. Older sister and parents living in city	Self-esteem needs
8. Intermittent pain on right side for several months following certain foods: pizza, cheese, ice cream, cheesecake, butter	Self-actualization needs—2
9. "I have lots of gas, several hours after eating."	
10. Two days ago had "excruciating pain" from right side to back and shoulder	
11. Nausea and vomiting past two days	
12. "I'm really scared. I haven't slept or eaten well since I decided to have the surgery."	
13. "I've never been in the hospital except for the birth of the children."	
14. "The anesthetic scares me most. What if I can't breathe with that mask over my mouth. Or what if I choke on the tube in my throat? Do people 'talk' when they are 'under'?"	
15. "I've never had an IV. Does it feel like a needle in your arm constantly?"	
16. "Can my husband stay with me until I have to go to surgery?"	

nurse admitting Mrs. L. Johnson. These data will be used throughout the chapter to illustrate the steps of the nursing process.

Analysis of Data

Having completed data collection, the nurse begins to analyze the data. One approach that has been helpful for many nurses is to use the basic needs of Maslow. This may be done by placing data about a particular need under the need category as in Table 17–2. Note that an additional category of growth and development has been added to accommodate the nurse's notation of data in this area. (Chapters 11 through 14 discuss growth and development.) Hospitalization may have an effect on growth and development. Some individuals regress (go backward) to an earlier level of development with the stress of hospitalization. This is frequently seen in children who are completely toilet-trained at home and during hospitalization begin to require diapers. An adolescent who demonstrates mature behavior at home may demand that "Mommy" stay at the bedside during hospitalization. The growth and development of other individuals may be arrested during hospitalization. This may not be significant if the illness is brief, but if the illness is lengthy, the problem may require nursing intervention. The nurse uses a knowledge of growth and development to assess the level of patient functioning and then compares them to chronological norms. Most often, the nurse encourages the patient to be as independent as possible in order to foster growth and development. Sometimes, however, it is necessary for the nurse to accept dependency to enable the patient to feel safe and secure in the hospital environment. Some adults express this need by requesting that "my nurse stay with me," by requesting a bed bath when they are capable of a shower, by the desire for an inflexible schedule. The nurse attempts to meet these needs in order to assist the patient to progress.

Using Maslow's categories of needs (food, fluid, oxygen, and so forth) also assists the nurse to identify omissions in data collection. For example, if all the data are in the physical need category, the nurse may need to review the content of the initial interview or perhaps spend more time with the patient in order to get to know the patient better. The data in a category may reveal either that a need is met or that a need is unmet. Consider the following examples:

Need for love and belonging

"I wish my wife could come but there is no one to stay with the children." (Data indicating unmet need.)

"The visit from my children really made me feel better. They are so thoughtful." (Data indicating need satisfaction.)

Need for safety and security

"I'm afraid to get out in winter. If I fell on the ice it would mean another broken hip." (Data indicating unmet need.)

"With my tripod cane and rubber-soled shoes, I'm pretty steady on my feet and able to get around easily." (Data indicating need satisfaction.)

Formulating Nursing Diagnoses

The formulation of nursing diagnoses is the final activity in the assessment step of the nursing process. A *nursing diagnosis* is a statement of a present or potential problem that requires nursing intervention in order to be resolved or lessened.

The nursing diagnosis must first be a patient problem. Either the nurse or the patient may define a problem. The patient may complain of pain, may state a fear of falling when walking, or may be unable to read the small-print labels on medicine bottles. This data would indicate problems defined by the patient. The nurse may note that the patient does not wash hands after using the toilet, that teeth brushing is inadequate, that only food of a soft texture is selected from a menu. All these observations may indicate a problem to the nurse, although further data are needed in each case.

Occasionally, the patient and the nurse may define a problem differently. For example, a patient who has experienced a heart attack may have an altered self-image which includes having total self-imposed activity restrictions and no sexual activity. The nurse may interpret the problem as a lack of knowledge about recovery from a heart attack and a problem that will require substantial teaching. The nurse listens to the data the patient reveals and bases the statement of the problem on this data. The problem stated in the nursing diagnosis can be either present or potential. A present problem is a current problem, it exists in the here and now for the patient. Examples of present problems are:

Bowel elimination: Constipation related to dietary intake

Alteration in comfort: Gas pain related to lack of peristalsis

Alteration in nutrition: Eats more than body requirements associated with depression

A potential problem refers to one that may cause difficulty for the patient in the future. The nurse who

Table 17–3. **Examples of Nursing Diagnoses**

PROBLEM	+	CAUSE IF KNOWN
Difficulty breathing		associated with increased secretions
Potential for skin breakdown		related to incontinence
Unable to feed self		related to right hemiparesis
Confusion		related to sensory deprivation
Frustration		associated with lack of independence in activities of daily living
Boredom		associated with prolonged traction
Potential for bladder infection		related to indwelling catheter
Anorexia (loss of appetite)		associated with medication therapy

has an understanding of physical and behavioral sciences is able to identify problems the patient is prone to develop in the future. By identifying potential problems, the nurse is able to plan nursing interventions to prevent the development of the problem or lessen its effects. Examples of potential nursing diagnoses include:

Potential impairment of skin integrity related to decreased circulation
Potential fluid volume deficit related to inadequate oral intake
Potential for injury related to unfamiliar hospital environment (patient is blind)

A tentative nursing diagnosis is written when the nurse has insufficient data to support a firm present or potential nursing diagnosis. Writing a tentative diagnosis helps to ensure that data collection continues with regard to a specific problem. With additional data, the nurse is able to eliminate the problem or further clarify the problem and establish a plan of care to resolve it. Tentative diagnoses are comparable to the physician trying to make a medical diagnosis when confronted by the possibility of two or three related diseases with similar symptoms. The physician may write: Rule out (R/O) myocardial infarction (MI) and then perform diagnostic tests to gather more data to prove or disprove the diagnosis. The nurse proceeds in the same manner. The nurse may write:

Possible lack of knowledge related to home care of juvenile diabetes (patient is a six-year-old child whose mother is also diabetic)
Possible altered self-concept related to loss of hair (patient is a teenager beginning cancer treatment which will result in the loss of hair)
Possible minimal self-esteem related to lack of muscular coordination associated with extreme obesity (patient is high-school student who is 25 percent overweight)

Writing Nursing Diagnoses

The use of the following formula will assist the nurse to write a nursing diagnosis:

Nursing diagnosis = Patient problem + Cause if known

Nothing else belongs in the nursing diagnosis. Table 17–3 gives examples of nursing diagnoses written using this formula. When beginning to write a nursing diagnosis, it may be helpful to identify the data upon which the

Table 17–4. **Example of Medical Diagnoses that Suggest Nursing Diagnoses**

MEDICAL DIAGNOSES	NURSING DIAGNOSES
Cholelithiasis	Abdominal pain associated with stones in the duct or gallbladder
Cerebrovascular accident	Unable to express self verbally related to cerebrovascular accident
Staphylococcus-infected incision	Loneliness related to isolation procedure
Fracture of the neck at C-7	Prone to decubiti related to immobility
Juvenile diabetes mellitus	Knowledge deficit related to diabetic diet

Table 17–5. **Guidelines for Writing Nursing Diagnoses**

1. Keep the nursing diagnosis brief.
2. Keep the nursing diagnosis specific.
3. Identify one problem in each nursing diagnosis.
4. Base the nursing diagnosis on the patient's data base.
5. Make sure that the problem is not the same as the cause. Example: Alteration in comfort associated with pain in the right hip. This is better stated: Alteration in comfort related to fracture of right hip.
6. Select problems that require nursing intervention rather than problems related to other areas, such as financial services or physical therapy.
7. State nursing diagnoses in a way that directs nursing interventions. For example, ''Sleep pattern disturbance related to hospitalization'' does not give direction to nursing care. The same problem stated, ''Sleep pattern disturbance related to disruption of home bedtime routine,'' gives a great deal of direction to nursing intervention.

Exhibit 17–2. **List of Nursing Diagnoses Accepted at The Fourth National Conference of North American Nursing Diagnosis Association**

- Airway clearance, Ineffective
- Bowel Elimination, Alterations in: Constipation
- Bowel Elimination, Alterations in: Diarrhea
- Bowel Elimination, Alterations in: Incontinence
- Breathing Patterns, Ineffective
- Cardiac Output, Alterations in: Decreased
- Comfort, Alterations in: Pain
- Communication, Impaired Verbal
- Coping, Ineffective Individual
- Coping, Ineffective Family: Compromised
- Coping, Ineffective Family: Disabling
- Coping, Family: Potential for Growth
- Diversional Activity, Deficit
- Fear
- Fluid Volume Deficit, Actual
- Fluid Volume Deficit, Potential
- Gas Exchange, Impaired
- Grieving, Anticipatory
- Grieving, Dysfunctional
- Home Maintenance Management, Impaired
- Injury, Potential for
- Knowledge Deficit (specify)
- Mobility, Impaired Physical
- Noncompliance (specify)
- Nutrition, Alterations in: Less than Body Requirements
- Nutrition, Alterations in: More than Body Requirements
- Nutrition, Alterations in: Potential for More than Body Requirements

- Parenting, Alterations in: Actual
- Parenting, Alterations in: Potential
- Rape-Trauma Syndrome
- Self-Care Deficit (specify level: Feeding, Bathing/hygiene, Dressing/grooming, Toileting)
- Self-concept, Disturbance in
- Sensory Perceptual Alterations
- Sexual Dysfunction
- Skin Integrity, Impairment of: Actual
- Skin Integrity, Impairment of: Potential
- Sleep Pattern Disturbance
- Spiritual Distress (Distress of the Human Spirit)
- Thought Processes, Alterations in
- Tissue Perfusion, Alteration in
- Urinary Elimination, Alteration in Patterns
- Violence, Potential for

New Diagnoses Accepted for Clinical Testing 1982: Fifth National Conference on Classification of Nursing Diagnosis

- Activity Intolerance
- Anxiety
- Family Processes, Alteration in
- Fluid Volume, Alteration in: Excess
- Health Maintenance Alteration
- Oral Mucus Membrane, Alterations in
- Powerlessness
- Social Isolation

Source: North American Nursing Diagnosis Association. Reproduced with permission.

Table 17–6. **Case Study—Mrs. L. Johnson**

Nursing Diagnoses PROBLEM	+	CAUSE	DATA NUMBER
Pain	associated with	cholelithiasis	8–10
Knowledge deficit	related to	hospitalization and surgery	13, 15, 16
Fear	associated with	anesthesia	14

*Numbers refer to data in original data collection, page 000.

nursing diagnosis is based. This helps to assure the accuracy of the nursing diagnosis. If it is not possible to identify these data, the nurse may need to review the data collection again, to consult with other nurses, or to continue the data-collection process with the patient. At times, the cause of the problem may be uncertain. The nurse then attempts to identify related or contributing factors. When writing nursing diagnoses, the nurse uses the terms "associated with" or "related to" in order to identify causative or contributing factors. This is preferable to saying "due to" since it is not always possible to show a direct cause-and-effect relationship.

The nursing diagnosis is not the same as the medical diagnosis. The nursing diagnosis focuses on the patient's perception of the health problem, the patient's response, and the patient's ability to cope with the problem. It may also include the patient's response to health care. These things are all concerned with the caring role of the nurse. In contrast, the medical diagnosis focuses on the disease process. However, the medical diagnosis may suggest nursing diagnoses as in Table 17–4. A nursing diagnosis

Is not a medical diagnosis
Is not a nursing action
Is not a patient need (but may be an unmet need)
Is not a physician's order
Is not a therapeutic treatment or medication.

The guidelines in Table 17–5 may be helpful to the nurse beginning to write nursing diagnoses. Exhibit 17–2 lists the nursing diagnoses currently accepted by the North American Nursing Diagnosis Association. This listing is an attempt to standardize nursing diagnoses and is not complete. Nurses are encouraged to add to the list and develop their own statements of nursing diagnoses that are useful in the clinical areas in which they work. At the end of this chapter in Self-Assessment is an exercise to assess understanding and application of a nursing diagnosis. The student may choose to complete this exercise before continuing to the second step of the nursing process.

Table 17–6 lists the nursing diagnoses for Mrs. Johnson, the patient whose care plan will be used to illustrate the nursing process throughout this chapter.

Planning

Once the assessment phase is completed, the nurse is ready to begin planning patient care. The planning phase consists of three activities: setting priorities, writing goals, and planning nursing actions.

Setting Priorities

Priority setting is a decision-making process in which the nurse determines the order in which the patient's problems are approached. The nurse assigns number "one" to the nursing diagnosis given the highest priority, and so on. This does not mean that one problem must be totally resolved before another problem can be undertaken. Nursing intervention for several

problems may be initiated simultaneously. Sometimes, however, it is crucial that the nurse correctly identify the order of priority of nursing diagnoses so maximum effort can be directed toward resoltuion of the most urgent problem.

One approach to priority setting which has been used extensively is based on Maslow's theory of basic needs. Maslow states that the lower physiological needs must be met to some degree before the higher level needs can be met. Using this theory, the nurse reviews the nursing diagnoses for those that relate to survival needs. Any problem that is life threatening must be met first. Examples of this might include problems related to oxygenation, such as the patient who is hemorrhaging after being involved in an automobile accident. The patient whose lung has been punctured by a stabbing has a life-threatening need for oxygenation, and this must be met first. Once life-threatening needs have been met or partially met, the nurse can continue setting priorities using Maslow's theory by focusing on the remaining lower needs before higher needs. For example:

> The nursing student who has studied all night (need for rest and sleep) may be unable to listen and absorb a lecture about the nursing process (self-actualization need) the next morning.
> The patient who is in pain (lower need) must have relief before learning about self-care for diabetes (need for self-esteem).
> The patient with a full bladder (elimination need) who is unable to void may need to be catheterized before wanting visitors (love and belonging need).

Once the physical needs are met to some degree, the nurse can consider higher needs. At this point, a higher need can take priority over a lower need or at least be equal to it. For example, once the patient in the emergency room has been stabilized and is not in danger of death from hemorrhage, the patient may begin seeking information about other family members involved in the accident. At this point, the need for love and belonging is equal to physiological needs. Unless this need is met, it can have negative effects on the satisfaction of physiological needs. For example, the patient may be so concerned over family members that rest and sleep are impossible.

In setting priorities, it is also necessary that the nurse consider the patient's choices. However, at times, safety needs take precedence over patient preferences. The patient who was in the automobile accident may prefer to rest undisturbed throughout the night, but the nurse must check pulse and blood pressure and make a complete neurological assessment every half hour. In this case, the physical-safety need takes precedence over the preference of the patient.

If there are no contraindications, the nurse and the patient mutually set priorities. This has several advantages. The nurse may overlook or minimize the importance of a problem which is consuming the patient's energy. If patients participate in determining priorities, they have another opportunity to bring their concerns to the attention of the nurse. Mutual goal setting also enhances the nurse-patient relationship because the patient is assured that the nurse will attempt to accomplish what is important to the patient. This also increases the cooperation of the patient.

The nurse considers the potential for future problems when setting priorities. It may be necessary to take early action in order to prevent the development of problems, even though the patient may not see this as

important. Frequently, for example, patients do not wish to begin early ambulation after surgery. The nurse is aware of the serious problems which can develop as a result of bed rest and establishes the prevention of complications related to bed rest as a high priority.

In summary, when setting priorities the nurse considers

- Maslow's hierarchy of needs
- Effect of lower needs on satisfaction of higher needs and the reverse
- Fulfillment of patients' preferences
- Potential for future problems
- Medical problem and treatment

Nursing Goals

Nursing goal: the desired outcome of nursing care; that which you hope to achieve with your patient; that which is designed to remedy or lessen the problem identified in the nursing diagnosis.

A *goal statement* is needed to identify clearly what it is that the nurse strives to achieve through nursing action. For each nursing course the student takes, a list of course objectives is given to the student by the faculty. The objectives are the goals of the course. If the student successfully completes the course, the student has achieved the goal, that is, has accomplished the objectives. Similarly, the nursing goals are statements of what the nurse hopes to achieve through nursing intervention. Some goals for patients are also learning objectives. This is the case when the patient has a need to learn certain information or skills related to health care. The process of patient teaching is discussed in Chapter 9. Other nursing goals have to do with such things as prevention of problems, pain relief, and body responses to nursing intervention.

Types of Goals

There are two categories of goals: short-term goals and long-term goals. Short-term goals are those that can be met in a relatively short period of time—a few days or even a few hours. These are used most frequently in a hospital where patient conditions change often and stays are not long. Examples of short-term goals are

Patient will walk the length of the hall three times a day by 9/22.
Oral intake will be 1,800 ml/24 hours by 7/16.
Patient will demonstrate correct procedure for wrapping ace bandage by 9/16.

A series of short-term goals may be used to reach a long-term goal. The frequent achievement of short-term goals may help to motivate a patient toward a long-term goal. Such an example is

Long-term goal: Patient will lose 25 lb by 9/26.
Progressive short-term goals:
    Patient will weigh 148 lb, 5/7.
    Patient will weigh 146 lb, 5/16.
    Patient will weigh 144 lb, 5/23.

Another example of this might be

Long-term goal: Patient will be able to safely and correctly administer own insulin within one week, 6/13.
Progressive short-term goals:

1. Patient will verbalize feelings related to giving self-injection, 6/7.
2. Patient will demonstrate which parts of equipment are sterile and nonsterile, 6/8.
3. Patient will demonstrate correct procedure for drawing up the prescribed amount of insulin and injecting it into an orange, 6/9.
4. Patient will correctly and safely administer own daily dose of insulin under the supervision of nurse three times before discharge, 6/10, 6/11, 6/12

Long-term goals are outcomes that take an extended period of time to accomplish and require nursing actions dealing directly with that goal. Such a goal for a nursing student might be

Long-term goal: I will complete this nursing course with a grade of B or better by January.

The student must then do many actions to assure this goal, such as reading the textbook, attending clinical laboratory, and practicing nursing skills.

An example of a long-term goal for a patient is

Prevention of skin breakdown while on bed rest.

The nurse then plans nursing interventions that deal directly with this goal. These might include massage, frequent change of position, and the use of an alternating air mattress.

Beginning to Write Goals

When the student first attempts to write a goal statement, the following suggestions may be helpful:

1. First, refer back to the nursing diagnosis. The goal statement is a patient behavior or response which demonstrates reduction or alleviation of the problem identified in the nursing diagnosis. If the nursing diagnosis has to do with pain, the goal must have to do with the relief of pain. If the nursing diagnosis has to do with threats to physical safety, the goal statement must relate to providing safety or protection from injury. At times, it can almost be said that the goal is the opposite of the nursing diagnosis.

2. The goal must be realistic for both the patient's and the nurses's capabilities. For example, it is not realistic to set a goal that expects the patient to lose 5 lb per week, nor is it realistic to expect a beginning student nurse to provide sexual counseling to a couple unable to conceive a child. These goals exceed appropriate expectations for each individual.

3. The goal should be congruent with and supportive of other therapies. This means that the goals should not conflict or undermine the goals of other profes-

Table 17–7. **Examples of Goal Statements**

SUBJECT	+	VERB	+	CRITERIA	+	CONDITION, IF RELEVANT
The patient		will sit in a chair		for 15 minutes three times each day		
The patient		will select		three days' menus by 10/6		using diabetic exchange diet
The patient		will give own insulin		using sterile technique by 11/3		
The patient		will drink		1000 ml liquid by 8 P.M. 6/3		
Blood pressure		will be		110/65 or greater by 7 P.M. 11/6		
The patient		will lose		1 lb per week (9/3)		while on a 1200-calorie diet
Child's PaO_2		to be		within normal limits by 2 P.M.		while in 28% O_2

Table 17–8. **Guidelines for Writing Goal Statements**

---

1. Write goals in observable, measurable, objective terms. Avoid the use of words such as "improved," "adequate," "normal," since these all mean different things to different people and tend to make the goal unclear.
2. Write goals in terms of patient responses, outcomes, and behaviors, not in terms of nursing actions.
3. Each goal is related to one nursing diagnosis. The goal is short and specific.
4. Include a time for the response, behavior, or outcome in the goal. This is done by including either the date the goal was written or the date the goal is to be evaluated. The latter format is more common.

---

sional members of the health team. For example, if the physical therapist has determined that the patient is to use crutches for ambulation at the time of discharge, the nurse does not set a goal that the patient will use a three-footed cane.

4. Whenever possible, the goal should be valued by the patient, the nursing staff, and the physician. This will help to assure the patient's commitment to the goal, as well as assuring that the medical treatment is not in conflict. If other nurses value the goals, they are more likely to carry out the written plan of care.

When nursing students begin to write goals, it is recommended that they focus on short-term goals related to the amount of time they will be with the patient. If the students' goals are time-limited, the student will also be able to gain experience in completing the other steps of the nursing process: implementation and evaluation.

A nursing goal consists of

1. Subject. This is the patient or any part of the patient—a noun. The subject may not always be stated in the goal, but it is assumed to be the patient unless otherwise indicated.

> The patient's pulse
> The patient
> The patient's temperature

2. Verb. This is the action that the subject (the patient) will perform

> Will not exceed
> Will walk
> Will remain

3. Criteria of acceptable performance. These indicate the level at which the patient will perform the specified behavior. How long? How far? How much? The criteria also contain a date or time for evaluation of the behavior.

> 90 beats per minute
> The length of the hall by 9/22
> 99°F or less during hospitalization

4. Condition. This indicates the circumstances, if important, under which the behavior will be performed. Not all goals have a condition that is necessary to include.

> After walking 50 ft
> Using a tripod cane

In summary, the goal statement includes a subject, verb, criteria of performance, and condition of performance if necessary. Table 17–7 lists correctly written goal statements.

Some general guidelines to follow in writing goals are included in Table 17–8. Table 17–9 includes the goals written for Mrs. Johnson, the patient whose care plan is being used throughout this chapter to illustrate the use of the nursing process.

Table 17–9. **Case Study—Mrs. Johnson**

Nursing Diagnosis	Goal
Pain associated with cholelithiasis.	Patient will state pain has decreased to a #2 (on a scale of 1 to 10) within 45 minutes after nursing intervention

Knowledge deficit related to hospitalization and surgery.	Patient will state accurate understanding of what will happen
	   The morning of surgery
	   During stay in recovery room
	   After return to room, (IV, nursing care), 8/26

Fear associated with anesthesia.	Patient will state fear of anesthesia has decreased, 8/26

Planning Nursing Actions

Nursing actions are all those things the nurse does in order to help the patient achieve the goals established in the nursing care plan. Nursing actions are written on the care plan in a sequence that describes the order in which the actions are to be carried out.

Nursing orders are a form of nursing action used in some hospitals or agencies. The nurse writes a nursing order to communicate specific instructions for nursing care. Nursing personnel then have the obligation to complete the ordered care. The nursing order includes the date it is written, the specific instructions, the time, frequency, or duration of the action, and the signature of the nurse writing the order. Some examples of nursing orders are

> 9/15—Reposition every hour with left leg elevated at 30-degree angle from bed.
> 9/16—Reassess for pain every 2½ hours through midnight 9/18.
> 9/16—Encourage daily fluid intake to
> 7 a.m.–3p.m., 1,000 ml
> 3 p.m.–8p.m., 500 ml

The nurse begins this activity of the nursing process by selecting nursing actions. The nurse has skills and a knowledge base from which to select nursing actions. This base grows with additional experience and education. The nurse may also consult other more experienced nurses or search the nursing literature for ideas. At times, the patient who has lived with a particular condition for a long time may be a valuable source of information. When writing a care plan, the nurse reviews the range of available nursing interventions and selects those best suited to the particular patient situation and the particular goals of nursing care. Several factors influence the choice of the nurse:

1. The nursing actions must be safe for the patient.

2. Nursing actions must be congruent with other therapies. For example, if the dietitian has placed the patient on a calorie-restricted diet, the nurse does not offer unplanned, between-meal snacks to the patient.

3. One set of nursing actions is written to accomplish each goal.

4. Nursing actions are chosen that are most likely to accomplish a stated goal.

5. Nursing actions should be realistic:

For the patient. If the patient is unwilling to follow a weight-reduction diet, for example, the nurse does not plan that action.

For the nurse. Are there enough nurses available to carry out the plan, and do the nurses have the necessary skills?

For the available equipment. The nurse works with the equipment available in the hospital.

6. Nursing actions should be acceptable to the patient. If, for example, the goal is to have the patient drink 1,500 ml of fluid per day, the nurse might begin by asking patient preferences. If the patient enjoys iced tea, the nurse may offer this to the patient.

7. List the nursing actions in the sequence in which they should be done, if it matters. For example, nursing actions based on assessing and relieving pain precede the nursing action of getting the patient out of bed to walk. Reviewing medical orders, hospital routine, and Maslow's hierarchy of needs may also give the nurse an indication of the sequence of nursing actions.

8. Nursing actions must be based on principles and knowledge from behavioral and physical sciences. This knowledge forms the explanation or rationale for nursing actions. For example:

Nursing diagnosis: Muscle weakness associated with prolonged bed rest
Nursing goal: Increased muscle strength as evidenced by ability to walk the length of the hall 9/17

1. Nursing action: Complete passive range-of-motion exercises in bed three times each day for two days
Explanation: Increased blood circulation to the muscles. Maintain joint mobility. Prevent muscle deterioration.

2. Nursing action: Complete active range-of-motion exercises three times each day.
Explanation: Use of muscle maintains and increases muscle strength and mass.

3. Nursing action: Assist patient to sit on the edge of the bed and then, with the aid of two people, assist patient out of bed to sit in chair up to a half hour three times a day.
Explanation: Sitting on the edge of the bed helps the patient to get sense of balance in upright position while still remaining in a safe position if dizzy. Two nurses assisting provide the maximum support and safety for the patient. Sitting upright requires increased muscular activity.

4. Nursing action: Assist patient to walk in room, increasing distance as tolerated.
Explanation: Increased muscle use will increase the strength of the muscle and increase the distance that the patient is able to walk.

Students are often required to write the rationale or explanation in their initial care plans, but this is a learning tool. Written rationale is not included in the patient's care plan although it is part of the thought process used by the nurse.

Implementation

The implementation phase of the nursing process consists of several activities: validating the care plan, documenting the care plan, giving the nursing care, and continuing data collection.

Validating the Care Plan

When the student nurse first begins writing nursing care plans, the student probably writes out a worksheet before writing the shortened form of the care plan on a hospital form. Similarly, the staff nurse who is planning complex care may choose to write out a "rough draft" of the nursing care plan. At this point, the student or the staff nurse may take the proposed care plan to another nurse for validation. It is important that an appropriate person be selected to validate the care plan. For example, nursing assistants who have worked in an area for a long period of time are often very knowledgeable about certain aspects of patient care, but although they may make a valuable addition to the care plan, writing and validating care plans are functions of the professional nurse. The nursing student will probably review the care plan with the nursing instructor. Staff nurses may not always seek validation, depending on their nursing skill and experience with the nursing process. The staff nurse may select a nurse colleague who has experience in the care of this type of patient or perhaps a nurse clinician. In either case, the validation process is not a formal or lengthy process. The nurse who wrote the care plan is just seeking a quick "second opinion." The second nurse may validate the care plan by answering the following questions:

1. Does the plan assure the patient's safety?
2. Are the nursing diagnoses supported by data?
3. Is the plan based on nursing knowledge and scientific principles?

4. Does the goal describe behavior or a condition that lessens or alleviates the problem described in the nursing diagnosis?
5. Is the goal stated in such a way that it can be observed or measured?
6. Can the planned nursing actions realistically be expected to assist the patient to achieve the intended goal?
7. Are the nursing actions arranged in a logical sequence, if it matters?
8. Are the patient's preferences being considered?
9. Is the plan individualized to the unique needs and capabilities of the patient?

In summary, the second nurse is reviewing the care plan for safe, individualized nursing practice.

Documenting the Care Plan

The completed care plan is intended as a communication tool for members of the nursing staff and the rest of the health care team as well. In many institutions, the nursing care plan is retained as a part of the patient's permanent record. For this reason, it is recommended that nursing care plans be written in ink and signed with the name and title of the responsible nurse.

Nursing care plans may be written following the format of problem-oriented medical records (see Chapter 8). In such a system, the nurse writing the care plan writes the nursing diagnoses sequentially on the numbered problem list.

Many hospitals use some form of a nursing Kardex to organize the care plans of a group of patients. Often, a Kardex is a flip file of 6 × 11-inch index cards which are preprinted with spaces for nursing diagnoses, goals, nursing action, and evaluations. Some institutions have

Table 17–10. Guidelines for Writing an Abbreviated Care Plan

1. The headings on the written plan include nursing diagnoses, goals, nursing actions, and evaluations.
2. Abbreviate whenever possible, using only standardized English or medical symbols.
3. Use key words or phrases to communicate ideas; do not write entire sentences.
4. Refer to procedure books for procedure rather than trying to list all the steps.
5. Include a date for the evaluation of each goal.
6. When goals are evaluated, sign with name and title.
7. All long-term goals are written. It is not necessary to write a short-term goal that will be met during the nurse's eight-hour duty period. Short-term goals that cannot be met within the shift of one nurse should be written in order that other nurses can continue the plan of care.

PATIENT CARE PLAN CARD

ROCHESTER METHODIST HOSPITAL

Contact Person(s)

Relationship

Local Address

Local Tel. No. Home Tel. No.

Admitting Diagnosis

Smoking ____ Non-Smoking ____

Medications brought in: Yes No

Medical Problems

Medications sent to:

Valuables:

Surgical Procedure(s), Date(s)

X-rays brought in: Yes No

X-rays recorded:

Dismissed: Date Init. Time

PATIENT PROFILE

DIET

Intake

Output

Food Sensitivities/Intolerances

Age ______ Ht ______ cm Wt ______ kg

CODE STATUS

Special Needs B____ L____ D____

Beverages

Physician

Received by RN

RELIGIOUS PREFERENCE

INTERDISCIPLINARY TEAM

Anticipated Dismissal Date

Destination

REFERRAL: Yes No Started date

Phone Call date , Init. RN, Person Contacted

Referral Completed date

Sent to

TEAM MEMBER COMMENTS/DISMISSAL PLANNING COMMENTS

DISCIPLINES(name, telephone and/or page number)

Admitting Officer

Pharmacist

Chaplain

Physical Therapist

Dietitian

Public Health Nurse

Nurse Specialist

Respiratory Therapist

Occupational Therapist

Social Worker

Other

DISMISSAL RN

PRIMARY SERVICE Page No.

ON CALL PHYSICIAN Page No.

RMH-601-005-6/81

Figure 17–1. A. Example of patient care plan card. (Courtesy of Rochester Methodist Hospital, Rochester, MN.)

adopted 8½ × 11-inch care plan forms, since these correspond to a standard chart size and facilitate permanent storage. (See Figure 17–1.)

The written nursing care plan is abbreviated as much as possible. The nurse writes down those plans that need to be communicated to the following shifts of nurses. If the nurse has identified and resolved a nursing diagnosis during a duty period, it is noted in the charting of that day. It is not necessary to add it to the nursing care plan, although it is reported to other staff. The written care plan is used to communicate care plans that cover an extended period of time and require the coordination of several nurses.

Table 17–10 contains some suggestions to assist the nurse to write a care plan on a Kardex or similar form. It is helpful if the care plan form includes an area for treatments that the patient is to receive while in the hospital. Treatment orders by physical therapists, nurses, physicians can all be written in this area. Some of the nursing actions selected for goal achievement will be

PATIENT NAME _____

APPOINTMENTS/CONSULTS

Monday	Tuesday	Wednesday	Thursday	Friday	Saturday	Sunday

DIAGNOSTIC STUDIES/X-RAYS

Test Date	Time	Location of Test	Comp. Date	TEST	Special Preparation

NURSING/PHYSICIAN ORDERS

Start Date	ORDERS	Times	Eval. Date	Start Date	ORDERS	Times	Eval. Date

Weight (frequency)	Bed	Standing	ACTIVITY and/or POSITION
T.P.R.	BP.P.R.		
Type of Bath	Prefer AM	PM	
Last BM			

ALLERGIES/SENSITIVITIES (Reaction)	SAFETY MEASURES

Figure 17–1. B.

treatments. They are then identified by number in the "Planned Action" section of the care plan.

Figure 17–2 is an abbreviated care plan for Mrs. Johnson as it might appear in the nursing Kardex.

Giving Nursing Care

The nurse now uses the care plan to give patient care. However well the care plan may have been written, situations occur in the hospital to interfere with implementing the care plan. The patient may be out of the unit for several hours for a diagnostic procedure and may want only to sleep upon returning. Another patient may be in severe pain and unable to participate in the teaching plan the nurse has devised. Frequently, spending time with unanticipated visitors is a priority for the patient. In each of these situations, the nurse remains flexible and open to modification of the care plan.

| NURSING CARE PLAN | | | BETHESDA HOSPITAL | CINCINNATI, OHIO |

OPTIMAL OUTCOME: (1) COMPLETE RECOVERY   (2) RECOVERY WITH LIMITATIONS   (3) DIGNIFIED/PEACEFUL DEATH

DATE NAME	ASSESSMENT INDIVIDUAL NEEDS PROBLEMS OR CONCERNS	PLAN GOALS: NUMBER EQUALS LONG RANGE LETTER EQUALS SHORT RANGE	IMPLEMENT NURSING APPROACH & ORDERS	EVALUATION ACTUAL OUTCOME	DATE RESOLVED NAME
8/25	Pain / cholelithiasis	A. Patient will state pain has decreased to a #2 on a scale of 1–10 within 45 min. p nsg. intervention.	A. # Assess pain: activity at onset, location, severity on scale, comparison # Pain medication as ordered # Provide distraction: TV reading materials # Guide systematic relaxation # Backrub # Reassess pain 30 min.		
8/25	Knowledge deficit / hospitalization & surgery.	B. Patient will state accurate understanding of: – AM of surgery – stay in recovery room – return to room, I.V., nursing care, 8/26	B. Preop teaching to include: # NPO p MN, med before surgery to relax, dry mouth, no jewelry, family wait in room, pt. gown, no hairpins. # Return to room: NPO, Breathing exercises, vital signs, ambulation, pain med.		
8/25	Fear / anesthesia	C. Patient will state fear of anesthesia has decreased 8/26	C. # Request anesthetist to visit # Convey pt. fears to above # Stay c pt. during visit to be able to reinforce teaching.		

DISCHARGE PLANNING

CONDITION	NEXT OF KIN OR SIGNIFICANT OTHER	HOME TELEPHONE	OTHER TELEPHONE	CONSULTS		ISOLATION	LANGUAGE
	John B. Johnson	639-1518	691-1813				ENG
ADMIN DATE 8/25	PRIMARY DIAGNOSIS Cholelithiasis		SECONDARY DIAGNOSIS OR SURGICAL PROCEDURES			OCCUPATION Bank officer	AGE 42
ROOM NO 603	LAST NAME JOHNSON,	FIRST NAME Louise	SEX F	HOSPITAL NO. 68294	RELIGION RC	SACRAMENT OF SICK no	PHYSICIAN B. L. Trim

Figure 17–2.   Abbreviated care plan for Mrs. Johnson as it might appear in a nursing Kardex. (Courtesy of Bethesda North Hospital, Cincinnati, OH.)

Continuing Data Collection

The activity of data collection continues throughout the time the patient receives nursing care, from admission until discharge. As the patient's condition changes and as the nurse spends more time with the patient, the data collection becomes more extensive. The ongoing data collection is the basis for evaluating the effectiveness of the care plan and for revisions of the care plan.

Evaluation

The final step in the nursing process is *evaluation*. When the nurse writes a care plan, evaluation includes the activities of evaluating goal achievement and the reassessment of nursing care.

Evaluation of Goal Achievement

The purpose of evaluation is to determine if the stated goal has been achieved as of the time or data

Table 17–11. **Case Study—Mrs Johnson**

Goals	Evaluation
1. Patient will state pain has decreased to #2 (on a scale of 1 to 10) within 45 minutes after nursing intervention.	1. Goal met. Patient states she is free of all pain, 0. *M. Knedle, RN*
2. Patient will state accurate understanding of what will happen The A.M. of surgery, During stay in recovery room After return to room, IV, nursing care	2. Goal partially met. Patient understands surgical and recovery room experience, but is too tired to continue and asks to rest. *M. Knedle, RN*
3. Patient will state fear of anesthesia has decreased, 8/26.	3. Goal met. Patient states, "I'm not nearly so worried about the anesthesia anymore. It really helped to talk to Dr. Sulman." *M. Knedle, RN*

specified in the care plan. The nurse reviews the goal and determines the behavior or criterion to be measured. For example, was the patient able to perform the behavior specified in the goal? What were the objective or subjective data specified in the goal? Using current data, the nurse makes a decision about whether the goal was met, partially met, or not met. Table 17–11 shows the evaluations of Mrs. Johnson's care plan.

Reassessment of the Care Plan

Reassessment is the process of changing or eliminating previous nursing diagnoses, goals, and actions based on new patient data. While giving care, the nurse gathers additional data which may show a need to alter the nursing care plan. Each of the following situations demonstrates a need to change the care plan:

1. The patient's condition changes, and new problems or priorities are identified.

2. The nursing actions were effective in meeting the goal, but the problem continues. This is the situation in which there are a long-term goal and a series of short-term progressive goals. Each short-term goal is met, but the problem continues.

3. The goal may be only partially met or not met at all. The nurse then checks to be sure that the nursing diagnosis was based upon correct data, that the goal was realistic, that the nursing actions selected were likely to accomplish the goal. Changes may be necessary in any or all of these areas. Table 17–12 shows reassessment of Mrs. Johnson's care plan.

Table 17–12. **Case Study—Mrs. Johnson**

1. Goal met.
   Patient states she is free of all pain, 0
2. Goal partially met.
   Patient understands surgical and recovery room procedures but it too tired to continue and asks to rest.
   Reassessment:
      New data: Patient is tired
      New nursing diagnosis: Inadequate rest and sleep related to cholelithiasis.
      New action: Provide patient with uninterrupted rest.
      Schedule two short teaching periods during next eight-hour shift.
3. Goal met.
   Nursing diagnosis resolved.

Summary

The nursing process is an approach that can help to ensure quality nursing care. It is similar to a problem-solving approach and consists of four steps: assessment, planning, implementation, evaluation. During each step, the nurse performs certain activities which focus on the identification of the patient's health problems and planning effective nursing interventions to resolve the problems. The nursing process is the way the nurse thinks as a nurse. One outcome of the nursing process is a written patient care plan.

Both the patient and the nurse benefit from the use of the nursing process. The patient is given the opportunity to participate in planning care. The patient also gains experience in problem solving in matters related to health care. With a written care plan, omissions and duplications can be avoided. The nurse gains increased job satisfaction when nursing care is positively evaluated, as well as a sense of confidence that nursing actions are based on correctly identified patient problems.

Terms for Review

assessment	implementation	nursing history	reassessment
evaluation	nursing action	planning	signs
goal statement	nursing diagnosis	priority setting	symptoms

Self-Assessment

I. Select the correctly written nursing diagnoses and identify what is wrong with the incorrectly written diagnoses.
   1. Prolonged bed rest related to immobility
   2. Anxiety related to unfamiliar hospital environment
   3. Fear and pain associated with surgical incision
   4. Alteration in body-image associated with loss of breast
   5. Cerebrovascular accident

Answers
1. Incorrect. The problem and the cause are the same. Also, the real patient problem is the result of the prolonged bed rest. A better nursing diagnosis would be: Prone to skin breakdown related to prolonged bed rest.
2. Correct.
3. Incorrect. Two problems are included in one nursing diagnosis. A better nursing diagnosis would be: Fear associated with anesthesia. Pain associated with surgical incision.
4. Correct.
5. Incorrect. This is a medical diagnosis. A better nursing diagnosis would be: Inability to communicate verbally associated with cerebrovascular accident.

II. Select the correctly written goal statements and identify what is wrong with the incorrect goal statements.
1. Patient will demonstrate changing dressing on surgical incision.
2. Patient will walk the length of the hall three times each day using a tripod cane by 8/16.
3. Pain will be less by 8/12.
4. Teach the patient self administration of insulin by 8/12.
5. Patient will plan two day's menus that meet the requirements for a low-fat diet using own food preferences by 6/3.

Answers
1. Incorrect. What is the criterion of performance? No date. A better goal would be: Patient will demonstrate changing dressing on surgical incision using sterile technique by 6/3.
2. Correct.
3. Incorrect. Not possible to measure. A better goal would be: Patient will state pain has decreased by 8/12. Another goal would be: Patient will state pain is less than 3 on a scale of 1 to 10 by 8/12.
4. Incorrect. This is a nursing action. A goal would be: Patient will correctly demonstrate self-administration of insulin by 8/12.
5. Correct.

Learning Activity

In a clinical laboratory, read the care plan of an assigned patient before beginning to plan or provide nursing care. Respond to the following questions after giving care to the patient:

1. What were the major problems identified in the care plan?
2. Was the care plan current?
3. What information would have helped you provide better care to the patient if it had been included in the care plan?
4. Write the additions you will make to the care plan.

Review Questions

1. The nursing process is most accurately described as
   a. An individualized nursing care plan
   b. An approach the nurse uses to plan, implement, and evaluate the care of patients
   c. The systematic evaluation of nursing care
   d. A method of physical assessment
2. During the assessment phase of the nursing process, the nurse focuses on
   a. Collection and analysis of data
   b. Selecting nursing actions
   c. Validating the care plan
   d. Planning patient care conferences
3. The nurse who validates the care plan is reviewing it for
   a. Creativity
   b. Nonsexist language
   c. Safety and individualized nursing practice
   d. Presence of judgments and conclusions
4. Which of the following data relate to the need for love and belonging?
   a. "It's hard to breathe sitting up."
   b. "It's scary to go out alone. I'm not as steady on my feet as I used to be."
   c. "The pain goes down the back of my leg like a streak."
   d. "My children live over 500 miles away so I don't see much of them."
5. Which of the following data relate to safety and security needs?
   a. BP 120/72
   b. Ambulates with use of tripod cane
   c. "I was a mail carrier for the Post Office for 28 years."
   d. Three-inch scar on right hand from prior tendon surgery
6. Objective data is to a sign as subjective data is to
   a. Analysis
   b. Conclusion
   c. Fact
   d. Symptom
7. The purpose of writing a tentative nursing diagnosis is
   a. To ensure continued data collection related to the problem
   b. To direct preventive nursing measures
   c. To provide for safe nursing care
   d. To document the nursing care being given
8. "Patient will complete active range-of-motion exercises two times each day. 6/1" is an example of
   a. A nursing diagnosis
   b. A nursing action
   c. A goal statement
   d. An evaluative statement
9. Using Maslow's hierarchy of basic needs, which of the following problems should be the highest priority for the nurse?
   a. Loneliness for husband
   b. Loss of appetite
   c. Depression
   d. Bleeding from severed artery
10. Which of the following are objective data?
    a. Blood loss of approximately 500 ml
    b. Moderately severe blood loss
    c. Patient states, "I lost a lot of blood."
    d. Ambulance driver reports blood loss minimal.

Answers

1. b
2. a
3. c
4. d
5. b
6. d
7. a
8. c
9. d
10. a

Suggested Readings

McConnell, L.: How Nursing care plans help you. *Nursing Life,* **2**:55–59, 1982. A nursing consultant offers practical suggestions for writing and using nursing care plans.

References and Bibliography

American Nurses' Association: Standards of Nursing Practice. Publication Code No. NP–41 20M 8/81R, Kansas City, 1973.

Atkinson, L., and Murray, M.: *Understanding the Nursing Process* 2nd ed. Macmillan, New York, 1983.

Gordon, M.: *Manual of Nursing Diagnosis.* McGraw-Hill, New York, 1982.

Griffith, J., and Christensen, P.: *Nursing Process: Application of Theories, Frameworks, and Models.* Mosby, St. Louis, 1982.

Joint Commission On Accreditation of Hospitals: *Standards for Accreditation of Hospitals.* Chicago, 1981.

Maslow, A.: *Toward a Psychology of Being,* 2nd ed. Van Nostrand, New York, 1968.

National Group for Classification of Nursing Diagnoses: List of Nursing Diagnoses Accepted at Fourth National Conference, St. Louis, 1982.

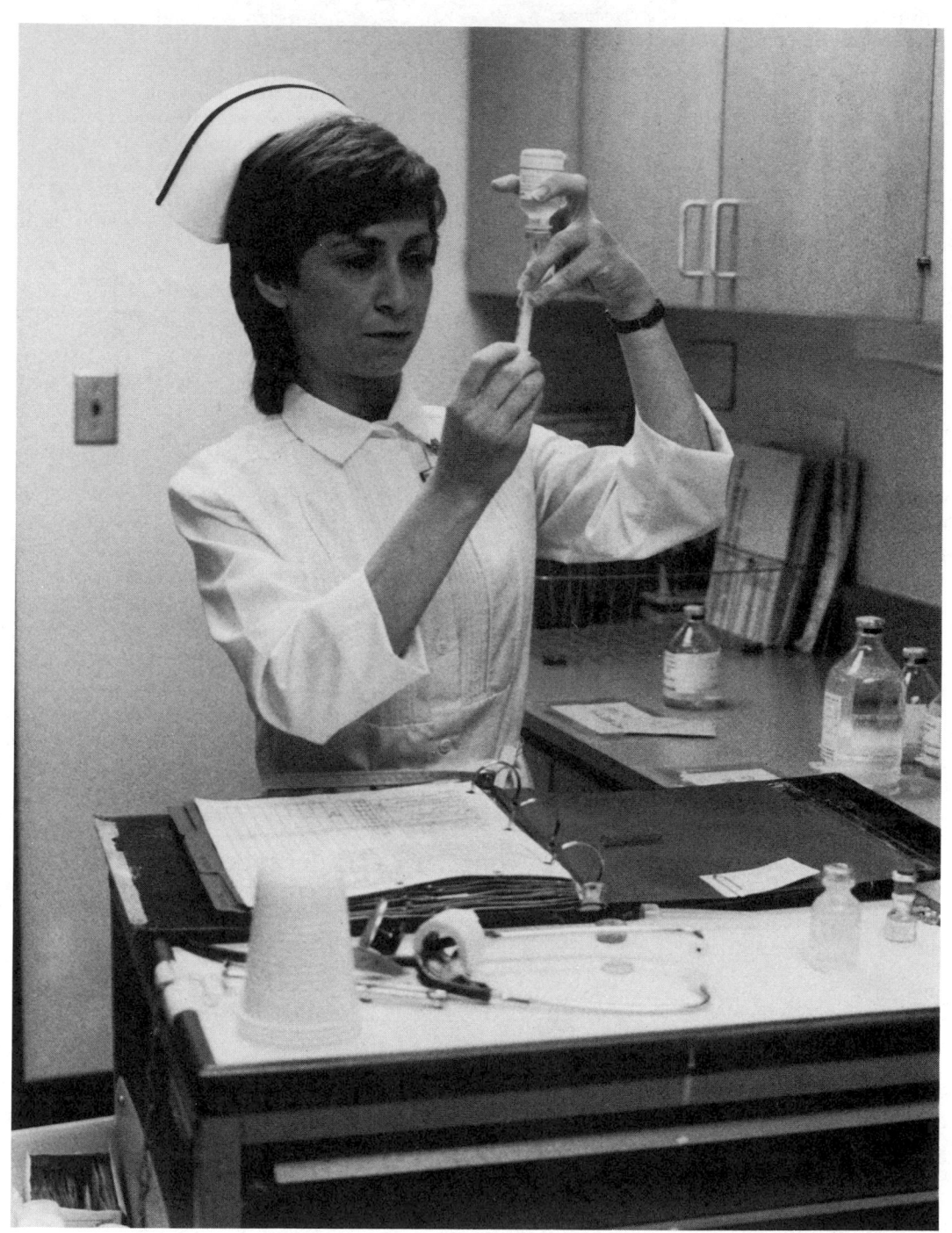

UNIT **V**

THE PROCESS OF ENVIRONMENTAL MANAGEMENT

PROVIDING A BIOLOGICALLY SAFE ENVIRONMENT

Objectives

1. Discuss why a knowledge of biological safety measures is important for the nurse.

2. Describe the steps in the chain of infection.

3. Discuss what is meant by specific and nonspecific defenses of the body against foreign matter.

4. List the primary characteristics of inflammation.

5. Describe the sequence of events comprising the inflammatory response.

6. Contrast antibody-mediated specific defenses to cell-mediated specific defenses.

7. Explain the following types of immunity: innate, acquired, active acquired, passive acquired.

8. Discuss factors that affect the need for biological safety.

9. Discuss reasons why hospitalized patients have an accentuated need for biological safety.

10. Describe the ethical requirements of the Code for Nurses as it applies to biological safety.

11. Explain the relationship between the need for biological safety and other basic human needs.

12. List data that may indicate the presence of infection.

13. Explain the two systems of isolation precautions: category-specific and disease-specific.

14. Contrast medical asepsis to surgical asepsis.

15. Discuss requirements for nurses' uniforms related to the need for biological safety.

16. Demonstrate safe performance of the following skills: medical handwashing, giving a bed bath, giving a towel bath, making an unoccupied bed, making an occupied bed, surgical handwashing, opening a sterile pack, putting on sterile gloves and gown, pouring sterile liquids, changing sterile dressings, strict isolation technique.

The Importance of Biological Safety

Minute, living organisms, called microorganisms, exist everywhere in the environment, on the human body, and within the human body. Most of these microorganisms are harmless or even beneficial to the human body. Others, called *pathogens*, have the potential to cause disease. When the body is unable to defend against them successfully, pathogens multiply within the body. This is called infection. Biological safety is the protection of the individual from disease-producing microorganisms.

Many especially strong (*virulent*) types of pathogens exist within the hospital environment. The nurse is exposed to the pathogens of each patient and, in turn, the nurse caring for several patients can spread micoorganisms from patient to patient. If, for example, a nurse caring for a patient with an infected surgical incision does not carefully wash hands after changing bandages on the wound and then proceeds to give care to a second patient, the second patient is exposed to the pathogen and is at risk for developing the infection. Later, if an accident results in a scratch or cut on the nurse's hands, the nurse is at risk for developing an infection. Procedures that provide for bacteriological safety must consider the patient and the care-giver. Handwashing before giving care protects the patient from pathogens on the nurse's hands. After giving care, the nurse washes to protect both self and the next patient from the microorganisms acquired from the first patient.

Threats to Biological Safety

Disease or infection does not necessarily result each time pathogens are present in or on the human body. A series of several steps, called the infection cycle or the *chain of infection*, must precede the onset of disease. First, a pathogen must be present in a place where it can live and multiply (*reservoir*). For example, the skin or nostrils of the nurse may serve as a reservoir for a particular bacterial pathogen called *Staphylococcus*. Next, there must be a way for the pathogen to leave or exit the reservoir. In the example, the nurse may sneeze while changing the dressing covering the incision of a patient. The pathogen, to cause disease, must then be able to move to the organism it will invade (called a *host*). In this example, the host is the patient. The pathogen may be spread by air currents, by food, or by insects. These are called *vehicles of transmission*. If the nurse sneezes over the patient, the pathogen may be transmitted by droplets carried in the air. Next, the pathogen must gain access or entry to the host (*portal of entry*). This may be done, for example, via a break in the skin, through the nose, mouth, or urinary tract. The patient with a surgical incision provides a readily available portal of entry for the pathogen. Finally, the pathogen seeks a *susceptible* host. Many hosts are able to defend against pathogens, but the hospitalized patient, already in a weakened state, has lowered resistance to disease. If the host cannot destroy the pathogen, an infection or disease may result. In the example, the patient may develop an infection of the incisional site. The susceptible host, in this case, the patient, often becomes the reservoir for the pathogen, and the cycle can be repeated.

In summary, the cycle of infection consists of presence of a pathogen, reservoir, portal of exit, vehicle of transmission, portal of entry, susceptible host.

The control of infection consists of eliminating any step in the cycle or chain. In the example, if the incision had been covered with sterile dressings or if the incision had been well healed, the pathogens would have had no portal of entry and the chain of infection would have been interrupted. Although it is not possible to avoid all infections within the hospital setting, thorough handwashing by nurses effectively eliminates a frequent vehicle of transmission for pathogens.

Normal Means of Body to Provide a Biologically Safe Environment

The human body has the ability to distinguish substances that are part of the body from those that are foreign to the body. This ability to discriminate "self from nonself" is the basis of the body's defense against foreign matter. When the body recognizes a microorganism as foreign, physiological processes are initiated that destroy, eliminate, or neutralize it. The person is resisting the process of infection and, if successful, the person is said to be resistant (*immune*) to that particular organism. At other times, the defenses of the body are not sufficiently strong to resist the pathogen. In this case, the person is considered *susceptible*, and infection or disease results. Although this ability to recognize and destroy foreign matter is essentially a protective mechanism, it may also function to the detriment of human beings. For example, the body may reject a heart transplant because the body recognizes the new organ as nonself. Body defenses against foreign substances are divided into two groups: nonspecific and specific.

Nonspecific Defenses Against Foreign Matter

All nonspecific body defenses have a common characteristic: all defend against any microbe or any foreign substance that invades the body. Hence, they provide a very general protection for the host.

Mechanical Defenses.   Unbroken skin and intact mucous membranes are the first line of defense against microorganisms. The skin encases the body and provides a thick, tough seal for vital body organs. Because the skin is in constant contact with the external environment, it is covered with microorganisms, particularly on the hands, the anal area, and in cracks between fingers and toes which are difficult to wash and which are not exposed to light and air. Microorganisms grow best in warm, moist, dark areas. Although the skin can be *cleaned* (freed of many disease-producing microorganisms) by washing, using careful scrubbing and rinsing methods, the number of microorganisms can only be reduced. The skin surface cannot be made *sterile* (free of all microorganisms) because this would require conditions of extreme heat and pressure or damaging chemicals. When patient conditions require sterility, nurses wear sterile gowns and gloves, as well as protective masks and hair coverings to avoid transferring microorganisms from nurse to patient. Sterile conditions are required during surgery.

Membranes lubricated with a secretion called mucus line body openings to the outside such as the eyes, mouth, and vagina. When these membranes are unbroken by sores or cuts, they are a strong defense against microorganisms. Mucus secretions are thick and thus function to trap foreign matter. Within the nose, there are mucus-covered hairs that filter and trap pollutants, dust, and microorganisms. Mucous membranes are also richly supplied with blood vessels and thus can rapidly circulate other defense mechanisms produced by blood cells to the area of injury.

In addition, the mucous membrane of the respiratory tract, specifically the nose, pharnyx, larynx, trachea, and bronchi, contains cells covered with microscopic, hairlike projections which wave only in one direction (ciliated epithelial cells). Cilia protect the body by moving foreign matter, such as dust or pus, out of the respiratory tract.

Tears, a watery solution of mucus, salts, and a bacteria-killing (bactericidal) enzyme called lysozyme, also serve a protective function. Tears clean and moisten the eye. Normally, about 1 ml of tear solution is produced per day. This solution is drained from the eye through ducts or is evaporated. When an irritant is present in the eye, tearing is increased, and the irritant can be diluted and washed away. This washing action prevents the establishment of microorganisms in the eye. When a person wears a contact lens for the first time, the body treats the lens as foreign matter and attempts, by excessive tearing, to get rid of the object.

Saliva is another washing mechanism to keep microorganisms from the mouth and teeth. In a similar manner, the outward flow of urine washes microorganisms from the urinary tract. Diarrhea and vomiting, although abnormal processes, are protective mechanisms of the body to remove products from the body.

Chemical Defenses.   Within the body, certain chemicals also contribute to immunity to disease. For example, the digestive juices within the stomach are highly acidic. There is sufficient acidity to destroy most bacteria and most poisons (toxins) produced by the bacteria.

Lysozyme is a substance found in tears, perspiration, saliva, nasal secretions, mucus, internal fluids, and cells. This enzyme is capable, under certain conditions, of breaking down the cell walls of bacteria, thus, destroying them.

The skin is also acidic, thus discouraging microbial growth. In addition, the oil glands of the skin produce sebum. One of the components of sebum is unsaturated fatty acid which kills certain pathogenic bacteria. One microorganism that is killed by the action of fatty acids is *Streptococcus pyogenes* which causes "strep throat" and scarlet fever.

Vaginal secretions have an acid environment created by harmless acid-producing bacteria. This environment is not favorable for the growth of pathogenic bacteria. In fact, when the normal acid-producing bacteria are either lessened or eliminated, as is the case when certain medications are taken, disease-producing microorganisms may be able to multiply rapidly and cause harm. The acid-producing bacteria of the vagina are normal and reasonably constant in the healthy individual. They are called normal or *resident flora*, in contrast to other bacteria which are occasionally present for a brief period (*transient flora*).

Inflammatory Response. Whenever the body sustains an injury or infection, many physiological processes are initiated by the body. Collectively, these processes are called the *inflammatory response*. Microorganisms, heat, chemicals, broken bones, or a severe cut from a sharp object may all stimulate the inflammatory response. It is important to note that not all inflammations involve infection. The inflammatory response is a protective device of the body which serves the following functions:

1. To destroy the injurious agent, if possible, and to remove it and its by-products from the body
2. If destruction is not possible, to confine or wall off the injurious agent and its by-products to limit the effects on the body
3. To repair or replace tissue damaged by the injurious agent or its by-products (Tortora *et al.*, 1982).

In order to illustrate the physiology and symptoms of a *local* (at the site of injury) inflammatory response, consider the example of a child who has fallen while roller-skating and reports for first aid with a bloody knee. The child complains of pain. Later, redness, heat, and swelling will be present at the site. These are the four primary characteristics of inflammation. Sometimes a fifth characteristic, loss of function, may be present if the injury is severe. In this example, the child may have a stiff knee and have difficulty walking for a few days.

PROCESS OF INFLAMMATION. The processes of inflammation are not yet completely understood, but all seem to involve injury and death to a number of body cells. These dying cells release chemicals which start the changes occurring during inflammation. The processes comprising the inflammatory response involve the blood vessels, specialized actions of cells, and tissue repair.

RESPONSES OF BLOOD VESSELS. After an injury has occurred (such as the child falling on roller skates) or some irritant (perhaps a bacteria or a chemical) has entered the tissue, changes in the blood vessels occur (the vascular response). There is a very brief period of narrowing of the diameter of blood vessels (vasoconstriction) followed by an increase in the diameter of the blood vessels (vasodilation). There is also increased ability of the blood vessels to permit passage of fluid and protein substances normally retained within the blood into the tissue (increased permeability). Vasodilation increases the blood flow to the injured area and increases the delivery of white blood cells (leukocytes) which are capable of ingesting and destroying (*phagocytosis*) substances such as bacteria, cells, particles.

Vasodilation and the increased permeability of blood vessels is caused by the release of chemicals, mainly histamine, bradykinin, serotonin, and prostaglandin from the injured cells. These chemicals are also thought to irritate local nerve endings and contribute to pain sensation. The increased blood flow (hyperemia) to the area which occurs as a result of vasodilation is responsible for the symptoms of heat and redness. The swelling or edema is caused by the increased fluid and protein leaking out of the blood into the tissues. The pressure of the swelling on local nerve endings also causes pain.

SPECIALIZED ACTIONS OF CELLS. Shortly after the injury, usually within an hour, phagocytic white blood cells are present at the site. Neutrophils are the first type of white blood cell to arrive at the injured tissue. These cells migrate out to the tissue to surround the irritant and become part of the mass of cells, fluid, and proteins in the tissue (*inflammatory exudate*). This cellular movement is dependent upon the attraction of neutrophils by chemicals generated in the inflamed cells. The whole response is called *chemotaxis*. Neutrophils then begin phagocytosis. Their main role occurs early in the inflammatory response, and they tend to die off rapidly.

Later, monocytes (another type of white blood cell) follow neutrophils into the tissue where they are transformed into phagocytic cells called wandering or free macrophages. These cells are more strongly phagocytic than neutrophils. How phagocytic cells "know" which objects to attack is thought to be determined by the presence of certain characteristics on the surface of the foreign or injured cells. What these characteristics are remains unclear. After phagocytes ingest large numbers of microorganisms and dead tissue, they eventually die and fill a cavity in the inflamed tissue. This debris is called pus. Frequently, the pus cavity opens to the body surface and empties. Sometimes, the pus cavity remains closed and is absorbed. At other times, the pus cavity is walled off by a fibrous protein of connective tissue (collagen) and cells that produce connective tissue (fibroblasts). This pus cavity is called an abscess and must be drained for healing to occur.

The blood also contains a soluble protein called fibrinogen which is converted to fibrin when it is released into the tissues. Fibrin is an elastic, thick, stringy, netlike substance which serves to form a barrier against the invading organisms, wall off the infectious process, and prevent its spread.

The exudate produced as a result of the inflammatory response varies in both consistency and character. It is called *purulent* exudate when it is composed of dead neutrophils and macrophages and is thick and yellow. A *serous* exudate contains mostly the liquid part of the blood and lymph and appears watery or clear. A *fibrin-*

ous exudate contains a fibrin clot and is sticky. A *hemorrhagic or sanguineous* exudate contains many red blood cells and appears red.

Tissue Repair.   The final process in the inflammatory response is tissue repair, that is, the replacement of dead or injured cells. Tissue repair begins even during inflammation, but healing cannot be completed until the inflammation has ceased and pus and dead or necrotic tissue have been removed. Tissue healing may occur by replacement of the injured cells with cells that have the same structure and function as injured cells (regeneration). Whether or not regeneration occurs depends upon the tissue involved. The skin, bones, and liver are organs that are capable of regeneration. Muscle cells such as those of the heart or the nerve cells of the brain do not regenerate.

New cells used in tissue repair are produced by supporting connecting tissue (stroma) and the functioning part of the tissue called parenchyma. The quality of the tissue repair depends on which type of cell, stromal or parenchymal, dominates the repair. If only parenchyma is involved, the repair may be excellent. If the stroma is active in the repair, scar tissue, which cannot perform the functions of the destroyed tissue, is produced. Sometimes, in the case of a severe injury, both elements are involved. Initially, a fragile pink or red (due to the presence of small blood vessels) framework of actively growing connective tissue, called granulation tissue, is produced. This is replaced in a matter of days by fibrous connective tissue which later results in a scar.

In summary, inflammation is a nonspecific defensive response of the body which is composed of several phases:

1. Vasodilation and increased vascular permeability
2. Chemotaxis and phagocytosis
3. Tissue repair

Inflammation is characterized by four local signs: redness, heat, swelling, and pain.

In addition to the signs of inflammation present at the point of injury or infection, characteristics of inflammation are also present throughout the body (*systemic*). All systemic signs are not necessarily found in all inflammatory responses. Fever is the most common sign and is frequently the result of bacterial or viral infection. Fever is caused when neutrophils release a protein called pyrogen. Pyrogen is thought to cause the movement of iron out of the plasma and into the liver. Since bacteria require high concentrations of iron to multipy, this is benefifical to the body (Vander *et al.*, 1980). Other systemic signs of inflammation may include lethargy, tiredness, and loss of appetite (anorexia), which may be an attempt of the body to conserve energy for

the healing process. Nausea, vomiting, and diarrhea may be present. There may also be an increased production of white blood cells (*leukocytosis*) in amounts exceeding 10,000/cu mm. (Normal is 5,000 to 10,000/cu mm.) Swollen, painful lymph nodes in the neck, underarm, or groin may develop as phagocytes, bacteria, and destroyed tissue accumulate.

There may also be an elevated *sedimentation rate.* This is a blood test done on venous blood placed in a 1-mm-diameter tube and allowed to settle for one hour. Test results are the distance that the red blood cells descend or settle in one hour. The normal rates are

Men: up to 15 mm/hour
Women: up to 20 mm/hour

The sedimentation rate is increased in infections, inflammations, tumors, and diseases causing the death of tissues. As the disease improves, the sedimentation rate decreases, and as the disease worsens, the sedimentation rate increases.

Interferon.   Another nonspecific defense of the body is interferon, a protein produced by cells infected by a virus. Interferon binds to the surface of uninfected cells and stimulates cells to produce antiviral proteins. The antiviral proteins then prevent the multiplication of the virus. The interferon produced by animal cells is of little value to human beings, that is to say that interferon is host-cell-specific. It is effective only in the species that produced it. However, interferon is active against many different viruses.

Complement System.   This is a group of 11 proteins, designated C1 (a complex of three proteins) to C9, found in normal blood serum in an inactive state. They are called "complement" because they function to complete certain immune reactions involving antibodies. These will be discussed later as a form of a specific defense of the body, but here complement is considered a nonspecific defense. Upon stimulation, the system's proteins change from an inactive to an active state. The change can be stimulated by the presence of a foreign substance (antigen) which, in turn, can stimulate the production of antibodies, which are proteins that protect the body by combining with antigens. In the inflammatory response, the complement system functions in chemotaxis, the release of histamines, and the release of substances that facilitate phagocytosis (opsonins).

Properdin System   This is a group of three serum proteins which functions to destroy certain bacteria, to enhance phagocytosis, to activate the complement system, and stimulate the inflammatory response.

Specific Defenses

Specific defenses of the body are directed against a particular foreign body, either microbial or chemical, and are generally ineffective against others. Specific defense mechanisms depend upon the ability of the cell to distinguish a particular foreign matter to be destroyed or neutralized. These defenses can be divided into two groups: antibody-mediated defenses and cell-mediated defenses.

Antibody-Mediated Defenses. The body produces specialized proteins called *antibodies* in response to the presence of either microbes or foreign chemicals which are called *antigens.* When an antigen comes in contact with a certain type of lymphocyte (called B cells), they cause the B cells to differentiate into either plasma cells which secrete antibodies or into memory cells which serve to strengthen the body response to invasion by the same antigen at a later date. This defense is alternatively called the B-cell system or humoral-mediated defense. Antigens stimulate the production of specific antibodies (immunogenicity) and react specifically with the antibody produced (reactivity). The unique structure of antibodies accounts for the specificity of the antigen-antibody reaction.

Antibodies belong to a group of proteins called immunoglubulins which contains five classes. Each class contains thousands of antibodies. Immunoglobulins are designated by the symbol Ig followed by a class letter G, A, M, D, or E. Each class performs certain functions within the body. Antibodies, in general, serve the following functions within the body:

1. Initiate the complement system
2. Enhance phagocytosis
3. Neutralize bacterial toxins or viruses
4. Neutralize some bacteria directly

When an individual is exposed to antigenic substances and antibodies are produced as a response, the individual is said to have an *active* or *acquired immunity.* While the original antigen-antibody response develops over several days, subsequent contact with the same antigen will result in a much more rapid defensive response of the body. Active immunity may be developed not only through contracting a specific disease such as measles but also through the injection of small amounts of dead or weakened microbes, as in the case of Salk polio or tuberculosis vaccines. *Passive immunity* is conferred by giving actively formed antibodies from

---

Table 18–1. **Summary of Types of Immunity**

I. *Innate Immunity (present at birth; depends on nonspecific defenses of the host)*
   a. Species immunity. Certain species are resistant to specific diseases.
     Example: Human beings are resistant to canine distemper.
   b. Individual immunity. Certain individuals are resistant to certain diseases which affect other individuals of the same species.
     Example: Some individuals may be resistant to influenza while others are not.
II. *Acquired Immunity (obtained during life; results from production of antibodies)*
   a. Active. Results from the production of antibodies by the body in response to the presence of an antigen.
     1. Naturally acquired active immunity. Results from the presence of active infection.
       Example: Scarlet fever immunity
     2. Artificially acquired active immunity. Inactivated or weakened microorganisms are introduced into the body in an amount that does not cause disease but does stimulate antibody production.
       Example: Vaccines against German measles, mumps, polio
   b. Passive. Results when antibodies produced by a source are transformed to a second person who needs them.
     1. Naturally acquired passive immunity. Results from transfer of antibodies from an immunized donor to a susceptible recipient.
       Example: Through breastfeeding the mother passes antibodies to an infant.
     2. Artificially acquired passive immunity. Results from injection of antibody containing serum into a second person.
       Example: Antisera against diphtheria, rabies, and botulism.

Source: Gerard J. Tortora; Berdell R. Funke; and Christine L. Case: *Microbiology: an Introduction* Benjamin Cummings, Menlo Park, Calif., Copyright 1982. Reproduced with permission.

Table 18–2. **Summary of ABO Blood Type System**

| | BLOOD TYPE | | | |
	A	B	AB	O
Agglutinogen	A	B	A and B	Neither A nor B
Antibodies	Anti-B	Anti-A	Neither anti-A nor anti-B	Both anti-A and anti-B
Compatible blood types for transfusions	O and A	O and B	O, A, B, AB (universal recipient)	0 (universal donor)
Percent of U.S. population	43	10	3	44
Percent of black population	30	20	3	47
Percent of Oriental population	35	23	12	30

one person to another, as in the case of infants who receive antibodies through the breast milk of the mother. This immunity is very temporary. Table 18–1 summarizes different types of immunity.

Although the antigen-antibody responses of the body are most often protective in nature, they can also work to harm the body. This is the case in an allergic reaction or an *autoimmune disease* (a disease in which the body produces the immune response against itself). Both of these conditions involve malfunctions of the specific defense system of the body.

Blood transfusion reactions are an unusual example of the antigen-antibody response since antibodies against a specific antigen are present without exposure to the specific antigen. Blood types are identified by the antigens (called agglutinogens) present on the red blood cell. These may be of the type A, B, O, or AB. Unlike the typical antigen-antibody reaction, a person with the blood type A, for example, has a high amount of anti-B

antibodies, even without an exposure to the B antigen. Why this occurs is not known. Table 18–2 shows the antibodies present in the four blood types. Thus, if a patient with blood type B were to receive a transfusion of blood type A, the patient would experience a reaction because

1. The patient's blood contained anti-A antibodies causing the donated blood to be attacked, and

2. The donated blood contains anti-B antibodies which attack the recipient's blood.

Number 2 is of little problem since the antibodies are diluted in the recipient's plasma, but number 1 causes the allergic reaction (Tortora and Anagnostakos, 1981). Signs of an allergic reaction may include hives, itching, and difficulty in breathing. This may worsen and even lead to death if the reaction is severe.

Cell-Mediated Defenses. T cells are a second type of lymphocyte cell. There are three classes of T cells:

Table 18–3. **T-Cell Lymphokines and Their Actions**

LYMPHOKINE	ACTION
1. Cytotoxic factor	Destroys microorganisms directly
2. Transfer factor	Causes nonsensitized lymphocytes at the site of the invasion to act as sensitized cells
3. Chemotactic factors	Attracts macrophages and monocytes
4. Macrophage-activating factor (MAF)	Increases phagocytosis of macrophages, polymorphs
5. Migration-inhibition factor	Prevents migration of cells away from site
6. Interferon (also produced by cells other than lymphocytes)	Blocks virus infection of tissue cells

1. Cell-destroying (cytolytic) cells
2. "Helper" cells, which enhance the production of antibodies by B cells
3. "Suppressor" cells, which decrease the production of antibodies by B cells

The helper-suppressor function is not well understood at this time. Cytolytic cells are of primary importance in cell-mediated defenses.

T cells do not produce antibodies. Rather, in response to an antigen, T cells become *sensitized*. This means that the T cell enlarges and splits into specialized cells. Some of the T cells are now called killer T cells. They travel to the invading antigen where they give off a powerful group of chemicals called lymphokines which serve to enhance the nonspecific inflammatory response. Table 18–3 summarizes the action of the lymphokines.

Like the B cells, some of the T cells function as memory cells which greatly accelerates the defense reaction to a second invasion by the same antigen.

Finally, cell-mediated defenses (T cells) function against cancer. Cancer cells are thought to arise from changes in normal body cells and thus act as foreign cells. T cells then become sensitized to the antigens of the foreign cells and destroy them. Only when the T cells fail to recognize the foreign cell, or when T cells are ineffective in destroying them, is detectable cancer produced.

Factors Affecting the Need for Biological Safety

Under normal conditions, the healthy body has sufficient defenses to protect against pathogenic microorganisms. In addition to the specific and nonspecific defenses already discussed, the following factors affect resistance to pathogens:

1. Nutritional status. In general, an inadequate nutritional status decreases the body's ability to respond effectively against disease. Why this is so is not completely understood, but it is suggested that since antibodies are proteins, it is possible that the severe depletion of body proteins reduces the ability of the body to make antibodies (Beland and Passos, 1981). Conversely, there is little evidence to suggest that excessive nutrition enhances resistance to disease.

2. Preexisting disease conditions may weaken the ability of the body to respond to pathogens. For example, the patient with multiple sclerosis is prone to developing kidney or respiratory infections.

3. Tissue injury decreases resistance of the involved tissue. The patient with a broken leg is more susceptible to infection than a patient who has not sustained the injury.

4. Inability of the body to produce a substance needed for defense, such as gamma globulin (IgG, the most abundant immunoglobulin in plasma), increases susceptibility to infection.

5. Inability of the body to produce functional white blood cells lowers resistance.

6. Reduced activity of lymphocytes decreases resistance.

7. Age. The lowered resistance of elderly people may be due to reduced activity of lymphocytes. Infants under the age of three months are dependent upon the antibodies passed to them from the mother, either before birth or via breast milk, as their immune system matures. The normal newborn begins to produce antibodies between the ages of three and six months. Adult levels of antibodies are not produced until adolescence.

8. Presence or absence of immunities. Some individuals are immune to certain disease (individual immunity), and some races are immune to diseases (racial immunity). Caucasians are more immune to tuberculosis and smallpox than are blacks and American Indians. Persons who have been vaccinated against such diseases as polio, diphtheria, or tetanus have an artifically acquired long-lasting immunity.

9. Use of antibiotics. Although antibiotics are effective and beneficial drugs against many pathogens, they are not without potential dangers and are not to be taken indiscriminately. Antibiotics may change the normal bacteria within the body and permit other pathogens to grow which resist the action of antibiotics. There is also the danger that antibiotics are no longer effective against certain pathogens. This is what is meant by the term *antibiotic resistance*.

10. Hormones. These substances are secretions of the ductless glands of the body which are carried in the blood. Individuals who have an unusually high level of hormones, either due to a disease process where they are hypersecreted or due to receiving hormones from an external source as in a medication, all have a decreased resistance to infection. One group of hormones, corticosteroids, is known to decrease the production of antibodies and interferon. Another group of hormones,

the glucocorticoids, is an extremely effective anti-inflammatory drug which suppresses the inflammatory response. If glucocorticoids are given as a medication or are produced by the body at abnormally high levels, an infection caused by bacteria will not be localized by the inflammatory response but will spread throughout the body.

Problems Related to the Need for Biological Safety

Hospitalized patients have an accentuated need for microbial safety due to the very nature of the hospital environment. Patients are exposed to pathogens that they might not normally contact in the course of everyday life. Hospitalized persons are also generally in a physically weakened state due to a disease process or trauma and are thus less likely to be able to produce strong body defenses. Within the hospital setting, there are four major causes for microbial safety problems: personnel and environmental factors, disease conditions, diagnostic and treatment procedures, and medication therapy.

Problems Related to Personnel and Environment

It has been estimated that 5 to 10 percent of patients, as many as 1,500,000 people each year, acquire infections during their hospitalization. These infections were not present at the time of admission. Such hospital-acquired infections are called *nosocomial infections*. Both very old patients and very young patients (newborns and infants) are particularly susceptible to these infections. Hospital rooms, bathing, and toilet facilities are shared with strangers who, in turn, have visitors. All of these persons carry microorganisms to the patient. The large numbers of hospital·personnel who come in contact with each patient are also responsible for the spread of microbes. Consider that each patient may be seen daily by nurse aides, nurses, physicians, dietary staff, housekeepers, laboratory technicians, and perhaps other health team members. Now multiply this by the number of shifts, usually three, that comprise a hospital day of 24 hours. In addition, consider that each of the hospital staff members may see as many as 10 to 20 patients per day. Thus, it is easy to see the potential for the spread of microorganisms. Often a person may be apparently healthy and show no evidence of a disease state but still harbor a pathogen. Such a person is a called a *carrier* and may be one cause of nosocomial infections. Another cause of hospital-acquired infections may be cross-contamination by care-givers. If a nurse changed the dressings on an infected surgical incision and then gives care to a second patient without adequate handwashing, the nurse may pass the pathogens to the second patient. This is one example of cross-contamination. *Contamination* means that microorganisms are introduced into an area where they are not normally present. Supplies, equipment, and medications may all be contaminated in a similar manner.

Problems Related to Disease Conditions

Certain disease conditions increase the need to provide biological safety for patients. The patient who has particular allergies has a high need for protection from those substances. The allergic patient is overly sensitive to a particular antigen which is now called an allergen. Consider the patient who is allergic to a bee sting. Initially, the patient is stung and the *allergen*, the chemical from the sting, enters the body as an antigen. The body produces antibodies against it. This is called *sensitization*. Memory cells also develop. After a second bee sting, the antigen-antibody reaction functions to destroy both the cells and the allergen. When the injured cells release histamine, the inflammatory response is activated, and the resulting symptoms occur. If the reaction is severe, the patient may experience difficulty breathing, severe edema, and a decrease in circulating blood. This condition is known as *anaphylactic shock* and can lead to death if untreated. It is important to remember that almost any substance can be an allergen to a particular person. Foods, medications, certain fabrics, plants, and cosmetics are all frequent allergens. The nurse who admits a patient to the hospital must carefully question the patient for the presence of allergies and document the response. The nurse then places identification of the allergen such as "codeine allergy" on a prominent tag on the patient's wrist.

In some diseases, the body begins to respond to its own tissue as it would respond to an antigen. The body produces antibodies or sensitized T cells which destroy body tissues. The damage to the body cells which results is called *autoimmune disease*. Rheumatoid arthritis and multiple sclerosis are thought to be examples of such diseases. The theory of causation and prevention of autoimmunity is the subject of much research.

Problems Related to Medication Therapy

The intended purpose of medication therapy related to biological safety is to combat pathogens and restore the health of the individual. Certain medications, however, produce side effects (actions other than those that are desired or intended). One side effect of some anti-infective drugs is the destruction of resident flora. In some cases, this makes the body susceptible to other types of pathogens which would not be able to grow and multiply in the body under ordinary conditions. This infection is called a suprainfection (one infection on top of another infection). The pathogen causing the suprainfection is called an opportunist.

Some types of pathogens have become increasingly resistant to certain antibiotics and may require alternative drug therapy. Hospitalized patients require diagnostic testing to determine the most effective drug against a particular pathogen.

Many drugs used to treat cancer also have the effect of decreasing the production of leukocytes, thereby reducing the inflammatory response. These drugs also suppress lymphocyte production and thereby decrease the production of antibodies. Patients receiving these drugs are very susceptible to opportunist organisms that can cause serious antibiotic-resistant infections.

Problems Related to Diagnostic and Treatment Procedures

Although the benefits of medical treatments are intended to outweigh the side effects, many therapeutically effective procedures cause actual or potential harm to the patient. Patients with cancer often receive drugs that are immunosuppressive as a side effect. This means that the normal protective responses of the body are incidently decreased. The white blood cell count of the patient is radically decreased, limiting the ability of the body to resist infection. Patients with leukemia (cancer of the blood-forming tissue) are also at severe risk due to a low production of normal white blood cells and the side effects of drug therapy. It is essential that nurses working with patients with low white blood cell counts use biologically protective techniques such as frequent, thorough handwashing. These patients may require a special room in which purified air can be circulated.

Patients receiving radiation treatments are also at risk since radiation has the effect of destroying lymphocytes, thus decreasing the ability of the body to produce the immune response. This may be the case in patients with cancer or in patients who are to receive an organ transplant. In transplant patients, the suppression of immunity is a desirable effect which should lessen the chances that the body will reject and destroy the new organ because it is recognized as foreign. At the same time, however, the patient is also at increased risk for developing infection.

Diagnostic procedures, while very necessary, also predispose the patient to infection. Those examinations that involve breaking the skin to administer intravenous dyes or medications or entering sterile body cavities to insert drainage tubes or to perform internal visualization all carry the risk of infection. The risk is minimized by the sterile technique used by the persons conducting the procedures.

Surgical procedures all involve breaking the skin, the body's first defense against microorganisms. If the surgery involves opening the intestine or bowel, areas considered grossly contaminated, the risk is further increased.

Ethical and Legal Considerations Related to Biological Safety

Protecting the patient by using clean or sterile technique is a nursing intervention which is part of the care of all patients although it is more crucial to some patients than it is to others. Much of the conduct of the nurse regarding aseptic (free of disease-producing microorganisms) technique is undetectable to either patients or other nurse colleagues. For example, if a nurse inadvertently contaminated a sterile needle by touching it to the surface of the countertop, the patient would not be able to detect that the needle was no longer sterile. The nurse must acknowledge the error, if only to self, and discard the contaminated needle, replacing it with a sterile one. Maintaining clean or sterile technique requires time. Adequate handwashing between patients takes time. Yet, this basic skill can prevent the transfer of microorganisms from nurse to patient. The Code for Nurses requires that the nurse safeguard the patient when health care is affected by incompetent practices. Violations of aseptic technique are such practices. The nurse has an ethical responsibility to maintain the technique of self and others. If others violate sterile technique and do not recognize their error, the nurse is obligated to point this out for the protection of the patient.

In addition to the ethical considerations, there are

also legal implications. Cheifetzin (1978) cites several situations where violations of aseptic technique could be a basis for legal action:

1. Nurses' failure to wash hands
2. Use of improperly sterilized equipment

3. Improper wound care
4. Reusing an article intended to be disposable

Using strict aseptic technique when needed is the best defense the nurse has against such lawsuits.

Effect of Unmet Need for Biological Safety on Other Needs

When an infection or inflammation is present, other needs are also affected, depending on the severity of the disease process. Oxygen consumption is increased as the body temperature rises. The patient will have an increased pulse and respiratory rate. Fluid needs are increased in order to replace those lost in the sweating response to fever and to replace circulating fluids. If fluid needs are not maintained, urine production will decrease, and urine will appear dark and concentrated. Nutritional needs change as the body metabolism rises and causes increased caloric use and protein breakdown. The metabolic rate increases approximately 7 percent for each degree of fever. Therefore, additional protein and carbohydrates are required to aid in tissue repair. The mobility of the patient may be limited during the acute phase of the illness and exercises in bed may be needed to minimize the effects of bed rest. The need for rest and sleep is increased since most of the available body energies are directed toward the healing process.

In addition to the effect on physiological needs, the process of infection or inflammation also affects higher level needs, although in a less predictable manner. Many patients may experience fear and loss of control of their lives related to the uncertainty of the infection. For example, a diabetic patient with an infected foot may be facing the possibility of an amputation. If it is necessary to isolate the patient as a protective measure, the patient may feel the loss of support of family and visitors, even though this is not the attitude of the family. Some patients withdraw and experience some degree of depression. The patient's energy level may be so low as to decrease the desire for social contact or the ability to perform work. The effect of the disease process on both the survival needs and the higher level needs is considered in planning nursing care.

Assessment of Biological Safety

Objective Data

Objective data indicating the presence of infection are obtained by tests and measurements of body functions and by clinical signs.

Body temperature greater than 98.6°F or 37°C when taken orally.
Skin hot to touch, reddened area, or red streaks.
Unexplained fever (called FUO—fever of unknown origin).
Unexplained diarrhea.
Foul odor.
Purulent drainage.
Skin rashes.
Coughing or sneezing.
Areas of localized edema.
Limited movement of the affected part.

Possibly weight loss.
Elevated sedimentation rate (normal rates: men, up to 15 mm/hour; women, up to 20 mm/hour).
Urine or blood cultures positive for the presence of microorganisms.
Altered white blood cell (WBC) count (5,000 to 10,000/cu mm is normal for an adult). The WBC is generally increased (*leukocytosis*) during infection or inflammation. In addition, the numbers of different white blood cells present (called a *differential white blood cell count*) aid in the diagnosis of the causative agent.

A differential white blood cell count is done to measure the percentage of each type of leukocyte in a blood sample. This is important diagnostic information since certain types of white blood cells are elevated or decreased in certain diseases. The normal levels for an adult's differential white blood cell are as follows:

Neutrophils. Normal, 55 to 70 percent. Increased neutrophils (neutrophilia) are present in acute suppurative infections and myelocytic leukemia. Neutrophils are decreased (neutropenia) in certain drug therapies, in acute bacterial infection, especially in the aged, or as a side effect of radiation therapy.

Lymphocytes. Normal, 20 to 40 percent. Lymphocytes are increased (lymphocytosis) in chronic bacterial infections, viral infections, infectious mononucleosis, lymphocytic leukemia. Lymphocytes are decreased (lymphopenia) in leukemia, immune deficiency diseases, and some drug therapy.

Monocytes. Normal, 2 to 8 percent. Monocytes are increased (monocytosis) in tuberculosis, some protozoal and rickettsial infections, Hodgkin's disease (a form of cancer), and monocytic leukemia.

Eosinophils. Normal, 1 to 4 percent. These are increased in allergic reactions, autoimmune diseases, and leukemia.

Basophils. Normal, 0.5 to 1.0 percent. Because there are so few basophils in the circulating white cells, a decrease is difficult to detect, but an increase (basophilia) is readily apparent. Basophilia is seen in Hodgkin's disease and chronic myelocytic leukemia. Decreased basophils are seen in an acute allergic reaction (Pagana and Pagana, 1982).

Subjective Data

Some complaints of the patient are subjective data that suggest the presence of infection.

Pain localized to the site of infection.
Loss of appetite.
Tiredness, loss of energy.
Headache
Nausea
Complaints of burning on urination

Nursing Intervention Related to a Biologically Safe Environment

Medically Safe Environment

A major function within the role of the nurse is maintaining an environment for the patient that is free of pathogens. Together, all of the skills the nurse uses to establish and maintain this environment are called *medical asepsis, aseptic technique*, or *clean technique*. These techniques do not make the environment completely free from all microorganisms but limit the spread of pathogens or confine them to a particular area.

Nurses' Uniforms. Nurses' uniforms vary according to the setting in which nurses are employed. Whatever the uniform requirement of the employing institution, the nurse has responsibilities regarding the uniform which are related to the concept of a biologically safe environment.

For this reason, the nurse wears a clean uniform while on duty. The uniform is laundered daily and is not worn in public prior to its use in the hospital. Uniforms must be loose enough and long enough to permit ease of movement and safety. Long sleeves may become snagged in machines and also do not permit ease of handwashing and thus are discouraged. Because a nurse's shoes (and shoelaces) are easily soiled, they require frequent cleaning and polishing. Long hair must be worn off the collar since hair is a source of microor-

ganisms and a potential source of contamination to sterile areas. It is also possible to snare long hair in hospital equipment. Dangling jewelry is also avoided for the same reason. Detailed rings and long fingernails trap microorganisms and are difficult to wash adequately. They may also scratch patients as the nurse gives care, creating skin openings for bacteria. Also, like long-sleeved uniforms, they make it difficult to perform adequate handwashing. Unless sweaters are laundered after each use, they have the potential to transfer microorganisms to patients. Nurses' caps are a source of microorganism transfer and are discouraged in clean areas of the hospital such as surgery or obstetrics.

Medical Handwashing. Handwashing is the single most important means of preventing the spread of infection. It is frequently, however, incorrectly or inadequately done in an attempt to save time. Unfortunately, this may cause increased infections and longer patient hospitalizations at increased cost. Handwashing is recommended at the following times:

1. Upon arriving at the clinical unit prior to beginning a period of duty. This will serve to decrease the microorganisms transported to the hospital from the external environment. Nurses also wash their hands prior to leaving the clinical area for rest and meal breaks in order to decrease the spread of microorganisms to other areas of the hospital and to themselves.

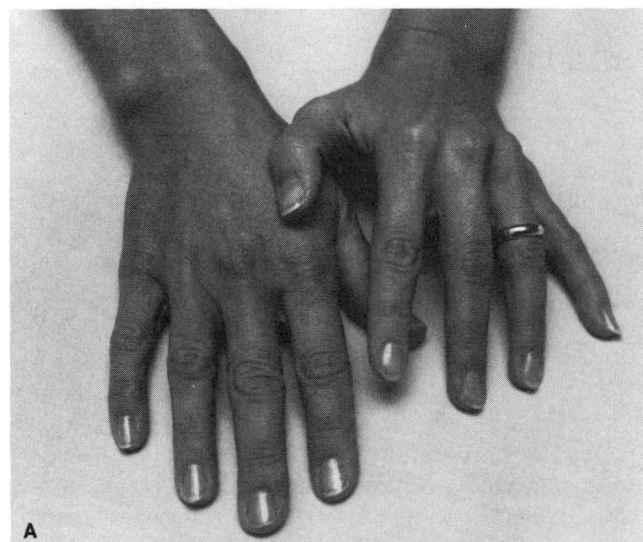

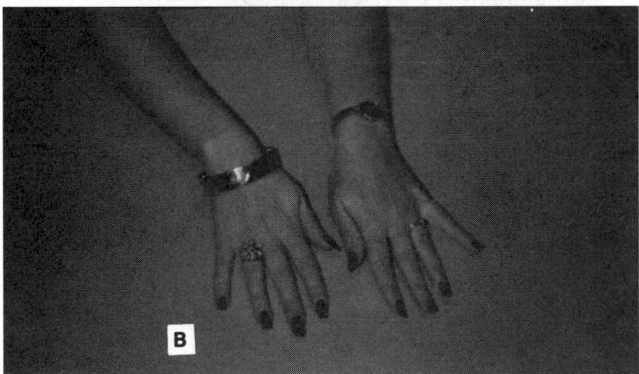

Figure 18-1. The nurse's hands could be a source of microorganisms. Long fingernails and ornate jewelry are difficult to cleanse adequately.

2. Before and after giving patient care in order to prevent the spread of micoorganisms between patients.

3. Prior to performing any clean duties such as preparing medications, handling food trays, assembling equipment, or selecting clean linen.

4. After performing any duties involving contaminated articles such as bedpans, surgical dressings, soiled tissues, or dirty linen.

Nursing Skill 18-1 is one method of medical handwashing.

Patient Hygiene Needs. The hospitalized patient may be unable to meet basic needs for hygiene without assistance. It is the responsibility of nurses to assess the level of independence of which the patient is capable. The health and recovery of the patient are promoted by encouraging the patient to be as independent as possible in care. This is not done to save the nurse work or because the nurse is unwilling to provide care for the patient. It is because the ability of the patient to be as independent

as possible is a goal for adult patients. The level of independence of the patient changes as the condition of the patient changes. A patient who has been admitted to the hospital for surgery two days later may initially require little assistance in meeting hygiene needs. Immediately after surgery, the same patient may need complete hygiene care provided by the nurse.

Prior to beginning hygiene care, the nurse offers the patient who is on bed rest the bedpan or urinal. Ambulatory patients may be assisted to the bathroom. This will assure the patient's comfort during the procedure. Both the nurse's and the patient's hands are washed after the nurse assists the patient with elimination. In addition, it may be necessary to offer pain-relief measures before giving care.

Oral Care. On admission of the patient, the nurse has noted whether the patient has any removable dentures. Some hospitals permanently label the inside of the denture with the patient's name if they are not constantly worn by the individual. All dentures are to be placed in a labeled denture cup, when they are not in the patient's mouth, in order to prevent loss.

If the nurse is to clean dentures, which is done before and after meals if the patient is unable to clean them, they are removed and taken in a basin to a sink. Because dentures are easily broken, the sink is lined with a washcloth to protect the dentures if dropped. All surfaces of the dentures are brushed with a dentifrice. They are then rinsed well. Before returning dentures to the

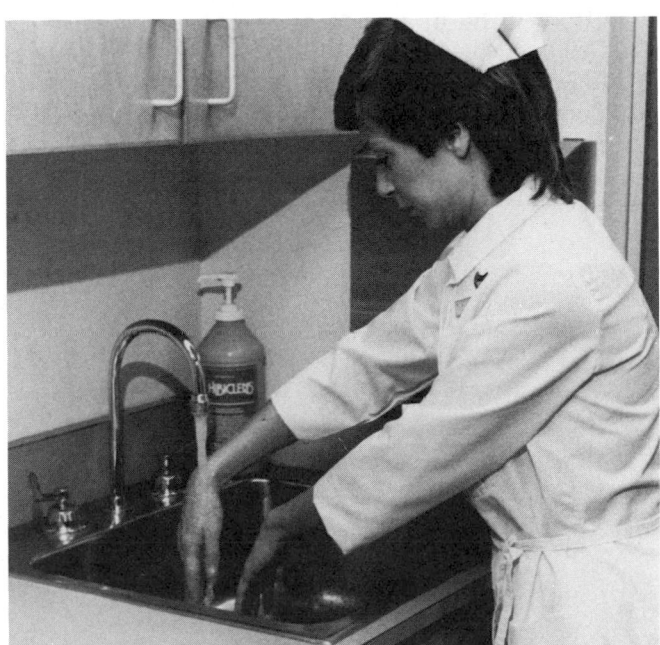

Figure 18-2. Medical handwashing.

Nursing Skill 18–1. **Medical Handwashing**

Supplies

Soap as provided by the hospital. This may be liquid in a foot-controlled dispenser, bar soap, or a paper sheet with soap in it.

Stick or brush for cleaning fingernails

Warm running water, preferably with foot or knee control

Disposable towels or warm air dryer

Procedure	Explanation
1. Remove jewelry. Rings may be pinned inside uniform pocket, watches pinned where visible to nurse.	1. Jewelry harbors microorganisms and is difficult to clean. Remove watch rather than push up on the arm since repositioning the watch on the clean wrist will contaminate the wrist area.
2. Adjust water to comfortable temperature.	2. Comfort and protection of the nurse. Heat opens pores and also removes protective oils on the nurse's hands.
3. Holding hands below the level of the elbows, wet the hands thoroughly.	3. In this manner, the water will flow from the least contaminated area (arms) to the most contaminated area (fingertips).
4. Apply soap. If bar soap is used, the bar is rinsed prior to returning it to the soap dish.	4. Most hospital soap kills some microorganisms, that is to say, it is bacteriostatic. Soap is rinsed to prevent the spread of microorganisms since microbes grow on the wet surface of the soap.
5. Wash each hand, finger, and nail separately paying special attention to the webbed areas between the fingers. Wash for one full minute.	5. These are areas frequently missed. Washing times will vary. A full minute is required for the first washing of the duty period and for heavily soiled hands.
6. Rinse so the water flows down from the wrist area off the fingertips.	6. Water flows from the least contaminated area (wrist) to the most contaminated area (fingertips).
7. Dry hands beginning at the wrist and moving to the fingertips. Use warm air dryer if provided.	7. Move from area of least toward most contamination.
8. Turn off the water using a new, dry paper towel. Discard paper towel properly.	8. Avoids contaminating clean hands by touching contaminated hand control.

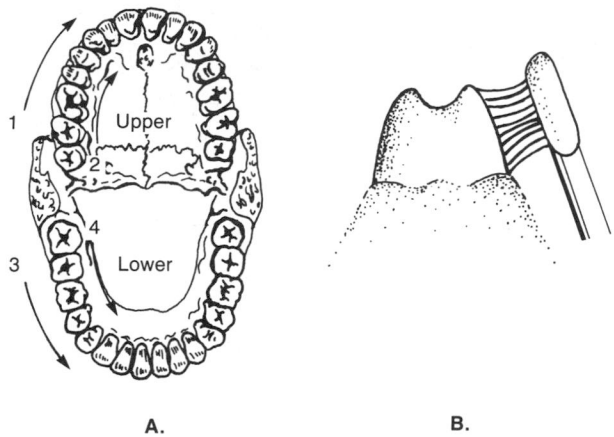

A.   B.

Figure 18–3. Techniques for brushing teeth. **A.** Brush upper teeth, then lower teeth. **B.** Brush thoroughly, especially where neck of tooth joins gum.

patient's mouth, offer the patient mouthwash to rinse the mouth. If mucous secretions are very thick, it may be necessary to wipe the mouth gently with sponge-tipped swabs. If the patient is able to cleanse the dentures, the nurse brings the supplies (brush, dentifrice, basin, glass, water, and towel) to the bedside and positions the patient comfortably in a sitting position.

It will be necessary for the nurse to brush the natural teeth of many patients confined to bed. If possible, the patient is in a back-lying (supine) position with the bed raised to a comfortable working height for the nurse and the head of the bed elevated. (See Figure 18–3.) The nurse places supplies on the tray table and assists the patient to turn slightly toward the nurse. A towel is placed under the patient's chin. After wetting the toothbrush with water and applying toothpaste on it, the nurse holds the brush at a 45-degree angle to the teeth. Beginning on the back top and cheek-side teeth, the nurse brushes the outer surfaces of the teeth, using a back-and-forth motion and being careful to brush the area where the teeth enter the gum. The same method is used to brush the tongue-side of the teeth. The inside surfaces of the front teeth are brushed, using the tip of the brush. The top of the tongue and the roof of the mouth directly behind the front teeth are also brushed to help remove

bacteria and reduce mouth odors. The nurse stops frequently to permit the patient to spit into the basin. If the patient must remain absolutely flat, the nurse gives the patient a straw to assist in removing the liquid. After brushing is complete, the patient is given fresh water to rinse the mouth.

Flossing Teeth.   Since food trapped between the teeth can cause tooth decay in a matter of hours, it is important that flossing of the teeth be continued while in the hospital. Flossing is usually done along with brushing. For some patients, the nurse need only provide the patient with the floss. At other times, the nurse may perform flossing for the patient. The patient may be unaccustomed to flossing or find it painful because of sensitive gums. The nurse may offer to floss but accepts the decision of the patient. Occasionally, disease conditions may contraindicate flossing, such as in patients having blood-clotting disorders.

Before beginning flossing, the nurse washes hands, and secures supplies (floss, glass of clean, tepid water, a basin, tissue). The nurse positions the patient as for brushing the teeth, if possible. (See Figure 18–4). Using approximately 12 to 16 inches of floss, wrap the ends around the second finger of each hand, leaving a length

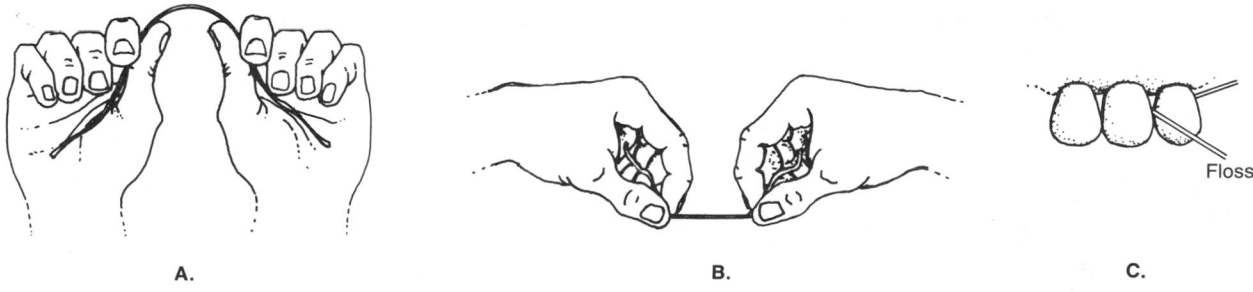

A.   B.   C.

Figure 18–4.   Techniques for flossing teeth. **A.** Upper teeth. **B.** Lower teeth. **C.** Wipe around tooth with floss.

Nursing Skill 18–2.   Giving a Bed Bath

Equipment
    Wash basin
    Bath blanket
    Washcloth and two towels
    Clean patient gown
    Grooming aids as desired: soap, bath oil, deodorant, comb, brush, lotion,
       shaver, powder
    Hamper for soiled linen

Preparation
    Assess if patient is having pain, and intervene as necessary.
    Explain the procedure to the patient.
    Provide for privacy by closing the door and pulling the curtains.
    Offer the patient the bedpan or urinal. Completing elimination at this time adds
       to the patient's comfort and makes the bath as clean a procedure as possible.
    Wash hands and gather clean equipment.
    Offer assistance with shaving, for male or female patients.

Procedure	Explanation
1. Adjust the bed to a comfortable working height for the nurse.	1. Eliminate unnecessary muscle strain for the nurse.
2. Place a bath blanket over the patient and ask the patient to hold the top edge of the blanket, if able.	2. Provide privacy for patient.
3. Remove the top linen from the bed, folding it if it is to be reused. If the linen is dirty, roll the linen and place it in the hamper.	3. This will keep the linen dry during the bath. Rolling the linen will limit the spread of the microorganisms.
4. Remove patient's gown while keeping covered with bath blanket.	4. Provides for privacy. Keeps patient warm.
5. Place side rails up and fill basin with warm (43–46° C or 110–115° F) water.	5. Side rails prevent the patient from falling out of bed. Water is comfortably warm without risk of burning.
6. Make a mitt of the washcloth. (See Figure 18–5.)	6. A mitt retains heat and water and protects patient from fingernails of nurse.
7. Wipe the patient's eyes with clean, damp cloth, moving from the inner corner of the eye (inner canthus) to the outer canthus. Use a clean area of the cloth for each eye.	7. Cleansing from inner to outer canthus prevents substances from entering the tear ducts. Using clean areas of the cloth prevents the transfer of microorganisms between eyes.
8. Offer patient choice of using soap. Using the mitt, wash the patient's face and neck. Pat dry.	8. Many patients do not like soap. Wash from cleanest area of body to the most contaminated area. Patting dry is less abrasive to skin tissue.
9. Place a towel under the arm which is extended at the patient's side. Using the mitt, wash the arm using long strokes from the wrist toward and including underarm. Cover arm with towel. Rinse and pat dry. Repeat for other arm. Offer deodorant	9. Towel keeps the bed dry and provides warmth when used as cover. Heat is lost from the evaporation process of wet skin drying. This may make the patient cold and uncomfortable.
10. With towel under basin on bed, wash both patient's hands in basin. Rinse and dry.	10. Towel is protection for bed.

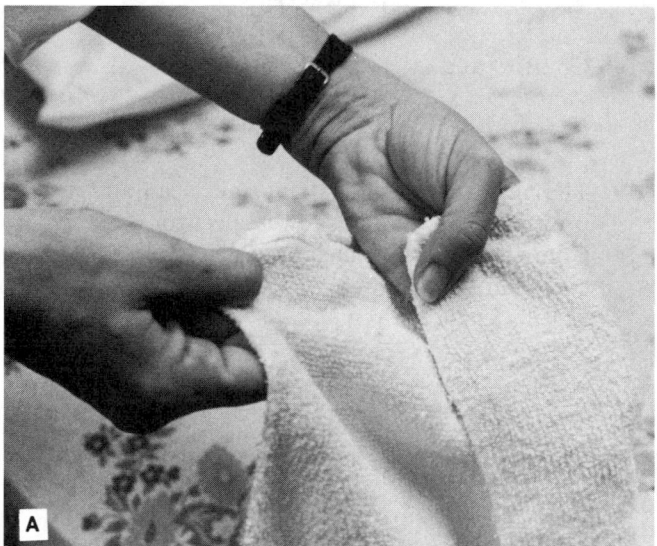
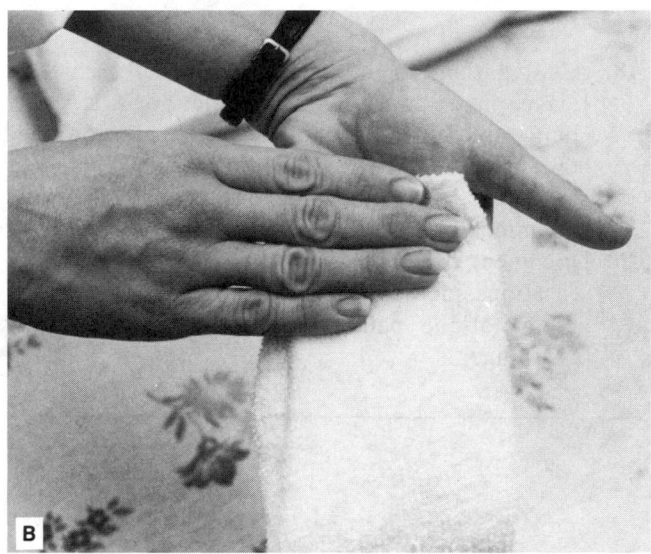
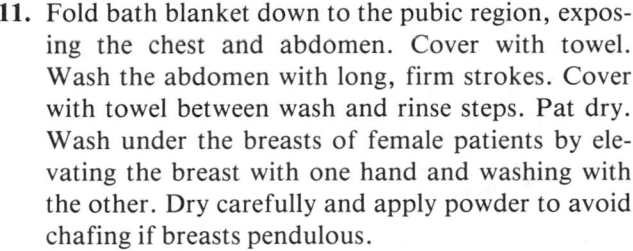

Figure 18–5. Making a mitt of a washcloth.

11. Fold bath blanket down to the pubic region, exposing the chest and abdomen. Cover with towel. Wash the abdomen with long, firm strokes. Cover with towel between wash and rinse steps. Pat dry. Wash under the breasts of female patients by elevating the breast with one hand and washing with the other. Dry carefully and apply powder to avoid chafing if breasts pendulous.

12. Expose one leg at a time, groin to toes, by pulling the bath blanket under the leg to be washed and tucking under at the hip.
    Place towel under calf of leg. Place basin near the leg. Flex the leg at the knee and, while supporting the heel in the cup of your hand, place the foot in the basin. Wash the leg with long, firm strokes.
    Cleanse foot. Rinse. Remove basin while supporting flexed leg with heel in cup of hand. Place leg on extended towel; dry. Repeat for other leg.

13. Assist patient to side-lying position.

14. Obtain clean, warm water.

15. Position the towel on the bed parallel to the patient. Fold the bath blanket on the patient, exposing the back and buttocks. Wash with long, firm strokes. Cover back with towel. Rinse and dry.

16. Back massage (see Chapter 25) may be given at this time. Assist patient to turn to back.

17. Complete perineal care. Obtain clean water. Assess how much assistance the patient requires and assist as necessary. (See discussion on pages 349, 352.)

11. The nurse provides privacy for the patient but at the same time must expose the patient for skin care and assessment.
    Same as #9.

    Chafed skin is portal of entry to infection.

12. Same as #9.

13. Restful position which permits cleansing, massage, and visualization of the back.

14. Water cools off quickly. Warm water provides comfort. Soap film left on skin is irritating and drying.

15. Same as #9.

16. Long period of bed rest causes discomfort which can be reduced with massage.

17. Many patients prefer to wash their own genital area. The nurse may either assist or do the entire procedure as required.

Procedure	Explanation
18. Assist patient to put on clean gown; brush hair. Leave patient in a comfortable position. May change linen at this time. (See discussion on page 000.)	**18.** Comfort and safety of the patient.
19. Wash, dry, and put away basin, soap dish, and grooming aids.	**19.** The nurse leaves the patient unit clean and neat to prevent accidents and show respect for patient.
20. Document the procedure, noting any unusual observations such as reddened areas of the skin, degree of fatigue, pain upon movement, or difficulty breathing.	**20.** Contribute to continued data collection of nursing care plan. Fulfills legal requirements.

of about 3 inches between the two index fingers. Most of the excess floss is wrapped around one finger, which is then unwound as needed. Used floss is wrapped around the opposite finger. Grasping the floss between the thumb and forefinger for the upper teeth, work the floss between the upper teeth from the crown to the gum line and as far along the gum line as possible. For the lower teeth, use the index fingers to push down on the stretched floss and move it between the teeth. The teeth are wiped with the floss, rather than using a sawing motion which might injure the gums. When all the teeth have been flossed, offer the patient water to rinse the mouth since the flossing has loosened food particles trapped between the teeth.

Bathing Patients. Giving a patient a bath provides the nurse with the opportunity to perform several important functions. Bathing is intended to cleanse the skin and reduce the number of microorganisms present. This is especially important when the patient is on bed rest and must both urinate and have bowel movements in bed. The exercise of bathing also increases circulation. Second, hygiene measures provide comfort and relaxation for the patient. Patients frequently comment on how much better they feel having had their teeth brushed and a bed bath. Third, giving this care gives the nurse the opportunity to observe and assess the patient. The nurse observes the skin condition, noting especially any areas that appear reddened and prone to skin breakdown. Scars and rashes are also noted. The nurse observes the ability of the patient to move, as well as the presence of pain upon movement. All of these things contribute to the ongoing data collection of the nursing care plan. Finally, the time that the nurse spends in providing this care, especially giving a bed bath, helps to establish the therapeutic relationship between the nurse and the patient. This time is usually quiet and uninterrupted. Patients may use the opportunity to discuss serious concerns with the nurse.

All hospitalized patients require some type of bath, and the determination of which type is often a nursing decision. The nurse must consider the patient's strength, condition, and level of independence. A patient with an IV or new surgical dressings is usually limited to a bed bath since sterile dressings must be kept dry. Microorganisms multiply rapidly in wet dressings. The facilities available for bathing also influence the nurse's decision. If shower stalls which accommodate chairs with wheels are available, many patients prefer showers. Patient preferences regarding the type of bath and the time of bath are taken into consideration when possible. Many patients prefer bathing before bed in the evening since this is the routine they follow at home. If the nurse is able to meet this patient choice, it may be that the pa-

tient will rest better since the home routine has been preserved. Whatever type of bath is selected, it must be safe for the patient. The patient's chart or nursing care plan is reviewed for activity restrictions.

Many hospitalized patients will choose to take a tub bath or a shower. In this case, the nurse gives minimal assistance. The nurse is responsible for assuring that the shower or tub area is clean and has been washed with disinfectant according to hospital procedures. Since the disinfectant may be harmful to the patient's skin, the shower or tub must be thoroughly rinsed.

Other patients may require a bed bath. Again, it is a nursing decision how frequently baths need be given. When skin is extremely dry, such as in elderly patients, the frequency of bathing is reduced to preserve the oil on the skin. At other times, baths are given more frequently, such as to a patient with an elevated temperature who is perspiring profusely.

The procedure for bathing a patient in bed follows. A word of caution is in order. Procedures are intended as general guidelines which must be adapted to meet the individual needs of a patient or nurse. At all times be guided by common sense. If an alternative method is safe, is more comfortable for the patient, does not violate principles of asepsis, or is preferred by the patient, it is usually acceptable. When considering an alternative approach, the nurse may wish to consult a nurse colleague to discuss the measure. Nursing Skill 18–2 is one method of bathing a patient in bed.

An alternative to the traditional bed bath above is the towel bath procedure described in Nursing Skill 18–3. This procedure is thought to be more comfortable for the patient and more efficient for the nurse. In addition, nursing research has indicated that the towel bath is more effective in reducing anxiety than the conventional bed bath. This is thought to be due to the relaxing combination of heat and massage used in the towel bath (Barsevick and Llewellyn, 1982). Some nurses use a towel bath when it is necessary to restrict all activity of the patient, such as after a severe heart attack.

Although baths are given primarily for their cleansing purpose, they can also be given for therapeutic purposes when, for example, medication for a skin condition may be added to the bath water. Back rubs, which relieve tension and stimulate circulation, are often given along with a bath. (See Chapter 25.)

Perineal Care. Having the nurse bathe the genital area is often an embarrassing procedure for the patient and also for some nurses. However, this procedure must be done thoroughly and unfailingly if the patient is to be clean and comfortable. The more matter of fact the attitude of the nurse, the more comfortable will be the patient. The nurse must determine how much assistance

Nursing Skill 18–3. Giving a Towel Bath

Supplies
Cleansing, conditioning agent
½ gal (approximately 2 liters) water 115–117° F (46–47° C)
Large plastic bag
Large terry-cloth towel: fold towel in half top to bottom twice, fold in half side
   to side, roll towel beginning at folded edge, place in large plastic bag
Clean patient gown
Two washcloths and bath towel

Preparation
Explain the procedure to the patient.
Provide for privacy by closing the door and pulling the curtains.
Offer the patient a bedpan or urinal. Completing elimination at this time adds to
   the patient's comfort and makes the bath as clean a procedure as possible.
Wash hands and gather clean equipment.

Procedure	Explanation
1. Adjust the bed to a comfortable working height for the nurse.	1. Eliminate unnecessary muscle strain for the nurse.
2. Remove spread and blanket, fold if they are to be reused. Loosen sheet at foot of bed. Remove patient gown, cover patient with sheet or bath blanket. Raise the side rails.	2. This will keep the linen dry during the bath. Rolling soiled linen will limit the spread of microorganisms. Provide privacy for the patient. Provide safety.
3. Add measured amount of cleansing conditioning agent to water. Pour solution into plastic bag, quickly knead the solution into the towel. Squeeze out excess into sink. Close bag and take immediately to the patient's bedside.	3. Measure agent to prevent waste or excessive use of product. Retain warmth of towel.
4. Remove sheet to patient's waist, placing towel, unrolled and unfolded once, on the patient's chest (towel edges down and at the neck). While removing the sheet, unfold the towel, covering the patient, including the feet. Leave approximately 1-ft overlap folded down above the shoulders to allow for washing the face. (See Figure 18–6**A**)	4. Provide for patient privacy. Towel provides warmth. Leaves clean area of the towel for the face, the cleanest area of the body.
5. Wash the patient's face, ears, and neck with the overlapped portion of the towel. Then, beginning at the feet, moving upward, and using a clean section of the towel for each part of the body, cleanse with gentle massaging strokes. As the towel is moved toward the patient's head, leaving a space of 4–6 inches to allow for drying, pull the sheet up to cover the patient. (See Figure 18–6**B**)	5. Wash the face while the exposed surface of the towel is warm. Begin at the feet in order to facilitate recovering of patient with the sheet. A clean area of the towel is used for each part of body, thus reducing the transfer of microorganisms. Solution will dry in 2–3 sec.
6. Remove the towel and fold soiled side in, in quarters. Place on clean surface. Turn patient to side-lying position. Drape sheet below buttocks. (May also drape front of patient with sheet.) Place towel with fold on shoulders, edges on buttocks. (See Figure 18–6**C**)	6. Outside of the towel is clean and will be used to minimize the transfer of microorganisms. Position facilitates washing back and buttocks. Provide for privacy and warmth.

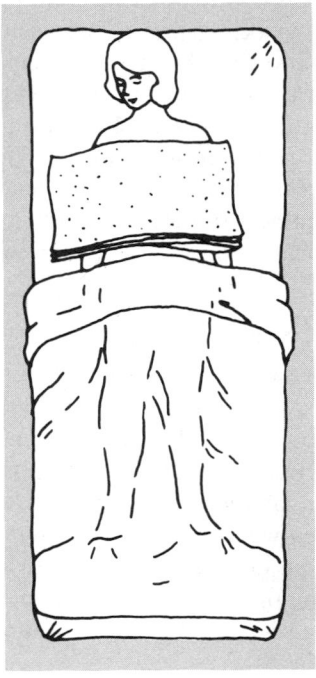 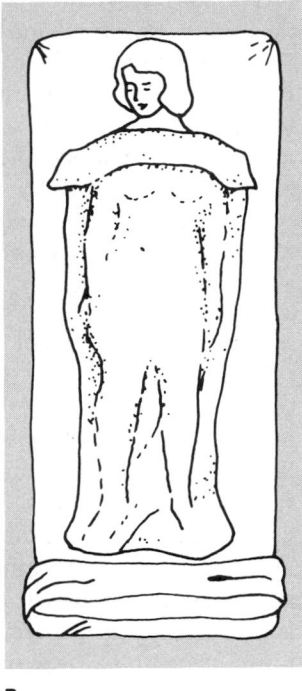

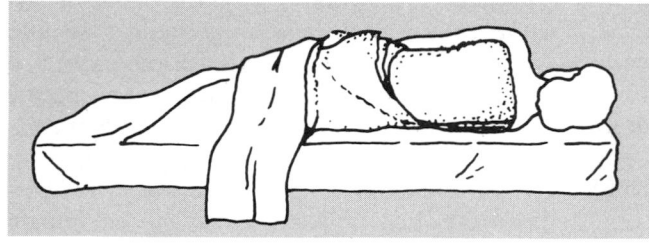

Figure 18–6. Towel bath. **A.** Unroll towel across chest and unfold downward. **B.** Begin bathing at the feet, moving upward. **C.** Turn patient to the side, and bathe from the shoulders down. (Reproduced with permission: Vestal Laboratories, Chemed Corporation, St. Louis, MO.)

7. Cleanse from shoulders down.
8. To cleanse the buttocks, fold three edges of the towel up, and use the fourth to begin. Use a clean section of the towel for each wipe. As a section is used, tuck it underneath, and use one of the remaining sections.
9. Place the bath towel in the linen hamper.
10. Assist the patient to put on clean gown, brush hair, offer grooming aids. Leave patient in a comfortable position. May change linen at this time. Return bed to low position.
11. Put away any supplies and grooming aids.
12. Document the procedure.

7. Clean from the cleanest area to the dirtiest.
8. The buttocks are a very contaminated area and re-use of a section of the towel would spread many microorganisms.

9. Remove soiled towel from clean environment.
10. Comfort for the patient.

11. Leave the patient unit clean and neat.
12. Contribute to continued data collection for patient care plan.
Fulfills legal requirement.

the patient will need in order to wash the perineum. At times, the nurse may provide clean water and washcloth within safe reach of the patient and ask the patient to finish the bath. The nurse may need to be very specific in giving clear directions to the patient in words the patient understands. The nurse may say, for example, "I will leave for a few moments while you wash your bottom." For other patients, the nurse may need to remain at the bedside to assist as necessary. For some patients, the nurse must do complete perineal care. Because the area contains many microorganisms, many nurses choose to wear clean gloves during this procedure. The gloves can then be thrown away, and the nurse does not risk transmitting the microorganisms to other patients. Other nurses maintain that, with good handwashing, the risk of cross-contamination is minimal and that wearing gloves suggests to the patient that this is a dirty and offensive procedure.

Perineal Care for Female Patients.

The nurse assists the patient to her back, legs slightly flexed at the knees, and drapes the patient with a bath blanket. A towel is placed under the patient's hips. With clean water and a washcloth, the nurse first cleans the area between the legs and the labia. Next, the labia are spread, and the nurse washes with a clean washcloth using one downward stroke, and then taking a clean area of the washcloth for each further stroke. The nurse first wipes from the urethral orifice to the vaginal orifice. Then the nurse wipes between the labia majora and the labia minora on each side. In this way, the nurse is moving from "clean to dirty," preventing the spread of microorganisms. Some nurses prefer to put the patient on a bed pan so clean water may be poured over the area. The area is then dried thoroughly. The patient is turned to her side, and the buttocks are thoroughly washed and dried, with particular attention to the anal area. Powder or ointments can then be applied as the patient wishes.

Male Perineal Care.

When the nurse gives perineal care to the male patient, it is possible that the patient will have an erection. This is due to the manipulation of the penis during washing. The patient may be very embarrassed by this, as may the nurse. Both will be helped by the professional attitude of the nurse. At such a time, the nurse may choose to continue and complete the procedure, to leave the room for a time, simply to explain to the patient what has happened, or to ask the patient what he prefers.

The male patient is positioned on his back, legs apart, and slightly flexed. The nurse also drapes the male patient with the bath blanket. The thighs are washed first. If the patient has not been circumcised, the foreskin is retracted. The penis is washed next. Holding the penis in one hand and using a clean part of the washcloth for each wipe, the nurse washes the tip of the penis with a circular motion, then the shaft of the penis with lengthwise strokes. The scrotum must be held so all surfaces can be cleansed. The area is thoroughly dried. The foreskin is replaced by sliding it back over the end (glans) of the penis in uncircumcised male patients. The buttocks and anal area are washed in the same manner as for a female patient.

Making a Patient's Bed.

A well-made bed can greatly contribute to the comfort of the patient. It is helpful if the patient can be out of bed while the nurse changes linen. Many nurses choose to make the bed while the patient is sitting up in a chair. Because it is not always possible to have the patient out of the bed, the nurse develops skill in making the bed while the patient remains in it. This procedure must be done quickly because it may cause discomfort for the patient. Whether the bed is occupied or not, there are several guidelines that apply to all bed-making activities.

1. Raise the bed to a comfortable working height (hip level) for the nurse. This will prevent unnecessary strain on the nurse's back. The bed is then made completely on one side before moving to the second side. This saves the nurse multiple trips around the bed.

2. Do not touch soiled linen to the uniform. Used linen is contaminated, and this causes the transfer of microorganisms, first to the nurse's uniform and then to other patients.

3. Soiled linen is not placed on the floor. The floor is one of the most contaminated areas in the hospital. Linen hampers are provided for the disposal of soiled linen.

4. Use all the linen necessary to provide care to the patient but do not use excess. Frequently, nurses bring clean linen into the patient's room without checking to see what is already in the room. This contaminates the linen, and it cannot be used for another patient. Linen costs are a large expense in the hospital which nurses can help to contain.

5. The patient is left in a safe position when the linen change is complete. If the patient requires side rails, they are up. The signal for the nurse is within the patient's reach. The bed is returned to a low position.

6. When the linen change is complete, the room is left in order. Soiled supplies are promptly removed. The nurse may offer to remove old newspapers, soiled paper cups, or dead flowers. Although not all of these tasks are strictly nursing responsibilities, they show a concern for the comfort and well-being of the patient.

Nursing Skills 18–4 and 18–5 describe two methods of bed-making.

Nursing Skill 18–4.   **Making an Unoccupied Bed**

Supplies

Mattress pad
Two sheets, bottom one fitted, if available
Draw sheet if used
Blanket
Bedspread
Hamper for soiled linen

Preparation

Check the patient's room to see what clean linen is available there. Do not bring unnecessary linen into the patient's room since it cannot then be used for other patients. Wash hands before securing clean linen from supply area. This decreases the transfer of microorganisms between patients.

Procedure	Explanation
1. Bring required clean linen into room and place on bedside chair.	1. Do not place clean linen on second patient's bed. This causes cross-contamination.
2. Raise the bed to comfortable working level for the nurse. Screen bed if there is a second bed in the room.	2. Avoid unnecessary muscle strain and bending for nurse. Limits transfer of microorganisms.
3. Loosen the linen, working from the side of the bed where you are standing to the other side, including all four corners.	3. Conserve number of times walked around bed.
4. Starting at the head of the bed, fold the top edge of the blanket over to the bottom edge. Fold in half and hang over back of chair. Repeat for each article of linen. While doing this, be alert for such articles as lost dentures, jewelry. etc. Do not shake linen.	4. Reduce the transfer of microorganisms This method gives nurse the opportunity to look for articles which often are lost in hospital laundry. Shaking linen spreads microorganisms.

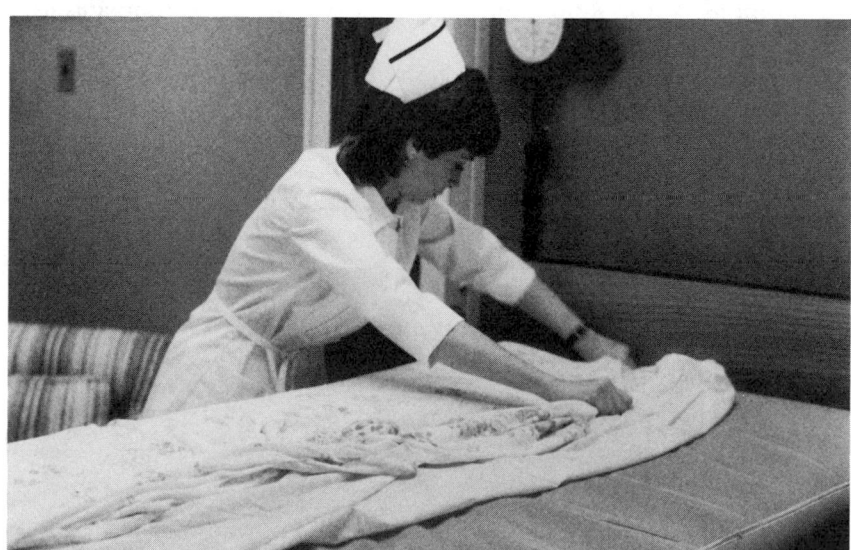

Figure 18-7. In making an unoccupied bed, one side is made completely before moving to make the second side.

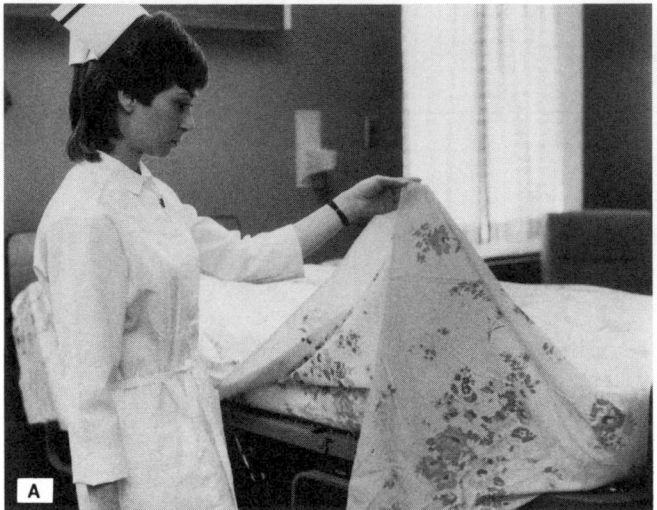

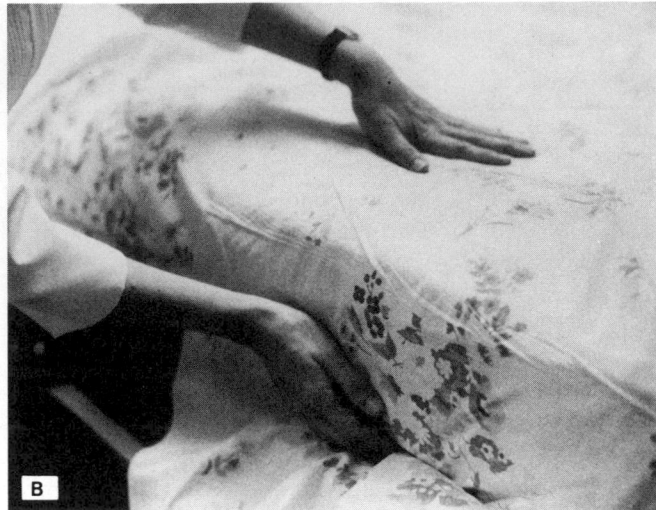

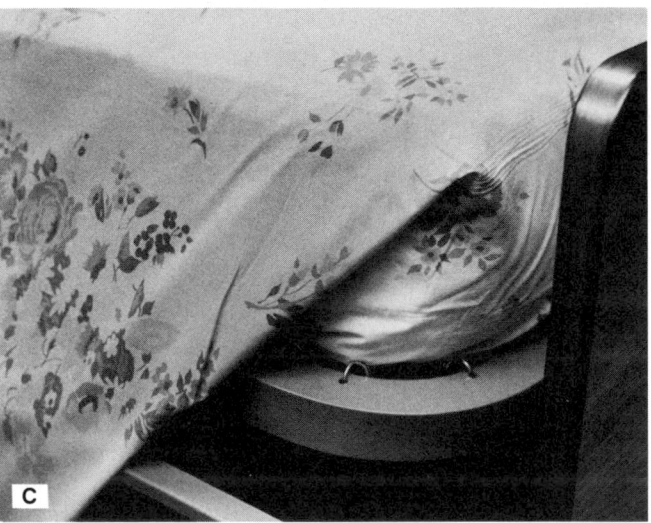

Figure 18–8. A, B, C. Making a mitered corner.

Procedure	Explanation
5. If linen is not to be reused, it can be rolled one piece at a time and placed in dirty linen hamper.	5. Rolling linen limits the transfer of microorganisms.
6. Move the mattress to the head of the bed. Beginning at the foot of the bed, place the fitted sheet on the bed, securing all four corners. If no fitted sheets are available, place the sheet at the foot of the bed, so the center fold of the sheet is at the center of the mattress, the edge of the sheet even with the end of the mattress. Unfold the sheet over the bed.	6. With electric beds, mattresses tend to slide to the foot of the bed. Fitted sheets are secured on all four corners before other linen is added because it is difficult to secure corners without wrinkling entire bed if done later. Nurse's energy is conserved by making one side of the bed completely before moving to the other.
7. Moving to the head of the bed on the same side, fold the sheet under the mattress and miter the corner. (See Figure 18–8.) Tuck the sheet under the foot end.	7. Mitering firmly anchors the sheet.
8. Working from the same side, place the draw sheet on the center third of the bed, fold of the sheet on the center line of the bed. Unfold the sheet and tuck in on near side.	8. Conservation of energy. Decreases number of times nurse must walk around bed. Draw sheet protects the bottom sheet from soiling or is used in moving and lifting.

9. From the same side, place the top sheet at the top edge of the mattress, center fold of the sheet at the center line of the bed. Unfold the entire sheet. Tuck in at foot end.

9. Conservation of energy.

10. Place top edge of blanket about 6–8 inches below top edge of sheet, center fold of blanket to center line of bed. Unfold blanket and tuck under foot end of bed.

10. The sheet will form a cuff over the edge of the blanket and spread which will be soft in contact with the patient's skin.

11. Place bedspread in same manner as blanket. Miter all three layers together. Fold top of sheet over spread and blanket.

11. Same as #7.

12. Walk around to other side of bed and make second side in the same manner.

12. Conservation of energy.

13. Loosen covers slightly at foot of bed if patient desires.

13. Tight sheets may rub on the patient's feet and cause discomfort.

14. Fanfold back the covers by grasping all three layers from the top and fold in thirds over the foot of the bed.

14. Fan-folded covers are out of the way when the patient enters the bed, yet easily pulled up.

15. Replace clean pillow case by holding the bottom center of the case with one hand and gathering the case from top to bottom with the second hand. This makes a mitt over the first hand. Grasp the center of one end of the pillow with the mitt and pull on the case with the other hand. Replace pillow on bed.

15. The clean pillow case does not touch the nurse's uniform, thereby decreasing the transfer of microorganisms from the nurse's uniform to the clean pillow case.

16. Replace patient's call light. Lower bed to usual level. Put furniture in order. Remove soiled linen.

16. Provide safety for the patient.

Nursing Skill 18–5.   **Making an Occupied Bed**

Supplies

Clean linen as necessary

- Mattress pad
- Two sheets, bottom one fitted, if available
- Draw sheet if used
- Blanket
- Bedspread
- Hamper for soiled linen

Preparation

This procedure will usually take place at the completion of the patient's bath. Assess the patient to determine if able to tolerate the procedure, or if a rest will be necessary before changing the bed. Clean linen should be in the room if this is after the bath, or, wash hands and secure clean linen from supply area. Explain the procedure to the patient. Close door and pull curtains around bed.

Procedure	Explanation
1. Remove spread, blanket, and top sheet in same manner as when bathing a patient. Cover patient with bath blanket. Slide mattress to head of bed.	1. Limit the transfer of microorganisms. Provide for privacy and warmth for the patient. With electric beds, mattresses tend to slide to the foot of the bed. (May need help moving mattress)
2. Move the patient, while on back, to the far side of the bed. (See Nursing Skill 28–3.) Reposition in side-lying position on far side of bed. Place pillow comfortably. Place side rail up in front of patient.	2. Moving the patient to the far side of the bed gives the nurse room to make one side of the bed first. Provide safety for the patient.
3. Working from side of bed away from patient, loosen linens and fanfold, moving linen as close to the patient as possible.	3. Conserve nurse's energy by completing one side of the bed before moving to the other side. Space is now clear to put on clean linens.
4. Place clean mattress pad with center fold at the center of the bed. Smooth half of the pad on the exposed mattress. Fanfold the remaining half of the pad lengthwise as close to the patient as possible.	4. Replace mattress pad only if soiled. Nurse now makes half of the bed at a time with the patient remaining in the unmade half.
5. If sheet is fitted, place on foot end of mattress corner, then on head corner. Smooth to the center of the bed and fold as close to the patient as possible. If sheet is not fitted, place the sheet at the foot of the bed so the center fold of the sheet is at the center fold of the mattress, the edge of the sheet even with the edge of the mattress. Moving to the head of the bed, fold the sheet under the mattress and miter the corner. Tuck the sheet under the side to the foot end. Smooth sheet to the center of the bed and fanfold the remaining sheet as near to the patient as possible. (See Figure 18–9A)	5. As above.
6. Place the draw sheet on bed in the same manner, if one is being used.	6. Not all patients require draw sheets.

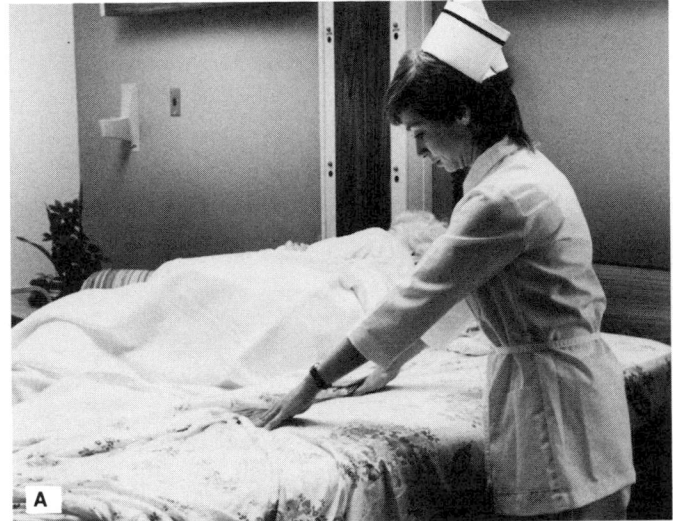

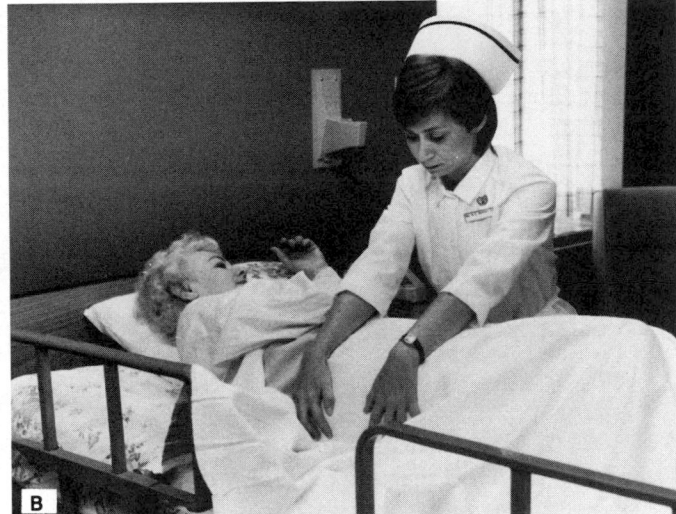

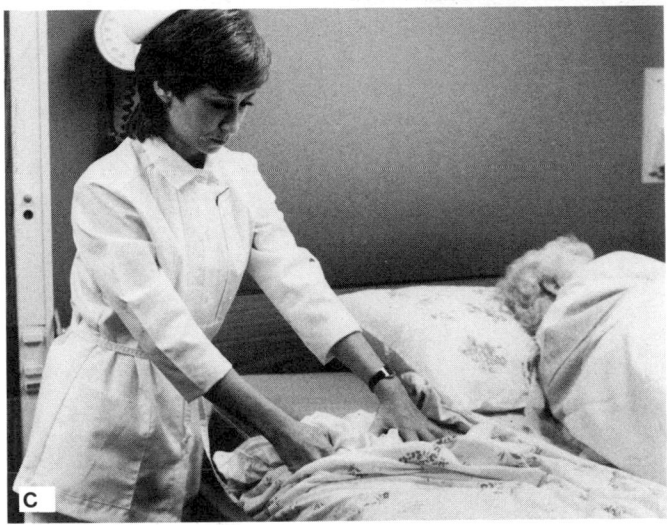

Figure 18-9. A. With the patient on the opposite side of the bed, the nurse makes the bottom of one side of the bed, folding clean and dirty linens to the center of the bed.
B. The nurse assists the patient to move to the clean side of the bed.
C. The nurse removes the soiled linen and makes the second side of the bed, pulling the linen from the center of the bed. The top of the bed can then be made while the patient is in any comfortable position.

7. Assist patient to turn on back. Then assist patient to the clean side of bed in side-lying position. (See Figure 18-9**B**)

8. Put up the side rail facing the patient, then move to the second side of the bed.

9. Loosen soiled linen and roll to the foot of the bed. Place in hamper if within reach or leave rolled at the foot of the bed.
Pull the clean linen toward the nurse. Smooth the mattress pad.

10. Beginning with the head end of the bottom sheet, smooth the sheet, tuck it around the top of the mattress, and miter the corner. Tighten and tuck in the sheet down the side, working toward the feet. Secure the draw sheet. The patient may now turn back if desired.

7. Patient will have to move over the pleated pile of linen to the made side of the bed. This will permit the nurse to make the second side of the bed.

8. Provide safety for the patient.

9. Limit the transfer of microorganisms. Do not place soiled linen in hamper at this time if it means it is necessary to walk away from the bed creating a safety hazard.

10. Make the bed as free of wrinkles as possible to protect the patient's skin.
Patient may be tired from the procedure and position

Procedure	Explanation
11. Place top sheet over patient with middle of sheet at middle of bed. Leave sufficient sheet to form cuff for spread and blanket. Request the patient to hold sheet or secure by tucking under patient's shoulders. Remove the bath blanket, folding if it will be reused.	11. Provide privacy and warmth for the patient.
12. Tuck the foot end around the mattress. Put on the blanket and spread in the same manner, but place top edge of each at approximate shoulder level. Miter the three layers together.	12. Complete making second half of bed.
13. Put on clean pillow case as in Nursing Skill 18–4, step 15.	13. Limits the transfer of microorganisms.
14. Verify that patient is in comfortable position and can reach nurse signal light. Lower the bed.	14. Before leaving, be sure the patient is in a comfortable position. Leaving a patient without a signal light creates a safety hazard. Bed must be in low position whenever the nurse is not present for safety in case patient gets out of bed.

Surgically Safe Environment

The condition of the hospitalized patient often requires an environment or procedures that are free from all microorganisms. This is called *surgical asepsis* or *sterile technique*. Surgery, for example, is performed under strict surgical asepsis. Nurses use sterile technique daily in less dramatic skills such as changing sterile dressings, urinary catheterizations, and the preparation of intravenous medications. Because skills involving surgical asepsis are used daily by nurses, it is important that every nurse be competent in sterile technique. It is not necessary or even desirable for the nurse to memorize all of the steps in a sterile procedure. Rather, the nurse needs to understand the principles of sterile technique and be able to apply them in a variety of situations.

Several guidelines apply to every skill that requires sterile technique:

1. The purpose of sterile technique is to protect the patient from micoorganisms which may be present on the patient's own body or which are transferred by caregivers. For example, during an operation, only the operative area is exposed. The rest of the patient's body is covered with sterile towels (called drapes) which serve to protect from microorganisms on the patient's own body.

2. If a sterile object touches an unsterile object, the sterile object may now have some micoorganisms on it and must considered unsterile, or contaminated. This may occur when the nurse accidentally touches a sterile needle with a finger when drawing up an insulin injection.

3. Sterile objects that touch other sterile objects are still sterile. For example. The nurse wearing sterile gloves counts sterile bandages. Both the gloves and the bandages are sterile unless, of course, something else has contaminated either of them.

4. A sterile field is the area considered free from all micoorganisms. Frequently, a nurse sets up a sterile field on a table by opening a sterile drape over the table, much as a tablecloth is over a table. Sterile objects may then be placed on the sterile field and still be sterile.

5. The sterile field must be within the vision of the nurse at all times. This means that objects below the level of the waist (as in the operating room) are considered contaminated. The nurse does not walk away from a sterile field because it is then impossible to determine whether it has been contaminated. The nurse also avoids reaching over a sterile field in order to decrease the risk of contamination from microorganisms falling from the nurse onto the sterile field by gravity.

The following skills require knowledge and application of surgical asepsis.

Surgical Handwashing. Many patient care situations require a more thorough handwashing than the medical handwashing described above. Prior to entering a newborn nursery, assisting in the operating room, or performing sterile procedures, the nurse completes surgical handwashing. This is different from medical handwashing in that here the elbows are considered most contaminated and the fingertips least contaminated. This handwashing also takes more time and may be required for as long as 10 minutes with three separate lather-and-rinse cycles. This will vary with institutional policy and the specific work area. This is described in Nursing Skill 18–6.

In order to determine whether medical or surgical handwashing is appropriate, the nurse questions who is "clean" and who is "dirty." In the above examples, the nurse, physician, and other members of the surgical team are "dirty." That is, they have more microorganisms than the sterile field. In this case, the "dirty" nurse does a surgical handwashing. The closer one moves to the trunk of the nurse, the greater the number of micoorganisms. For surgical handwashing, the hands are considered less contaminated with microorganisms than the elbows of the individual nurse.

If the nurse is considered "clean" compared to the patient, a medical handwashing is done. This is most often the case in the general areas of the hospital. In medical handwashing, the elbows are considered to have fewer microogranisms than the hands which have been in direct contact with patients.

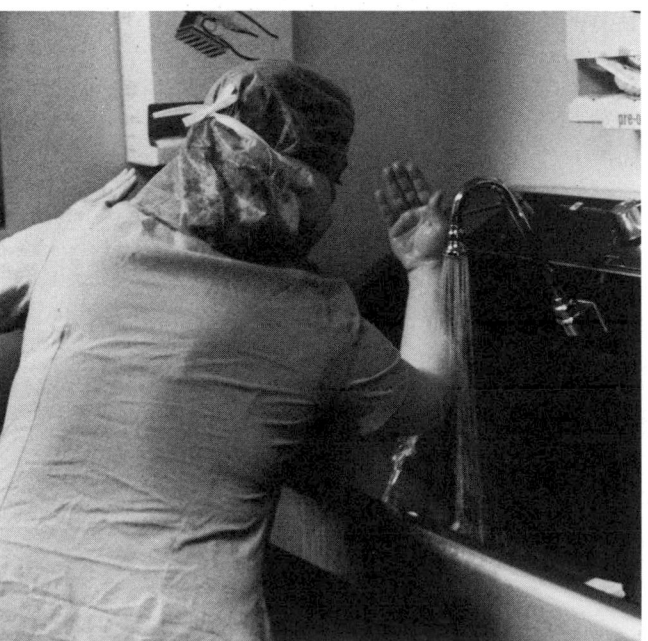

Figure 18–10. Surgical handwashing.

Nursing Skill 18–6.   Surgical Handwashing

Supplies
   Soap as provided by the hospital
   Stick or brush for cleaning the fingernails
   Warm running water with foot or knee control
   Brush or sponge for cleaning the skin
   Towels (frequently sterile towels are provided in the operating room)

Preparation
   Nurse must be in a short-sleeved uniform or scrub suit to perform this procedure since it involves scrubbing to the elbows.

Procedure	Explanation
1. Remove all jewelry.	1. Jewelry harbors microorganisms and is difficult to clean.
2. Adjust water to comfortable temperature.	2. Comfort of nurse. Excessively hot water opens pores to bacteria. Warm water enhances action of the soap.
3. Holding hands above the level of the elbow, wet hands thoroughly. Apply soap.	3. Water flows from area of least contamination to most contamination. Soap is mildly bacteriostatic.
4. Beginning at the fingertips, lather and wash, using both circular and interlaced-fingers technique. Move from fingertips to the elbows of one hand and repeat for the second hand. Use brush if available.	4. Friction and lather raise microorganisms. Wash from area of least contamination to area of most contamination. Use of brush maximizes friction.
5. Rinse each arm separately, fingertips first, holding hands above the level of elbows.	5. Do not let rinse water flow over clean area. Water should flow from area of least contamination to area of most contamination.
6. Wash for the length of time and the number of times as required.	6. Different sterile procedures will require different handwashing times.
7. Using a separate towel for each hand, wipe from the fingertips to the elbow, and then discard the towel.	7. Do not contaminate clean hand by using contaminated towel. Move from least to most contaminated during drying.
8. *If donning sterile gloves and gown*: hold hands above the level of the waist and do not touch anything. Immediately get into sterile garb.	8. Contact with contaminated object renders clean object contaminated. Area below the level of the waist is considered contaminated.
9. If the nurse's hands touch any "dirty" object during the procedure, steps 3 through 8 must be repeated.	9. Same as #8.

Nursing Skill 18–7.   **Opening a Sterile Pack**

Supplies
Sterile pack
Clean table or surface to hold pack

Procedure

1. Wash hands.
2. Set pack on clean dry surface. Position so the top flap of the wrapper is facing you. Remove tape on pack.
3. Pinching the top flap at the corner, open the pack away from yourself, bringing your arm back around the outside of the open pack.
4. Open side flaps one at a time.

5. Open flap nearest to you last.
6. Inside of wrapper is considered sterile and may be used as base for sterile field. Other sterile objects may now be added.

Explanation

1. Decrease the transfer of microorganisms.
2. Same as #1. Wet surface under sterile field will contaminate it as solution is absorbed. Pack can be opened without reaching over a sterile field.
3. Hands do not touch the inside of the wrapper which would contaminate it or cross sterile field.

4. Being able to watch each flap being opened decreases the risk of contamination.
5. Same as #4.
6. Sterility is maintained when sterile objects are placed within a sterile field.

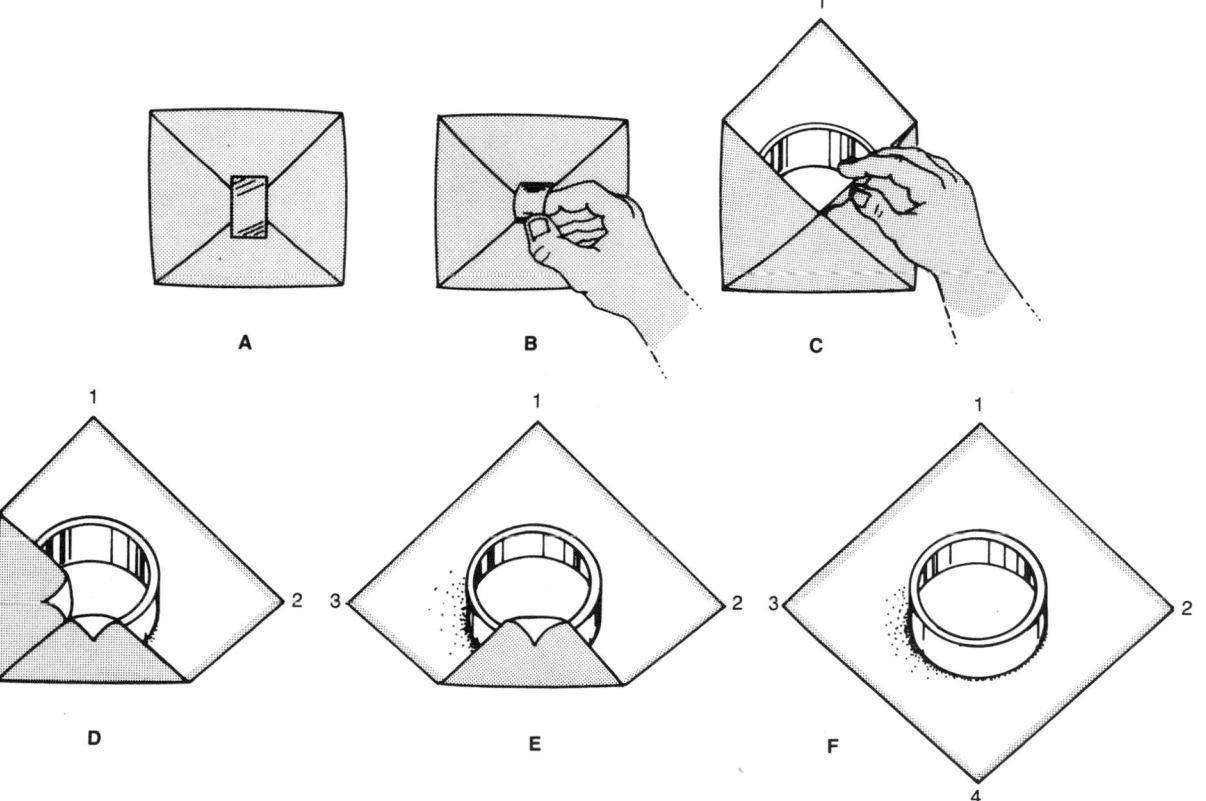

Figure 18–11. Opening a sterile pack. (*Note*: all shaded areas are considered contaminated.)

Opening a Sterile Pack. All sterile supplies come wrapped in some type of pack, either paper or cloth, to protect the contents from environmental microorganisms. Many packs, such as the type that sterile gloves come in, contain an inner and an outer package. The outer package can be peeled apart using both hands. The inner pack may then be added to a sterile field or opened to form the base of a sterile field. Cloth packs are sealed with a tape which indicates that the contents are sterile. These are opened in the manner described in Nursing Skill 18–7. Once opened, a sterile pack may not be reclosed and considered sterile for another use.

Putting on a Sterile Gown. The nurse wears a sterile gown under conditions of surgical asepsis when the pur-pose is to protect the patient from organisms which may be carried by the nurse. If protective cap, mask, and shoe coverings are required, they must be put on prior to donning the gown. These items are not sterile and may not be touched after handwashing is complete. Putting on a sterile gown must always be preceded by a surgical handwashing. Because the hands are never sterile, even after a surgical scrub, the sterile gown may be touched only at the neckband when put on. Thereafter, the nurse does not touch the neckband which is now considered contaminated. Nursing Skill 18–8 describes one method of putting on a sterile gown.

Putting on Sterile Gloves. The nurse wears sterile gloves not only in the operating room but anywhere a

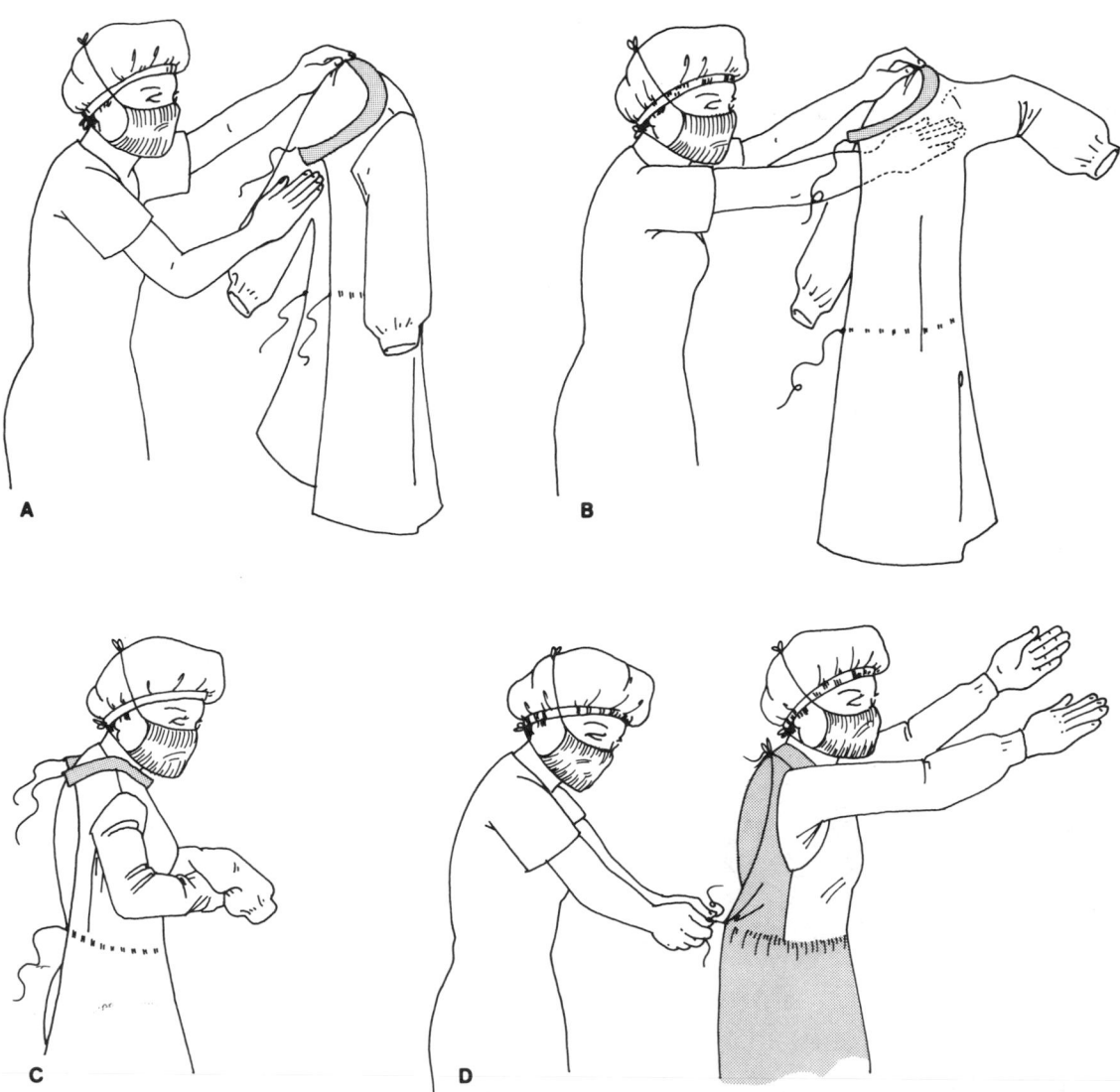

Figure 18–12. Putting on a sterile gown. (*Note*: all shaded areas are considered contaminated.)

Nursing Skill 18–8.   **Putting on a Sterile Gown**

Supplies
    If required: Shoe covers, face mask, protective cap.
    Sterile gown

Procedure	Explanation
1. Wash hands.	1. Decrease transfer of microorganisms.

2. If required put on
  a. Protective cap.
  b. Face mask—secure mask with four ties, above the ears and at the nape of the neck. Paper masks are adjusted by bending a flexible nosepiece and by elastic straps.
  c. Shoe covers.
	2. Putting on cap, mask, and shoe covers is intended to cover parts of the nurse's body that are sources of contamination. These are not sterile. Proceed from area of least contamination to most contamination: hair, face, shoe covers.

3. Complete surgical handwashing. (See Nursing Skill 18–6.)	3. This is a sterile procedure.
4. Open sterile pack containing gown (see Nursing Skill 18–7). Grasp gown by the neck band and hold away from the body and at shoulder level to unfold.	4. Pack containing gown is sterile. Neckband of gown is considered unsterile.
5. While holding neckband, slide one arm into sleeve.	5. Neckband is considered unsterile
6. With the first arm encased in the sleeve and holding the gown, slide second arm into the gown. Do not touch the outside of the gown with hands.	6. The gown acts as a sterile "mitt" which assists in movement into the gown. Hands are not sterile and touching would contaminate the gown.
7. A second person who is not in sterile garb will now, touching only the inside surface of the gown, pull the gown into place and tie the neckties. The gowned nurse then bends forward to make the waist ties (located waist level on side of gown) fall away from gown. These are then tied by the second person who is careful not to touch the front of the gown. If the waist ties are on the back of the gown, they are simply tied by the second nurse.	7. The inside of the gown is considered contaminated and thus may be touched by the unsterile person. Care must be taken not to permit neck ties to fall forward to the front of the gown as this would contaminate the gown. Waist ties are sterile until touched by the second person.
8. If the gown is contaminated at any point, it is discarded and steps 3 through 7 are repeated.	8. Contact with any unsterile object makes the gown unsterile.

Nursing Skill 18–9.   **Putting on Sterile Gloves**

Supplies
Package of sterile gloves in correct size
Clean table or surface to hold open glove package

Procedure	Explanation
1. Remove all jewelry and wash hands.	1. Decrease transfer of microorganisms.
2. Open glove package without contaminating and lay on flat surface. Open inner wrapper and, touching only the outside, secure both flaps in open position.	2. The outside of inner wrapper is contaminated. The inside of the inner wrapper is sterile.
3. Remove first glove from the package by grasping the inside fold of the cuff. Lift the glove, holding away from the body, above the waist, fingers of the glove down.	3. The inside of the first glove is now contaminated because it has been in contact with the nurse's hand. The outside of the glove remains sterile.
4. Slide glove on first hand, still touching only the inside of the glove.	4. Same as #3.
5. Remove second glove from the package by sliding three fingers of the first hand, now gloved, under the cuff of the second glove. Lift the glove away from the body, above the level of the waist. Slide the second hand into the second glove, touching only the inside of the glove with the second hand.	5. Same as #3.
6. Pull glove over wrist with first hand which is gloved, without touching second arm.	6. Both outside surfaces of the gloves remain sterile.

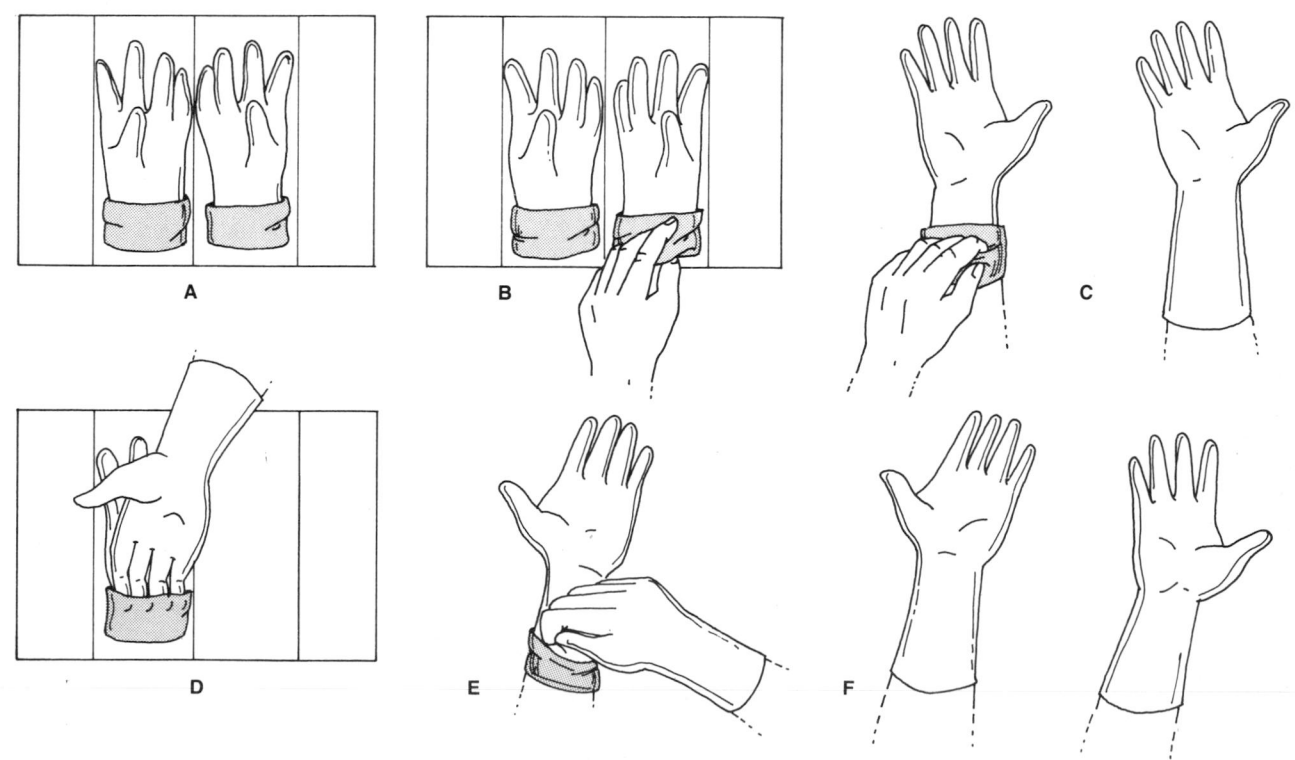

Figure 18–13.   Putting on sterile gloves. (*Note*: all shaded areas are considered contaminated.)

7. Adjust fingers of both gloves using opposite gloved hand. (See Figure 18–13)

8. If contamination occurs at any point in steps 1 through 7, discard the gloves and begin again, using new gloves.

7. If a sterile object (first gloved hand) touches a second sterile object (second gloved hand), both objects remain sterile.

8. Use of any nonsterile object in a sterile procedure introduces microorganisms and is potentially dangerous.

Nursing Skill 18–10.   **Pouring Sterile Liquids**

Supplies
   Sterile liquid
   Sterile container in which to pour

Procedure	Explanation
1. Wash hands.	1. Decrease the transfer of microorganisms.
2. Carefully read and check the label on the bottle.	2. Safety: prevent error of using wrong solution.
3. Remove the cap from the bottle without touching the inside of the cap. Set the cap, top down, on a clean surface.	3. Outside of the cap is unsterile. Inside of the cap is sterile.
4. If this is a previously unopened bottle: pouring away from the label, pour the required amount into the sterile container without touching bottle to container.	4. Lip of the bottle is sterile. Outside of the bottle is considered contaminated. Prevents solution from running over label, making reading difficult.
5. If the bottle had been previously opened: pour a small amount of the liquid away from the label into a waste receptacle without permitting the bottle to touch the receptacle. Pouring away from the label, pour the required amount into the sterile container. (See Figure 18–14)	5. Cleanses the lip of the bottle. Keeps the label of the bottle clean and readable. Same as #4.
6. Replace the cap tightly on the container, being careful not to touch the sterile inside surface. Label the bottle with the date it was opened.	6. Maintain sterility of the bottle. The next person using the bottle will know if it can be used. Opened sterile solutions are usually kept only 24 hours.

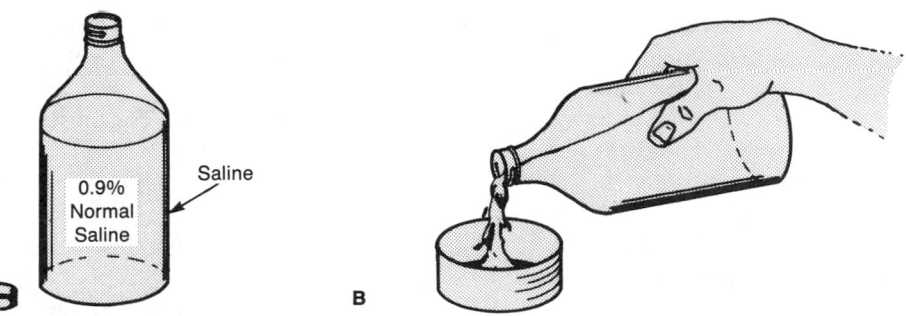

0.9% Normal Saline   Saline

A   B

Figure 18–14.   Pouring sterile liquid into a sterile container. (*Note:* all shaded areas are considered contaminated.)

sterile procedure is performed. It is the responsibility of each nurse to ascertain the best-fitting glove size for personal use, and then select gloves accordingly without the need to try on several pairs. Gloves range from a small size 6 to a large size 8½. Gloves must be large enough to put on with ease, but small enough to fit snugly. Nursing Skill 18–9 lists this skill.

Pouring Sterile Liquids. The nurse may need to add sterile liquids to a sterile field, as when sterile normal saline is poured into a sterile container as part of a surgical procedure. The nurse is careful to pour the liquid without spilling on the sterile field, as well as not to reach over the sterile field. The outside of the bottle is not considered sterile so the nurse must not place the bottle on the field. Usually, a second nurse who is not in sterile garb performs this task. Nursing Skill 18–10 describes this procedure.

Sterile Dressing Change. Anytime the patient has a break in the skin, due either to surgical incisions or to trauma, the wound is covered with sterile dressings. Covering the wound results in faster wound healing with less scarring than if the wound is left open (Strand, 1978). The disadvantage is that covered wounds have a greater danger of bacterial infection. The nurse uses techniques of surgical asepsis to change sterile dressings. Although sterile gloves are always worn, a face mask may be optional. Some institutions require that face masks be worn to protect the wound from droplet infection from the nurse's respiratory tract. For some patients, a dressing change is a painful procedure. The nurse assesses the patient's pain and attempts to make the patient more comfortable before starting the dressing change.

The decision when to change a sterile dressing depends upon several factors. If the patient has had surgery, the physician may wish to change the dressing the first time. If the incision is draining, the nurse may leave the original surgical dressing in place and apply additional dressings on top of the original. This is called reinforcing the dressing. The nurse documents the type of drainage observed and reports as appropriate. Excessive drainage could be an indication of a severe problem.

Frequently, dressing changes are done by physicians. This permits the nurse and the physician to observe the wound and take any necessary intervention. The dressing may also be changed if it is causing discomfort to the patient. Occasionally, dressings are loose, and the patient may feel they are going to fall off during ambulation. Because it is essential that patients exercise to enhance recovery, the nurse makes certain that the dressing is secure. Dressings may be changed when a medication is to be applied to the wound, or if the dress-

ing becomes wet or soiled. The nurse uses judgment in selecting the amount and size of the dressings necessary.

Some wounds are irrigated at the time of the dressing change. The purpose of irrigation is to cleanse the wound and to flush out the remains of dead cells or broken-down tissue. This procedure must be done gently in order not to disturb newly formed healthy tissue. Nursing Skill 18–11 includes this procedure.

Determination of the Presence of Infection

In order to determine the presence of an infection, as well as the specific pathogen causing the infection, samples of body secretions, excretions, fluids, or tissues (called specimens) may be taken. It is often a nursing responsibility to collect these specimens. Once obtained, specimens are taken to the hospital laboratory where they are grown (cultured) in a nutritive substance, usually agar. Most organisms take at least 24 hours to grow, after which a preliminary report can be made. When a request is made for a culture, it will also include a request for sensitivity testing (called *C & S testing*) to determine which antibiotics will be most effective in destroying the organism. In this procedure, a plate of microorganisms cultured in the laboratory is used. Disks treated with different agents, some of which are antibiotics, are placed on the plate. Since the drugs move out into the agar, the diameter of the ring of no growth around the disk is an indication of the effectiveness of the drug. In this way, the physician has information with which to select appropriate medications.

To collect a specimen, the nurse first completes handwashing, then selects the correct container for the specimen and determines if anything needs to be added to the container before it is used. Some specimens require the addition of preservatives or fixatives to the container. The nurse then explains the procedure to the patient, indicating what the patient is to do. In collecting the sample, the nurse is careful not to touch the inside of the container for this would contaminate the sample. The container is then closed securely. The outside of the container is cleaned. After handwashing, the nurse labels the container with the patient's name, room number, date, time, and contents. The specimen is then sent directly to the laboratory. The nurse documents specimen collection in the patient's record.

The nurse may be required to secure cultures such as wound, throat, and nose cultures. The procedure involves using a sterile swab to wipe the suspected area on the patient's body. Then, the swab is placed directly in a sterile, sealed container and taken to the laboratory. When a wound culture is taken, the nurse uses sterile technique to avoid contaminating the specimen.

Nursing Skill 18-11.   **Sterile Dressing Change**

Supplies

Sterile dressings of correct size
Tape
Clean gloves
Sterile gloves
Sterile basin, sterile cleansing solution (sterile forceps optional)
If irrigating the wound:
- Sterile syringe (at least 30-ml size)
- Sterile basin, irrigating solution (90-95° F)
- Waterproof pad
- Prepackaged irrigation tray may be available to which the nurse need only add irrigating solution

Face mask if required
Plastic or lined bag for soiled dressings

Preparation

Explain the procedure to the patient. If the patient is experiencing pain, it may be necessary to relieve the pain before proceeding. Many methods of pain relief are available to the nurse. (See Chapter 26.) Provide for patient privacy, closing the door and pulling the curtains around the bed. Position the patient comfortably and expose as necessary to permit access to the wound.

Procedure	Explanation
1. Put on mask, if necessary. Wash hands.	1. Limit the transfer of microorganisms.
2. Position bag for soiled dressings, open and convenient.	2. Nurse will need to place soiled dressings into the bag without contaminating anything else in the environment.
3. Loosen tape holding dressing, pulling tape toward the wound. If Montgomery ties are used, untie the straps and open.	3. Montgomery tapes remain in place and secure dressings without the use of tape.
4. Put on clean gloves and remove soiled dressings. If dressings adhere to the wound, it may be necessary to moisten with sterile saline in order to loosen. If pouring solution for another to use, repeat name and concentration of solution to verify correctness.	4. Prevents the transfer of microorganisms from the wound to the nurse's hands. Moistening the dressing permits the dressing to be removed without disturbing healing process. Prevention of medication error.
5. Cleanse the wound, using swabs moistened in sterile cleansing solution. Wipe only once with each swab, moving in outward direction from the center of the wound (see Figure 18-15). Discard swabs in bag. If no wound irrigation is to follow, gloves may be removed by peeling off inside out and placing in bag.	5. Cleanse moving from cleanest to least clean area. Even if the wound is not contaminated, this direction prevents microbes present on the skin from entering the wound. Gloves are considered soiled and are not used for sterile procedure.
6. Wound irrigation if ordered: a. Place waterproof pad to protect the bed and the patient. b. Position sterile basin to catch the solution. c. Using sterile syringe, draw up irrigating solution and release over the wound with gentle pressure, so the solution flows from the cleanest area to the least clean area.	6. Wound irrigation requires physician order. a. Keep bed and patient dry. b. As above. c. Water flow must be at gentle pressure to avoid disrupting the healing process. Direction of water flow decreases the spread of microorganisms.

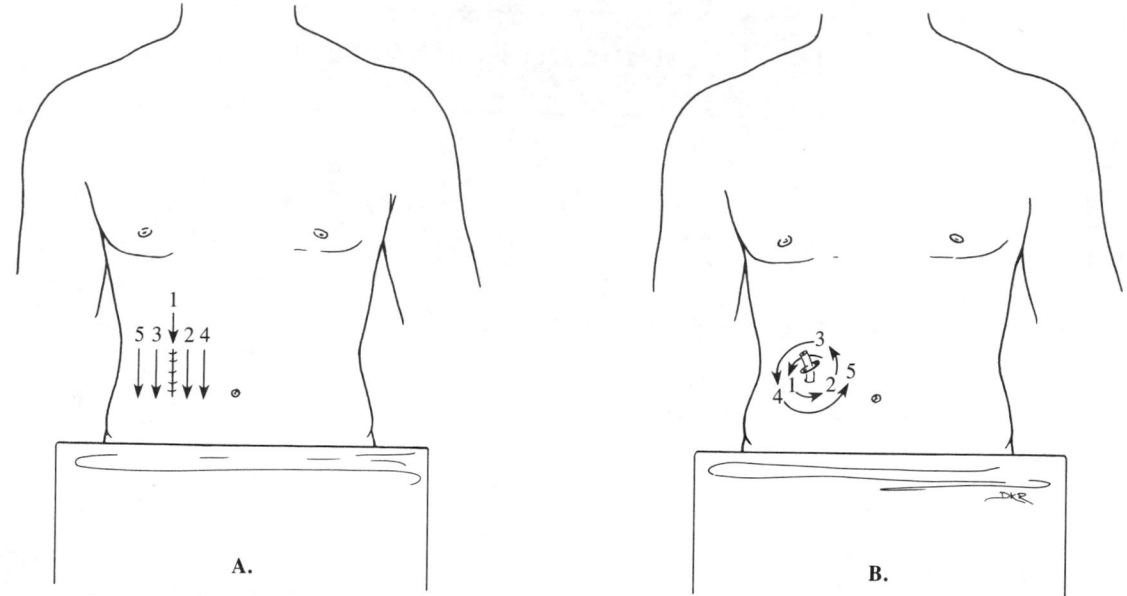

Figure 18–15.   The wound is cleaned from the cleanest area toward the most contaminated area.

Procedure	Explanation
d. Dry the area with sterile gauze, using new gauze for each wipe, and moving out from the center of the wound.	d. Limit the spread of microorganisms. Same as #5.
7. Put on sterile gloves.	7. Use sterile gloves to keep the procedure as clean as possible.
8. Apply sterile dressings to the wound, using sterile forceps or sterile gloved hand. Cover with large dressing or abdominal pad.	8. Maintain sterility of dressings. Large dressing helps to secure smaller dressings and closes off the dressing from the environment.
9. Secure dressing with tape or ties. Remove gloves.	9. Patient will be ambulating and moving in bed so dressings must be secure.
10. Assist patient to comfortable position.	10. Demonstrates concern for the patient.
11. Remove soiled equipment.	11. Decrease microorganisms in the patient's environment.
12. Document the precedure: a. Time and date of dressing change. b. Amount and type of drainage on soiled dressing. c. Appearance of wound—size, shape, depth, odor. d. Wound irrigation if done. e. Type of replacement dressing. f. Condition of the patient during the procedure: pain, nausea, movement, response to teaching.	12. Continued data collection for patient care plan. Fulfill legal requirements.

While awaiting the results of the culture, the physician may decide to initiate isolation precautions. These can later be discontinued if the results indicate an absence of pathogens. Once begun for an identified pathogen, isolation precautions are usually continued until a later culture is negative for the organism.

Protection from Infection

The hospital environment contains many microorganisms, some pathogenic. The presence of these organisms may require special care for some patients. The patient who has a communicable infection poses a threat to the safety of the nurse and to other patients as well. For the protection of others, isolation procedures (also called barrier procedures) are begun. The patient is isolated from other patients and extra precautions are taken by all who come in contact with the infected patient. The precautions are undertaken in an effort to interfere with the transmission of the microorganisms, thus breaking the chain of infection. The precautions taken depend upon the pathogen causing the infection.

The Center For Disease Control (1983) identifies two systems of isolation precautions from which hospitals may select one. In System A (*Category-Specific Isola-*

Table 18–4. System A: Category-Specific Isolation Precautions

CATEGORY	PRIVATE ROOM	MASK	GOWN	GLOVES	HANDWASHING	EXAMPLES
1. Strict	Yes—door closed	Yes	Yes	Yes	After touching patient or contaminated articles. Before caring for another patient	Diphtheria Plague Chickenpox
2. Contact isolation	Yes	Yes	Yes—if soiling is likely	For touching infective material	Same as above	Acute respiratory infections in infants Impetigo Scabies
3. Respiratory isolation	Yes	Yes	No	No	Same as above	Measles Meningitis Mumps
4. Tuberculosis isolation	Yes	Only if patient is coughing	Only if needed to prevent contamination of clothing	No	Same as above	Pulmonary tuberculosis
5. Enteric precautions	If patient hygiene is poor	No	Yes—if soiling is likely	For touching infective material	Same as above	Amebic dysentery Cholera Poliomyelitis
6. Drainage/secretion precautions	No	No	Yes—if soiling is likely	For touching infective material	Same as above	Wound infection Infected decubitus ulcer Conjunctivitis
7. Body/fluid precautions	If patient hygiene is poor	No	Yes—if soiling is likely	For touching blood or body fluids	Must be washed immediately if they are potentially contaminated with blood or body and before taking care of another patient	Acquired immune deficiency syndrome (AIDS) Hepatitis B Malaria

Source: Summarized from J. Garner and B. Simmons, CDC: Guideline for isolation precautions in hospitals. *Infect. Control,* **4**: Issue 4, 1983.

tion Precautions) diseases for which similar precautions are required are grouped together. There are seven such groupings. Each disease within the group is treated by the same set of precautions. Although this system has the advantage of being simple and easy to teach to hospital personnel, more precautions are applied to certain patients than are required by the specific disease. Other diseases within the group require the full range of precautions of the group designation. This system is summarized in Table 18–4. Exhibits 18–1 and 18–2 give examples of category-specific isolation precaution cards which may be placed on the patient's chart and door.

In System B (Disease-Specific Isolation Precautions) each infectious disease is treated separately and only those precautions that are required to interrupt transmission of the disease are applied. This system saves time, supplies, and expense since only the measures ac-

tually needed are begun. However, since isolation precautions are often begun before a specific diagnosis is confirmed, it may be necessary to use the category-specific isolation precautions. Exhibit 18–3 is a sample card which may be placed both on the door and on the chart of the patient in disease-specific isolation. The necessary precautions would be indicated.

Patients with certain conditions, such as those receiving total body irradiation prior to organ transplant, cancer, leukemia, or steroid therapy, are very susceptible to infection. At times a procedure known as protective isolation (or reverse isolation) may be instituted in an attempt to protect the patient from microorganisms in the environment. Nurses caring for a patient in protective isolation use surgical aseptic technique. Hair covering and mask are required. A surgical handwashing is completed prior to donning sterile gown and

---

Exhibit 18–1. Sample Instruction Card for Category-Specific Isolation Precautions

(Front of Card)

Contact Isolation

Visitors—Report to Nurses' Station Before Entering Room

1. Masks are indicated for those who come close to patient.
2. Gowns are indicated if soiling is likely.
3. Gloves are indicated for touching infective material.
4. HANDS MUST BE WASHED AFTER TOUCHING THE PATIENT OR POTENTIALLY CONTAMINATED ARTICLES AND BEFORE TAKING CARE OF ANOTHER PATIENT.
5. Articles contaminated with infective material should be discarded or bagged and labeled before being sent for decontamination and reprocessing.

(Back of Card)

Diseases or Conditions Requiring Contact Isolation

Acute respiratory infections in infants and young children, including croup, colds, bronchitis, and bronchiolitis caused by respiratory syncytial virus, adenovirus, coronavirus, influenza viruses, parainfluenza viruses, and rhinovirus.
Conjunctivitis, gonococcal, in newborns
Diphtheria, cutaneous
Endometritis, group A Streptococcus
Furunculosis, staphylococcal, in newborns
Herpes simplex, disseminated, severe primary or neonatal

Impetigo
Influenza, in infants and young children
Multiply-resistant bacteria, infection or colonization (any site) with any of the following:
1. Gram-negative bacilli resistant to all aminoglycosides that are tested. (In general, such organisms should be resistant to gentamicin, tobramycin, and amikacin for these special precautions to be indicated.)
2. Staphylococcus aureus resistant to methicillin (or nafcillin or oxacillin if they are used instead of methicilin for testing)
3. Pneumococcus resistant to penicillin.
4. Haemophilus influenzae resistant to ampicillin (betalactamase positive) and chloramphenicol
5. Other resistant bacteria may be included in this isolation category if they are judged by the infection control team to be of special clinical and epidemiologic significance.
Pediculosis
Pharyngitis, infectious, in infants and young children
Pneumonia, viral, in infants and young children
Pneumonia, Staphylococcus aureus or group A Streptococcus
Rabies
Rubella, congenital and other
Scabies
Scalded skin syndrome (Ritter's disease)
Skin, wound, or burn, infection, major (draining and not covered by a dressing or dressing does not adequately contain the purulent material), including those infected wiht Staphyloccus aureus or group A Streptococcus
Vaccinia (generalized and progressive eczema vaccinatum)

Source: J. Garner and B. Simmons, CDC: Guideline for isolation precautions in hospitals. Infect. Control, 4: Issue 4, 1983.

gloves. The nurse may then enter the room and give care to the patient. The protective isolation procedure is no longer included in the Center for Disease Control Guidelines. The publication states that protective isolation does not appear to reduce the risk of infection any more than strong empahsis on appropriate handwashing during patient care. Moreover, these highly susceptible patients are often infected by their own microorganisms or by nonsterile items such as food, air, or water used in protective isolation. The CDC Guidelines (Garner and Simmons, 1983) state that the care of these patients requires frequent and appropriate handwashing before, during, and after patient care.

When isolation procedures are begun, the nurse must explain the procedure to the patient, both in terms of what will be done and why it is done. The patient in isolation may feel very lonely and rejected. Teenagers

---

Exhibit 18-2. Sample Instruction Card for Category-Specific Isolation Precautions

(Front of Card)

Strict Isolation

Visitors—Report to Nurses' Station Before Entering Room

1. Masks are indicated for all persons entering room.
2. Gowns are indicated for all persons entering room.
3. Gloves are indicated for all persons entering room.
4. HANDS MUST BE WASHED AFTER TOUCHING THE PATIENT OR POTENTIALLY CONTAMINATED ARTICLES AND BEFORE TAKING CARE OF ANOTHER PATIENT.
5. Articles contaminated with infective material should be discarded or bagged and labeled before being sent for decontamination and reprocessing.

(Back of Card)

Diseases Requiring Strict Isolation

Diphtheria, pharyngeal
Lassa fever and other viral hemorrhagic fevers, such as Marburg virus disease§
Plague, pneumonic
Smallpox§
Varicella (chickenpox)
Zoster, localized in immunocompromised patient, or disseminated

Source: J. Garner and B. Simmons, CDC: Guideline for isolation precautions in hospitals. *Infect. Control,* **4**: Issue 4, 1983.

Exhibit 18-3. Sample Instruction Card for Disease-Specific Isolation Precautions

(Front of Card)

Visitors—Report to Nurses' Station Before Entering Room

1. **Private room indicated?** _____ No
   _____ Yes
2. **Masks indicated?** _____ No
   _____ Yes for those close to patient
   _____ Yes for all persons entering room
3. **Gowns indicated?** _____ No
   _____ Yes if soiling is likely
   _____ Yes for all persons entering room
4. **Gloves indicated?** _____ No
   _____ Yes for touching infective material
   _____ Yes for all persons entering room
5. Special precautions indicated for handling blood? _____ No
   _____ Yes
6. **Hands must be washed after touching the patient or potentially contaminated articles and before taking care of another patient.**
7. Articles contaminated with _____ infective material(s) should be discarded or bagged and labeled before being sent for decontamination and reprocessing.

(Back of Card)

Instructions

1. On Table B, Disease-Specific Precautions, locate the disease for which isolation precautions are indicated.
2. Write disease in blank space here: _____
3. Determine if a private room is indicated. In general, patients infected with the same organism may share a room. For some diseases or conditions, a private room is indicated if patient hygiene is poor. A patient with poor hygiene does not wash hands after touching infective material (feces, purulent drainage, or secretions), contaminates the environment with infective material, or shares contaminated articles with other patients.
4. Place a check mark beside the indicated precautions on front of card.
5. Cross through precautions that are *not* indicated.
6. Write infective material in blank space in item 7 on front of card.

Source: J. Garner and B. Simmons, CDC: Guideline for isolation precautions in hospitals. *Infect. Control,* **4**: Issue 4, 1983.

Nursing Skill 18–12.   Strict Isolation Technique

Supplies
Disposable gown (preferably) or reusable gown
Masks
Clean gloves
Double bag for soiled linen

Preparation
Prior to entering the isolation room, the nurse gathers all the equipment which will be needed to provide care for the patient. Once in the room, the nurse may not leave the room without removing all garb and washing hands. In order to maximize efficiency, the nurse attempts to anticipate needs for equipment and supplies. The patient in isolation must be prepared for the initiation of the procedure since all persons coming into the room will be wearing gowns, gloves, and masks. Signs must be posted on the door to the patient's room which state that the patient is on isolation precautions and anyone entering the room must first check with the nurse for assistance.

Procedure	Explanation
To Enter the Isolation Room	
1. Remove watch and rings.	1. Jewelry traps micoorganisms and is difficult to clean effectively.
2. Put on clean mask. Wash hands.	2. Limit the transfer of microorganisms.
3. Put on gown.	3. The purpose of this is to protect the nurse from the microorganisms of the patient.
a. If gown is reusable, pick up gown from the inside, slide arms into sleeves, tie gown at neck, and overlapping the gown at the back, tie the gown at the waist.	a. The inside of the gown and the neckband and ties are considered clean from the patient's microorganisms.
b. If gown is disposable there is no special way to get into the gown.	b. The entire gown is clean at this point. The purpose of the gown is to protect the clean uniform of the nurse.
4. Put on gloves.	4. Gloves protect the hands of the nurse and limit transfer to other patients.
5. Upon entering room, identify yourself for the patient.	5. Garb conceals identity of nurse.
To Double-Bag Soiled Linen	
1. The gowned nurse places all linen in linen bag inside the room.	1. All contaminated linen is handled within the room to decrease the transfer of microorganisms.
2. Ungowned assistant outside the room holds second linen bag, cuffing hands with the bag.	2. Outside of first linen bag is contaminated. The second nurse's hands are protected by the cuff of the clean bag.
3. Gowned nurse comes to the doorway of the isolation room and places first bag into the second. (See Figure 18–16)	3. The gowned nurse does not leave the isolation room while in gown as this would spread microorganisms.
4. Assistant seals the bag and disposes of it according to institutional policy.	4. Bag must be sealed in such a manner as not to transfer the microorganisms to the environment and be identified as contaminated to protect laundry workers.

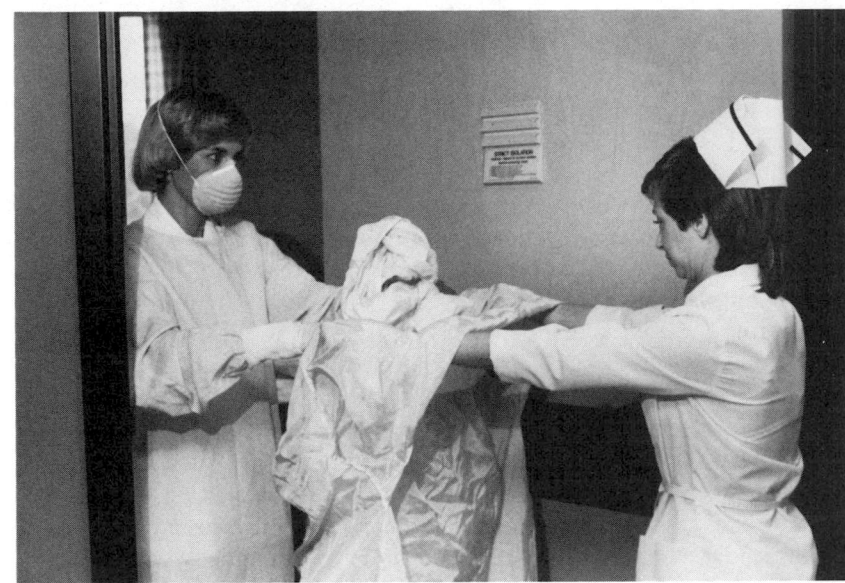

Figure 18–16. Soiled linen is double-bagged when it is removed from an isolation room.

To Exit Isolation Room

1. Remove gloves by peeling off inside out and disposing of properly.
   Remove mask (only touching ties).

2. If gown is to be reused:
   a. Untie waist ties.

   b. Wash hands if waist ties are in front of gown.

   c. Untie neck ties.
   d. Place fingers of one hand under the cuff of the opposite sleeve and pull the sleeve over the opposite hand. With the second hand covered by the sleeve, pull the outside of the opposite sleeve down over arm and off, being careful not to let the neck ties fall forward to the front of the gown.
   e. Fold the gown with the inside in and hang gown contaminated side out.

3. If gown is disposable:
   a. Untie waist ties.

   b. Place clean hands under the neckband and peel off the gown over the shoulders.
   c. Touching only the inside of the gown, roll the gown up inside out and dispose of it.

4. Wash hands.

1. The contaminated outside surface of the gloves is contained within the glove.
   Removing mask with clean hands limits the transfer of microbes to the face.

2.
   a. The waist ties are contaminated but not as much as the gloved hands.
   b. Hands were contaminated by the waist ties if near patient contacts.
   c. Neck ties are clean.
   d. Inside of the gown is clean.

   Neck ties are clean and touching the contaminated front side of the gown would contaminate them.
   e. Protect the clean inside of the gown.

3.
   a. Waist ties are considered less contaminated than gloved hands.
   b. The inside of the gown is clean.

   c. Same as above.

4. Wash hands upon leaving isolation room because contamination may have occurred without your awareness. This will also decrease the possibility of spreading the microorganisms to the next patient of the nurse.

may feel the separation especially keenly. Very young children may feel that isolation is a punishment. Nursing intervention includes meeting the patient's needs for social contact. This is done by instructing visitors about how to enter and exit the room. The nurse also tries to spend time with this patient beyond the time required for physical care. This may even include playing a game of cards or a board game with the patient as a form of recreation.

Isolation procedures are expensive, inconvenient, time-consuming, and often complex. Nurses must complete multiple handwashings in the course of a day, may be in exclusive contact for long periods of time with a patient who may be irritable and may have to wait for assistance to complete procedures. The nurse caring for a patient in strict isolation may also experience real concern about personal safety. This may create additional stress for the nurse at a time when patient care demands are already high. The nurse caring for patients in isolation needs the support of colleagues. It is also important for the nurse to take regularly scheduled rest and meal breaks in order to meet personal needs for refreshment and human contact. These provide relief from stress for the nurse.

Strict isolation. The patient in strict isolation must be placed in a private room. Signs on the patient's door clearly indicate the precaution and the measures which must be carried out. Visitors are directed not to enter the room without contacting the nurse for assistance. All persons entering the room must wear protective haircovers, masks, shoe covers, gown, and gloves. Depending on hospital policy, some of these items may be omitted. Some hospitals use disposable gowns. Although this is expensive, it gives maximum protection. Reusable gowns may be used, if necessary, but this is a less desirable technique because of a greater chance of microorganism transfer.

All items in contact with the patient must be sterilized or thrown away. For this reason, patients in strict isolation usually receive meals with paper or plastic supplies. All soiled linen must be double-bagged (see Nursing Skill 18–12) to protect the laundry workers from contamination. Gowns worn by the nurse and visitors must also be discarded. Nursing Skill 18–12 describes procedures used in strict isolation. Other types of isolation involve modifications of this skill. (See Exhibits 18–1, 2, 3).

Summary

Biological safety is the protection of the body from foreign bodies, both chemical and microorganisms. The basis of the body's defense system is the ability of the body to distinguish self from nonself. Body defenses are divided into two groups:

Nonspecific defenses: defenses that react to all microorganisms and foreign substances in the same manner,
Specific defense mechanisms: defenses that are directed against particular foreign substances or microrganisms.

Examples of nonspecific defenses are skin, tears, acid environment, inflammatory response, and interferon. An example of a specific response is the antigen-antibody response.

Hospitalized patients have an accentuated need for microbial safety due to:

Their weakened physical status
The nature of the hospital setting—the great numbers of people in contact with them
Certain disease conditions and diagnostic procedures, and some types of medication therapy

Nursing interventions focus on providing a biologically safe environment. The primary preventive skill is handwashing. Other nursing intervention focuses on the identification of infection and protecting patients from infection. Category-specific and disease-specific isolation precautions are methods of enhancing biological safety for hospitalized patients.

Terms for Review

active immunity	antibodies	C & S testing
allergen	antigens	carrier
anaphylactic shock	aseptic technique	category-specific isolation precautions
antibiotic resistance	autoimmune disease	chain of infection

chemotaxis

clean

contamination

differential white blood cell count

disease-specific isolation precautions

exudate

  fibrinous

  hemorrhagic (sanguineous)

  purulent

  serous

host

immune

inflammatory response

interferon

leukocytosis

local

medical asepsis

nosocomial infection

passive immunity

pathogens

phagocytosis

portal of entry

reservoir

resident flora

sedimentation rate

sensitization

sterile

surgical asepsis

susceptible

systemic

transient flora

vehicle of transmission

virulent

Self-Assessment

1. Complete the following data collection for yourself and any minor for whom you are responsible. It is recommended that this information be carried with you.

```
Name _____

Blood type_____

Food allergies _____

Drug allergies _____

Current medications _____(as of date) _____

Date of last:

    Tetanus booster _____

    Tuberculin test_____

Childhood vaccinations completed (year):

    Polio _____

    Diphtheria, pertussis, and tetanus (DPT) _____

    Measles, mumps, and rubella (MMR)_____
```

2. In the nursing laboratory, apply Glo-germ (or a similar clear liquid which when dry is visable under black light) to your hands. Then perform a medical handwashing. Next, observe your hands under a black light. White areas on your hands indicate areas that have been missed during handwashing. How effective is your skill?

Learning Activities

1. Select a partner and practice the nursing skills in Chapter 18. For those skills that require sterile technique, direct the partner to observe while you demonstrate the procedure, stopping you anytime a contamination occurs. Then, reverse roles so each partner has the opportunity to observe and demonstrate. This is an effective method of practicing any nursing skill.
2. In a public restroom observe persons washing their hands.

    How often is soap used?

    How long is the average handwashing?

    Do people recontaminate their hands when turning off

      the faucets?

    How do these practices spread microorganisms?

Review Questions

1. Which of the following illustrates the sequence of the chain of infection?

    a. Pathogen→portal of entry → susceptible host → reservoir → portal of exit

    b. Pathogen → reservoir → portal of exit → vehicle of transmission → portal of entry → susceptible host

    c. Pathogen → reservoir → portal of exit → susceptible host → vehicle of transmission

    d. Microorganism → portal of exit → vehicle of transmission → portal of entry → susceptible host

2. Before giving direct patient care, the nurse washes hands in order to

    a. Protect self from the pathogens of the patient

   b. Protect the patient from pathogens that the nurse might carry
   c. Sterilize hands prior to giving care
   d. Remove potential antigens from the skin surface.
3. The basis of the body's defense against invasion is
   a. Based on chemicals known as lymphokines
   b. Primarily nonspecific in nature
   c. Enhanced by the administration of glucocorticoids
   d. The ability to distinguish self from nonself.
4. Which of the following is the common characteristic of nonspecific body defense mechanisms?
   a. All involve chemically mediated responses.
   b. All protect against any microbe or any foreign substance in the same way.
   c. All are weakened by the presence of antibodies.
   d. None is fully operative until adolescence.
5. The body's first line of defense is
   a. Unbroken skin and mucous membrane
   d. Tears
   c. Acid environment
   d. Lysoenzyme
6. Which of the following statements best defines the inflammatory response?
   a. All the localized responses initiated by the presence of microorganisms
   b. The series of changes occurring in blood due to invasion by pathogens
   c. All local and systemic responses of the body initiated by injury or infection
   d. Process by which infection is walled off to limit the effect on the body
7. A nurse must put on the following items: (1) hair covering, (2) face mask, (3) sterile gown, (4) gloves, then (5) open sterile pack containing sterile gown and gloves. Indicate the order in which this is done.
   a. 5, 1, 2, 3, 4
   b. 2, 1, 5, 3, 4
   c. 5, 2, 1, 3, 4
   d. 1, 2, 5, 3, 4
8. The primary local symptoms of infection include
   a. Pain, redness, heat, swelling
   b. Loss of mobility, redness, swelling, heat
   c. Fever, pain, redness, swelling
   d. Elevated WBC, pain, fever, heat
9. During infection, the white blood cell count is
   a. Increased
   b. Decreased
   c. No change is seen
10. Procedures for skills in nursing fundamentals textbooks are intended as
   a. A recipe for how to do it
   b. Steps to be followed in unvaried sequence
   c. General guidelines to be adapted to individual patient needs
   d. The proven, most efficient method of accomplishing a skill

Answers

1. b
2. b
3. d
4. b
5. a
6. c
7. d
8. a
9. a
10. c

References and Bibliography

Barsevick, A., and Llewellyn, J.: A comparison of the anxiety reducing potential of two techniques of bathing. *Nurs. Res.,* **31**:22–27, 1982.

Beland, I. L., and Passos, J. Y.: *Clinical Nursing,* 4th ed. Macmillan, New York, 1981.

Dubay, E. C., and Grubb, R. D.: *Infection Prevention and Control.* Mosby, St. Louis, 1978.

Garner, J., and Simmons, B.: CDC guideline for isolation precautions in hospitals, *Infect. Control,* **4**: 245–322, 1983.

Griffiths, M.: *Introduction to Human Physiology.* Macmillan, New York, 1981.

Guyton, A. C.: *Textbook of Medical Physiology.* 6 ed. Saunders, Philadelphia, 1981.

Jacob, S. W.; Francone, C. A.; and Lossow, W.: *Structure and Function in Man,* 5th ed Saunders, Philadelphia, 1982.

Pagana, K. and Pagana, T. J.: *Diagnostic Testing and Nursing Implications.* Mosby, St. Louis, 1982.

Phipps, W.; Long, B. C.; Woods, N.; and Fugate: *Medical Surgical Nursing,* 2nd ed. Mosby, St. Louis, 1983.

Smith, A. L.: *Microbiology and Pathology,* 12th ed. Mosby, St. Louis, 1980.

Strand, F. L.: *Physiology: A Regulatory Systems Approach.* Macmillan, New York, 1978.

Tortora, G. J., and Anagnostakos, N.: *Principles of Anatomy and Physiology,* 3rd ed. Harper & Row, New York 1981.

Tortora, G. J.; Funke, B. R.; and Case, C. L.: *Microbiology: An Introduction.* Benjamin/Cummings Publishing Co., Inc., Menlo Park, Calif., 1982.

Vander, A. J.; Sherman, J. H; and Luciano, D. S.: *Huamn Physiology,* 3rd ed. McGraw-Hill, New York, 1980.

Wilson, M. E.; Mizer, H. E.; and Morello, J. A.: *Microbiology in Patient Care,* 3rd ed. Macmillan, New York, 1979.

CHAPTER 19

PROVIDING A CHEMICALLY SAFE ENVIRONMENT: MEDICATION ADMINISTRATION

Objectives

1. Discuss how the nurse uses a knowledge of pharmacology to provide chemical safety for patients.

2. List the five rights of medication administration.

3. Discuss how the following factors influence chemical safety related to medication administration: age, body size, sex, body organ system function, psychological factors, individual drug history, disease conditions.

4. Discuss the ethical responsibilities of the nurse related to medication administration.

5. Discuss the legal responsibilities of the nurse related to medication administration.

6. Describe precautions the nurse takes to protect the patient with a known food or drug allergy.

7. Describe the three safety checks the nurse completes in preparing any medication.

8. Demonstrate the use of a drug reference text to obtain the following information for a specific drug: generic and trade names, route, usual dose, action, side effects, contraindications, nursing implications.

9. Safely perform the following skills:
   Accurate calculation of drug dosages

Administration of
   Oral medication
   Subcutaneous injections
   Intramuscular injections
   Intravenous medications
   Intradermal medications
   Medications via the skin and mucous membrane

The Importance of Chemical Safety: Medication Administration

Medication (drug) *therapy* (the administration of chemical substances that alter body function in order to achieve therapeutic effect) is part of the care of many patients given by members of the health team. Thus, it is part of the nursing role. It is helpful and often necessary for nurses to understand the actions of a medication in order to administer it in such a way as to enhance the *therapeutic effect* (intended effect of the drug) and to prevent or minimize *side effects* (effects of medications other than those intended). Some medications, for example, must be taken when the stomach is empty because food inhibits the absorption of the drug. Other medications must be taken with food to decrease irrita-

tion to the lining of the stomach. Using their knowledge of *pharmacology* (the study of drugs), nurses make decisions about the scheduling of medications, assess the patient's response to medications, observe for side effects, and teach patients about medication therapy. The nurse communicates these data to other members of the health team and shares in the responsibility of implementing and evaluating medication therapy. Because nurses provide care 24 hours a day to hospitalized patients, they are in a unique position to assess the patient's response to medication and to make a significant contribution to this aspect of patient care.

Threats to Chemical Safety

Although medications correctly given have enormous potential benefit to patients, medications given in error can cause harmful, if not lethal, effects. Medications can be given in the wrong amount, to the wrong patient, or at the wrong time. Another error may result if the medication is given by the wrong *route* (method of administration), such as giving the drug in a pill form when an injection was ordered. An error of omission may also occur if a nurse does not give an ordered medi-

cation. Accidental poisoning poses another threat to chemical safety.

Nurses protect patients by applying their knowledge of pharmacology to the decisions they make during medication administration and by following procedures designed to result in safe medication administration. These procedures will be discussed as part of the skills of medication administration.

Providing Chemical Safety During Medication Administration

Physicians and nurses share the responsibility for medication therapy. However, it is usually the nurse who actually gives the medication to the patient and is thus responsible for assuring patient safety. Like other nursing skills, medication administration requires both knowledge and practice in order to achieve competent, safe performance. A consideration of several factors helps the nurse to develop this skill.

Knowledge of the Drug

It is unreasonable to expect that the nurse memorize hundreds of drugs and the related information necessary for giving them safely. It is reasonable to expect that the nurse knows how to look up a drug in a reference available on the clinical unit. Several reference sources are described in Table 19–1. The nurse may use

Table 19-1. **References for Drug Administration**

Source	Publisher	Contents
United States Pharmacopeia (USP)	United States Pharmacopeia Convention—nonprofit, nongovernmental, corporation.	Official listing of drugs designated by Federal Food, Drug & Cosmetic Act. Drugs are described according to source, chemical and physical composition, tests for purity and identity, method of storage and usual dosages.
British Pharmacopoeia (BP)	British Pharmacopoeia Commission	Official listing of drugs including standards for purity, identification, and formulas.
Canadian Formulary (CF)	Official publication of the Canadian Food and Drug Act	Listing of drugs which are used in Canada but which are not necessarily in the BP.
American Hospital Formulary Service	Two volumes published by the American Society of Hospital Pharmacists. Updated with annual supplements.	Contains monographs on every drug entity available in the United States. Includes information about chemistry, absorption, mechanisms of action, uses, excretion, dosage. Cross-referenced by generic and brand name.
Physicians' Desk Reference	Published annually by Medical Economics, Inc., Oradell, N.J.	Contains manufacturers' indexes by brand name and generic name, therapeutic classification index (such as analgesic, antibiotics, etc.), and product information section.
Handbook of Non-Prescription Drugs	American Pharmaceutical Association, Washington, D.C.	Contains information on over-the-counter medications in the United States. Chapters are divided by therapeutic activity such as antacid products, cold and allergy products, etc.

the *trade name* of the drug (the name used by a specific manufacturer of a specific brand and designated by the symbol ®, also called the proprietary name) or the *generic name* (the common name of a drug which may be used in all countries by all manufacturers) to look up a particular drug. Occasionally, some drugs are so new that they are not included in reference texts. Often literature describing the drug is printed by the manufacturer and packaged with the drug providing the nurse with the necessary information for safe administration. At other times, the nurse may call the hospital pharmacist for information. Most nurses find that, through experience, they develop a knowledge of the drugs most frequently given in the clinical area in which they work.

Once the nurse has located a particular drug in a reference book, the listing of information about that drug may be overwhelming. The nurse may note the following information in order to condense the listing: generic name of the drug, common trade name, route of administration and usual dose, action (how the drug works), side effects, *contraindications* (conditions under which the drug should not be given), nursing implications. Nursing students often find it helpful to write this information on small index cards, which may then be used for study purposes.

Preparation of the Drug

When preparing drugs for administration to patients, it is recommended that the nurse work in a quiet area where distractions are at a minimum. There are two usual methods of administering medications to patients. In the traditional method, the nurse prepares the medications for several patients in a central medication area. Each medication is then placed on a large tray and delivered to the various patients. In the second method, called the unit dose system, all medications are placed in a large movable cart which has a separate drawer for the medications of each patient. The medication for each patient is prepared as the cart is wheeled from room to room. This system eliminates errors made when medications of several patients are prepared at the same time or are placed on the same tray. In the unit dose system, each patient's medications are prepared separately and administered before the nurse begins preparation of a second patient's medications.

Whatever the system of medication administration, the nurse uses some written form of a medication order originally written by the physician in the patient's chart to prepare medications. This may be the written drug order in the unit dose system, or it may be a medication

NAME	ROOM
John R. Smith	642'
DRUG	METHOD
Cimetidine 300mg	O
HOURS	FREQ.
8ᵃ 12noon 6ᵖ hr	qid
INITIALS	DATE
L. K.	1/9/85

Figure 19–1. Example of a medication card.

card or Kardex prepared from the original order as shown in Figure 19–1. All forms contain the same information: name of patient, date, drug, dose, route, frequency and duration of drug, and name of physician or nurse practitioner ordering the drug. In two states, Oregon and Washington, nurses can legally prescribe medication independently. Other jurisdictions have statutes that allow nurse practitioners to write prescriptions when this authority is delegated by a physician (Baker, 1981).

Five Rights of Medication Administration

There are five rights of medication administration which the nurse considers to ensure safe administration of any chemical substance:

1. Right patient. Each hospitalized patient wears some form of identification, usually a wristband. The nurse checks the medication card or the record sheet from the unit dose cart against the wristband of the patient. They must match exactly. In a nursing home where the residents do not wear identification bands, some other form of identification is necessary. The nurse may also ask the patient, "What is your name please?" This is preferable to calling the patient by name as a form of identification. If the nurse says, "Mr. Jones, I have your medication for you," the patient is likely not to listen carefully and correct the nurse who has made an error. Few patients will give a wrong name, however, when asked a direct question.

2. Right drug. The nurse reads the label on the drug when removing it from the shelf or storage area, before pouring or removing it to a container for the individual patient, and when placing it back in storage. The nurse compares the medication card or unit dose sheet to the label with each reading. They must match exactly, or the nurse must know that they are the same drug if the order has the generic name and the drug has a trade name or vice versa. If the nurse is unsure that acetaminophen is the same as TYLENOL, the nurse uses a drug reference book to find out BEFORE administering the drug.

3. Right dose. The nurse has a knowledge of the drug and knows what would be a reasonable amount of the medication, given the age and body weight of a particular patient. The nurse uses this knowledge to evaluate the dose ordered for the patient. If the dose appears to be inappropriate, the nurse seeks clarification of the medication order from the physician who ordered the drug. If the nurse must calculate the dosage, the mathematics are done carefully and rechecked with a second nurse if there is any question of accuracy. Some medications, such as insulin or those administered intravenously, are always checked by a second nurse prior to administration. When asking another nurse to double-check a medication, the first nurse presents the second nurse with the medication card, the bottle or vial of medication, and the prepared medication. The first nurse then asks, "What do I have?" In this manner, the nurse checking the preparation of the dose has the original information to use in evaluating correctness.

4. Right route. Many medications may be given in a variety of ways: orally, intramuscularly, intravenously, topically, or rectally. The nurse reads the label on the medication to determine if the preparation of the drug is intended for the use which is ordered. The person ordering the drug designates the route for administration.

5. Right time. Drugs are ordered to be given at specified times. For some medications, it is important that a blood level of the drug be established and maintained. It is therefore important to divide the doses evenly throughout the day. Thus, if four doses of the drug are required, they may be given at 6 A.M., 12 noon, 6 P.M. 12 midnight. Other drugs may be given before meals; others withheld until after diagnostic blood tests are completed. Errors in the timing of medications may result in harm to the patient as well as lengthened hospital stay and added expense to the patient.

It is generally acceptable practice to give medications a half hour before or after the time they are due. This means that a medication scheduled for 8:00 A.M. could be given any time between 7:30 A.M. and 8:30 A.M. Exceptions to this rule include certain medications that must be given prior to surgery or other diagnostic tests, since it is important that the patient receive these for a specified time prior to the operation or examination. Other medications are ordered "stat," meaning they are to be given immediately. Some medications are to be given hourly, and rigid adherence to a schedule is necessary to enhance the effectiveness of these medications.

Factors Affecting Chemical Safety During Medication Administration

Each individual has both shared and unique manifestations of the need for chemical safety as it relates to medication administration. All persons receiving medication therapy share the need to receive the correct medication in the prescribed amount at the correct time. Factors that influence the unique safety needs of an individual follow.

Age

People who are very old or very young have unique needs related to medications. The fetus and the neonate have immature organs which make them more vulnerable to the effects of drugs. The elderly and the very young person may have an impaired ability to absorb, circulate, and excrete drugs. Both of these persons usually require smaller doses than an average adult.

Body Size

The weight of the average adult is considered to be 150 lb. Thus, dosage for persons smaller or larger must be adjusted upward or downward to achieve the same blood level of a medication.

Sex

The female body has a higher percentage of fatty tissue than does the male body. Fatty tissue has fewer blood vessels than, for example, muscle tissue. Thus, women may require larger dosages of a drug to achieve the same result as in a man who does not have the same amount of fatty tissue. Another consideration related to chemical safety is a determination of pregnancy. Pregnancy is a contraindication for almost any drug. Some drugs are able to cross the placenta and affect the developing fetus, particularly during the first trimester. After delivery, some drugs may be passed in the breast milk to the infant. The effects of many drugs on the fetus during pregnancy are still unknown.

Body Organ System Function

The physiological functioning of body systems determines how drugs affect the body. The circulatory system, the elimination system, and the respiratory system are all involved. The circulatory system brings the drug to the tissues where it produces its effect. The liver metabolizes drugs. The waste products of the drugs are then excreted primarily via the kidneys, but also by the lungs and intestines. If the circulatory system is impaired, there may be a build-up of toxic chemicals within the blood. Thus, the effectiveness of drug therapy depends in large part on the level of functioning of these systems.

Psychological Factors

Although difficult to measure objectively, it appears that the emotional state of the individual affects response to medication. Patients who "expect" that a medication will help them frequently experience more positive results than those who do not have this expectation. This is an example of the mind-body reciprocal influence that is described in holistic health care.

Individual Drug History

A drug history may be helpful in identifying unusual reactions to a drug. Some individuals may report *idiosyncratic effects* (highly unusual and unexpected results) of a drug. The person may report signs or symptoms that are rarely associated with the particular drug. Drug allergies may be also identified in a drug history.

Disease Conditions

Disease pathology affects the response of the body to drugs. Antibiotics have little effect on the healthy person but are very effective against sensitive bacteria. Different degrees of pain may require different medications. A headache is often relieved by aspirin, while severe postoperative pain from a surgical incision would be unrelieved by such treatment.

Problems Associated with Chemical Safety: Medication Administration

Problems Related to the Administration of Drugs

The nursing literature, as well as the medical-legal literature, contains many articles which report the medication errors of nurses, physicians and pharmacists. In most instances the error could have been avoided if the health care professional had followed exactly the correct procedure for medication administration. The correct procedure includes the five "rights" of medication administration: the right patient, right drug, right dose, right route, and the right time.

Problems Related to the Effect of Drugs

Side Effects. These are responses unrelated to the therapeutic use of the drug. They are observed and reported by the nurse. Mild side effects, such as slight nausea, may be acceptable if they are outweighed by the benefits of the drug. If the side effects are serious, the dosage of the medication may need to be reduced, or the medication may need to be discontinued, temporarily or permanently.

Drug Toxicity. Harmful effects that are related to the purpose for which the drug was given are called drug *toxicity*. These may occur as a result of high circulating blood levels of a drug, slowed metabolism, inability of the body to excrete the drug, or administration of excessively high dosage. One example of drug toxicity is excessive slowing of the heart from digitalis. In therapeutic amounts, digitalis slows the heart rate and increases the effectiveness of the contraction of the heart muscle.

Allergic Reactions. Some persons have been sensitized to a drug, that is, they have an allergy to certain medications. This means that the drug acts as an antigen in the body and stimulates the production of antibodies against it. If the individual is given the drug a second time, an allergic reaction results. This reaction may vary from hives, itching, redness, tearing, and a feeling of apprehension to anaphylactic shock and death. (See Chapter 18 for further discussion.)

Drug Tolerance. An individual who has developed a drug tolerance requires successively larger doses of the drug in order to produce the same therapeutic effect as the original dose.

Drug Interactions. An *interaction* occurs when the effects of a drug are altered by a second drug. This may be a beneficial result, or it may be harmful. *Addition* is the interaction effect obtained by giving two drugs at a low dose rather than one drug at a higher dose. This method may avoid harmful effects of a higher dose of one medication. *Potentiation* is the effect that occurs when the action of one drug is enhanced by the administration of a second drug. The action of the first drug is greater than it would be if it had been administered alone. Promethazine (PHENERGAN) is frequently given to potentiate the effects of meperidine, a medication for pain relief.

A negative example of drug interaction is drug *antagonism*, one drug working to negate the effects of a second. This may occur inadvertently when the patient is taking nonprescription medications of which the physician is unaware. For example, a patient who is taking THORAZINE, a prescribed tranquilizer, may begin to take antacid. The antacid interferes with absorption of the THORAZINE. Drug *incompatibility*, another negative interaction, refers to medications that may not be mixed without causing chemical changes. This usually refers to two medications that are mixed in one syringe or one intravenous infusion before administration. It is sometimes possible to see small particles in the solution. This is extremely dangerous and is never administered to a patient.

Drug Addiction. The physical and/or psychological dependence of a person on a drug for a feeling of well-being or relief of pain is called *addiction*. Not all drugs that relieve pain produce addiction, but some of the most potent *analgesics* (drugs that relieve pain) do. Most patients receive these drugs for only a limited period of time so addiction does not become a problem. At other times, patients with lengthy illnesses with severe pain are at risk for becoming dependent on these drugs. Nurses may then face a serious ethical dilemma: to relieve pain knowing of the risk of addiction, or to withhold medication allowing the patient to experience excessive pain. Refer to Chapter 26 for a discussion of pain control using drugs, addiction, and placebos.

Problems Related to the Medication Order

Since the nurse is the person directly administering the drug to the patient, it is the responsibility of the nurse to understand clearly the medication order. If the handwriting of the physician or nurse practitioner is unclear, the nurse seeks clarification rather than making an "educated guess." Although this may incur the wrath of the writer, it may also encourage legibility. It is indefensible for the nurse to claim that the handwriting was unclear and "I gave what I thought it said."

At other times, the medication order may be incomplete. For example, the route of administration may have been omitted. Again, the nurse seeks clarification from the writer of the order.

Medication orders may be expired. Frequently, antibiotics may be written for only seven days and are then automatically discontinued. The nurse faced with an expired order is unsure if the physician or nurse practitioner meant to discontinue the drug or merely forgot to reorder it. Because this could have serious consequences for the patient, the nurse clarifies the order. Similarly, orders for *narcotics* (medications with addictive effects) are good only for a limited time period and must then be renewed.

Problems Related to prn Orders

The inclusion of the term "prn" in a medication order means "as necessary." Medications for pain or sleep are often ordered prn, meaning to be given as needed by the patient. It has been said that these letters (prn) account for much of the pain of hospitalized patients. Nurses have been known to comment, "He can't be in that much pain. His surgery was a week ago," or "She can't have pain. I gave her pain medication only two hours ago." When administering prn medications, nurses who are expert in the field of pain control recommend that pain be considered "whatever the patient says it is." All prn medications require that the nurse document the data that indicated a need for the medication, as well as the patient's response to the medication. These data will be needed to evaluate the effectiveness of the drug for the patient and to adjust the drug dose or schedule, if necessary. (See Chapter 26 for a complete discussion of pain-relief methods.)

Ethical Considerations Related to Medication Administration

During their professional careers, it is probable that nurses will make mistakes while giving medications. This is a consequence of being human. Although individual nurses occasionally claim that they have never made a medication error, it is more likely that the medication error had not been discovered and therefore nothing could be done to correct it or lessen any negative consequences. When acting in accord with the Code of Ethics, the nurse accepts accountability and responsibility for nursing actions. Applied to this situation, this means that the nurse acknowledges the medication error and reports it to the responsible physician or nurse practitioner. It also means that the student in nursing reports an error or a suspected error to the nursing instructor without delay for fear of criticism or loss of a "good grade." Ethical behavior also includes completing the required documentation. (See Figure 19-2.)

Another ethical situation involves the administration of a *placebo*, an inert substance that produces its effect because of the patient's belief in its efficacy, rather than its chemical or physical properties. Placebos may be injections of normal saline or pills of sugar. Studies have shown that they do produce an effect in many cases. (See Chapter 26.) Many nurses question the ethics of administering placebos. They state that to give a placebo is a deception and a violation of the trust within the nurse-patient relationship. There is no right or wrong to this issue, and each nurse must resolve this issue individually.

A difficult ethical issue facing nurses concerns reporting nurse colleagues suspected of drug abuse. While this is a difficult task, it is necessary, both to protect the patient and to assure that the colleague receive the necessary health care. One nurse addict offered the following advice to nurses who suspect a colleague of drug abuse, "Confront the nurse, her family, and her superiors with your suspicions. And the sooner the better" (Mereness, 1981).

Legal Considerations Related to Medication Administration

Nurse Practice Act

Professional nurses are licensed and authorized to administer drugs, that is, to give a single dose of a medication to a patient according to the order of a licensed medical doctor or another licensed practitioner. Nurses are not licensed to dispense drugs. Preparing drugs from large bulk containers, relabeling drugs, or preparing compounds is the legal role of the pharmacist. The nurse working the evening or night shift (when many hospital pharmacies are closed) may occasionally find it necessary to open the hospital pharmacy to secure one dose of a drug for a particular patient. Although this is within the limits of the law, to do so repeatedly and as a matter of routine practice leaves the nurse in a vulnerable position. In such circumstances, institutions need to develop procedures to provide the required professional pharmacist services to patients for extended hours.

The final responsibility for the administration of a medication rests upon the nurse who gives it. It is the right and responsibility of the nurse to refuse to give any medication that appears to be in error or unreasonable. The statement, "That was the way the physician's order was written," is no defense for a medication error. If the nurse questions a medication order, the nurse reports the question to the nurse in charge or to the physi-

UNIVERSITY OF MINNESOTA HOSPITALS & CLINICS
INCIDENT REPORT

NAME OF PERSON INVOLVED		AGE	SEX	INCIDENT DATE	INCIDENT TIME	INCIDENT LOCATION (AREA AND ROOM)
Grass Susan L.		48	F	1/29/83	9:00 ☒AM ☐PM	Room 146²

CATEGORY OF PERSON INVOLVED	[X] PATIENT →	UH# 368-2954-02	CONDITION [X]AMBULATORY [ ]UP WITH HELP [ ]BEDREST [ ]SEDATED
	[ ] EMPLOYEE →	JOB TITLE	DEPARTMENT
	[ ] OTHER →	SPECIFY (E.G.,VISITOR, VOLUNTEER, ETC.)	HOME PHONE (AREA CODE) ( )

GENERAL TYPE OF INCIDENT	[ ] INJURY · FATALITY	☐ PROPERTY /FACILITY DAMAGE	☒ MEDICATION ERROR	☐ ADVERSE DRUG REACTION
	[ ] THEFT (CALL SECURITY IMMEDIATELY)	☐ PATIENT PROPERTY OR VALUABLES	☐ DEFECTIVE PRODUCT ☐ POTENTIAL HAZARD	☐ OTHER (SPECIFY)

DESCRIPTION OF INCIDENT - PLEASE OBJECTIVELY <u>DESCRIBE ALL INCIDENTS</u> IN THIS SPACE. IN ADDITION, A CHECKLIST HAS BEEN PROVIDED FOR MEDICATIONS, FALLS AND LABORATORY-RELATED INCIDENTS FOR YOUR CONVENIENCE. CONTINUE ON REVERSE IF NECESSARY.

Patient was to receive Lanoxin 0.125 mg at 9am. The patient was scheduled for diagnostic procedures off of the clinical area and the dose was forgotten. The error was discovered at 4pm. Physician notified & medication given at 4³⁰ as per order of Dr. Samuels.

CHECK HERE IF CONTINUED ON BACK [ ]

	TYPE (CHECK ALL THAT APPLY)	STEPS WHICH MAY HAVE CONTRIBUTED TO INCIDENT (CHECK ALL THAT APPLY)	INTRAVENOUS FLUIDS (CHECK ALL THAT APPLY)
MEDICATION RELATED INCIDENTS	[ ] DIFFERENT MED/DOSE/SOLUTION ARRIVED ON STATION [ ] DIFFERENT MEDICATION GIVEN [ ] DIFFERENT DOSAGE GIVEN [ ] MED. GIVEN TO DIFFERENT PATIENT [ ] MED. GIVEN AT DIFFERENT TIME [ ] MED. GIVEN BY DIFFERENT ROUTE [X] MEDICATION OMITTED [ ] OTHER	☐ ORDERING MEDICATION ☐ TRANSCRIBING ORDER ☐ LABELING MEDICATION ☐ READING MEDICATION LABEL ☐ COMPARING LABEL W/MED KARDEX ☐ CHECKING PATIENT I.D. BAND ☐ GIVING MEDICATION ☐ PATIENT DISREGARDED INSTRUCTIONS ☐ OTHER	☐ TOO FAST ☐ TOO SLOW ☐ DIFFERENT SOLUTION ☐ DIFFERENT ADDITIVE ☐ DIFF. ADMINISTRATIVE APPARATUS ☐ I.V. INFILTRATED ☐ OTHER
	TYPE OF FALL	ACTIVITY AT TIME OF INCIDENT	CIRCUMSTANCES (CHECK ALL THAT APPLY)
INCIDENTS INVOLVING FALLS	[ ] FROM COMMODE [ ] FROM WHEELCHAIR [ ] FROM CHAIR [ ] FROM BED [ ] OTHER	☐ WALKING ALONE ☐ WALKING ASSISTED ☐ TRANSFER ALONE ☐ TRANSFER ASSISTED ☐ SITTING UP ☐ LYING DOWN ☐ OTHER	☐ SLIPPERY WALKING SURFACE ☐ TRIPPED ☐ FAINTED ☐ LOSS OF BALANCE ☐ SEIZURE ☐ DISREGARDED INSTRUCTIONS ☐ OTHER
LABORATORY RELATED INCIDENTS	TYPE OF INCIDENTS [ ] RESULTS REPORTED INCORRECTLY [ ] SPECIMEN HANDLED IMPROPERLY	☐ RESPONSE TIME ☐ MISLABELED SPECIMEN → ☐ UNLABELED SPECIMEN →	[ ] OTHER _____ STATION/CLINIC SENDING SPECIMEN WAS	PHLEBOTOMIST WAS
PHYSICIAN NOTIFIED? [X] YES [ ] NO	IF YES, NAME Dr. E. J. Samuels SIGNATURE X	PHYSICIAN'S FINDINGS	CHECK HERE IF CONTINUED ON BACK [ ]
PERSON COMPLETING	SIGNATURE X L. Lind, R.N.	TITLE Clinical Nurse II	DATE 1/29/83	PHONE 642-1718

UH 1038, APR 81

Please forward to Box 708 Mayo within 24 hours.

Figure 19–2. Example of an incident report which documents a medication error. (Courtesy of the University of Minnesota Hospitals, Minneapolis, MN.)

cian who ordered the drug. Often this communication will resolve the problem for the nurse. If the nurse still questions giving the medication after this communication, the nurse documents the situation and reports to nursing supervisors. This is a serious situation requiring accountability and responsibility of the nurse.

Controlled Substance Act

In 1970, Congress passed the Comprehensive Drug Abuse Prevention and Control Act. This act, which repeals almost 50 other laws written since 1914, is intended to improve the administration and regulation of drugs found necessary to control (Squire and Clayton, 1981). The Canadian Control Act of 1961 provides for similar controls.

Narcotics are kept under lock on the clinical unit using keys or combination locks. Keys to the narcotic storage areas are carried by the nurse on duty at all times. Federal law requires an accounting of all narcotics administered within the hospital. Usually, this includes recording the patient's name, the medication, date, time, dosage, the physician prescribing the drug, and the nurse administering the drug. If a narcotic must be wasted for some reason, perhaps the nurse contaminated a sterile needle, a second nurse must sign the record to indicate that the drug was in fact wasted. At the end of each shift, the narcotics are counted, usually by one nurse who is completing the shift and by a second nurse who is coming on duty. If the amount of narcotics on hand does not correspond to the record, this must be reported immediately. Frequently, this is merely a case of a nurse forgetting to complete the record at the time the medication was given. Because of the inconvenience this causes, it is recommended that nurses complete this record immediately after preparing the drug.

Patient's Rights

A final legal consideration involves the patient's right to refuse a medication. When this occurs, the nurse does not attempt to force the patient to take the medication. To do so could result in a charge of assault and battery against the nurse. The nurse seeks, through communication, to determine why the patient refuses the medication and the possible consequences of omitting the medication. Frequently, the patient requires additional information and/or teaching to make a decision to accept treatment. If the patient continues to refuse the medication, the nurse documents the events and reports to the physician.

Assessment of Chemical Safety

Admission Data

The nurse admitting a patient to a health care facility completes a careful drug history. The following questions are included in this assessment:

1. Are you currently taking any medications? If so, what is the name of the medication? How frequently do you take it? What is the reason you are taking this medication? By asking these questions, the nurse is alert to any current drug therapy the patient may be receiving.

Table 19-2. **Poison Checklist for the Home**

Kitchen

1. Do all harmful products have child-resistant caps?
2. Are all potentially harmful products in their original containers with the original label? (Labels often contain first aid information in case the substance is ingested.)
3. Are harmful products stored away from food?
4. Are cabinets that hold potentially harmful products locked, or are the products stored high out of the reach of children?

Bathroom

1. Do aspirins and other potentially harmful products have child-resistant closures?
2. Have you thrown out all out-of-date prescriptions?
3. Do you give medicines only to the person for whom it was prescribed?
4. Are all medications in their original containers with their original labels?

Garage/Basement/Storage Area

1. Are all harmful products locked up out of sight and out of reach? Consider paint, paint thinner, gasoline, oil, swimming pool chemicals, insecticides, antifreeze, cleaners.
2. Do poisons have child-resistant caps?
3. Have you made sure that no poisons are stored in pop bottles or food jars?
4. Are the harmful products stored in their original containers with their original label?

Source: United States Consumer Product Safety Commission.

The nurse also learns the patient's understanding of medications and thus may identify needs for patient teaching. Most hospitals require that patients who are admitted do not keep any of their own medications and give any that were brought to the hospital into the care of the nurse. The purpose of this is to assure physicians and nurse practitioners planning treatment regimes that the patient is receiving only those medications ordered. This is important in determining the effectiveness of the regime or if an allergic reaction should result. It also protects other patients who might take another patient's medication in error.

2. Do you have any food or drug allergies? If the patient has known allergies, the nurse follows hospital procedure for safeguarding the patient. This usually involves special identification procedures, such as a red wristband, and labeling the patient's chart and medication administration record.

During Hospitalization

The nurse is responsible for observing and documenting the patient's response to drugs. In order to do this competently, the nurse needs to understand the intended actions of drugs and their possible side effects.

Related to Poison Control

Poisonous agents within individual homes in the community are also a threat to chemical safety. As part of a teaching role, the nurse works to educate the public about poison control. An essential part of preventing poisoning involves a careful assessment of the environment. Poisons are identified, labeled, and placed in a safe area, preferably one that can be locked. One such poison assessment list is included in Table 19–2.

Nursing Diagnoses Related to Chemical Safety: Medication Administration

The following list includes possible nursing diagnoses related to chemical safety.

Drug toxicity associated with barbiturates.
Potential drug toxicity related to decreased liver function
Idiosyncratic drug reaction related to digoxin (a drug to increase the strength of contraction of heart muscle)
Drug intolerance to codeine (an individual may be intolerant of any specific drug)

Potential drug dependence related to prolonged use of diazepam (drug used as muscle relaxant, antianxiety drug)
Difficulty ingesting potassium in liquid form
Inaccurate therapeutic drug management associated with self-medication
Altered respirations associated with ingestion of poison
Inadequate information related to drug abuse
Inadequate information related to self-medication

Nursing Interventions Related to Medication Administration

General Guidelines for Medication Administration

The responsibility for safe medication administration primarily depends upon the nurse, since it is the nurse who actually gives and assesses the effectiveness of most drugs. A review of Table 8–2 (medical abbreviations) may be helpful prior to studying medication administration. The following guidelines will help the nurse assure patient safety and nursing competence in this skill.

1. Know each drug you administer. Use available drug references, the hospital pharmacist, or package insert to determine the usual dose of the drug, route of ad-
ministration, action, side effects, contraindications, and any nursing care that the use of this drug might require. Some drugs require that certain assessments (such as taking blood pressure or apical pulse) be done before the medication is given A decision is then made to give or withhold the drug.

2. Know how to calculate the required amount of medications from the available supply. Table 19–3 lists a conversion table for different units of measurement used in calculating dosages. Table 19–4 shows methods of calculating various dosages and examples of problems the nurse might encounter. Some nurses choose to carry a small pocket calculator to use for this purpose.

3. Check the five rights of medication administra-

Table 19-3. **Equivalents for Different Measurement Systems**

(Conversions are given for equivalents most frequently used by the nurse.)
Metric: International system of measurement which is organized around units of ten.
Apothecaries': Original system of measurement brought to colonial United States from England.
Household: System of measurement commonly used within the home. Not as accurate as the other systems.

	METRIC	APOTHECARIES'	HOUSEHOLD
Fluid Equivalents	1 milliliter (ml)	= 15 minims (m)	= 15 drops (gtt)
	15 ml	= 4 fluid drams (℥)	= 1 tablespoon
	30 ml	= 1 fluid ounce (℥)	= 2 tablespoons or 8 teaspoons
	500 ml	= 1 pint	= 2 glassfuls
	1,000 ml	= 1 quart	= 4 glassfuls
	4,000 ml	= 1 gallon	
Weight Equivalents	60 milligram (mg)	= 1 grain (gr)	
	30 mg	= $1/2$ gr	
	15 mg	= $1/4$ gr	
	1 mg	= $1/60$ gr	
	0.6 mg	= $1/100$ gr	
	0.5 mg	= $1/120$ gr	
	0.4 mg	= $1/150$ gr	
	1 gram (gm)	= 15 gr	
	4 gm	= 1 dram	
	30 gm	= 1 ounce	
	500 gm	= 1.1 pound (lb)	
	1,000 gm	= 2.2 lb	

tion. These are the right patient, drug, dose, route, time.

4. Avoid distractions while preparing drugs.

5. Give medications in accordance with institutional policy. This may involve having a second nurse check certain medications or checking all mathematical calculations.

6. Remove any outdated drugs according to institutional procedure. This usually means returning them to the pharmacy. The purpose is to avoid the risk of giving ineffective drugs to patients.

7. If a patient questions a medication, resolve the question *before* giving the drug. A patient may say, "That doesn't look like the pill I received yesterday." At this point, the nurse *stops* until the issue is resolved. The nurse may know that the drug was changed and be able to give this information to the patient. It may also be that the nurse is in error and it is necessary to go back and check the drug. Listening to patients is one way to avoid errors.

8. Check for the presence of allergies each time you prepare and give medications.

9. Name the drug and state its intended purpose for the patient. The nurse may state, "Mr. Smith, this is your penicillin. This is an antibiotic to help clear up your skin infection." In this way, the nurse is teaching the patient. Mr. Smith will know that he has taken a specific antibiotic, that he is not allergic to it, and what it was intended to do for him. As a secondary benefit, the nurse has again identified the patient and offered the patient a chance to correct a possible error. Mr. Smith may say, "The doctor said this morning that that medication was to be changed."

10. Document all medications as soon as possible after giving them. Figure 19–3 is an example of recording medications. This is always done in ink and signed in such a manner that the full name and title of the nurse administering the drug are readily legible.

11. Do not give medications prepared by someone else. The nurse who gives the medications is responsible for their accuracy, and this is not possible if another nurse has prepared the medication. The possible exception to this guideline is intravenous fluids to which are added medications by the pharmacist. These are often prepared in the pharmacy under special conditions to protect their sterility.

Table 19-4. **Calculating Medication Doses**

A simple method of calculating doses is with the use of a ratio and proportion. In the proportion, the ratio on the left-hand side is what is known, in this case, the medication available. On the right side of the proportion is the desired dose, represented by X.

Example 1. The order reads: 60 mg phenobarbital bid, oral, 8 A.M. and 8 P.M.
Phenobarbital is available in 15-mg tablets. How many tablets does the nurse give?

$$\text{Known} = \text{Desired}$$
$$15 \text{ mg}: 1 \text{ tablet} = 60 \text{ mg}: X \text{ tablets}$$
$$\frac{15}{1} = \frac{60}{X}$$

Cross-multiply $15 \times X = 60 \times 1$

Divide $X = \dfrac{60}{15}$

$X = 4$ tablets

The same method can be applied to more difficult problems.

Example 2. The order reads: 600,000 units procaine penicillin IM stat.
Procaine penicillin is available in 500,000 units per ml.
Using the same method:

$$\text{Known} = \text{Desired}$$
$$500,000 \text{ units}: 1 \text{ ml} = 600,000: X \text{ ml}$$
$$\frac{500,000}{1 \text{ ml}} = \frac{600,000}{X \text{ ml}}$$

Multiply $500,000 X = 600,000$

Divide $X = \dfrac{600,000}{500,000}$

$X = 1.2$ ml

Example 3. At times, it may be necessary to add sterile water, sterile saline (or other diluent) to a powdered drug for injection.
Order: crystalline penicillin, 350,000 units, IM q3h.
Available: 20-ml vial containing 1,000,000 units of crystalline penicillin in dry form. The label reads on the vial: Adding 3.6 ml of diluent yeilds 250,000 units per ml. After adding the diluent as ordered, the nurse makes the following calculation:

$$250,000: 1 \text{ ml} = 350,000: X \text{ ml}$$
$$\frac{250,000}{1} = \frac{350,000}{X}$$
$$250,000 X = 350,000$$
$$X = \frac{350,000}{250,000}$$
$$X = 1.4 \text{ ml}$$

Administration of Oral Medications

The nurse prepares oral medications using medical asepsis or clean technique. Since the medication is to be taken by mouth, which is not a sterile cavity, sterile technique is not necessary. When preparing medications, the nurse notes any nursing actions required by the particular drug to be most effective. For example,

some medications must be given with milk. The nurse would provide this for the patient.

A single dose of a tablet or capsule is prepared by pouring the medication into the cover of the multiple-dose bottle and then into the medication cup. This prevents the nurses' fingers from contaminating drugs. If the drug requires an assessment of the patient prior to administration, the nurse prepares the drug in a separate

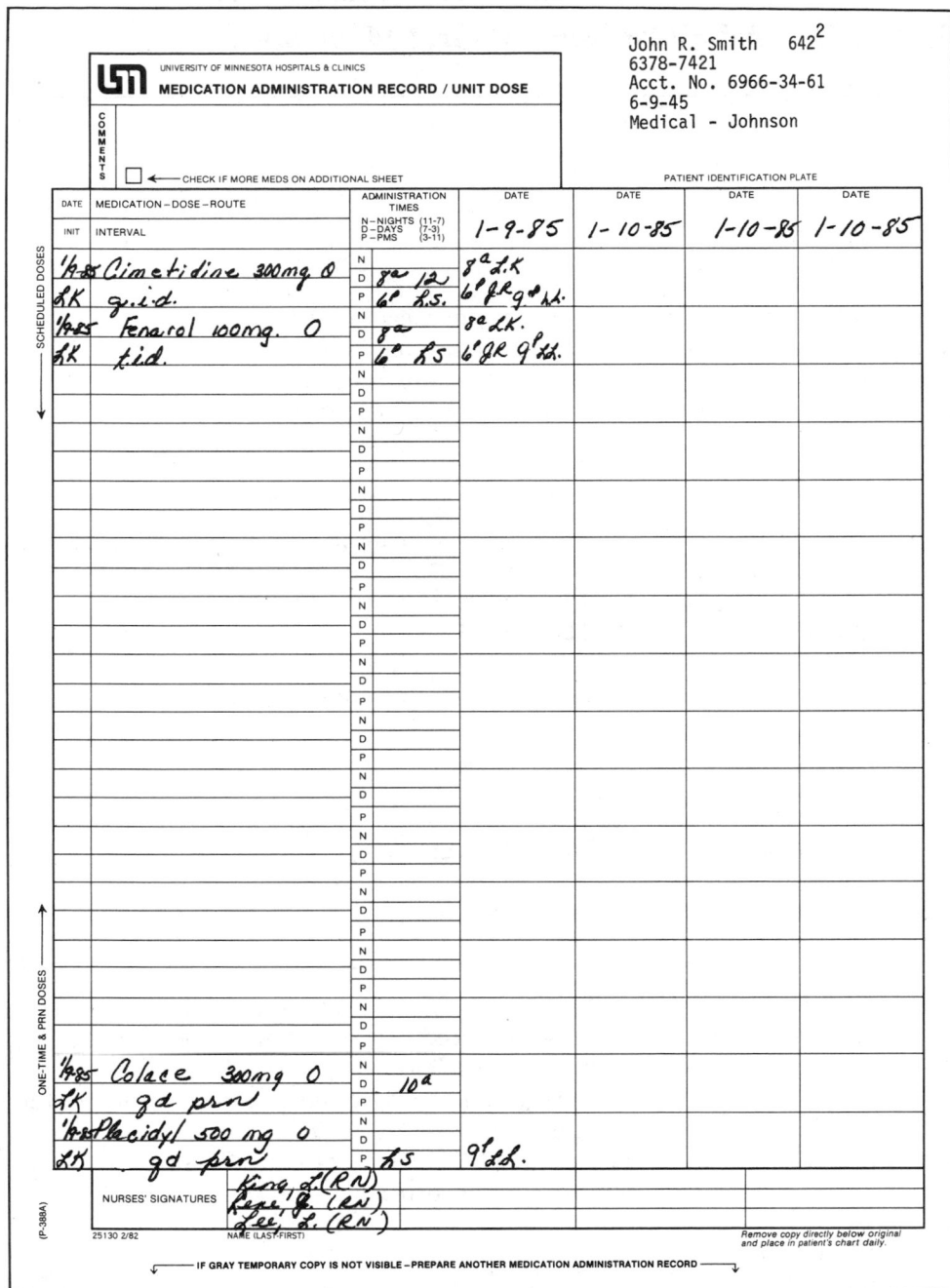

Figure 19-3. Documentation of medication administration using unit dose system. (Courtesy of the University of Minnesota Hospitals, Minneapolis, MN.)

medication cup. An example of this is digoxin, which is not usually given if the apical heart rate is less than 60 beats per minute. Thus, the nurse must assess the apical pulse prior to giving the drug. It is easy to identify and withhold the drug since it has been kept separate from any other medications the patient is receiving at the same time. Any medications that have been prepared and are not administered are considered contaminated and may not be returned to the original bottle. They are discarded according to hospital policy.

Many oral medications come individually labeled and packaged in a clear plastic bubble. These are taken still packaged to the patient's room. If for any reason they are not administered, they are not contaminated and may be used later by the patient. Some oral tablets are scored (a line dividing the tablet in half) in order that

Nursing Skill 19–1.   Administration of Oral Medication

Supplies
Medication cups
Clean medication tray
Straws and paper cups as needed

Preparation
Verify the accuracy of the medication by checking the medication card against the medication Kardex, or against the original order, or on the unit dose sheet. Verify the medications in the order in which they are listed. A random order may lead to errors of omission. Wash hands and clean the medication tray. An alcohol wipe may be used for this purpose.

Procedure	Explanation
1. Begin the preparation of the first listed medication the patient is to receive. Read medication order and select the correct medication.	1. Preparing medications in an ordered sequence helps to avoid errors of omission. This is check #1
2. Compare label on the medication card or unit dose sheet with label on the container for: a. Right patient b. Right medication c. Right dose d. Right route e. Right time	2. This is check #2. Five rights of medication administration.
3. Pour the individual dose of the medication without contamination.	3. Maintain medical asepsis.
4. Compare the bottle and the medication card or unit dose sheet for the "five rights" again. Return the multiple dose container to the shelf.	4. This is check #3.
5. Repeat 1 through 4 for each medication. Keep medications separate that require special assessments before administration. Do not mix liquids.	5. Provides safe medication administration. The nurse may need to withhold medication if indicated by the assessment. Mixing liquids may result in extremely distasteful solution.
6. Sign for any controlled substances as required.	6. Required by the Federal Controlled Substance Act.
7. Identify the patient by a. Asking the patient's name. b. Comparing the medication card or unit dose sheet to the patient's identification band.	7. Provides for correct identification of patient.
8. Assist the patient to a comfortable position and provide with water to take the medication.	8. Demonstrates concern for patient.
9. Administer the medications and stay with the patient until the medications are taken.	9. Prevents error of another patient taking the drug. Assures that the drug was taken.
10. Document medications on the patient's record including a. Drug b. Dose and route c. Time and date d. Signature of nurse and title e. Any response to medication	10. Legal responsibility.

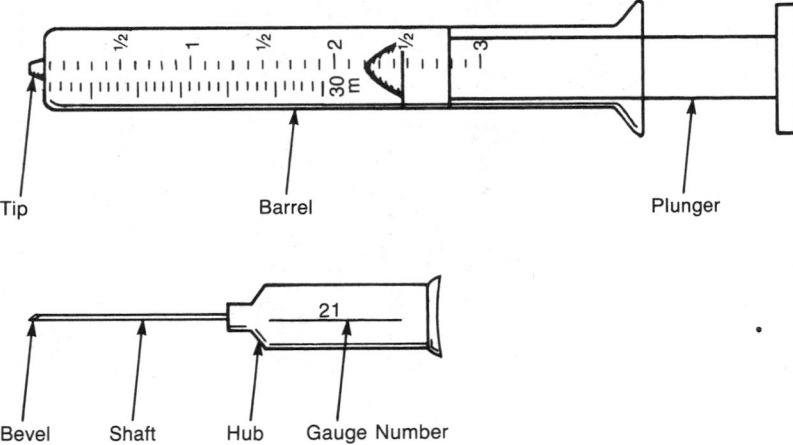

Figure 19-4.   Parts of a needle and syringe.

the tablet can be broken equally to give a partial dose. If the tablet is not scored, it should not be divided since an accurate measurement is not possible.

When a liquid medication is prepared, the bottle must be thoroughly shaken or rotated in order to assure that the medication is uniformly distributed in the liquid. When the bottle is opened, the cover is placed on the counter with the inside facing up to avoid contamination. The liquid is poured away from the label to avoid smudging the label and making it difficult to read should medication drip over the label. Liquid medications are poured into a single-dose, clear plastic measuring cup which has measurement markings. The nurse reads the measurement at eye level at the dip of the *meniscus* (fluid curve). Before the bottle is recapped, the outer rim of the bottle is wiped with a clean paper towel. After administering a small dose of a liquid medication to a patient, the nurse may rinse out the medication cup with a small amount of water and ask this patient to take this also. This assures that the patient receives the full dose of the medication.

The nurse assists the patient to take the medication, pouring fresh water and helping the patient to a comfortable position. The nurse stays with the patient until the medication is taken. Medication is not left at the the bedside of the patient. This protects other patients from taking the drug in error and assures the nurse that all prescribed medications were taken. Nursing Skill 19-1 gives one method of administering oral medications.

Administration of Parenteral Medications

Parenteral medications are those administered by a route other than the alimentary canal (the digestive tube from the mouth to the anus). Parenteral injections are medications administered through a needle. The most

frequent parenteral routes are *intramuscular* injections (medications are put into a muscle), *subcutaneous* injections (medications are deposited into subcutaneous tissue), *intravenous* (medications are placed into the vein). All of these routes have the advantage of more rapid absorption than the oral route. The disadvantage is that they are irretrievable once given, and because they are so rapidly absorbed, considerable damage can be done in a brief period by a drug given in error. Because the skin is broken in each of these routes, there is also some risk of infection. For this reason, all parenteral medications are prepared and administered by sterile technique.

Equipment.   Most of the parenteral equipment used today in health care facilities is disposable and individually packaged for single use. Although this is an added

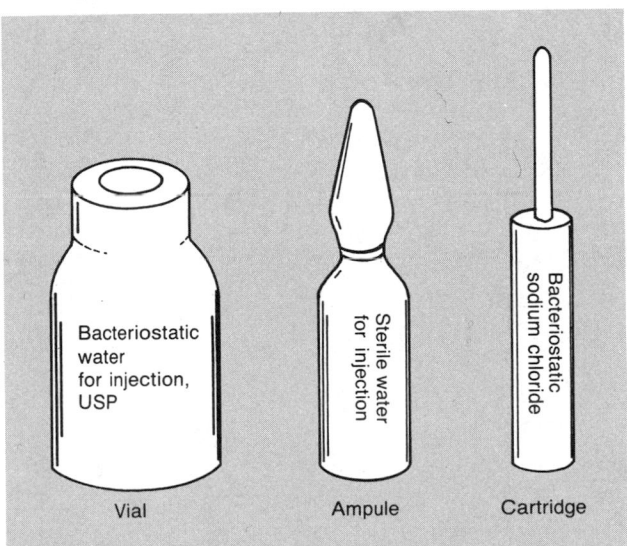

Figure 19-5.   Containers for parenteral medications.

cost to the patient, it increases biological safety. Patient comfort is also increased since needles are not dulled from multiple use and resterilization. Syringes are available in sizes which range from 1 to 50 cc. Most syringes are callibrated in units of minims (m, approximately equal to a drop) and/or milliliters (ml). Special syringes are available for the preparation of insulin. These are calibrated in units that correspond to the type of insulin being used. A 1-cc syringe is also available with calibrations down to 1/16 of a minim or hundredths of a milliliter. This is used primarily for tuberculosis testing or when extremely precise measurements are required. Figure 19–4 illustrates the individual parts of a syringe and needle.

Needles are numbered according to the size of the lu-

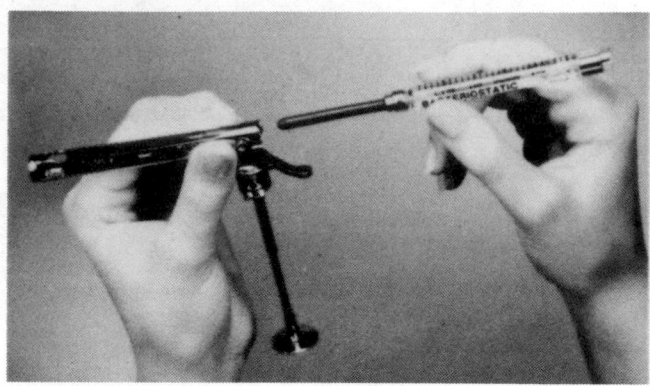

Figure 19–6. A prepackaged cartridge of medication is inserted into a syringe-type holder. After administration, the cartridge is discarded. (Courtesy of Wyeth Laboratories, Philadelphia.)

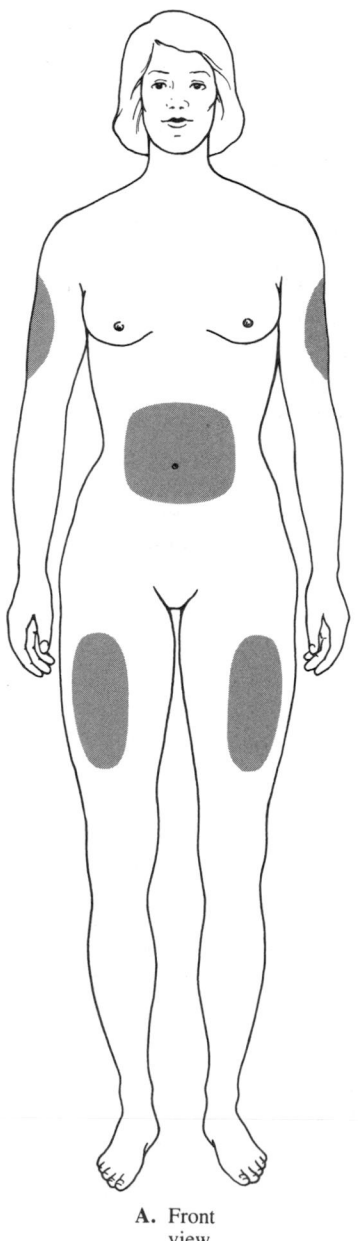

A. Front view

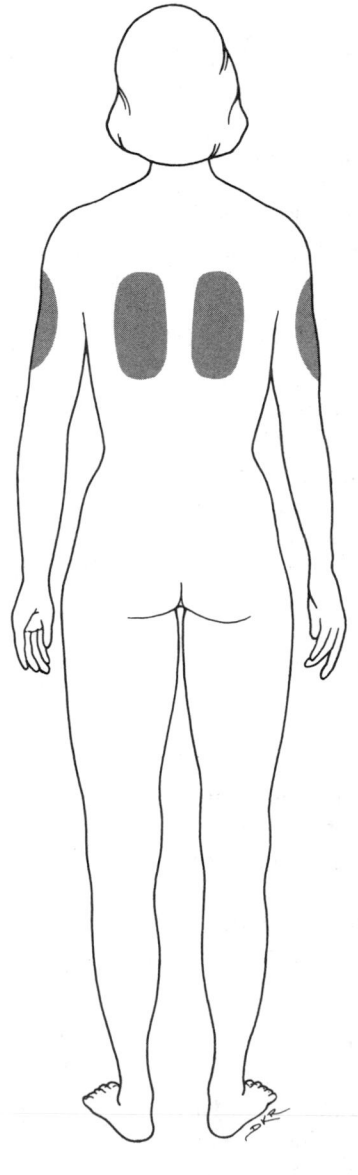

B. Back view

Figure 19–7. Subcutaneous injection sites.

men. This is called the gauge of the needle. The larger the number, the smaller is the lumen of the needle. A large lumen (example, 18 or 20 gauge) is required for the administration of thick viscous medications, while an aqueous (water-based) solution may be administered with a small-lumen needle (example, 26 gauge). Needles also range in length of the shaft from ¼ inch to 5 inches or more. The length of the shaft is selected according to the route of administration with consideration of the size of the patient. A ⅜-inch needle is generally sufficient for a subcutaneous injection, but if the patient is obese, a 1-inch or larger needle may be required.

A vial is a glass bottle covered with a rubber seal which can be penetrated by a needle. (See Figure 19-5.) Vials may contain either single or multiple doses of a medication. The nurse who opens a multiple-dose vial labels it with the date it was opened in order that it can be discarded when it is no longer safe for patient use. The length of time a vial may be stored and used is determined by both the nature of the drug and institutional policy.

An ampule is a glass bottle containing a single dose of a medication. The neck of the bottle is scored so it is easily snapped off with quick pressure. The medication is then withdrawn with a needle and syringe.

A cartridge is a prepackaged dose of medication contained in a glass or plastic unit with a needle attached. The cartridge is then inserted into a syringe-type holder. After administration, the cartridge is discarded, but the holder is retained for multiple use. (See Figure 19-6.)

Subcutaneous Injections. This route of drug administration permits rapid absorption of the drug. Since there are many alternative subcutaneous *sites* (places on the body where injections can be safely given), medication can be given via this route for extended periods of time, as in the case of insulin administration. Figure 19-7 illustrates common subcutaneous injection sites. The nurse is careful to select a site for the injection that has adequate circulation and is not damaged by previous injections or scar tissue. Nursing Skill 19-2 presents a method of administering subcutaneous injections.

SPECIAL CONSIDERATIONS FOR GIVING INSULIN. Insulin is a medication which diabetic patients frequently administer subcutaneously to themselves. Because this medication is taken daily, the sites must be rotated in order to prevent damage to the tissue from repeated use of the same site. Figure 19-8 shows common sites for injection of insulin. The numbers on the site indicate a suggested order in which the sites are used. Thus, the nurse who has given a patient insulin would indicate that on that date it was given in site 22. When the patient is hospitalized and the nurse is administering the insulin, the nurse may select sites that the patient is unable to use, in

order to rest the other sites if this is agreeable to the patient.

Insulin comes in concentrations U-40 and U-100. The terms refer to the number of units per milliliter. Thus, U-40 insulin contains 40 units per milliliter. Each type of insulin must be given in the corresponding type of syringe. To use the wrong syringe would result in an error in the dosage. For example, if the patient were to receive U-100 insulin and the nurse administered it in a U-40 syringe, an overdose would result. Similarly, insufficient dosages may also result if undersized syringes are used. U-100 insulin is gradually replacing other concentrations as the single standard type.

Some patients receive what is referred to as a "mixed" dose of insulin. This means that two types of insulin, usually one fast acting and one slow or interme-

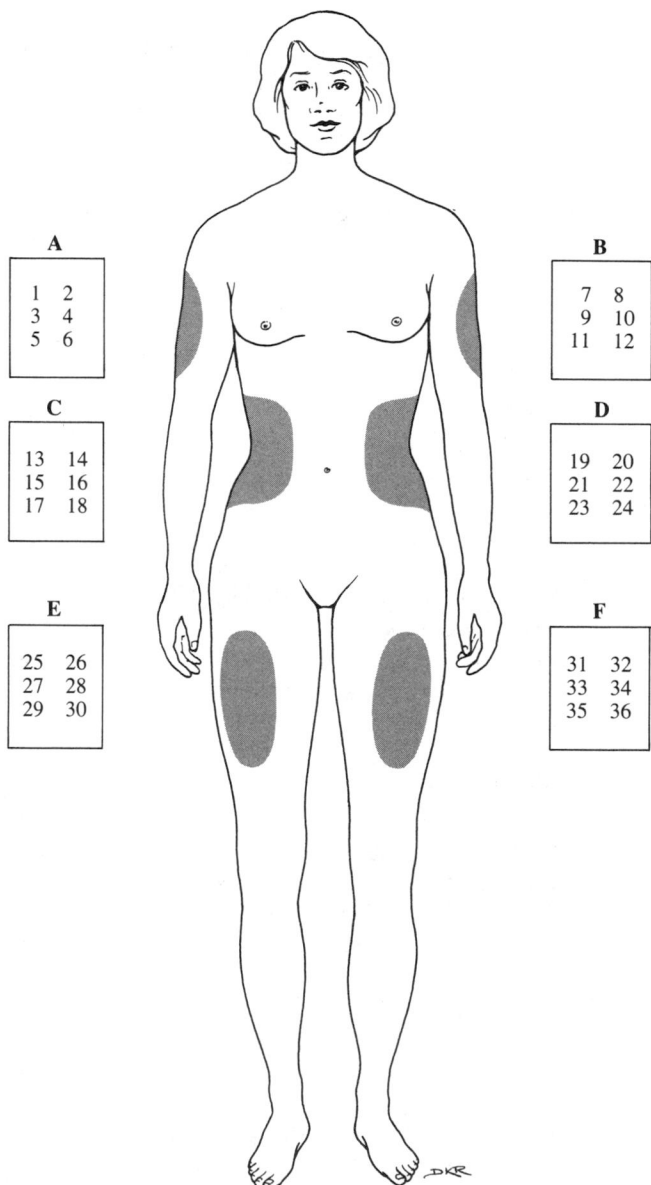

Figure 19-8. Injection sites for insulin administration.

Nursing Skill 19–2.   The Administration of Medications: Subcutaneous Route or Intramuscular Route

Supplies
Alcohol swabs
Select correct needle size
- For subcutaneous: usually ⅝ inch, 25 guage
- For intramuscular—deltoid site: ⅝ to 1 inch long, 23–25 gauge
- Large muscle sites: 1½ to 3 inches long, 20–23 gauge

Select correct syringe size
- For subcutaneous: usually 1 ml
- For intramuscular: usually 2–5 ml, depending upon the amount of the medication

Medication tray if used in the area

Preparation
Verify the accuracy of the medication order by checking it against the medication Kardex, or against the original order, or on the unit dose sheet. Wash hands and clean the medication tray. This may be done with an alcohol wipe.

Procedure | Explanation

1. Read the medication as ordered and select the medication from the supply.

1. This is check #1.

2. Compare the label on the medication card (or unit dose sheet) to the label on the supply for:
a. Right patient
b. Right medication
c. Right dose
d. Right route
e. Right time

2. This is check #2.

3. Assemble the syringe using sterile technique.

3. The needle will penetrate the skin, thus opening the tissue to possible infection. Sterile technique reduces the transfer of microorganisms.

4. Draw up the medication into the syringe.
a. From an ampule: Tap the tip of the ampule to drain the neck of the bottle into the base. Cover the neck of the ampule with an alcohol wipe and, holding the base of the ampule in one hand, snap the neck of the ampule by breaking it with the thumb and index finger in a direction away from the nurse. A special needle with a filter may be used in some institutions to prevent drawing up glass particles with the solution. This needle is then removed and the injection needle is attached. Insert the needle into the medication and draw up the medication.

4.
a. Protects the hands of the nurse.

b. Vial: Cleanse the cover of the bottle with an alcohol wipe. Draw up an amount of air into the syringe which is equal to the amount of medication to be withdrawn.
Place the needle into the vial and inject the air. Withdraw the required amount of medication.

b. A multiple-dose vial is cleaned before each use in order to decrease the transfer of microorganisms. Injecting air creates a positive pressure on the inside of the container, making it possible to withdraw the dose. If this was not done, a vacuum would be created inside the container, making it difficult to withdraw the medication.

c. Cartridge: Secure the cartridge of medication in the syringe holder.

5. Holding the syringe upright, tap any air bubbles to the surface of the medication. Expel any excess air or medication. Check the amount of medication in the syringe.

6. Pull back on the plunger of the syringe to create small air bubble. Place sterile needle cover over the needle.

7. Compare supply and medication card or unit dose sheet for 2, a–e, as above.

8. Sign out any controlled substances as required.

9. Identify the patient by
   a. Asking the patient's name
   b. Comparing the patient's identification band to the medication card or unit dose sheet.

10. Provide for the patient's privacy and assist the patient to a comfortable position for the injection.

11. Cleanse the injection site with an alcohol wipe by
    a. Wiping in a downward direction with one stroke, or
    b. Wiping in a circular motion from the center to the outside.
    Permit the skin to dry before injecting.

12. To hold the skin:
    a. For a subcutaneous injection: The nurse may either spread the skin with the nondominant hand or pinch a fold of the patient's skin. (Caution: spreading the skin on a very thin person could result in the medication being injected into the muscle.)

    b. For an intramuscular injection: With the nondominant hand, the nurse spreads the skin taut at the site.

13. With the dominant hand, the nurse inserts the needle:
    a. For a subcutaneous injection: At a 45-degree angle or a 90-degree angle to the skin with a rapid motion.

    b. For an intramuscular injection: At a 90-degree angle to the skin with a rapid motion.

14. The nurse pulls back on the plunger (*aspirates*). If there is no blood return, the medication is slowly injected.
    Caution: Do not aspirate heparin, as this could cause tissue damage.

15. Placing an alcohol swab over the site and applying slight pressure, the nurse withdraws the needle.
    The site may then be massaged if required.

5. Eliminating the air bubble helps the nurse to check the accuracy of the dose.

6. The injection of the air bubble helps to clear the shaft of the needle of medication and assures that the patient receives the full dose. It also serves to seal the medication in the tissue. Maintains sterility of the needle.

7. This is check #3.

8. Required by Federal Controlled Substance Act.

9. Provides for correct identification of the patient.

10. The position will depend upon which site is selected for the injection.

11. This method decreases the transfer of microorganisms.

Liquid alcohol is not introduced into the injection site since it burns.

12.
    a. Spreading the skin makes it firmer and easier to insert the needle, while pinching may decrease the sensation of pain.

    b. This makes the skin easier to enter and ensures the needle will reach the muscle.

13.
    a. Either injection angle is acceptable, although a 90-degree angle is recommended when there is more adipose tissue.
    A rapid motion lessens the sensation of pain.

14. The nurse aspirates in an attempt to determine if the needle is in a blood vessel. If blood returns, the nurse may either withdraw the needle slightly and check again, or withdraw completely and begin again if there is a large amount of blood returned. This is a safety check to prevent the injection of medication directly into blood vessels.

15. Slight pressure helps to seal the site.

Procedure	Explanation
Caution: Do not massage heparin. This could rupture small blood vessels and cause damage. *Do not* massage insulin.	Massage helps to distribute the medication in the tissue.
16. Assist the patient to a comfortable position.	16. Demonstrates concern for the patient and provides physical comfort.
17. Document the administration of the medication on the patient's record including: a. Drug b. Dose, route, and site c. Time and date d. Signature of the nurse and title e. Any response to the medication	17. Legal responsibility.
18. Dispose of equipment as directed by institutional policy.	18. Contaminated needles are a source of infection.

Nursing Skill 19–3. **Preparing a Mixed Dose of Insulin**

Supplies
    Alcohol swabs
    Insulin syringe with correct markings for ordered type of insulin
    Medication tray

Preparation
    Same as for any subcutaneous injection. (See Nursing Skill 19–2.)

Procedure	Explanation
1.–3. Steps 1–3 same as 1–3 of Nursing Skill 19–2.	**1.–3.** Insulin is administered by subcutaneous injection.
4. Cleanse the top of each vial, using a new alcohol wipe for each vial.	**4.** Drawing up parenteral medications is a sterile procedure. This reduces the transfer of microorganisms.
5. Draw up an amount of air equal to the longer acting insulin and inject it into the vial of longer acting insulin. This is done with the vial in an upright position.	**5.** This creates a positive pressure which makes it possible to withdraw medication. This is done at this point in the procedure since later there will be regular insulin in the syringe and to do so then would risk contamination. Holding the bottle upright prevents contamination of the needle with medication.
6. With the same syringe, draw up an amount of air equal to the amount of regular insulin ordered and inject it into the bottle of regular or fast-acting insulin. Invert the bottle and withdraw the required amount of regular or fast-acting insulin. Before removing the needle, tap out any air bubbles that may be in the syringe, and withdraw additional medication as necessary to make the required dose.	**6.** This creates a positive pressure making it possible to withdraw a medication. The fast-acting insulin is withdrawn first to avoid any contamination with long-acting insulin. Assures accurate dose.
7. Insert the needle into the longer acting insulin and withdraw the required amount. Cover the needle with the protective cap.	**7.** Air has previously been injected into the vial so the insulin can be readily withdrawn. Maintain sterility of the needle.
8. If institutional policy requires that nurses check mixed doses of insulin, this check should be made after steps 6 and 7.	

The nurse may now proceed as with Nursing Skill 19–2 for subcutaneous injection.

diate acting, are mixed in the same syringe. In this manner, the patient need only receive one injection. It is important that a mixed dose be drawn up out of multiple dose vials without contaminating the rapid-acting insulin with intermediate- or slow-acting insulin. Nursing Skill 19-3 gives instructions for drawing up a mixed dose of insulin. After injecting insulin, the nurse does not massage the site. With that exception, the procedure for administering insulin follows Nursing Skill 19-2.

SPECIAL PRECAUTIONS FOR GIVING HEPARIN. Heparin is an anticoagulant, a medication that inhibits blood clotting. It may be given subcutaneously or by other routes. It is also important to remember that when administering heparin, the nurse does not aspirate the syringe before injecting the medication or massage the site after injection. Both of these actions could result in tissue damage. A ½-inch needle is used, and the skin is pinched prior to inserting the needle at a 90-degree angle into the fold. The remainder of the procedure is the same as that in Nursing Skill 19-2.

Heparin is injected subcutaneously into an abdominal site above the level of the anterior iliac spine, but below the navel. The area covered by a belt is not used to avoid tissue irritation.

Intramuscular Injections. Medications injected into the muscle are absorbed more rapidly than subcutaneous injections. Large doses of medications (up to 5 ml) can be administered by this route. It is also possible to give medications intramuscularly that do not come as oral preparations because they are irritating to the gastric mucosa. The chief disadvantage is the damage to

nerves, tissue, or blood vessels which may result. These risks are minimized by the skill and knowledge of the nurse.

SITES FOR INTRAMUSCULAR INJECTIONS. There are four primary sites, as illustrated by Figures 19-9 to 19-12, for intramuscular injections. The site chosen depends upon several factors:

1. Condition of the muscle. If the patient has already received multiple injections in a site and hard masses can be felt upon palpation, the nurse selects an alternate site.

2. The volume of the medication. The deltoid site is a small muscle suitable for injecting small amounts, whereas the dorsogluteal site can absorb up to 5 ml (though it is recommended to split a dose this large).

3. The type of the medication. Iron preparations are usually administered only into the dorsogluteal sites.

4. Patient preference. If there are no medical reasons to deny it, the patient's preference is considered.

There are clear anatomical landmarks for locating safe injection sites. The location of the site requires knowledge of anatomy and practice. It is somewhat easier to find the landmarks on persons of normal weight, but it is necessary to be able to locate them on obese individuals also. The injection site will determine the position of the patient during the administration of the injection. The nurse does not administer intramuscular injections to a patient in a standing position because patients may faint or become weak during the injection, creating a safety hazard.

The *deltoid* site is not often used because it is a small muscle and is in close proximity to the radial nerve. The

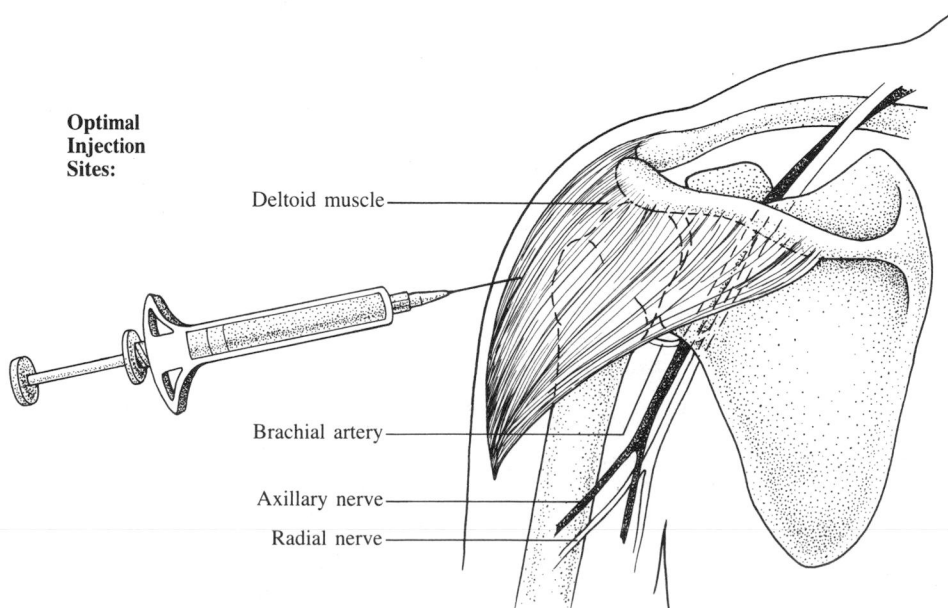

Optimal
Injection
Sites:

Deltoid muscle

Brachial artery

Axillary nerve

Radial nerve

Figure 19-9. Deltoid intramuscular injection site. (Courtesy of Winthrop-Breon Laboratories, New York.)

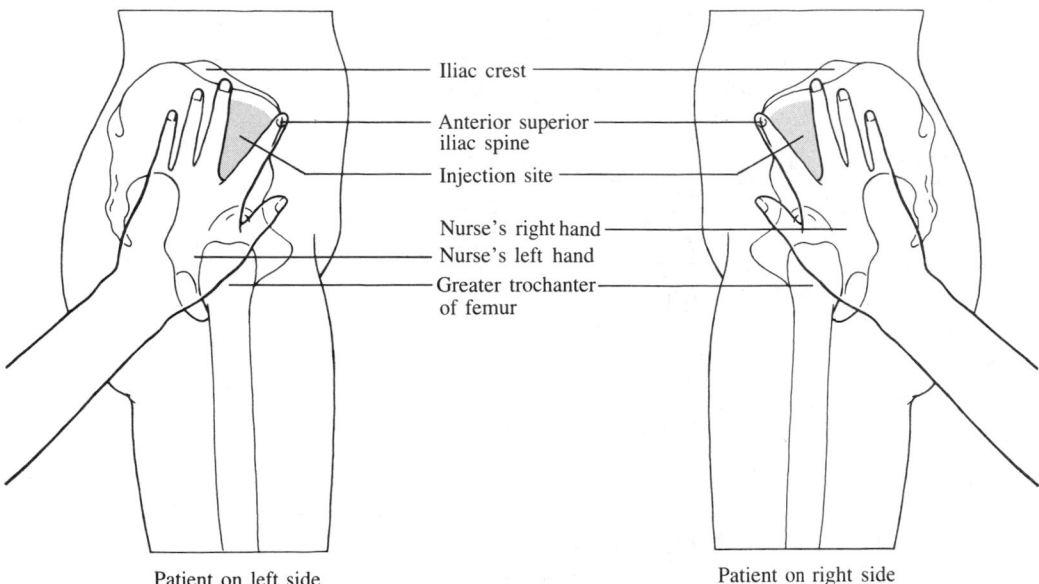

Iliac crest

Anterior superior
iliac spine

Injection site

Nurse's right hand
Nurse's left hand
Greater trochanter
of femur

Patient on left side

Patient on right side

Figure 19–10.   Ventrogluteal intramuscular injection site.

deltoid site is located on the outer (lateral) aspect of the arm, with the top boundary approximately two finger-widths beneath the acromial process, and the midpoint at a level with the axilla. The patient receiving an injection in this site may be either sitting or lying. (See Figure 19–9.)

The *ventrogluteal* site is a very desirable site for IM injections because it is free of large nerves and blood vessels and has less fat tissue than the buttocks. It is located (on the patient's right side) by placing the left hand of the nurse with the palm on the head of the trochanter. The index finger is placed on the anterior superior iliac spine. The second finger then traces the curve of the iliac crest up forming a V. The injection site is in the gluteus medius and gluteus minimus muscle which is located within the V formed by the first and second fin-

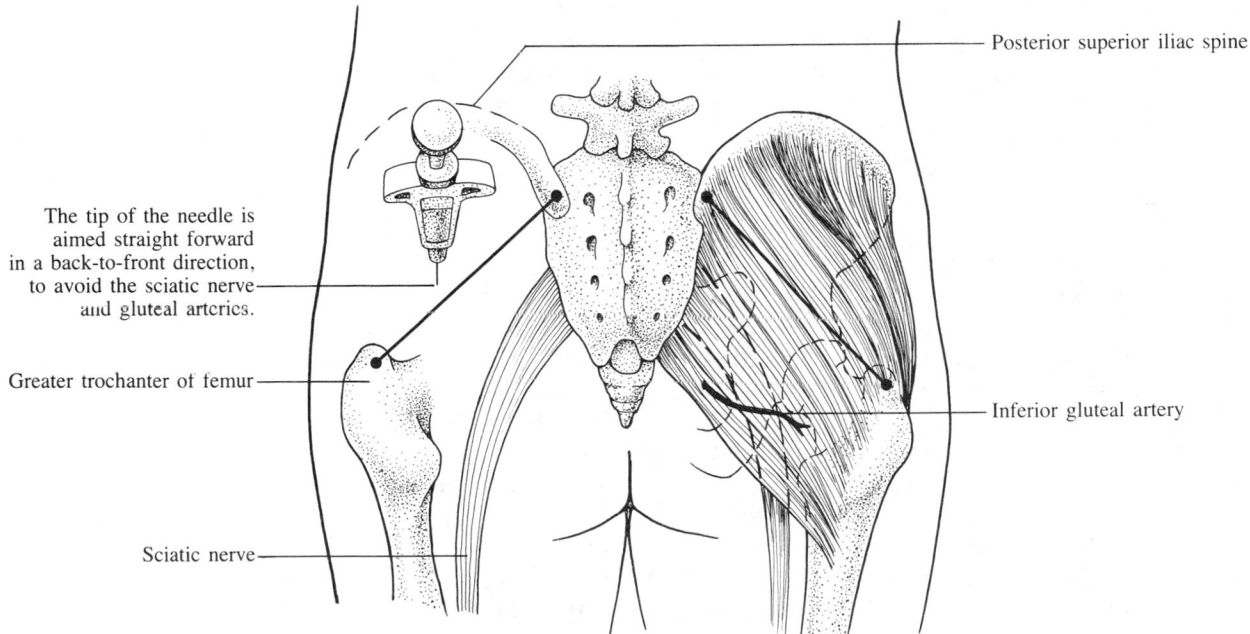

Posterior superior iliac spine

The tip of the needle is
aimed straight forward
in a back-to-front direction,
to avoid the sciatic nerve
and gluteal arteries.

Greater trochanter of femur

Inferior gluteal artery

Sciatic nerve

Figure 19–11.   Dorsogluteal intramuscular injection site. (Courtesy of Winthrop-Breon Laboratories, New York.)

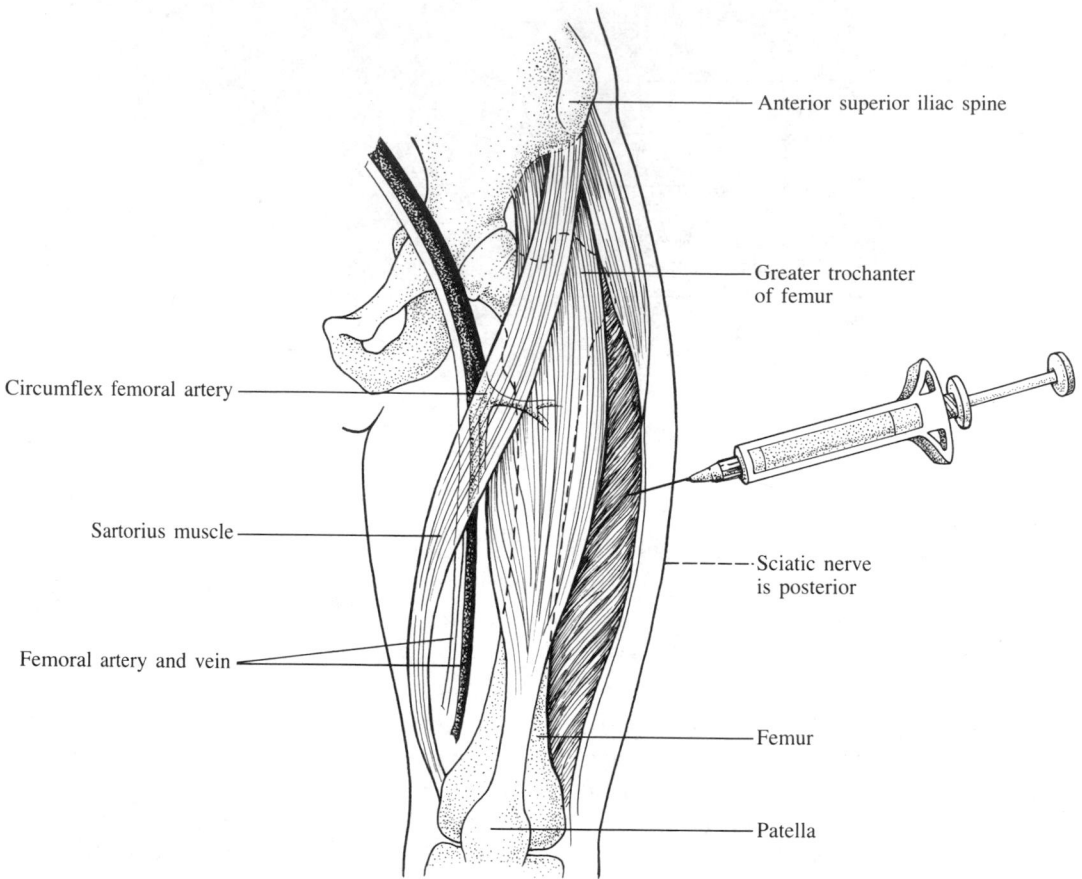

Anterior superior iliac spine

Greater trochanter of femur

Circumflex femoral artery

Sartorius muscle

Femoral artery and vein

Sciatic nerve is posterior

Femur

Patella

Figure 19–12. Vastus lateralis intramuscular injection site. (Courtesy of Winthrop-Breon Laboratories, New York.)

gers. A patient receiving an injection in this site is positioned on the back or side. (See Figure 19–10.)

The *dorsogluteal* site is acceptable for adults but is not recommended for children who can not yet walk since their muscle mass is not large enough. The large gluteus maximus muscle makes this a good site, although it is near to the sciatic nerve, large blood vessels, and bone. The site is identified by palpating the posterior superior iliac spine with one hand and the greater trochanter with the other. An imaginary line is drawn connecting these two landmarks. The imaginary line is above but parallel to the sciatic nerve, a large nerve which is to be avoided in giving injections. The injection may safely be given lateral to the line and approximately 2 inches below the iliac crest. Patients receiving injections in this site are positioned prone (on their stomach), with the toes pointed inward, or on their side.

The *vastus lateralis* site is used for infants, children, and adults. It is a safe site because there are no major blood vessels or nerves nearby. It is located on the anterior lateral aspect of the thigh. The site is identified by dividing the area between the knee and the greater trochanter into thirds. The injection is given in the lateral

aspect of the middle third. The patient receiving this injection may be in a sitting or lying position. (See Figure 19–12.)

Nursing Skill 19–2 is a procedure for administering intramuscular injections.

THE Z-TRACK METHOD OF INTRAMUSCULAR INJECTION. This variation of an intramuscular injection is used to administer drugs that are irritating to the skin and subcutaneous tissues. The parenteral administration of iron requires this technique. The nurse draws up the medication in the syringe using the same procedure as in Nursing Skill 19–2. After the correct amount of medication and an air bubble of 0.3 cc to 0.5 cc have been drawn up, the nurse replaces the needle used to draw up the medication with a new sterile needle. This is done in order to protect the skin from any medication on the needle. The site used for this medication is the large dorsogluteal site. To administer the medication, the nurse identifies the site, cleanses the site, and retracts the skin laterally (approximately 1 to 2 inches) away from the intended site. This assures entry of the needle into the muscle. The medication is then slowly injected into the site. After the medication is injected,

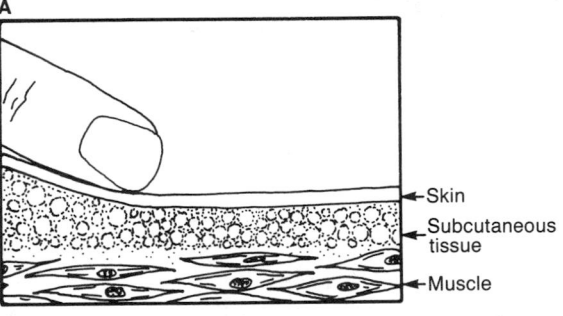

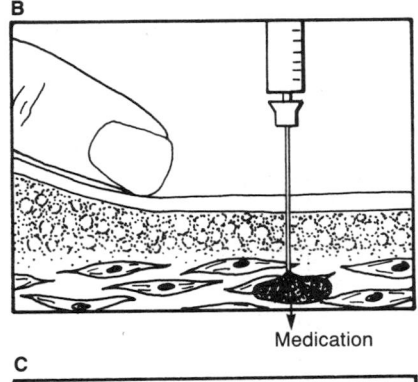

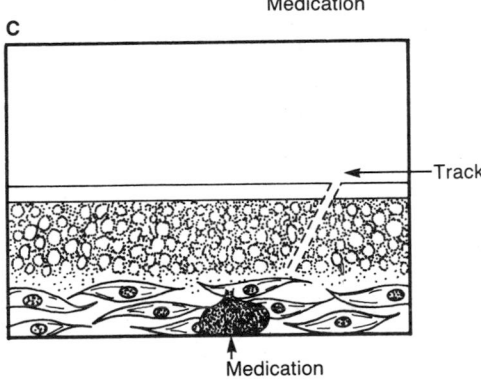

Figure 19-13. Adminstration of medication using Z-track technique. **A.** The nurse retracts the skin laterally. **B.** The nurse injects the medication and maintains the retraction for 10 seconds. **C.** The needle is withdrawn, and the skin; is released.

with the needle still in place, the nurse maintains the retraction for 10 seconds to prevent the medication from leaking into the tissue. The needle is then withdrawn and the skin released. This injection is not massaged for to do so would cause irritation to the tissue. Figure 19-13 illustrates the Z-track method.

Intravenous Administration of Medication. The major advantage of administering medications by the intravenous (IV) route is the rapid speed of absorption. In this route, the medications are injected directly into the bloodstream. This is especially important in an emergency situation where the patient requires immediate medications. When repeated doses of parenteral medi-

cations are required, this system also eliminates the pain of repeated injections for the patient. A disadvantage of this route is that a drug injected in error is effective immediately. Similarly, if a patient has an allergic reaction to the drug, the effect is immediate and full blown. For this reason small test doses may be given to check for reactions. There is also the potential of infection since each administration breaks the body defense of the intact skin. Each of these disadvantages can be minimized by appropriate nursing actions. The nurse administers all intravenous drugs slowly and repeatedly assesses the patient's responses. Sterile technique is used throughout the preparation and administration of intravenous medications in order to reduce the risk of infection.

Intravenous medications can be administered diluted in a bag or bottle in the patient's IV fluids, by adding a secondary container of medication or "piggyback" set-up, or by direct injection into the vein (called *bolus* or IV push). The same principles of medication administration apply to this route as were described for other parenteral medications with slight modifications. The site of administration is now changed, and additional safety precautions are taken. If required by hospital policy, the nurse checks all dosages of bolus intravenous medications with a second nurse. The student administering an intravenous drug is supervised by a nursing instructor throughout preparation and administration. Intravenous drugs are not mixed unless the nurse consults with a pharmacist regarding any potential drug incompatibility. The nurse may also have questions about the rate since the administration of IV medications may be different than that of IV fluids. These questions can be resolved using a reference text or consulting the hospital pharmacist, charge nurse, or nursing instructor. Other questions are referred to the physician as with any other medication.

ADDING MEDICATION TO AN IV BOTTLE OR BAG. In this method, the patient already has an IV infusion in place, and the nurse is required to add medications to an existing or new bottle or bag of fluid. This method dilutes the concentration of the medication. The medication order will specify the amount of the medication, the amount and type of fluid into which the medication is added, and the time over which it is to be administered. Using Nursing Skill 19-2 as a guide, the nurse draws up the required medication. At this point, the nurse or student nurse checks the medication with a registered nurse or nursing instructor, if this is required by hospital or school policy.

To insert the medication into a bottle of intravenous fluid, the nurse first correctly identifies both the IV fluid and the medication, using the five rights of medication administration. Then the nurse removes the metal cover from the IV bottle and the latex seal, cleanses the rubber stopper with an alcohol wipe, and injects the medication into the bottle using the larger hole of the two holes in the cover. (The second hole is an air vent.) If this is a vacuum bottle, the medication will be drawn into the bottle by the vacuum. If the nurse is to insert the medication into an already hanging IV bottle, the nurse must first be sure that there is sufficient fluid remaining to dilute the medication. Then the nurse closes the flow regulator. This is essential since failure to do so would result in giving the drug undiluted. After cleansing the rubber stopper covering the bottle, the nurse administers the medication through the triangular marked area or the injection port which is marked by the word "add." Each bottle is now gently rotated to mix the medication. The flow regulator is then opened and the rate adjusted. The bottle is labeled with the name and dose of the medication, and markings to indicate amount of flow per hour or other time unit, and the signature of the nurse. Drugs may be added to bags of intravenous fluid in the same manner. Bags of fluid have a medication port, a special rubber-stoppered point of entry to the contents. It is located on the front of the bag. If the bag is already hanging, the nurse turns off the flow regulator and injects the medication into the port. The bag is rotated to mix the medication. The nurse then proceeds to hang the bottle or bag as in Nursing Skill 23–2. The rate of flow is then regulated. (See Nursing Skill 23–1). The entire procedure is then documented, usually both on the medication record and on the parenteral fluid administration record.

USING ADDITIVE SETS TO ADMINISTER INTRAVENOUS MEDICATIONS. There are many variations of intravenous tubing that enable the nurse to administer IV medication while leaving an existing IV bottle in place. One such method is called "piggyback." Medication is prepared in IV solution according to the procedure described above. The nurse next inserts the special piggyback IV tubing into the prepared bottle and, uncovering the needle at the end of the tubing, fills the tubing with fluid as with any other IV set-up. (See Nursing Skill 23–2.) The needle is recovered to maintain sterility. The bottle is then labeled. After correct identification of the patient, the nurse cleanses the piggyback port on the primary IV tubing which the patient has infusing. The needle on the piggyback line is then inserted into the tubing and secured with tape. If using an extending hanger, the existing primary bottle is lowered on the IV pole, and the piggyback bottle is hung in the regular manner so it is higher than the other bottle. The rate of flow of the piggyback is then regulated. When the piggyback is completed, the primary bottle will begin to flow due to the presence of a valve in the piggyback tubing. However, at the completion of the piggyback, the primary bottle is returned to its normal position and the flow

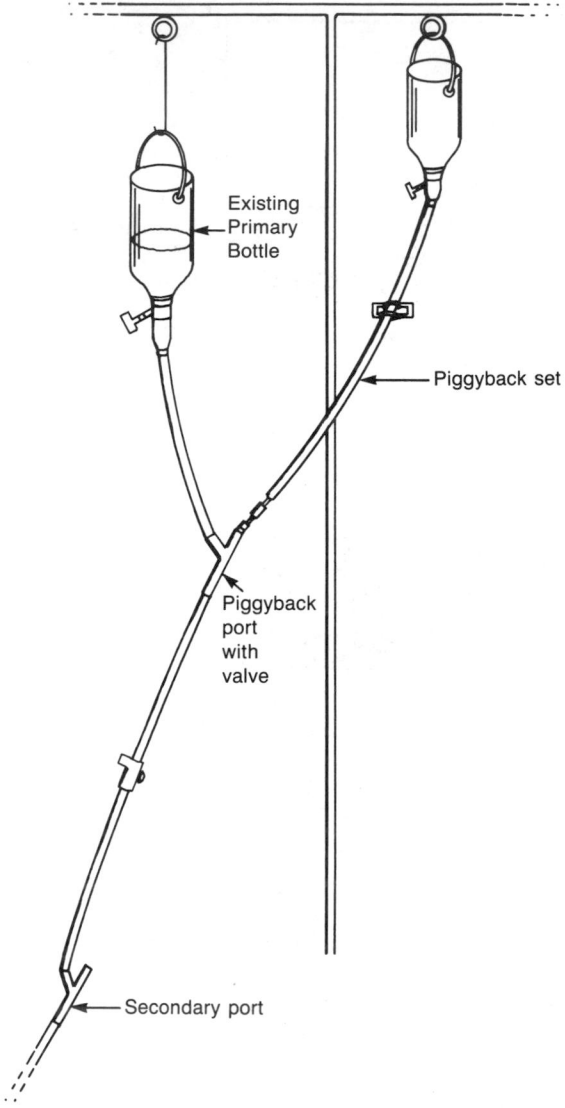

Figure 19–14. Piggyback administration of IV medication.

rate regulated. (See Figure 19–14.) The procedure is then documented.

Another method of IV medication administration is the use of a volume control device. (See Figure 19–15.) This consists of a small chamber connected to the primary line IV tubing via a port site. The chamber may be filled with any amount of fluid prescribed. The medication is then added to the chamber. This system has the advantage of enabling the nurse to dilute IV medication precisely in a small amount of fluid.

INTRAVENOUS ADMINISTRATION BY IV BOLUS. The bolus method is also known as IV push. It refers to the administration of a drug directly into a vein. Medications administered in this way are not diluted. This method is used in emergencies to achieve the most rapid effect. It is also used to achieve the maximum level in the patient's blood. It can also be used to avoid the trauma of repeated injections. Medications to be administered by this route are drawn up in the same manner as any parenteral medication. It is especially important that the nurse recheck the accuracy of the preparation with a registered nurse if this is institutional policy. If there is no IV existing, the nurse must complete a venipuncture prior to injecting the drug. (The skill of venipuncture is considered beyond the fundamental level of nursing, and students are referred to medical-surgical nursing texts for this procedure.) If there is an existing IV line, the nurse first closes the clamp to turn off the primary line to prevent the medication from flowing up into the tubing. The nurse then cleanses the port with an antiseptic swab. The needle is inserted into the port. The nurse then aspirates to assure that the needle is in the blood vessel. The nurse then injects the medication at

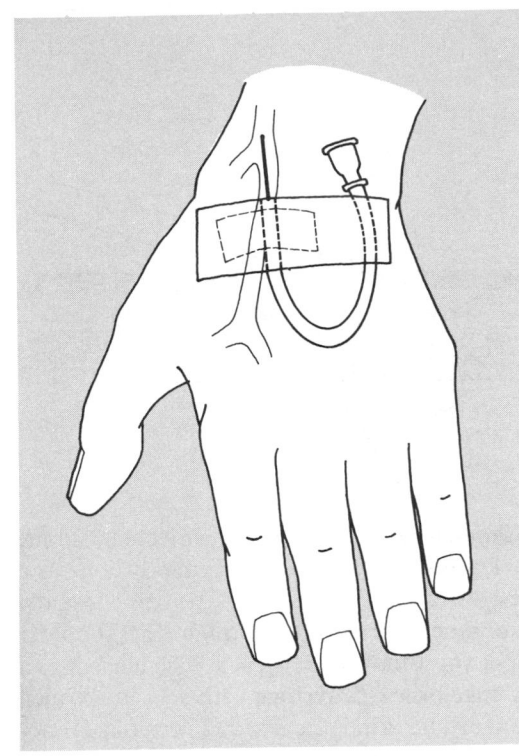

Figure 19-16. A heparin lock is used for intermittent infusion of IV medications.

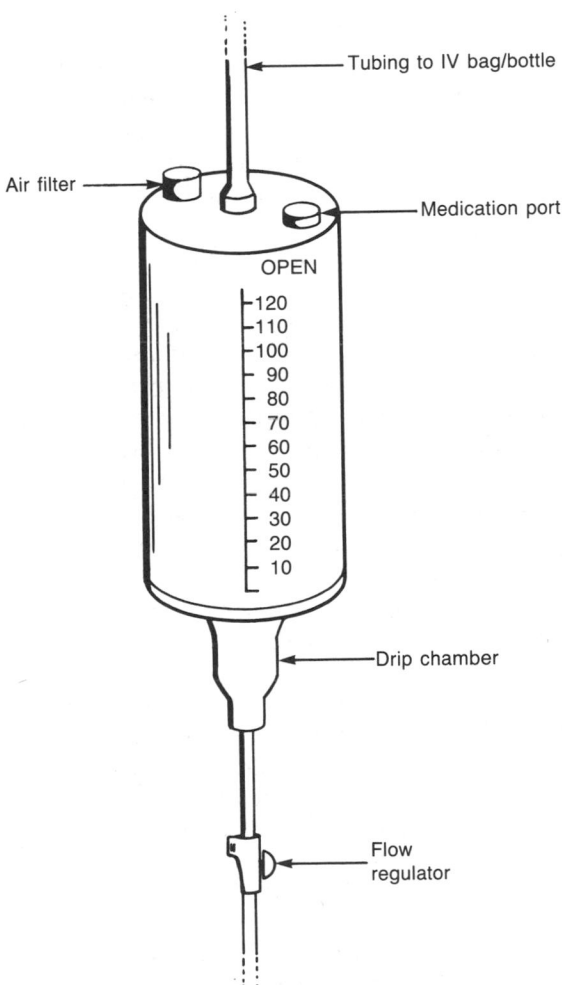

Figure 19-15. A volume control device is used to dilute medication in small amounts of fluid.

the prescribed rate. When this is completed, the needle is withdrawn, and the regulator on the primary bottle is reopened. The rate of flow of the primary bottle must then be regulated. Documentation is then completed.

The nurse can also administer an IV bolus through an intermittent infusion set (also called a heparin lock or INT needle, see Figure 19-16). The heparin lock consists of a needle secured in place, tubing, and a port. This method is used for patients who require frequent IV drug administration without the volume of IV solution. It also permits maximum mobility for the patient. The nurse prepares the IV medication as above. The port is then cleansed, and the nurse inserts the needle into the port. The nurse aspirates to assure that the needle is in place in the blood vessel. The medication is then injected at the prescribed rate. After the injection is complete, the needle is removed, and the port is again cleansed. The nurse then injects 1 ml of *heparin flush* (a solution of 100 units of herparin per milliliter of sterile normal saline) into the port. This will keep the system free of clots. Institutional policies vary regarding this procedure. Some agencies heparinize before and after the medication is injected. Some flush the system with saline after the medication is injected but prior to heparinizing. The nurse follows the procedure of the institution and then completes documentation. (See Figure 19-16.)

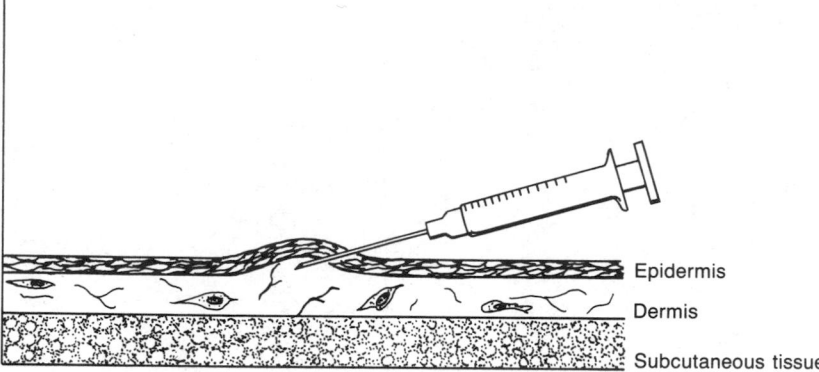

Figure 19-17. Medication is inserted under the epidermis in an intradermal injection.

Intradermal Injections. This form of injection is done primarily in skin testing. It is most frequently done as a tuberculin test or for allergy testing. The test is usually given on the inner forearm, although the shoulder blades or upper chest may also be used. The nurse uses a tuberculin syringe or a 1-cc syringe with a ¼- to ⅝-inch needle, 26 gauge. The skin is cleansed. The syringe is positioned almost flat (about a 15-degree angle) against the skin with the bevel of the needle up. (See Figure 19–17.) The needle is inserted just below the surface of the skin. (Some nurses say this feels like lifting the skin to remove a splinter.) The medication is then injected, and a small raised welt (called a bleb) forms. The area is not massaged since this might spread the medication. The area is then assessed periodically as directed, depending on the medication injected. Tuberculin tests are read in 48 to 72 hours by measuring the hardened or reddened area and comparing it to control charts.

Administration of Medications via the Skin or Mucous Membranes

The skin and mucous membranes offer a safe and effective route for the administration of medications. Although absorption is slower than in parenteral routes, there are fewer side effects and allergic reactions than with other routes.

Sublingual Route. Medication given by the *sublingual* route is placed under the patient's tongue where it is absorbed by the blood vessels on the back of the tongue. The patient is instructed not to swallow the medication as a pill. Nitroglycerin (a drug used to relieve pain around the heart) is given by this route.

Buccal Route. *Buccal* medications are placed in the pocket between the patient's gums and cheek. The patient is instructed not to swallow the medication as a pill, but to let it slowly dissolve.

Topical Route. The *topical* route refers to the application of a medication directly to a specific body site where the drug exerts its effects.

DERMATOLOGIC PREPARATIONS. These substances are applied direclty to the skin. Powders are used to dry the skin and prevent chafing. Ointments are used to soften the skin, retain body heat, and increase the length of contact between the medication and the skin. Creams and lotions are used to lubricate, soothe, and soften the skin. Alcohol is used to cool and dry the skin. A paste is a thick compound of ointment and powder which evenly distributes the medication and acts to repel water.

Before applying any of these preparations, the nurse makes certain the skin is clean and dry. Any medication remaining from a previous application is removed, unless it is specifically ordered not to do so. Patients with unsightly skin conditions may feel a low sense of self-esteem and embarrassment. For this reason, the nurse makes a careful decision whether or not to wear gloves when applying these medications. The use of gloves may further enhance the patient's negative feelings. The nurse does wear gloves if the patient's condition is contagious, if the nurse is allergic to the medication, if a sterile procedure is required, or if the nurse's skin might absorb the medication. A brief explanation is made to the patient. The nurse is careful to maintain eye contact with the patient. Lotions are shaken before application to distribute the ingredients evenly. Medications are warmed, if possible, before application. This is done by holding them in the hands for a few moments before application.

Skin preparations are applied as directed. Some may be massaged into the skin, while others must be patted on without rubbing. Some require the cover of dressings or heat to enhance absorption.

OPHTHALMIC MEDICATIONS.   Before giving any ophthalmic (eye) preparation, the nurse carefully reads the label to make certain the medication is intended for ophthalmic use. If the label does not indicate this, it is not given. The patient's head is tilted back slightly, and the patient is requested to focus on an object on the ceiling. With an index finger, the nurse retracts the skin under the eye to expose the conjunctival sac. Medication is then placed into the lower edge of the sac, taking care not to touch the medication container to the eye. The nurse is also careful not to place the medication on the cornea, thus causing discomfort for the patient. The patient may then close the eye and move the eyeball (unless this is contraindicated) to distribute the medication. Any excess medication is wiped away with a clean tissue or a cotton ball with the patient's eye closed and wiping from the inner to the outer canthus. Eye ointment is squeezed along the lower ridge of the conjunctival sac in the same manner. Approximately ½ inch (about 2 cm) of medication is applied, rotating the tube to disconnect the ointment. The patient may be asked to keep the eye closed for a minute or two to enhance absorption of the medication. The patient may also move the eye to spread the medication, unless this is contraindicated.

OTIC MEDICATIONS.   Otic (ear) medications are given at room temperature to minimize discomfort. The external ear is cleansed with a cotton-tipped swab moistened with saline if necessary. The patient who is to receive eardrops is positioned lying on the unaffected side or sitting with the head tilted so the affected ear is uppermost. The nurse gently pulls the auricle of the ear upward and back in order to straighten the ear canal of an adult. (In a child, the auricle is pulled down and back.) The drops are then placed to the side of the ear canal without touching the ear with the dropper. The ear is then released. The patient is asked to remain in this position for 3 to 5 minutes to distribute the medication. A cotton ball is then loosely put in the ear to help in retaining the medication. The procedure may then be repeated for the other ear if ordered.

Occasionally, the nurse may be required to irrigate a patient's ears. This may be done to remove an accumulation of earwax. The nurse uses a warmed irrigating solution (hydrogen peroxide or saline as ordered) and a large irrigating syringe. The patient is in a sitting position and holds a basin under the ear to catch the returned solution. The nurse gently pulls the auricle up and back and, holding it in this position, directs the irrigating stream with gentle pressure toward the top of the ear canal. The returned solution is assessed and documented. The ear is cleansed and dried.

NASAL MEDICATION.   To receive nosedrops intended to relieve nasal congestion, the patient is seated upright with the head tilted back. If the medication is intended to relieve a sinus condition, the patient is positioned in a back-lying position with the head tilted straight back to treat the sphenoidal and ethmoidal sinuses; tiled to one side to treat the maxillary and frontal sinuses. The patient is instructed to breathe through the mouth. The nurse inserts the dropper about ⅓ inch inside the nares, avoiding touching the nares with the dropper in order to avoid contamination. The dropper is directed toward the midline of the superior concha of the ethmoid bone and the medication released. The patient is asked to remain in this position for a few minutes to enhance distribution of the medication. The patient is provided with tissue for any secretions.

VAGINAL MEDICATION.   Drugs to be inserted into the vagina may come as a suppository or as a cream, foam, or jelly in a prepackaged dose. Privacy is provided, and the patient is positioned on her back with the knees flexed and spread apart. The nurse opens the suppository or the applicator of the preparation and lubricates the tip, usually with a water-soluble jelly or plain water, in order to make insertion easier. This is then placed on the clean inside of its wrapper. The nurse then puts on clean gloves and spreads the labia to visualize the vaginal opening. If it is necessary to cleanse the area due to contamination from the anal area, this is done using forceps and cotton balls moistened in warm water. The nurse's glove on the dominant hand is still considered clean. The suppository is then inserted as far as it will go along the posterior wall of the vagina. An applicator is inserted toward the sacrum in a downward and backward path about 2 inches. The plunger is depressed and the applicator removed. The nurse removes gloves by pulling them off inside out to decrease the spread of microorganisms. The patient is asked to remain lying on her back, hips slightly elevated on a pillow to distribute the medication. A perineal pad may be applied for drainage.

RECTAL MEDICATIONS.   The rectal route can be used for medications which are irritating when given by other routes. It is also used when the patient is nauseated, unconscious, or unable to swallow. However, the absorption of the drug is uncertain so the nurse carefully assesses the patient's response. These medications are most frequently given in the form of a rectal suppository. Privacy is provided for the patient. The patient is in a side-lying position with the top leg flexed. The nurse puts on either a finger cot on the index finger or a clean glove. The nurse unwraps the suppository and lubricates the tip with a water-soluble jelly. With the ungloved hand, the nurse separates the patient's buttocks in order to visualize the patient's anus. The patient is instructed to take a deep breath while the nurse inserts the suppository, narrow end first, using the index finger to direct it against the rectal wall. The suppository must be inserted approximately the length of the index finger so it is beyond the internal anal sphicter. The glove or finger cot is removed by turning it inside out to contain the microorganisms. The patient is then told to squeeze the buttocks together or the nurse may press the buttocks together to reduce the urge to expel the suppository. The patient holds the suppository for a time, which depends on the type of medication administered, usually 15 to 20 minutes. If the suppository was administered to relieve gas, the patient may expel it at any time.

INHALATION MEDICATIONS. The lungs are richly supplied with blood vessels which enable them to be used as a route for medications. Devices, called nebulizers or atomizers, break the liquid medication into particles by the force of compressed air or oxygen. The smaller the particles of medication, the farther down the respiratory tract they will be effective. Many of the medications prepackaged in small hand-held nebulizers are accompanied by specific instructions for their use. General instructions for use include having the patient sit upright and exhale. The patient's lips are then closed around the mouthpiece. While the patient slowly inhales, one dose of the medication is released. The mouthpiece is removed, and the patient is instructed not to breathe momentarily. Then the patient exhales slowly through pursed lips. The procedure is repeated as ordered.

Nursing Interventions Related to Chemical Safety: Poison Treatment

Prevention is the single best method of providing chemical safety as it relates to poison. The nurse teaches parents and families about the need for safe storage and use of medications, as well as other potentially harmful products. In this teaching, the nurse stresses:

1. All medications are to be given only to the person for whom they were prescribed. A medication that is beneficial to one person may harm another.

2. All medications are kept in their original containers with the original label. If an accident occurs, it is possible to identify the substance. The label may also have first aid instructions in case of an emergency.

3. All medications are kept in child-resistant containers, out of the reach of children, and preferably locked.

4. Medications that are no longer needed are discarded.

5. Emergency telephone numbers for the local poison control center need to be readily available. In an emergency, be able to tell the poison control staff member what was taken and how much.

Although the above instructions were related to medications, they apply equally to any other potentially harmful substances in the environment. Dishwasher detergent, toilet bowl cleaner, bleach, turpentine, and insecticides may all be harmful.

The initial step in the treatment of poisoning is to call the poison control center. The decision about how to treat a specific type of poisoning requires judgment and medical diagnosis. At times, no treatment is necessary, and to treat the victim would only cause unnecessary trauma and discomfort. Therefore, the first step is to call the poison center.

There is no one treatment (universal antidote) that is an effective treatment for all poisons. One poison treatment method is the induction of vomiting. (This *is not done* if the ingested poison was a corrosive or caustic agent. Caustic agents burn as they are being ingested. To have the victim vomit them would cause more burning and increase the possibility of some of the agent being aspirated into the lungs.) One method of inducing vomiting is by the administration of syrup of ipecac, a nonprescription medication which is readily available. The adult dose is 30 ml, the child's dose (over one year of age) is 15 ml. This is given with about 200 ml water or milk to promote complete emptying of the stomach. Note that it is essential that syrup of ipecac is given. This is easily confused with ipecac fluidextract. Ipecac fluidextract is 14 times more potent and could result in death.

Another effective poison treatment is the use of activitated charcoal. This substance is usually given after the victim has vomited from the syrup of ipecac. The activated charcoal absorbs the drug and prevents it from being absorbed into the gastrointestinal tract. It is particularly effective against certain drug overdoses, such as aspirin, barbiturates, morphine, and amphetamines. It is also used to treat ingestion of poisonous mushrooms. The adult dose is 600 mg to 5 gm orally. A child's dose is based on body weight: 0.5 to 1 gm/kg. Activated charcoal is given with water.

If a corrosive (such as lye or bleach) has been ingested, *do not induce vomiting*. Treatment is directed at neutralizing the poison. A small amount of milk or water may be given, but emergency medical care is necessary immediately.

When a poisoning occurs, both the patient and the family need the support of the nurse. Communication skills then become an important part of intervention.

Summary

The provision of chemical safety, as it concerns nurses, is largely related to medication administration. Nurses use a knowledge of pharmacology to plan, implement, and evaluate nursing care related to medication therapy.

Whenever nurses administer medication, five "rights" are checked in order to maximize patient safety: right patient, drug, dose, route, and time. The nurse checks these five items as the drug is removed from storage, before the medication is poured, and as the drug is returned to storage. If the nurse does make an error in administering medications, it is promptly reported, documented, and the condition of the patient thoroughly assessed.

There are three primary routes for medication administration: oral, parenteral, and the skin and mucous membranes. The oral route is the most convenient but has slower absorption time than parenteral medications. Parenteral medications are rapidly absorbed but have the disadvantage of being irretrievable if given in error. Medications given via the skin or mucous membranes have the advantage of being applied directly to the surface where they exert their effect, but absorption is somewhat uncertain. The route of administration is dependent on the nature of the drug and the disease condition of the patient.

Parenteral medications can be given in many sites. The site selected for intramuscular injections depends upon the nature of the medication, the amount of the medication, the condition of the muscle, and the patient's preference if there is no medical contraindication. Subcutaneous sites may be alternated, as is done in the administration of insulin.

Intravenous medications have the most rapid effect. This route is often used in emergencies. Medication may be given intravenously through an existing IV line or by using additional equipment. Some patients receive medications through an intermittent infusion system. This enables the patient to receive IV medications without a large volume of IV fluid. Since medications given by the bolus method are not diluted, the nurse takes additional safety precautions, such as checking the prepared dosage with a second registered nurse.

The principles of providing chemical safety apply to all routes of administration and to all medications. Principles include correct identification of the patient and the medication (including the dose, route, time), correct documentation, and thorough assessment of the patient's response to the medication.

Terms for Review

addiction, addition, analgesic, antagonism, aspirate, bolus, contraindication, generic name, heparin flush, idiosyncratic effect, incompatibility, interaction, medication therapy, meniscus, narcotics, parenteral, patent, pharmacology, placebo, potentiation

route: buccal, intradermal, intramuscular, intravenous, ophthalmic, oral, otic, subcutaneous, sublingual, topical, Z track

site: deltoid, dorsogluteal, vastus lateralis, ventrogluteal, therapeutic effect, tolerance, toxicity, trade name

Self-Assessment

Use the ratio and proportion method to calculate the following dosages.

1. Order: sodium pentobarbital 150 mg, IM stat.
   Available: ampule containing 100 mg sodium pentobarbital for injection per 2 ml
   Correct dosage is:

2. Order: chlorpromazine hydrochloride 50 mg, oral tid
   Available: chlorpromazine 25 mg per tablet
   Correct dose is:
3. Order: RITALIN 15 mg, oral bid
   Available: RITALIN 10 mg per (scored) tablet
   Correct dose is:
4. Order: diphenhydramine hydrochloride 50 mg, oral tid
   Available: 12.5 mg per 5 ml oral
   Correct dose is:

5. Order: meperidine hydrochloride 75 mg, IM q3–4 h, prn for pain.
   Available: ampules containing 50 mg meperidine hydrochloride per ml for injection
   Correct dose is:
6. Order: digoxin 0.250 mg, oral 8 A.M. qd
   Available: digoxin 0.125 mg per tablet
   Correct dose:
7. Order: heparin 1500 units, 8 A.M. subq injection
   Available: heparin 5000 units per ml for injection
   Correct dose (using a tuberculin syringe):
8. Order: nystatin 750,000 units, oral tid
   Available: nyatatin 500,000 units per oral (scored) tablet
   Correct dose:
9. Order: NATERETIN 7.5 mg, oral qd
   Available: NATURETIN 2.5 mg per (scored) tablet
   Correct dose:
10. Order: penicillin G benzathine 1.2 million units, IM today only, 1/9/85
    Available: penicillin G benzathine 300,000 units per ml for injection
    Correct dose is:

Answers

1. 3 ml
2. 2 tablets tid
3. 1 ½ tablets bid
4. 20 ml tid
5. 1.5 ml
6. 2 tablets qd
7. 0.3 ml
8. 1 ½ tablets tid
9. 3 tablets
10. 4 ml

Learning Activities

1. For the following list of drugs, prepare a medication card which includes the following information for each medication: generic name, trade name, route of administration and usual dose for that route, action, side effects, contraindications, and nursing implications. Use at least three different references. Record the information on a 3- × 6- inch index card.
   ampicillin sodium
   aspirin
   methocarbamol
   magnesium magma
   Hydrocortex
   ALDOMET
2. Select one of the above medications to look up in each of the three references you used in the above activity. Read the information given by each reference. Then respond to the following questions in order to help you evaluate the helpfulness of the references.
   Which reference was the easiest to use in locating the information?
   In which reference was the information most clearly written and easy to understand?
   In which reference were the contraindications most clear and easy to pick out of the text?
   In which reference were drug interactions identified clearly?
   In which reference were major side effects easiest to pick out?
   Which references gave the most clear nursing implications?

Review Questions

1. Side effects are
   a. Considered sufficient reason to stop the administration of a medication
   b. Evaluated as a possible reason for discontinuing a medication
   c. To be expected to some degree with all medications
   d. Caused by incompatible properties of medications
2. The five rights that the nurse checks for in medication administration are
   a. Generic name, proprietary name, dose, route, time
   b. Name, action, route, time, dose
   c. Patient, drug, dose, route, time
   d. Patient, drug, dose, expiration date, time
3. A medication scheduled for 11:30 A.M. may be given
   a. Between 11:00 A.M. and 12:00 noon
   b. Anytime before the noon meal is served
   c. Between 10:30 A.M. and 12:30 A.M.
   d. Immediately after the patient has finished the noon meal
4. A contraindication for almost all drugs is
   a. Surgery scheduled within the next four hours
   b. Blood type B-positive
   c. Pregnancy
   d. Being over 65 year of age
5. Waste products of drugs are excreted primarily by
   a. The liver
   b. The circulatory and respiratory systems
   c. The kidneys, lungs, intestines
   d. The skin and lungs.
6. Which of the following nurse statements indicates a knowledge of holistic health care principles when the nurse administers medications?
   a. "Mr. Jones, this is your medication for pain. It is very strong, and you will feel much better in about 15 minutes."
   b. "Mr. Jones. This is your DEMEROL."
   c. "Mr. Jones, this is your pain medication. Let me know if it doesn't help in about 15 minutes."
   d. "Mr. Jones, this is the pill you asked for."

7. The nurse is preparing to hang an IV infusion to which has been added medications. The nurse observes small particles in the bottle. Which is the most appropriate nursing action?
   a. The nurse vigorously shakes the bottle to dissolve the particles.
   b. The nurse hangs the bottle, regulates the infusion at a very slow rate, and observes the patient for any possible effects.
   c. The infusion is not used, and the nurse calls the hospital pharmacy to question drug incompatibility.
   d. The infusion is not used, and the nurse tries to mix the same medication a second time.

8. When the physician's or nurse practitioner's handwriting on the medication order is unclear, the nurse
   a. Calls the nursing supervisor to ask for assistance
   b. Calls the physician or nurse practitioner who wrote the order and asks for clarification
   c. Consults a drug reference to look for hints
   d. Reviews past handwriting of the nurse practitioner and physician to see if it can help.

9. When the nurse is giving a medication, and the patient asks, "What is the name of this medication and what does it do?" The nurse most appropriately responds
   a. "You'll have to ask your doctor for that information."
   b. "Are you concerned about taking drugs?"
   c. "This is your medication for your infection."
   d. "This is penicillin. It is an antibiotic that will work to clear up the infection around your incision."

10. Nurse A. is in a rush and asks Nurse B., "Would you please help me. My meds are all prepared. Could you just pass them out?" An appropriate response from Nurse B. is
    a. "I'd by happy to."
    b. "I'm not allowed to give medications I didn't prepare."
    c. "I can't give your meds, but can I help by doing something else?"
    d. "I'll do it just this once because you're so rushed."

Answers

1. b
2. c
3. a
4. c
5. c
6. a
7. c
8. b
9. d
10. c

Suggested Readings

Fink, J.: Medication errors to avoid. *Nurs. Life.* 3:26–29, May/Apr., 1983. The author presents malpractice cases involving nurses. Ten safeguards are given as a means of avoiding medication errors.

Hayter, J.: Why response to medication changes with age. *Geriatr. Nurs.* 2:411–16, Nov./Dec. 1981) The author discusses the physiology of aging which affects medication therapy. Nursing implications are included.

Skeist, R., and Carlson, G. Storing medications safely. *Geriatr. Nurs.* 2:429–32 Nov./Dec., 1981. Two brief vignettes are presented to illustrate the effects of incorrect drug-storage methods. The authors discuss the effects of heat, light, humidity, and age on medications. Suggestions are given for safe storage which will protect the efficacy of the drug.

Todd, B. How a drug gets to market. *Geriatr. Nurs.* 2:434–35, Nov./Dec., 1981. A brief summary of the procedures it takes to get a drug from research laboratories to Food and Drug Administration approval.

References and Bibliography

Baker, N.: Prescriptive authority for nurse practitioners. *Geriatr. Nurs.* 2:420–21, 1981.

Fink, J.: Medication errors to avoid. *Nurs. Life.* 3:26–29, 1983.

Hayes, J.: Normal changes in aging and nursing implications of drug therapy. *Nurs. Clin. N. Am.,* 17:253–61, 1982.

Mereness, D.: Protect your patients from nurse addicts. *Nurs. Life,* 1:71–73, 1981.

Nursing Photobook, West, R. ed.: *Giving Medications.* Nursing '82 Books, Intermed Communications, Pa. 1982.

Nursing Photobook, West, R. ed.: *Managing I.V. Therapy.* Nursing '83 Books, Intermed Communications, Pa. 1983.

Scott, M.: *Calculations of Medications Using the Proportion.* Prentice-Hall, Englewood Cliffs, N.J. 1982.

Sheridan, E.; Patterson, H.; and Gustafson, E.: *Falconer's the Drug, the Nurse, the Patient,* 7th ed. Saunders, Philadelphia, 1982.

Squire, J., and Clayton, B. *Basic Pharmacology for Nurses,* 7th ed. Mosby, St. Louis, 1981.

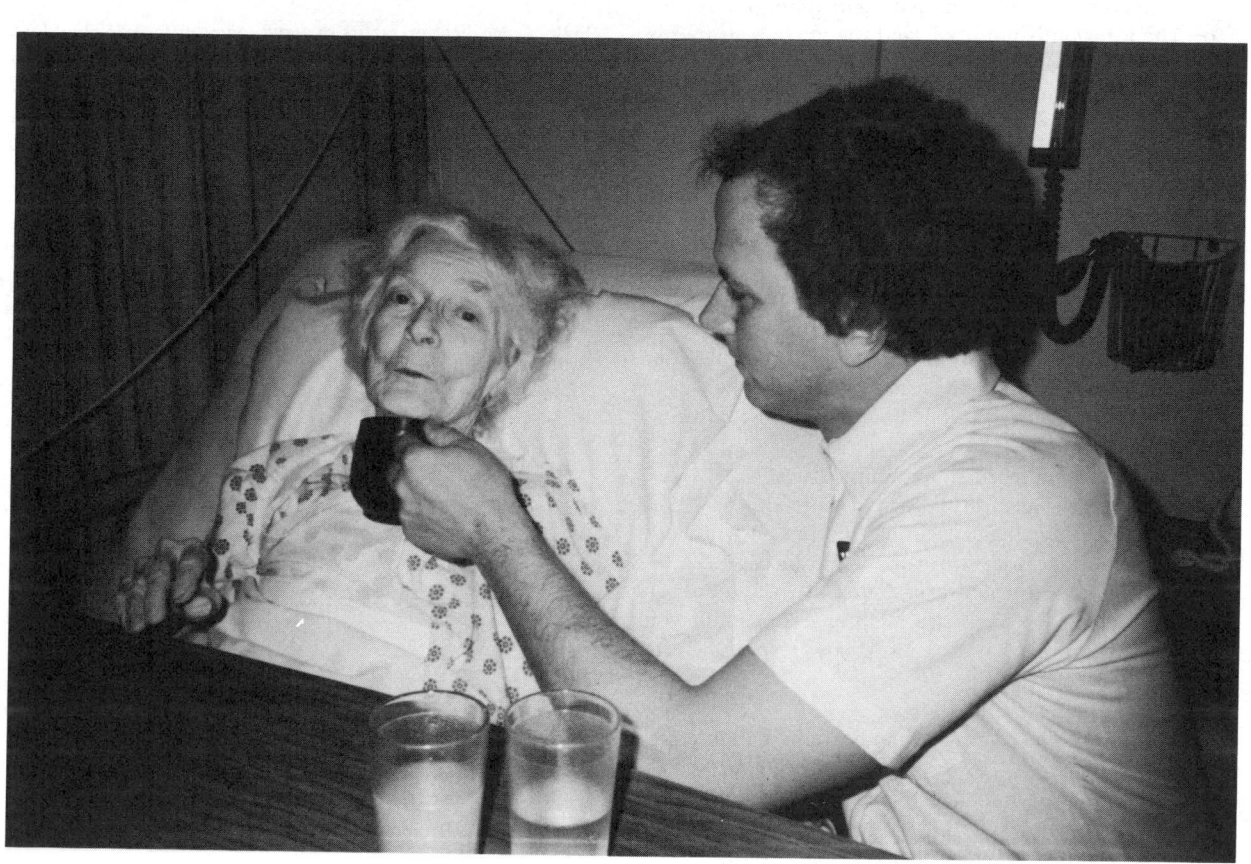

UNIT VI
BASIC HUMAN NEEDS: A FRAMEWORK FOR NURSING INTERVENTION

THE NEED FOR OXYGEN

Objectives

1. Explain why the body needs oxygen.
2. Describe how the body normally brings oxygen from the air to the individual cells within the body.
3. Explain how the body regulates the level of oxygen in the arteries (PaO_2).
4. Explain how specific areas of the body are able to regulate their local oxygen supply.
5. Identify factors that may interfere with satisfaction of oxygen needs.
6. Identify data indicating satisfaction of oxygen needs in the body.
7. Identify data associated with unmet oxygen needs.
8. Identify general nursing diagnoses associated with unmet oxygen needs.
9. Describe nursing interventions designed to prevent problems with adequate oxygenation from developing.
10. Describe nursing interventions to assist patients who are having difficulty meeting their oxygen needs.
11. Safely perform the following skills:
    Assessment of heart and lung sounds
    Assessment and documentation of pulse, respirations, blood pressure
    Application of elastic bandages or stockings
    Postural drainage
    Percussion and vibration of chest
    Suctioning airways
    Care of tracheostomy
    Oxygen administration
    Abdominal thrusts/Heimlich maneuver
    CPR (Cardiopulmonary resuscitation)
    Artificial respirations

Oxygen as a Basic Survival Need

The body's need for oxygen is the most basic and pressing of the physiologic needs. Without oxygen for even short periods, the body's cells will suffer irreversible damage and quickly die. The brain is permanently damaged when deprived of oxygen for more than a few minutes. A block in the oxygen supply to the heart causes severe muscle damage and possible cessation of the vital pumping action. Why is oxygen so important? A constant supply of oxygen is needed because it cannot be stored in the body as many other essential elements are. The need for oxygen lies at the level of the individual cells within the human body. In order for the living cell to function and survive, it must have fuel. The source of fuel for the cell is the molecule *ATP (adenosine triphosphate)*. This molecule provides the cell with the energy it needs to perform the various activities necessary to keep the entire body functioning effectively. Muscle contractions, synthesis of organic molecules,

and transport of materials across the cell membrane all require energy. Various substances can be utilized to produce ATP such as lipids, proteins, glucose, and other nutrients. The one essential component in the normal production of ATP is oxygen. Since oxygen is not stored in the body, it must reach the cell and be available to structures within the cell, called mitochondria, for the production of ATP. ATP cannot be made by the mitochondria in the absence of oxygen. Formation of ATP accounts for almost all the oxygen utilized by the cell. If enough cells lose the ability to function becaues of inadequate ATP (and oxygen), tissues and organs lose function. When tissues and organs lose function, the life of the individual is in danger. All body physiology is ultimately dependent on a continuous, adequate oxygen supply for the formation of ATP to fuel the body's life processes.

Normal Means for Meeting Oxygen Needs

In order to meet the body's need for oxygen, three basic activities must occur. First, there must be effective ventilation. *Ventilation* is the exchange of air between the atmosphere and the alveoli within the lung. It consists of *inspiration* (breathing air into the lungs) and *expiration* (exhaling air out of the lungs). The air travels through the nose or mouth to the oropharynx and then into the lungs by way of the trachea. From the trachea, it flows into the left and right bronchi and from there into smaller and smaller tubes called bronchioles until it reaches the alveoli, which are small elastic sacs at the end of the smallest airway tubes. (See Figure 20–1.) There are approximately 300 million alveoli within the adult lung, and it is here that the gas exchange between the air and blood occurs.

The second element necessary in meeting oxygen needs is effective diffusion of gases between the alveoli and the blood. Oxygen must move from the alveoli across the cell membrane, through the interstitial fluid, across the cells forming the walls of the capillaries, and into the blood.

The third element essential in meeting oxygen needs involves the transport of the oxygen from the capillaries in the lungs to the cells throughout the rest of the body. This requires an adequate blood volume, an adequate number of red blood cells containing sufficient amounts of the hemoglobin molecule, and an effective heart action to pump the blood throughout the body. When the oxygen finally reaches the cell, true *respiration* oc-

curs, which is the exchange of gas molecules across the cellular membrane. (See Figure 20–2.)

In summary, the three activities needed to meet oxygenation needs are:

1. Ventilation
2. Diffusion of oxygen from the alveoli into the blood
3. Transport of oxygen to the individual cells where cellular respiration occurs

Ventilation

Ventilation is achieved by pressure changes within the lung. The respiratory system is composed of the following structures involved in ventilation: mouth and nose, pharynx, larynx, trachea, two bronchi, bronchioles, and alveoli. During inspiration, air is drawn into the lungs because the pressure within the lungs is less than the atmospheric pressure. This decreased pressure within the lungs is accomplished by increasing the size of the chest and drawing the lung tissue out into the expanded volume. Boyle's law of physics indicates that the pressure of a gas varies inversely with its volume, so as volume decreases, pressure increases; when the volume of the gas increases, pressure decreases. During inspiration, the lung volume increases, therefore, the pressure

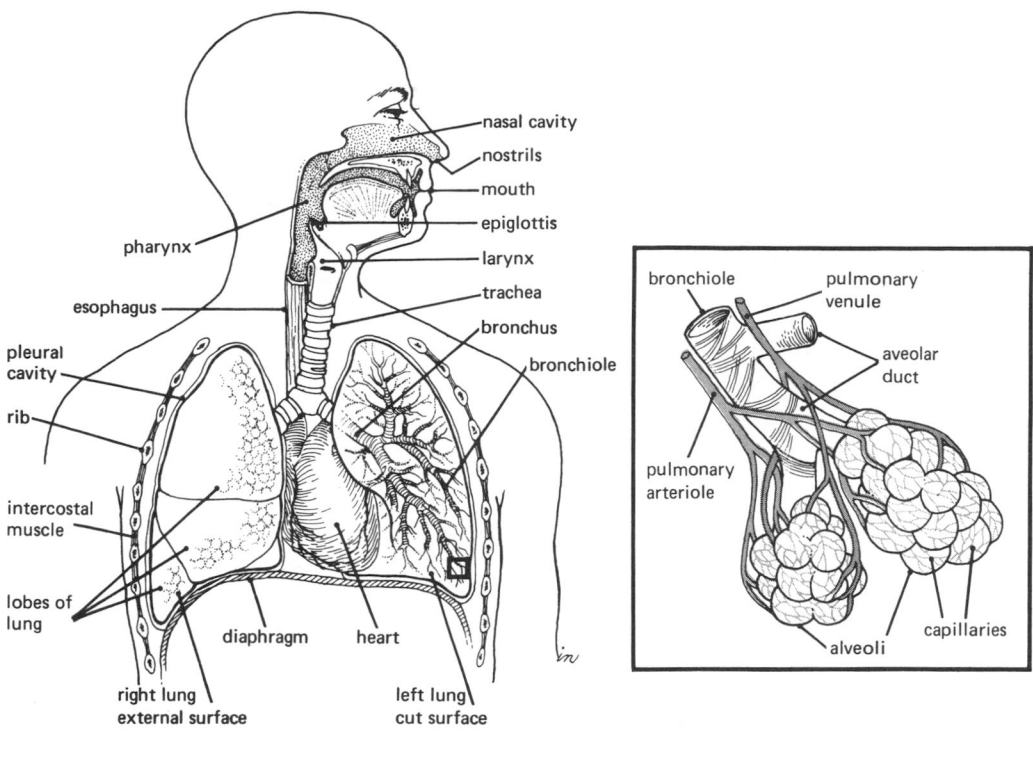

A. Respiratory system   B. Alveoli of the lungs

Figure 20-1. Structures of the respiratory tract. (From M. Griffiths: *Introduction to Human Physiology*, 2nd ed. Macmillan, New York, 1981, p. 162.)

of the air within the lungs decreases and air is drawn into the respiratory system until the pressure within the alveoli is equal to the atmospheric pressure.

Several activities occur during inspiration to increase the volume of the lungs. The diaphragm contracts and moves down toward the abdomen. The intercostal muscles of the chest contract and pull and ribs upward and outward. Both of these activities expand the chest. The ribs move away from the lungs with the contraction of these respiratory muscles. This expansion of the thoracic cage decreases the intrapleural pressure. This is the pressure between the two layers of the pleura, one lining the internal chest wall (parietal pleura) and the other lining the surface of the lung and diaphragm (visceral pleura). As the chest wall expands, it pulls the parietal pleura with it, creating a negative pressure between the two pleural walls. This negative pressure pulls the visceral pleura out toward the expanded chest. Since the visceral pleura is attached to the lung, the negative pressure also pulls the lung tissue out, expanding the volume. The expanded volume decreases the pressure within the alveoli, creating a negative pressure (less than atmospheric pressure), and air is drawn into the respiratory tract. Air continues to move into the alveoli until the alveolar pressure equals the atmospheric pressure.

At that point, air movement ceases. Inspiration is an active process involving muscle contractions.

Expiration is a passive process in the normal lung involving recoil of the elastic tissue within the lung, as the muscles of the diaphragm and the intercostal muscle relax and chest volume decreases. This decreased volume of the chest increases and pressure within the alveoli, and air is forced out of the lungs until the alveolar pressure is again equal to atmospheric pressure.

The *tidal volume* is the term given to the amount of air involved in a normal inspiration or expiration. In an adult, this is approximately 500 cc of air. Of that 500 cc, approximately 150 cc of air is not involved in gas exchange at the alveolar level. This amount of air is in the airway structures above the alveoli. The space within these structures is termed the *anatomical dead space.* This leaves 350 cc of air entering the alveoli during a normal inspiration. For a particular individual, the tidal volume can be calculated at the rate of 5 to 7 cc per kilogram of body weight. Normally, an additional 3,000 cc can be inspired during a maximum inhalation. This is called the *inspiratory reserve volume.* There is also an *expiratory reserve volume* of approximately 1,000 cc of air left in the lungs after a normal expiration. This can be exhaled and still leave the individual with a *residual*

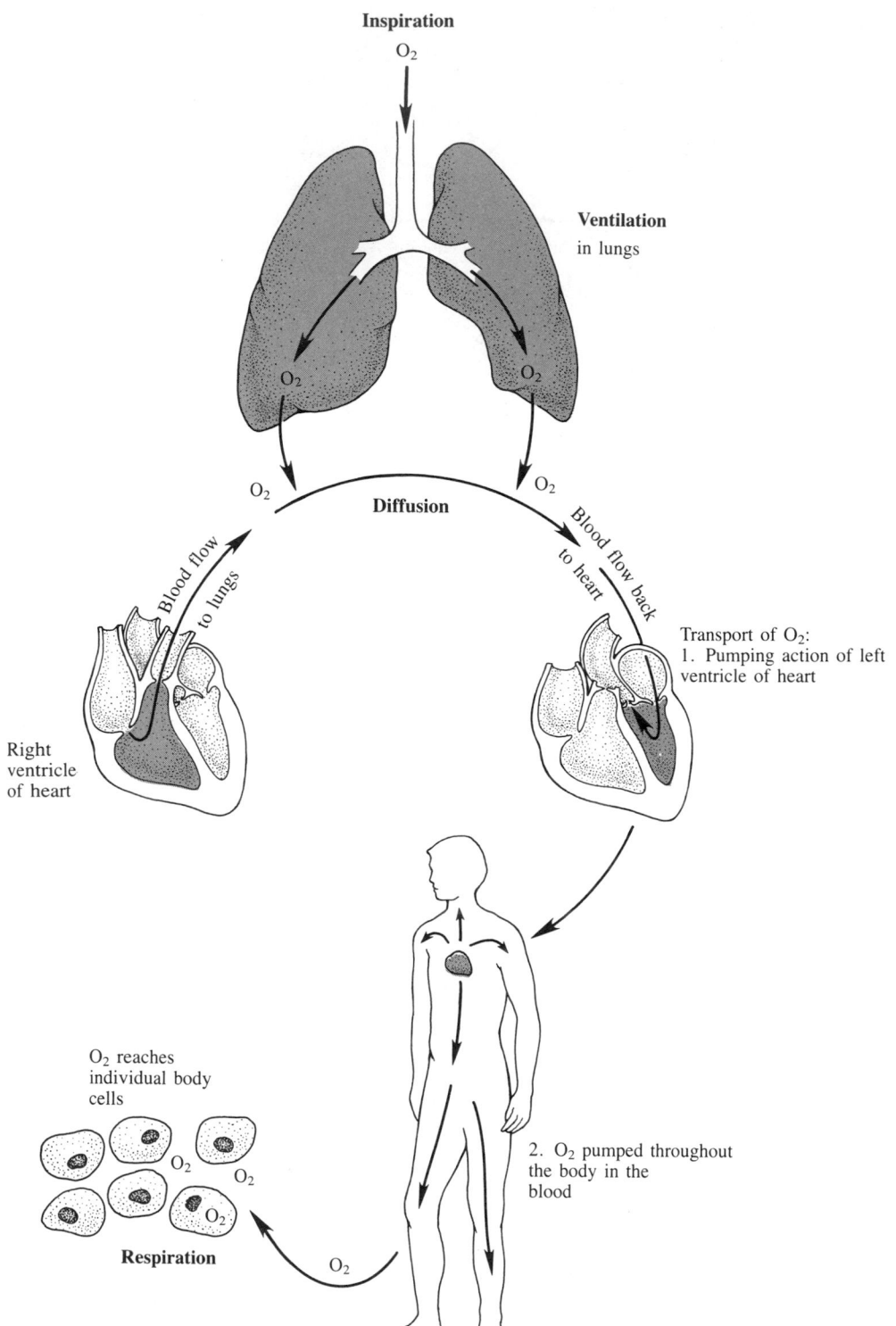

Inspiration

O_2

Ventilation
in lungs

O_2 O_2

O_2 O_2
Diffusion

Blood flow
to lungs

Blood flow back
to heart

Transport of O_2:
1. Pumping action of left
ventricle of heart

Right
ventricle
of heart

O_2 reaches
individual body
cells

O_2 O_2

O_2

Respiration O_2

2. O_2 pumped throughout
the body in the
blood

Figure 20-2. Movement of oxygen from the inspired air to the individual body cells.

air volume of 1500 cc in the lungs. This permits gas exchange between the alveoli and the blood to continue between breaths. The *vital capacity* of the lungs is equal to the inspiratory reserve volume (3,000 cc) and the tidal volume (500 cc) plus the expiratory reserve volume. It represents the maximum volume of air that can be expelled following a maximum inspiration and is used to measure lung function. In the normal adult, it represents a volume of approximately 4,500 cc of air. From these figures, it is obvious that a normal inspiration rep-

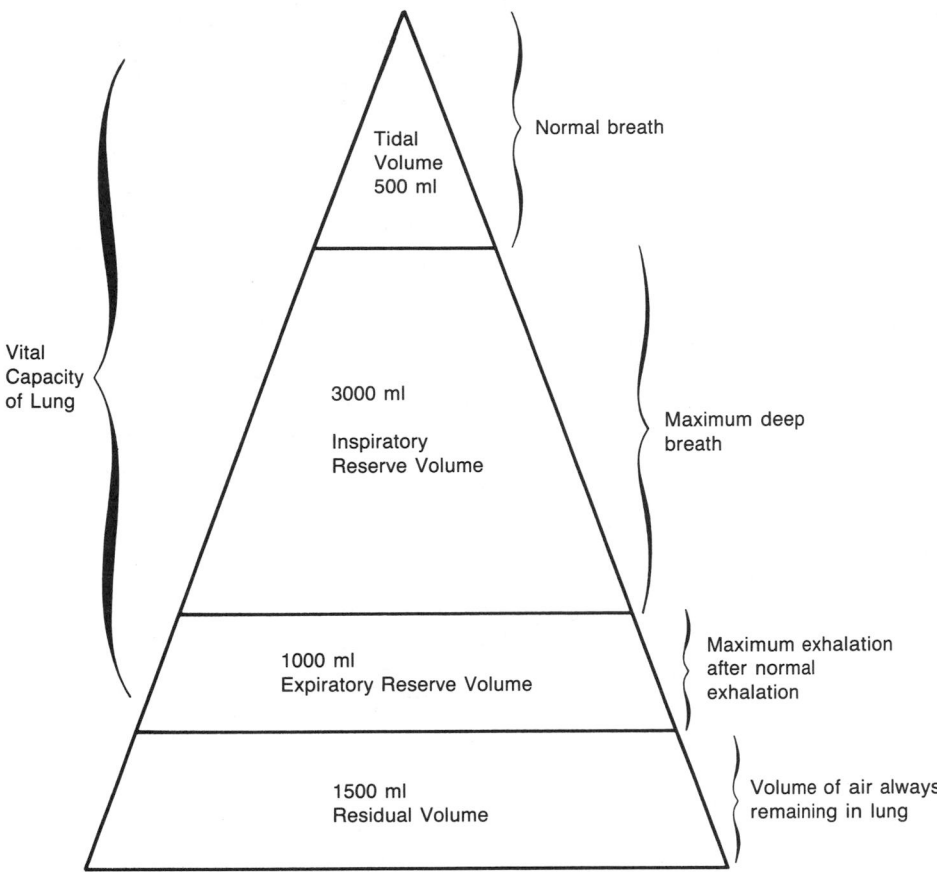

Figure 20-3. Volume capacities of the lungs.

resents only a small air exchange compared to the maximum capabilities of the lung. (See Figure 20-3.)

Normal ventilation depends on a normal chest anatomy, an intact and compliant (elastic) chest wall, functioning respiratory muscles, normal nerve stimuli for contraction and relaxation of the respiratory muscles, an intact pleural membrane to move the lungs in and out with the chest wall, an open and intact upper airway, and compliant lung tissue with alveoli that inflate during inspiration and recoil during expiration. Alterations in the structure or function of any of these components can interfere with normal ventilation.

Diffusion of Gases Between Alveoli and Blood

In order for oxygen to diffuse from the alveoli into the blood, the concentration of oxygen in the alveoli must be higher than the oxygen concentration in the blood. Normally, the blood circulated to the alveoli within the lungs has had oxygen removed during cellular respirations. This makes the oxygen concentration in the blood much less than that in the inspired air. Air contains 21 percent oxygen. Well-oxygenated arterial blood has a partial pressure of oxygen (PaO_2) ranging from 80 to 100 mm Hg. The *partial pressure* of a gas, according to Dalton's law, is the pressure the gas would exert if it were alone in the container. The total pressure of gases in the blood is equal to the sum of all the partial pressures exerted by each gas, primarily oxygen and carbon dioxide. The oxygen pressure of inspired air is approximately 159 mm Hg. As deoxygenated blood moves back to the lungs from the body, the partial pressure of oxygen is in the range of 40 mm Hg. The oxygen then readily moves from the area of higher concentration (159 mm Hg in alveoli) to the area of lower concentration (40 mm Hg in deoxygenated blood) present in the blood circulating around the alveoli.

Carbon dioxide, which is a waste product of cellular metabolism, is brought back to the lungs for excretion, which is accomplished by simple diffusion. The partial pressure of CO_2 within the alveoli of the lung is 40 mm Hg. The partial pressure of carbon dioxide in deoxygenated *venous* blood circulated to the alveoli is 46 mm Hg. The carbon dioxie moves from the blood into the alveoli because of this concentration difference. Well-oxygenated arterial blood pumped from the heart has a $PaCO_2$ (partial pressure of carbon dioxide in *arterial* blood) of 40 mm Hg, equal to the pressure within the alveoli. (See Figure 20-4.)

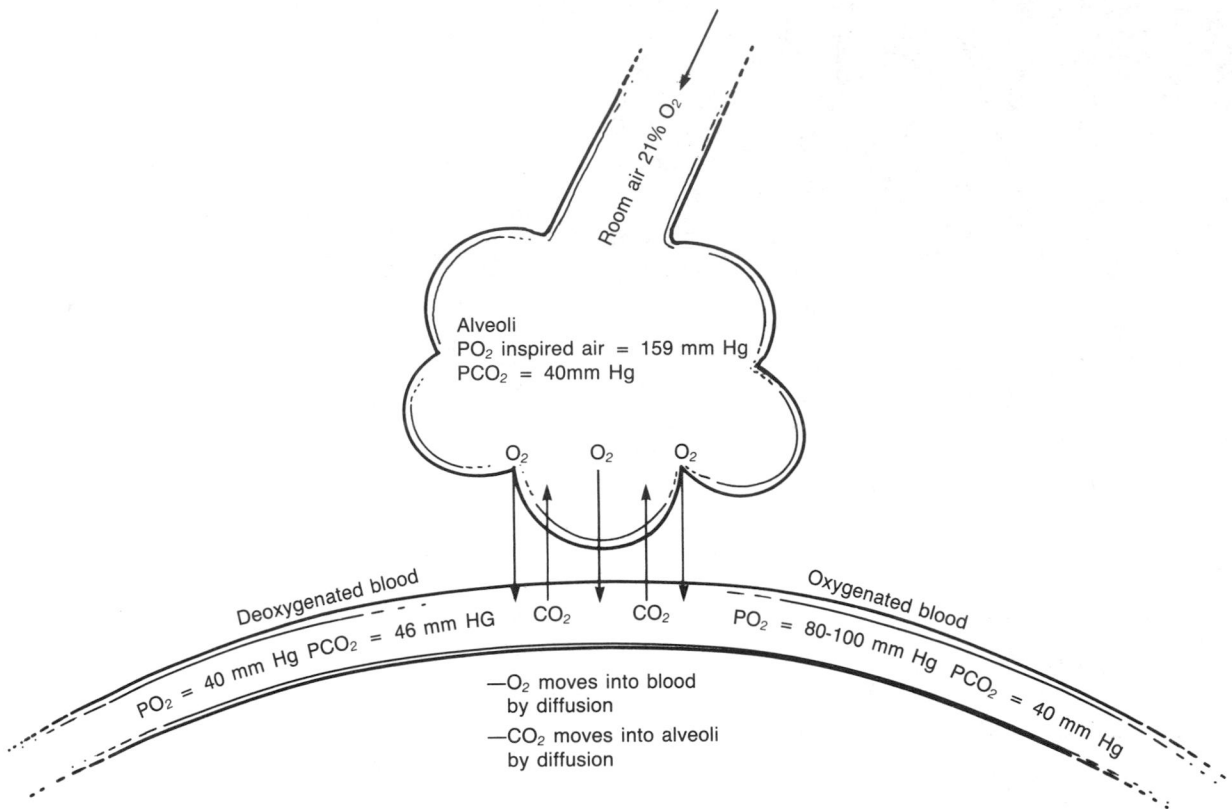

Figure 20-4. Diffusion of gases between capillaries and the alveoli of the lung.

These figures represent the values found in blood gases and are used as a guide in assessing the adequacy of oxygen need satisfaction. PaO_2 (partial pressure of oxygen in *arterial* blood) equals 80 to 100 mm. Hg. $PaCO_2$ (partial pressure of carbon dioxide in *arterial* blood) equals 35 to 45 mm. Hg. Diffusion of oxygen and carbon dioxide into and out of the blood depends on an adequate oxygen concentration in the inspired air (normally 21 percent), thin-walled alveoli to allow gases to diffuse across their cell membranes, a capillary system supplying an adequate blood flow to the alveoli, and well-functioning alveoli which inflate during normal inspiration.

Transport of Gases

The need for oxygen is created by the individual cells within the body, and it is at this level that respiration takes place. Oxygen moves from the blood through the walls of the capillaries, through the interstitial fluid, and then through the cell wall where it is used to create ATP. All of this movement occurs because the concentration of oxygen outside the cell is greater than the concentration within the cell. Movement of both oxygen and carbon dioxide is by diffusion from the area of higher concentration to the area of lower concentration.

Transport of oxygen to the cell and carbon dioxide away from the cell depends on several factors. There must be an adequate blood supply to reach all of the capillaries throughout the body. The heart must be able to pump the blood effectively, and the blood flow must be uninterrupted to reach all areas of the body.

Hemoglobin and the Red Blood Cell (RBC). Ninety-eight percent of the total oxygen in the blood is attached to the hemoglobin molecule within the RBCs. The remaining 2 percent is dissolved in the fluid part of the blood, and it is this dissolved oxygen plus the dissolved carbon dioxide that determine the value of the blood gases. Some of the carbon dioxide resulting from cellular metabolism is carried back to the lungs attached to the hemoglobin molecule. Most of the carbon dioxide (81 percent) undergoes a chemical change, being converted to bicarbonate and free hydrogen ions. The hydrogen ions then combine with the hemoglobin molecule for transport back to the lungs. The bicarbonate ions are dissolved in the fluid part of the blood. (See Figure 20–5.)

In the lungs, the oxygen diffuses into the blood and

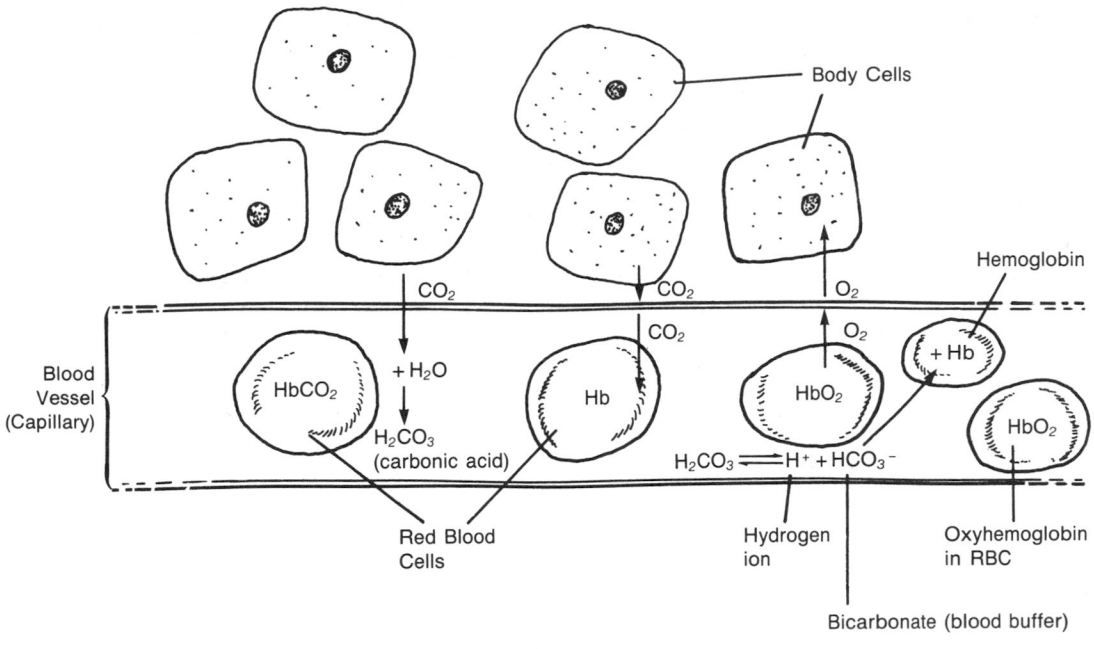

Figure 20–5. Action of the hemoglobin molecule in buffer systems of blood.

Blood Buffer System

Hb (hemoglobin) + H^+ = buffer to prevent excessive
                                             acidity and ↓pH of blood

Hb — binds with O_2 or CO_2 for transport

HCO_3^- — formed when Carbonic acid dissociates
                              act as a buffer preventing ↑pH

then rapidly combines with the hemoglobin. After releasing oxygen to the cells, the hemoglobin molecule remains about 75 percent saturated with oxygen when the body is at rest. During times of increased cellular activity with increased oxygen consumption by the cells, the hemoglobin molecule is capable of releasing almost all of the oxygen carried for use by the cell. Inadequate numbers of red blood cells or inadequate hemoglobin within the RBCs will interfere with the ability of the blood to transport oxygen and carbon dioxide to and from the lungs.

The adult has a blood volume of approximately 8 percent of total body weight. An adult weighing 155 lb (70 kg) has 5½ liters of blood or 11 to 12 pints. Blood is normally 45 percent cells and 55 percent fluid. The *hematocrit* is the measurement of the percentage of cells in the blood. A low hematocrit indicates a reduced number of cells in the blood. Since 99 percent of the cells in the blood are red blood cells (erythrocytes or RBCs), a low hematocrit would indicate a reduced ability to carry oxygen and carbon dioxide. The erythrocytes within the blood also give the blood its typing as O, A, B, or AB, depending on the proteins contained on the cell membrane.

Normal erythrocytes have a life span of 120 days and cannot reproduce. They are produced in the bone marrow and destroyed by macrophages in the liver, spleen, bone marrow, and lymph nodes. Normally, RBC pro-

Table 20–1. **Normal Blood Values (Adult)**

	MALE ADULT	FEMALE ADULT
Hgb (hemoglobin)	13–18 gm/100 ml	12–16 gm/100 ml
Hct (hematocrit)	45–52 %	37–48%
WBC (white blood cells)	4,500–11,500/mm	
PaO₂ (oxygen in arterial blood)	75–100 mm Hg	
PaCO₂ (carbon dioxide in arterial blood)	35–45 mm Hg	
pH (hydrogen ion concentration)	7.35–7.45	

duction is equal to RBC destruction. Production can be increased sixfold in times of stress, such as hemorrhage.

The measurement of blood *hemoglobin* indicates the amount of hemoglobin in each erythrocyte. Normally, if the erythrocyte has an adequate amount of hemoglobin, the hematocrit value is three times the hemoglobin value. (See Table 20–1 for normal blood values.) A decrease in the hematocrit value may indicate bleeding, decreased production of RBCs, abnormal formation of RBCs, or increased destruction. A decrease in hemoglo-

bin values may indicate any of the conditions associated with a low hematrocit. If hematocrit is normal, but hemoglobin is low, anemia is often the problem. In all cases, the ability of the blood to transport oxygen and carbon dioxide is jeopardized.

The Route Oxygen and Carbon Dioxide Follow.   There are two circuits for carrying blood within the body, and the oxygen molecules travel through both circuits to reach the individual cells. The two systems are the *pul-*

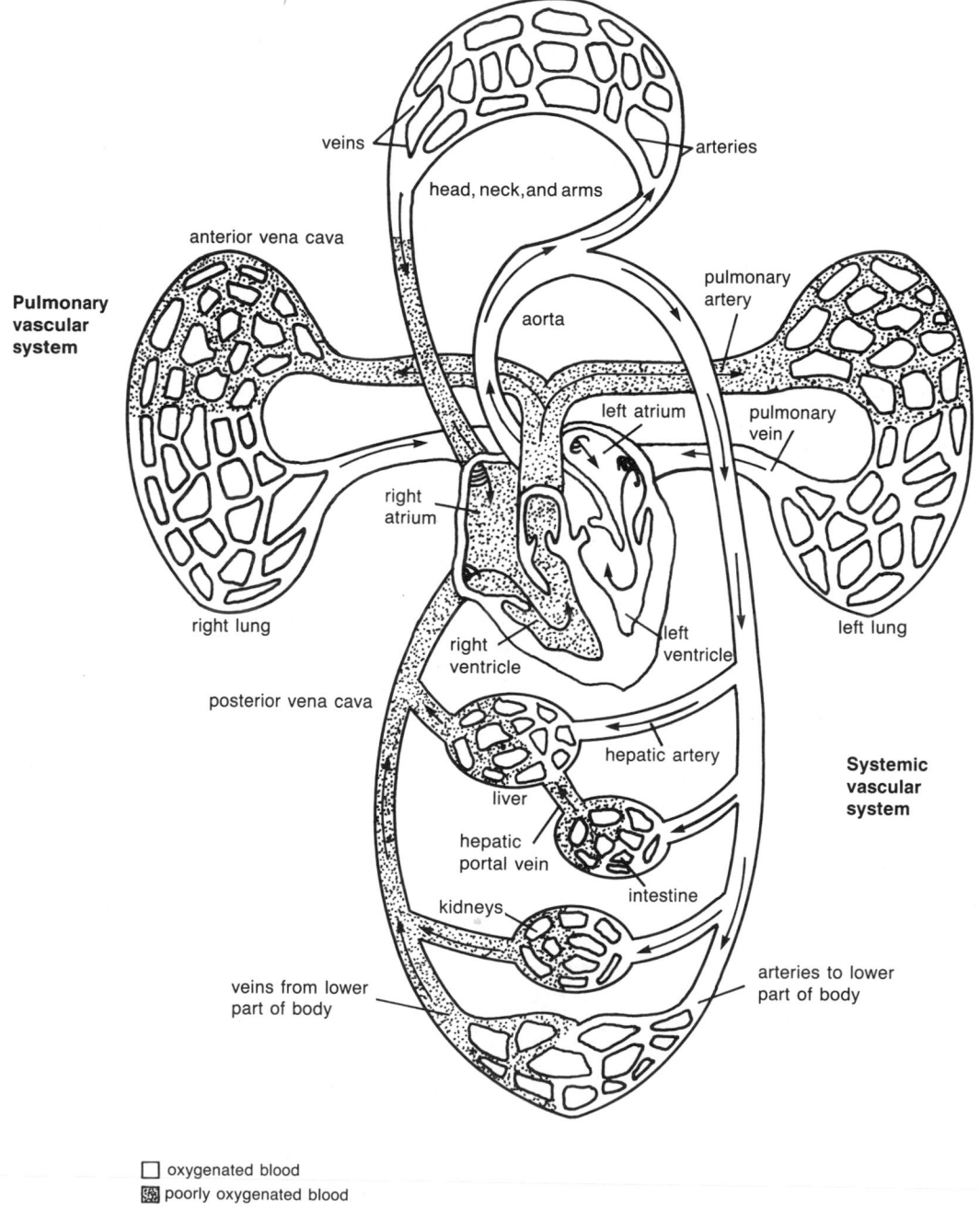

Figure 20–6.   Pulmonary and systemic circulatory systems. (From M. Griffiths: *Introduction to Human Physiology*, 2nd ed. Macmillan, New York, 1981, p. 112.)

Table 20-2. **The Circuits for Oxygen and Carbon Dioxide**

The Path Through the Body for the Oxygen Molecules

Respiratory System: Inhalation through nose or mouth → pharynx → larynx → trachea → two bronchi → bronchioles → alveoli →
Pulmonary Vascular System: interstitial fluid → capillaries around lung alveoli → venules → veins → large pulmonary veins → left atrium of heart → mitral valve →
Systemic Vascular System: left ventricle of heart → aortic valve → aorta → arteries → arterioles → capillaries → interstitial fluid → cell.

The Path Through the Body for Carbon Dioxide

Systemic Vascular System: Cell → interstitial fluid → capillaries → venules → veins → inferior or superior vena cava → right atrium of heart →
Pulmonary Vascular System: tricuspid valve → right ventricle of heart → pulmonary valve → pulmonary trunk → two pulmonary arteries → arterioles → capillaries → interstitial fluid →
Respiratory System: lung alveoli → bronchioles → two bronchi → trachea → larynx → pharynx → exhaled through the nose or mouth.

monary system and the *systemic system*. (See Figure 20-6.) The pulmonary system circulates blood from the heart to the lungs and back to the heart where the blood enters the systemic circulation. The systemic system circulates blood from the heart throughout the body and then back to the heart. Table 20-2 shows the path of the oxygen molecule.

The Pump.   At rest in the healthy adult, the right and left ventricles of the heart each pump approximately 5 liters of blood per minute into the two circuits at a rate of 60 to 90 beats a minute. Normally, the right heart pumps the same amount of blood as the left heart. Blood flow can increase more than three times the resting rate when the individual is involved in exercise. The increased flow from the heart can be routed to the cells performing the work, such as muscle cells. During heavy work or exercise, the muscle cells receive ten times their normal blood flow, while other cells may receive less than their normal blood flow. Blood flow to the brain remains fairly constant, regardless of activity level, but blood flow to the heart increases and decreases, depending on how hard the cardiac muscle is working.

Heart muscle is capable of self-excitation. This means no nervous stimulation from the central nervous system is needed to create a contraction in cardiac muscle. The sinoatrial node in the right atrium is the center for coordinating stimulation, causing atrial and ventricular contractions in sequence.

Cardiac output is the amount of blood the heart pumps into the systemic circulation each minute. The two components of cardiac output are heart rate and stroke volume. *Stroke volume* is the volume of blood pumped by the left ventricle of the heart with each contraction (systole). The total blood volume is usually fairly constant, so to increase blood flow to an area, the blood vessels dilate and the rate of circulating that volume is increased.

Regulation of Cellular Oxygen Supply

Regulation of cellular oxygen supply depends on the coordination of many factors. Control of ventilation, heart action, blood volume, RBC production and destruction, and blood flow to various areas of the body are all important elements in regulating the oxygen supply to the cells. These elements are all internally controlled by the body. External factors, primarily the concentration of oxygen and carbon dioxide in inspired air, can also greatly affect the amount of oxygen reaching the cells.

Neural Control

Involuntary Control of Ventilations.   The brain and nervous system are the primary controllers of oxygen in the systemic circulation. The center for control of the respiratory and cardiovascular systems is in the medulla of the brain located just above the spinal cord. The medulla regulates rate and depth of ventilations, rate and strength of cardiac contractions, and diameter of the blood vessels, which affects blood flow and blood pressure. The inspiratory neurons within the medulla are responsible for stimulating the muscles of respiration and causing inspiration. It is believed they have the capacity for self-excitation and maintain a constant rate of activity to cause regular inspirations. Nervous input from various areas of the body will affect the rate of firing of these neurons and thus the respiratory rate. Control of the heart rate and force of heart contractions are regulated by the medulla which increases or decreases the rate of stimulation to the heart from the sympathetic and parasympathetic nervous systems. Sympathetic stimulation causes an increased heart rate and increased force of each contraction, resulting in more blood being pumped from the heart each minute (increased cardiac output). Parasympathetic stimulation of the heart causes the heart to slow and pump less forcefully. Increased stimulation of the sympathetic system will also cause *vasoconstriction* (narrowing of the diameter of the blood vessels) to most areas except the brain and heart. Decreased stimulation of the sympathetic system results in vasodilation (widening of the diameter of the blood vessels). The extent of vasoconstriction or vasodilation in the systemic vascular system will affect the blood pressure. A minimal blood pressure is required to circulate blood to all areas of the body. If blood pressure in the arterial system drops too low (*hypotension*), some areas of the body will not be perfused (receive an adequate blood flow). If pressure in the system is too high (*hypertension*), tissue damage to organs or ruptured blood vessels may result.

The medulla receives input from the following key areas in order to regulate oxygen supply to the cells:

1. *Pulmonary stretch receptors in the lungs.* These receptors indicate when inspiratory depth is sufficient so that relaxation of the diaphragm and intercostal muscles can begin to terminate inspiration.

2. *Carotid and aortic chemoreceptors.* These cells, in the carotid and aortic arteries, become increasingly active as PaO_2 decreases. This stimulation is received by the medulla, indicating a reduced oxygen concentration in arterial blood.

3. *Carotid and aortic baroreceptors.* These cells act as pressure sensors for the medulla in regulating the degree of vasoconstriction and vasodilation of the blood vessels. An increased arterial blood pressure causes an increased rate of firing of these cells, communicating an elevated pressure to the medulla. In response to this input, the medulla decreases sympathetic stimulation to the heart and blood vessels and increases parasympathetic stimulation of the heart. This results in a slowing of the heart rate, decreased force of contractions, and varying degrees of vasodilation, thus, lower blood pressure. The opposite response occurs with decreased pressure. Sympathetic stimulation increases cardiac output and constricts the blood vessels to raise blood pressure.

4. *Large arteries and veins.* Other large veins and arteries also contain baroreceptors providing feedback on blood pressure for the medulla.

5. *Central chemoreceptors in the medulla.* These receptors monitor the hydrogen ion concentration in the fluid surrounding the brain and spinal cord (cerebrospinal fluid). Increasing concentrations of hydrogen ions (H^+) stimulate the medulla's respiratory centers to increase ventilation. This response to hydrogen ions is the primary sensing mechanism for supplying oxygen to the body's cells. It is based on carbon dioxide levels in the blood. As cellular oxygen usage increases because of an increased metabolic rate within the cell, the production of carbon dioxide as a waste product also increases. Inadequate ventilation, or breathing air with an increased CO_2 concentration, causes $PaCO_2$ to rise. This elevated level of $PaCO_2$ diffuses into the cerebrospinal fluid. It undergoes the reaction to create free H^+ and bicarbonate molecules. Since there are no RBCs in cerebrospinal fluid, therefore, no hemoglobin, the H^+ remains in this free state rather than attaching to the hemoglobin molecules as it does in the blood. The increased concentration of H^+ stimulates the central receptors in the medulla to increase ventilation which returns the $PaCO_2$ to normal. "The control of breathing (at least at rest) is aimed primarily at the regulation of brain hydrogen ion concentration" (Vander *et al.*, 1980).

Voluntary Control of Ventilations. Another neural control for respirations resides in the cerebral cortex of the brain and is under voluntary control. The cerebral cortex sends impulses directly to the muscles of respiration, completely bypassing the medulla, and allowing voluntary control of the rate and depth of respirations. Voluntary control of ventilation is essential during activities such as singing, speaking, swimming, and drinking. However, as $PaCO_2$ rises and H^+ concentration in the cerebrospinal fluid increases, voluntary control is lost and control of respirations is returned to the medulla.

Chemical Control

Various hormones and chemicals within the body can affect both local and systemic blood flow, quantity of RBCs, and ventilation.

Erythropoietin is a hormone normally secreted by the kidney. It stimulates RBC production in the bone marrow. Increased erthropoietin production in response to inadequate oxygen supply to the kidney causes increased erythrocyte production and, therefore, increased capacity for carrying oxygen to all areas of the body.

Epinephrine, produced by the adrenal medulla above the kidney, increases the rate of cardiac contractions, thus increasing cardiac output and distribution of oxygen-carrying blood. This hormone also causes vasoconstriction to most systemic arterioles, raising the blood pressure. Epinephrine causes dilation of the airways which decreases the resistance to air flow and promotes increased ventilation of the alveoli. Epinephrine is released in increased amounts in response to stress, fear, anger, and excitement.

Pulmonary surfactant is produced by the alveoli within the lungs. This lipoprotein coats the internal surface of each alveoli and reduces the surface tension cre-

ated by two wet surfaces coming in contact with each other. Less energy or force is needed to inflate the alveoli and overcome the surface tension when surfactant is present. Without adequate surfactant in the alveoli, the force created by the inspiratory muscles is unable to overcome the resistance of the alveoli surface tension. This results in a gradual progressive loss of functioning in the lung as more and more alveoli fail to open with each inspiration.

Histamine is a chemical released by white cells in the blood known as basophils. Histamine causes airway constriction and reduced air flow during ventilation. It also causes local vasodilation, increasing the blood flow

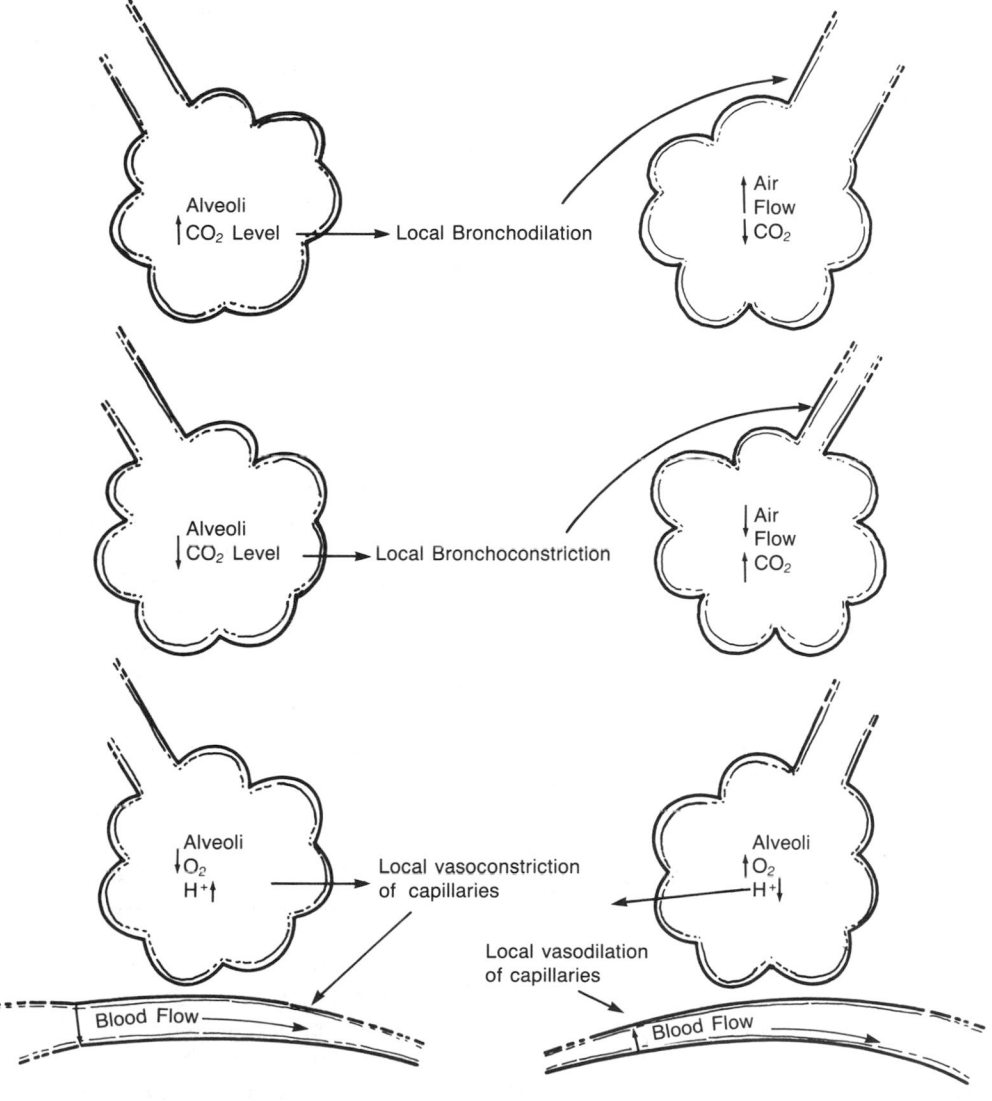

Purposes of Local Control: Keep well-ventilated alveoli perfused for maximum gas exchange.
Reduce perfusion of poorly ventilated alveoli.

Figure 20-7. Local control of alveoli blood flow and air flow.

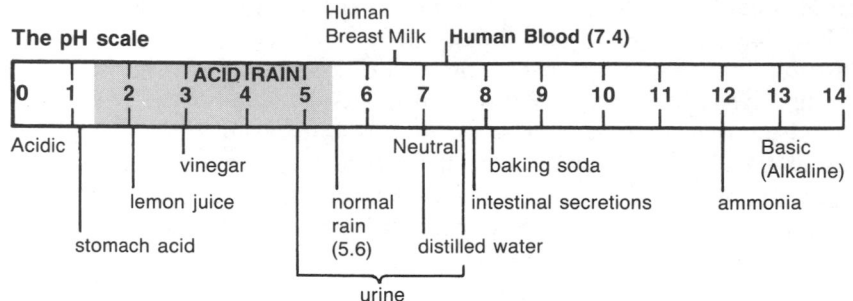

The pH scale

| 0 | 1 | 2 | 3 | 4 | 5 | 6 | 7 | 8 | 9 | 10 | 11 | 12 | 13 | 14 |

Acidic — vinegar — lemon juice — stomach acid — normal rain (5.6) — urine — distilled water — Neutral — baking soda — intestinal secretions — ammonia — Basic (Alkaline)

Human Breast Milk   Human Blood (7.4)   ACID RAIN

Figure 20–8. The pH scale and human blood.

to injured or irritated tissues. Histamine is released in response to tissue trauma or allergic reactions.

Local Control

Local autoregulation by organs and tissues is another way of increasing the blood flow, thus the oxygen supply, to specific areas of the body with an increased metabolic rate. Decreasing concentrations of oxygen or increasing concentrations of carbon dioxide and hydrogen ions in the tissues stimulate local vasodilation. The net blood flow to an area is the combined effect of local control and systemic control. These two may work together or may oppose each other. Increasing CO_2 in the alveoli causes local bronchodilation to increase air flow. Decreasing CO_2 in the alveoli causes local bronchoconstriction and reduced air flow. Decreasing oxygen concentrations within the alveoli cause local vasoconstriction of the capillaries supplying those poorly oxygenated alveoli. Increasing concentrations of alveolar oxygen cause local pulmonary capillary vasodilation to match blood flow to air flow. Increasing hydrogen ion concentrations in alveoli within the lung cause local capillary vasoconstriction, while low hydrogen ion concentrations cause local capillary vasodilation. (See Figure 20–7.) The purpose of this local control within the lung is to keep well-ventilated alveoli perfused with blood and reduce blood flow to alveoli receiving an inadequate air flow.

Blood Acidity—pH

As the concentration of hydrogen ions in the blood increases, it becomes more acidic. The pH is a measurement of the level of blood acidity. It indicates the concentration of hydrogen ions: the greater the hydrogen ion content in the blood, the more acidic the blood and the lower the pH measurement. The normal pH of human blood is 7.40, with a range of 7.35 to 7.45. The pH of the blood varies little during health, but when oxygen needs are unmet, hydrogen ions increase and lower the pH into the acidic range. A pH value of blood below 7.0 or above 7.8 is not compatible with life. (See Figure 20–8.)

The concentration of hydrogen ions in the blood also affects the hemoglobin molecule. As H+ concentration rises, there is a decrease in the affinity of hemoglobin for oxygen at the cellular level. This results in more oxygen being released from the hemoglobin molecule, so more oxygen is available to the cells. Increased activity in a tissue or organ increases the local concentration of hydrogen ions, affecting the amount of oxygen available locally. Temperature also affects the hemoglobin molecule. Active tissue has an increased local temperature. This increased temperature decreases the affinity of hemoglobin for oxygen, and it is quickly released to the tissue, complementing the effect produced by increased hydrogen ion concentrations.

Alterations in Cellular Oxygen Needs

Cellular metabolism requires oxygen to produce the fuel ATP to drive the chemical reactions representing work done by the cells of the body. Anything that increases the metabolic rate of the cell will automatically increase that cell's oxygen requirements. Muscle activity in the form of exercise, work, or play will greatly increase the body's need for oxygen. Rest and inactivity will minimize the body's need for oxygen.

Temperature greatly affects oxygen needs. For every 1° F rise in body temperature, oxygen need increases by 7 percent. Fevers and chilling both have the same effect on the cell's oxygen need. They both increase the metabolic rate and oxygen need. Chilling causes increased muscle tone and shivering which accelerates the metabolic rate within the muscle cells. Severe chilling which lowers the body temperature significantly will decrease cellular metabolism and thus reduce the body's oxygen need.

Illness, trauma, and tissue damage all increase the need for oxygen, either at a local level or throughout the body, as rebuilding and healing activities within the body are stimulated. Medications such as stimulants or thyroid preparations increase the cellular metabolic rate. The effects of stressors, such as fear, continuous noise, sleep deprivation, and anxiety, tend to increase the metabolic rate of the cells and increase oxygen needs. Pain is another stressor that causes chemical changes within the body to increase cellular metabolism and oxygen needs. Pain may also interfere with normal breathing patterns as the person overrides medullary control and does not breathe deeply, sigh, or cough because of the pain. This voluntary shallow breathing decreases the tidal volume during inspiration and decreases the air flow to the alveoli.

Factors That May Interfere with Oxygen Need Satisfaction

This section will look at problems affecting oxygen supply to the cells in four basic areas:

1. Problems related to ventilation
2. Problems with alveolar/blood diffusion
3. Problems related to transport of oxygen and carbon dioxide
4. Problems related to regulation of oxygen supply

Problems Related to Ventilation

Obstructions.   Obstruction to air flow into and out of the lungs will interfere with alveolar air supply in varying degrees. A complete obstruction eliminates all air flow, and hypoxemia (lowered PaO_2 of the arterial blood) develops rapidly. Food lodged in the trachea or further down in the lungs causes obstruction to air flow and may result in death if not removed within several minutes. The Heimlich maneuver for removing foreign material aspirated into the lungs is presented later in this chapter under "Nursing Interventions." Tumors of the respiratory tract will also obstruct air flow progressively as they grow. Swelling of the lining of the respiratory tract can obstruct air flow because the airways become narrower and, therefore, offer more resistance to the flow of air. This is the problem in childhood croup, asthma, and inhalation of irritating chemicals or hot smoky air by victims of a fire. The tissues of the respiratory tract may become so swollen that air flow is completely blocked, and an artificial opening (*tracheostomy*) below the obstruction becomes necessary.

Secretions may collect in the airways and obstruct the flow of air to and from the alveoli. Normally, a "mucus escalator" works within the lungs to move secretions and foreign particles up toward the pharynx where they can be coughed out or swallowed, keeping the airway clear. The airways are lined with small hair structures, called cilia, and epithelial glands which secrete mucus. The mucus traps foreign particles not trapped by the mucus and hairs in the nose. The cilia move the mucus up toward the pharynx. If excess mucus is produced, as in bronchitis, the airways will be narrowed by the added secretions.

Diseases such as asthma, emphysema, and bronchitis are grouped together under the term *chronic obstructive pulmonary diseases* (COPD), because they all involve some form of obstruction or increased resistance to the normal flow of air during inspiration or expiration or both. Emphysema is a progressive disease where air flow is obstructed by narrowing of the bronchioles. This leads to air being trapped in the alveoli, which can become overstretched and eventually rupture. This reduces diffusion of gases with the blood.

Atelectasis.   Atelectasis is a condition in which the alveoli collapse and fail to reopen during inspiration. This obstructs air flow into the alveoli, and since they fail to inflate, no gas exchange can be made with the blood. The more alveoli that are affected by atelectasis, the more obstruction to air flow develops at the alveolar level. If enough alveoli fail to inflate, the body's oxygen supply can be greatly reduced since no gas exchange is taking place within the affected part of the lung. Atelectasis is a very common postoperative complication following abdominal or chest surgery since the patient avoids breathing deeply because of the pain. Periodic deep breathing is essential to keep all alveoli open. Shallow breathing and failure to take periodic deep breaths, both common in the postoperative patient, can lead to progressive atelectasis in a matter of hours. The occasional sustained maximum lung inflation (SMI), occurring with a sigh or a yawn, along with normal volumes of inspired air (500 cc) during each breath, are effective in preventing major atelectasis. One hour of shallow breathing without any sustained maximum lung inflations is sufficient to cause microatelectasis and decreased arterial oxygen concentrations.

Physical Problems.   Other problems with ventilation can be caused by interferences with the physical aspects of ventilation. If the chest is unable to expand or the lung loses its elastic properties, the normal volume changes within the lung will be affected. Air accidently entering the intrapleural space will eliminate the negative pressure which normally causes the lung to expand with the chest. When this negative pressure is lost, the natural elastic properties of the lung plus the atmospheric pressure between the chest wall and the lung will cause the lung to collapse. Trauma to the chest, stab wounds, or rupture of alveoli with air escaping into the intrapleural space (*pneumothorax*) will cause the lung to collapse.

Problems with Alveolar-Blood Diffusion of Gases

Anything that affects the concentration of gases within the alveoli or constriction of capillaries circulating blood around them will interfere with the diffusion of gases from the one to the other. Inadequate oxygen in the blood as measured by blood PaO_2 is called *hypoxemia*. Inadequate oxygen at the cellular level is called *hypoxia*. These two conditions may occur together or separately. The person with emphysema has altered gas diffusion because of a loss of some of the normal elasticity of the lung. The lung does not recoil as it should during expiration, so air tends to be trapped within the lung. This air has already been involved in cellular respirations and is high in carbon dioxide. The inspired air mixes with this trapped air during inspiration so the emphysema patient has air in the lungs that is higher in CO_2 levels. This elevated CO_2 concentration in the alveoli increases the level of arterial CO_2; an elevated arterial CO_2 ($PaCO_2$) is called *hypercapnia*. Exposure to smoke and other air pollutants over time is thought to be the primary causative agent in this disease.

Pulmonary consolidation is a condition in which the alveoli become partially filled with fluid or become solidified with secretions and debris from pulmonary infections or tumor growth. This prevents air from entering the alveoli or, in less severe cases, compromises diffusion across the alveolar membrane. Inflammation from pneumonia, tumor growth, and pulmonary edema (fluid in the alveoli) secondary to heart or kidney disease can reduce or eliminate diffusion of gases across the alveolar membrane.

Gas exchange will be reduced if the capillaries surrounding the alveoli are not well perfused. Heart disease, pulmonary vessel vasoconstriction, and pulmonary emboli (clots lodged in a pulmonary vessel) can all decrease the blood flow to the alveoli in varying degrees.

Another factor affecting the diffusion of gases within the alveoli and the blood is the concentration of gases in the inspired air. Excessive amounts of oxygen in the inspired air will increase the concentration of oxygen in arterial blood. This may be a necessary therapy to bring the oxygen concentration in arterial blood up to normal values in patients with compromised lung function or heart disease. Excess oxygen in the inspired air can lead to oxygen toxicity if PaO_2 becomes greatly elevated beyond normal levels. This is termed *hyperoxia*. Oxygen becomes toxic to the human cells at PO_2 values double the normal or in the 200 mm Hg range. Excessive oxygen interferes with the normal chemical reactions occurring within the cells. It also promotes vasoconstriction, thus decreasing blood flow to the cells. Local damage occurs within the lung tissue with the chronic use of oxygen concentrations above 21 percent (normal room air). Pulmonary edema results from overuse of therapeutic oxygen concentrations and is termed chronic O_2 toxicity. People who use oxygen under pressure such as deep sea divers, astronauts, and patients receiving hyperbaric oxygen treatments run the risk of acute oxygen toxicity. Visual disturbances and ocular damage (retrolental fibroplasia) also occur in the preterm newborn exposed to oxygen concentrations that raise the PaO_2 above normal. The high O_2 levels damage the maturing optic nerve and retina in the preterm newborn. The adult may experience pulmonary congestion and edema, twitching, and visual disturbances with elevated PaO_2 levels. As the PaO_2 rises in the blood, seizures and coma may result.

High levels of carbon monoxide (CO) in the inspired air will decrease the amount of oxygen that diffuses into the blood. The hemoglobin molecule has a greater affinity for CO than for O_2 by 210 times. This means that the hemoglobin molecule picks up CO but not O_2. The O_2 is still dissolved in the plasma of the blood, but this normally accounts for only 2 percent of the oxygen available to the cells. The PaO_2 remains normal in CO inhalation, so no hypoxemia is present. However, CO inhalation is a form of hypoxia because there is inadequate oxygen at the cellular level.

There may also be cases where the O_2 concentration of inspired air is less than 21 percent, and this will reduce the concentration differences between oxygen in the pulmonary capillaries and the alveoli. This results in less oxygen diffusing into the blood and a lowered PaO_2. In this case, hypoxemia and cellular hypoxia are present.

Problems Related to Transport of Gases

In this category fall all problems associated with an ineffective pump to circulate blood, vascular problems affecting the integrity and function of the blood vessels, and abnormal or inadequate blood formation or volume.

Problems Related to the Blood as a Transport Medium for Gases.   *Anemic hypoxia* occurs when there is an inadequate number of RBCs, an inadequate amount of hemoglobin, or ineffective RBCs to transport the gases to and from the cells. Competition for the hemoglobin molecule by CO was already discussed as affecting the amount of oxygen that diffuses into the blood. Blood loss temporarily reduces the number of RBCs in the circulating blood volume. The fluid part of the blood is replaced quickly, but RBCs are not as rapidly replaced. When the number of RBCs is significantly reduced, the ability to carry oxygen is diminished. Blood replacement may be necessary to restore this oxygen-carrying capacity. A rapid, massive blood loss associated with shock results in an inadequate volume of blood to circulate to all areas of the body, and vasoconstriction begins in various areas of the body in an effort to keep the heart and brain perfused with blood. The local hypoxia resulting from this vasoconstriction may be so severe that cell damage and death of tissues result. This is a form of *ischemic hypoxia* because too little blood is reaching the tissues to meet their oxygen needs, even though the blood may have a normal PaO_2.

Anemia is associated with a lower-than-normal hemoglobin or hematrocrit blood measurement or both, since the problem relates to inadequate numbers of RBCs or hemoglobin. *Sickle cell anemia* affects the hemoglobin molecule, interfering with its ability to carry oxygen. The red blood cells break apart or clump together, obstructing capillary blood flow and resulting in tissue ischemia. *Ischemia* is a local reduction in the number of red blood cells reaching an area of the body because of an obstructed blood flow. Anemia is also associated with leukemia and Hodgkin's disease, an inadequate diet, use of some medications, kidney disease (decreased erythropoietin), bone marrow damage from drugs, radiation, or lead poisoning, some gastrointestinal problems affecting absorption of nutrients, and hereditary factors.

Cardiac Problems—The Pump.   Cardiac problems may arise from various causes, but the end result, affecting oxygen supply, is inadequate pumping of blood through either or both of the two circuits (pulmonary and systemic). Inadequate pumping of blood into the pulmonary system leads to lowered PO_2 and elevated PCO_2 in arterial blood. This also occurs when there are defects in the heart or circulatory system which allow mixing of blood from the two circuits. For example, when an atrial septal defect exists (an opening between the two atria of the heart through the septum which normally separates them). Heart damage from tissue ischemia after a heart attack is a leading cause of death in adults in the middle and later years.

Vessel Problems—The Route.   Vascular problems affect the blood vessels by causing obstruction of flow. Any decreased delivery of blood to the tissues has the potential for creating hypoxia at the cellular level. Disease processes that narrow the blood vessels and make them more rigid will reduce the volume of blood delivered to tissues supplied by the affected vessels. Narrowing will also raise the blood pressure since there is more resistance to flow. Coronary artery disease is a major problem for people in middle age and beyond. The vessels become narrowed by the deposition of plaque along the inner walls. This process, called atherosclerosis, can lead to complete obstruction of a major coronary vessel supplying oxygen to the heart. When the oxygen needs are suddenly unmet, the person experiences a myocardial infarction (heart attack). If a large area of the heart is without its oxygen supply for a significant time, the cells begin to die and the total heart function is jeopardized. If enough tissue becomes hypoxic, the heart ceases functioning and the person experiences a cardiac arrest (cessation of the heart's pumping action). This type of hypoxia is ischemic, since the problem lies with the vessels supplying certain tissues rather than with the blood quality.

Inadequate perfusion of the brain may also occur when blood vessels are affected by atherosclerosis. Loss of short-term memory, confusion, uncoordinated movements, and loss of control in regulating and integrating body functions and conscious thought may all be affected by cerebral hypoxia. A complete obstruction to blood flow in particular areas of the brain is called a cerebrovascular accident (CVA), commonly known as a stroke. The cause of this hypoxia is local vascular ischemia. The problems created by a CVA relate to the amount and type of tissue involved and the extent of the damage done.

Forty million Americans have some form of heart disease requiring medical or surgical treatment. An estimated 60 million Americans have high blood pressure, reflecting an increased resistance to the flow of blood in the arteries. Americans have 1.5 million myocardial infarctions each year, with two-thirds of the victims surviving. One million people in the United States die of heart disorders or stroke-related problems each year. The basic problem in most of these disorders is unmet cellular oxygen needs (hypoxia) because of problems with the vessels supplying blood to an area of the body (ischemia).

Problems Related to Regulation of Oxygen Supply

In this category are problems affecting the neural and chemical control systems of the cardiovascular system and the respiratory system. Trauma or damage to systems delivering input to the brain will affect the medulla's ability to maintain normal cellular oxygen supply and optimal vascular functioning. Damage to the brain from disease, hypoxia, or trauma may affect the ability of the medulla to regulate lung function, heart activity, and blood vessel diameter for routing of blood.

Problems in the nervous conduction system of the heart may result in altered contraction patterns and failure to respond to medullary control. The sinoatrial node within the right atrium of the heart is the site of initiation of impulses causing contraction of the atrium followed by contraction of the ventricles. (See Figure 20-9.) Without a normally functioning SA node, the heart contracts in an uncoordinated manner and becomes ineffective in pumping blood through the body. A pacemaker is a battery-operated device that provides the initiating electrical impulse to the heart, causing atrial contraction followed by ventricular contraction. This external electrical signal from the pacemaker replaces the ineffective SA node function. The electrical signal triggers contractions at a set rate to maintain a heart rate in the normal range. Some 500,000 Americans have had significant problems with their SA node in the heart to require implantation of artificial pacemakers. The new battery systems last for approximately five years.

Trauma or disease within the spinal cord may sever the nervous connections between the medulla and the nerves communicating with the muscles of respiration. Spinal cord damage at the level of the third cervical vertebrae, as occurs in a broken neck, will terminate impulses to the diaphragm, and the victim will cease

breathing (*respiratory arrest*). Some forms of polio paralyze the muscles of the body, rendering them incapable of responding to nervous control. Paralysis of the diaphragm by this disease required the use of a mechanical device called an iron lung, which created pressure changes around the chest to cause chest expansion and relaxation in order to maintain ventilation.

General anesthesia and spinal anesthesia for surgical procedures also affect medullary control and muscle response to nervous stimuli. The muscles of respiration may become completely paralyzed during anesthesia, and artificial ventilation may be temporarily required. Abuse of narcotics can also affect the control of ventilation, possibly resulting in a respiratory arrest if blood levels become excessively elevated.

Sudden infant death syndrome (SIDS) is another tragedy created by a failure in the normal controls of ventilation. In this condition, the infant stops breathing during sleep. The theories related to causes of SIDS are all speculative at this point and range from hypoxia to the fetus during a critical time in the pregnancy to some form of allergic reaction from the immunizations infants receive beginning at two or three months of age.

Hypertension, which is a blood pressure above the upper limit of normal (usually considered to be 140/90 mm Hg), is a problem of increased resistance to the flow of blood in the arteries. This increased pressure is caused by a combination of factors such as decreased elasticity within the vessel walls, increased vasoconstriction, and atherosclerosis causing narrowed vessel lumens. Most often, there is no specific disease or problem, such as kidney disease, causing the elevated blood pressure. High blood pressure is a significant contribut-

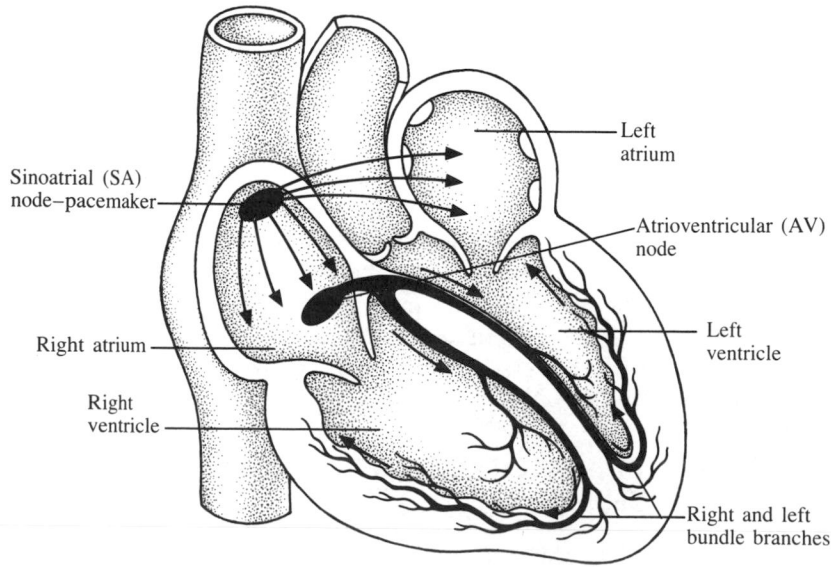

Figure 20-9. The conduction system of the heart. Impulses originating in the SA node spread across both atria, causing them to contract. Impulses reach the AV node from the SA node and spread through the ventricles, causing them to contract following atrial contraction.

ing factor in 68 percent of all first heart attacks and 75 percent of first strokes (Ramsey, 1982). Elevated blood pressure can cause damage to the capillary system throughout the body. This leads to damage in specific organs and interferes with normal exchange of gas and nutrients at the cellular level. During pregnancy, elevated blood pressure can result in retarded fetal growth, abortion, or stillbirth. The term "essential hypertension" is applied to the condition of elevated blood pressure with no specific diagnosable cause and is the most common form of high blood pressure. According to Ramsey (1982), "In most cases of well established hy-

pertension, the major abnormality is believed to be increased peripheral blood flow resistance due to arteriole diameters that remain abnormally reduced." Nervous and chemical control of the vessels causing this vasoconstriction seems to regulate the blood pressure at an elevated pressure for unknown reasons. High blood pressure can exist for a long time, causing vascular and tissue damage before the person is aware of any symptoms. Regular monitoring of the blood pressure and interpretation by qualified health personnel are important in maintaining optimum health and ultimately in meeting cellular oxygen needs.

Assessment of Oxygen Need Satisfaction

In this section of the chapter, the processes of assessment, planning, intervention, and evaluation will be applied to patients experiencing potential or identified problems in meeting their oxygen needs.

Data Indicating Satisfaction of Oxygen Need

Objective Data. The following data, for an apparently healthy adult, are objective measurements indicating satisfaction of oxygen need:

Respiration in normal range of 12 to 18 breaths each minute (Nursing Skill 20–1)
Respiratory pattern is regular in rhythm; breathing appears effortless
Normal lung sounds heard over chest and back

Lung Sounds

1. *Vesicular sounds* are heard over the normal lung and are created by the movement of air in and out of the smaller airways and alveoli of the lung. (See Figure

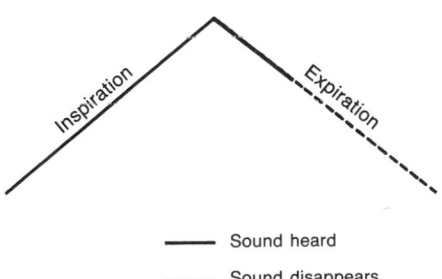

Figure 20–10. Normal vesicular sounds. Sounds heard during entire inspiration and first third of expiration.

20–10.) Inspiration is accompanied by continuous vesicular sounds similar to a low-pitched, rustling sound. Vesicular sounds during expiration normally last during the first third of the expiration, making inspiration sound much longer than expiration.

2. *Bronchial sounds* are normally heard over the larger airways and are created by air movement in and out of the trachea and larger bronchi. Bronchial sounds are harsher than vesicular sounds and are heard higher up over the chest and back and more over the midline. Listening with a stethoscope over the trachea of a healthy adult will give the learner a loud version of bronchial sounds.

3. *Vocal resonance* is heard with a stethoscope while listening over the chest and back as the person repeats the numbers "99." In normal lungs, the sound seems to be produced at the diaphragm (flat part) of the stethoscope. The sound is quite audible, but the numbers being repeated are unclear.

4. *Absence of adventitious lung sounds* (no added breath sounds during inspiration or expiration).

ASSESSING LUNG SOUNDS. When auscultating lung sounds, the following suggestions may prove helpful. Always begin by explaining to the patient that you are listening to the movement of air in the lungs to help you assess adequacy of the air flow and any problems that may interfere with the patient's oxygen supply. Ask the patient to breath through the mouth to avoid any possible sounds from the nasal passages confusing your interpretation of lung sounds. Have the patient breathe in a regular pattern, at a comfortable rate, and slightly deeper than normal. Use the diaphragm (flat part) of the stethoscope during auscultation and hold it firmly to the skin, without pushing it to the point that you are leaving marks on the patient's skin. Warming the stethoscope by holding it between your hands before placing

Nursing Skill 20–1.   Taking Respiration

The respiratory rate is the number of ventilations occurring each minute. One inspiration plus one expiration equals one respiration, more accurately called a ventilation. Respiratory rates may be over 100 breaths each minute or as slow as 12 breaths or less each minute, depending on the age and health status of the patient. Respirations can be assessed by visual inspection, watching the chest rise and fall. The respiratory rate can also be obtained by auscultation of air movement in the lungs while listening with a stethescope. Respirations can be counted by palpation if the nurse places a hand on the chest and feels the movement. Most patients have their respiratory rate assessed by visual inspection because this method makes the patient least conscious of what the nurse is doing. When people know someone is counting their respirations, they find it difficult to breathe normally and will often alter the rate and depth of their breathing efforts. For this reason, the nurse tries to assess respirations without making the patient aware of the observations of rate, depth, pattern or character and rhythm. The *rate* is the number of breaths in one minute. The *depth* of respirations refers to the volume of air being exchanged with each breath, compared to the normal volume of 500 cc per breath at rest. Depth is usually described as normal, shallow, or deep. *Rhythm* of respirations refers to the time interval between each breath. When respirations are regular, the time interval is similar between each breath. When respirations are irregular, this time interval varies. The *character* or pattern of the respirations refers to an observable, repetitive pattern of respirations. These patterns are described at the end of this nursing skill and are used in documenting respiratory character. The character of normal respirations is termed *eupnea*. Table 20–3 defines words used to describe respirations. Table 20–4 identifies factors affecting respirations.

Table 20–3. **Words Commonly Used to Describe Respirations**

Eupnea—normal respirations: normal rate, depth, and rhythm for age

Dyspnea—difficult or *labored* breathing; may be accompanied by other signs of labored breathing such as nasal flaring, retractions of the skin around the ribs and above and below the sternum, noisy breathing, and increased rate of breathing

Tachypnea—increased rate of breathing above normal for age group

Bradypnea—decreased rate of breathing below normal for age group

Apnea—absence of breathing; may be periodic so respirations occur with periods of apnea lasting 10 seconds or more

*Hyperventilation—*increase in *rate* and *depth* of respirations

*Hypoventilation—*decreased *rate* and *depth* of respirations

Hyperpnea—increased depth of breathing with normal rate

*Cheyne-Stokes breathing—*a cycle of ventilation with increasing rate and depth to a point, then decreasing rate and depth, followed by a period of apnea (20 seconds or more). The breathing cycles last approximately 30 to 40 seconds before each apnea episode; related to increased intracranial pressure, congestive heart failure, renal disease, meningitis, and drug overdose.

*Kussmaul's—*increased rate and depth; appears labored and similar to panting; related to renal failure and metabolic acidosis

*Biot's—*similar to Cheyne-Stokes breathing because of intermittent periods of apnea; breathing episodes are of the same depth; related to central nervous system problems

Table 20–4. **Factors Affecting the Respiratory Rate**

Respirations decrease with age until adulthood.
Severe hypothermia decreases respiratory and pulse rates.
Reduced hydrogen ion concentrations and low CO_2 in the blood tend to decrease the rate and depth of respirations to decrease the alkalosis.
Emotions increase respiratory rate.
Discomfort and pain increase respiratory rate.
Temperature elevation increases respiratory rate.
Elevated hydrogen ion concentration and CO_2 in the blood increase rate and depth of respirations to decrease the acidosis.
Illness, tissue damage and infections tend to increase respiratory rate.
Reduced blood volume and anemia increase respirations and pulse.
Pregnancy increases respiratory rate.

Equipment Needed

A watch with a second counter
A stethoscope if respirations are to be auscultated.

Preparation for Taking Respiration

1. Determine need for measuring the respiratory rate based on the patient's condition or symptoms, a physician's order, or the recommendations of a more experienced nurse. Generally, whenever the pulse is measured, the respirations are checked, since oxygen need satisfaction is dependent on both the respiratory and cardiovascular systems. Patients in unstable condition, febrile (elevated body temperature), strongly medicated, or recovering from anesthesia require frequent monitoring of their respiratory status for signs of hypoventilation (inadequate ventilation in rate and depth).
2. Make sure the patient is resting and has not just been involved in muscular activity that would increase the pulse rate and respiratory rate.
3. Wash hands.
4. Explain procedure as necessary to patient (explaining that you are going to take the patient's pulse, without mentioning that you will be counting respirations after taking the pulse, is useful in preventing the patient from altering respiratory rate).
5. Provide privacy as necessary.

Procedure	Explanation
1. Take the pulse for 30 seconds. (See Nursing Skill 20–2.)	1. Pulse and respirations together provide better data on oxygenation than either alone.
2. Continue to hold the patient's wrist and count respirations for 30 seconds (1 minute if rate irregular or rapid).	2. Patient unaware respirations being assessed; normal pattern preserved; accuracy increases when counting rate over longer time (1 minute).
3. Note rate, depth, and character.	3. Indicates possible problems with ventilation or O_2 supply to tissues.
4. Leave patient in comfortable position.	4. Communicates respect for individual, increases patient comfort.
5. Wash hands.	5. Decreases spread of microorganisms.
6. Document and report data on pulse and respirations as requested by institution; report any unusual data to responsible nurse and nursing instructor; recheck any unusual findings. Include rate, depth, rhythm, and character if other than eupnea.	6. Communication among members of the health team; legal responsibility; verifies competent nursing care.

it on the patient's skin increases comfort. Listen to the front of the chest with the patient lying in the supine position (on the back) or leaning back in a slightly reclined sitting position (high Fowler's position). Listen to the back of the chest with the patient in a sitting position if possible or on the side if the patient is unable to sit. Auscultate over the anterior, posterior, and lateral chest walls, moving from side to side in order to compare lung sounds in the same area on the left and right lung. Try to have the room as noise-free as possible during auscultation. Be aware that shivering by the patient can block lung sounds, and moving the stethoscope over a patient's hairy chest may sound like extra (*adventitious*) lung sounds.

PALPATION AND PERCUSSION. Palpation of the chest is another assessment activity the nurse may use to collect data on ventilatory status. The chest normally expands out and up during inhalation. In an adult male with normal ventilatory function, an expansion of 6 to 9 cm or 2.4 to 3.6 inches measured over the nipple line is expected. When the patient has exhaled maximally, place your hands around the patient's chest with the thumbs touching at the lower edge of the sternum. You can now assess lung expansion during inhalation. Ask the patient then to inhale as deeply as possible and watch for separation of your thumbs as the chest expands. The movement and expansion should be equal on both sides of the chest. Observe for any indications of pain while palpating a maximum inhalation, and question the patient about any pain with deep breaths. The trachea is also palpated in the suprasternal notch, and it should be located in the midline.

Assessment of vibrations in the lung is called *tactile fremitus* and is another type of palpation. While the patient repeats the numbers "99," place your hand on the chest wall and you should feel a tickling sensation from the normal lung. Increased or decreased fremitus may indicate lung problems. Normally, there is no fremitus felt over the heart.

Percussion of the chest wall can also provide information on lung integrity. It will help determine if the lung is full of air as it should be or has fluid-filled areas or areas with solid material (*consolidation*), such as occur in tumors. The third fingers of both hands are used to percuss the chest. The nondominant hand is placed on the chest, and the third finger of the dominant hand briskly taps the third finger of the hand on the patient's chest. The tapping finger is swung from the wrist rather than the elbow or knuckle. The sound created by tapping will travel 5 to 7 cm or 2 to 2.8 inches into the chest and can be helpful in detecting lung problems up to this depth. The patient's chest is percussed at approximately 2-inch intervals over the front, down to the level of the top of the sternum and also across the back. There is normally a resonant sound in healthy lung tissue. This sound will vary from person to person and in different areas within the same person. The area of the clavicle is not usually percussed because it produces a dull sound. If this same dull sound is heard over other areas of the chest, it may indicate that fluid rather than air is filling the alveoli and small airways. Consolidation of lung tissue will also decrease the resonance in an area when compared to the resonance in the same area on the other lung. *Hyperresonance* occurs when an area filled with excess air is percussed. It sounds like the sound made when you percuss a puffed cheek, and it may indicate problems such as an air cavity in a patient with emphysema or a pneumothorax.

In summary, objective data from lung assessments indicating satisfaction of oxygen needs would include:

- Normal vesicular and bronchial lung sounds, no adventitious lung sounds
- Normal chest expansion of several inches during maximum inspiration
- Midline position of trachea in suprasternal notch
- Normal tactile fremitus felt over chest
- Normal resonance from percussion of the chest

Other objective data indicating a patient's ability to meet oxygen needs are:

Absence of a cough
Ability to speak at a normal pace and not have to stop to catch a breath
Normal body temperature in the range of 97° to 99° F, orally (36.2–37.2°C)
Hemoglobin of 12 to 14.2 in women and 14 to 16.5 gm/100 ml in men
Hematocrit of 37 to 48 percent in women and 45 to 52 percent in men
Normal skin color with pink mucous membranes
Alert and oriented to time, place, and person
Coordinated body movements
A pulse rate of 60 to 90 beats per minute (Nursing Skill 20–2)
Blood pressures in the range of 90/60 to 140/80 mm Hg (Nursing Skill 20–3)
A pulse rhythm that is regular
A pulse quality that is palpated as strong at the radial site
Pulse to respiratory rate ratio of 5:1
Apical and radial pulse identical in rate and rhythm
Urine output of at least 30 ml per hour (indicates adequate hydration and perfusion of the kidney)
Normal electrocardiogram (see Figure 20–12)
Normal heart sounds

Nursing Skill 20-2 **Taking a Pulse**

There are two ways of taking a pulse. One is by using a stethoscope and listening over the apex of the heart. This is called an *apical pulse*. The other way of taking a pulse involves palpation of an artery between your fingers and a bony surface within the patient. By trapping the pulsing artery between your fingers and a hard surface, the heart rate can be determined in a peripheral site. The pulse that is palpated at any of a number of sites on the body is caused by the contraction of the left ventricle which forces a bolus of blood into the aorta. The aorta distends to accommodate the surge of blood and then recoils as the ventricles relax and the blood moves on down the artery. The surge of blood acts on the elastic arteries to cause a wavelike distention and recoil all the way down the artery. This is what is palpated as the pulse. The pulse is normally easily palpated and feels strong and regular. Variations from this may indicate problems with perfusion of tissues because of conditions in the cardiovascular system and should be reported and documented. Table 20-5 presents words used to describe different types of pulses. Table 20-6 identifies factors affecting the pulse rate.

Equipment Needed
A watch with a second indicator
A stethoscope for apical pulse auscultation

Table 20-5. **Words Used to Describe a Pulse**

Regular—interval between the beats is equal
Irregular—the inerval between each beat is uneven
Tachycardia—pulse (heart rate) is above normal range for patient's stage of growth and development (150 beats per min is normal for a newborn but is considered tachycardia in an adult)
Bradycardia—pulse rate is below normal range for stage of growth and development; slow heart rate
Weak, feeble, thready—all indicate a reduced force or volume in a peripheral pulse; easily obliterated by pressure
Bounding—indicates an increased force or volume of a peripheral pulse; difficult to obliterate by pressure
Bigeminal pulse—pulse has occasional premature beats, resulting in a shorter interval between beats followed by a longer interval. Beats in groups of two with pause before next beat
Paradoxical pulse—the force or volume of the peripheral pulse is reduced when the patient inhales (if pronounced, may indicate critical situation called cardiac tamponade where blood fills the sac around the heart, the pericardial sac, and interferes with the pumping action of the heart)
Chaotic pulse—the pulse is completely irregular with no pattern to the irregularity
Sinus arrhythmia—pulse speeds up at peak of inspiration and slows down as the person exhales; common in children; disappears if pulse taken while child holds breath
Intermittent pulse—a pulse with normal rhythm intermixed with periods of irregular rhythm
Pulse deficit—the difference in number of beats each minute between the apical and radial (or peripheral) pulse when measured simultaneously; apical rate is always higher if there is a pulse deficit
Apical-radial pulse—one nurse takes the radial pulse, while another nurse simultaneously takes apical pulse; taken whenever pulse rates are known or suspected of being different. Record pulse deficit in chart

Table 20-6. **Factors Affecting the Pulse Rate**

Increased emotions (fear, excitement, anxiety, joy) increase pulse rate	Drugs—stimulants will increase rate; depressants will decrease rate
Pain increases pulse rate	Hypoxemia and hypoxia increase pulse rate
Pulse rate decreases with age until adulthood	Illness, injury, large wounds tend to increase pulse rate
Exercise and physical activity increase pulse rate	Bed rest—over time, bed rest increases the pulse rate
Elevated body temperature increases pulse rate	Obesity increases pulse rate
Eating a meal increases pulse rate	Pregnancy increases pulse rate

Preparation for Taking a Pulse

1. Determining the need for measuring a patient's pulse may be an independent nursing decision based on the patient's condition, or it may be ordered by the physician or another nurse on a set schedule, such as every four hours (q4h). Whenever there is any change in the patient's condition based on objective or subjective data, take the pulse, blood pressure, respiration, and temperature since many changes will be reflected in these measurements. Remember that an order for vital signs (pulse, respirations, BP, and temperature) on a set schedule is not based on the patient's current condition but on a previous evaluation. It is the responsibility of the nurse caring for the patient at the time to decide if more frequent measurements of pulse and other vital signs are needed. Generally, a pulse is taken at least twice a day on a hospitalized patient and may be taken as often as every 5 to 15 minutes if the patient is in an unstable condition, such as upon return from the recovery room following surgery.

   Determine which method is appropriate for taking a patient's pulse. Generally, most pulses are taken at the radial site on the wrist. This minimizes exposure of the patient and is usually very easy to palpate. Figure 20-11 indicates the various sites available for taking a pulse. If one site is unavailable because of injury or treatments, select another site. If an apical pulse is needed, it is usually specifically ordered. If the order is for vital signs or pulse on a set schedule, the palpation of an available artery is the usual method chosen rather than taking an apical pulse. If you have any trouble counting or palpating a peripheral pulse, take the apical pulse to verify the accuracy of your measurement. Also, if there is any irregularity in the pulse, take an apical pulse. Sometimes the heart will contract abnormally, and an extra beat will be heard at the apex but will not be palpable on a peripheral pulse site. This is called an *apical-radial deficit* and indicates a potential problem with the pumping effectiveness of the heart and should be reported and documented. Newborns and infants have very small arteries, and palpation of peripheral pulses is difficult compared to taking an apical pulse to determine heart rate.

   Anytime a patient has had surgery, trauma, or diagnostic tests that might affect blood flow to certain areas of the body, the pulses below the possible obstruction are palpated to assure circulation of blood to the tissues below. For example, in knee or leg surgery, the pulses in the feet would be palpated to assure continued perfusion. Normal color and temperature would also be assessed as an indication of oxygen need satisfaction to the area. Invasive treatments or diagnostics involving the femoral artery would be an indication to the nurse for frequent monitoring of pulses in the foot to confirm that no obstruction to blood flow in the leg was occurring as a postprocedure complication.

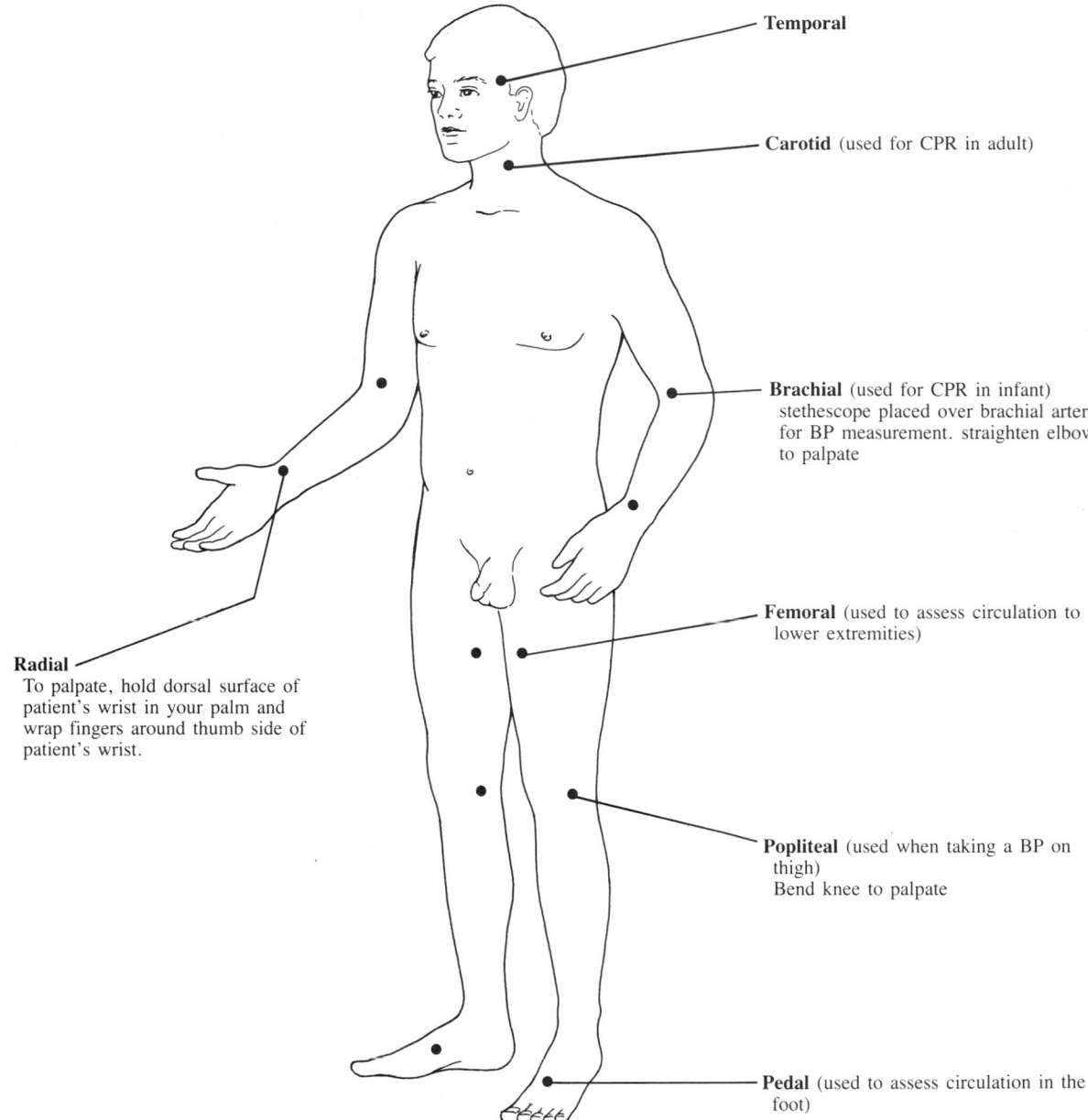

Temporal

Carotid (used for CPR in adult)

Brachial (used for CPR in infant) stethescope placed over brachial artery for BP measurement. straighten elbow to palpate

Femoral (used to assess circulation to lower extremities)

Radial
To palpate, hold dorsal surface of patient's wrist in your palm and wrap fingers around thumb side of patient's wrist.

Popliteal (used when taking a BP on thigh) Bend knee to palpate

Pedal (used to assess circulation in the foot)

Figure 20–11. Peripheral pulse sites.

2. Make sure the patient has been resting for several minutes since exercise increases pulse rate.
3. Clean off the stethoscope diaphragm to reduce transfer of microorganisms.
4. Wash hands.
5. Explain procedure to the patient.
6. Provide privacy as necessary (apical pulse should not be taken over clothing, peripheral pulse should not be palpated over clothing).
7. Eliminate as much room noise as possible if you are auscultating the apical pulse.

Procedure	Explanation
Radial or Peripheral Pulse	
1. Place three fingers over the pulsing artery and hold hand steady on body area.	1. The nurse's thumb has a pulse of its own which may confuse the measurement of a patient's pulse.
2. Apply light pressure until the pulse is palpated and maintain pressure.	2. Excessive pressure will occlude the blood flow and eliminate the pulse. Inadequate pressure on the artery will make the pulse difficult to feel.
3. Count pulse for 1 min if rate is rapid, irregular, or very slow. Count for 30 sec and double the number if pulse regular and seems to be of an average rate.	3. Degree of error is reduced by counting the pulse for longer times.
4. Note the rhythm and volume of the pulse.	4. Indication of possible problems with cardiovascular system and tissue perfusion.
5. Leave the patient in a comfortable position.	5. Communicates respect for individual and provides comfort.
6. Document pulse rate as desired by institution; report any abnormal findings to the responsible nurse and nursing instructor.	6. Communicates data for further assessment; legal responsibility; verifies competent nursing care.
Apical Pulse	
1. Warm diaphragm with hands.	1. Increases patient comfort.
2. Place over the apex of the heart (just below left nipple and 3 inches to left of sternum).	2. Site of maximum sound for assessing rate.
3. Count the rate for 1 min.	3. Maximum accuracy.
4. Assess rhythm and any unusual sounds.	4. Indication of possible cardiac problems.
5. Leave patient in comfortable position.	5. Communicates respect for individual; protects modesty and provides comfort.
6. Document pulse rate, rhythm, and any additional sound as indicated by institution; report any unusual findings to the responsible nurse and nursing instructor.	6. Communicates data for further assessment; legal responsibility; verifies competent nursing care.

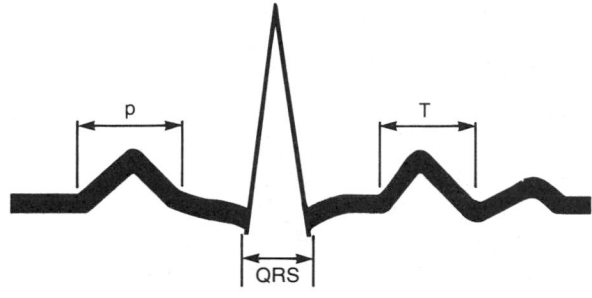

Electrical nervous activity in heart:
p   = Electrical activity moving through atria (depolarization
       precedes contraction of right and left atrium
QRS = Electrical activity moving through ventricles (depolarization
       precedes contraction of right and left ventricles
T   = Recovery period as electrical status in
       ventricles returns to normal (repolarization

Figure 20-12.   Normal electrocardiogram (ECG) tracing for one heartbeat.

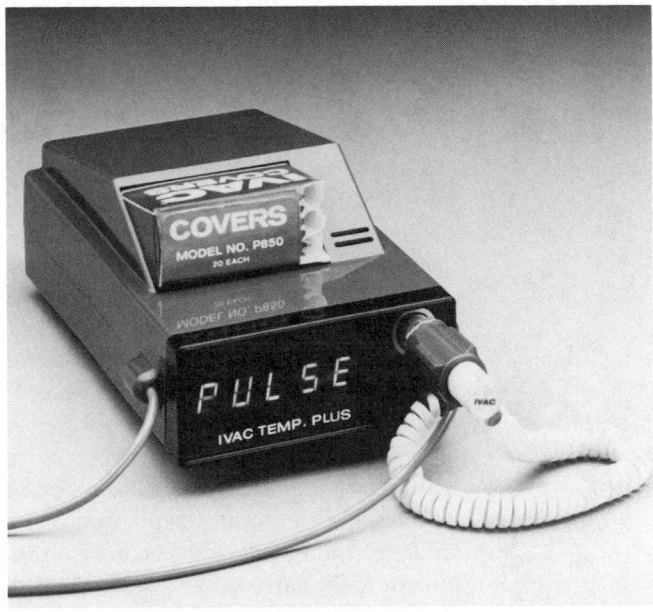

Figure 20-13. Electronic vital signs monitor for measuring pulse and temperature. (Photograph courtesy of the IVAC Corp., San Diego, CA.)

ASSESSING HEART SOUNDS.   Auscultation of heart sounds with a stethoscope is a nursing skill that provides information on the pumping action of the heart and may indicate problems if abnormal sounds are heard. Normal heart sounds are caused by the closing of the valves between the atrium and ventricles at the beginning of systole (a ventricular contraction) and by the closing of the aortic and pulmonary valves during ventricular diastole (relaxation). The first sound is designated S_1 and is the "lub" sound. The second sound is designated S_2 and is the "dub" sound heard through the stethoscope. Both are heard best with the diaphragm of the stethoscope. In adults, there are normally only these two sounds. In children, there are four heart sounds, with S_3 being created by the rapid flow of turbulent blood into the ventricle. It is heard during ventricular diastole and after S_2. It sounds like the rhythm in the word "Ken(S_1)-tuck(S_2)-y(S_3)." The S_4 sound is caused by the flow of turbulent blood into the ventricle from the contracting atrium. It is heard before the S_1 sound in children. It sounds like the rhythm in the word "Ten(S_4)-nes(S_1)-see(S_2)." S_3 is sometimes referred to as ventricular gallop and S_4 as atrial gallop. Both are heard more clearly with the bell part of the stethoscope at the apex of the heart. Additional sounds can be caused by partial obstruction or narrowing of the usual openings through which the blood moves, by an abnormally large blood flow, by abnormal connections between the blood vessels routing blood to the lungs and systemic circulation, or by openings within the heart which are normally closed, as when valves leak or an atrial septal defect is present.

As when listening to lung sounds, explain to the patient what you are doing and why you are doing it before beginning. Provide privacy and warmth for the patient, and eliminate as many noises in the room as possible. Clean and warm the stethoscope before auscultating. Listen for one sound at a time in each of the four areas of the heart indicated in Figure 20-14. The

Stethoscope Placement for Heart Sounds

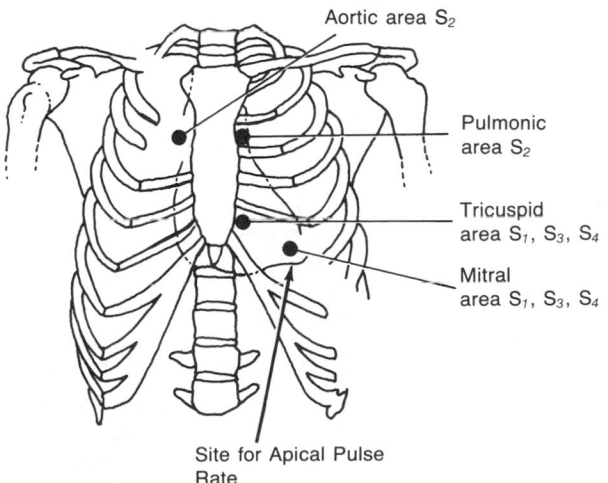

Aortic area S_2

Pulmonic area S_2

Tricuspid area S_1, S_3, S_4

Mitral area S_1, S_3, S_4

Site for Apical Pulse Rate

Figure 20-14. Sites for stethoscope placement when assessing heart rate apically or when auscultating individual heart sounds.

Nursing Skill 20–3   Taking a Blood Pressure

A blood pressure consists of two measurements: a systolic blood pressure and a diastolic blood pressure. The *systolic pressure* is the maximum pressure to which the arteries are subjected during left ventricular contraction of the heart (systole). The *diastolic pressure* is the remaining pressure within the arterial system when the ventricles are relaxed and filling with blood (diastole). A *pulse pressure* is the numerical difference between the systolic and diastolic pressure measurements. Normally, the systolic, diastolic, and pulse pressures are in the ratio of 3:2:1. For example, in a blood pressure of 120/80, the ratio is 120/80/40 or 3:2:1. The pulse pressure is an indicator of adequate cardiac stroke volume. In shock, the systolic blood pressure tends to fall before the diastolic pressure, and this decreases the pulse pressure, indicating an inadequate volume of blood is being pumped from the heart. Perfusion of the tissues with blood is dependent on blood pressure to move the blood through the capillaries and back to the heart. If pressure drops too low, some body tissues will be inadequately perfused and hypoxia will result. If blood pressure is too high, tissue and capillary damage can occur. The effectiveness of the pumping action of the heart and the amount of resistance to blood flow offered by the vascular system will determine blood pressure. As the vessels constrict, blood pressure rises. As the vessels relax and dilate, blood pressure goes down. Table 20–7 identifies factors affecting the blood pressure, and Table 20–8 identifies factors that affect blood pressure measurement.

Equipment Needed
   A stethoscope
   A sphygmomanometer

Several types of sphygmomanometers are available for use by nursing personnel. The mercury gauge contains a column of mercury, and the height of the column corresponding to the first and last sounds heard with the stethoscope gives the BP reading. The aneroid gauge has a needle which points to different numbers when a blood pressure is taken, and it is considered less accurate compared to the mercury gauge,

Table 20–7. **Factors Affecting Blood Pressure**

Exercise increases blood pressure.
Patients who are talking before and during blood pressure recordings tend to have an elevation in BP above their normal value (Sandroff, 1982).
Discomfort, pain, anxiety, stress, and cold tend to increase blood pressure.
Medications may affect blood pressure, causing increases or decreases.
Obesity tends to increase blood pressure.
Changing from a sitting or lying position to a standing position may temporarily lower the systolic blood pressure by 10 to 15 mm Hg, but it should return to normal within several minutes.
Increasing age is related to an increasing blood pressure.
Before menopause, women tend to have lower BPs than men of similar ages.
Black people tend to have a higher incidence of hypertension (50 percent) than Caucasians and Asians; people of Philippine extraction tend to have a BP in the hypertensive range more frequently than Caucasians and less frequently than blacks; people of Asian, Chinese, and Japanese heritages have the lowest incidence of hypertension (Leonard *et al.,* 1981).
Blood pressure taken in lower extremities is usually higher (10 mm Hg).

Table 20-8. **Factors Affecting Blood Pressure Measurement**

Falsely High Measurement

Cuff too narrow for extremity
Cuff applied too loosely to extremity
Tilting mercury manometer away from you
Arm used for measurement is below heart level
Taking blood pressures in rapid succession on the same extremity
Pumping cuff back up after missing a systolic or diastolic reading without letting all the air out and waiting 30 sec
Dropping pressure too rapidly—falsely high diastolic reading
Irregular heart rate—falsely high diastolic reading
Difficulty hearing sound—falsely high diastolic reading
Not placing stethoscope over artery—falsely high diastolic reading

Falsely Low Measurement

Cuff too wide for extremity
Cuff applied too tightly to extremity
Clothing rolled up on arm and constricting blood flow
Tilting the mercury manometer toward you during measurement of BP
Arm used for measurement is above heart level (BP may be as much as 13 to 17 mm Hg lower)
Pressing too hard into the patient's skin with the stethoscope so blood flow is partially obstructed
Putting stethoscope under the cuff during auscultation
Dropping pressure too rapidly—falsely low systolic reading
Irregular heart rate—falsely low systolic reading
Difficulty hearing sounds—falsely low systolic reading
Not placing the stethoscope over the artery—falsely low systolic reading
Not pumping cuff up high enough—falsely low systolic reading

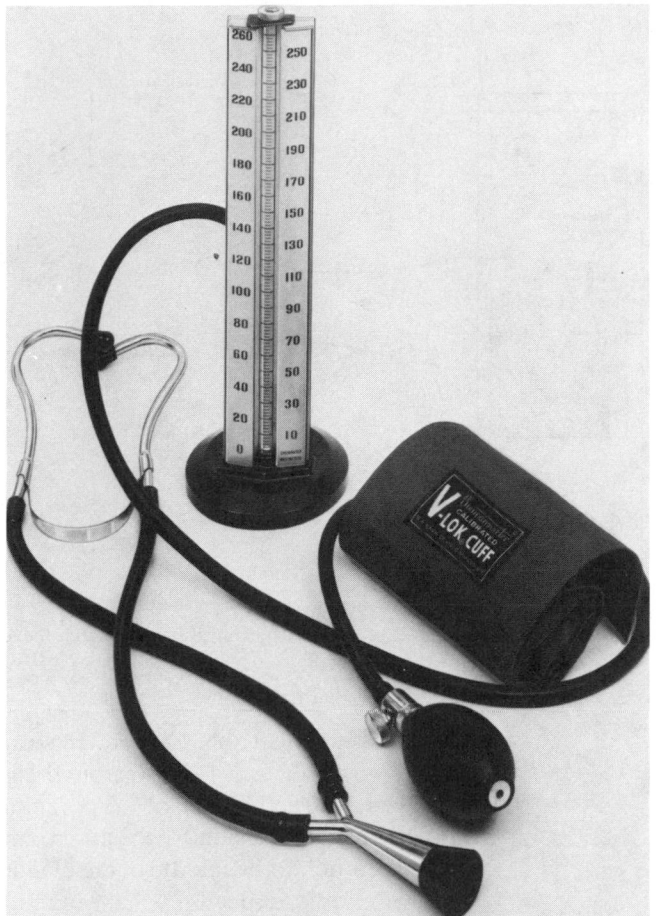

Figure 20-15. Blood pressure equipment. Equipment needed to measure a person's blood pressure includes a stethoscope, a blood pressure cuff of the correct size, and a manometer (mercury manometer as pictured) or aneroid manometer. Digital display models are also available. (Photograph courtesy of W. A. Baum Co., Inc., Copiague, NY.)

but less cumbersome. A third type of sphygmomanometer is electronic or battery operated and takes the blood pressure automatically, so no stethoscope is needed. (See Figure 20-15.)

All of these types of equipment have a cuff which is wrapped securely around the patient's arm above the elbow or the leg above the knee. The cuff has a bladder in it located in the first part of the cuff. This is inflated with air and puts pressure on the arm, eventually occluding the artery when the external pressure is great enough. As the pressure is released, the systolic and diastolic readings are heard or displayed (on the electronic models). The tubing from the cuff to the gauge or machine must not be kinked or the blood pressure reading will be inaccurate. The American Heart Association recommends the bladder within the cuff be 13 × 24 cm for most adults. This provides a bladder width which is greater than 40 percent of the arm circumference and a length that is 80 percent of the circumference of the arm (Kirkendall *et al.,* 1981). (See Figure 20-16.) To select a proper size cuff, compare the bladder's width to the diameter of the patient's arm. It should extend slightly beyond the arm diameter. A cuff with a bladder that is too wide will give a falsely low blood pressure reading, and a cuff with a bladder that is too narrow will give a falsely high blood

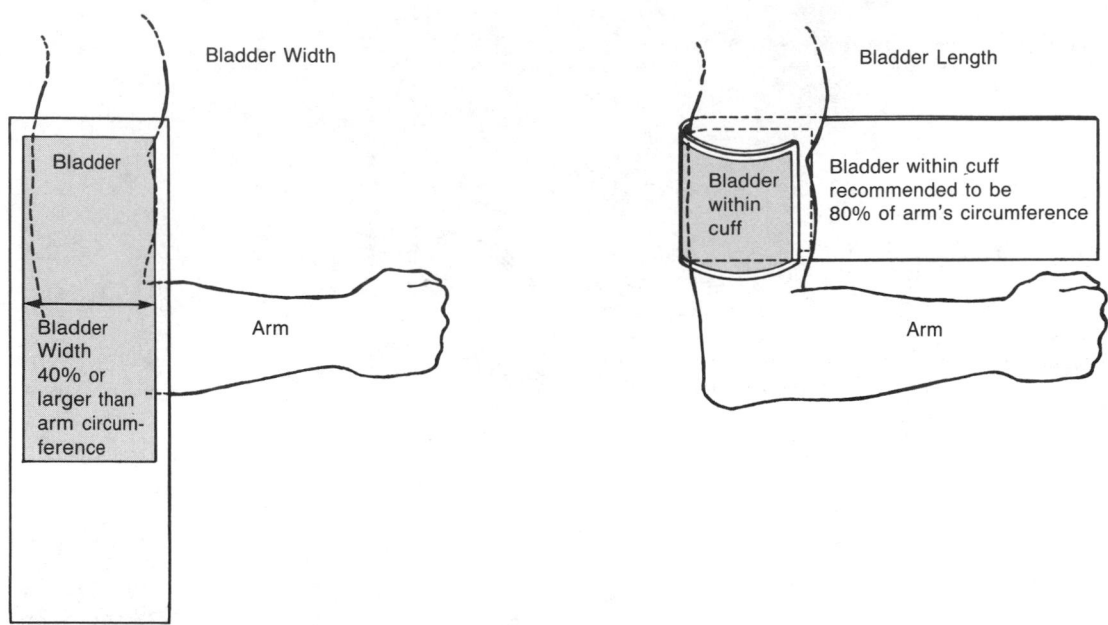

Figure 20-16.   The blood pressure cuff is measured to match the size of the patient's arm for maximum accuracy in blood pressure assessment.

pressure reading. Table 20–9 presents various cuff and bladder measurements. If the cuff is wrapped too loosely around the arm, the blood pressure reading will be falsely high. The bladder of the cuff should also be centered over the artery to give maximum compression to the artery beneath. The tubes coming from the bladder are sometimes in the middle of the bladder, sometimes left of middle, and sometimes right of middle, depending on the manufacturer.

The manual sphygmomanometers have a bulb to pump up the cuff and a valve where the tubing connects to the bulb for holding or releasing the air. Some valves screw open and closed, and some operate by pressing a release switch.

Preparation for Taking a Blood Pressure

1. Determining need to take a blood pressure reading is guided by the patient's current condition, the physician's orders, and advice from more experienced nursing personnel. Generally, a patient's blood pressure is taken at least once or twice a day, but if the patient is unstable, it may be taken every few minutes. One blood pressure reading in isolation is not as helpful in assessing the patient's condition as a series of readings. The patient's normal blood pressure, usually considered to be an admission BP unless the patient was unstable when admitted, provides a baseline value for comparison of current and future readings. For example, an isolated reading of 100/70 mm Hg seems normal, but if the patient normally has a blood pressure in the 150 to 160/90

Table 20–9. **Approximate Range of Cuff Sizes**

	LIMB CIRCUMFERENCE (CM)	BLADDER SIZE (CM)		LIMB CIRCUMFERENCE (CM)	BLADDER SIZE (CM)
Newborn	6–11	2.5 × 5	Adult	25–35	12 × 23
Infant	10–19	6 × 12	Large arm	33–47	15 × 33
Child	18–26	9 × 18	Thigh	46–66	18 × 36

mm Hg range, this lower reading indicates a significant drop in pressure and probably inadequate blood flow to the tissues. A patient experiencing an elevation or decrease from normal blood pressure values should have more frequent blood pressure measurements than a patient who remains within personal normals.

2. Clean off the stethoscope diaphragm or bell with an antiseptic to decrease the spread of microorganisms.
3. Wash hands.
4. Select an appropriate-size BP cuff.
5. Explain procedure to patient. Ask patient not to talk and just relax during procedure. BP may be significantly elevated by talking (Sandroff, 1982).
6. Provide privacy as necessary. (BP should not be taken over clothes, so unless the sleeve or pant leg can be rolled up above the area where the cuff will be wrapped, the clothing will have to be removed. If the sleeves are rolled up and are too tight, they can obstruct blood flow to the arm and cause an inaccurate reading.)
7. Eliminate as much room noise as possible when using a manual sphygmomanometer.

Procedure	Explanation
1. Position arm at heart level.	1. If arm above heart level, falsely low reading; below heart level, falsely high.
2. Have gauge at eye level and close enough to read (within 3 ft), make sure mercury manometer is not tilted. (See Figure 20–17.)	2. Necessary for accurate reading of aneroid or mercury manometer; tilting mercury gauge gives false BP reading.
3. Palpate brachial artery.	3. To locate site for stethoscope placement.
4. Place center of bladder in cuff over brachial artery.	4. Maximum compression of artery.
5. Wrap cuff securely around arm; have cuff 2 cm or almost 1 inch above antecubital space.	5. Loosely wrapped cuff gives falsely high BP reading; placement above antecubital space provides room for stethoscope placement without touching cuff or going under cuff.
6. Ask patient what normal blood pressure is and inflate 20 mm Hg above normal value; if patient does not know normal value, inflate 30 mm Hg above expected normal value for that patient's age group.	6. Identification of health learning need; pumping the cuff up to pressures significantly above the patient's normal BP is needed to detect elevations from normal; pumping cuff more than 30 mm Hg over normal BP is usually unnecessary and is uncomfortable for the patient.
7. Place diaphragm of stethoscope over brachial artery.	7. Turbulence in blood flow created by obstructed artery as it slowly opens is heard as a heartbeat through the stethoscope.
8. Tighten valve and inflate cuff rapidly (7 sec or less) by pumping up bulb to desired pressure.	8. As bulb is pumped, air is forced into cuff and compresses arm at the pressure indicated on gauge; reduces time for development of venous congestion.
9. Loosen valve slightly so air escapes and pressure decreases at the rate of 2 to 4 mm Hg per heartbeat (for normal adult).	9. Slow air release reduces compression on the arm gradually so the sound when blood first enters the artery can be read on the gauge.
10. Record systolic BP when first sound heard (Korotkoff's I sound). See Table 20–10 on Korotkoff's sounds.	10. Sound created when blood first enters compressed artery at peak of ventricular systole.
11. Record diastolic BP at cessation of sound (Korotkoff's V sound), if sound continues to very low reading, record muffling (Korotkoff's IV sound) of sound and cessation (muffling is often recorded for children).	11. Sound when blood flow is completely unobstructed and vessel open during entire cardiac cycle; muffling occurs when artery first stays open during entire cardiac cycle, but artery still partially occluded by cuff.

Table 20–10. **Korotkoff's Sounds in Blood Pressure Measurement**

   I. Tapping sound when blood first enters the constricted artery during ventricular systole; starts out as faint clear tapping which increases in amplitude; first sound is systolic BP.
   II. Sound changes to a swishing or murmur sound as cuff continues to be deflated.
   III. Sound changes to a knocking quality and is louder than Korotkoff's II sound.
   IV. Sound becomes muffled; artery is remaining open during systole and diastole but is still partially occluded by the cuff pressure; taken as the diastolic BP in children and in adults who have audible sounds down to a zero reading or slightly above because of abnormal blood turbulence at the site of measurement.
   V. Sound disappears and nothing is heard through the stethoscope; artery completely open in systole and diastole with no occlusion from the remaining pressure in the cuff; blood flows unobstructed with no turbulence to create the pulsing sound; taken as the diastolic reading in most adults.

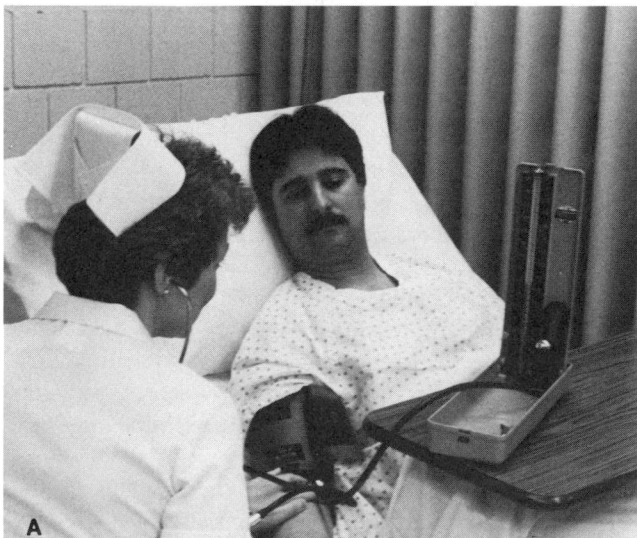

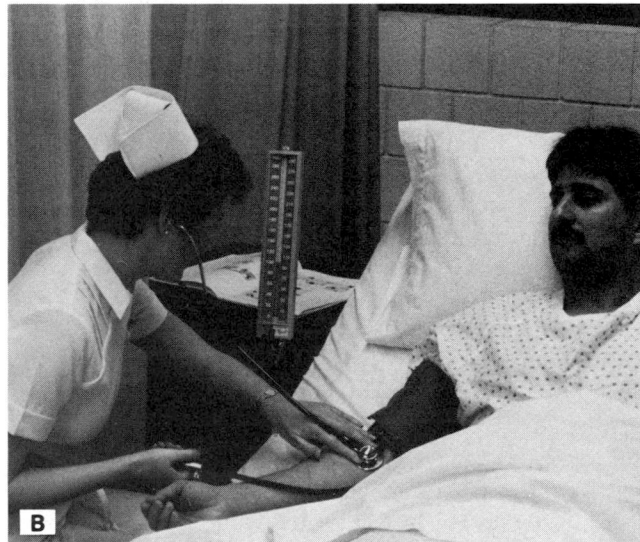

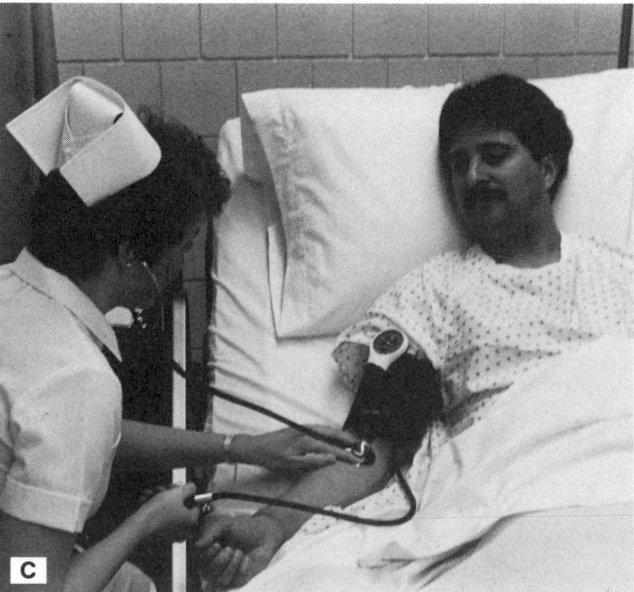

Figure 20–17. Measuring blood pressure. Correct viewing angles using various forms of equipment. **A.** Tabletop model of mercury manometer. **B.** Floor model of mercury manometer. **C.** Aneroid manometer.

Procedure	Explanation
12. Release all air from cuff after sound ceases.	12. Maintaining pressure in the cuff is uncomfortable for the patient and obstructs venous return from the lower arm.
13. If unsure of BP readings, wait a minimum of 30 sec before retaking.	13. Waiting allows venous blood to leave the arm and return to the heart; venous congestion increases the BP reading by increasing the resistance to flow.
14. Leave patient in comfortable position.	14. Communicates respect and promotes comfort.
15. Clean diaphragm of stethoscope with antiseptic and replace equipment.	15. Decreases the spread of microorganisms from patient to patient.
16. Wash hands.	16. Decreases patient-to-patient and patient-to-nurse spread of microorganisms.
17. Record and report BP as appropriate in institution; report any unusual finding to responsible nurse and nursing instructor. Recheck unusual readings to assure accuracy.	17. Communication among health team; legal responsibility and verification of competent nursing care.

second and third intercostal spaces on both sides of the sternum are auscultated for the S_2 sound which should be most loud in these two areas. The fifth intercostal space at the left edge of the sternum and also further off to the left on an imaginary line drawn down from the middle of the clavicle are areas where S_1, S_3, and S_4 can best be heard. (See Figure 20–17.) Any additional sounds or the presence of S_3 or S_4 in adults should be reported and documented. When documenting heart sounds that are abnormal, try to indicate when they occur in the cardiac cycle in relation to S_1 and S_2, the site where they are most easily heard, the loudness and quality of the sound, and the effect of inspiration or expiration on the sound.

Subjective Data. Satisfaction of oxygen needs is indicated when the patient reports the following subjective data:

Normal amount of energy and physical activity
No shortness of breath during normal activity
No pain associated with ventilation or in chest area
Absence of cough or sputum production prior to admission
No history of chronic or acute respiratory or cardiovascular problems
Has not smoked for at least one year
Reports that normal blood pressure is similar to current reading (this indicates the person is knowledgeable about personal blood pressure values and that no significant elevation or decrease in BP is occurring)

Documentation of Vital Signs

Documentation of the pulse, respirations, and blood pressure will vary depending on the form used by the institution. Most forms found in a patient's chart have pulse and temperature charted on the same graph, with respirations and blood pressure written separately or charted in another place. When patients are on frequent vital signs (more than every four hours), different forms for documentation are often used to provide the additional space compared to the six to twelve spaces provided by standard forms with times written in ahead of time, such as 4–8–12–4 or 3–7–11–3. Several chart forms are presented below as examples of how vital signs may be charted. All chart forms are done in dark blue or black ink since the patient's chart is a permanent legal document. The following vital signs are charted on the graphs in Figures 20–18 and 20–19:

Vital Signs

1/15
8 A.M.: BP, 120/60; P 64; R 20; T 98.4° F
12 P.M.: BP 126/68; P 60; R 18; T 98° F
4 P.M.: BP 120/58; P 60; R 18; T 98° F
8 P.M.: BP 120/62; P 62; R 16; T 98.2° F

1/16
1 P.M.: BP 100/60; P 90; R 24; T 99° F
1:05 BP 100/58; P 88; R 24
1:10: BP 98/60; P 89; R 24
1:15: BP 100/60; P 86; R 22
1:30: BP 102/54; P 84; R 24; T 98.8° F
1:45: BP 106/60; P 84; R 21
2 P.M.: BP 110/62; P 82; R 20
2:15 BP 116/62, P 84; R 20
2:30: BP 120/64; P 78; R 18; T 98.6° F

Data Indicating Inadequate Oxygenation of Tissues

Objective Data. Inadequate oxygenation of tissues may be indicated by the following objective observations:

Respirations above 18 or below 12 per minute in an adult
Irregular respirations
Patient exerting varying degrees of effort to breathe (dyspnea)
Abnormal lung sounds heard over chest and back

Lung Sounds
1. *Absent or reduced vesicular sound* will indicate inadequate ventilation of alveoli and small airways, unless patient is breathing very quietly. There may be an abnormal layer of air or fluid between the lung and the stethoscope, reducing the transmission of normal vesicular sounds. An obstruction in the air flow into a section of the lung will also reduce or eliminate vesicular sounds in the affected lung section. Atelectasis is a common cause of reduced vesicular sounds over affected areas of lung.

2. *Presence of bronchial sounds where vesicular sounds should normally be heard* indicates that lung tissue has been altered in some way to conduct sound more readily: the more dense the tissue, the more it conducts sound. Tumors, consolidation of lung tissue by pneumonia or tuberculosis, and atelectasis are all examples of problems producing changes in the lung which will eliminate vesicular sounds and promote the transmis-

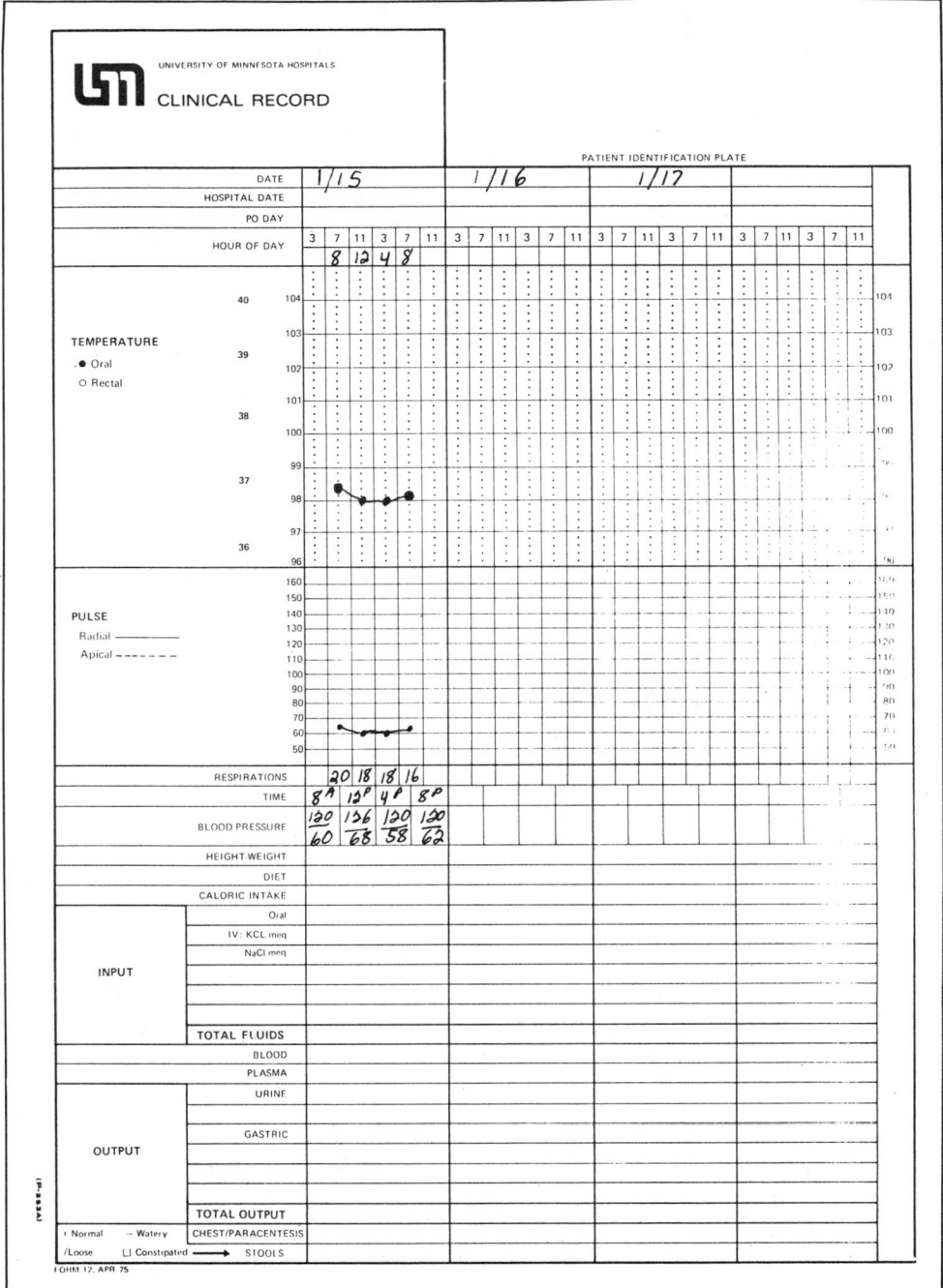

Figure 20–18. One example of a chart form and documentation of assessments made every four hours or less. (Courtesy of the University of Minnesota Hospitals and Clinics, Minneapolis, MN.)

sion of bronchial sounds down into deeper areas of the lung.

3. *Reduced vocal resonance* indicates some alteration in the tissues between the lung and chest wall. Air, fluid, or a thickened pleura will all tend to reduce vocal resonance.

4. *Increased vocal resonance* indicates possible changes in the lung tissue between the bronchioles and

the chest wall, making it more dense, such as tumors, consolidation, or increased secretions.

5. *Rales* as adventitious lung sounds indicate the presence of secretions in the airways. The sound is created by the air during inspiration moving through fluid or secretions in the lower airways as it opens the small bronchioles and alveoli. The sound created by rales can be simulated by rolling a few strands of hair together

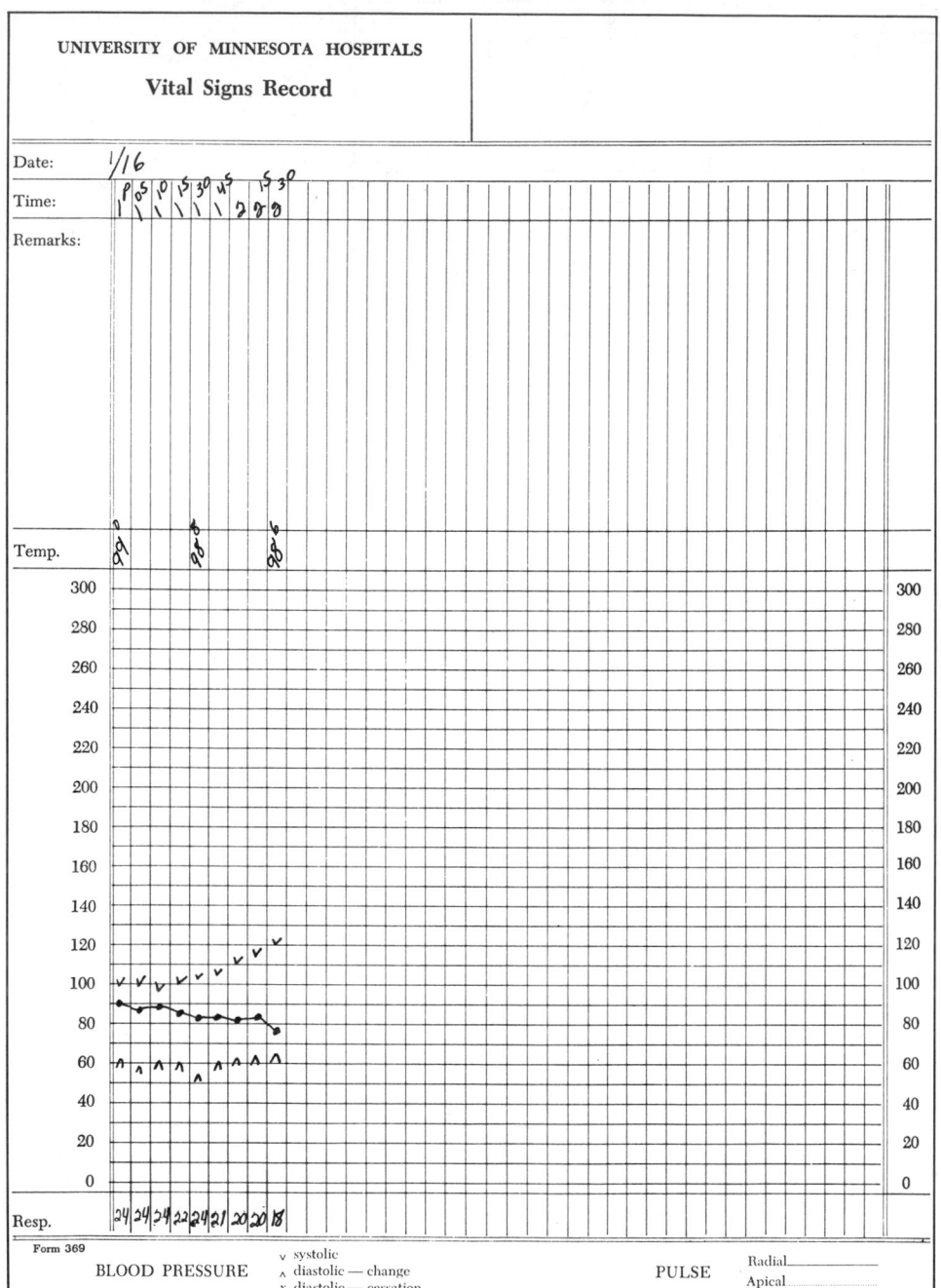

Figure 20-19. One example of a chart form and documentation of vital signs when assessment is made more often than every four hours. (Courtesy of the University of Minnesota Hospitals and Clinics, Minneapolis, MN.)

next to your ear. This is the sound you will hear through the stethoscope when a patient has rales. The word is French and actually means ''rattle''; it was coined by Rene Laeñnec who invented the stethoscope in 1819. The term ''crepitations'' (*creps*) is sometimes used as a synonym for rales. Moving a stethoscope over a hairy chest creates sounds like rales, so don't be fooled. Rales have been described as sounding crackling, moist, interrupted popping, and explosive. *Fine rales* sound like a crackling and are caused by moisture in the lower respiratory structures and by the opening of collapsed alveoli. They are commonly heard in early or resolving pneumonia and at the base of the lung in congestive heart failure. The opening of the alveoli will sound more like pops than crackles. *Medium rales* involve fluid in larger airways, and they are louder, rougher noises heard during midinspiration. *Coarse rales* are louder yet, with more of a gurgling noise caused by secretions in major bronchi. If rales clear up with coughing, the congestion in the lung is less severe than if the patient continues to have rales after effective coughing.

6. *Rhonchi* are another type of adventitious lung sounds indicating possible problems with ventilation and gas exchange in the lung. Rhonchi are caused by something within the airway acting like a reed on a musical instrument such as a clarinet. The material within the airway vibrates with the movement of air, creating a sound described as wheezy, musical, continuous, and dry. A partial airway obstruction by secretions, swelling, tumors, and conditions such as asthma and croup produces a high- or low-pitched, continuous sound heard on expiration in mild obstruction, and during inspiration and expiration in severe obstructions.

7. *Pleural friction rub* is another abnormal lung sound which occurs when the two pleural walls rub together, as occurs in pleurisy. The sound can be simulated by scratching the back of the hand held over the ear. It is a rubbing or grating sound which does not change when the patient coughs but may be audible intermittently. A pleural rub sounds louder and closer than rales or rhonchi.

Chest Assessment

1. *Unequal chest expansion during inspiration* can be another sign of problems with ventilation. Conditions such as tumors, pneumonia, pneumothorax, atelectasis, and collapsed lung will all decrease expansion of affected lung tissue.

2. *Reduced chest expansion* during a maximum inhale and a maximum exhale is common in the patient with emphysema since the chest is already enlarged and barrel shaped.

3. *A trachea palpated to the right or left of midline* in the suprasternal notch can also be a sign of respiratory problems. In pleural effusion (excess fluid in the pleural space) or pneumothorax, the trachea is displaced away from the affected lung. In a fibrotic or collapsed lung or atelectasis, the tachea is pulled toward the affected lung.

4. *Decreased fremitus* is a sign of an obstructed bronchus or laryngitis. Fremitus is absent in pleural effusion or pneumothorax.

5. *Increased fremitus* may indicate an area of consolidation within the lung or an air-filled cavity near the lung surface.

6. *Hyperresonance* is observed when air is present in abnormal places or amounts within the lung, such as in pneumothorax or emphysema.

7. *Diminished resonance* is present when a solid area has replaced normal lung tissue, such as in a thickened pleura, lung consolidation, or lung collapse.

8. *A dead note termed "stony dullness"* is heard when fluid fills areas of the lung normally filled with air.

Other objective data indicating possible problems with oxygenation include the *nurse's observation* of:

- Presence of a persistent cough
- Increased production of sputum
- Positioning for optimal chest expansion—leaning back with hands clasped behind neck or leaning over table with arms upon table (orthopneic position)
- Unusual color, odor, or thickening of sputum or secretions
- Inability to cough effectively (too weak, unable to cooperate, too painful)
- Increased size or abnormal shape of chest
- Frequently stopping to catch a breath when speaking
- Dyspnea upon mild-to-moderate exertion
- Retractions and nasal flaring (nostrils flare out during inspiration; skin over chest drawn in between bones on chest)
- Elevated temperature
- Hemoglobin below 10 to 12 gm/100 ml in women; below 13.5 in men
- Hematocrit below 30 to 34 percent in women; below 39 percent in men
- PaO_2 below 70 mm Hg in adult; $PaCO_2$ above 45 mm Hg
- Cyanosis, dark or dusky appearance to skin, mucous membranes pale or gray
- Restless, confused, agitated, disoriented, drowsy (may be one of earliest signs of hypoxia)
- Uncoordinated body movements
- Urine output less than 30 ml per hour
- Distended neck veins (back pressure in vein from inadequate pumping of blood by heart)
- Slow refilling of capillary nailbeds following blanching
- Systolic blood pressure measured during inspiration is more than 10 mm Hg lower than systolic measurement on expiration (this may indicate a serious condition called cardiac tamponade where blood fills the sac around the heart, and the pressure can block the pumping action of the heart in a patient with unobstructed breathing)
- Hypotension or hypertension for that·particular individual
- A pulse rate below 60 beats per minute or above 90 beats per minute

- An irregular pulse rhythm
- An abnormal electrocardiogram tracing
- A weak or bounding pulse quality
- A pulse deficit between apical and radial pulses
- Absence or disappearance of a peripheral pulse, with cool feel to skin and pale, dusky, or cyanotic color to area
- Abnormal heart sounds: *Muffled heart sounds* may indicate cardiac tamponade. *Murmurs and additional sounds* within the heart indicate increased turbulence of the blood, and this may be a sign of compromised pumping effectiveness of the heart.

Subjective Data. Possible problems in meeting oxygen needs are indicated when the *patient reports* the following subjective symptoms:

Fatigue and lack of energy or strength
Dyspnea upon exertion or during normal activity
Painful ventilations
Increased sputum production, unusual color or odor
History of respiratory, cardiovascular, or hematological problems
Smokes cigarettes
Unaware of normal blood pressure

Sleeping with several pillows placed under head to elevate head and chest to ease breathing
Shortness of breath

Nursing Diagnoses Related to Unmet Oxygen Needs*

General Diagnoses. Examples of general nursing diagnoses related to unmet oxygen needs are:

Activity tolerance, decreased
Airway clearance, ineffective
Breathing pattern, ineffective
Cardiac output, alterations in: decreased
Gas exchange, impaired
Tissue perfusion, chronic alterations in

Specific Diagnoses. Some examples of more specific nursing diagnoses based on a particular patient's situation are given below:

Hyperventilation related to inappropriate use of breathing exercises for childbirth
Anxiety related to dyspnea when in physical therapy
Increasing atelectasis related to reluctance to deep breathe and cough following abdominal surgery
Prone to personal injury related to confusion and restlessness from hypoxia

---

Nursing Interventions to Facilitate Adequate Oxygenation

Maintaining Oxygen Need Satisfaction—Preventive Nursing Care

Prevention of problems with oxygenation is usually easier on the patient and the nurse, and definitely healthier for the patient, than trying to correct a problem after it develops. Knowing which patients are high risk for developing respiratory and circulatory problems on admission will enable the nurse to develop specific plans to reduce a patient's risk.

All of the things that increase oxygen requirements may tax a patient's ability to provide an increased oxygen supply to the tissues. A healthy individual can normally tolerate increases in oxygen need with little difficulty over short periods of time. The real problem occurs when oxygen needs are increased over an extended period of time or when the patient is in a compromised state of health.

High-Risk Situations—Anticipating Problems with Oxygenation

SURGERY. Preoperative patients are in varying degrees of respiratory, cardiovascular, and hematological health. During and following surgery, medications, anesthesia, pain, decreased activity, and shallow breathing all put a patient at risk for adequate oxygenation.

BED REST AND IMMOBILITY. Any patients with restricted activity, for whatever reasons, are at risk for developing problems meeting their oxygen needs. Both the respiratory and cardiovascular systems are affected by short- and long-term bed rest or minimal activity levels. Bed rest and immobility result in a deterioration of the regulatory mechanisms provided by the sympathetic and

---

*North American Nursing Diagnosis Association: List of Nursing Diagnoses Accepted at the Fourth National Conference of North American Nursing Diagnosis Association.

parasympathetic nervous systems leading to decreased muscle tone and slowed venous bloodflow (venous stasis). One of the results is a condition called *orthostatic hypotension* in which the patient experiences a severe drop in blood pressure when changing from a lying to a standing position as blood pools in the legs. The drop in blood pressure is accompanied by feelings of dizziness and weakness, and the patient may lose consciousness. This condition can occur within a matter of days and is to be anticipated when getting a patient out of bed the first few times following a period of bed rest.

One nursing intervention that is very helpful in combating decreased muscle tone in the legs is to apply some form of elastic stockings or wraps to the legs while the patient is on bed rest or when activity is restricted because of surgery, illness, or injury. Elastic stockings come in various sizes and may extend to the knee or to the groin. (See Figure 20–20.) Elastic wraps to the leg accomplish the same result of increased muscle tone and improved blood flow in the legs. Elastic bandages and elastic stockings both maintain normal blood flow in the legs, thereby preventing inflammation of a vein (*phlebitis*) and formation of a blood clot in the vein (*thrombus*). Another name for elastic stockings is antiembolism stockings. Application of elastic bandages is discussed in Nursing Skill 20–4.

Other changes occurring with bed rest include an increased blood volume for the heart to circulate because gravity is no longer holding blood in the legs. Heart rate tends to increase progressively with extended immobility and bed rest. Using the arms and upper body to move in bed increases the intrathoracic pressure when the patient holds a breath. This interferes with venous return to heart, first decreasing it during breathholding and movement, and then suddenly increasing the blood flow to the right atrium with relaxation and breathing. In a damaged heart, the results of this *Valsalva maneuver*, as it is called, can cause cardiac arrest as the most serious response, and in many patients there is a transient tachycardia. Encouraging patients to keep breathing while moving in bed and assisting their efforts can greatly reduce the blood flow changes.

External pressure from pillows under the knees or one leg on top of another during bed rest can interfere with venous blood return to the heart and affect oxygen supply in the legs. Support the entire lower leg with a pillow rather than placing a pillow behind the knee.

Respiratory function is also affected by bed rest. Respirations are generally more shallow because of the resistance of the bed to deep inhalations, general weakness, or positions in bed that interfere with chest expansion. This leads to an increased risk for atelectasis and excess fluid in the lungs.

Nursing Interventions to Maintain Oxygenation

DEEP BREATHING—SUSTAINED MAXIMAL INSPIRATIONS. The most important part of deep-breathing exercises is to encourage sustained maximum inhalations (SMI) by the patient. Maximum exhalations, as occur with the use of blow bottles, are of questionable value as a technique in maintaining lung function because the exhalations may actually increase the number of alveoli that deflate and fail to reopen, thereby, worsening or encouraging the development of atelectasis (Fuchs, 1983). Encouraging the patient to take in as deep a breath as possible, hold it for several seconds, and then relax and exhale seems to be most beneficial in preventing atelectasis. The activity is repeated at least every hour while the patient is awake, and the patient should be encouraged to take at least five deep inspirations during each deep-breathing session. A single deep breath held for at least 3 seconds at the point of maximum inspiration has been found more effective in preventing and reducing lung complications than several deep breaths without holding at peak inspiration. The term *sustained maximal inspiration (SMI)* is used to describe a deep inhalation held for at least 3 sec to allow time for alveoli inflation.

Incentive spirometers are devices used to promote SMI in patients at risk for developing respiratory problems. There are numerous devices on the market, but basically they all reward the patient by creating some visible sign of an SMI. Some devices measure the patient's effort by measuring the flow of air created when the patient inhales. (See Figure 20–22.) Usually, the reward is seeing one or more Ping-Pong type balls move inside the spirometer. Another type of spirometer which measures the volume of air inspired by the patient is usually more expensive and often requires nursing assistance or assistance from respiratory therapy personnel. (See Figure 20–23.) The cost of the flow spirometers usually is under $15.00. The volume spirometers may cost several hundred dollars, but measure pulmonary exercise more precisely.

COUGHING. Another important technique in maintaining optimum lung function is to encourage the patient to cough if an assessment indicates the accumulation of secretions. However, encouraging coughing when the patient has no secretions or adventitious lung sounds may acutally increase the risk of atelectasis because coughing causes forced expiration and deflation of alveoli which may not reopen. However, if secretions are present, the patient should be encouraged to cough at least every hour in an attempt to move the secretions higher in the bronchial airways so they can be expelled as sputum or swallowed. For an incisional area that causes pain, bracing with a pillow firmly pressed against

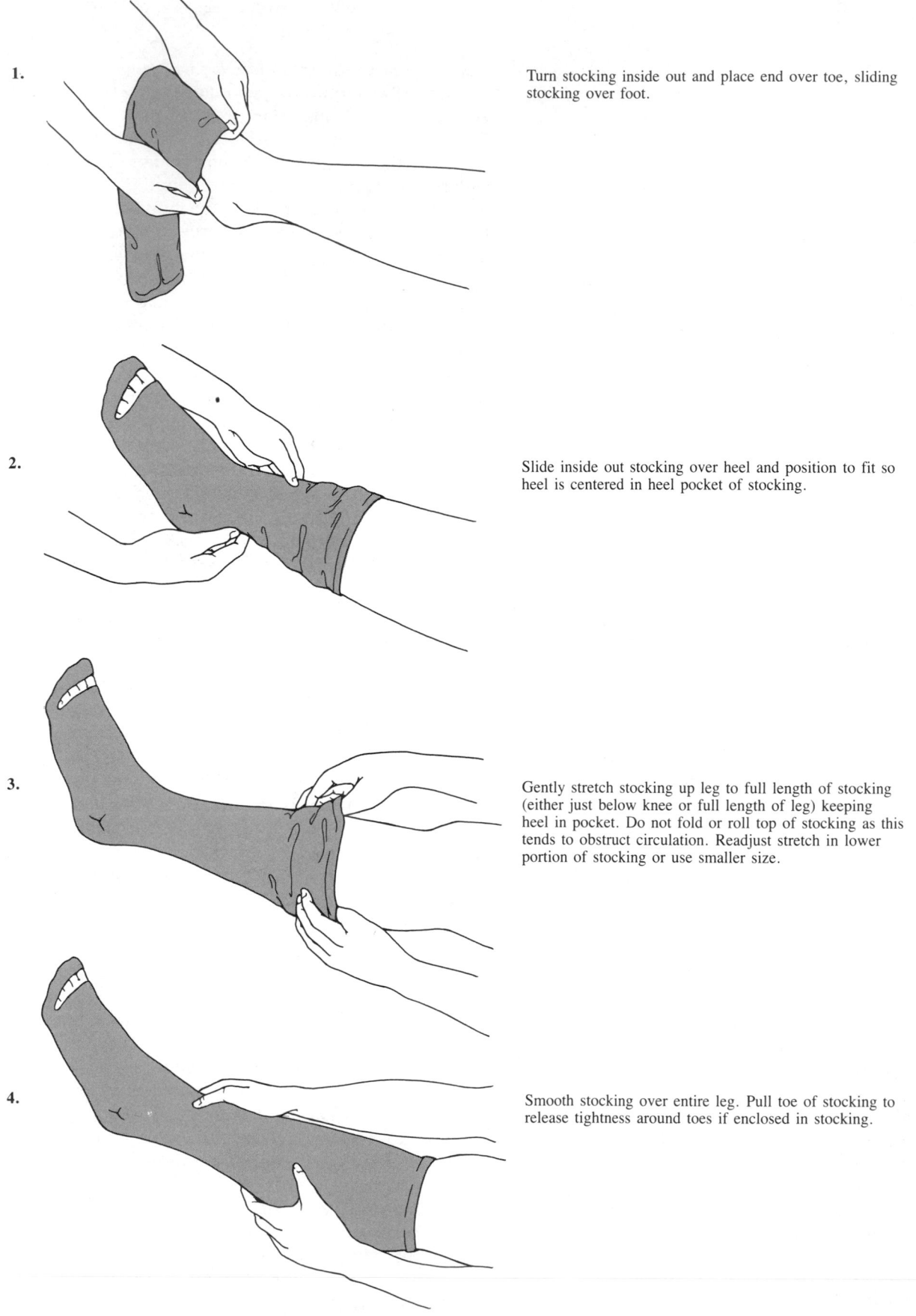

1. Turn stocking inside out and place end over toe, sliding stocking over foot.

2. Slide inside out stocking over heel and position to fit so heel is centered in heel pocket of stocking.

3. Gently stretch stocking up leg to full length of stocking (either just below knee or full length of leg) keeping heel in pocket. Do not fold or roll top of stocking as this tends to obstruct circulation. Readjust stretch in lower portion of stocking or use smaller size.

4. Smooth stocking over entire leg. Pull toe of stocking to release tightness around toes if enclosed in stocking.

Figure 20-20. Technique for putting on elastic stockings.

Nursing Skill 20–4   Application of Elastic Bandages to the Legs

Applcation of elastic bandages to the legs will promote return of venous blood to the heart and prevent pooling of blood in the legs during inactivity or early ambulation. These bandages have been largely replaced by the use of elastic stockings covering the leg to the knee or groin, depending on the type of stocking. Support after strains or sprains of the ankle represent more common usage of elastic bandages.

Equipment Needed
Several 2- to 4-inch (width) bandages, tape, or metal clips

Preparation for Procedure
1. Determining need may be based on patient behavior and symptoms when attempting ambulation. If the patient becomes weak and faint, elastic bandages applied to the legs will prevent the pooling of blood and may relieve the symptoms so the patient can get out of bed. The physician may order elastic bandages to the knee or groin for a preoperative patient, one with circulatory problems in the legs, or someone on prolonged bed rest.
2. Wash hands.
3. Explain procedure to patient.
4. Place patient in a position so that the legs are not in a dependent position. Apply before the patient gets out of bed to prevent pooling of blood.
5. Have legs clean and dry before applying bandages for patient comfort and to decrease chances of skin irritations.
6. Provide privacy for the patient.

Procedure	Explanation
1. Begin at foot and anchor bandages with two circular turns. Each turn covers the bandage underneath exactly.	1. Promotes venous return by applying support up the leg rather than down the leg.
2. Use a figure-8 wrap around the ankle joint, oblique turns that alternate ascending and descending after encircling the leg or foot. (See Figure 20–21.)	2. Allows joint movement for walking; provides maximum support to leg, and stays in place better than other patterns when walking.

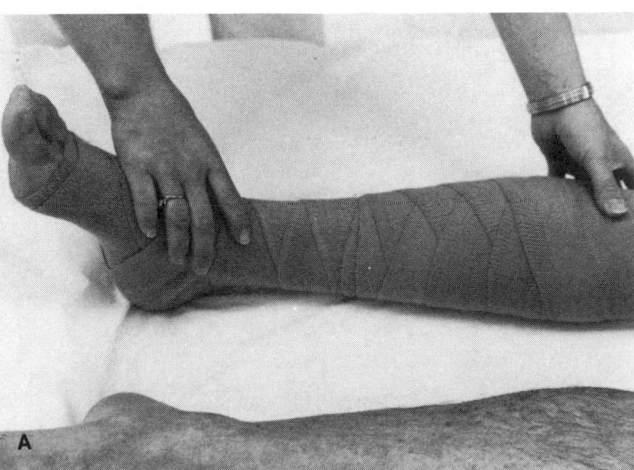
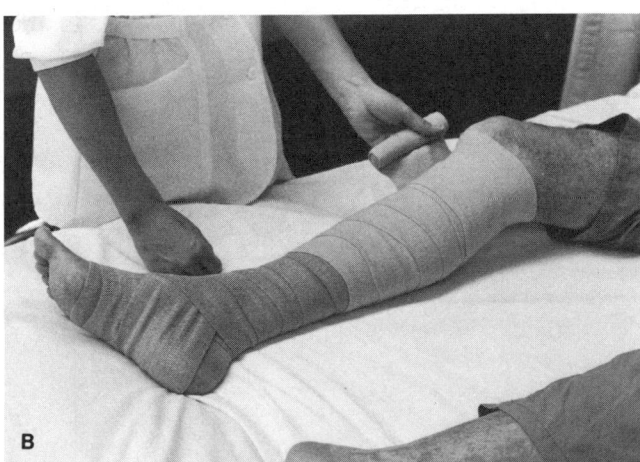

Figure 20–21.   Applying elastic bandages. **A**. Figure-eight wrap. **B**. Spiral wrap.

Procedure	Explanation
3. Continue until bandage used up; secure next bandage over first bandage with two circular turns.	3. Two to three bandages needed to wrap a large leg with a figure 8.
4. Wrap to desired height and fasten bandage with a circular wrap and tape or clip.	4. The circular wrap uses up remaining bandage and provides thickness so pins and clips do not go through to the skin.
5. Check for presence of pedal pulses in both legs.	5. If the bandages are applied too tightly, they may interfere with blood flow in the leg and foot. If pulse absent, rewrap bandages more loosely.
6. Rewrap bandages as needed if they become unwrapped or slip down on leg or foot.	6. If bandages slip, they may put excess pressure on some areas of the leg and interfere with blood flow; maximum support for venous return is lost if bandages become loose.
7. Remove bandages at least every 8 hr and air legs for 10 to 20 min before rewrapping.	7. Allows inspection of leg for any skin problems, evaporation of moisture from skin, and time for cleaning legs.
8. Leave patient in comfortable position.	8. Communicates respect for the individual and promotes comfort.
9. Wash hands.	9. Decreases spread of microorganisms.
10. Document application of elastic bandages to specific height; indications for bandages and pedal pulses.	10. Legal responsibility; verifies competent nursing care; communication among health personnel.

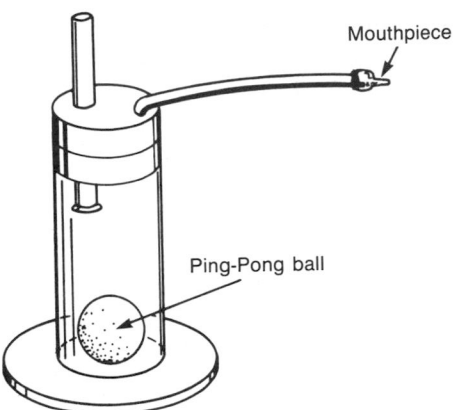

Figure 20–22. Flow spirometer. Ball moves up in the tube as patient inhales on the mouthpiece.

the area will help to reduce the pain when a new postoperative patient tries to cough. Applying counterpressure with the hands is also effective in decreasing pain from coughing if the patient has an incision on the chest or abdomen. The patient should be encouraged to take several sustained maximal inspirations before, and especially after, any coughing efforts to promote opening of the small airways and alveoli in the lung. Provide the patient with tissues for any secretions coughed out, and ask the patient to report to the nurse any unusual color, odor, or thickness of expelled secretions. A waste receptacle for contaminated tissues should be within the pa-

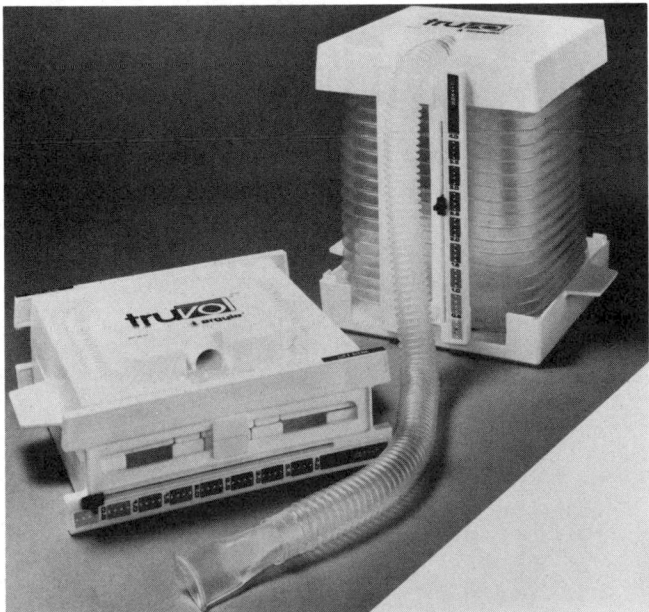

Figure 20–23. Volume spirometer. (Photograph courtesy of Argyle, Division of Sherwood Medical, St. Louis, MO.)

tient's reach, and it should be changed frequently to decrease the risk of microorganism transfer.

Patients who have secretions they cannot expel because they are unable to cough effectively will need additional help in the form of suctioning to remove these secretions. Suctioning is discussed later in this chapter. Listening to the patient's lung sounds before and after coughing will help the nurse assess the effectiveness of the patient's efforts to clear the airways of secretions, based on reduced or changed adventitious lung sounds. Pain relief may also be necessary for the patient prior to deep breathing and coughing, since this activity will increase the pain for a brief time. The pain a patient feels when coughing may be very intense. Analgesics taken at least 15 to 30 min before attempting these activities may take the edge off the pain enough so the patient is willing to try to remove lung secretions.

ACTIVITY. Early ambulation following any surgical procedure is especially helpful in reducing lung complications from accumulated fluid and atelectasis. The physician will usually indicate how soon after surgery or after a procedure a patient may begin getting out of bed and walking. This will be based on the patient's previous condition, the type of anesthesia or analgesia used, and the surgery or procedure performed. A patient may feel unready to begin ambulating when the physician orders, but an explanation of the benefits of early, progressive ambulation on the respiratory and cardiovascular systems will often motivate the patient to attempt the ambulation. Assuring safety is of primary importance when getting a patient out of bed for the first few times. More than one nurse may be needed to assist the patient if muscle strength is greatly reduced. Increase the activity level by having the patient sit on the edge of the bed for a few seconds to standing at the edge of the bed. If the patient tolerates this, walking in the room can be attempted. If the patient feels dizzy or has any unusual complaints when attempting to ambulate or get out of bed, do not advance the activity level but have the patient sit or lie down until the feeling subsides. Elastic stockings or wraps when put on the patient before getting out of bed are very helpful in preventing the dizziness associated with orthostatic hypotension. Before the patient is able to get out of bed, a turning program can be implemented to reduce collection of fluid in dependent (lower-most) areas of the lung. A patient on bed rest should be encouraged and reminded to turn and reposition every two hours until ambulation begins. Help achieving comfortable positions is offered every two hours as needed. Various positions for the bed patient are discussed in Chapter 28.

MOISTURE AND HYDRATION. Inspiration of air without much humidity tends to dry out the secretions of the respiratory tract, making them more viscous (thick). The more viscous the secretions, the more difficult it is to move them up along the ciliary elevator to the pharnyx. It also takes increased effort to remove thick secretions through coughing. Hospitals and similar institutions providing medical and nursing care are not known for keeping the humidity in the air at a level for optimal respiratory function. Dry air is a frequent problem for patients and staff. Dry nasal and oral passages, sore throats, and viscous lung secretions may all be related to inadequate room humidity. Humidity can be provided to the patient in many ways. Room humidifiers may be ordered for a patient experiencing problems with dry air. If the nurse anticipates that a patient may have problems with inadequate humidity entering the lungs, humidification devices can be ordered before a problem exists. (See Figure 20–24.) Institutions using heating and cooling systems continuously in climates where environmental air is too warm or cold will be most at risk for reduced room humidity levels. Humidity can also be provided to a patient through a mask attached to a wall humidifier or nebulizer. (See Figure 20–25.) A nebulizer provides a visible mist of water particles for the patient to inhale. A nebulizer or humidifier used with a mask frequently accompanies the administration of oxygen, which is discussed later. The nebulizer can provide 100 percent humidity at room temperature. Humidity can be provided to patients in the form

of a tent fitting over the bed into which humidified air or oxygen is circulated. These are often used on children with croup and are called croup tents or croupettes in some areas.

Maintaining hydration is another way of enhancing respiratory and cardiovascular function. When a patient is poorly hydrated, secretions in the lung become more viscous and difficult to remove. Blood volume may be decreased in the dehydrated patient which increases the work load on the heart. The blood will have to be circulated more rapidly (increased heart rate) to reach all areas of the body, and vasoconstriction and decreased perfusion of some areas may be needed to maintain adequate blood pressure. These adaptations to dehydration will reduce oxygen supply to the tissues of some areas of the body and increase the oxygen needs of the heart, since heart activity is increased. Hydration can be assessed by the adequacy of the urine output (greater than 30 ml per hour), by oral intake of fluid (in range of 1,000 to 2,000 ml per 24 hr in an adult), by weight changes (loss of weight may indicate dehydration, gained weight may indicate excess hydration and retained fluid in the tissues in the form of edema), and by tissue turgor (dehydrated patient's skin feels loose, and when pinched up, it recoils slowly compared to normally hydrated skin). Chapter 23 discusses fluids and hydration assessment more thoroughly.

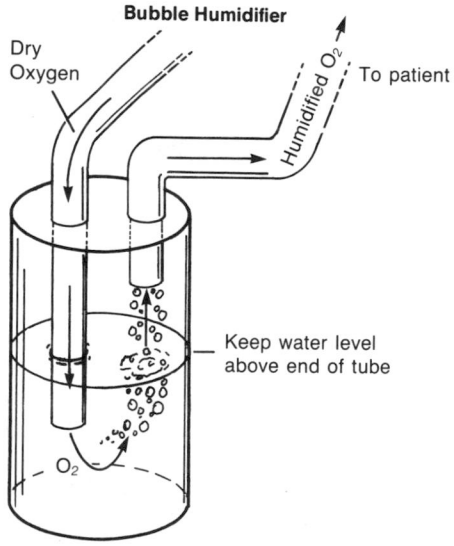

Bubble Humidifier

Dry Oxygen

Humidified O$_2$ → To patient

Keep water level above end of tube

O$_2$

A. Humidification—adding molecular size water to air—unable to see humidity
Used with all low-flow oxygen delivery systems. (Cannula and masks).

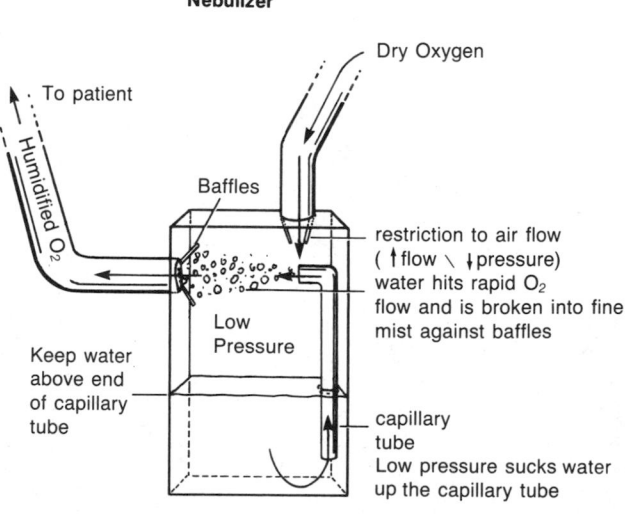

Nebulizer

Dry Oxygen

To patient

Humidified O$_2$

Baffles

restriction to air flow (↑ flow \ ↓ pressure) water hits rapid O$_2$ flow and is broken into fine mist against baffles

Low Pressure

Keep water above end of capillary tube

capillary tube
Low pressure sucks water up the capillary tube

B. Nebulization—adds molecular water and particulate water— a visible mist is formed. 100% humidity at room temperature (used with tracheostomy patients, croup tents, and head boxes for newborns).

Figure 20–24. **A.** Humidifying unit. **B.** Nebulization unit.

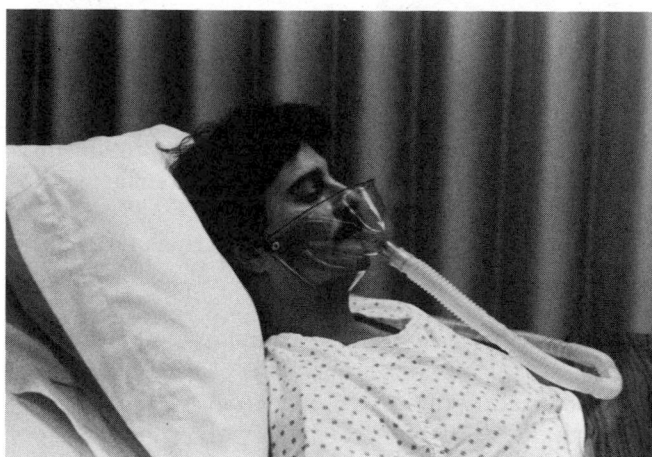

Figure 20-25. Providing moisture to the respiratory tract with a face mask.

The physician will usually indicate when a patient can begin taking fluids and food following a procedure or surgery. Oral intakes significantly below normal will result in progressive dehydration, unless supplemental fluid in some form, such as an intravenous infusion, is provided to the patient. Encouraging the patient to drink fluids and maintain hydration cannot be overlooked as an intervention for assisting the patient to meet oxygen needs.

TEMPERATURE MAINTENANCE. Providing patients with adequate warmth or appropriate environmental temperatures is another important technique in preventing increased oxygen need. As body temperature rises, oxygen consumption rises. When a patient is chilled, muscle tone increases, as does cellular metabolism, and shivering may begin. These activities increase oxygen consumption at the cellular level. Providing blankets, heat, air conditioning, and removing excess blankets and covers when a patient is too warm will all help maintain a normal body temperature, thus minimizing oxygen need.

MAINTAINING NUTRITION. Adequate nutrition is essential for the formation of blood. It also provides the materials needed for the manufacturing of ATP and other cellular products. Patients with inadequate diets may become anemic because of a reduced ability to produce normal red blood cells. This decreases the blood's ability to transport oxygen to the cells. Assessment and interventions to assist patients meet their nutritional needs are discussed in Chapter 22.

ENCOURAGING REDUCTION OR ELIMINATION OF SMOKING. Smoking causes some degree of temporary bronchial constriction, which increases the resistance of air flow in the lungs. Smoking also contributes to cancer and chronic obstructive pulmonary diseases. Educating and encouraging patients to abstain or reduce smoking activities, especially when activity levels are reduced or after surgery, will help reduce complications from atelectasis.

TURNING AND REPOSITIONING. Tactile stimulation to an area of skin through massage increases the flow of blood to that area. By increasing the blood flow, the available oxygen to the tissues is also increased. A patient who has been putting pressure on one area of skin for several hours because of an unchanging position in a chair or bed will have a reduction in blood flow to the area under pressure. If this pressure is continued or repeated often enough, cellular death and skin damage can result. The formation of a bedsore (decubitus ulcer or pressure sore) indicates an area of tissue where a patient is having difficulty meeting current body oxygen needs. A decubitus ulcer can develop very rapidly, within a matter of hours. Turning a patient frequently will alter the pressure areas and help blood recirculate in the areas of the body in contact with the bed or wheelchair. Areas over bones are especially likely to have oxygen needs unmet when the patient is in a position putting pressure on the skin over the bone.

DECREASING ABDOMINAL DISTENTION. Abdominal distention puts pressure on the diaphragm and prevents it from descending completely. Severe abdominal distention may affect ventilation to the point that the patient is exchanging inadequate volumes of air, and is not maintaining a normal PaO_2 level. Assessment and nursing interventions to prevent or relieve abdominal distention are discussed in Chapter 22 with problems of digestion and transport of food. Children and infants receiving liver transplants from larger children will have similar problems with respirations because the transplanted liver is large and puts pressure on the diaphragm. These infants are frequently ventilated by respirators for several days to avoid respiratory problems from shallow, labored breathing.

In summary, the following nursing interventions are recommended to help patients maintain their ability to meet oxygen needs:

1. Encouraging several sustained maximal inspirations every hour
2. Turning and repositioning every two hours, or more frequently
3. Applying elastic stockings to the legs of patients with limited activity
4. Promoting good nutritional intake
5. Encouraging adequate fluid intake
6. Discouraging smoking
7. Assisting patients to maintain a normal body temperature

8. Providing room humidity for dry air

9. Encouraging early ambulation and progressive activity as physical status permits

10. Encouraging coughing when there are adventitious lung sounds and increased secretions in the lungs

11. Encouraging patients to continue breathing while moving in bed rather than performing the Valsalva maneuver

12. Preventing pressure under knee of immobile patient by supporting entire leg with pillow

13. Encouraging active exercises in bed to promote venous blood return to the heart

14. Preventing excess abdominal distention.

Assisting Patients with Unmet Oxygen Needs

There are two basic ways of assisting the body to meet oxygen needs. One way is to decrease the oxygen need to the point that the patient is able to meet it unassisted. The other way is to increase the amount of oxygen available to the cells. At times, both techniques may be utilized in a severely compromised patient.

Reducing Oxygen Need

In order to reduce oxygen need, cellular activity must be decreased. This can be accomplished by helping a patient reduce activity levels, by decreasing the stress and pain a patient is experiencing, and by reducing a patient's temperature if that patient is febrile. Activity may have to be curtailed greatly to the point of bed rest with nursing help in positioning, feeding, and other activities normally done independently. Analgesics and sedatives may be needed to reduce the patient's reactions to pain and stress. Some patients will require help in adjusting their life-style as respiratory or cardiovascular problems progress and activity levels must be simultaneously decreased to avoid severe hypoxia. The nurse may have to provide total care to assist the patient to avoid hypoxia and extreme fatigue from even minimal activity when oxygen need satisfaction is severely compromised. Avoiding the use of caffeine and other stimulants is helpful in decreasing oxygen needs since caffeine increases cellular metabolism.

Increasing Oxygen Supply

Nursing interventions for increasing oxygen available to a patient at the cellular level are presented in several broad categories:

1. Improving efficiency of ventilations

2. Improving diffusion of gases between alveoli and blood

3. Improving transport of gases

4. Assisting regulation of oxygen supply

IMPROVING EFFICIENCY OF VENTILATIONS.   Ventilations can be improved in many ways. Interventions that decrease the resistance to air flow in the lungs will increase efficiency of ventilation.

Bronchodilators.   Medications, such as bronchodilators, may be prescribed by the physician and administered by the nurse to decrease bronchial constriction and increase air flow. This is very common in patients with asthma. Inhalation of bronchodilators usually results in rapid relaxation of some constriction and varying degrees of relief. Very frequent use of bronchodilators may constitute abuse, and the importance of following the directions and the physician's recommendations related to home use of these medications should be emphasized in discharge teaching. A certain amount of strength is also required to depress the applicator to release the medication in the form of a mist. The nurse should be sure the patient is strong enough to use the aerosol device if one is ordered.

Postural Drainage.   Postural drainage is an intervention designed to remove secretions collecting within the smaller airways of the lungs. Postural drainage uses gravity to assist the patient in moving secretions up into the larger airways where they can be removed by coughing or suctioning. The patient is placed in a position where the upper airway is below the lower airways, and the lobe of the lung to be drained is the most elevated part of the lung. Auscultation of rales in one area of the lung which do not clear with coughing might be one indication of the need for postural drainage. Often institutional policy requires that the physician order postural drainage. A patient receiving postural drainage will often have this treatment several times each day until the lungs sound clear of secretions. Postural drainage done on a full stomach is often uncomfortable and may cause nausea and vomiting. Work with the patient to identify times distributed through the day when postural drainage would be preferred.

There are a number of different positions for draining each lobe of the lung, and these are described in Figure 20–26. Each position is usually maintained for approximately 5 to 15 min. Postural drainage is done only for the part of the lung with accumulated secretions. Assessment of respiratory status is performed before and after postural drainage to evaluate effectiveness of the treatment. The patient is instructed to cough as needed during the time in each position and is asked to try to cough up secretions at the end of each draining position before repositioning. Make sure the patient has tissues or a basin available for secretions while in each of the needed positions.

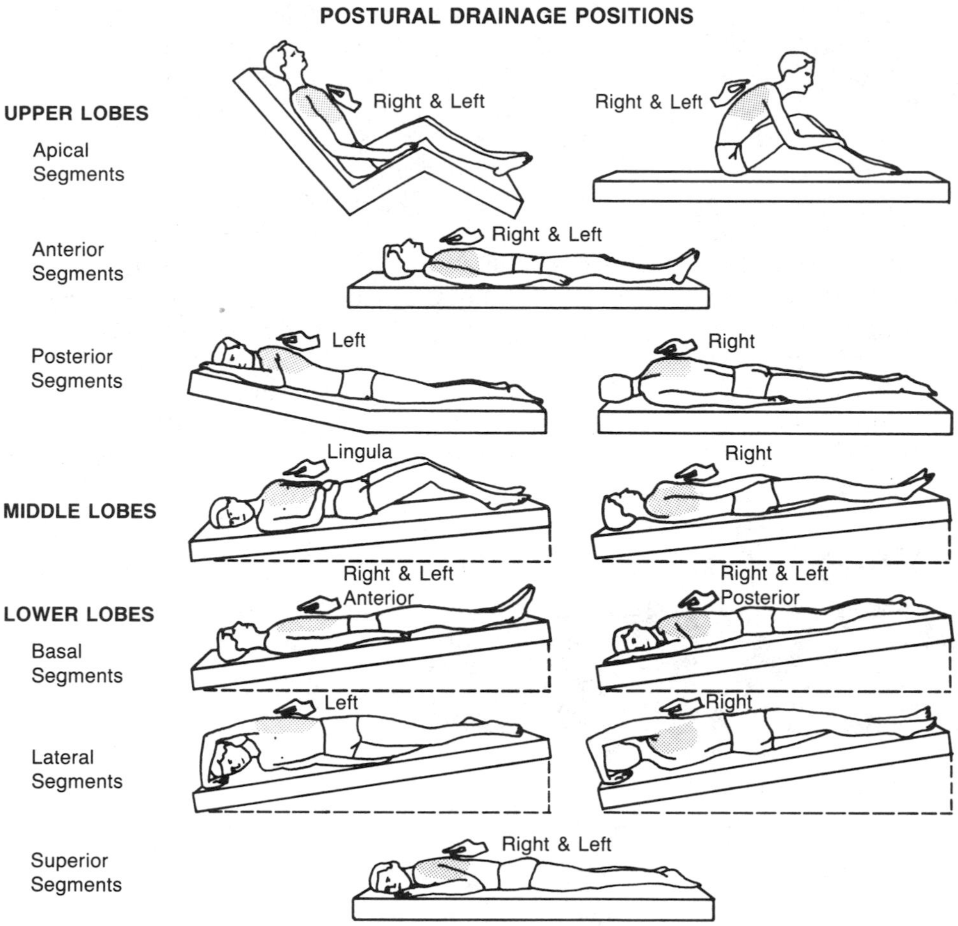

POSTURAL DRAINAGE POSITIONS

UPPER LOBES

Apical Segments — Right & Left / Right & Left

Anterior Segments — Right & Left

Posterior Segments — Left / Right

MIDDLE LOBES — Lingula / Right

LOWER LOBES

Basal Segments — Right & Left Anterior / Right & Left Posterior

Lateral Segments — Left / Right

Superior Segments — Right & Left

Figure 20-26. Postural drainage positions. Hand indicates procedure of clapping over area, followed by vibration during several exhalations to loosen secretions. The patient coughs as needed to clear secretions from lungs and follows this by several sustained maximal inspirations. (Reprinted with permission from the May issue of *Nursing 83*, p. 49. Copyright © 1983, Springhouse Corporation. All rights reserved.)

Postural drainage can be performed on infants, children, and adults, but each patient's tolerance for this procedure may be different. Infants and small children are often held by the nurse or parent during postural drainage, while adults are positioned in the bed or in a chair. As long as the area of the lung which is filling with secretions is above the larger airways, gravity will promote drainage. Positions can be adapted for individual patient's conditions and comfort. The techniques of percussion and vibration may be used during postural drainage to loosen secretions and enhance drainage. Following postural drainage and coughing, the patient should be instructed to take in several sustained maximal inspirations to reinflate any collapsed alveoli. Humming, singing, or reciting rhymes to children during postural drainage may make it seem more of a game than a therapeutic treatment. Providing adults with music or other diversions may make the time in an uncomfortable position pass more quickly.

Percussion and Vibration of the Chest. Percussion and vibration over the chest are designed to loosen secretions within various areas of the lung and promote their removal by coughing. A physician's order may be necessary depending on the institutional policy. *Percussion* involves repeated striking of an area of the chest over the congested lung section with cupped hands. The cupped hands trap air which exerts force over the chest and sets up vibrations, which are transmitted to the airways and loosen secretions. The hands are moved at the wrists to avoid too much force to the patient, and the nurse alternates hands in striking the chest at as rapid a rate as possible. Arms and shoulders are kept relaxed. Percussion is usually done for several minutes to each congested area, and care is taken to avoid hurting breast tissue or percussing over the spine or other internal organs. The smaller the patient, the less force is applied, so that minimal force is applied while percussing an infant and maximal force is applied when percussing an adult of sturdy build.

Vibration is a technique of shaking the chest over the congestion. It is done by placing one hand over the other on the patient's skin and vibrating the area by shaking the arms and hands back and forth in rapid, short movements, without moving the hand's position on the patient's skin. The wrists remain stiff. It is done as the patient exhales, and it increases the turbulence of the air flow within the alveoli and small airways and dislodges accumulated secretions. Percussion is done first, followed by vibration. Practice vibrating by exhaling and producing a tone with your voice. Then try vibrating an area of your own chest, and the sound produced by your voice should also vibrate. Sessions of percussion and vibration may be performed as frequently as hourly in severely congested patients, but whenever possible, each session should be followed by several attempts to cough and remove secretions and then by several sustained maximal inspirations. A patient who is unable to cough may need to be suctioned following percussion and vibration.

Preventing Aspiration or Removing Foreign Material from the Airway.   When foreign material is sucked into the trachea, bronchi, or other airways during inspiration, it is called *aspiration*. Food is the most common material to be aspirated, and if the piece of food is large enough, the entire airway can be obstructed, eliminating all air flow. This is called *obstructed apnea* because the person is trying to breathe, but the upper airway obstruction blocks all air flow. The *Heimlich maneuver* (manual thrusts) is presented in Figure 20–27 for removing food and other objects from an obstructed airway.

Preventing aspiration of food, secretions, and other objects requires careful assessment of each patient's respiratory status, level of growth and development, level of consciousness, and general strength. If respirations

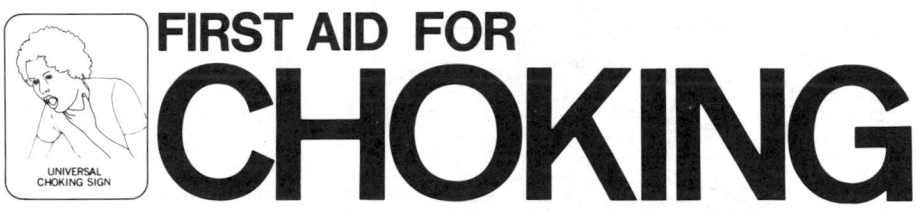

FIRST AID FOR CHOKING

UNIVERSAL CHOKING SIGN

If victim can cough, speak, breathe ➡ Do not interfere

If victim **cannot** cough speak breathe

Have someone call for help. Telephone : _____ (Number)

⬇

TAKE ACTION: FOR CONSCIOUS VICTIM

4 QUICK BACK BLOWS   4 MANUAL THRUSTS

Repeat steps until effective or until victim becomes unconscious.

TAKE ACTION: FOR UNCONSCIOUS VICTIM

TRY TO VENTILATE   4 BACK BLOWS   4 MANUAL THRUSTS   FINGER PROBE

Repeat steps until effective.

Continue artificial ventilation or CPR, as indicated.

Everyone should learn how to perform the above first aid steps for choking and how to give mouth-to-mouth and cardiopulmonary resuscitation. Call your local Red Cross chapter for information on these and other first aid techniques.

Caution: Abdominal thrusts may cause injury. Do not <u>practice</u> on people.

AMERICAN RED CROSS

Poster 1030 (5-76) (Sept. 1978 Prtg.)

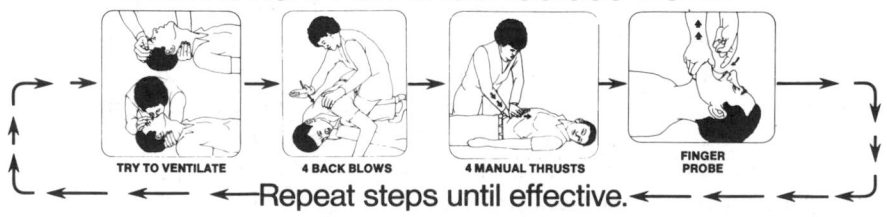
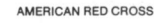

Figure 20–27. Actions to take when breathing becomes obstructed. (American Red Cross Poster.)

are rapid, coordination of eating and breathing becomes more difficult. If breathing is labored or the patient is in some form of respiratory distress, aspiration during eating is more likely. Infants and toddlers will put anything small in their mouth, so any object capable of fitting in the child's mouth could be aspirated and should be removed from the environment. Patients who are very weak are also more likely to aspirate food while chewing and swallowing. A patient who is coughing while eating can easily aspirate food during the maximal inspirations associated with coughing. Patients with a decreased level of consciousness from medications, anesthesia, disease, or a medical condition will have an increased risk of aspiration. Patients with coordination problems following a stroke or a muscle-nerve disease are also at increased risk for aspiration.

Preventing aspiration is a primary responsibility of the nurse who can assess the patient on a continuous basis. Withholding feedings is a very appropriate intervention when the nurse feels aspiration is likely. Discussing concerns about aspiration with the patient's physician and alternate ways of maintaining hydration and nourishment on a temporary or permanent basis is essential whenever feedings are withheld for more than a few hours. Placing the patient in an upright position uses gravity to assist the movement of food and fluid into the stomach. Waiting until the patient is alert and oriented before offering food or fluids following administration of medications or anesthesia will reduce the chance of aspiration. Keeping the patient's head slightly forward rather than extended backward will also help keep food out of the trachea. Other suggestions can be found in Chapter 22 in the section on assisting patients meet nutritional needs. Positioning an unconscious patient on either side will assist the drainage of secretions out of the mouth rather than having a collection of secretions in the mouth and pharynx where they can be easily aspirated.

Teaching Breathing Technique to Reduce Dyspnea. A breathing technique called *pursed lip breathing* is helpful in preventing premature closure of the small airways and trapping of air within the alveoli and bronchioles. It is especially helpful in patients with COPD. The patient is taught to exhale slowly through the mouth with lips pursed as if blowing out a candle. This creates a back pressure to the airflow in the lungs during expiration and holds the small airways open. It also prolongs the time needed for expiration, slowing the flow of air and keeping airways open. This type of breathing is combined with abdominal breathing, using the muscles of the abdomen to assist the diaphragm during exhalation. The patient inhales with relaxed abdominal muscles and exhales with contracted abdominal muscles. Relaxation techniques can also be helpful in decreasing

dyspnea by decreasing the oxygen need in relaxed muscles compared to that in tense muscles.

Teaching the dyspneic patient to relax for ten minutes using comfortable positioning and imagery may reduce the symptoms and ease breathing. *Imagery* involves clearing the mind of current thoughts and problems and visualizing a relaxing place. The patient tries to image the self in this quiet, peaceful place. Ask the patient to think of someplace he or she has been that was totally relaxing and to hold that image in the mind while letting the body relax for 5 to 10 min. This is a helpful technique for any kind of stress or anxiety for the patient, the nurse, or the student.

Suctioning Secretions from the Lungs.   Suctioning is a nursing intervention to remove secretions from the upper airways, trachea, and bronchi when the patient is unable to remove them through normal means, such as coughing or swallowing. It is generally uncomfortable for the patient and has the risk of causing tissue damage, cardiac arrhythmias, infection, and creating hypoxemia in the patient. Other less aggressive techniques are used before suctioning, since the risk of causing additional harm is greater with suctioning. Suctioning of the upper airways may involve the nose, mouth, and back of the throat (pharynx). Suctioning on the adult patient is usually accomplished using various electrical devices to create varying amounts of suction. A catheter is used with the suction device and is put in through the patient's nose or mouth and advanced down the pharynx to the trachea prior to applying suction. Suction is then applied as the catheter is slowly withdrawn, removing secretions along the way. (See Nursing Skill 20–5.)

Tracheostomy.   The tracheostomy is a surgically created opening into the trachea to allow ventilation when there is an upper airway obstruction. Trauma, tumors, surgery, and edema of the upper airways are conditions that may reduce air flow to the point that ventilations are not effective. Tracheostomies may be temporary or permanent, depending on the patient's problem with the upper airway. The patient with a tracheostomy has some type of tube (tracheostomy tube) keeping the incision into the trachea open for air exchange. (See Figure 20–29.) Should the tube become dislodged, a recent tracheostomy will close spontaneously and obstruct air flow. The patient is unable to make sound with a tracheostomy tube in place because the air flow enters and exits at a site below the larynx, and there is no vibration of the vocal folds in the absence of air flow. When the tracheostomy is occluded, the patient is able to speak if air will move through the upper airways. The tracheostomy bypasses the natural defense system of the upper airways, increasing the risks of respiratory infections. Secretions are more likely to become dry and viscous in the patient with a tracheostomy because the

Nursing Skill 20–5   **Suctioning the Respiratory Tract**

Suctioning is the application of suction to the patient's respiratory tract to assist in the removal of fluid secretions from the upper or lower airways when the patient is unable to remove these secretions independently. Suctioning of the upper airways may involve the nose, mouth, and oropharynx. Suctioning the lower airways involves primarily the trachea, and occasionally deep suctioning will involve the right and left bronchi. The risks of suctioning include infection of lower airways, tissue trauma from excessive suction on the lining of the respiratory tract, hypoxemia from removal of air with secretions during suctioning and the removal of oxygen therapy during the procedure, bronchospasms and vagal stimulation causing slowing of the heart from irritation of the airways and possible cardiac arrhythmias, anxiety, and discomfort. The patient may be suctioned through either nostril, the mouth, or through a tracheostomy tube.

Equipment Needed

A stethoscope, sterile suction catheter, sterile saline solution, sterile container for solution, sterile gloves. Much of this equipment is prepackaged in sterile, disposable kits for suctioning. Read what equipment is included in each kit before gathering duplicate equipment and taking it into the patient's room.

Preparation for Respiratory Suctioning

1. Determining the need for suctioning is a nursing responsibility. Assessment of the patient's respiratory status, including lung sounds, will provide data on secretions within the airways. Less invasive techniques for removal of secretions are usually implemented and evaluated for effectiveness in removing secretions before suctioning is used. Patients who are unable to cough and deep breathe using the SMI breathing techniques because of their medical condition or age are more likely to require some form of suctioning for removal of secretions. This is especially true if their activity level is minimal. Patients with tracheostomies are often unable to cough out mucus and require suctioning assistance. The physician may write an order to suction the patient prn (as needed), but this activity may also be left up to the individual nurse's judgment. The development or worsening of moist lung sound in the form of rales or rhonchi, which do not clear with coughing and deep breathing, indicates a build-up of secretions and the need for suctioning. Gurgling, which can be heard without a stethoscope in a patient's throat or trachea during ventilations, is an obvious sign that the patient needs immediate suctioning. Coughing, which is weak and ineffective in bringing secretions high enough in the airways so they can be expelled or swallowed, is another indication that a patient may need suctioning assistance.
2. Assemble equipment.
3. Wash hands.
4. Explain procedure to the patient.
5. Provide privacy.

Procedure	Explanation
1. Auscultate lung sounds.	1. Provides baseline for evaluation of effectiveness of suctioning.
2. Open suction kit on clean, dry, flat surface, touching only corners of wrapper. Open far side first.	2. Prevents contamination of sterile field (inside of wrapper is sterile field, once unwrapped).

3. Put sterile glove from kit on dominant hand.

4. Using gloved hand, set up container for solution on sterile field.

5. Using ungloved hand, remove cap from sterile saline and pour solution into container on sterile field (½ full).

6. Using sterile, gloved hand, attach sterile suction catheter to suction tubing (held in ungloved hand).

7. Turn on wall suction with ungloved hand.

8. Remove humidity cup from tracheostomy.

9. Insert catheter into saline and suction small amount of solution by placing thumb of ungloved hand over hole near attachment of catheter to tubing.

10. Ask the patient to take several SMIs, if able.

11. Catheter is inserted at peak of inspiration.
No suction is applied during insertion.
Insert catheter into tracheostomy as far as it will go until resistance is felt.

or

Insert through nose or mouth to desired depth depending on level of secretions needing removal.

3. Optimum control of catheter and prevention of microorganism transfer.

4. Prevents transfer of microorganisms

5. Prevents transfer of microorganisms.

6. Prevents the transfer of microorganisms.

7. Prevents the spread of microorganisms.

8. Humidity keeps secretions liquefied.

9. Lubricates catheter to reduce friction on tissues; tests functioning of equipment.

10. To provide maximal oxygenation before suctioning to reduce the risk of hypoxemia from procedure.

11. Allows gas exchange before obstructing air flow with catheter.
Suction during insertion causes trauma to tissues above secretions and removes excess air, increasing risk of hypoxemia.
Pushing past point of resistance likely to cause tissue damage.
Suctioning only as deep as necessary reduces risk of complications.

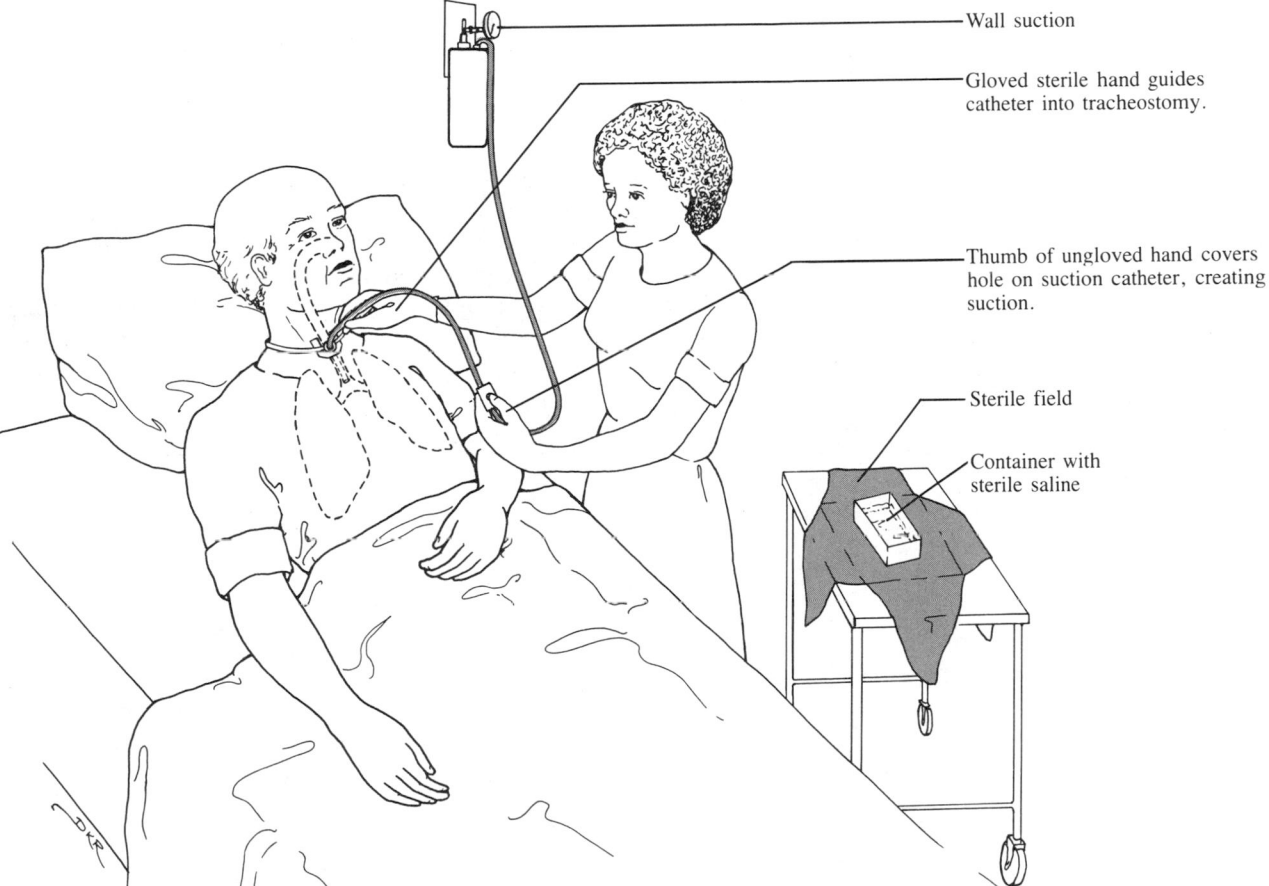

Wall suction

Gloved sterile hand guides catheter into tracheostomy.

Thumb of ungloved hand covers hole on suction catheter, creating suction.

Sterile field

Container with sterile saline

Figure 20–28.   Tracheal suctioning using sterile technique.

Procedure	Explanation
12. Pull tip of catheter back slightly from point of resistance and apply suction. Roll catheter in gloved hand and simultaneously withdraw during 10 to 20 sec; periodically (2 to 3 times) break the suction during the withdrawal (*make-break suctioning*). (See Figure 20–29.)	12. Prevents tissue damage. Removal of secretions on all sides of airway; longer time for suctioning increases risk of hypoxemia; intermittent suction decreases risk of tissue damage and hypoxemia.
13. Wait approximately 1 min before reinserting catheter if more suctioning is needed.	13. Gives the patient time to take several breaths and relax; decreases risk of hypoxemia.
14. Insert catheter in sterile saline before each suctioning pass and apply brief suction.	14. Clears the catheter of secretions to prevent gravity from draining secretions from catheter back into airway during insertion of catheter.
15. Continue suctioning until no mucus or minimal mucus is obtained; stop suctioning if bradycardia develops and wait until heart rate back up to normal; give O_2.	15. Increases interval between suctionings. Bradycardia decreases oxygen supply to tissues and may lead to cardiac arrhythmias or arrest if stimulus continues. O_2 will reduce hypoxemia.
16. Replace humidity cup over tracheostomy.	16. Humidity keeps secretions liquefied.
17. Suction the mouth and oropharynx after suctioning the tracheostomy.	17. Removes accumulated secretions, decreasing risk of aspiration; prevents spread of microorganisms to lower airways as would occur if upper airway suctioned before tracheostomy.
18. Rinse suction catheter and tubing with remaining saline.	18. Decreases growth and spread of microorganisms.
19. Turn off suction.	19. No longer needed.
20. Have patient take several SMIs.	20. Inflates alveoli, decreases hypoxemia and risk of atelectasis.
21. Remove glove with catheter bunched up inside hand to trap catheter within inside-out glove; dispose of equipment. (Clean or change suction bottle and tubing every 12 to 24 hr.)	21. Decreases spread of microorganisms.
22. Wash hands.	22. Decreases spread of microorganisms.
23. Auscultate lung sounds.	23. Data for evaluation of effectiveness of procedure.
24. Leave patient in comfortable position.	24. Conveys respect for individual and increases comfort. Helps patient relax after stressful procedure.
25. Document need, procedure, and evaluation of effectiveness; note color, odor, and consistency of mucus, and patient's reaction to procedure.	25. Legal responsibility; verifies competent nursing care; communication among other health personnel. Data may indicate infection, trauma, or dehydration.

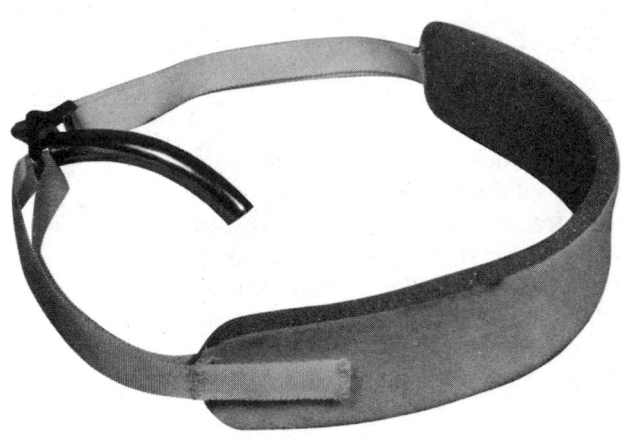

Figure 20–29. Tracheostomy tube with neck collar. The collar goes around the patient's neck to hold the tracheostomy tube in place in the trachea. (Photograph courtesy of J. T. Posey Co., Arcadia, CA.)

normal warming, filtering, and humidification of inspired air provided by the upper airway is missing. Humidification is replaced for the patient by a nebulizer or humidifier attached by tubing to the patient's neck or fastened directly to the tracheostomy tube.

The patient with a tracheostomy may be extremely apprehensive and feel isolated because of the inability to communicate verbally. Finding an alternate method of communication is very important to the patient's physical and psychological well-being. The patient's self-esteem may be compromised because of the artificial opening and the alteration in appearance created by it. The reactions of significant others in the patient's environment affect personal acceptance of the tracheostomy, and the nurse can help by preparing the patient and family for the appearance and care of the tracheostomy and explaining activities before giving tracheostomy care.

Sterile technique is essential whenever suctioning or tracheostomy care is performed to protect the patient from respiratory infections. Many tracheostomy tubes have an inflatable cuff to seal the area between the trachea and the tracheostomy tube. This prevents the aspiration of secretions above the inflatable cuff and reduces the chance that food will be aspirated. Directions on each type of tube should be closely followed in regard to the inflatable cuff. Too much pressure on the walls of the trachea over an extended period of time will interfere with oxygenation of the cells in the mucous lining of the trachea, and tissue necrosis (death) can result. Deflating the cuff periodically, as suggested by the manufacturer and the institutional policy on tracheostomy care, will reduce the chances of this complication. Keeping a minimal amount of pressure in the cuff, as sug-

gested by the manufacturer, is designed to reduce the risk of tissue damage to the trachea. The cuff should always be inflated when the patient eats or drinks to prevent aspiration. The area above the tracheostomy cuff should also be suctioned before deflating the cuff to prevent aspirations of any accumulated secretions into the lungs. See Nursing Skill 20–6 on care of a tracheostomy.

Improving the Diffusion of Gases Between Alveoli and Blood.

OXYGEN THERAPY. The most common intervention to improve gas exchange between the alveoli and the blood is to increase the concentration of oxygen in the inspired air. *Oxygen therapy* is the administration of oxygen above 21 percent to assist the patient to meet cellular oxygen needs. It may be initiated by the nurse if the patient begins experiencing respiratory distress, but therapy is usually ordered by the physician. A notification of the physician by the nurse is essential when the patient's condition changes, and the nurse initiates oxygen therapy. The physician will order the concentration of oxygen and often the flow rate and type of equipment for administering oxygen. Room air is 21 percent oxygen, and a concentration up to 100 percent may be ordered by the physician, based on the patient's condition and the values of the blood gases. Measurement of blood gases is the most accurate means of assessing the need and effectiveness of oxygen administration at a particular concentration. Arterial oxygen concentrations can be measured by either invasive (taking a blood sample through venipuncture) or noninvasive techniques, using a device called an oximeter. The oximeter is an electrode that measures the amount of oxygen diffusing through the skin. It is used in neonates whose thin skin makes it especially effective. In the adult, it is used on the ear.

Hazards of Oxygen Therapy. Exposure to high concentrations (80 to 100 percent) of oxygen has been associated with development of respiratory complications in the adult. The alveoli cells do not tolerate high oxygen concentrations over an extended period of time and may become edematous, hemorrhage, and necrose. The alveolar capillary membrane is susceptible to damage during high concentrations of oxygen. High concentrations of oxygen in the preterm newborn are associated with destruction of optic nerve growth and retinal capillary damage, causing varying degrees of vision loss or blindness.

Absorption atelectasis may develop if high concentrations of oxygen are administered and absorbed into the alveolar capillary system. Room air is 79 percent nitrogen which is not involved in gas exchange within the

Nursing Skill 20–6   Care of a Tracheostomy

Because the tracheostomy is an opening into the trachea, secretions may accumulate around the tube and skin during coughing and suctioning. The opening on the skin is usually protected from the irritation of the tracheostomy tube by an absorbent, sterile dressing. The tube is held in place by ties made of material which also absorbs moisture and can become soiled, as can the dressing. Tracheostomy care is designed to keep the tube free of secretions, the dressings and ties clean and dry, and the skin surface clean and intact. Remember dark, warm, and moist conditions, as are present under a tracheostomy dressing, will encourage the growth of microorganisms and increase the risk of skin breakdown.

Equipment Needed

A tracheostomy kit (4×4 dressings, brushes for cleaning inner cannula, two containers for solutions, sterile gloves, tracheostomy ties), a scissors to cut the tracheostomy ties, hydrogen peroxide (H_2O_2), and sterile normal saline, waste receptacle for contaminated dressings

Preparation for Giving Tracheostomy Care

1. Determine the need for tracheostomy care based on observations of the patient. The physician will not order this procedure. It is expected as part of competent nursing care for a patient with a tracheostomy. If the dressings are damp or soiled or if the patient is coughing up a lot of mucus into the humidity cup over the tracheostomy, there is probably a need to do tracheostomy care. Helping patients look their best for visiting hours by doing tracheostomy care just before visiting hours may be especially appreciated by the patient and visitors. At a minimum, tracheostomy care should be done every eight hours to assess the area under the dressing and the patency of the inner cannula of the tracheostomy tube (if this is the type the patient has in place).
2. Assemble equipment.
3. Wash hands.
4. Place patient in a semi-Fowler's position (reclined sitting position) to have tracheostomy at working level.
5. Explain procedure to the patient.
6. Suction as necessary before cleaning tracheostomy tube and site since secretions often accumulate in the tube and on the dressings during suctioning and the coughing it stimulates.

Procedure	Explanation
1. Open tracheostomy care kit keeping inside of wrapper sterile. Remove soiled dressing and dispose of it; rewash hands.	1. Prevents the spread of microorganisms.
2. Put on one sterile glove. With the ungloved hand, pour hydrogen peroxide into one container in the kit and normal saline into the other container. (If solution packets contained within kit, put on both sterile gloves after opening tray wrapper.)	2. Allows nurse to set up containers with sterile hand and pour from unsterile surface of bottles without contaminating sterile field.
3. Put cleaning utensils in hydrogen peroxide solution.	3. Container with cleaning utensils identified as containing H_2O_2, since both solutions are clear and could be confused.

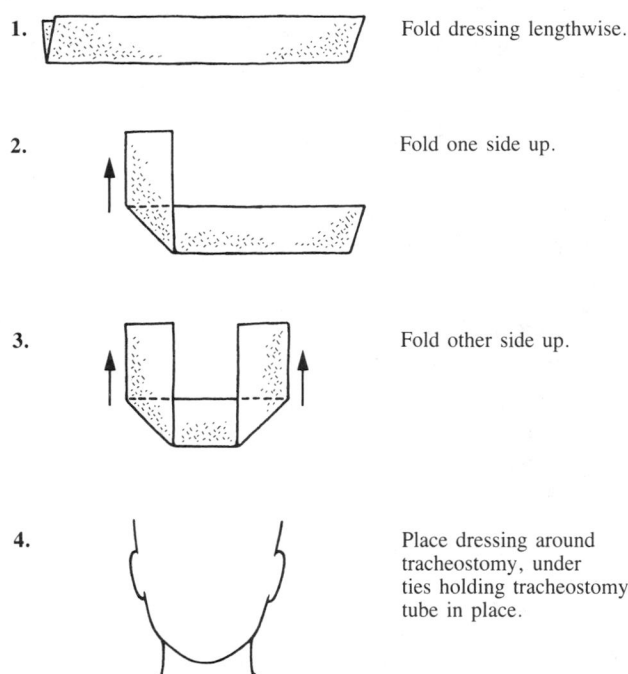

1. Fold dressing lengthwise.

2. Fold one side up.

3. Fold other side up.

4. Place dressing around tracheostomy, under ties holding tracheostomy tube in place.

Figure 20-30. Folding a tracheostomy dressing. It is better technique to fold the dressing to fit rather than cutting it, since cutting the dressing may separate material fibers which could be aspirated into the trachea.

4. Put on other sterile glove.
5. Remove inner cannula, if present, and place in H_2O_2; clean with brushes/pipecleaner on inside and outside surfaces.
6. Rinse in normal saline and drain on dressing; dry with gauze and reinsert.

7. Clean skin area around tracheostomy with swabs dipped in H_2O_2 and rinse with swabs dipped in NS.
8. Blot skin dry with sterile gauze.
9. Fold dressing to fit around tracheostomy. (See Figure 20–30.)

10. Change tracheostomy ties with 2 nurses: one nurse holds tracheostomy tube in place with sterile gloved hand, while other nurse removes soiled ties and replaces them with clean ones.
    With one nurse: old tracheostomy ties are left tied while clean ties are put on (patient now has two sets of ties around neck). After new ties are secured in place on side of patient's neck, old ties are removed.

4. Decreases spread of microorganisms.
5. H_2O_2 foams off secretions; brush removes any remaining secretions.

6. H_2O_2 would irritate the mucus lining of the trachea if drops drained from the cannula after reinsertion. Normal saline does not irritate tissues; drying reduces surface tension between inner and outer cannula, making removal easier.

7. Same as #5 and #6.

8. Moisture increases risk of skin breakdown.
9. Cutting the dressing releases small threads which may be inhaled into the trachea and cause problems.

10. The risk of the patient coughing out the tracheostomy tube when the ties are removed is always present. Occlusion of the tracheal opening would result. For this reason, the tube must remain securely held or tied while changing ties.

Procedure	Explanation
New ties secured at each side of tracheostomy tube in slits on side of tube and fastened with a square knot at side of neck. Ties are tight enough to hold tracheostomy tube stable without obstructing blood flow in skin. Poke hole in tie about ½ inch from end and thread through slit. Next, thread other end of tie through hole on opposite end and tighten around slit.	Prevents accidental untying; knot on side easier to tie than at back of neck. Placing a finger under the ties when securing will help achieve proper degree of tightness. Prevents loose fibers from entering trachea, as might happen if ties were cut to make a hole.
11. Replace humidity cup after cleaning.	11. Humidity essential to prevent drying and thickening of secretions in lungs.
12. Remove gloves and dispose of equipment.	12. Decreases spread of microorganisms.
13. Leave the patient in a comfortable position.	13. Conveys respect and promotes rest and relaxation.
14. Wash hands.	14. Decreases spread of microorganisms.
15. Document care; report any skin changes or problems.	15. Legal responsibility; verifies competent nursing care; communication with other health personnel.

alveoli. The unabsorbed nitrogen remains in the alveoli and keeps them open. In high concentrations of inspired oxygen, the nitrogen concentration is greatly reduced to the point that if most of the inspired oxygen diffuses into the blood, nothing is left to keep the alveoli patent (open), and they begin to close and fail to open on inspiration.

In COPD, patients experience the risk of apnea with oxygen therapy. The driving force for respirations is varying degrees of hypoxia rather than CO_2. This occurs because the patient with COPD adapts to increased CO_2 and H^+ over time. By administering oxygen to these patients, the drive to breathe is reduced, and they may hypoventilate or develop apnea.

Other side effects include anorexia, nausea, irritation to the cornea and lens of the eye, and anemia due to increased destruction of red blood cells. At hyperbaric pressures (greater than 2½ atmospheres of pressure), oxygen can cause central nervous system toxicity and seizures.

Safety Considerations in Oxygen Administration

1. Use oxygen only as needed, based on signs of respiratory distress and blood gases. PaO_2 below 70 mm Hg is considered hypoxemia and indicates the possible need for oxygen. Signs of respiratory distress include increased rate of respirations, retractions, nasal flaring, a grunting sound on expiration, pallor or cyanosis, mental confusion or lethargy, agitation, tachycardia, and possibly hypotension.

2. Concentrations above 40 to 50 percent oxygen for several days pose an increased risk to the adult patient compared to higher concentrations of oxygen for brief periods of several hours.

3. Respiratory status can change very quickly, and changes in a patient's appearance or behavior should be evaluated with blood gases to assess the need to increase, decrease, or maintain oxygen concentrations.

4. Use techniques such as suctioning, postural drainage, deep breathing with SMI, coughing, and percussion and vibration to improve respiratory status and shorten the length of time a patient will require oxygen.

5. Monitor the concentration of oxygen in the inspired air every one to two hours and maintain at ordered concentration. Make sure the sensing device is measuring oxygen concentration around the nose and mouth if patient is in an oxygen hood, incubator (Isolette) or croup tent.

6. Report changes in blood gases to the physician as soon as possible for any changes in ordered oxygen concentration.

7. Oxygen is flammable! Keep all electrical devices at least 5 ft from the bed and from the primary source of oxygen. Prevent smoking by the patient and visitors. Patients should wear cotton pajamas rather than silk or synthetics which may create static electricity. The patient should not use oil or alcohol-based products such as cosmetics or petroleum jelly because of the potential for explosion in the presence of oxygen. Have fire extinguishers available and know how to operate them.

8. Patients on oxygen through a mask may feel isolated because of the difficulty communicating with a mask over the nose and mouth. They may also be depressed about requiring assistance to meet a basic need most people take for granted. The activity restrictions imposed by oxygen therapy may further reduce a patient's self-esteem and interaction with others. Spending time with patients, encouraging visitors, and making oxygen therapy as portable as possible will help meet some of your patient's higher level needs during oxygen therapy.

OXYGEN DELIVERY SYSTEMS. Oxygen delivery systems are divided into two categories, based on the amount of inspired air provided by the oxygen system. A *low-flow device* provides part of the amount of inspired air, with the rest coming from room air. The room air mixes with the oxygen provided by the low-flow device and is usually used to deliver low concentrations of oxygen. The concentrations of oxygen in the inspired air are affected by the rate and depth of the patient's inspirations, with deep breathers drawing in more room air and decreasing the oxygen concentration compared to shallow-breathers. Hyperventilation also decreases the concentration of oxygen inspired with low-flow devices. Low-flow devices should not be used if the respiratory rate is above 25 breaths per minute or the volume of each breath is greater than 700 cc. *High-flow devices* provide the total volume of inspired air, and oxygen concentrations can be more accurately maintained. High-flow devices are less affected by abnormal breathing patterns and are the chosen method for patients with rapid or very deep breathing.

Low-Flow Devices for Oxygen Administration. Low-flow devices currently used today are the nasal cannula, nasal catheter, and oxygen mask. The *nasal cannula* (or *nasal prongs*) has almost replaced the use of the nasal catheter because it is more comfortable for the patient and has fewer undesirable side effects. The nasal cannula consists of oxygen tubing anchored around the head with two prongs opening into the nostrils through which oxygen is flowing into the nose and sinus area. (See Figure 20–31.) Room air mixes with the oxygen flowing from the prongs and is stored in the nose and sinus space during the time between expiration and inspiration. The maximum flow rates for nasal cannulas are 6 liters per minute since this fills the space in the nose and sinuses and provides maximum oxygen concentrations. Flow rates above this are wasted and may cause

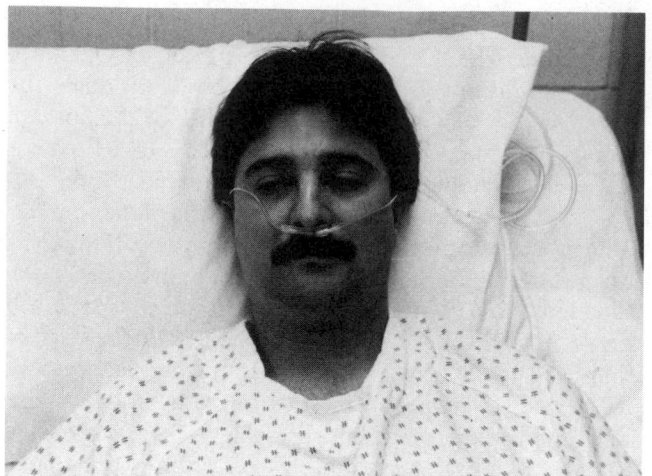

Figure 20-31. Nasal Cannula (prongs) for oxygen administration. The nasal cannula is a low-flow device providing part of the volume of air for each inspiration.

discomfort. The patient can talk, eat, drink, sleep, and have vital signs taken without removing the nasal cannula and disturbing the oxygen therapy. This device does require that the nostrils be open to be effective, and it may cause slight irritation to the nares which can be relieved by application of a water-soluble lubricant.

Mouth-breathers can still use the nasal cannula for oxygen therapy if the nares are patent, but they receive a lesser concentration of oxygen than if breathing through the nose. The concentration of oxygen achieved through the nasal cannula during a normal respiratory pattern ranges from 24 percent oxygen at 1-liter-per-minute flow rate to 44 percent at a 6-liter-per-minute flow rate. The concentration of oxygen increases approximately 4 percent with each step increase in the flow rate from 1 to 6 liters per minute.

The *nasal catheter* is a piece of oxygen tubing with holes in the end through which oxygen flows into the oropharynx. The tubing is threaded through the patient's nostril and taped in place on the nose when the catheter is visible in the oropharynx through the patient's open mouth. The nasal catheter can cause gastric distention, irritation of the nostril, and patient discomfort. The catheter is rotated between nostrils each eight hours to avoid excess irritation to one side of the nose. Room air mixes with oxygen during inspiration as with the nasal cannula.

The *oxygen mask* uses the mask and the nasal sinuses as a reservoir for oxygen which is then mixed with room air drawn in through the holes in the mask during inspiration. The mask covers the nose and mouth, interfering with speaking and preventing eating, drinking,

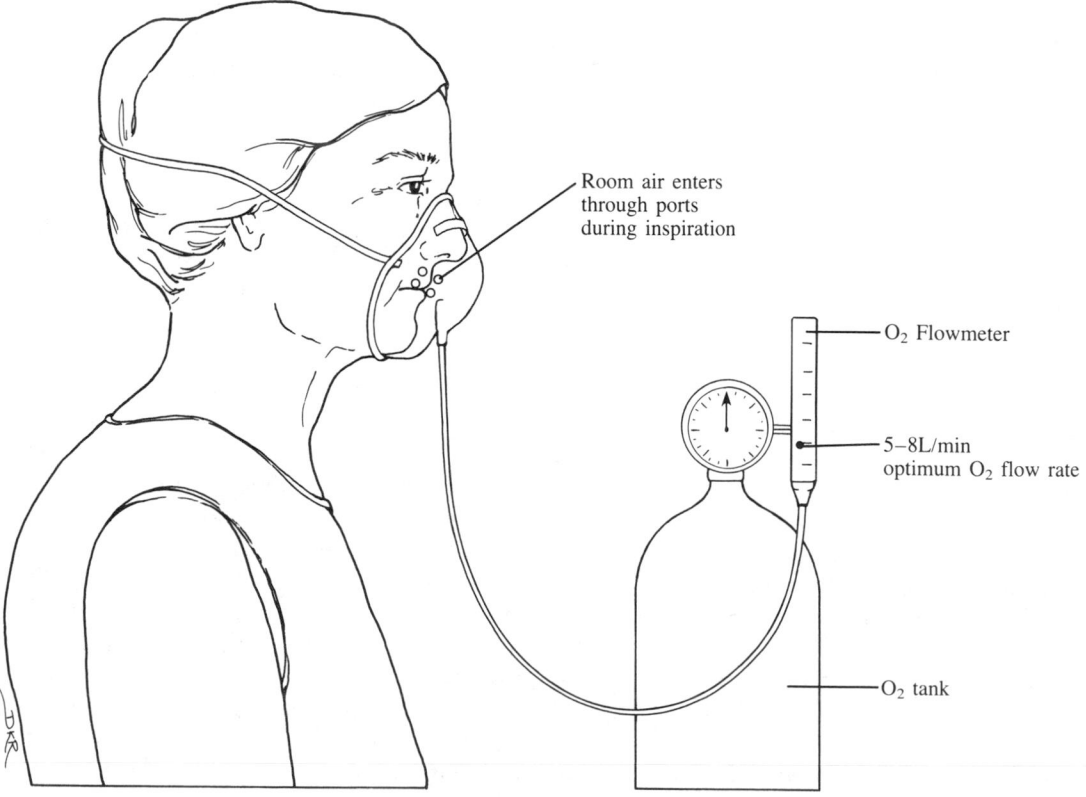

Room air enters through ports during inspiration

O_2 Flowmeter

5–8L/min optimum O_2 flow rate

O_2 tank

Figure 20-32.   Oxygen mask. The oxygen mask is a low-flow device providing part of the volume of air for each inspiration.

and possibly temperature taking. (See Figure 20-32.) The flow rate minimum with the mask is 5 liters per minute since this flow is needed to clear the expired CO_2 from the mask. The maximum flow rate is 8 liters per minute which fills the reservoirs. At this flow range, oxygen concentrations of 40 to 80 percent can be achieved in inspired air. Again, respiratory rates above 25 breaths per minute or deep inspirations greater than 700 cc greatly alter the concentration of inspired oxygen and make the mask an unreliable system for oxygen therapy. The mask is used for patients with a regular respiratory pattern who need higher concentrations of oxygen than can be provided by the cannula or for patients with occluded nares. The patient may feel claustrophobic and need reassurance that there is sufficient air and oxygen for ventilations.

High-Flow Devices for Oxygen Administration. High-flow devices commonly used for oxygen administration include the *air entrainment mask (Venturi mask),* the *nonrebreathing mask,* and the *partial rebreathing mask.*

The *Venturi mask* passes air through a restriction in the tubing which then draws room air into the moving stream of air at a specific rate. (See Figure 20-33.) The concentration of inspired oxygen is maintained at a constant concentration, as long as the only air entering the system is through the air vents around the restriction. The flow of air coming from the portholes in the mask should not stop or reverse during inspiration. If it does stop or reverse, the flow rate is inadequate for proper functioning of the device and should be increased until only air flows out of the mask portholes during inspiration. The room humidifier is recommended for use with the Venturi mask, rather than adding humidity directly to the system, because of the risk of moisture interfering with function. As with any mask that covers the nose

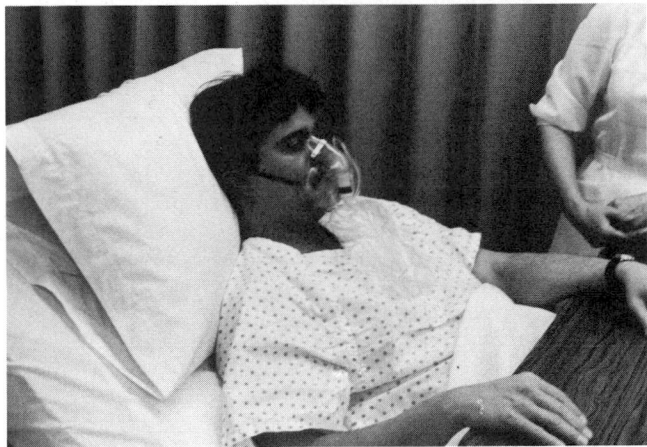

Figure 20-34. The partial rebreathing mask for oxygen administration. This is a high-flow device providing the total volume of air for each inspiration.

and mouth, some activities are prevented. When the patient must remove the mask to eat, drink, or perform other activities involving the nose and mouth, an alternate oxygen administration method, such as the nasal cannula, should be put on the patient so the oxygen level in the blood does not drop too low.

A *nonrebreathing mask* has a bag below the mask which acts as a reservoir for oxygen. Oxygen is inhaled from the mask, but exhaled air is prevented from entering the bag and exits out valves of the mask. If the mask has a snug fit around the face, it can provide concentrations of oxygen up to 90 or 100 percent. When the patient inhales, the bag below the mask should remain partially filled with oxygen. If the bag collapses during inspiration, room air is being drawn in through the mask safety valves because the air flow in the mask and bag is less than the volume of air inspired by the patient. This decreases the concentration of oxygen in the inspired air, but also prevents the patient from suffocating should the air flow to the bag be completely blocked. One disadvantage of the nonrebreathing mask is that humidification of the oxygen in the system is not recommended because the reserve bag tends to fill with water, and the valve regulating air flow from the bag to the mask begins to stick with the condensation. For this reason, the nonrebreathing mask is usually only used for short periods of time. Room humidification, which is used in the Venturi mask, is ineffective since room air is not normally drawn into the administration system during inspiration as it is in the Venturi mask.

The *partial rebreathing mask* is similar to the nonrebreathing mask in appearance, but the first one-third of the patient's expired air is returned to the bag for rebreathing. (See Figure 20-34.) The air returned to the bag is still the desired oxygen concentration, since this is

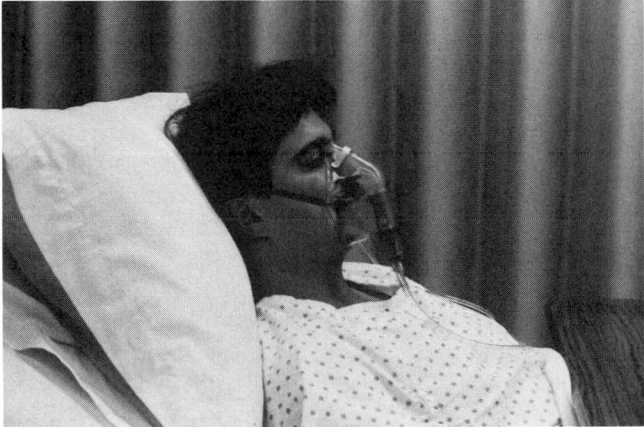

Figure 20-33. The Venturi mask for oxygen administration. The Venturi mask is a high-flow device providing the total volume of air for each inspiration.

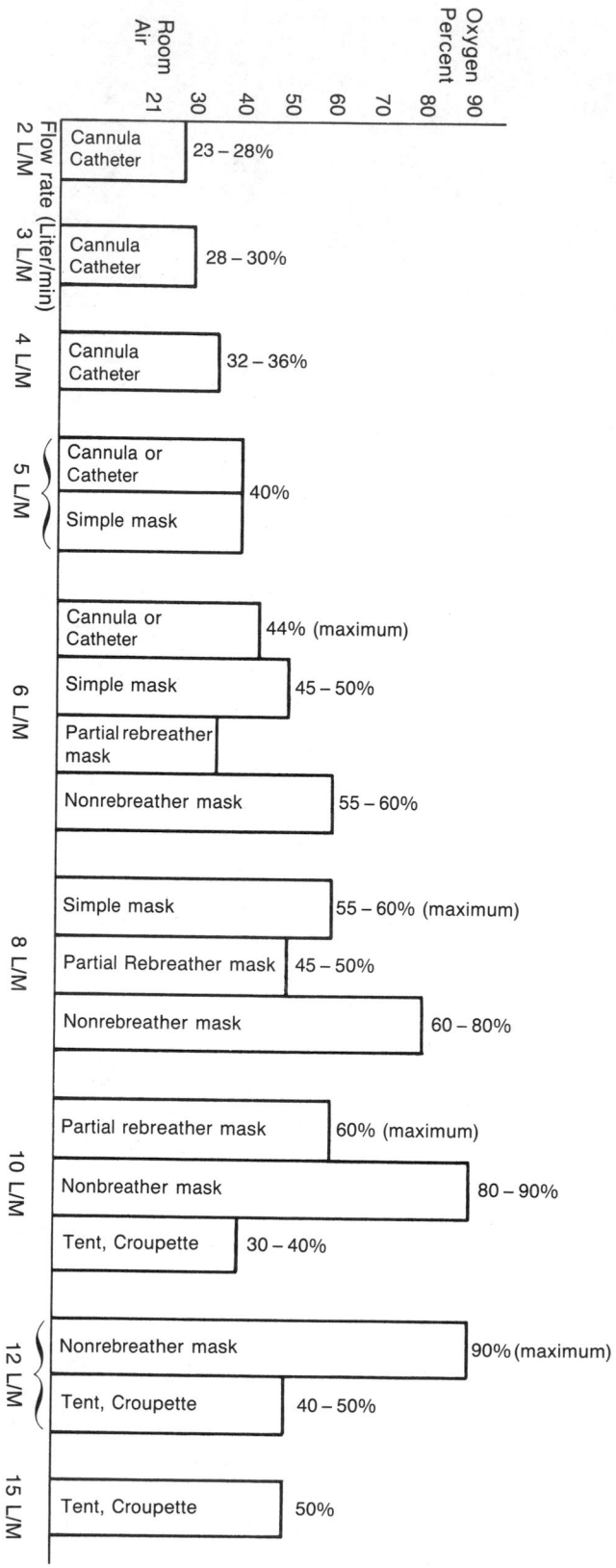

Figure 20–35. Comparison of the oxygen concentration capacities of various oxygen delivery systems.

the air which filled the dead space and was not involved in gas exchange in the alveoli. The advantage of this system is that there is some conservation of oxygen and some natural humidification provided by the expired air from the upper airways. Again, the snugness of the mask's fit determines the oxygen concentrations achievable with this mask: the better the fit, the higher the concentrations of oxygen. (See Figure 20–35.) As with the nonrebreathing mask, the partial rebreathing mask's bag should remain partially filled during inspiration. The partial rebreathing mask delivers slightly lower concentrations of oxygen compared to the nonrebreathing mask, with the concentration of oxygen increasing in direct relationship to an increased flow.

Improving Transport of Gases

BLOOD ADMINISTRATION.   In addition to the nursing interventions of elastic stockings, turning, and early ambulation discussed in the previous section on maintaining oxygenation and preventing complications, the administration of blood to the anemic or hypovolemic (inadequate blood volume) patient will improve transport of oxygen to the cells. Each institution will have specific policies related to blood administration, and these should be reviewed before giving blood to a patient. The amount of blood to be given may seem small, as when a preterm infant receives 30 ml of blood to replace lost volume from repeated blood sampling. However, the amount of blood is significant considering the total blood volume of the infant may be 200 ml or less. In an adult, blood is usually replaced in amounts called units consisting of approximately 250 ml of blood. Administration of blood is similar to administering any intravenous medication in volume. The main IV line is established, and the blood administration set is added into the intravenous line at a point close to the patient through the inline entry ports. One set of tubing may be used if the IV is to be discontinued after the patient receives the blood.

All systems have several common elements. There is a filter for the blood which should be completely covered with blood during administration to be effective in filtering the blood and to prevent damage to the red blood cells. There is another bottle of solution hanging to fill the IV tubing before adding the blood and to flush the tubing following completion of the transfusion, so the patient receives all available blood. The IV solution also serves as a safety factory in case the patient would have a reaction to the blood, since the blood can be discontinued without removing the IV line, which may be needed for fluids or medications. Normal saline (NS) is usually used when administering blood. Some other solutions may damage RBCs or cause clumping of the cells, so check with pharmacy or the physician before running any solution other than NS with blood.

There are several different types of blood products which may be ordered by the physician, but nursing responsibility remains fairly constant. Identification of the blood as the correct type for a particular patient, identification of the correct patient, and careful monitoring of the patient during administration of blood are important when blood products are administered. Identification of correct blood and correct patient are usually done with another R.N. In most institutions, students in nursing are not permitted to administer blood, so make sure you check with the responsible staff nurse and your nursing instructor before administering blood to a patient. Care of the blood during the interval between removal from the institution's blood bank to administration to the patient is also important to preserve the integrity of the blood. Putting blood in a refrigerator which is too cold, storing it at room temperature for too long a time, or overheating it during administration can damage the red blood cells and cause a negative reaction in the patient.

Synthetic Blood. There is a synthetic blood product on the market available on an experimental basis. It contains no living cells but has the capacity to carry large amounts of oxygen to the cells and transport CO_2 back to the lungs. The product, called Fluosol-DA, requires concurrent administration of 70 to 100 percent oxygen to be effective. No blood typing is necessary, and the product may be frozen, refrozen, and autoclaved. It is also less expensive than blood, costing approximately $15.00 a unit, which is half the price of blood. The risks of oxygen toxicity, lung damage, and liver and spleen damage from the product make its use limited to acute emergencies or to patients whose religious beliefs prevent the receiving of blood.

Assisting Regulation of Oxygen Supply

APNEA MONITORS. The use of apnea and cardiac monitors in patients having trouble meeting their oxygen needs is very common. Cardiac monitors are used prior to birth in assessing indications of fetal hypoxia during the stress of labor and birth. Apnea monitors are used for infants at risk for sudden infant death syndrome (SIDS) at home to prevent death from problems with respiratory control. These monitoring devices are used for people of all ages during surgery and recovery to alert the nursing and medical personnel to any developing problems. Stimulation to the patient will sometimes restore normal control and respirations or heart contractions will resume. This is the basis for the *precordial blow* to the chest in a witnessed heart attack.

The inactive heart will sometimes respond with a normal beat to a blow on the midsternum area of the chest if it is given soon after heart action has stopped. Similarly, stimulation to the patient with apnea usually causes inspiration and resumption of ventilations. This is especially true in the preterm newborn and the potential SIDS victim. The stimulation usually takes the form of gentle shaking or jarring of the body.

MEDICATION ADMINISTRATION. Medications may also be effective in restoring control to the medulla if there is swelling within the brain interfering with function. Medication is used to stabilize the blood pressure at lower levels, to strengthen heart activity, and improve problems with blood formation. Generally, when medications are necessary, the normal control systems within the body are inadequate to maintain optimal function. Table 20-11 identifies various drug classifications used to promote satisfaction of oxygen needs.

Resuscitation. The technique of cardiopulmonary resuscitation (CPR) is a skill becoming increasingly known and used among the general population. Many lay people are trained each year in the techniques of CPR. People who have sudden heart attacks are surviving because of the skills of other people in the community who can provide immediate assistance to the victim in meeting oxygen needs. *Cardiopulmonary resuscitation* is needed when both the heart and respirations have ceased. *Artificial respiration* or *ventilation* is needed when the person is in complete apnea, but a heart rate is still present. You will not find a person breathing when heart action has stopped. CPR can be performed successfully on people of all ages from a newborn to the elderly. Adaptations are necessary, depending on the age and size of the person. The idea behind resuscitation is to ventilate the lungs and compress the chest and heart at a rate similar to the low normal range for that age group. A newborn may need to be ventilated at a rate of 40 breaths per minute, while 10 breaths per minute may be adequate for the adult. The same is true with chest compressions. The newborn normally has the highest heart rate compared to all ages and may need compression rates of 100 or more to adequately perfuse the vital organ, while an adult will do well with compressions in the range of 60 per minute. The techniques of artificial respiration (Nursing Skill 20-7) and CPR (Nursing Skill 20-8) are presented as recommended by the American Heart Association and the American Red Cross. In the hospital, people experienced in resuscitation are quickly available to take over the nurse's initial efforts if an arrest is witnessed. Getting a second person to call for help while a nurse begins immediate resuscitation efforts is critical for maximum recovery of the patient.

Nursing Skill 20-7   **Artificial Respiration**

WHEN BREATHING STOPS

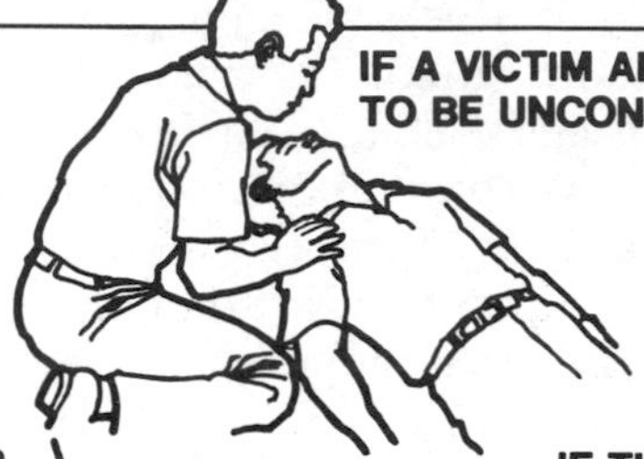

IF A VICTIM APPEARS TO BE UNCONSCIOUS TAP VICTIM ON THE SHOULDER AND SHOUT, "ARE YOU OKAY?"

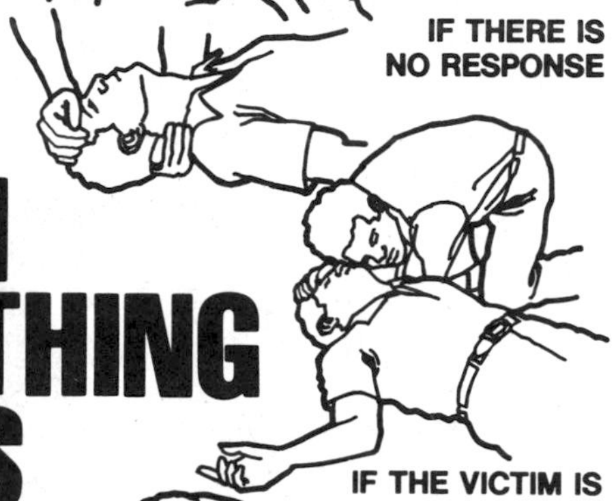

IF THERE IS NO RESPONSE TILT THE VICTIM'S HEAD, CHIN POINTING UP. Place one hand under the victim's neck and gently lift. At the same time, push with the other hand on the victim's forehead. This will move the tongue away from the back of the throat to open the airway.

IMMEDIATELY LOOK, LISTEN, AND FEEL FOR AIR.
While maintaining the backward head tilt position, place your cheek and ear close to the victim's mouth and nose. Look for the chest to rise and fall while you listen and feel for the return of air. Check for about 5 seconds.

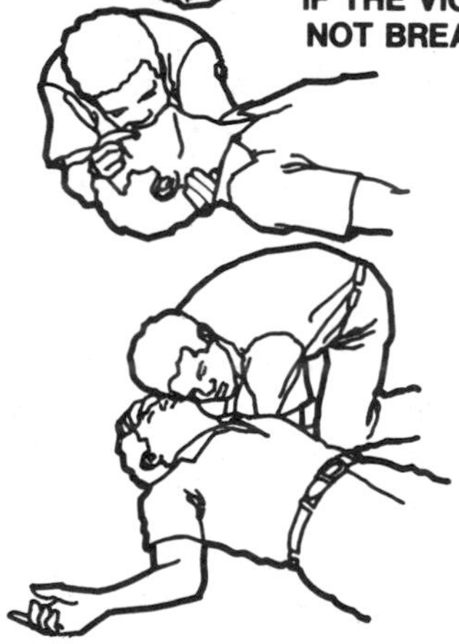

IF THE VICTIM IS NOT BREATHING GIVE FOUR QUICK BREATHS.
Maintain the backward head tilt, pinch the victim's nose with the hand that is on the victim's forehead to prevent leakage of air, open your mouth wide, take a deep breath, seal your mouth around the victim's mouth, and blow into the victim's mouth with four quick but full breaths just as fast as you can. When blowing, use only enough time between breaths to lift your head slightly for better inhalation. **For an infant,** give gentle puffs and blow through the mouth *and* nose and do not tilt the head back as far as for an adult.

If you do not get an air exchange when you blow, it may help to reposition the head and try again.

AGAIN, LOOK, LISTEN, AND FEEL FOR AIR EXCHANGE.

IF THERE IS STILL NO BREATHING CHANGE RATE TO ONE BREATH EVERY 5 SECONDS **FOR AN ADULT.**

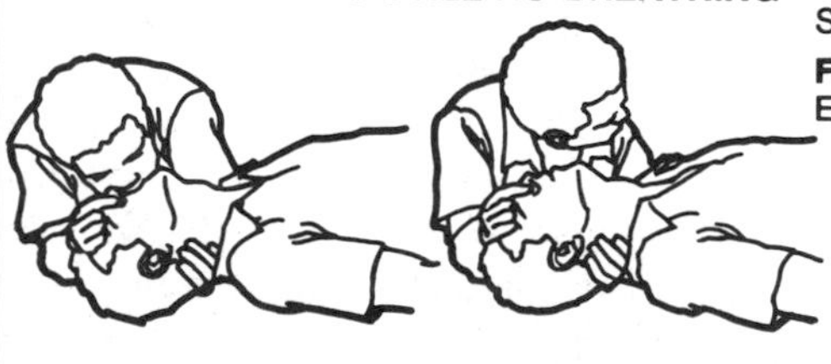

FOR AN INFANT, GIVE ONE GENTLE PUFF EVERY 3 SECONDS.

MOUTH-TO-NOSE METHOD

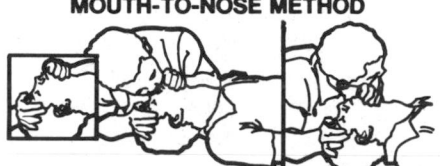

The mouth-to-nose method can be used with the sequence described above instead of the mouth-to-mouth method. Maintain the backward head-tilt position with the hand on the victim's forehead. Remove the hand from under the neck and close the victim's mouth. Blow into the victim's nose. Open the victim's mouth for the look, listen, and feel step.

For more information about these and other lifesaving techniques, contact your Red Cross chapter for training.

Nursing Skill 20-8 **Cardiopulmonary Resusitation**

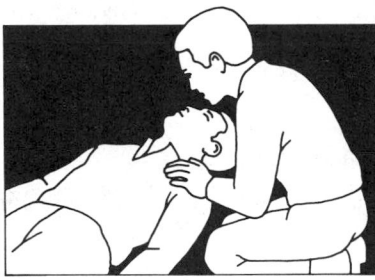

1. DETERMINE IF VICTIM IS UNCONSCIOUS
Tap or gently shake the victim's shoulder. Shout, "Are you O.K.?" If no response shout "HELP!" (Someone nearby may be able to assist.) Do the AIRWAY step next.

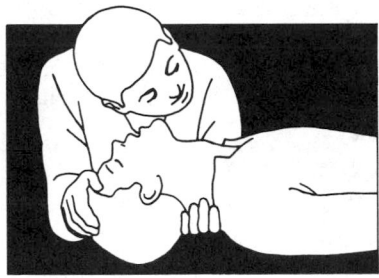

2. AIRWAY STEP
Place one hand on the forehead and push firmly backward. Place the other hand under the neck near the base of the skull and lift gently. Tip the head until the chin points straight up. This should open the airway. Place your ear near the victim's mouth and nose. LOOK at the chest for breathing movements, LISTEN for breaths and FEEL for breathing against your cheek. If no breathing occurs do the QUICK step next.

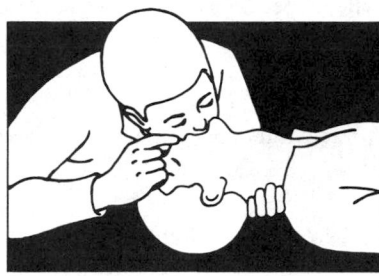

3. QUICK STEP
Give 4 QUICK full breaths, one on top of the other. To do this keep the head tipped and pinch the nose. Open your mouth wide and take a deep breath, making a good seal. Now, give the 4 breaths without waiting in between. Do the CHECK step next.

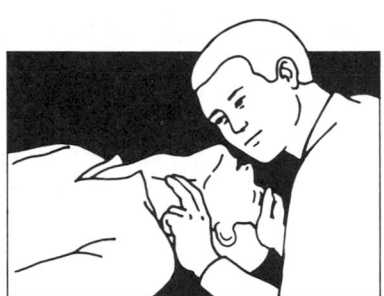

4. CHECK STEP
CHECK the pulse and breathing for at least 5 seconds but no more than 10. To do this, keep the head tipped with the hand on the forehead. Place the fingertips of your other hand on the adam's apple, slide your fingers into the groove at the side of the neck nearest you. If there is a pulse but no breathing give one breath every 5 seconds. If no pulse or breathing is present send someone for emergency assistance (dial 911 or operator) while locating proper hand position. Begin Chest Compressions.

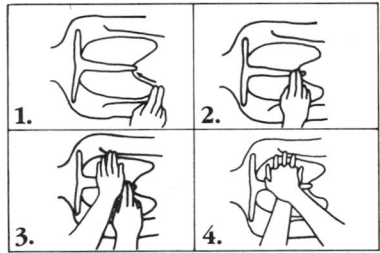

5. HAND POSITION FOR CHEST COMPRESSIONS
1. With your middle and index fingers find the lower edge of the victim's rib cage on the side nearest you.
2. Trace the edge of the ribs up to the notch where the ribs meet the breastbone.
3. Place the middle finger **on** the notch, the index finger next to it. Put the heel of the other hand on the breastbone next to the fingers.
4. Put your first hand on top of the hand on the breastbone. Keep the fingers off the chest.

YOU CAN LEARN CPR
When a person's heart and lungs stop functioning because of a heart attack, shock, drowning or other causes, it is possible to save that life by administering CPR, or cardiopulmonary resuscitation.

CPR provides artificial circulation and breathing for the victim. External cardiac compressions administered manually are alternated with mouth-to-mouth resuscitation in order to stimulate the natural functions of the heart and lungs.

This brochure contains an overview of CPR training and is not intended as a complete guide. Contact your local chapter of the AMERICAN RED CROSS for further information on how you can learn this life-saving procedure.

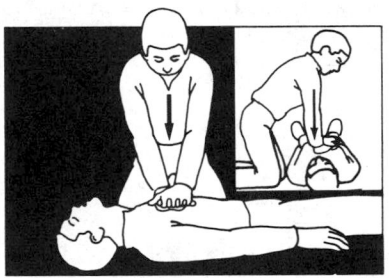

6. CHEST COMPRESSIONS
PUSH straight down without bending your elbows while maintaining proper hand position. Keep knees shoulder width apart. Shoulders should be directly over victim's breastbone. Keep hands along midline of body. Bend from the hip not the knees. Keep fingers off the chest. Push down about 1½ to 2 inches. Push smoothly Count, "1 and, 2 and, 3 and, etc.".

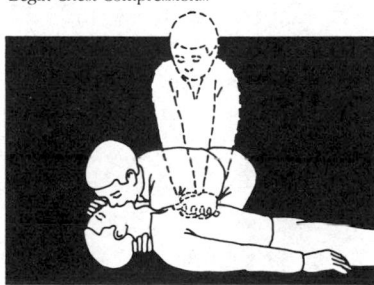

7. PUSH 15—BREATHE 2
Give 15 compressions at a rate of 80 per minute. Tip the head so the chin points up and give 2 quick full breaths. Continue to repeat 15 compressions followed by 2 breaths. Check the pulse and breathing after the first minute and every few minutes thereafter.
NOTE: **Do not practice** chest compressions on people as it could cause internal injuries.

THIS INFORMATION DOES NOT TAKE THE PLACE OF CPR TRAINING. CONTACT YOUR LOCAL RED CROSS CHAPTER ON HOW YOU CAN LEARN THIS LIFE-SAVING PROCEDURE.

Table 20–11. **Classifications of Drugs Used to Promote Oxygen Need Satisfaction**

Antihistamine Drugs

Inhibit the action of histamine: provide symptomatic relief from allergic reactions, especially nasal allergies, decrease resistance to air flow in upper nasal passages

Anti-infective Agents

Used to treat pulmonary infections; tuberculosis

Blood Derivatives

Used to expand blood volume in shock from excessive blood loss

Antianemic Drugs

Used to reduce anemia from inadequate numbers or quality of red blood cells (iron preparation)

Coagulants and Anticoagulants

Used to alter blood clotting to prevent blood loss or to prevent thrombus formation

Cardiovascular Drugs

Used to increase strength of cardiac contractions; reduce irregularity in heartbeat rhythm; reduce elevated serum triglyceride and cholesterol levels in patients with hyperlipidemia and a risk of atherosclerotic vessel changes; reduce hypertension; control angina pain

Synthetic Blood (Perfluorochemicals)

Used to carry O_2 to the cells when RBCs critically low and human blood not available or not acceptable to patient

Spasmolytics

Used to treat spasms of blood vessels and increase collateral circulation in severe vascular obstructions; used as a bronchodilator in asthma and bronchospasms

Expectorants and Cough Preparations

Used to suppress coughs; liquefy secretions in airways so they can be removed through coughing

Nursing Care Plan for a Patient with Unmet Oxygen Needs

Assessment

Data: Mrs. Price is a 69-year-old widow who was admitted to the hospital following a CVA (stroke) in her home. She had been living by herself for the last five years since her husband died. She is unable to respond verbally and has no control of voluntary movement. Her eyes are open frequently, but she does not follow movement with her eyes. She makes no effort to speak or communicate. She responds to pain with a facial grimace. A tracheostomy was done to assist with removal of secretions from her lungs when pneumonia developed. She is unable to follow directions or cooperate with her care. Her temperature has been elevated for seveal days in the range of 102 to 103° F. She has gurgling sounds audible without a stethoscope and requires frequent suctioning. She is receiving nourishment through a gastrostomy tube into her stomach with feedings given every four hours. Lung sounds over the lower lobes on both sides of the lung are diminished, and moist rales are very loud and coarse over most of her chest. Bronchial sounds are audible in place of vesicular sounds in the lower lobes, and resonance upon palpation is dull. she has much thick mucus which she can partially cough out. Her PaO_2 is 70 mm Hg, and she is receiving 28 percent oxygen to her tracheostomy. Urine output is 900 ml/24 hours. Pulse is 88/minute; respirations are 28/minute and slightly irregular; BP is 130/70 mm Hg. She is diaphoretic (sweating).

Nursing Diagnoses

1. Ineffective gas exchange in lungs related to increased secretions and developing atelectasis
2. Ineffective airway clearance related to excess mucus and ineffective cough
3. Prone to skin breakdown (inadequate PaO_2 + bed rest + immobility + diaphoresis)
4. Prone to anxiety related to inability to communicate and altered mental and physical state

Planning

Goals of Nursing Care

1. PaO_2 will be above 80 mm Hg within 24 hours while on oxygen therapy.
2. Rales will decrease in intensity within the next 24 hours.
3. Skin will remain intact during hospitalization.
4. Patient will show no significant changes in behavior or vital signs prior to any nursing interventions which might indicate anxiety.

Nursing Actions (Interventions)
Goals 1 and 2

1. Suction patient every half hour until minimal secretions obtained.
2. Provide warmed, nebulized oxygen at 28 percent as ordered. Check concentration q1hr.
3. Clean inner cannula of tracheastomy every two hours or more frequently prn.
4. Talk with physician about increasing fluid intake through gastrostomy feedings.
5. Turn and reposition every hour.
6. Percuss and vibrate lower lobes of both lungs every two hours and suction following procedure.
7. Maintain temperature below 100° F through the use of ordered antipyretics and use of cooling blanket (discussed in Chapter 21).
8. Discuss with physician the need for breathing exercises with respiratory therapy personnel and equipment. (SMI are impossible for this patient without specialized equipment, since she is unable to cooperate.)

Goal 3

1. Obtain alternating pressure air mattress for increasing blood supply to skin (type will vary with hospital supply—all reduce the pressure on skin areas in contact with the bed)
2. Turn and reposition every hour.
3. Massage skin areas in contact with the bed after repositioning.
4. Keep skin clean and dry.
   (All actions from goal #1 will also help goal #3 and improve gas exchange.)

Goal 4

1. Introduce yourself to patient prior to any interventions. Make eye contact when possible.
2. Explain where she is and why she is in hospital.
3. Explain procedures to her in simple language before beginning.
4. Reassure her during procedure.
5. Encourage visits from family and have them reassure her during procedures.
6. Encourage family to bring in a few familiar possessions from home.

Evaluation

Goal 1 not met. Patient's PaO_2 increased to 76 mm Hg from 70 mm Hg during 24 hours.
Goal 2 met. Rales are less coarse and quieter after 24 hours.
Goal 3 met for today. No signs of skin breakdown present.
Goal 4 partially met. The patient is beginning to show an arching of her back in response to preparation to suction her. This is relieved by stroking her arm and slowly explaining she will be able to breathe easier after suctioning.

Reassessment

Goal 1—continue actions since gas exchange improved. New goal: patient's PaO$_2$ to be 80 mm Hg within next 24 hours while on 28 percent oxygen.

Goal 2—continue current interventions. New goal: rales to be mild or absent within 72 hours.

Goal 3—continue goal and actions until discharge. Assess skin every turning.

Goal 4—continue goal and actions but include touching during explanation as an aid to communication and a comfort measure.

Summary

Oxygen is needed by the cells of the body to create the ATP molecules which are the fuel for cellular activity. Oxygen is not stored in the body, therefore, a continuous supply is needed if the body's cells are to function.

Oxygen is provided to the cells through the coordinated activities of ventilation of the lungs, diffusion of gases between blood and lung alveoli, and transport of gases to the cells in the blood. Transport requires an effective cardiac pump, blood with adequate numbers of red blood cells containing hemoglobin, and a system of blood vessels leading to the cells throughout the body.

Ventilation is achieved through physical changes of pressure within the lung. During inspiration, pressure within the alveoli is less than atmospheric pressure, and air moves into the lungs through the nose and mouth. During expiration, the pressure within the alveoli increases as the diaphragm relaxes. This forces air out of the alveoli until the pressure is equal to atmospheric pressure.

The primary control for ventilation is the concentration of hydrogen ions in the cerebrospinal fluid. Sensors respond to a rising hydrogen ion concentration by increasing activity in the respiratory center of the medulla within the brain, which then increases ventilations. There are also sensors in the arterial system for oxygen concentration (PaO$_2$) and for blood pressure. Specific areas of the body are capable of increasing blood flow by vasodilation when O$_2$ concentration decreases, CO$_2$ concentration increases, and H$^+$ concentration increases. Increased local temperature created by increased cellular metabolism reduces the affinity of hemoglobin for oxygen, making it more rapidly available to the cells.

Factors interfering with oxygen need satisfaction are many and varied, affecting ventilation, gas diffusion, gas transport, and regulation of oxygen levels.

Patients at risk for developing respiratory problems include those experiencing surgery, especially of the chest or abdomen, and people with activity restrictions, especially bed rest, elevated temperatures, stress, pain on deep inspiration, and anesthesia. All may compromise a patient's ability to continue to meet oxygen needs.

Data indicating satisfaction or lack of satisfaction of oxygen needs are presented with nursing diagnoses related to unmet O$_2$ needs.

Nursing interventions designed to prevent patients from developing problems with oxygenation include turning and repositioning; encouraging SMI's; encouraging coughing for excess secretions; maintaining adequate nutrition, hydration, and temperature; early and progressive ambulation; exercises in bed to promote venous return; providing room humidity; discouraging: smoking, the Valsalva maneuver, and abdominal distention.

Nursing interventions to assist clients currently having problems meeting their oxygen needs, in addition to those listed above, include oxygen administration, medication, postural drainage, percussion and vibration of the chest, preventing aspiration, removal of material obstructing airway, teaching breathing techniques to reduce dyspnea, suctioning respiratory secretions, care of a tracheostomy, administration of blood, use of apnea monitors, and resuscitation measures.

Terms for Review

adventitious lung sounds	anatomical dead space	apnea	atelectasis
alveoli	apical-radial deficit	aspiration	ATP

bradycardia
bronchial sounds
CPR
cardiac output
diastolic pressure
dyspnea
eupnea
expiration
Heimlich maneuver
hematocrit
hemoglobin
hypertension
hyperventilation
hypotension
hypoventilaton
hypoxemia

hypoxia
inspiration
ischemia
"make-break" intermittent suctioning
nasal cannula
nonrebreathing mask
orthostatic hypotension
partial rebreathing mask
percussion
phlebitis
pneumothorax
pulse pressure
rales
respiration
rhonchi
SMI

systolic pressure
tachycardia
tachypnea
tactile fremitus
thrombus
tidal volume
tracheostomy
vasoconstriction
vasodilation
ventilation
Venturi mask (air entrainment mask)
vesicular sounds
vibration
vital capacity
vocal resonance

Self-Assessment

One quick assessment technique for ability to satisfy personal oxygen needs is the step test. Only students who have no cardiac or respiratory problems should attempt self-assessment using this test. The test uses exercise as a stressor to the cardiac and respiratory systems as they provide oxygen to the body cells. The more rapidly the heart rate returns to your normal resting rate, the better is your ability to meet your oxygen needs both at rest and during activity. The procedure for the step test is presented below, along with suggestions for improving your own cardiopulmonary fitness.

Step Test

1. Obtain a bench, chair, or other object that will support your weight which is approximately 16 to 18 inches off the floor.
2. Step up and down from the bench for 3 min, using the following pattern and rate: one foot up, second foot up, first foot down, second foot down; this is done at a rate of 120 steps for men and 96 steps for women each minute (each leg movement counts as a step).
3. After 3 min of this exercise, sit down on the bench.
4. Count your pulse for ½ min after resting for 1 min.
5. Count your pulse for ½ min after resting for 2 min.
6. Count your pulse for ½ min after resting for 3 min.
7. Add the numbers you obtained in #4, 5, 6 (gives 1½ min of pulse).
8. Compare to Table 20-12.

Table 20-12. **Heart Rate Recovery Ratings for the Step Test**

	HEART RATE (MEN) (PER MIN)	HEART RATE (WOMEN) (PER MIN)
Super	97–117	95–118
Excellent	122–132	126–135
Good	137–147	141–153
Average	152–162	158–170
Fair	167–177	176–186
Poor	182–192	193–204
Very poor	197–217	210–233

Source: Adapted from B. Getchell: Physical Fitness—A Way of Life, 2nd ed. Wiley, New York, 1979. Reprinted with permission.

Three factors are important in improving your own cardiopulmonary status:

1. Exercise regularly, at least four times each week.
2. Exercise for at least 30 min during each exercise session.
3. The form of exercise should be vigorous enough to raise you pulse into the range of 150 to 170 if your body is in average physical condition and you are under 30 years of age. If you are older, the desired heart range decreases gradually with advancing age, so older adults (above 65) would aim for exercise heart rates in the 130 to 140

beats-per-minute ranges. Of course, before any vigorous exercise program your general health should be assessed by your physician.

Learning Activities

1. Measure your own vital signs and those of some other nursing students:
   a. Measure someone's pulse and respirations after two consecutive cigarettes and compare to the individual's baseline measurements.
   b. Run in place for several minutes and assess BP and pulse and compare to baseline values.
   c. Measure your vital signs before going to your next test, and consider the effect of stress on oxygen needs.
2. Discuss with other students how you might respond to a nurse who insisted that you quit smoking for health reasons but smelled of smoke and was seen smoking in the cafeteria. Is it ethical to give patients health advice that you as their nurse have chosen not to follow in your personal life?
3. Accompany a respiratory therapist on hospital rounds and discuss how the interventions used facilitate O_2 need satisfaction for various patients. Discuss adaptations needed in the interventions to treat various age groups.
4. Enroll in a community CPR course and identify the extent of CPR training for the general public in your area.

Review Questions

1. What is the main use for oxygen within the body?
   a. Manufacturing proteins for body growth
   b. Production of ATP within the cell
   c. To hold the alveoli open during gas exchange
   d. To regulate respirations
2. Which of the following conditions is *not* essential if cellular oxygen needs are to be met?
   a. Well-perfused alveoli
   b. Ventilations that inflate the alveoli with each inspiration
   c. PO_2 in alveoli lower than PO_2 in deoxygenated blood circulated to lungs from right ventricle
   d. PaO_2 higher than concentration of oxygen in the cells
3. Which of the following statements correctly explains some aspect of normal ventilation?
   a. Inspiration moves more air than expiration
   b. The intrapleural pressure during inspiration is greater than atmospheric pressure
   c. The normal tidal volume is approximately 500 cc of air in the adult
   d. Expiration requires contraction of the diaphragm and intercostal muscles.
4. During a maximum inhalation, how much air is drawn into the respiratory system in an adult?

   a. 800 cc
   b. 1,000 cc
   c. 1,500 cc
   d. 2,500 cc
   e. 3,500 cc
5. The major factor controlling respiratory rate is
   a. PaO_2
   b. $PaCO_2$
   c. H^+ concentration in fluid surrounding the brain (CSF)
   d. Aortic and carotid baroreceptors
6. The control center for respiratory and cardiovascular activity is located in which of the following structures?
   a. Cerebral cortex
   b. Hypothalamus
   c. Medulla
   d. Bone marrow
   e. Aortic and carotid chemoreceptors
7. The risk of atelectasis is increased by which of the following factors?
   a. Pain on normal inspiration
   b. Sustained maximum inhalations
   c. Occasional sighs and yawns
   d. Production of surfactant within the alveoli

Matching

8. _____ A low PaO_2
9. _____ Hypoxia caused by inadequate blood flow to certain cells
10. _____ Hypoxia caused by inadequate RBCs or decreased hemoglobin
    a. Anemic hypoxia
    b. Ischemic hypoxia
    c. Hypoxemia

11. When listening to lung sounds, which of the following data indicate potential problems with oxygenation?
    a. Vesicular sounds that are three times as long on inspiration as on expiration
    b. Absence of adventitious lung sounds
    c. Coarse rales
    d. Vesicular sound heard in all lobes of lungs
12. Which of the following findings indicate possible hypoxia?
    a. Confusion, lethargy, anxiety
    b. Urine output of 40 ml/hr
    c. Heart rate of 72 beats/min
    d. Respiratory rate of 14/min
    e. Normal amount of energy
13. Which of the following events is occurring in the artery when the diastolic reading is taken?
    a. Artery is completely occluded.
    b. Artery is first open at peak of systole.
    c. Artery is open during systole and disastole but remains partially constricted.
    d. Blood flow in artery is unrestricted by cuff pressure.
    e. Pressure during contraction of left atrium.

14. Based on the following data, select the most appropriate nursing diagnosis:
    T 99° F, P 110, R 28, BP 110/80, age 28 yr, agitated, audible wheezing on inspiration, vesicular sounds present, no rales, labored breathing, history of asthma
    a. Dyspnea related to fever
    b. Inadequate ventilations related to complete airway obstruction
    c. Inadequate cardiac output due to ischemia
    d. Hypoxemia
    e. Dyspnea related to probable asthma attack

15. Sustained maximal inspirations are effective in reducing or preventing atelectasis for which of the following reasons?
    a. Holding a maximum inspiration for several seconds is needed to inflate alveoli.
    b. They exercise the muscles of respiration.
    c. They increase the concentration of oxygen in the inspired air.
    d. The SMI is followed by forceful expiration of all air possible, and it is this emptying of the air from the lung that reduces the risk of atelectasis.

16. The "make-break" techique for applying intermittent suction to the patient's respiratory tract is recommended for all of the following reasons *except*
    a. Decreases risk of tissue damage
    b. Decreases risk of hypoxemia
    c. More effectively clears suction catheter of mucus

Answers

1. b
2. c
3. c
4. e
5. c
6. c
7. a
8. c
9. b
10 a
11. c
12. a
13. d
14. e
15. a
16. c

References and Bibliography

Benson, A.: The challenge of the gram-negative rod in today's hospitals. *Nurs. Clin. North Am.,* **16**:285–92, 1981.

Breslin, E.: Prevention and treatment of pulmonary complications in patients after surgery of the upper abdomen. *Heart Lung* **10**:511–19, May–June, 1981.

Brown, I.: Trach care? Take care—infections on the prowl. *Nursing 82,* **12**:45, May, 1982.

Bull, S.: Vascular pressures and critical care management. *Nurs. Clin. North Am,* **16**:225–39, 1981.

Burke, M.; Towers, H.; O'Malley, K.; Fitzgerald, D.; and O'Brien, E.: Sphygmomanometers in hospital and family practice: problems and recommendations. *Br. Med. J.,* **285**:469–71, Aug. 14, 1982.

Burns, K., and Johnson, P.: *Health Assessment in Clinical Practice.* Prentice-Hall, Englewood Cliffs, N.J., 1980.

Corbett, J.: *Laboratory Tests in Nursing Practice.* Appleton-Century Crofts, Norwalk, Ct. 1982.

Davida, J.: Pulmonary rehabilitation, *Nurs. Clin. North Am.,* **16**:275–83, 1981.

Ellmyer, P., and Thomas, N.: A guide to your patients' safe home use of oxygen. *Nursing 82,* **12**:56, Jan., 1982.

Fink, J.: The challenge of high blood pressure control. *Nurs. Clin. North Am.,* **16**:301–308, 1981.

Fuchs, P.: Getting the best out of oxygen delivery systems. *Nursing 80,* **10**:34, Dec., 1980.

Fuchs, P.: Before and after surgery stay right on respiratory care. *Nursing 83,* **13**:47–50, May, 1983.

Graham, H.: Making a match. *Nurs. Mirror,* **154**:32, Jan. 13, 1982.

Graham, H.: First the bad news. . . . *Nurs. Mirror,* **154**:46, Jan. 6, 1982.

Grim, C.: Nursing assessment of the patient with high blood pressure. *Nurs. Clin. N. Am.,* **16**:349–64, 1981.

Hellman, R., and Carlo, S.: Effects of talking on diastolic blood pressure readings. *Am. J. Nurs.* **80**:2190, 1980.

Humbrecht, B., and Van Parys, E.: From assessment to intervention—How to use heart and breath sounds as part of your nursing care plan. *Nursing 82,* **12**:34, Apr. 1982.

Hunter, P.: Bedside monitoring of respiratory function. *Nurs. Clin. North Am.,* **16**:211–24, 1981.

Iveson-Iveson, J.: Respirations. *Nurs. Mirror,* **154**:31, Mar. 10, 1982.

Iveson-Iveson, J.: Pulse taking. *Nurs. Mirror,* **154**:28, Feb. 24, 1982.

Kinnebrew, M.: Add paradoxical pulse to your assessment routine. *RN,* **44**:32, Nov., 1981.

Kirkendall, W.; Feinleib, M.; Freis, E.; and Mark, A.: Recommendations for human blood pressure determinations by sphygmomanometers. *Hypertension,* **62**:509, Mar., 1981.

Kozier, B., and Erb, G.: *Techniques in Clinical Nursing.* Addison-Wesley, Reading, Mass., 1982.

Leonard, A.; Igra, A.; and Hawthorn, A.: Status of high blood pressure control in California: A preliminary report of a statewide survey. *Heart Lung,* **10**:255–60, Mar.–Apr. 1981.

Lester, D.: Synthetic blood: A future alternative. *Am. J. Nurs.* **82**:452, 1982.

Matheny, L.: Emergency: First aid for cardiopulmonary arrest. *Nursing 82,* **12**:34, June, 1982.

Newton, K.: Comparison of aortic and brachial cuff pressures in flat supine and lateral recumbent positions. *Heart Lung,* **10**:821–26, Sept.–Oct., 1981.

Pepler, C.: Your fingers on the pulse. Evaluating what you feel. *Nursing 80,* **10**:34, Dec., 1980.

Peterson, G.: Application and assessment of oxygen therapy devices. *Nurs. Clin. North Am.,* **16**:241–57, 1981.

Pfester, S.: Respiratory arrest—are you prepared? *Nursing 82,* **12**:34–41, Sep., 1982.

Pinney, M.: Foreign body aspiration. *Am. J. Nurs.,* **81**:521, 1981.

Popkess-Vawter, S: Reducing cardiac risk factors in the obese patient. *Nurs. Clin. North Am.,* **17**:233–44, 1982.

Rambo, B., and Wood, L.: *Nursing Skills for Clinical Practice.* Saunders, Philadelphia, 1982.

Ramsey, J.: *Basic Pathophysiology—Modern Stress and the Disease Process.* Addison–Wesley, Reading, Mass., 1982.

Roberts, A.: Systems and signs: Respirations: Auscultation. *Nurs. Times,* **77** (Jan. 1), Center Section, 1981.

Roberts, A.: Systems and signs: Respirations: Palpation. *Nurs. Times,* **76** (Dec. 4), Center Section, 1980.

Roberts, A.: The cardiovascular system. *Nurs. Times,* **76** (Oct. 2), Center Section, 1980.

Rokosky, J.: Assessment of the individual with altered respiratory function. *Nurs. Clin. North Am.,* **16**:195–209, 1981.

Sandroff, R.: Blushing on the inside—A new look at hypertension. *RN,* **45**:40, Feb., 1982.

Schare, B., and Stephlen, C.: What those breath sounds are telling you to do. *RN,* **44**:48, Dec., 1981.

Trafford, A.: America's $39 billion heart business. *U.S. News and World Report,* **92**:53, Mar. 15, 1982.

Vander, A.: Sherman, J.; and Luciano, D.: *Human Physiology: The Mechanisms of Body Function.* McGraw-Hill, New York, 1980.

Weaver, T.: Refreshers on pulmonary studies. *RN,* **45**:64, Oct. 1982.

THE NEED FOR TEMPERATURE MAINTENANCE

Objectives

1. Explain a human being's need to maintain constant temperature and consequences of hyperthermia and hypothermia on body functioning.
2. Describe how body oxygen needs are affected by a person's temperature.
3. Describe how the body normally loses heat; conserves heat, and increases heat production to maintain a constant core temperature.
4. Explain how body temperature is regulated by the nervous system.
5. Identify risk factors for problems with temperature maintenance.
6. Identify subjective and objective data indicating satisfaction of temperature maintenance needs.
7. Identify subjective and objective data associated with alterations in thermal regulation leading to varying degrees of hypothermia or hyperthermia.
8. Identify purposes for applying heat or cold to the body.

9. Describe nursing interventions designed to help a patient maintain normal temperature.

10. Describe nursing interventions designed to reduce total body temperature or the temperature of a specific body area.

11. Discuss nursing interventions designed to raise total body temperature or the temperature of a specific body area.

12. Discuss safety considerations in the use of heat or cold.

13. Demonstrate safe performance of the following skills:
    Taking an oral, axillary, or rectal temperature
    Applying dry heat
    Assisting a patient take a sitz bath
    Applying moist heat
    Using a cooling blanket
    Giving a cooling sponge bath

Temperature Maintenance as a Basic Need

"Humans can go without water for days at a time and do without food for several weeks, if need be, but they cannot do without warmth for more than a few hours" (Pozos and Born, 1982). The body's need to maintain its core temperature within a very narrow range, for optimal functioning, makes human beings *homoiothermic*. Unlike some other animals whose temperature fluctuates within a wide range depending on the environmental temperature, humans are homoiothermic and do not allow their temperatures to vary

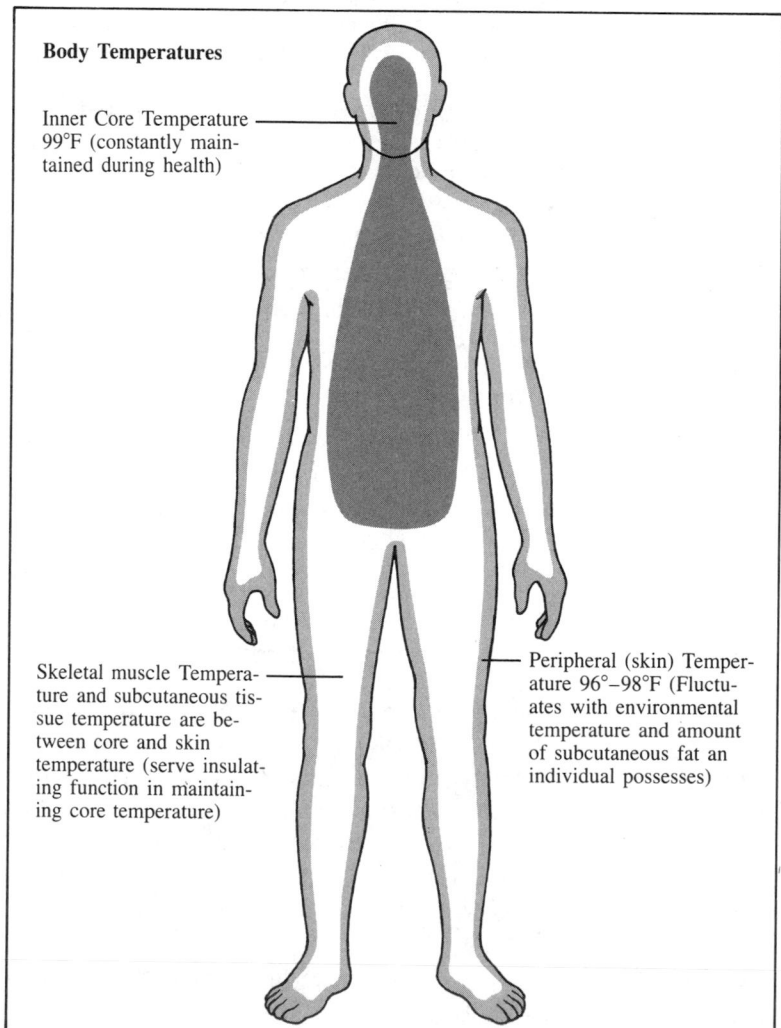

Body Temperatures

Inner Core Temperature 99°F (constantly maintained during health)

Skeletal muscle Temperature and subcutaneous tissue temperature are between core and skin temperature (serve insulating function in maintaining core temperature)

Peripheral (skin) Temperature 96°–98°F (Fluctuates with environmental temperature and amount of subcutaneous fat an individual possesses)

Figure 21-1. Body temperatures. Core temperature around the vital organs tends to be several degrees warmer than the peripheral (skin) temperature.

Table 21–1. **Temperature Variation and Effect on Body Function**

°F		°F	
114		82	Ventricular fibrillation may begin
113	Death from hyperthermia almost always inevitable	81	
112		80	Voluntary motion ceases, pupils dilated and nonreactive, no reflexes
111			
110	Considered upper limit for life	79	
109		78	
108	Cells begin to be damaged and die, especially brain cells	77	Ventricular fibrillation or cardiac arrest, absolute limit for life without medical intervention
107	Hypothalamic ability to regulate temperature is impaired and difficult to return temperature to normal	76	
106	range without help	75	Pulmonary edema
105	Febrile seizures, heat stroke	74	
104		73	
103		72	
102		71	Maximum risk of ventricular fibrillation
101		70	
100	Hard exercise in adult, actively playing children	69	
99		68	Cardiac arrest
98	Normal body temperature (measured by oral route)	67	
97	Shivering may begin	66	
96	Early morning temperatures in some individuals	65	Lowest accidental hypothermia victim to recover
95	Point of maximum shivering	64	
94	Impaired ability of hypothalamus to regulate temperature	63	
93	Person still conscious; normal blood pressure	62	
92	Muscle rigidity starts to develop with loss of manual dexterity	61	
		60	
91	Severe hypothermia	59	Therapeutic cooling for medical purposes, as in open-heart surgery
90	Therapeutic hypothermia for medical purposes, such as cardiac surgery	58	
89	Consciousness altered, pupils dilated but respond to light, BP faint	57	
		56	
88		55	
87	Shivering ceases, death from hypothermia unless rewarming begins	54	
		53	
86	Unconscious, pulse and BP hard to assess, respirations decreased	52	
		51	
85	Hypothalamus loses ability to regulate temperature	50	
84		49	
83		48	Lowest artificially cooled hypothermia patient to recover
		47	

Source: Reprinted from *HYPOTHERMIA: Causes, Effects, Prevention* by Robert S. Pozos and David O. Born © 1982. By permission of New Century Publishers, Inc., Piscataway, New Jersey.

more than a few degrees, regardless of the environmental temperature. If body temperature becomes excessively high or low, all body systems are affected, and death will result unless temperature can be returned to a more normal range. Temperature is a measure of heat concentration. The normal temperature range for men and women is approximately 97 to 99° Fahrenheit (36 to 37.3° Celsius) measured using the oral route. This is a measure of the body's optimum core temperature, and

body efforts are exerted to maintain it at this level. *Core temperature* refers to the temperature of the body's core, or inner mass. The brain, heart, and other vital organs, including the spinal cord, have thermal receptors to monitor the core temperature within the body. The core temperature usually remains the same, within small limits of 2° F, regardless of age, sex, or environmental temperature. If the core temperature rises above this level, the body adapts by increasing heat loss. If the core temperature drops below this level, the body adapts by increasing heat production and decreasing heat loss. Temperature is maintained at a constant level when heat production and absorption equal heat loss. Excessive elevation of body temperature causes nerve malfunction, breakdown of body protein, accelerated cellular activity, and eventual death. Excessive low temperatures cause progressively decreasing cellular activity, significant slowing of nerve conduction, loss of thermal regulation, coma, and death. The limits for human life are approximately 109° F for temperature elevation and 77° F or below for reduced body temperature. The length of time an individual remains at these temperature extremes and restorative activities during rescue will affect survival. People at lesser extremes of body temperature may also be risking other problems, permanent damage, and death if they remain outside the body's normal core temperature range for extended periods of time. See Table 21–1 for a range of temperatures and the effect on body function.

The body's need to maintain temperature within the narrow limits of 97 to 99° F relates to the needs of the individual cells which comprise all body parts. The cells are designed to work effectively within this narrow range. Temperature increases accelerate the rate of chemical reactions occurring within the cell (metabolic rate). Temperature reduction will initially increase the metabolic rate as the body tries to increase heat production. Eventually, with further cooling, metabolic rate will decrease in proportion to the degree of cooling. Either situation jeopardizes the normal functioning of the cell. If enough cells are unable to function normally or are actually damaged due to extremes of temperature, vital tissues and organs within the body will lose ability to function. This places the total body at risk for permanent or fatal consequences. Preservation of the core temperature is regulated very carefully by the body, sometimes to the detriment of tissues in contact with the environment. This is what occurs in frostbite or when entire extremities are allowed to freeze as the body tries to maintain the core temperature.

The surface, or peripheral temperature, of the body does fluctuate somewhat with the environmental temperature. The *peripheral temperature* is the temperature of the skin and superficial tissues directly under the skin. Peripheral temperature may be several degrees cooler than the core temperature, when the external environment is cold. Peripheral temperature may also be several degrees warmer than the core temperature when a person is exposed to heat sources such as the sun, a fire, or warm objects. Generally, the skin temperature is lower than the core temperature.

Temperature Measurement

The three methods of taking a temperature involve either a skin temperature taken in the arm pit (axillary), an oral temperature (at the base of the tongue), or a rectal temperature (1½ inches into the rectum through the anal opening in an adult). Each of these routes may be expected to give a slightly different reading. Axillary temperature is usually in the range of 96 to 98° F in the adult, about one degree lower than a temperature taken by the oral route. A rectal temperature is often one degree higher than an oral temperature, measuring 98 to 100° F. The oral route for temperature measurement is the most common in the adult and is the method used when talking about temperature, unless another route is specified. In newborns and infants, especially preterm newborns, the axillary temperature may be very close to the rectal temperature because of the reduced amount of subcutaneous fat. This allows more heat to be lost through the newborn's skin compared to an adult. A newborn or an emaciated older person may run an axillary temperature similar to the oral range of 97 to 99° F, when the core temperature is normal. A newborn with an axillary temperature below 98° F is considered cold, and heat conservation activities are begun by the nursing personnel.

Effect of Temperature on Other Needs

Temperature has a very direct effect on other basic needs. The primary need affected is the body's oxygen requirements. An increase or a decrease in body temperature will initially increase the need for oxygen by the cells. The rate of chemical reactions within the cell will accelerate in either case, and this increases the cells' need for oxygen. If the body temperature is raised 1.8° F (1° C), the oxygen needs of the individual will increase approximately 7 percent. The nutrition and fluid needs are also affected because, as cellular activity increases, so do the needs for fuel and water to run these reactions. The body gets fuel for cellular activity through the food and fluids consumed. In very severe chilling, the cells of the body become cooler and gradually lose their ability to function as the body temperature drops. The reduced activity within the cell now requires less oxygen and nutrition to survive. However, unless rewarming occurs fairly soon under carefully controlled conditions, the decreased activity within the cells can be fatal to individual cells and the body as a whole.

Heat Loss and Gain

To maintain a stable temperature, heat lost from the body must equal the amount of heat produced within the body. The body can lose heat in four ways: conduction, convection, radiation, and evaporation. The body can gain or absorb heat in three ways: conduction, convection, and radiation.

Conduction

Conduction is the loss or gain of heat through direct transfer with a cooler or warmer object. The person must be touching a cooler or warmer object for this heat transfer to occur. Holding a warm cup of coffee transfers heat, by conduction, to the person's cooler hands. Placing a person on a surgical table causes heat to be lost from the individual's skin surface to the cooler operating room table. Heat flows down a temperature gradient, meaning it always moves from warmer objects to cooler objects. Some material conducts heat more effectively than other material and is termed a good conductor. Water and metal objects are good conductors and will rapidly transfer heat from warmer to cooler objects. Some objects are poor conductors and thus good insulators. Good insulators are such things as human fat tissue, feathers, and fur. Because conduction through these materials is so slow, heat loss is reduced. Cells within the core of the body are usually losing heat through conduction to the cells around them as heat moves out from the core to the surface of the body. The cells of the skin are usually cooler than the cells within the body's organs and inner tissues, and heat moves down this gradient. Heat can also be gained if the cells on the skin are warmer than the inner cells. Conduction would then transfer heat toward the cells in the core of the body. Very little heat is gained or lost through cell-to-cell conduction, since it is slow and offers minimal control for the body's thermal regulatory system.

Convection

Convection is another method by which the body can gain or lose heat. Generally, heat is lost through convection, but it is possible to gain heat. Heat loss or gain through convection depends on the temperature of the air or water around the individual's body. When the body is warmer than the air or water, heat is lost to the molecules in direct contact with the skin through radiation. Convection occurs when air currents or water currents move this now warmer water or air away from the body, replacing it with cooler molecules which again draw heat from the body through radiation. Breezes on hot days will assist the body in losing heat through convection. Breezes on cold days will do the same thing, increasing the risk of excessive heat loss. The wind-chill index (see Table 21–2) indicates how convection can affect heat loss. A wind-chill index gives people an under-

Table 21–2. **Wind-Chill Index**

WIND SPEED (MPH) 0	AIR TEMPERATURE °F							
	45°	35°	25°	15°	5°	0°	−5°	−15°
5	43°	32°	22°	11°	1°	−5°	−10°	−20°
10	34°	22°	10°	−3°	−15°	−20°	−27°	−40°
15	29°	16°	2°	−11°	−25°	−32°	−38°	−52°
20	25°	11°	−3°	−17°	−32°	−39°	−46°	−60°
25	23°	8°	−7°	−22°	−37°	−44°	−52°	−66°
30	21°	5°	−10°	−25°	−41°	−48°	−56°	−71°

standing of the combined effects of cold and wind by giving the equivalent temperature if there were no wind. For example, if the outside temperature is 25° F, a breeze of 5 mph would make it equivalent to a temperature of 22° F. Yet, if that wind were blowing at 20 mph, the equivalent temperature would be − 3° F.

Convection is the primary way that the body transfers heat from one area to another. The blood moves through the body gaining heat from the cells in the core. As it moves through the extremities and the skin, heat is lost to cooler cells as the blood moves by. In order to accelerate heat loss, the body increases the blood flow to the surface. This is called *peripheral vasodilation*, since it is accomplished by increasing the dilation of the vessels within the skin, allowing more blood to flow through these cooler areas. The moving blood then loses heat to the cells in the skin. Vasoconstriction reverses this process when heat conservation is important to preserve core temperature. During vasoconstriction, the opening within the peripheral blood vessels is narrowed, and blood flow to the area is reduced. The reduction of blood flow to an area can be as great as 99 percent, and the body can bypass the cold areas completely in an effort to conserve heat. By keeping the heat in the core of the body, less heat is lost through convection and conduction. The body fat reduces conduction of heat from the core to the skin.

Radiation

Radiation is the third way in which the body can gain and lose heat. Radiation involves the transfer of heat between the body and the air. If the air is cooler than the body, heat will be lost to the air as heat radiates from warmer body surfaces. The rate of this heat loss from the body is determined by the temperature difference between the body and the air. If the air is cold, heat will be lost at a faster rate than if the air were warm. Above temperatures of 96 to 98° F, no heat can be lost from radiation since air temperature is equal to skin temperature. Above temperatures in the middle 90s, heat may be gained from the environment as heat moves to the cooler body from the air. This is especially true if an individual is exposed to the radiant heat from the sun. Wood-burning stoves and portable space heaters provide heat to the body through radiation.

Evaporation

Evaporation of water from the body in the form of perspiration is one of the primary ways the body has of cooling itself. Above air temperatures of 96 to 98° F, it

is the only way the body can lose heat. Sweating is initiated by the hypothalamus when skin temperatures or core temperatures begin to rise. As the water in the sweat vaporizes from the skin, heat is drawn away from the body. The faster sweat is vaporized, the more heat will be drawn away from the body. Air currents and low humidity increases the rate of evaporation from the skin. At a humidity of 100 percent, no evaporation will occur, and no heat will be lost from the body by this means. Hot, humid days with no breezes are times when the body has the most difficulty losing heat. If enough heat is not lost, the individual will begin to have a temperature rise and may have heat-related illnesses.

Water is vaporized into the environment by any moist area of the body exposed to the air. The respiratory tract loses approximately 10 percent of the body's heat through water vapor during normal respirations. If respirations are increased in rate or depth, more water will be vaporized and more heat will be lost. The average water loss from the skin and respiratory tract, without active perspiration, is 600 to 900 ml each day. This is accomplished as water molecules diffuse through the skin and vaporize on the skin's surface. It is termed *insensible water loss*.

The body of an adult has approximately 2.5 million sweat glands. During active perspiration, water and sodium chloride are lost from the body in the form of sweat. The upper limits of perspiration in a well-hydrated individual have been measured at the rate of 4 liters an hour, which equals 9 lb of water lost through perspiration in one hour. Active perspiration can draw a

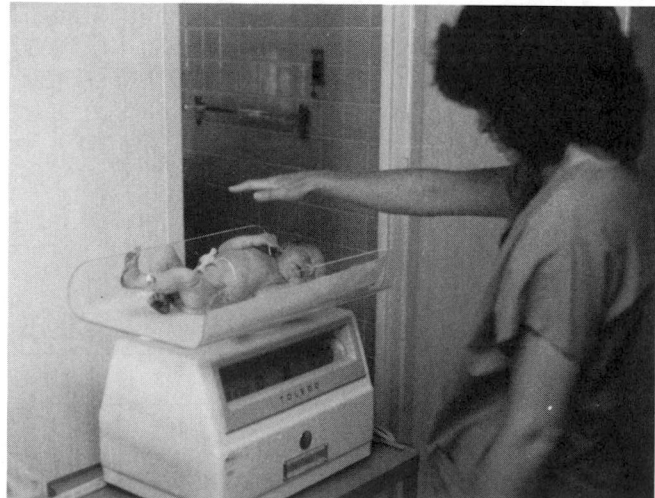

Figure 21-2. Heat loss. The newborn on the scale is demonstrating heat loss through conduction (direct contact with the cold surface of the scale), radiation from the body to the cooler air, convection as air currents in the nursery carry the warmed air away from the body, and evaporation from moist skin surfaces.

great deal of fluid out of the circulating blood volume as the body tries to maintain its temperature. Loss of too much fluid from the blood volume can lower the blood pressure (hypotension) and cause weakness and fainting.

A person who is acclimated to hot climates has an increased rate of sweating which begins at cooler body temperatures than an individual unaccustomed to hot weather. The loss of sodium is also reduced in an acclimated individual. An acclimated individual may produce 1,500 ml of sweat each hour to stay cool in hot weather. An individual who is not acclimated may produce 700 ml of sweat each hour as an upper rate. Newborns and infants are unable to perspire effectively to reduce their temperature and are, therefore, at risk for problems with temperature regulation in hot weather.

Normal Means of Maintaining Body Temperature

As in any heating and cooling system, there are three factors to consider when examining the body's ability to maintain a constant temperature:

1. Heat production
2. Heat loss
3. Insulation

In cold climates, people are acutely aware of the functioning of the furnace in their homes, the amount of insulation in their walls and ceiling, and the cracks around doors and windows where heat is lost. A stable temperature can be maintained by decreasing heat loss, improving insulation, and increasing heat production. As rising fuel bills show us, however, reducing heat loss and adding insulation are less costly in the long run than increasing heat production by the furnace. This is also true within the body. Adding extra clothing for insulation and reducing heat loss through *vasoconstriction* (narrowing) of the blood vessels near the skin put less physical demands on the body than increasing cellular activity, thereby increasing oxygen and nutrition needs at the cellular level.

Heat Production

Inability to produce enough heat may result in varying degrees of hypothermia. *Hypothermia* is a subnormal temperature in the body to the point that there is an inability to maintain normal cell functioning.

Production of excessive heat may result in varying degrees of hyperthermia. *Hyperthermia* is an abnormally elevated body temperature where heat production exceeds heat loss, and cellular function is increased to the point of risking integrity of the cell.

The body has several ways of increasing heat production when temperature sensors in the skin or core report cooler temperatures. *Shivering* is one activity in which all energy within the cell is converted to heat. No actual work is done by the contracting muscles. Shivering involves muscle tremors at the rate of 10 to 20 each second. This activity can increase the body's heat production several fold in seconds to minutes. Shivering usually begins when the core temperature falls below its normal set point. This set point varies slightly between different individuals and fluctuates within a degree or two, depending on the time of day in the same individual. Most people are shivering when their core temperature reaches 96.8° F. Maximum shivering is reached at a core temperature of 95° F and ceases when body temperature drops below 86° F. When body temperature gets this low, the ability to regulate temperature is lost by the hypothalamus within the brain. The hypothalamus is responsible for initiating and maintaining the shivering response by the muscles, and when the cold interferes with hypothalamic function, the message to shiver is lost. After this point, heat is lost rapidly, and death is certain without immediate attention to rewarming.

Increased muscle tone is another way the body has of producing heat. Muscle tone increases before shivering begins, and the accelerated activity within the cell caused by the increased tone results in greater heat production. This increased cellular activity may be enough to return the temperature to its normal set point without initiating shivering. If the temperature continues to drop, shivering will begin.

The metabolic rate within the cell is increased to produce more heat. All chemical reactions within the body produce heat. The metabolic rate refers to the total number of these reactions occurring at one time. As the metabolic rate increases, more chemical reactions occur within a given time period. As the metabolic rate decreases, the number of chemical reactions occurring within the cells also decreases. The metabolic rate is increased when epinephrine and thyroxin are released and transported in the blood to the individual cells. The release of these two hormones is initially triggered by the hypothalamus in response to sensing a decreased temperature. Heat will also increase the metabolic rate, so as body temperature rises above normal, activity in the cells accelerates.

Voluntary activity will produce large amounts of heat. Physical work and play normally produce heat which is excessive and requires the body to lose it through activities to be discussed in the section on heat loss. When a person feels cold, behavior such as stamping the feet, running in place, blowing into the cold hands, and going into a warmer area is initiated. People will turn up the thermostats in their homes or build fires to keep warm. Many of these activities increase heat production through increased muscular activity. Some activities add heat to the body such as drinking hot fluids or standing close to a warm fire or stove. After many of the body's involuntary responses occur in an effort to maintain temperature, it is often an individual's ability to recognize problems and take appropriate action in response to heat and cold that will make the difference between maximum recovery and death. The person who panics in the cold is often lost, just as someone who continues working in the heat may suffer heat stroke unnecessarily.

Voluntary activity does a lot to prevent thermal stress to the body. Dressing appropriately for the weather and avoiding outside activity when it is extremely hot or cold is the body's first line of defense against thermal stress.

Chemical or *nonshivering thermogenesis* (heat production) is another method for increasing body temperature. In this form of heat production, the body's brown fat is used as fuel for chemical reactions within the cell, and heat is produced. Newborns and infants have much more brown fat, mostly over their shoulder blades and around internal organs, compared to the adult. The infant can increase heat production 100 percent through nonshivering thermogenesis, but in the adult, this method of heat production only accounts for a 10 to 15 percent increase in heat production. Shivering in the adult is much more effective in producing heat, while in the infant, who is unable to shiver, chemical thermogenesis is the primary method of heat production. Oxygen consumption is also greatly increased during nonshivering thermogenesis. Signs of respiratory distress may develop if the infant is unable to meet increased oxygen needs caused by trying to return a low body temperature to normal.

Reduced heat production is the body's response to sensing body temperature above the normal set point. To reduce heat production, shivering is stopped, and muscle tone is decreased to a point below normal. This means less activity within the muscle cells and less heat production. General metabolic activity throughout the body is also reduced to minimize heat production and help lower the temperature.

Heat Loss—Conservation and Dissipation

Decreasing Heat Loss—Conservation. In an effort to maintain normal body temperature, heat can be either conserved or dissipated. There are several ways the body has for conserving heat, both voluntary and involuntary:

1. Vasoconstriction of peripheral blood vessels
2. Decreasing body surface area exposed to cooler environment
3. Decreasing sweat gland activity
4. Piloerection
5. Adding insulation
6. Taking shelter from the wind and cold
7. Refraining from alcohol consumption

Vasoconstriction of the peripheral blood vessels to the skin will reduce heat loss through convection, conduction, and radiation. When the entire body is subject to cold stress, blood circulation to the skin will be reduced first, followed by reduced blood flow to the extremities. The major part of the blood is kept within the core of the body circulating to the vital organs. Blood pressure will rise, and hands, feet, and skin will feel cool to the touch. The body fat insulates the blood within the body's core to reduce further heat loss from conduction. If exposure to cold is extreme and body temperature continues to drop, the body will maintain vasoconstriction to the extremities and the skin. The cells within the extremities will cool, and cellular activity will be reduced. This lack of activity also decreases heat production in these areas. The lack of blood flow and reduced heat production in the extremities make it more likely that tissue damage and death will occur from freezing. The oxygen and nutritional needs of the cells are reduced because of decreased cellular activity, but even the reduced needs may be unmet when severe vasoconstriction occurs over an extended period of time. Vasoconstriction is initiated by the hypothalamus when a decreasing temperature is sensed in the skin or body core.

Decreasing body surface area exposed to the colder environment helps to reduce heat loss from radiation and convection. Crossing the arms in front of the chest and huddling down in a crouched position will reduce heat loss by decreasing body surface area. Drawing the knees up to the chest and wrapping the arm around them is another method of reducing heat loss in cold weather. This is a voluntary response rather than a reflex response to the cold.

Decreased sweat gland activity reduces further heat loss from evaporation. Sweat gland activity is under hypothalamic control. Vasoconstriction of the vessels within the skin also decreases sweat gland activity.

Piloerection is commonly known as "goose bumps." It is ineffective in humans as a heat conservation technique since it is designed to cause hair and fur to stand on end, thus becoming better insulators. Most people have inadequate body hair to make this an effective heat conservation behavior. It is an involuntary response to the cold and can serve as a warning that too much heat is being lost from the body.

Adding insulation is one of the best ways of preventing or reducing heat loss to a cooler environment. Goose-down feathers make an excellent insulator because the feathers are three-dimensional rather than flat like most other feathers. Layers of clothing are more effective for insulating the body than one heavy layer since more air is trapped within multiple layers. Insulation prevents heat loss through conduction from the skin surface to the environment or to cooler objects. A good insulator for cold weather should allow evaporation. If a person is active and perspiration begins, clothing may become damp and lose the majority of its insulating ability, since water is an excellent heat conductor. This is another reason layers of insulation are better than one heavy layer since layers can be removed to prevent sweating during activity and replaced when activity and heat production are reduced. Loose-weave hospital blankets are designed to trap air and require another less porous covering over them, such as a bedspread, to provide good insulation for the patient. Covering the head with some form of insulation is very effective in reducing heat loss, since the head receives a major flow of blood. When patients are cold, consider some form of insulation for the head. Caps in the nursery have been very effective for preventing heat loss in newborns.

Taking shelter from the wind and cold is one of the best protections against heat loss. Coming in from the cold is important in preventing further loss of body heat, when body signs such as goose bumps and shivering indicate chilling. In the opposite situation where the temperature is very hot, taking shelter from the sun in a well-ventilated, shady area is one way of increasing heat loss. Because the temperature difference is greater, more heat will be lost from the body to the cooler environment.

Refraining from drinking alcoholic beverages is another way to reduce heat loss to a cool environment. Alcohol causes peripheral vasodilation of the blood vessels, bringing warm blood to the skin surface and increasing heat loss. This vasodilation acts against the body's natural response to constrict the peripheral blood vessels in order to keep the warm blood insulated within the core of the body. Alcohol also depresses the hypothalamus and may interfere with thermal regulation. The thermal receptors within the skin lose some of their sensitivity and cold may not be as accurately perceived when a person is under the influence of alcohol.

The skin feels warm because of vasodilation, and the person no longer feels chilled. This may affect behavior, and the person may not put on additional clothing or move to a warmer area. The individual's judgment may also be impaired, especially if large amounts of alcohol have been consumed. A person may return to the cold area before rewarming is complete, dress inappropriately for the cold, or lose consciousness in a snow bank and freeze to death.

The kegs carried by the Saint Bernard rescue dogs in the Swiss Alps did not contain straight brandy as is often portrayed, but rather a sugary liquid with a small trace of brandy. The sugary fluid was important for the cold individual because it provided a quick source of energy and fuel for the cells of the body for increased heat production. The trace of alcohol may have been effective in reducing the panic and intense cold feeling that a hypothermic person can experience.

Providing added insulation in the form of clothing and blankets is critical in a person who is cold and who has been drinking alcohol to reduce heat loss from vasodilation. People who come in from the cold, feeling chilled, often have a hot alcoholic beverage to reduce shivering and make them feel warmer. Actually, by consuming alcohol, they are increasing heat loss and lengthening the time it will take the body to bring its temperature back up to the normal set point, even though cold symptoms lessen.

Increasing Heat Loss—Dissipation. The body has several ways of dissipating heat when body temperature begins to rise above normal. Ways of increasing heat loss:

1. Vasodilation of peripheral blood vessels
2. Increasing sweat gland activity
3. Increasing respiratory rate
4. Moving to a cooler environment; increasing air currents
5. Drinking extra fluids
6. Providing insulation from the radiant heat of the sun
7. Increasing body surface area exposed to the environment
8. Providing additional water on the skin to accelerate evaporation

Vasodilation brings the warm blood to the surface of the body where increased heat is lost through conduction, convection, and radiation. Vasodilation is initiated by the hypothalamus in response to increasing skin or core temperature. Extensive vasodilation tends to cause a lowering of the blood pressure. Smoking cigarettes interferes with this process and tends to cause vasoconstriction. Smoking in hot weather may prevent maximum heat loss.

Increased sweat gland activity promotes heat loss through evaporation. In order to increase sweat production, the person should be well hydrated. Sweating is triggered by the hypothalamus when temperature elevation is perceived. This is the body's most effective way of losing heat. However, when air humidity is high, evaporation from the skin is reduced and less heat is lost.

The respiratory rate increases in response to a rising temperature to help the cells meet their increased oxygen needs from an increased metabolic rate. The increased respiratory rate also increases heat loss from the respiratory tract through evaporation of moisture from the mucus membranes.

Moving to a cooler environment and increasing air currents are two additional ways of increasing heat loss. The cooler environment will increase heat loss through radiation, and the air currents will provide heat loss from convection and increased evaporation of sweat. Taking cool baths, turning on fans and air conditioning, moving indoors, and sitting in the shade are all behaviors that increase heat loss.

Drinking extra fluids is important for optimal sweating so that blood volume is not severely reduced. Cold fluids in the stomach will also cause heat loss through conduction as the tissues in the stomach, throat, and mouth lose heat to the cooler fluid.

Providing insulation from the radiant heat of the sun is a voluntary activity that may require knowledge of how the body gains and loses heat before it makes sense as a heat loss measure. Loose-fitting, light-colored clothing is cooler than no clothing when exposed to the heat of the sun. The light color reflects the heat of the sun away from the body more effectively than darker skin. The darker the individual's skin, the more heat that will be absorbed from the sun and the cooler that person will be with light-colored clothing covering the skin. The clothing traps cooler air next to the body, and this serves as insulation from the warmer environmental temperatures above 99° F. The clothing must allow evaporation of sweat from the body and be able to absorb perspiration.

Increasing the body surface area exposed to the environment will increase heat loss through radiation. If a breeze or air currents are present, accelerated heat loss will occur from convection. Evaporation will also occur more rapidly. This presumes that the person is lying in a shady area and not in direct sunlight. Lying on cooler objects will expose a maximum body surface area to heat loss through conduction. For example, a cool water bed will draw heat from the body by conduction.

Providing additional water to the skin will cool the body through conduction and evaporation. The water should be below body temperature if cooling by conduction is to be effective. Water that is too cold may cause the temperature sensors in the skin to trigger the hypothalamus, causing shivering. This will increase heat production and work against heat loss through evaporation. Newborns and infants who are unable to perspire may need this additional cooling technique in very hot weather. Applying cool or tepid water to the skin is also used to help reduce excessively high fevers or to reduce the temperature of a heat stroke victim.

Regulation of Body Temperature

Internal regulation of body temperature is maintained through the actions of the hypothalamus within the brain. The hypothalamus can be thought of as the body's thermostat which is preset within a very narrow range of acceptable temperatures. If the hypothalamus receives input from the various thermal receptors throughout the body indicating a decreased temperature, the hypothalamus initiates changes to decrease heat loss and increase heat production. If the hypothalamus receives signals from the temperature sensors indicating a rising temperature, it initiates changes to decrease heat production and increase heat loss from the body.

The hypothalamus loses its ability to function at extremes of body temperature. This occurs around 106 to 108° F in hyperthermia and 85° F and below in hypothermia. Death will occur rapidly after hypothalamic control of temperature maintenance is lost if there is no medical intervention. The hypothalamus seems to be able to anticipate potentially excessive temperature changes and react earlier to minimize the alterations in body temperature which can be caused by external heat or cold. When skin temperature is very high, the hypothalamus will initiate sweating at a lower core temperature than when skin temperature is only warm. The opposite is true of very cold skin. The hypothalamus will initiate shivering at a higher core temperature in anticipation of a rapid heat loss when there is a large temperature difference between the skin and the cold environment (Guyton, 1981).

The hypothalamus receives temperature information from the skin's thermoreceptors and from thermoreceptors within the core of the body. It sends information to the cerebral cortex, the sweat glands, the blood vessels within the skin, the skeletal muscles, the anterior pituitary, and the adrenal medulla in its effort to maintain a stable core temperature. (See Figure 21-3.) The cerebral cortex is the part of the brain where an individual's voluntary actions and thought processes are controlled. Voluntary behavior to gain or lose heat may be initiated from the cerebral cortex based on data from the hypothalamus. Hypothalmic communication with

the blood vessels in the skin will result in varying degrees of vasoconstriction or vasodilation, depending on whether heat is to be conserved or dissipated. Communication with the skeletal muscles will result in decreased or increased muscle tone and possibly shivering. Heat production will then decrease as muscle tone is reduced and increase as muscle tone is increased and shivering begins.

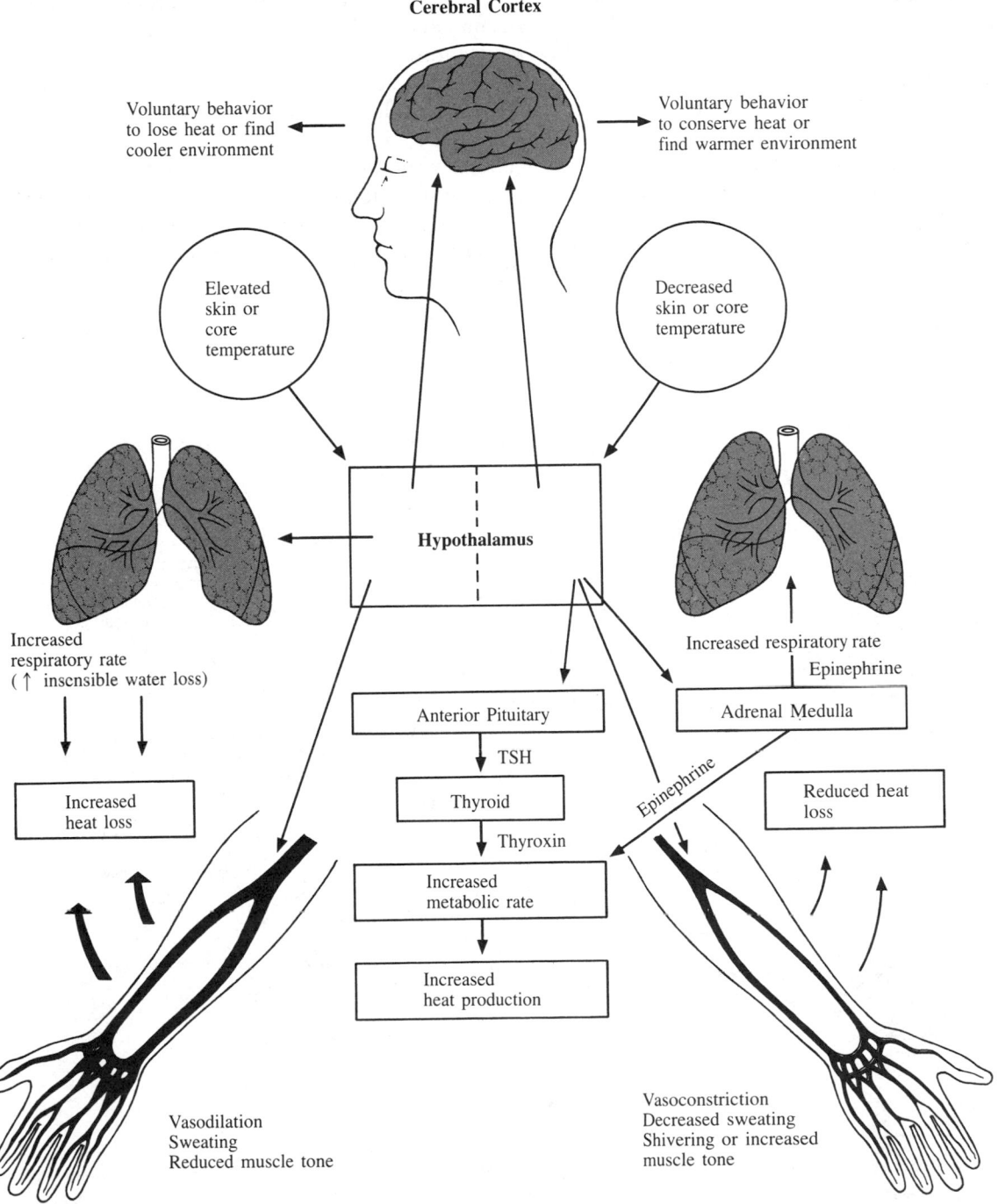

Figure 21-3.   Thermal regulation by the hypothalamus within the brain.

Communication with the anterior pituitary through the release of thyroid-stimulating hormone (TSH) releasing factor results in the anterior pituitary releasing TSH which is transported to the thyroid gland through the blood. The thyroid gland then releases increased amounts of thyroxin which accelerate the cellular metabolic rate, thus increasing heat production. Communication with the adrenal medulla through the sympathetic nervous system results in the release of epinephrine. Epinephrine increases the cellular metabolic rate, the heart rate, and the respiratory rate. More heat is produced, and the needs of the cells for increased oxygen and nutrition are met.

Other factors also affect body temperature, and these are discussed below:

1. Circadian rhythm. During a 24-hour period, the body will show consistent alterations in temperature within approximately 2° F. The maximum body temperature is reached between 4 and 8 P.M., and the lowest

body temperature occurs during sleep between 12 midnight and 4 A.M. This applies to an individual who sleeps at night and is active during the day. Someone who consistently is active at night and sleeps during the day may have this temperature pattern reversed.

2. Diurnal temperature fluctuations are related to sleep and awake states. During sleep, the temperature is generally lower than when awake, regardless of the time of day.

3. Sex of the individual will affect normal variations in temperature. Women have monthly changes in their temperature related to their menstrual cycle. (See Figure 21–4.) The temperature is lowest just before ovulation, about the 14th day of a 28-day cycle. The temperature then rises rapidly over the next day or two and remains elevated approximately ½ to 1° F until several days before menstruation, at which point it drops back down to normal. It remains above the lowest temperature until ovulation, where it again drops to a slightly subnormal

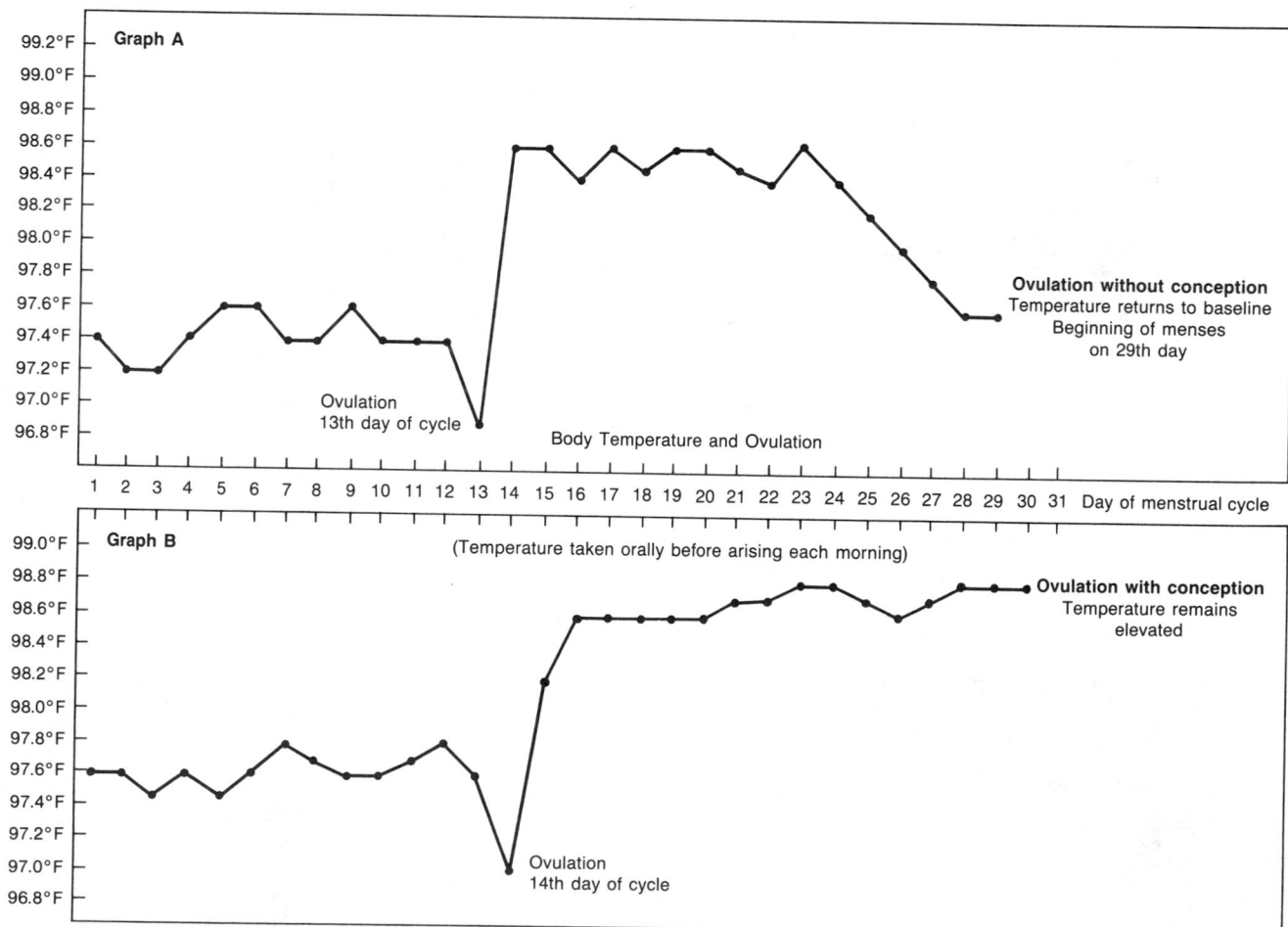

Figure 21–4.   Body temperature and ovulation. Temperature drops slightly before ovulation and increases from an individual woman's baseline temperature after ovulation. Graph **A** shows monthly temperature fluctuation when conception does not occur. Graph **B** shows the maintained elevation in temperature when conception occurs.

temperature for a brief time. The cause of this alteration in temperature with the monthly cycle is not solely the result of progesterone acting on the hypothalamus and is not completely understood at this time. When pregnancy occurs, the temperature remains slightly elevated past the time when menstruation normally occurs and can be very reliable as an indicator of conception, if other conditions affecting temperature are held constant. This fluctuation in temperature is also one component in natural family planning for fertility control.

4. Exercise is the fastest way of producing large amounts of heat within the body. Active children and adults doing hard exercise may have an elevation in temperature of several degrees, as measured using the oral route. When heat production through exercise exceeds heat loss for any length of time, the temperature will rise and the individual may begin to have signs of heat exhaustion or heat stroke. Exercise will also keep a person comfortably warm or even hot in cold environmental temperatures. Oxygen and fuel for the cells in the form of glucose and ATP are both needed to maintain this rate of activity. Exhaustion and rapid hypothermia will occur when the cells receive inadequate nutrition to perform their work in a cool or cold environment. Cellular activity will then slow down to a point below normal, with reduced heat production. The person who is inactive and poorly nourished is at risk for hypothermia because of reduced muscle tone and decreased ability to increase and maintain heat production through physical activity.

5. Stress, either physical or emotional, tends to increase the body temperature. The sympathetic nervous system is stimulated during stressful times, and epinephrine is released in an increased amount. This hormone will increase the metabolic rate within the cells of the body, producing more heat.

Factors Associated with Inability to Maintain Appropriate Temperature

There are three basic areas in which people may have problems affecting their ability to maintain body temperature. These are:

1. Problems with neural thermoregulation
2. Altered heat production (excessive or inadequate)
3. Altered heat loss (excessive or inadequate)

Neural Thermoregulation

Anything that interferes with the functioning of the hypothalamus, anterior pituitary, cerebral cortex, or communicating systems to and from the brain can affect thermoregulation. Brain lesions (tumors), cerebrovascular accidents (strokes), hypopituitarism (inadequate pituitary function), and spinal cord damage are problems that may interfere with thermoregulation. With spinal cord injuries, sensation from the area served by nerves below the damage can be altered or completely lost. The ability to cause vasoconstriction or vasodilation in the peripheral blood flow may also be lost in this part of the body.

Anesthesia for surgery will affect the body's ability to control temperature. Spinal anesthesia causes vasodilation of the peripheral blood vessels below the level of the block, removing control from the hypothalamus and increasing heat loss in this area of the body. General anesthesia also dilates the peripheral blood vessels and increases heat loss. The hypothalamus is depressed, and its regulating function over body temperature is compromised. A disease called *malignant hyperthermia* is a unique problem related to general anesthesia and temperature regulation. It occurs because an individual possesses a genetic trait which in some way alters thermal regulation during the use of general anesthesia. The trait has an incidence of 1 in 10,000 people, and any individual possessing this genetic tendency may die from uncontrolled temperature elevation during surgery with general anesthesia. The exact anesthetic agent is unknown but halothane (FLUOTHANE) is suspected, possibly in combination with other factors. The affected individual begins to show an elevation in temperature during surgery. The temperature rises rapidly, reaching 105.8 to 107.6° F (41 to 42° C), with muscle rigidity and cardiovascular and neurological problems. Efforts to cool the body are critical before permanent tissue damage and death occur.

Drugs and alcoholism can affect the function of the hypothalamus and its ability to initiate heat loss or heat conservation changes. Alcoholism may permanently damage the hypothalamus and jeopardize its functioning. See the chart on medications and their effect on temperature regulation, Table 21–3.

Temperature elevations related to bacteria or viruses are caused by the action of pyrogens on the hypothalamus. *Pyrogens* are substances released from the individual's white blood cells in response to infection or inflammation. This chemical affects the hypothalamus by resetting the thermostat at a higher level than normal.

Table 21–3. **Drugs Affecting Temperature Regulation**

1. Anti-infective agents help destroy bacteria causing elevated temperature; allergic reaction may increase temperature
   a. Antibiotics
      (1) Aminoglycosides (kanamycin, gentamicin, tobramycin)
      (2) Cephalosporins (cephalexin, cephalothin)
      (3) Erythromycins (erythromycin, erythromycin stearate)
      (4) Penicillins (amoxicillin, ampicillin, oxacillin)
      (5) Tetracyclines (tetracycline, methacycline)
2. Central nervous system drugs
   a. Antipyretics reset hypothalamic thermostat to lower level during fever related to pyrogens (acetaminophen, salicylates)
   b. Tranquilizers reduce or eliminate shivering response (phenothiazines, promazine)
   c. Sedatives reduce or eliminate shivering response (barbiturates, phenobarbital, alcohol)
3. Electrolytic and water balance agents
   a. Diuretics reduce ability to sweat by decreasing body fluid (thiazides, hydrochlorothiazide)
4. Hormones and synthetic substitutes
   a. Insulins ⎱ Increased levels increase metabolic rate and more heat produced
   b. Thyroid preparations ⎰
5. Autonomic drugs
   a. Sympathomimetic (adrenergic) agents
      Epinephrine (adrenaline) increases metabolic rate, resulting in more heat production
6. General anesthetics ⎱ Cause general or local vasodilation and loss of response to hypothala-
7. Spinal anesthetics ⎰ mic control; general anesthesia related to malignant hyperthermia
8. Cardiovascular drugs
   a. Cardiac drugs
      propranolol increases body heat loss, more susceptible to hypothermia

Pyrexia is another name for this type of temperature elevation. The hypothalamus recognizes that the body temperature is now below the newly altered thermostat setting, and it initiates changes to cause increased heat production and decreased heat loss. Shiverings, chills, vasoconstriction of the peripheral blood vessels, and increased metabolic rate all occur as the hypothalamus tries to raise the body temperature to the higher setting. Aspirin and acetaminophen will alter the effect of pyrogens on the hypothalamus and cause a temporary resetting of the thermostat at a lower level. As the effects of these medications wear off after several hours, the pyrogens will again reset the thermostat within the hypothalamus at a higher level. When the white blood cells are no longer releasing pyrogens, the thermostat will be reset at the normal body temperature, and heat loss changes will be initiated. Vasodilation, sweating, and removing insulation are behaviors seen when a fever "breaks" and the hypothalamic thermostat is reset to normal.

Altered Heat Production

Diseases of the thyroid gland may alter the production of thyroxin. Diseases of the adrenal medulla may alter the production of epinephrine. Both of these hormones affect the metabolic rate and heat production. Decreased amounts of these hormones reduce the metabolic rate, and less heat is produced within the body. Increased production of these hormones will have the opposite effect, and heat production will be accelerated.

People involved in very heavy physical activity, such as athletes or military personnel in basic training, are producing excessive heat. If the heat cannot be lost at a comparable rate, body temperature will rise. This is especially a problem on hot, humid days and can lead to heat stroke and possible death if heat production is not reduced, to allow heat loss to catch up. At the other extreme people who are very inactive have reduced heat production and are at risk for varying degrees of hypothermia. The elderly may be both inactive and have a decreased metabolic rate related to advanced age. The combination of these two factors can markedly decrease heat production and lead to hypothermia.

Paralysis of large body areas can also put a person at risk for hypothermia. Muscle tone and muscle mass are reduced, and the ability to generate heat through voluntary or involuntary activity is lost.

The ability to shiver is greatly reduced in the elderly and in children under five years of age. Newborns and infants are unable to shiver at all. This eliminates one of the body's best ways of increasing heat production in response to cold.

People who are malnourished or starving will have a reduced ability to generate heat through cellular activity. The oxygen is present, but the fuel is greatly diminished. Glucose or glycogen is essential for the chemical reactions occurring within an active cell. Inadequate nutrition or hypoglycemia (low blood glucose levels) from diabetes will limit the number of chemical reactions that can occur within the cell. This also limits the potential for heat production compared to an adequately nourished individual.

Altered Heat Loss

Problems with Inadequate Heat Loss. Heat loss can be either excessive or inadequate for thermal needs. Dehydration will decrease an individual's ability to sweat and lose heat. Obesity provides excessive insulation, and normal heat loss may be reduced. Cardiovascular disease may limit the ability to dissipate heat through vasodilation and increased pumping action of the heart. Young children, infants, and the elderly have an inadequate ability to sweat and may be unable to lose heat fast enough to maintain their temperature in hot weather.

Heat exhaustion occurs when the body's heat loss activities are being utilized to the maximum point, and the individual becomes unable to tolerate these activities. The person experiences decreased blood pressure from vasodilation of the peripheral blood vessels. The blood volume is often depleted because of profuse sweating. Body temperature is usually only slightly elevated because heat loss mechanisms have been effective. People with heat exhaustion often faint or feel dizzy and weak. They may experience nausea and vomiting, thirst, tachycardia (rapid heart rate), and headache. These symptoms are usually enough to force the person to alter voluntary behavior, thus reducing heat production. Additional heat loss measures may be needed until fluid loss is replaced. If symptoms of heat exhaustion are ignored or unrecognized and the body continues to produce heat faster than it can be lost, *heat stroke* may develop. In addition to the symptoms for heat exhaustion, the person with heat stroke has a very high temperature, in the range of 105° F. They are often confused and may be agitated, lethargic, or in a coma. It is essential to reduce the body temperature to a range close to 102° F within one hour to prevent cellular damage and possible death.

Heat cramps are a heat-related problem in actively working muscles. It is a local problem rather than a generalized problem affecting the entire body as in heat ex-

Table 21-4. **Nursing Interventions in Heat Illness**

Heat Cramps

Move to cooler area
Massage painful muscles
Rest muscle group
Increase fluid and salt intake

Heat Exhaustion

Move to cooler area
Have the victim lie down and elevate legs
Provide general rest
Increase intake of fluids and salt
Notify physician if nausea and vomiting occur and prevent
    fluid intake

Heat Stroke

Move to cooler area
Apply ice packs, cool baths to reduce temperature to 102° F
    within one hour
Fluid replacement (often IV is infused at a rate of several
    hundred ml/hr initially)
Massage extremities to maintain vasodilation and heat loss
    during treatment
Assess vital organ function

haustion or heat stroke. The person's temperature, pulse, respirations, and blood pressure are usually normal. See Table 21-4 for the treatment associated with these problems.

Problems with Excessive Heat Loss. Problems with excessive heat loss can lead to hypothermia or tissue damage from freezing. Individuals with skin problems, such as psoriasis or burns, will have accelerated heat loss through the skin. Skin irritations or damage increase the supply of blood to the affected area, thus increasing heat loss from vasodilation through conduction, convection, and radiation. Burn victims may have completely lost the skin over some body areas and, with it, the ability to decrease heat loss.

Alcoholics are also at risk for excessive heat loss from vasodilation, regardless of the environmental temperature. The emaciated individual has a reduced amount of subcutaneous fat, thus is inadequately insulated and loses heat more rapidly. Exposure of the body during surgery and earlier from evaporation of cleaning solutions from the skin in preparation for surgery puts the surgical patient at risk for accelerated heat loss and hypothermia.

Frostbite is a condition in which the skin and subcutaneous tissue is very cold or frozen. Any exposed body part is susceptible. Frostbite usually occurs in the fingers, toes, ears, cheeks, and nose. Joggers have experienced frostbite of breasts, nipples, and penis. Ice crystals begin to form in the area between the cells (interstitial fluid), and this causes fluid to be drawn out of the cell by osmosis. The cell may be damaged or destroyed as this process progresses. The body is often using vasoconstriction to conserve heat, and this increases the risk of frostbite to areas on the skin surface, since the cells are not being warmed by the blood. Severe frostbite can affect the skin, the blood vessels, nerves, muscle, and even bone. Rapid rewarming is the treatment of choice and is discussed in the section on nursing measures that provide heat. The extent of the damage from frostbite cannot be determined for several days to weeks.

The *dive reflex* is a response to excessive cold and anticipated heat loss. It is poorly understood, but it is known to be a rapid response to extreme cold on the face as occurs in cold-water submersion. Children are more likely to exhibit the reflex compared to adults. The following three responses occur very rapidly in the dive reflex: markedly decreased heart rate; vasoconstriction of peripheral blood flow; increased blood pressure as blood is rapidly rerouted to the core of the body. These responses protect the brain from severe anoxia. Children have survived cold-water submersion for nearly one hour when the dive reflex was triggered. The reflex occurs faster and lasts longer if the person is exhaling when the face goes under the water. The body cools very rapidly, and cellular metabolism is dramatically reduced, as are oxygen and nutrition needs. Resuscitation depends on an accurate diagnosis of life or death, which may not be easy since the heart rate may be only two beats each minute and respirations are absent. Resuscitation, once begun, continues until the victim has been rewarmed to a normal body temperature. This may take several hours, half a day, or longer. Rewarming applies to all cases of hypothermia in which resuscitation is necessary. The body temperature is to be restored using all recommended procedures available before the victim is pronounced dead. In severe hypothermia, a heartbeat of one to two beats per minute and a respiratory rate of two breaths per minute may be adequate for a brief time to sustain life and meet the oxygen needs of the barely active cells.

Assessment of Body Temperature Maintenance

This section of the chapter will provide the student in nursing with the signs and symptoms a patient may exhibit when thermal regulation is either adequate or inadequate. The skills of temperature taking are discussed in this section (Nursing Skill 21–1), and nursing diagnoses associated with altered thermal regulation are included. A comparison of the Celsius and Fahrenheit temperatures and calculations for converting one to the other are included in Table 21–5.

Data Indicating Adequate Temperature Maintenance

Objective Data. Objective data, for an apparently healthy adult, that indicate adequate temperature maintenance are:

- Oral temperature 97–99° F (36.3–37.4° C)
- Axillary temperature 96–98°F (35.8–37° C)

  Afebrile: absence of an elevated temperature

- Rectal temperature 98–100° F (37–38° C)
- Skin feels warm to the touch
- Normal skin color—neither pale or flushed
- Normal respiratory range of 16 to 20 breaths per minute
- Normal blood pressure for the individual, usually in the range of 100/68 to 140/90 mm Hg.
- Strong, regular pulse in the range of 60 to 90 beats per minute
- Normal sensation in the hands and feet
- Oriented to time, place, and person, mentally alert
- Absence of shivering, "goose bumps," or sweating
- Normal urine production of 1,000 to 2,000 ml per day
- Adequate fluid intake of 1,000 to 2,000 ml per day
- Appropriately dressed or covered for air temperature

Subjective Data. Person reports feeling comfortable: neither too warm nor too cool.

Data Indicating Potential Problems with Temperature Elevation

Problems with temperature elevation may be caused by excessive heat production or inadequate heat loss.

Objective Data. The following temperature elevations are significant:

Oral temperature above 99° F (37.4° C)
Axillary temperature above 98° F (37° C) (axillary
   or skin temperature may be almost as high as oral
   temperatures due to vasodilation)
Rectal temperature above 100° F (38° C)

Temperature may be slightly elevated or signifi-

Table 21-5. **Temperature Equivalents**

CONVERSION

Centigrade (celsius) to Fahrenheit Formula:
$9/5 \times$ temperature $C + 32 = F°$ Example:
To convert 38° C to F:

$$9/5 \times 38 + 32 = \frac{342}{5} + 32 = 100.4° F$$

Fahrenheit to centigrade Formula
(temperature $F - 32) \times 5/9 = C°$ Example:
To convert 100° F to C:
$(100 - 32) \times 5/9 = 37.8° C$

CELSIUS	FAHRENHEIT
34	93.2
34.2	93.6
34.4	93.9
34.6	94.3
34.8	94.6
35.0	95.0
35.2	95.4
35.4	95.7
35.6	96.1
35.8	96.4
36.0	96.8
36.2	97.1
36.4	97.5
36.6	97.8
36.8	98.2
37.0	98.6
37.2	98.9
37.4	99.3
37.6	99.6
37.8	100.0
38.0	100.4
38.2	100.7
38.4	101.1
38.6	101.4
38.8	101.8
39.0	102.2
39.2	102.5
39.4	102.9
39.6	103.2
39.8	103.6
40.0	104.0
40.2	104.3
40.4	104.7
40.6	105.1

cantly elevated, above 101° F. The temperature may remain consistently elevated within a narrow range or fluctuate by several degrees above normal. The temperature may return to the normal range periodically during 24 hours, or it may remain within the normal range for a day or more and then return to an elevated level.

- The skin may feel cool or hot. In the early stages of developing a fever, the body may use vasoconstriction as it tries to bring the temperature up to the new set point created by the action of pyrogens on the hypothalamus. This would cause the skin to feel cool and appear pale. If the body is trying to lose heat, the skin will feel warm from vasodilation and an elevated skin temperature.
- Skin may appear pale or flushed, depending on whether heat is being conserved or dissipated.
- Respiratory rate will be increased.
- Blood pressure may be increased or decreased, or normal, depending on the degree of vasodilation or vasoconstriction occurring in the body. Vasoconstriction to conserve heat may raise the blood pressure slightly. Vasodilation to dissipate heat may drop the blood pressure significantly from an individual's normal range.
- Pulse rate is elevated.
- Normal sensations in hands and feet.
- May be restless, confused about time, place, or person. Febrile seizures may occur with temperature elevations of 104 to 106° F and higher.
- May be unconscious.
- May be shivering or sweating. In the early stage of developing a fever, the person may be shivering to increase heat production. When a fever is coming down and heat production is greater than heat loss, the person will begin to perspire. There may be an absence of sweating at temperatures above 105° F since hypothalamic control of sweating is lost. Dehydration from earlier sweating may have depleted the fluid content of the blood to the point that sweating is greatly reduced or eliminated.
- Decreased urine output.
- Individual may be using excessive or inadequate insulation for air temperature.

Subjective Data.   During periods of elevated temperature, the patient may report subjective symptoms:

Person often feels too hot or chilled.
Person often is thirsty.
Dizziness and weakness may be reported, feeling
   faint.

Nursing Skill 21-1   Taking Temperatures (Oral, Axillary, and Rectal)

Available Equipment

MERCURY IN GLASS THERMOMETER.   This thermometer is made of glass and contains a bulb at one end which is filled with mercury. (See Figure 21–5.) As the mercury is warmed by the person's body heat, the mercury rises along a column within the glass. The thermometer has markings along its length to indicate temperature in either Fahrenheit or centigrade. If this thermometer is bitten or hit against a firm surface, it may break, and the mercury, which is poisonous if swallowed, can leak out. This thermometer takes 3 to 10 minutes to register, depending on whether the route is oral, axillary, or rectal.

ELECTRONIC THERMOMETER.   This battery-operated thermometer uses a heat-sensitive probe attached to a larger unit that displays the patient's temperature in either Fahrenheit or centigrade. (See Figure 21–6.) The metal probe is covered with a disposable plastic cover for each measurement. This cover is discarded after each use. The thermometer registers a person's temperature very quickly, usually in 10 to 30 seconds. It has a range from 94 to 108° F. If the probe is bitten, it will not break as the glass ones do. This is a suitable thermometer for assessing oral, axillary, or rectal temperatures. Separate probes are provided for oral and rectal routes.

DISPOSABLE THERMOMETERS.   These thermometers are made to be used one time and then discarded. They are made of nonbreakable material with chemicals that are sensitive to temperature. One common type gives a reading in Fahrenheit or centigrade by the number of circles which change color while the thermometer is in place. (See Figure 21–7.) Accuracy is in two-tenths of a degree. Another less accurate type indicates whether the temperature is normal, rising, or elevated by the color of the skin tape after being in place for 15 seconds. Each manufacturer's directions should be read and followed to assure maximum accuracy.

THERMOMETER SHEATHS.   The thermometer sheath is a disposable plastic bag which fits over a mercury-in-glass thermometer. (See Figure 21–8.) Since thermometers with mercury cannot be sterilized to assure destruction of all microorganisms, patient-to-patient transfer is a theoretical possibility, even after thorough cleaning. The sheath was designed to prevent this potential spread of microorganisms. The thermometer, with the plastic sheath covering it, is inserted into the person's mouth, axilla, or rectum, depending on the nurse's determination of appropriate route. The sheath for the rectal route is prelubricated. The sheath does not increase the time the thermometer must stay in place (Graves and Markarian, 1980). The sheath is removed, and the thermometer is read.

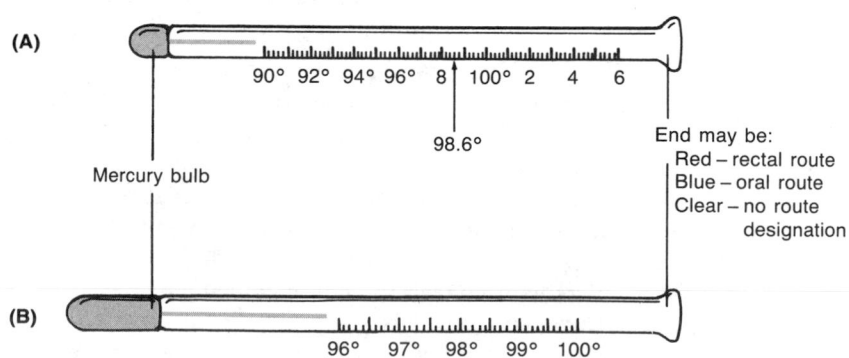

Figure 21-5.   Mercury thermometers. The mercury within the thermometer expands when it is heated and rises within the hollow tube inside the glass thermometer. **A** is a commonly used model recording temperatures above 90° F and below 106° F. **B** is a basal body temperature used to measure very small temperature changes of 0.10° F as were shown in Figure 21-4 for ovulation.

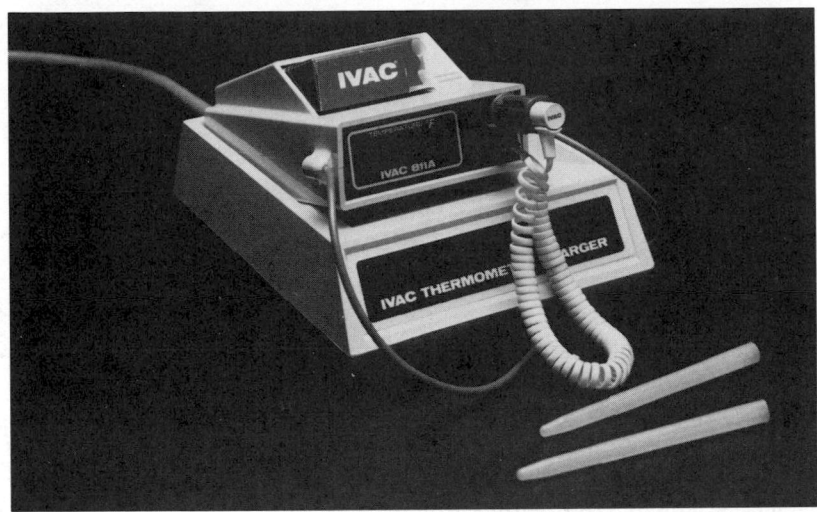

Figure 21-6. An electronic thermometer. The holder in which the thermometer sits charges the thermometer to keep it functioning optimally. (Photograph courtesy of IVAC Corp., San Diego, CA.)

Preparation for Taking a Temperature

Determine the need for temperature data is based on a physician's order or nursing judgment. Patient data indicating feelings of being chilled or hot, confusion, sweating, shivering, cold extremities, or a flushed face may indicate an altered thermal state and the need for assessment. Check the patient's last recorded temperature for unusually elevated or low readings. These patients should be assessed every 1 to 2 hours for temperature readings until they are consistently within the normal range.

Determine the best route for taking a particular patient's temperature. There are three routes available: oral, axillary or skin, and rectal. Generally, the oral route is preferred because it is quick and has minimum risks for causing the patient physical trauma or embarrassment. There are conditions when the oral route or the rectal route may be contraindicated.

Contraindications for Oral Route

a. Newborns, infants, and young children. Patients of these ages are unable to assist the nurse or parent with proper placement within the mouth. They may also bite the thermometer and break the glass type. Young children who are able to cooperate may have an oral temperature taken with the disposable or electronic type of thermometer. The preferred route for these age groups is the axillary route. It avoids the risk of damaging or perforating the bowel with the thermometer using the rectal route.

b. People with a recent history of seizures. The risk in taking oral temperatures with the glass thermometer is if the person should have a seizure and bite the thermometer. The electronic thermometer may be used for an oral temperature, as may the disposables.

```
100 OOOOO        .0.2.4.6.8
101 OOOOO    96  OOOOO
102 OOOOO    97  OOOOO
103 OOOOO    98  OOOOO
104 OOOOO    99  OOOOO
```

Figure 21-7. A disposable thermometer. Each dot represents 0.20° F. This thermometer will record temperatures above 96° F and below 105° F by chemical changes within the dots which change color in the presence of different temperatures.

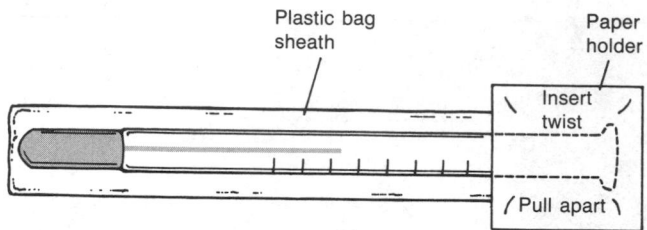

Figure 21–8. A thermometer sheath. The sheath encloses the thermometer while it is measuring the patient's temperature. The nurse removes the sheath to read the thermometer. Sheaths are used to reduce the spread of microorganisms from patient to patient.

c. Oral surgery, infections within the mouth, and patients with fractured jaws. These people will have a falsely elevated oral temperature because of oral inflammation and increased blood flow. In a fractured jaw, the teeth are wired shut, and proper placement of the thermometer is impossible, so a falsely low reading is likely to be obtained.

d. Mouth-breathers. People who are unable to breathe through their nose while their temperature is being taken tend to have a falsely low reading with a mercury thermometer. Electronic thermometers can be used since an open mouth does not affect the reading of the electronic thermometers (IVAC).

e. People receiving oxygen through a mask. Removing the mask for several minutes to check an oral temperature greatly reduces the blood level of oxygen and is, therefore, contraindicated for glass thermometers (Felton, 1978). Removing the mask for 10 to 30 seconds to use an electronic thermometer lowers the blood level of oxygen only slightly and may be appropriate, depending on the oxygen needs of the patient. The disposable thermometer may fit inside the patient's oxygen mask since it bends easily, making this method acceptable if the patient is nose breathing. The administration of oxygen through a nasal cannula is not a contraindication for oral temperatures (Lim-Levy, 1982).

f. Combative or confused patient. The risk here is biting and breaking the glass thermometer. Assistance may be needed, regardless of method, to reduce the risk of injury to patient and nurse.

g. Smoking, chewing gum, drinking, or eating warm or hot foods. This will cause a falsely elevated reading unless there is a 15- to 30- minute interval between the activity and the measurement.

h. Drinking or eating cold or frozen foods. This activity will cause vasoconstriction in the mouth and cool the mouth so a falsely low temperature reading is obtained. Waiting 15 to 30 minutes after consumption of cold foods will make the oral temperature accurate.

Contraindications for Rectal Route

a. Rectal surgery. Rectal surgery may result in local inflammation, increased blood flow to the area, and a possibly falsely high reading. The risk of damaging healing tissues also makes this route unacceptable. Women with fourth-degree lacerations into the rectum during childbirth should not have rectal temperature taken since the rectal area has been newly repaired.

b. Cardiac patients. Patients with heart problems may have rectal temperatures taken if the oral route is inaccessible. Rectal stimulation with a thermometer does not cause a reflex slowing of the heart or trigger arrhthymias from vagus nerve stimulation. This long-held belief of vagal nerve stimulation by taking a rectal temperature is unsupported by research (Kirchoff, 1981).

e. Diarrhea. Patients with diarrhea may have more loose stools in response to rectal stimulation with a thermometer.

f. Newborns and infants. After initial temperature is taken rectally to assess the patency of the rectum, temperatures using the axillary route are recommended to avoid the risk of perforating the bowel.

Consistency of route and equipment gives the most reliable data for assessment of an individual patient's thermal status. Whenever possible, use the same route and thermometer in measuring a patient's temperature.

1. Assemble equipment—For oral route:

Thermometer
Tissue } Mercury thermometer
Disposable sheath (optional)
Electronic thermometer } Electronic thermometer
Probe covers
Disposable thermometer

For rectal temperatures:

Water-soluble lubricant (all types of thermometers) (disposable rectal sheath is prelubricated)
Rectal probe for electronic thermometer
Disposable adapter for disposable thermometer

2. Wash hands.
3. Identify the patient.
4. Explain the procedure; ask about any contraindications such as recent consumption of hot or cold food or fluids, smoking.
5. Provide privacy as necessary for axillary or rectal route.

Procedure	Explanation
1. Prepare the thermometer. Oral route:	
Mercury thermometer	
a. Rinse thermometer under cold water.	a. Removes antiseptic soaking solution.
b. Wipe dry with tissue, moving from bulb toward fingers.	b. Prevents transfer of microorganisms from fingers to bulb; water on thermometer decreases visibility.
c. Shake thermometer down to 96° F (36.5° C).	c. To get current reading and avoid missing mild hypothermia.
d. Insert thermometer in disposable sheath (optional).	d. Reduce spread of microorganisms.
Electronic thermometer	
a. Remove probe and insert in clean probe cover.	a. Activates thermometer; reduces the spread of microorganisms.
b. Check that temperature on display is 96° F or less.	b. Machine working.
Disposable thermometer	
a. Read package directions.	a. Directions vary with manufacturers.
b. Open package as directed.	b. Prevents contamination from nurse's fingers.
Rectal route: Lubricate tip and 1½ inches up the thermometer.	Reduces friction and increases patient comfort.

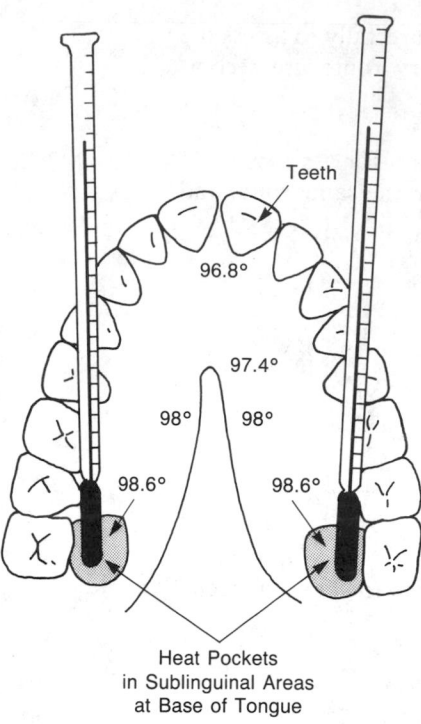

Teeth

96.8°

97.4°

98°   98°

98.6°   98.6°

Heat Pockets
in Sublinguinal Areas
at Base of Tongue

Figure 21-9. Heat pockets for thermometer placement in the mouth. (Adapted from W. Beck *et al.*: Clinical thermometry. *The Guthrie Bulletin*, Spring, 1975.)

Procedure	Explanation
2. Place thermometer correctly for accurate temperature assessment.	**2.**
Oral route:	
a. Place in right or left sublingual pocket. (See Figure 21-9.)	a. Warmest area of mouth with best blood flow.
b. Have patient close mouth around thermometer.	b. Air may cool mouth and give falsely low reading.
Axillary route:	
Place thermometer in axilla and position person's arm against side.	Skin encircles heat-sensitive part of thermometer; minimal exposure to environmental heat/cold; arm helps hold thermometer in place.
Rectal route:	
a. Position patient so clear visualization of rectal opening is possible (side-lying or prone; infants prone or supine).	a. Inserting thermometer in area other than rectum can cause pain and trauma.
b. Insert lubricated thermometer 1½ inches in adult rectum, ½ inch in infant rectum.	b. Length of rectum increases with age.
c. Hold in place during measurement.	c. Unexpected movements by patient may advance the thermometer to an unsafe depth if not held in place.
Hold electronic thermometer in place regardless of route since the weight may be uncomfortable for the patient to hold unassisted.	

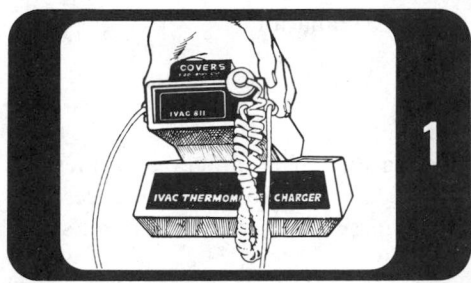

Remove the thermometer from the charger and place the carrying strap around your neck.

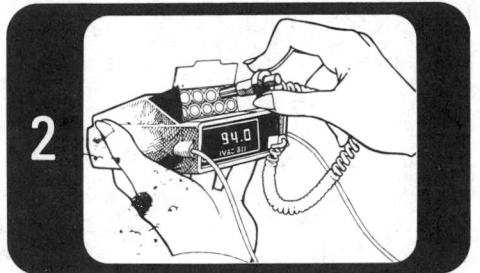

Grasp probe by the large ring at the top. Attach a disposable probe cover by inserting probe firmly into the probe cover. Do not push top — it is the ejection button.

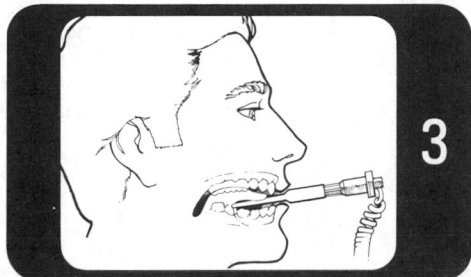

For oral temperatures*, *slowly* slide probe under the front of the patient's tongue and along the gum line, to the sublingual pocket at the base of the tongue. Patient's lips should come to rest at the step on the probe cover.

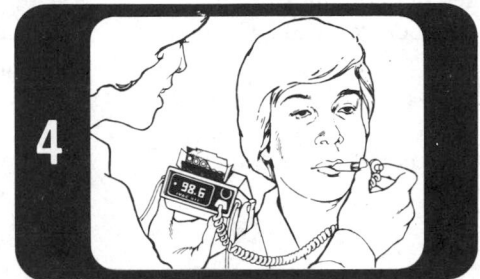

Hold the probe! Do not watch the digital display panel but watch the position of the probe in the patient until audible signal notifies you that the patient's temperature has been reached and is displayed.

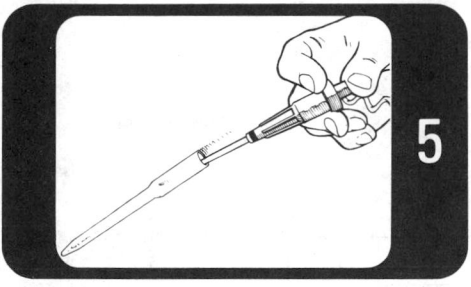

Remove probe from patient's mouth. Discard probe cover by pushing ejection button with thumb.

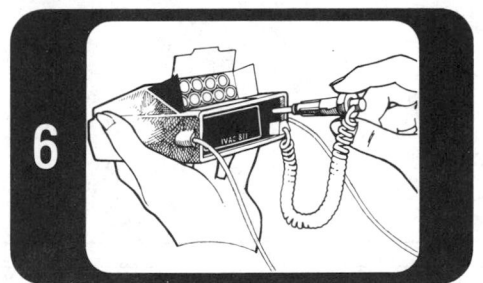

After reading and recording temperature, return probe to its storage well. This will automatically turn the thermometer off. After completing temperature rounds, return thermometer to charging base.

Figure 21-10. Procedure for using an electronic thermometer. (Reproduced with permission of the IVAC Corp., San Diego, CA.)

*For rectal temperatures, follow similar technique, except use red colored probe. Use current techniques for penetration.

3. Leave the thermometer in place long enough to obtain an accurate measurement.

Mercury-in-glass thermometer
Oral—3 min
Axillary—10 min
Rectal—3 min

Electronic thermometer (oral, axillary, or rectal)
Hold in place until tone or light on display indicates measurement is complete. (10 to 30 sec) (See Figure 21-10.)

Disposable thermometers (Oral, skin, or rectal)
Leave in place as recommended by manufacturer (often 15 to 45 sec)

3. Less than .2° F difference when taking oral temperature for 3, 5, 8, or 12 min, (Graves and Markarian, 1980). The greater the blood flow near the thermometer, the faster the mercury will rise; water conducts heat from the body to the mercury, heating it more rapidly than dry skin in axilla.

Manufacturer's recommendations. If tone or light does not appear, accuracy is questionable, and measurement should be repeated.

Varies with manufacturer and type of heat-sensitive material.

Procedure	Explanation
4. Remove the thermometer and read it.	**4.**

Mercury-in-glass thermometer

a. Wipe off secretions with tissue from fingers down toward bulb.

a. Better visualization of numbers and mercury column; wiping down toward bulb reduces contamination of nurse's fingers with patient's bacteria.

b. Do not touch bulb with fingers.

b. Touching bulb may add heat and falsely increase reading.

c. Read the height of the mercury column.

d. Remove sheath, if used, before reading thermometer.

d. Sheath interferes with visualization of mercury column.

Electronic thermometer
Number appearing on display is patient's temperature.

Disposable thermometers
Read as directed by manufacturer.

Varies with product.

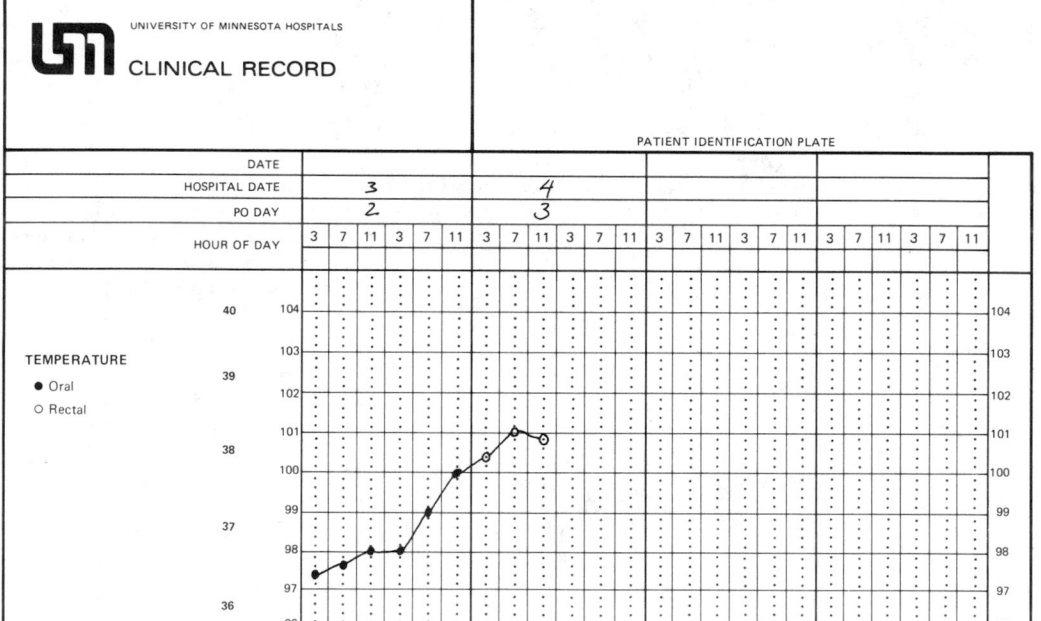

Charted Temperatures:

Hospital day #3		day #4	
3^A	97^4 Orally	3^A	100^4 Rectal
7^A	97^6	7^A	101
11^A	98	11^A	100^8
3^P	98		
7^P	99		
11^P	100		

Figure 21–11.   Recording temperatures in patient's chart. (Forms courtesy of the University of Minnesota Hospitals and Clinics, Minneapolis, MN.)

5. Return or dispose of equipment

Mercury-in-glass thermometer
a. Rinse in cold water.

b. Replace in patient's labeled container or return to supply area for cleaning.

Electronic thermometer
a. Eject probe cover into garbage.
b. Replace probe into thermometer.
c. Replace thermometer in charging unit.

Disposable thermometer
Dispose of thermometer or skin tape in garbage.

6. Leave patient in a comfortable, safe position.

7. Wash hands.

8. Record the patient's temperature. (See Figure 21–11).

9. If the patient's temperature is unusually low or elevated compared to previous readings, recheck the temperature immediately or within 30 min. Report low or elevated temperatures to nursing instructor, staff nurse, or physician.

5.

a. Removes secretion so antiseptic solution is in contact with glass.
b. Prevents transfer of microorganisms.

a. Prevents transfer of microorganisms.
b. Turns machine off.
c. Keeps batteries in thermometer charged for accurate measurement of later temperatures.

Reduces transfer of microorganisms.

6. Positioning for temperature taking may be uncomfortable or unsafe; redress to prevent unnecessary heat loss.

7. Reduces transfer of microorganisms from patient to patient and from patient to nurse.

8. Document in chart and temperature board if used in clinical area. Documentation provides information for assessment and diagnosis.

9. Measurement may have been inaccurate or thermometer may be defective. Changes or altered temperature is an indication for further evaluation and possible treatment.

Nursing Diagnoses Related to Temperature Elevation

Alterations in Thermal Regulation

CONSTANT FEVER.   The temperature does not vary more than 3.6° F and does not return to a normal range during a 24-hour period. This is characteristic of typhoid, brucellosis, pneumonia, and central nervous system infections such as encephalitis.

REMITTENT FEVER.   The temperature varies more than 3.6° F but does not return to normal during a 24-hour period. This is characteristic of acute viral and bacterial infections, typhoid, malaria, and tuberculosis.

INTERMITTENT FEVER.   Temperature fluctuates above and within the normal range during 24 hours. Rapidly changing temperature causes chills and sweats. This is characteristic of septicemia, infected abscesses, malaria, and allergic reactions to drugs, especially the penicillins. The allergic reaction often begins to affect the temperature on the seventh or eighth day of drug therapy.

LOW-GRADE TEMPERATURE.   This is a temperature elevation between 99 and 101° F. The cause is often unknown and may be referred to as FUO (fever of unknown origin).

HYPERPYREXIA.   This is an elevation in temperature above 105° F and is characteristic of heat stroke and malignant hyperthermia.

RELAPSING FEVER.   This is an elevation in temperature one or more times after a person has been afebrile (without a temperature elevation) for 24 hours or longer.

HEAT CRAMPS.   Normal temperature, but cramp in actively working muscle.

HEAT EXHAUSTION.   Temperature slightly elevated; active sweating; feels faint, weak, dizzy, thirsty; hot environmental temperatures, low blood pressure, increased pulse and respiratory rate.

HEAT STROKE.   Temperature significantly elevated; absence of active sweating; confused, disoriented, unconscious; hot environmental temperatures; often has been physically active in heat; low blood pressure; increased pulse and respiratory rate. Difficulty walking and slight paralysis of one side of the body may be present.

THERMAL BURN.   Area of the skin in contact with objects or water above 115° F may have cellular damage from the heat transfer. Areas with poor circulation due to vasoconstriction or blood vessel disease are especially susceptible since heat will not be carried away from the area through convection created by blood flow in the area. Healthy tissue usually requires hotter temperatures for burns to occur.

Data Indicating Potential Problems with Reduced Temperature Levels

Reduced temperature levels are caused by inadequate heat production or excessive heat loss.

Objective Data.   Reduced temperatures are significant at the following levels:

Oral temperature below 97° F
Axillary temperature below 96° F
(axillary and skin temperatures may be significantly lower than oral temperatures because of vasoconstriction)
Rectal temperature below 98° F
} Potential hypothermia

Other objective observations of the person with reduced temperature could be:

- Skin feels cool to the touch.
- Skin appears pale.
- Respiratory rate may be increased or decreased. In mild hypothermia, the respiratory rate is increased as heat production from chemical reactions in the cells are accelerated. In severe hypothermia, respiratory rate may be as slow as several breaths each minute.
- Blood pressure is elevated or decreased. In mild hypothermia, the blood pressure is increased because of the increased volume of blood caused by vasoconstriction of blood flow to the skin. In severe hypothermia, the blood pressure drops or may be unobtainable because of severe vasoconstriction of blood flow to the arms and legs and a greatly slowed heart rate.
- Pulse rate may be increased or decreased. In mild hypothermia, the pulse is increased due to the action of epinephrine. In severe hypothermia, the heartbeat will be reduced. The heartbeat may also be irregular.
- Sensations in the hands and feet are reduced.
- Oriented, disoriented, or unconscious. As hypothermia progresses, the level of cognitive functioning is reduced until unconsciousness occurs in severe cases.
- Shivering may be active or absent. In mild hypothermia, shivering is active. By the time the body temperature drops below 86° F, the ability to shiver is lost because of the effect of the cold on the hypothalamus.
- Urine production may be temporarily increased or

decreased. In mild hypothermia, vasoconstriction causes increased blood flow to the vital organs, including the kidney. This increased blood flow results in an increase in urine production, and the individual may have some spontaneous urination called "cold-induced diuresis." As hypothermia progresses, pulse and blood pressure drop, blood flow to the kidney is reduced, and urine production decreases.

- Clothing and insulation may be appropriate or inappropriate for the air temperature. An inactive elderly person may seem overdressed in temperatures which are comfortable to more active people wearing less clothing. In cold environments, an individual may have on as many warm clothes as are available. In severe hypothermia, judgment is impaired, and it is not uncommon to find hypothermic victims removing clothing and running around in the snow barely dressed or naked.

- Pupils will become dilated and fixed as severe hypothermia develops.

- Muscle activity, such as walking or swimming, will become awkward and eventually impossible in severe hypothermia; speech becomes slurred.

- Reflexes are lost in severe hypothermia.

Table 21-6. **Nursing Interventions in Cold Stress (First Aid)**

Mild to Moderate Hypothermia

Provide insulation.
Move to warmer area if possible.
Keep person flat during rewarming.
Provide warmth: two unclothed people in sleeping bag with unclothed victim; turn up thermostat; build fire; warm bath.
Provide warm or hot, sweet drinks.
Prevent person from smoking or drinking alcohol during rewarming (heat loss with alcohol; vasoconstriction interferes with rewarming with smoking).
Observe constantly during rewarming for further distress.

Severe Hypothermia

Assess carefully for life or death.
Insulate victim.
Allow victim to rewarm in comfortably warm environment—no external or internal heat as first aid (peripheral area of body may warm too rapidly and suffer hypoxia if respirations, blood flow, and brain control are inadequate).
Lay flat with legs and feet slightly elevated.
Watch constantly for respiratory and cardiac problems.
Initiate assistive ventilations if victim having trouble breathing or not breathing.
If any heartbeat present, no matter how slow, do not initiate chest compressions.
If no heartbeat, initiate CPR if rescuer in no danger of hypothermia. If victim did not suffer cold-water immersion or submersion, the question of initiating chest compressions is tending to be "no." Ventilate, do not compress chest, and get to the hospital as soon as possible.
Transport to hospital.

Frostbite

Do not begin rewarming until risk of refreezing ended (refreezing causes more damage than leaving frozen).
Rewarm: immerse part in warm water (100 to 110° F).
Prevent person from smoking (vasoconstriction).
Do not rub area (may damage tissue).
Check person for hypothermia; if temperature below 94° F, rewarm body before attending to frostbite.
Continue warm soaks or packs until area is flushed.
If frostbite is severe (part feels frozen solid), rewarm and transport to hospital.

Subjective Data. People with reduced temperatures may complain of the following symptoms:

The person feels cold or chilled.

The person may lose dexterity, especially in the fingers, and complain of being clumsy; muscles become rigid.

Response to pain is lost in severe hypothermia.

The hypothermic person may have amnesia for the time when body temperature was below 91° F (33° C).

Person may report "itching" or "burning" sensation on skin; pain on rewarming.

Person may complain of breathing difficulty during rewarming.

Nursing Diagnoses Related to Decreased Temperature

Alterations in Thermal Regulation

FROSTBITE. Skin may feel frozen to the touch and softer underneath or may feel frozen solid. Pale white in color; cold to the touch; prickly or itchy feeling; in severe case, no sensation felt.

MILD HYPOTHERMIA. Temperature between 95 and 98.6° F; shivering; person feels cold; alert and oriented; increased pulse, heart rate, and BP.

MODERATE HYPOTHERMIA. Temperature between 91.4 and 95° F, shivering; loss of dexterity, coordinated movement difficult; speech slurred; varying degrees of confusion; responds to pain; pulse, respirations, and BP slightly elevated.

SEVERE HYPOTHERMIA. Temperature is below 91.4° F (33° C); shivering gradually ceases; pupils dilate and gradually lose ability to react to light; pulse, respirations, and blood pressure decrease; mental confusion, amnesia, and eventual loss of consciousness; cardiac and respiratory arrest possible below 86° F (30° C); no response to pain.

Refer to Table 21–6 for nursing interventions associated with these diagnoses.

Nursing Interventions Associated with Temperature Maintenance

Maintaining Body Temperature—Prevention

The concept of a *neutral thermal environment* is important for the nurse to understand in assisting patients to maintain their normal body temperature with a minimum of adaptive effort. A neutral thermal environment is an environmental temperature in which the patient's oxygen consumption (thus, metabolic rate) is at a minimum, while body temperature is stable within the normal range. This means the person is exerting a minimum of effort toward temperature maintenance activities. The body is neither too warm nor too cool. Oxygen consumption will be increased in either case because cellular metabolism will increase. Shivering, increasing muscle tone, and heat all accelerate the metabolic rate in the body's cells. In the ideal thermal state, the oral, rectal, and axillary temperatures are within a few degrees of each other. When the body is working to conserve heat, skin and axillary temperatures are often much lower than oral temperatures. When the body is working to cool itself, the skin and axillary temperatures are often as high as the oral temperatures.

Providing an appropriately warm environment for each patient requires nursing judgment based on the age, physical build, activity level, and health of individual patients. A 3-lb newborn often needs an environmental temperature in the range of 93 to 95° F for minimum oxygen consumption. A larger newborn, up to 5 lb, usually requires a thermal environment in the range of 91 to 93° F, while an infant of normal birth weight is placed in an environmental temperature between 89 and 93° F. These are all considered neutral thermal environments, but are different temperatures based on a patient's thermal needs. Charts are available to suggest environmental temperatures when working with newborns and preterm infants. The very young and the elderly require more heat for a neutral thermal environment than younger adults. Emaciated patients tend to require more heat for a neutral thermal environment than adequately nourished individuals. Inactive or paralyzed patients also require more environmental heat, if heat production changes are not to be initiated.

Keeping patients adequately hydrated and nourished, as much as possible, is another nursing activity that will provide the patient with the reserves needed to maintain normal body temperature. This is especially important in a patient with a fever since fluid loss through sweating can be very great. Adequate nutrition and fluids are also essential in heat production.

Providing patients with appropriate insulation is another nursing responsibility aimed at temperature maintenance. Providing blankets for the patient's bed and also during transport to other areas of the hospital will add to the patient's thermal comfort. Asking patients periodically through the 24-hour day if they are warm enough or cool enough will enable the nurse to add or remove insulation for a patient before thermal regulation is greatly affected. Patients who are unable to communicate because of their stage of development or because of illness or disease conditions should be monitored closely for signs of overheating or underheating: too much insulation or environmental heat, and patients will begin to perspire, if they are able, and may develop an elevated temperature; too little insulation or environmental heat, and patients will feel cold, shiver, be unable to rest, and increase their need for oxygen and fuel to produce heat.

Taking patients' temperatures and observing for any signs of increased heat production or heat loss activities are among the best ways to assess each patient's thermal status. Talking with the patient about comfort levels will give the nurse additional data. Monitoring a patient's intake and urine output and weight will provide additional information about thermal regulation. Weight will not be gained if the calories are being used for heat production.

Providing Heat

Purposes for Providing Heat Locally or to Total Body. The use of heat in patient care can serve many purposes. Reasons for using local heat to a particular body area or generally to the whole body are listed below:

1. Heat can be used to promote a patient's comfort. Heat has long been used to increase comfort and reduce pain. The exact physiology involved is unclear at this time. Heat will trigger the thermoreceptors within the skin and may block transmission of pain from pain receptors. Heat is soothing to the muscles, and the added blood flow to the area may help reduce discomfort by providing oxygen and nutrients to the cells at an accelerated rate. Heating pads, aquathermia pads, and warm or hot soaks are common ways of providing heat for comfort and relaxation. See Nursing Skill 21-2.

2. Heat can be used to cause vasodilation to an area of the body, thus increasing blood flow. Heat for the purpose of causing vasodilation is effective in reducing edema in an area since the increased blood flow helps to draw the extra intercellular fluid back into the circulating blood. Increased blood flow to an area of tissue damage will promote healing by providing oxygen and nutrition to the cells at an accelerated rate and removing waste products from increased cellular activity. Heat will also dilate blood vessels, making venipuncture or blood drawing easier. Warm or hot moist packs and compresses, disposable hot packs, and sitz baths are

ways of applying heat for these purposes and are discussed in Nursing Skills 21-3 and 21-4. The heating pad and aquathermia pad are also used to promote vasodilation.

3. External heat can be used to rewarm a hypothermic patient or to rewarm an area affected by frostbite. Heat for rewarming the body's core temperature or peripheral skin areas is another general area in which heat is used. Heat for this purpose can be provided using several different routes. Heat can be applied directly to the cooler skin, as in frostbite. Warm, moist compresses or warm soaks are used to provide heat to frostbitten skin. Warm baths or body-to-body contact can be used to rewarm the victim of mild to moderate hypothermia. Heat can be administered orally in the form of hot drinks or gastric lavage. During gastric lavage, a tube is placed into the stomach through the mouth, and warm water (107° F) is placed into the stomach. This would be done for a severely hypothermic patient unable to swallow or who was unconscious. Heat can also be administered in the form of warmed, humidified oxygen which the patient breathes through a face mask. Heat may be administered through peritoneal lavage, in which an incision is made into the abdominal cavity and warm fluid, usually an intravenous solution of Ringer's lactate at 107° F, is run into the abdomen and drained out at the rate of 8 liters per hour (Lija, 1982).

The final route for rewarming the hypothermic patient involves the use of cardiopulmonary bypass, where the blood bypasses the heart and lungs through surgically created routes and is warmed and oxygenated by mechanical means. This method is used to rewarm patients following therapeutically induced hypothermia for major cardiac surgery and for patients in severe hypothermia or when the limbs are frozen solid.

Safety Considerations in Applying Heat. Always consider heat a potential source for further tissue damage if used inappropriately. The following precautions should be noted when applying heat:

1. Moist heat is more likely to burn than dry heat because water is a good conductor. Tissue burns and tissue hypoxia can result from application of heat. Heat can accelerate the rate of cellular activity, including cell division and growth. It is, therefore, contraindicated for areas with a malignant cell mass.

2. Appropriate temperatures for heat applications will be different for individual patients, based on age, reported comfort level, and medical problems. People who are very young or very old are more susceptible to tissue damage from heat application. Patients with circulatory problems may have difficulty with adequate vasodilation and blood flow to transport heat from the cells and are more susceptible to burns. Heat applied at

Nursing Skill 21–2   Applying Dry Heat

Heating Pad, Aquathermia Pad (AQUA-K PADS), Disposable Hot Packs

Heating pads, aquathermia pads, and disposable hot packs are all methods of applying dry heat to an area of the body. Dry heat will cause vasodilation and increase blood flow to an area. That is why hot packs are sometimes used prior to drawing a blood sample. The veins enlarge and are easier to see. Capillary blood samples are also easier to obtain from a well-perfused area following heat application. Heating pads are available in various sizes and shapes. Some are designed to wrap around extremities, and some are flat. The danger with a heating pad or aquathermia pad is the risk of burning the skin if the temperature is too hot. For this reason, many pads are preset in the hospital supply area so the temperature cannot be raised at the patient's bedside. The ''hot'' setting on many heating pads can reach temperatures that will burn. A special key is used to reset the amount of heat on many pads so the patient cannot increase the heat and risk burning. Many aquathermia pads have a maximum setting of 105° F. Heating pads usually provide heat in the area of 105 to 115° F; aquathermia pads provide heat in the range of 98 to 105° F (some brands do give more heat). Disposable hot packs, which are composed of chemicals that provide heat when they are mixed, provide heat in the range of 101 to 114° F. Some clinical settings try to discourage patients from using heating pads brought from home because of the risk of burning. Check institutional policies in regard to applying dry heat. Dry heat is used to reduce discomfort, increase relaxation, and cause vasodilation and increased blood flow to an area of the body.

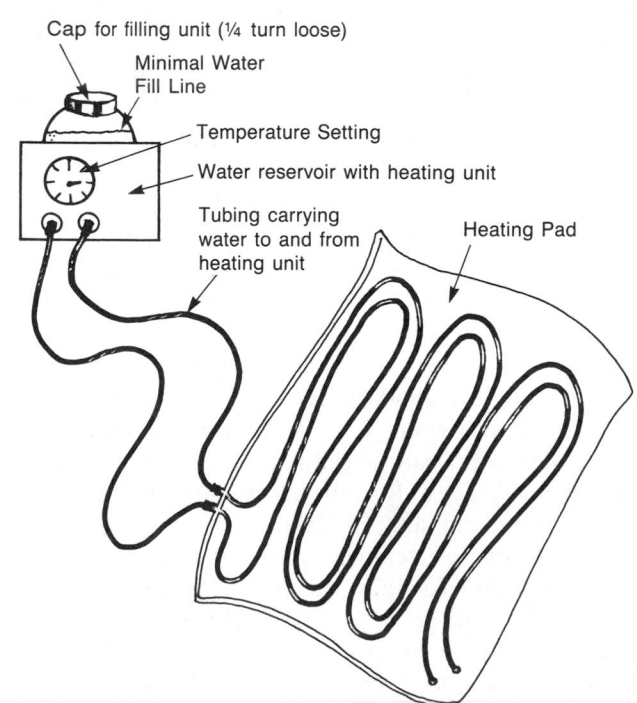

Figure 21–12.   Aquathermia (Aqua-K) heating pad.

Preparation

1. Determine need. Often a physician will order dry heat, specifying the type of equipment, the temperature, frequency of the treatments, and duration of each treatment. As an aid in drawing blood, laboratory technicians or nurses may apply a disposable hot pack for approximately 10 min prior to the drawing of the blood sample. Patients often request a heating pad, and in many institutions the physician is the only one who can order this form of dry heat, so the nurse will have to discuss the patient's request with the physician.
2. Wash hands.
3. Assemble equipment. Cover for heat source, distilled water for aquathermia pad, heating pad, aquathermia pad, or disposable hot pack.
4. Identify the patient.
5. Explain procedure to patient.
6. Provide privacy as necessary.

Procedure	Explanation
1. Prepare equipment. Disposable hot packs: follow directions to activate chemicals (often squeezing or striking the pack mixes the chemicals). Aquathermia pad: fill to indicator line with distilled water. Replace cap, leaving 1/4 turn loose. Plug in and recheck water level after pad has filled. Check temperature setting, and adjust if necessary. Cover with a cloth or pillowcase. Heating pad: plug in and cover, if not already done. Secure cover with tape rather than pins.	1. To promote safe operation Activation may vary with manufacturer. Water circulates in the pad after being heated in the main unit. Heats by conduction and convection. If the cap is tightened, a vacuum is created as water moves into pad and pad will not fill properly. Cloth protects patient's skin from burns, absorbs perspiration. Operates on electricity. Cover protects skin from heat and decreases perspiration. Pins conduct heat and may puncture pad or patient or burn the skin.
2. Dry body area to receive heat, if necessary.	2. Moisture conducts heat and is more likely to cause skin damage.
3. After pad warms, apply to skin area.	3. Once maximum temperature is reached, its effect on the patient can be evaluated.
4. Assess patient's reactions initially and during treatment. Observe skin for excess redness, blotchy areas.	4. Data collection for signs of patient discomfort or skin changes indicating burning.
5. Remove pad at appropriate time (as ordered by physician, after blood drawing, as requested by patient).	5. Heat no longer needed, or extended use may be unsafe.
6. Assess patient and skin area.	6. Sensations or skin changes will help in evaluating effectiveness of treatment and any complications.
7. Leave patient in comfortable position.	7. Patient comfort; conveys respect and caring for individual.
8. Wash hands.	8. Decreases spread of microorganisms.
9. Document treatment in patient's chart: reason for treatment, time, type of heat, appearance of skin, patient's reactions.	9. Communication among health team members; verification of safe nursing care.

Nursing Skill 21–3   Applying Moist Heat

Warm or Hot Packs/Compresses

Moist surfaces conduct heat more rapidly than dry surfaces. Compresses are moist dressings used to provide heat or cold to a small area. Packs are moist dressings used to cover large body areas and provide heat or cold. If the packs or dressings are warm, the temperature applied to the skin is in the range of 98 to 105° F. If the packs are to be hot, the temperature is above 105° F, often as hot as the patient will tolerate without discomfort or signs of skin damage. The packs or compresses may be sterile or unsterile, depending on the risk of infection to the area. If the skin is broken, the risk of infection is increased so sterile technique and supplies are usually used. Moist heat is more likely to burn than dry heat, but it is less drying to the skin and more penetrating.

Preparation

1. Determine need. Most warm or hot packs and compresses are ordered by the physician, who indicates frequency and duration for applications and temperature. Sterile or clean technique may be specified or left up to nursing judgment. Hot and warm packs are commonly used to soften crusty exudates from wounds, to cause vasodilation and increased blood flow to an area to promote healing and reabsorb fluid trapped in the tissues, for thrombophlebitis (inflammation of the vein), and for comfort.
2. Wash hands.
3. Assemble equipment. Dressings or material for packs/compresses, solution for moistening packs; plastic material to protect the bed and insulate packs; tape or gauze ties; bath thermometer; dry towels for insulation around pack; hot-pack machine (optional) and aquathermia pad (optional) to maintain heat in packs for longer time. Petroleum jelly or mineral oil may also be used to protect surrounding skin.
4. Identify the patient.
5. Explain procedure.
6. Provide privacy.

Procedure	Explanation
1. Place compresses/packs in solution at appropriate temperature. or Place packs in hot packer and turn on. Hot packer must be filled as indicated with appropriate solution (distilled water or sterile distilled water).	1. Moist heat at ordered temperature.
2. Assist patient to comfortable position in good body alignment; assess need for elimination before putting on packs/compresses.	2. Patient will have to remain inactive while packs are in place; promote patient comfort; warm, moist stimulation to skin may increase urge to void.
3. Remove dressings, if present; observe affected area.	3. Dressings insulate against heat transfer and cleaning; data collection.
4. Apply thin layer of petroleum jelly or mineral oil to surrounding skin area if it seems sensitive or delicate (for hot applications).	4. Insulates skin from heat transfer by conduction. Do not put on wound or damaged skin area which is to receive heat treatment.
5. Remove packs from hot packer and gently shake open.	5. Hot packer wrings out packs, dissipating some of heat as steam, decreasing risk of burns.

or

Wring out packs until they have stopped dripping (use sterile gloves for sterile packs).

6. Place compresses/packs on appropriate skin area and shape to fit

7. Assess patient's comfort level and appearance of the skin after several seconds.

8. Cover compresses with plastic wrap, then towels, and secure in place (aquathermia pad may be used between packs and plastic to maintain heat longer).

9. Assess patient after several minutes and periodically during treatment; check temperature, pulse, respirations, and blood pressure, if large body area covered.

10. Maintain heat level for appropriate length of time.

11. Remove packs/compresses and dispose of appropriately.

12. Pat area dry.

13. Assess area after treatment and patient's reaction.

14. Redress area if needed (wash hands first).

15. Assist patient into a comfortable position.

16. Wash hands.

17. Document treatment in patient's chart: time, appearance, amount of heat, duration, patient's response, any medication added to solution, any complications.

Water increases heat conduction and risk of burns.

6. Heat transferred through direct contact (conduction).

7. Perception of burning sensation may take a few seconds and indicates potential for skin damage. Extreme redness or blotchy area can indicate excessive heat.

8. Protects bed and clothes from becoming wet; towel insulates and decreases heat loss by conduction; aquathermia pad decreases heat loss by conduction by reducing temperature difference.

9. Data may indicate possible skin damage; a rising temperature, pulse, and respiratory rate or a dropping BP may indicate excessive heat or inadequate blood volume due to large-scale vasodilation.

10. Maintain as long as doctor's order or until signs of complications develop. To maintain heat level, hot compresses may have to be changed every 5 min; change hot packs every 10 to 30 min; with aquathermia pad, change every 15 to 60 min. (more often for hot treatments).

11. Packs may be cleaned for reuse or be disposable; decreases spread of microorganisms.

12. Patient comfort; reduce heat loss; rubbing may damage sensitive tissue.

13. Data collection.

14. Draining wounds will need dressings; dressings decrease spread of microorganisms.

15. Patient comfort; shows respect and concern for individual.

16. Decreases spread of microorganisms.

17. Communication with other health team members; verification of appropriate nursing care.

Nursing Skill 21–4   Assisting a Patient to Take a Sitz Bath

Equipment

Equipment for taking sitz baths consists of a plastic, disposable basin which fits in the toilet and a bag with tubing which is attached to the basin and provides flowing warm water to the perineal and rectal area. The bag is suspended above the patient on an IV pole or a hook on the back of the bathroom door. It has a clamp to regulate water flow. The basin has openings for the inflow of water from the tubing and outflow of water into the toilet. Patients have their own portable sitz bath, and they are discarded when sitz baths are no longer needed. Some clinical areas have sitz baths built into the bathroom area. These may look like tubs on the floor, about one-third the size of a bathtub, or they may be built at chair level so the patient's feet are on the floor and the patient is in a sitting position. These are cleaned between patients. They have a built-in water thermometer, and a safe thermal zone of 100 to 110° F is often labeled on the temperature gauge.

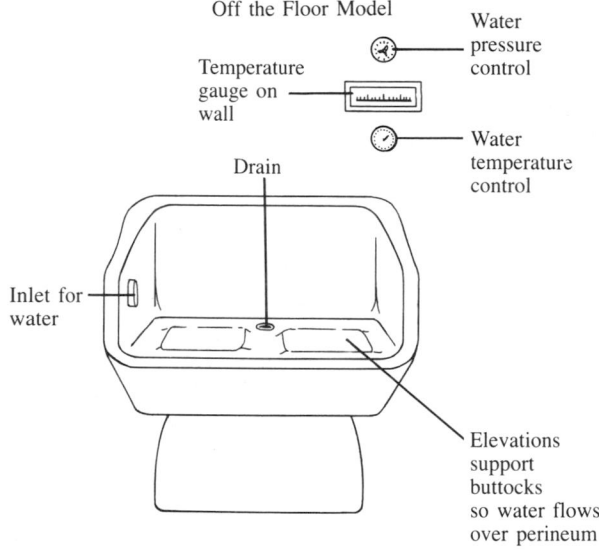

Off the Floor Model

Water pressure control

Temperature gauge on wall

Water temperature control

Drain

Inlet for water

Elevations support buttocks so water flows over perineum

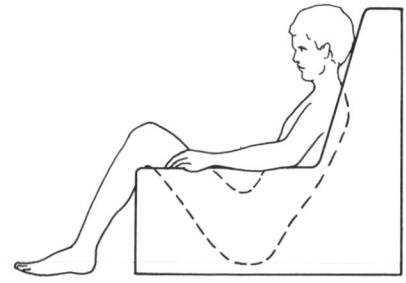

Floor Model

Figure 21–13. Sitz baths.

Preparation

1. Determine need. The physician will usually write an order for a patient to have a sitz bath, indicating frequency and number of days for the treatment. Sitz baths are frequently ordered after rectal or perineal surgery to promote healing through vasodilation, cleaning, and for patient comfort. Medication may be ordered by the physician for use in the water of the sitz. Sitz baths are also used to stimulate voiding.
2. Clean tub with disinfectant solution.
3. Wash hands.
4. Assemble equipment. Towel, bath mat, bath thermometer if not built in, medication for water if ordered, clean dressings and tape if needed, inflatable plastic ring for patient comfort (optional). If tension would be created on the newly sutured area by sitting on the ring, it should not be used.
5. Identify patient.
6. Explain procedure.
7. Provide privacy (curtains pulled and place "occupied" sign as needed).

Procedure	Explanation
1. For built in sitz bath, fill one-third to one-half full of water or provide a steady flow of water coming in and leaving sitz bath. Water should cover rectal/perineal area. Water temperature approximately 105° F.	1. Allow enough room for displacement of water when patient sits in sitz. Warm water causes vasodilation in affected area without risk of burning.
2. Folded towel or plastic ring may be placed in bottom of tub for patient comfort. Do not block drain.	2. Towel or ring provides a cushion between bottom of tub and skin.
3. Instruct patient how and when to use nurse call light and place within reach.	3. Circulation in legs may be obstructed in floor tub; vasodilation may cause weakness and faint feeling; tub may be difficult to get in and out of without risk of falling.
4. Remove dressing if present; inspect perineal area. (For portable sitz bath, fill container with water (several hundred ml.) at 105° and hang in bathroom. Insert basin sitz in toilet as directed on package instructions. Open and regulate flow clamp on tubing for slow steady flow of fluid into sitz.)	4. Dressings may loosen and obstruct drain and interfere with cleaning action of water. Data collection.
5. Assist patient into tub or on toilet sitz as necessary. Check on status during sitz.	5. Weakness or poor balance may make sitting into sitz difficult; minimize risk of falls.
6. Assist patient out of sitz after 10 to 20 min. Assess perineal area.	6. Reduce risk of falls; maximum effect obtained after 10 to 20 min without tiring patient.
7. Redress wound if necessary.	7. Dressings needed if wound draining or susceptible to infection by open skin surface.
8. Leave patient in comfortable, safe position.	8. Promotes patient comfort and shows respect for individual.
9. Clean sitz bath for next use.	9. Decreases spread of microorganisms.
10. Wash hands.	10. Decreases spread of microorganisms.
11. Document treatment: time, observations, and patient's reactions, any teaching done.	11. Communication with other health team members; verification of appropriate nursing care.

the same temperature is not perceived equally by all people, and subjective data of discomfort from a patient should be considered an indication of possible burning, and heat may have to be reduced. People who have had anesthesia of any form, or who are taking medication that reduces sensations, will be less perceptive of thermal discomfort and may be burned without reporting pain. These patients should be monitored very carefully for any signs of burning, as should any patient unable to communicate.

3. The temperature of the heat application should be checked frequently to guard against inadequate or excessive heat.

4. When large areas of the body are receiving heat applications, assess for signs of inadequate heat loss and rising temperature. The larger the body area receiving supplemental heat, the lower the temperature should be of that supplemental heat for patient comfort.

5. A cloth over hot packs will help protect the patient's skin from discomfort or burning.

6. Patient information and education should be included when heat is applied so the patient understands what should be reported to the nurse to prevent inadequate or excessive heat. The patient should also understand what degree of heat is being applied and the reasons behind this choice. Some people feel that heat applications have to be hot to be effective and will add more heat without medical approval and risk burning themselves. If a patient's perception of heat and cold is altered because of medications, surgery, or anesthesia, explain that the heat application may not feel as hot as it actually is and that no additional heat should be added.

7. Frequently observe the area receiving heat for pain, increased swelling, and extreme redness to detect the possibility of excessive heat and potential burning.

8. When using mechanical equipment and automatic temperature-regulating devices, consider the possibility that malfunctions or inaccuracies can develop. Objective and subjective data from the patient about heat applications may be the first clue that equipment is not working as it should, so check the patient initially and periodically during any heat treatments.

Promoting Heat Loss

Reasons for Promoting Heat Loss. Nursing activities to promote heat loss are used to assist the patient to reduce core temperature, when it is elevated, or for therapeutic reasons, such as cardiac surgery. When promoting heat loss, vasodilation causing heat loss through conduction, convection, radiation, and evaporation is used. If the nursing actions being used to assist the patient in losing heat cause the patient to shiver, heat production is increased, and heat loss activities may be inef-

fective until shivering can be eliminated. Medications may be necessary to decrease or stop shivering. Their need should be discussed with the physician. Medications, such as aspirin or acetaminophen, may be ordered to reset the hypothalamic thermostat, thus reducing body temperature. Frequent temperature checks are important in all activities causing accelerated heat loss in order to determine effectiveness of the treatment and need for additional measures or cessation of efforts.

Tepid or cool baths or sponge baths (Nursing Skill 21–5) are nursing measures that accelerate heat loss through conduction and evaporation. Turning on room fans or air conditioners will further increase heat loss through convection and radiation. Cooling blankets (Nursing Skill 21–6) draw heat away from the body through conduction and convection and are used to reduce elevated temperatures.

Safety Considerations. During nursing activities for heat loss or in providing cold, certain safety precautions should be observed.

1. Mild hypothermia should be considered as a possible negative side effect of promoting heat loss or applying cold.
2. Shivering is undesirable and can exhaust the patient and negate effectiveness of heat loss measures.
3. Check the patient's temperature frequently to assess effectiveness of treatment.
4. Place a cloth between the cold pack and the skin to protect skin from damage.
5. Explain to the patient what you are going to do and why you are doing it.
6. If using equipment, consider the possibility of malfunction. Check the patient's skin and core temperature using a different means to assure accuracy of data from the machine.
7. Check water temperature as appropriate to maintain desired temperature of treatment.

Providing Cold

Purposes for Providing Cold. Cold applications are used for the following reasons:

1. Nursing activities involving applications of cold are used to prevent swelling or prevent further swelling from an injury.
2. Cold is used to reduce pain in a superficial area.
3. Cold is used in the emergency treatment of burns.
4. Cold is used to preserve a severed part of the body for possible reattachment.
5. Cold is used in the treatment of some malignancies of the skin.

Nursing Skill 21-5   Giving a Cool Sponge Bath

Preparation

1. Determine need. A sponge bath to lower a patient's temperature by conduction, radiation, and evaporation often requires a physician's order but may also be ordered by a nurse in some clinical areas. Check the institutional policy. The patient's temperature is usually elevated several degrees above normal, and medications have usually been tried and found ineffective or inappropriate for lowering temperature.
2. Wash hands.
3. Assemble equipment. A basin, the patient's thermometer, several washcloths, a towel, a bath blanket, a thermometer to check water temperature. The use of alcohol in the water may be ordered by the physician to increase heat loss through evaporation, since alcohol evaporates at a lower temperature than water. The fumes and drying effect on the skin require added caution. The room must be very well ventilated, and lotion may be needed after the procedure to counteract drying of the skin. Inhalation of fumes by small children is not recommended. Ice may also be needed if a cool sponge bath (65 to 85° F) is given instead of a tepid sponge bath (80 to 90° F). The tepid bath is recommended over the cool bath because there is less incidence of shivering, and it is less distressing for the patient.
4. Identify the patient.
5. Explain the procedure to patient.
6. Provide privacy.

Procedure	Explanation
1. Take patient's temperature.	1. Provides baseline data for assessing temperature reduction.
2. Fill basin with water at appropriate temperature; tepid—80 to 90° F, cool—65 to 80° F, water with alcohol—85 to 95° F (no more than one-half of total volume of solution is alcohol).	2. Water should be below body temperature for heat loss by conduction. Water too cold will cause shivering. Alcohol cools by evaporation more effectively than water, so warmer water and alcohol provides comparable cooling to water alone at cooler temperatures.
3. Remove covers and patient gown; cover with bath blanket.	3. Expose body surface areas for bathing and evaporation. Provides privacy.
4. Begin with face, with plain water only. Wet skin and do not dry.	4. Alcohol can damage eyes and be unpleasant to smell or taste. Fumes around face will be inhaled. Wet skin looses heat through evaporation as it drys.
5. Place cool, moist washcloths in axilla and groin; remoisten when they feel warm.	5. Heat loss through conduction.
6. Sponge and massage body areas in rotation, doing neck, arms, legs, and back. Moisten for several minutes and allow to air dry. Then move on to another body area. Cover sponged area with bath blanket.	6. Massage brings warm blood to skin surface. Promotes heat loss because of difference between skin temperature and water being at maximum. Sponging chest and abdomen is more likely to initiate shivering and is often omitted but may be used unless shivering develops.

Procedure	Explanation
7. Check temperature, pulse, and respirations during bath. Assess every 15 min.	7. Sponging should be stopped when body temperature within 2° F of desired temperature or as ordered by the physician. Overcooling can occur which will trigger further heat production and conservation.
8. Discontinue bath when desired temperature is reached or as instructed by physician. Bath often lasts 20 to 30 min.	8. Assistance in heat loss no longer necessary.
9. Pat patient dry.	9. Wet skin areas will result in a damp gown. Rubbing the skin surface creates friction and heat.
10. Leave patient in a comfortable position. Put on clean gown; cover with sheet; dry linen on bed.	10. Promotes patient comfort and shows respect and caring for individual.
11. Remove equipment from room and dispose of properly.	11. Decreases spread of microorganisms.
12. Wash hands.	12. Decreases spread of microorganisms.
13. Document treatment: time, body temperature (before and after), type of solution, temperature of solution, patient's reactions.	13. Communication within health team. Verification of appropriate nursing care.
14. Recheck temperature in ½ to 1 hr, and every 1 to 2 hr at least three times.	14. Temperature may rebound and further treatment or medications may be necessary.

Nursing Skill 21–6 Using a Cooling Blanket— (Hypothermia/Hyperthermia Machine)

Equipment

A hypothermia/hyperthermia blanket is a machine that can be used for lowering a patient's temperature or raising it. The machine consists of a large, box-shaped cooling or warming unit, various size pads to put under and over the patient, and a rectal thermometer probe. Alcohol and water solution circulates from the machine through the pads and back to the machine. (See Figure 21–14.) The cooling/heating unit is on a stand with wheels and is portable, but it does require electricity for operation. There are a variety of machines and models on the market, so each machine should have the instruction manual attached, and it should be read by the nurse prior to operation. If the operating manual does not come with the machine from the hospital supply area, call supply and request a copy. Always check the hospital procedure book in each different clinical facility regarding the use of cooling blankets before initiating the treatment on a patient.

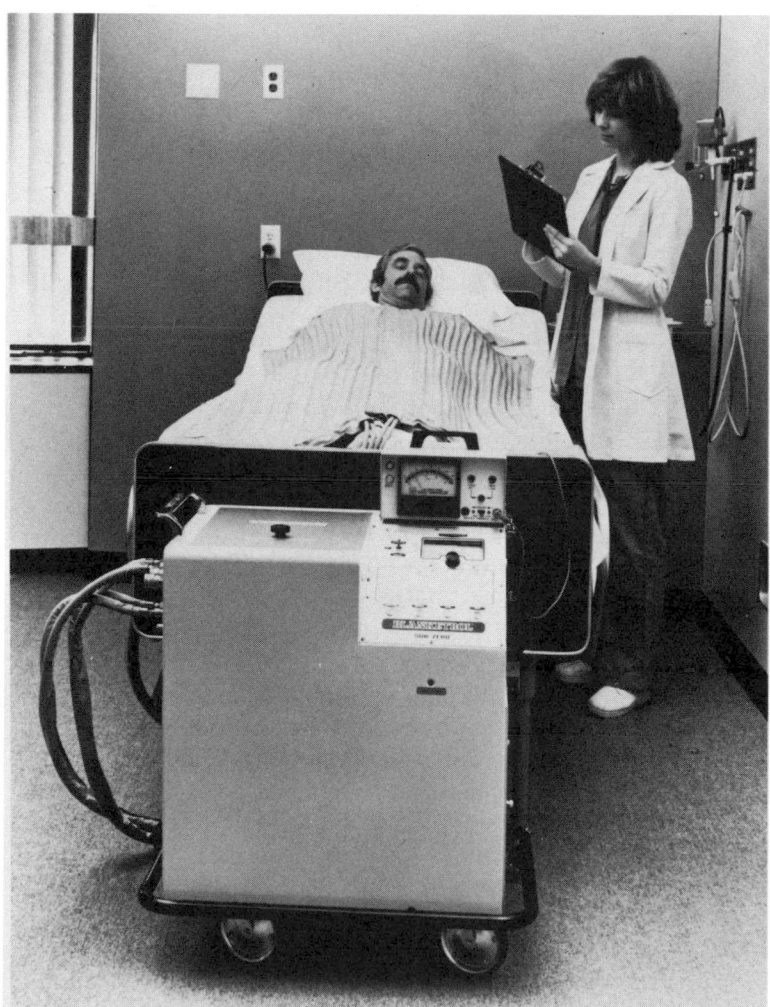

Figure 21–14. Hypothermia/hyperthermia machine. Water circulates within the blanket covering the patient and can be used to lower or raise the patient's temperature. (Photograph courtesy of Cincinnati Sub-Zero Products, Inc., Cincinnati, OH.)

Preparation

1. Determine need. A physician's order is usually required to initiate treatment to raise or lower a patient's temperature using this machine. The physician should specify the patient's temperature at which treatment is initiated and the temperature at which treatment is terminated. The cooling blanket is often used to bring a patient's temperature back to the normal range from elevations above 102° F after other activities such as medications have been ineffective. More frequently the patient has a very high fever which must be brought down to avoid possible cellular damage. The patient may be having repeated or continuous trouble with elevated temperatures as might occur when there are disturbances with the hypothalamus. Heat loss using the cooling blanket occurs through conduction and convection.
2. Assemble equipment. Order cooling blanket from hospital supply area. Ask personnel in supply if the machine comes ready for use or if the nurses will have to add the alcohol and water solution on the station. Pads and a patient temperature probe should come with the machine, along with the instruction manual.
3. Wash hands.
4. Take equipment into the patient's room and identify the patient.
5. Explain the procedure to the patient.
6. Provide privacy for the patient; ask patients if they wish visitors to leave or stay during treatment.

Procedure	Explanation
1. Plug in machine.	1. Operates on electricity.
2. Prepare machine as directed in manual, if not already done by supply staff. Set temperature.	2. Each machine may have slightly different preparation before use.
3. Attach pads to unit as directed.	3. The pads will cool the patient through conduction and convection; method of attachment may vary.
4. Turn on the pump as directed.	4. The pump will force the cooling fluid through the pads.
5. Loosen the cap on the reservoir while machine is pumping.	5. Failure to loosen cap will create a vacuum, and fluid will not flow to pads.
6. Add additional fluid to machine if fluid indicator is low (turn machine off before adding).	6. Pumping solution into the pad will lower the volume of fluid in the machine. A minimum amount of fluid is necessary for proper functioning.
7. Place cooling pads under and over patient as needed. A thin blanket or sheet may be used between the pad and the patient for comfort. Check institutional policy and instruction manual.	7. Placing pads under and over the patient exposes a maximum skin area for heat transfer and will bring a temperature down more quickly. A sheet or blanket insulates the patient from the cooling source and slows heat transfer, yet may protect delicate skin from trauma.
8. Attach thermometer sensor to machine. Lubricate rectal probe and insert into patient's rectum 1½ inches. Tape in place.	8. An accurate and continuous temperature reading from the patient will automatically regulate the amount of heat or cold in the pads so the patient is not overheated or overcooled.
9. Set patient temperature probe to desired rectal temperature. or Set machine 1° lower than patient's actual rectal temperature and recheck frequently, lowering temperature on machine by 1° F increments as patient's temperature drops.	9. This method will accomplish the most rapid cooling. Shivering may develop because of the large temperature difference between the patient's skin and the pad. This method is least likely to cause the patient to shiver because cold receptors in the skin are minimally stimulated. Frequent resetting of the machine is essential to lower temperature several degrees.

10. Assess patient's response. Check oral temperature at least every hour. If shivering develops, turn off machine and consult nurse in charge or physician. Assess skin area for any signs of pallor, blotches, or loss of sensation.

12. Turn patient every hour while on cooling blanket.

13. Wash hands.
14. Document treatment: time started, patient's temperature, temperature every hour on cooling blanket, patient's responses.

10. Oral temperature will help confirm accurate monitoring by machine. Shivering produces heat and works against cooling treatment. Medication may be needed to suppress shivering.
Skin damage may occur from pressure or prolonged contact with cold due to vasoconstriction.

12. Turning exposes warmer skin areas to the pads and increases total heat loss. Pressure to sensitive skin areas will be reduced and effects of prolonged vasoconstriction to an area will be avoided.

13. Decrease the spread of microorganisms.
14. Communication with other members of the health team. Verification of safe nursing care.

To Discontinue Treatment
Treatment is usually discontinued when patient's temperature is within 2° F of desired temperature because cooling effects of treatment continue for a while after termination.

1. Turn off machine.
2. Remove rectal probe from patient and machine. Return with machine.

3. Remove pads from connection with machine and replace caps to coupling outlets.

4. Remove pads from patient.

5. Leave patient in a comfortable position.

6. Remove equipment from patient's room and return to supply area.
7. Wash hands.
8. Document discontinuation: time, temperature, patient's response.
9. Recheck patient's temperature in 1 to 2 hr at least three times.

1. No further cooling desirable.
2. Leaving the probe in place when removing the pads could cause unnecessary discomfort. Probes are cleaned and reused.

3. This prevents solution from draining out of the machine. Easier to remove pads from patient if not attached to machine.

4. Cooling no longer necessary. Pads may sometimes be left in place for several hours if further problems with temperature elevation are expected.

5. Promotes rest and relaxation. Shows respect and concern for individual.

6. Cost control. Makes machine available to other patients after cleaning.
7. Reduces spread of microorganisms.
8. Communication with other health team members. Verification of appropriate nursing care.
9. Temperature may rebound after discontinuation of cooling blanket.

Application of cold to the skin causes vasoconstriction, decreased sensation, and reduced blood flow. Metabolic rate is slowed within the cooled cells. Tissue damage from excessive cold or prolonged application of cold can be both desirable and undesirable, depending on the purpose of the cold application. Cryotherapy is a medical technique involving freezing malignant growths on the skin in an effort to destroy the cells. This technique is being used on basal cell carcinomas, which are cancerous lesions of the skin, more often seen on people over 50 years of age.

Generally, the nurse is watching for signs of possible injury to the skin when using cold applications and takes actions to avoid it. Cold can be applied by using immersion in cold water, cold compresses, ice and ice packs, and disposable cold packs. These measures provide cold to the body through conduction. The cardiopulmonary bypass machine is also capable of cooling the patient's blood, returning it to the body, and thus lowering body core temperature during cardiac surgery.

Nursing Care Plan for a Patient with Unmet Temperature Maintenance Needs

Narrative Description

Data: Baby boy Johnson was born at 1:54 A.M. Birth weight was 5 lb, 1 oz. On admission to the newborn nursery, he was showing signs of respiratory distress: flaring of the nostrils on inspiration, a respiratory rate of 80 breaths per minute, and slight retractions. His heart rate was 160 beats per minute, and his rectal temperature was 96.2° F. His color was pink, and he was alert. The mother had received no medications during her labor.

Assessment: Nursing Diagnosis

Slight respiratory distress related to hypothermia.

Goals

Respiratory distress to be resolved within two hours.

Planned interventions: Nursing Actions

1. Place in warmed isolette at 93° F.
2. Monitor axillary temperature, pulse, and respirations every ½ hr until 98° F, then every 2 hr for 24 hr.
3. Delay bathing until temperature above 98° F.
4. Put cap on newborn's head (reduce further heat loss).
5. Check blood glucose level with blood sample from foot.
6. Delay oral feedings until respirations under 60 breaths per minute (danger of aspiration when respirations are very rapid).
7. Maintain patency of airway; clear nasal passages.
8. Notify pediatrician if respiratory distress increases or temperature does not begin to come up over the next hour.

Evaluation: Goal Met

Respiratory distress resolved within 1½ hr of admission to nursery.

(*Data.* No nasal flaring, no retractions, respiratory rate 48 breaths per minute, temperature 98.2° F. axillary.)

Reassessment: New Diagnosis

Potential for cold stress related to low birth weight.

New Goal

Newborn's axillary temperature will remain between 98 and 99° F during hospitalization.

New Actions

1. Keep hat on newborn until discharge.
2. Double-wrap in blankets when transferred to a standard open crib.
3. Keep in isolette for 12 hr and monitor temperature every 2 hr.
4. Talk with parents about keeping him wrapped when with mother for holding or breastfeeding.
5. Monitor temperature every 4 hr when transferred to standard newborn crib.

Summary

The human body is homoiothermic, and the individual cells are unable to function normally in temperatures more than a few degrees above or below a core temperature of 98.6° F. The chemical reactions occurring in the cell will accelerate or slow down as temperature rises or falls. Cell structures are damaged from temperatures either too high or too low. The need for a constant temperature is second only to the need for oxygen, for death will occur within several hours when severe hypothermia or hyperthermia develops. Body temperatures below 77° F or above 110° F for even brief periods of time will result in death of the total body, as more and more individual cells lose function and die. The ability of the body to regulate temperature is impaired at body temperatures above 106° F or below 94° F.

Temperature is measured by the oral, axillary, or rectal route. The oral temperature is the most common method. Temperature can be measured using a mercury-in-glass thermometer, an electronic thermometer, or various forms of disposable thermometers with chemicals reacting to different body temperatures.

As temperature initially increases or decreases, oxygen need increases. The added heat from a fever increases the metabolic rate in the cells spontaneously, resulting in increased heat production. With chilling, the body compensates by increasing cellular metabolic rate and by shivering, both heat-producing changes. The higher the temperature, the greater the O_2 need. As temperature continues to fall and hypothermia develops, metabolic rate and O_2 needs decrease, as do all body functions.

Heat is both gained and lost through conduction, convection, and radiation. The process of evaporation only results in heat loss from the body. The body responds in three basic ways to maintain temperature. Heat production may be increased. Heat conservation changes may be implemented. Heat loss may be accelerated. These activities are under hypothalamic control relying on data from skin temperature sensors and temperature sensors deep within the body. Core temperature is usually kept constant during health by these three mechanisms, while surface or skin temperature fluctuates with the environmental temperature. Skin temperature is cool when the body is trying to conserve heat by peripheral vasoconstriction. Skin temperature is warm when the body is trying to lose heat through peripheral vasodilation.

Inadequate temperature regulation can result in confusion, altered level of consciousness, dehydration, decreased urine output, weight loss, increased pulse and respirations, cool or hot skin, blood pressure changes, shivering or sweating, and feelings of being weak, dizzy, hot, cold, and thirsty and altered sensations in extremities.

Nursing interventions to assist a patient maintain

temperature during treatments, surgery, or while under nursing care focus on maintaining a neutral thermal environment for each individual patient based on unique needs. Adding or removing insulation is another intervention to assist patients avoid problems with temperature.

Interventions designed to assist a patient lose heat involve use of medications, cooling sponge baths, hypothermia cooling blankets, and cool or cold packs to specific body areas. Purposes for assisting a patient lose heat or for applying cold include:

1. Returning body temperature to normal
2. Reducing pain by cold applied to painful area
3. Reducing developing edema by causing local vasoconstriction to injured area

4. Preservation of severed body part for reattachment

Purposes for providing heat to the body include:

1. Returning body temperature to normal
2. Increasing comfort in sore muscles
3. Promoting healing through vasodilation
4. Rewarming cold body parts or skin
5. Reducing existing edema through vasodilation and reabsorption of intercellular fluid
6. Dilating local blood vessels for easier venipuncture when blood sample needed

Nursing interventions for providing heat include helping patients with a sitz bath, warm moist applications, and application of dry heat.

Terms for Review

afebrile	frostbite	hypothermia	peripheral vasodilation
conduction	heat cramps	insensible water loss	pyrexia
constant fever	heat exhaustion	intermittent fever	pyrogens
convection	heat stroke	low-grade fever	radiation
core temperature	homoiothermic	malignant hypothermia	relapsing fever
dive reflex	hyperpyrexia	neutral thermal environment	remittent fever
evaporation	hyperthermia	nonshivering thermogenesis	shivering
febrile	hypothalamus	peripheral temperature	vasoconstriction

Self-Assessment

Identify some of your risk factors for problems with local or total body alterations in temperature by answering the following questions:

1. My body build is
   a. Underweight for my height
   b. Overweight for my height
   c. Average for my height
2. I am
   a. A diabetic on insulin
   b. Taking sedatives or tranquilizers on a regular basis
   c. Taking medication to control my elevated BP
   d. A fairly heavy user of alcohol (three or four mixed drinks or more each night)
   e. None of the above
3. When I am engaged in outdoor activities in cold weather, I
   a. Put on several layers of clothing
   b. Wear one heavy jacket and shirt and pants

   c. Enjoy having hot, alcoholic drinks so I don't have to go inside to warm up as often
   d. Smoke frequently while outside
4. When the temperature is in the high 80s and 90s, I
   a. Continue to engage in heavy daily exercise as I normally do when it is cooler
   b. Increase my fluid intake
   c. Sweat profusely while doing heavy work or exercise
5. When I travel places in cold weather, I
   a. Put extra blankets in the car
   b. Dress for style, even though I know I should wear warmer clothes
   c. Put extra warm clothes in the car
   d. Always wear a hat
   e. Always carry jumper cables in the car
6. When I feel sick, I
   a. Usually assess my oral temperature periodically
   b. Put on extra covers if I feel chilled, even with a fever
   c. Keep blankets on when I have a fever, even though I feel hot and am sweating
   d. Try to maintain or increase my intake of fluids, especially with a fever.

Answers

These answers increase your risk:

1. a, b
2. a, b, c, d
3. b, c, d
4. a
5. b
6. c

These answers decrease your risk:

1. c
2. e
3. a
4. b, c
5. a, c, d, e
6. a, b, d

Learning Activities

1. Evaluate your own body temperature using the various routes discussed in this chapter. Take your temperature several mornings before getting out of bed, and compare this to your temperature between 4 and 8 p.m. Is the afternoon temperature consistently higher? Does your normal body temperature fall within the range of 97 and 99° F orally?
2. Compare your oral temperature using a mercury-in-glass thermometer, a disposable thermometer, and an electronic thermometer. Is there a significant clinical difference between the readings?
3. Consider the experiment with the effects of smoking, gum chewing, and drinking hot or cold fluids on oral temperatures. How long after these activities does it take for your temperature to return to the original baseline reading?
4. Take your oral temperature by placing the thermometer in the posterior area at the base of the tongue, and compare that reading to your temperature when the thermometer is placed in the front of the mouth, under the tip of the tongue.
5. Mouth-breathe and take your oral temperature using several devices. Compare this reading to one in which your mouth is kept closed around the thermometer.
6. Compare the temperatures of patients in the early morning to their temperatures in late afternoon. Is there evidence of fluctuations related to circadian rhythms?
7. Visit a nursing home or other care facility for older adults. Talk with the residents about feeling chilled. Are the patient's hands warm? Are there signs of heat conservation by the body? Are temperatures generally below normal ranges? Can added insulation and warm food or fluids restore a chilled patient's comfort level and body temperature after a few hours?

Review Questions

1. How do elevated temperatures within the cell affect the metabolic rate?
   a. It decreases slightly.
   b. It increases.
   c. It remains constant.
   d. It decreases dramatically.
2. When body temperature increases, what effect does this have on oxygen needs?
   a. O_2 needs decrease.
   b. O_2 needs increase.
   c. O_2 needs remain constant.
3. Which of the following are ways of increasing heat production?
   a. Piloerection
   b. Vasodilation
   c. Vasoconstriction of peripheral blood vessels
   d. Increasing muscle tone
   e. Putting a blanket over a patient
4. Which of the following activities is helpful in dissipating heat from the body?
   a. Vasoconstriction
   b. Drinking fluids
   c. Lying in the sun
   d. Release of epinephrine from adrenal medulla
5. Heat is conserved in the body by all of the following activities except
   a. Vasoconstriction of peripheral blood vessels
   b. Adding insulation
   c. Decreased sweat gland activity
   d. Drinking hot, buttered rum
   e. Decreasing body surfaces exposed to environment
6. Which of the following individuals is most at risk for problems with temperature maintenance?
   a. A 5-lb newborn in an isolette set at 92° F
   b. An emaciated man of 78 years, confined to a wheelchair, in a nursing home maintained at 68° F
   c. A well-nourished, middle-aged man who has worked for 20 years in a foundry where temperatures are between 85 and 95° F
   d. An infant whose axillary temperature is 98.4° F
7. When comparing the mercury to the electronic thermometer, which route for taking temperature has the most difference in time required for an accurate reading?
   a. Oral
   b. Rectal
   c. Axillary
8. When a person is cold or mildly hypothermic, which signs or symptoms would most likely be present?
   a. Decreased muscle tone
   b. Temperature of 98.6° F axillary in the adult
   c. Warm extremities
   d. Shivering
   e. Nausea and faintness
9. When a person is hyperthermic, which signs or symptoms would most likely to present?

a. Perspiration
b. Decreased respiratory rate
c. Increased urine production
d. Elevated blood pressure
10. When applying heat to a patient, which of the following activities may be unsafe?
a. Allowing the patient to regulate the amount of heat for personal comfort
b. Checking the physician's order for temperature and duration of treatment
c. Checking the appearance of the skin shortly after application of heat
d. Applying a thin layer of material between the heat source and the patient

Answers

1. b
2. b
3. d
4. b
5. d
6. b
7. c
8. d
9. a
10. a

References and Bibliography

Boyd, L.; Shurett, Pl; and Coburn, C.: Heat and heat-related illness. *Am. J. Nurs.,* **81**:1298, 1981.

Capobiaco, J.: How to safeguard the infant against life threatening heat loss. *Nursing 80,* **10**:64, May, 1980.

Castle, M.: Fever: Understanding a sinister sign. *Nursing 79,* **9**:26, Feb., 1979.

Davis, Sharts, J.: Mechanisms and manifestations of fever, *Am. Jr. Nurs,* **78**:1874, 1978.

DeLapp, T.: Taking the bite out of frostbite and other cold-weather injuries. *Am. J. Nurs.,* **80**:56, 1980.

DePalma, J.: Drug-induced changes in vital signs and blood pressure, *RN,* **40**:46, June, 1977.

Dowd, C., and Meyrick, R.: Cancer cells left out in the cold. *Nurs. Mirror,* **149**:32, July 19, 1979.

Drummond, G.: Hypothermia. *Nurs. Times,* **75**:2115, Dec., 6, 1979.

Erickson, R.: Oral temperature differences in relation to thermometer and technique. *Nurs. Res.,* **29**:157, May–June, 1980.

Felton, C.: Hypoxia and oral temperatures. *Am. J. Nurs.,* **78**:56, 1978.

Gedrose, J.: When cold can be a killer—Prevention and treatment of hypothermia and frostbite. *Nursing 80,* **10**:34, Feb., 1980.

Graves, R., and Markarian, M.: Three-minute time intervals when using an oral mercury in glass thermometer with or without J-Temp Sheaths. *Nurs. Res.,* **29**:323, Sept.–Oct. 1980.

Guyton, A. *Textbook of Medical Physiology.* 6th ed. Saunders, Philadelphia, 1981.

IVAC: IVAC electronic thermometer inservice presentation. IVAC Corp. San Diego, Calif., TWX 910–337–1281.

Iveson-Iveson, J.: Body temperature, *Nurs. Mirror,* **154**:32, Feb. 10, 1982.

Kirchoff, K.: An examination of the physiologic basis for "coronary precautions." *Heart Lung,* **10**:874, Sept.–Oct., 1981.

Kozier, B., and Erb, G.: *Techniques in Clinical Nursing.* Addison-Wesley, Reading, Mass. 1982.

Lija, G.: Emergency treatment of hypothermia. In Pozos, R., and Born, D. (eds.): *Hypothermia—Causes and Effect.* New Century, Piscataway, N.J., 1982.

Lim-Levy, F.: The effects of oxygen inhalation on oral temperature. *Nurs. Res.,* **31**:150, May–June, 1982.

Ozuna, J., and Foster, C.: Hypothermia and the surgical patient. *Am. J. Nurs.,* **79**:646, 1979.

Pozos, R., and Born, D.: *Hypothermia—Causes, Effects, Prevention.* New Century Publishers, Piscataway, N.J., 1982.

Rambo, B., and Wood, L.: *Nursing Skills for Clinical Practice.* Saunders, Philadelphia, 1982.

Riccardi, V.: *The Genetic Approach to Human Disease.* Oxford University Press, New York, 1977.

Vander, A.; Sherman, J.; and Luciano, D.: *Human Physiology—The Mechanisms of Body Function,* 3rd ed. McGraw-Hill, New York, 1980.

CHAPTER **22**

THE NEED FOR NUTRITION

Objectives

1. Discuss several reasons why nutrition is an essential need for survival.

2. Describe the processes involved in bringing food from the mouth to the internal cellular environment.

3. Explain the roles of the primary nutrients needed by the body for adequate nutrition.

4. Identify four food groupings and the recommended daily servings of each; list foods found in each group.

5. Calculate an individual's total daily energy utilization in kcalories and compare to total kcaloric intake.

6. Identify internal and external factors regulating nutritional intake.

7. Identify factors that increase and decrease an individual's nutritional needs.

8. Describe the possible effects of unmet nutritional needs on other human needs.

9. Describe common problems with food ingestion and possible nursing interventions to reduce them.

10. Describe patient data indicating possible problems with nutrition.

11. Identify situations and medical treatments that may interfere with a patient's ability to meet nutritional needs.

12. Describe ways of feeding patients that may increase their intake.

13. Contrast the commonly ordered therapeutic diets.

14. Describe the uses for nasogastric suction.

15. Demonstrate the following skills: insertion of a nasogastric tube, administration of a tube feeding, feeding a patient.

Nutrition as a Basic Human Need

Nutrients provided from adequate food intake are the building materials from which the body is made. They are essential for growth, tissue repair, and normal functioning of the cells of the body. Nutrients are used to produce energy in the form of ATP for all body activity. The sum total of all chemical reactions occurring within the body (*metabolism*) requires a continuous supply of nutrients. Muscle movement, transmission of nervous impulses, thinking, and heat production are all dependent on energy produced from the food the individual eats. The body is constantly removing aging cells and replacing them with new cells. This keeps the body in a constant state of good repair, rather than waiting until old cells die and function is lost. The body practices preventive medicine through this constant replacement of the old for the new. For example, the maximum life expectancy of a red blood cell is 120 days. The cells lining the digestive tract are replaced every three days. This maintenance activity requires both energy and raw materials for building. Both are supplied by the food an individual consumes. If the individual's diet is lacking in some of the essential nutrients, the body may be unable to grow, maintain, or repair itself. When total body nutrition is grossly inadequate, life itself is at risk.

Normal Means of Meeting Nutritional Needs

There are four processes effecting nutrition. These are ingestion, digestion, absorption, and elimination. The first three will be discussed in this chapter. Elimination is presented in Chapter 24 as a separate but related need.

Ingestion

Ingestion is the process of bringing food and fluids into the digestive tract. The digestive tract consists of a muscular tube, approximately 26 ft long. Food and fluids enter the digestive tract through the mouth and unused waste products exit from the tract through the anus. It is essentially outside the body, much in the way the hole in a doughnut is outside the doughnut. The digestive or gastrointestinal tract (GI tract) consists of the mouth, esophagus, stomach, small intestines, and large intestines. (See Figure 22–1.) It contains many bacteria from the environment which have taken up permanent residence in parts of the gut (intestines) and often serve an important function in nutrition. If these bacteria were to gain access to the inner body through a hole in the digestive tract, the individual would become very ill from infection. The digestive system is composed of the digestive tract plus the organs and glands that produce substances needed for digestion and absorption of the food consumed. The liver, pancreas, and salivary glands are part of the gastrointestinal system.

Ingestion of food involves several activities. Inability to perform these activities will reduce or eliminate food consumption, unless feeding help is available.

1. Coordination of the muscles of the hand and arm is necessary to bring food up to the mouth. Loss or restraint of hand and arm movement will prevent the individual from getting food into the mouth.

2. Chewing breaks large pieces of food into smaller ones which will pass down the esophagus without obstructing it. Chewing requires teeth or dentures and voluntary control of the muscles of the mouth. Chewing is both a voluntary and involuntary activity. Food against the gums, teeth, hard palate, and tongue will cause a reflexive chewing action. Central nervous system control allows an individual to chew as much or as little as desired.

3. Swallowing is the final step in ingestion as the food moves from the mouth down the esophagus to the stomach. Swallowing can be initiated reflexively or voluntarily. Pressure on the back of the pharynx causes a reflexive swallowing controlled by the medulla. Central nervous system control allows the individual to initiate swallowing when food is adequately chewed. Swallowing is a complex activity involving inhibition of respirations, raising the larynx, and closing the glottis to prevent food from moving into the lungs. Muscular contractions (*peristalsis*) in the esophagus move the food down into the stomach, usually with the help of gravity. The medulla in the brain coordinates these activities.

During ingestion of food, the salivary glands (parotid gland, sublingual gland, and submandibular gland) secrete saliva to moisten food and begin the digestion process. Saliva contains the enzyme, salivary amylase, which begins to break down carbohydrates, one of the nutrients. Saliva is 99 percent water and 1 percent salt and protein. Saliva keeps the mouth moist, lubricating

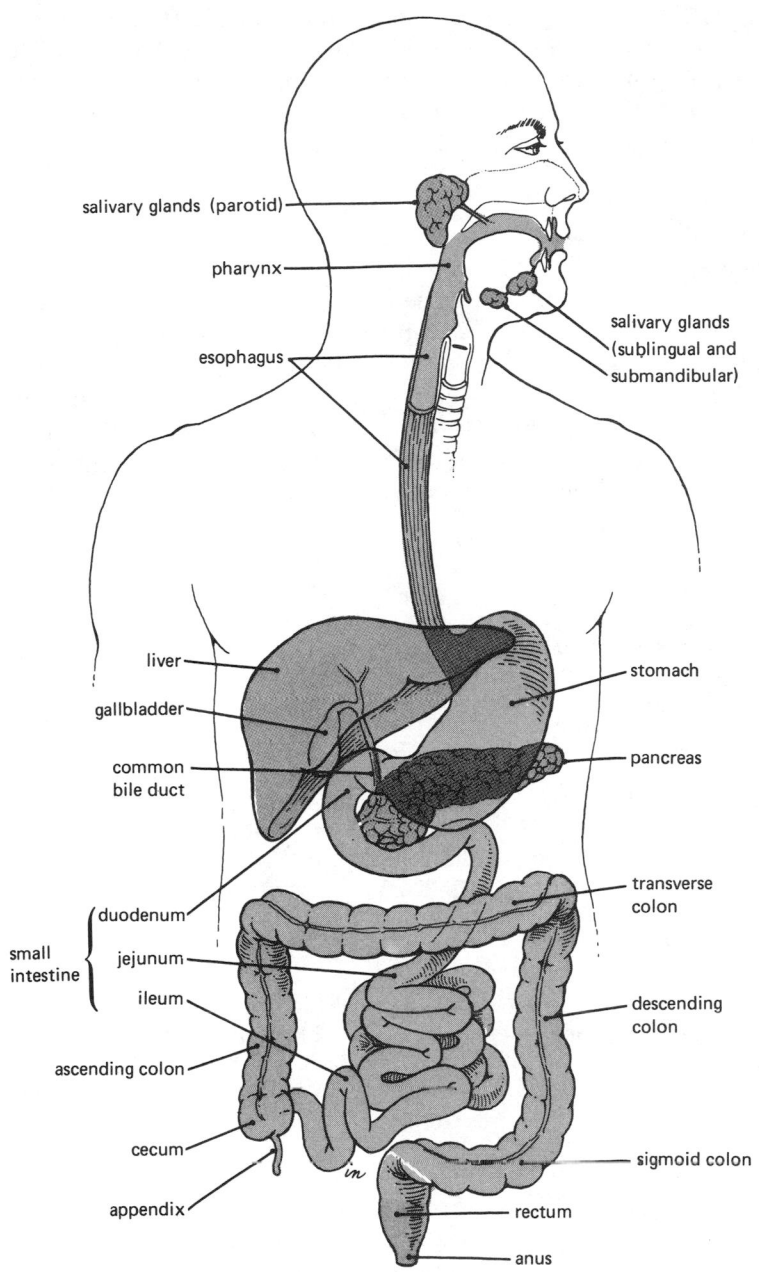

salivary glands (parotid)

pharynx

esophagus

salivary glands
(sublingual and
submandibular)

liver

stomach

gallbladder

common
bile duct

pancreas

duodenum

small
intestine

jejunum

ileum

transverse
colon

ascending colon

descending
colon

cecum

appendix

sigmoid colon

rectum

anus

Figure 22–1.   The digestive tract from mouth to anus with its associated glands (salivary glands, liver, pancreas). (From M. Griffiths: *Introduction to Human Physiology*, 2nd ed. Macmillan, New York, 1981, p. 214.)

food for swallowing and dissolving molecules of food in fluid for the sense of taste. It can be produced at a maximum rate of 4 ml per minute.

Digestion

Digestion begins in the mouth through the action of saliva on carbohydrates and continues in the stomach and small intestines. Digestion is the breaking-down process which changes large pieces of food into much smaller structures, which can then be absorbed through the bowel into the blood or lymph. In the stomach, hydrochloric acid (HCl) and gastric enzymes are secreted and mixed with the food to break the complex food molecules apart. The stomach reacts to food by increasing peristalsis to mix the food with the digestive enzymes and the HCl. The HCl dissolves the food particles into a liquid called *chyme*. It also kills most of the bacteria entering the stomach with the food. The HCl is quite strong and will cause burning of the esophagus if it is allowed to reflux up out of the stomach.

The stomach itself is protected from the strong acid by the secretion of thick mucus by the cells lining the inside of the stomach. The *cardiac sphincter* at the top of the stomach prevents the acidic chyme from flowing backward into the esophagus. The *pyloric sphincter* at the other end of the stomach prevents food from passing into the small intestine until it is well digested. The food leaves the stomach slowly as the pyloric sphincter relaxes and opens to allow small amounts of chyme to enter. It reflexively closes in response to the acidity of the entering chyme. This allows time for secretions from the pancreas and liver to neutralize the acidity of the chyme in the upper part of the small intestine (*duodenum*). When the chyme is neutralized, the pyloric sphincter relaxes, allowing more chyme to enter the small intestine from the stomach.

The presence of fats in the small intestine causes the reflexive release of bile stored in the gallbladder. The bile acts on the fats, promoting digestion and absorption of this nutrient by emulsifying the fats (mixing the fat with water molecules.)

Absorption

Absorption is the movement of digested food from the gastrointestinal tract into the blood or lymph for transport to the cells of the body. Absorption occurs primarily in the 20 ft of small intestine. Food is moved through this tube by peristalsis of the muscles forming it. The inner wall of the small intestine contains tiny projections called villi, providing over one-quarter acre

Table 22–1. **Basic Four Food Groups**

Food Group (Serving Size)	Servings/Day			Nutrients
	Child	Teen	Adult	
Milk Use low-fat milk (1 cup), cheese (1½ oz), yogurt (1 cup), ice milks (1¾ cup), cottage cheese (2 cups), pudding (1 cup)	3 (90–150 kcal/serving)	4	2	Protein; vitamins: riboflavin (B₂), A & D (in fortified milk); minerals: calcium
Meat Beef, pork, chicken, fish (2–3 oz), 2 eggs, cheese (2 oz), cottage cheese (½ cup), dried legumes—beans, peas, nuts (1 cup)	2 (165–220 kcal/serving) (55–110 kcal/serving for legumes)	2	2	Protein; carbohydrates; fat; vitamins: A, B (thiamin), B₂ (riboflavin), niacin; minerals: calcium, iron, zinc, (fiber for bulk)
Fruit/Vegetable Cooked (½ cup) Juice (½ cup) Raw (1 cup) One whole fruit	4 (25–80 kcal/serving)	4	4	Carbohydrates Vitamins A & C, B-complex Folic acid (fiber source for bulk), minerals: calcium, potassium
Grains 1 slice bread 1 cup ready-to-eat cereal ½ cup cooked cereal, pasta, grits	4 (55–110 kcal/serving)	4	4	Minerals: iron; vitamins: niacin, B₁ (thiamin), carbohydrates, (fiber)
Other Alcohol, soda, candy, cake, gelatin, jam, salad dressing, cooking oil				Fats, carbohydrates

of surface area for the absorption of the digested chyme. The villi draw the nutrient molecules into their structure, and from there they are transported into the blood or lymph. The villi contain enzymes that break down the nutrient molecules into even smaller units. In the small intestine, absorption of almost all nutrients occurs, leaving water and undigestible fiber to pass into the large intestine through the ileocecal valve. In the large intestine, almost all of the water is absorbed and some of the minerals. In addition to the water in foods and ingested fluid, the large intestine absorbs the 7,000 ml of fluid produced from the salivary glands, stomach, pancreas, and liver, leaving only about 100 ml to be eliminated with the stool. Within the large intestine, the action of bacteria on the remaining food material produces vitamin K which is then absorbed and used by the body in the process of clot formation. Excessive use of antibiotics can destroy these normal bacteria, leaving the individual with a potential deficit of vitamin K, unless food sources are providing adequate amounts.

Essential Nutrients

There are six classes of nutrients: carbohydrates, proteins, lipids (fats), vitamins, minerals, and water. All are essential to optimum health and are provided to the body through the foods that are eaten and digested. Almost all foods contain mixtures of carbohydrates, fats, and protein, but many foods are especially high in one or the other. Food groups, such as the basic four food groupings (meat, breads/cereals, fruits/vegetables, milk/dairy), contain foods high in one or more nutri-

ents. Eating a variety of foods from four food groups each day, in appropriate amounts, will meet the body's need for all six nutrients. Table 22–1 presents the food groups and recommended daily servings. Three of the nutrients (carbohydrates, lipids, and protein) are capable of producing energy which is measured in calories. A *calorie (kcal)* is a measure of the amount of heat energy it takes to raise the temperature of 1 kg of water 1° centigrade. The individual's caloric needs are determined by calculating the total energy utilized by that individual each day. An adequate diet then provides this number of calories through an appropriate balance of nutrients in food.

Carbohydrates. Carbohydrates are the body's preferred energy source in the form of glucose. This is the form utilized within the cell for the production of ATP. (See Figure 22–2) Complex carbohydrates (starch) are ultimately broken down into glucose for use in energy production. Stored glucose, in the form of *glycogen* in the muscles and liver, will be used for energy before fats and proteins. Glucose is essential for normal brain activity and is the only form of nutrient the central nervous system uses for energy. During starvation or inadequate intake, the carbohydrate reserves of glycogen are used up within several hours to 12 hours, depending on the individual's energy expenditure and initial state of nutrition. After the glucose and glycogen stores are depleted, the body will begin to break down fats and body protein for fuel. The average adult requires approximately 125 gm of carbohydrates each day, making up about 50 to 60 percent of the total caloric intake. Carbohydrates are either converted into energy, stored in the

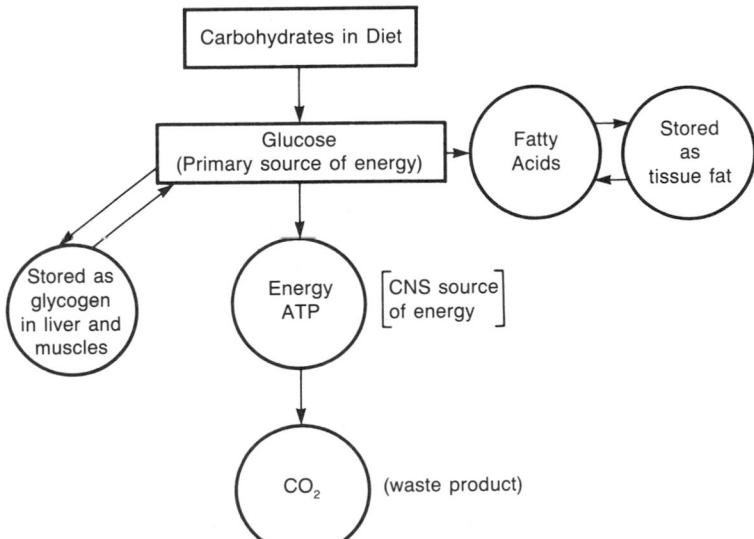

Figure 22–2. Carbohydrate metabolism. Formation of glucose from ingested carbohydrates is the body's primary source of energy through ATP production.

form of glycogen in the muscles and liver, or converted into fat and stored. Foods high in carbohydrates include milk, breads and cereals, fruits, and some vegetables. Sweets such as candy and soft drinks are high in carbohydrates but contain few, if any, other nutrients.

Lipids. Lipids are a nutrient required for normal cellular function. Lipids (or fats) in the diet contribute to skin and scalp oils for good complexions and healthy hair. Fats comprise the subcutaneous layer between skin and muscle which helps insulate the body from temperature extremes. Fat pads around the base of the kidneys protect them from jarring injury. Fat serves as the back-up energy supply when carbohydrates are not available for ATP production. The fat cells within the body seem to be able to store an almost limitless supply of fat for future body use. Unfortunately for the majority of people in developed countries, future utilization of stored fat never occurs. The fat continues to be stored and, over the years, weight is gained. *Obesity* (weight which is 20 percent or more above ideal weight for height) probably affects almost half of the population in the United States. While not obese, many more people are overweight. One pound of body fat produces 3,500 kcal. To lose 1 lb, a person must utilize 3,500 kcal more than are consumed. To lose 1 lb in a week, an individual would have to utilize 500 cal more than are consumed

each day. Fats should contribute approximately 30 percent of the daily caloric intake.

When body fat is being used for energy production instead of carbohydrates, ketones are formed. Many cells of the body are able to use ketones to produce energy, with the exception of the central nervous system (CNS).

Lipids are divided into two categories: saturated and unsaturated fatty acids. The unsaturated fatty acids have open areas in their chemical structure for bonding with other molecules. The saturated fatty acids do not. Cholesterol is a saturated fatty acid found in foods and also produced by the liver. Cholesterol is used to form bile which is necessary for digestion and absorption of ingested lipids. Cholesterol is associated with atherosclerosis because the plaque lining the affected vessels are composed primarily of cholesterol. The terms "high-density lipids" and "low-density lipids" are being used in association with atherosclerosis. An elevated blood level of high-density lipids (HDL), which are lipids being returned to the liver from other parts of the body, is associated with a reduced risk of heart attacks from atherosclerosis of coronary blood vessels. An elevation of low-density lipids (LDL) is associated with high serum cholesterol and an increased risk of coronary heart disease. Frequent, sustained physical exercise is also associated with an elevated HDL.

Proteins. Proteins are nutrients essential for all body activities from functioning of the immune system to normal body growth. Proteins are needed for the production of enzymes, cellular maintenance, and repair. Proteins help to maintain the balance of water within different compartments of the body. Inadequate protein in the diet leads to abdominal or generalized edema as body water leaks out of circulation and into the tissues.

All body cells contain protein. When protein intake is inadequate, growth is slowed or arrested. Muscle wasting begins as the body breaks down its own muscles to free the proteins for more critical uses, such as preservation of the immune system and maintaining adequate blood volume. In an adequate diet, protein is not used for energy, carbohydrate is used instead. The protein is used to build and maintain or repair all body structures.

Foods high in protein include lean meats, fish, eggs, legumes, and milk. At least 10 to 20 percent of the total calories consumed each day should come from foods high in protein.

Protein is 16 percent nitrogen. When nitrogen intake through ingestion of protein-rich foods is equal to nitrogen output, the body is in nitrogen balance. When intake exceeds nitrogen output, the body is in positive nitrogen balance. This occurs during times of growth,

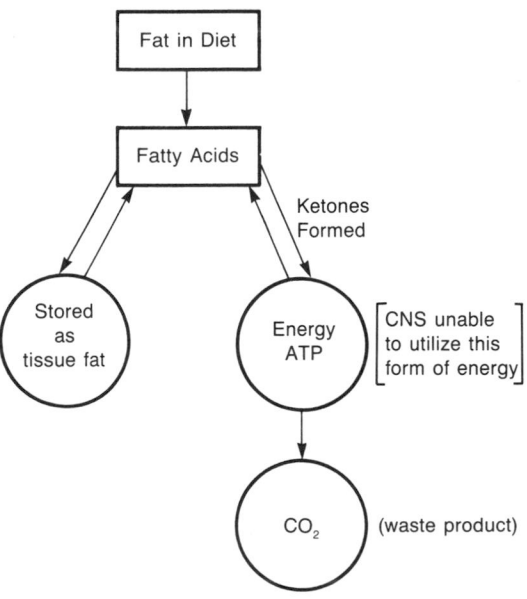

Figure 22–3. Lipid (fat) metabolism. Fats provide a back-up energy source when carbohydrate intake is inadequate and glycogen stores are exhausted.

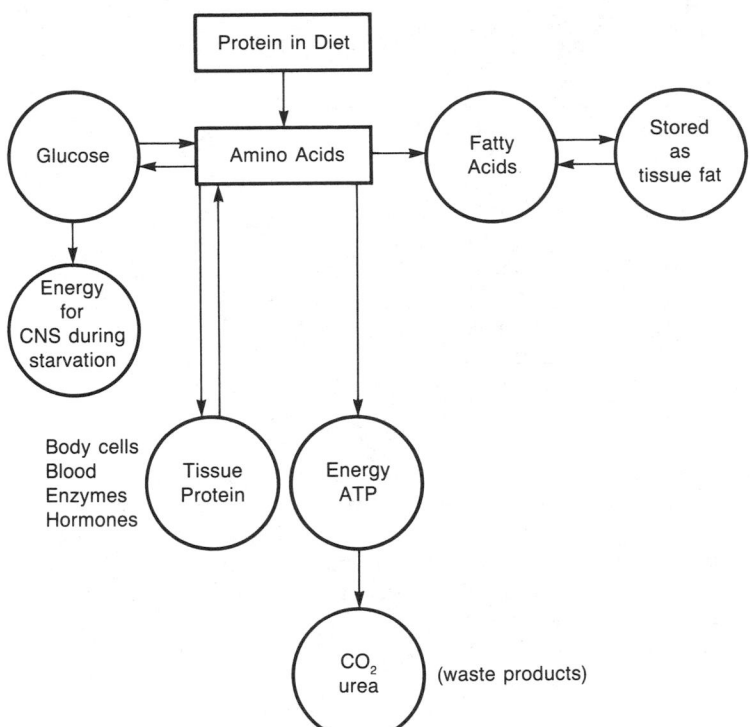

Figure 22–4. Protein metabolism. As proteins in the diet are broken down into amino acids, they are used to form new body structures and fluids. Amino acids obtained from the breakdown of body tissues can be used to form glucose for the energy needs of the nervous system (especially the brain) during times of inadequate nutritional intake.

tissue repair, muscle development, and pregnancy. When the body takes in less nitrogen than it puts out, the body is in a negative nitrogen balance and is losing body protein. Starvation, prolonged immobilization, and infections are states in which body proteins are being broken down faster than they are replaced. Elevations in the blood urea nitrogen level indicate a negative nitrogen balance and breakdown of lean body mass.

Body protein can be chemically converted to form glucose. Some body proteins must be broken into glucose when carbohydrate intake is inadequate to meet the energy needs of the CNS. During prolonged fasting, a person who is still overweight may die of starvation when too much of the body's lean muscle mass (proteins) is broken down for energy (Whitney and Hamilton, 1981.)

Vitamins, Minerals, and Water. These three nutrients do not provide the body with energy. Vitamins are essential for the absorption, digestion, and cellular use of carbohydrates, proteins, and fats. Some vitamins are soluble in water and some are soluble in fat. Vitamins A, D, E, and K are fat-soluble vitamins absorbed into the body with ingested fats. Vitamins C and the B-complex vitamins are water soluble and cross directly into the blood from the small intestine. Any excess amounts

of the water-soluble vitamins are excreted by the kidney. These vitamins are needed in small frequent doses as part of daily food intake. The fat-soluble vitamins can be stored with the fat, allowing less frequent ingestion of higher doses. Toxicity from very large doses of the fat-soluble vitamins is more likely because the body will store them rather than excreting the excess through the kidneys. Some vitamins improve the absorption of minerals. For example, vitamin C improves the absorption of iron.

The minerals are soluble in water and primarily help the body regulate the acid-base balance in the blood, interstitial fluid, and intracellular fluid. Minerals are also critical in regulation of fluid volume within the various compartments of the body.

Water is inorganic and contributes no energy, but it is the most important nutrient for survival. The body can tolerate a deficit of all other nutrients for fairly extended periods of time, but a continued intake of water is essential for survival. The body is a fluid medium containing three times as much water as any other nutrient. The body's need for fluids is further discussed in chapter 23.

Table 22–2 and 22–3 present sources and uses of the various vitamins and minerals. Table 22–4 presents some dietary guidelines and suggested food choices.

Table 22–2. **Summary of Vitamins**

Water Soluble

NOMENCLATURE	IMPORTANT SOURCES	PSYSIOLOGY AND FUNCTION	EFFECTS OF DEFICIENCY	RECOMMENDED ALLOWANCES
Ascorbic acid Vitamin C	Citrus fruits; tomatoes; melons; cabbage; broccoli; strawberries; fresh potatoes; green leafy vegetables	Very little storage in body Formation of intercellular cement substance; synthesis of collagen Absorption and use of iron Prevents oxidation of folacin	Weakened cartilage and capillary walls Cutaneous hemorrhage; sore, bleeding gums, anemia Poor wound healing Poor bone and tooth development *Scurvy*	Men: 60 mg Women: 60 mg Pregnancy: 80 mg Lactation: 100 mg Infants: 35 mg Children under 11: 0.7–1.2 mg Boys and girls: 50 mg
Thiamin Vitamin B_1	Whole-grain and enriched breads, cereals, flours; organ meats, pork; other meats, poultry, fish; legumes, nuts; milk; green vegetables	Limited body storage Thiamin pyrophosphate (TPP) is coenzyme for decarboxylation and transketolation; chiefly involved in carbohydrate metabolism	Poor appetite; atony of gastrointestinal tract, constipation Mental depression, apathy, polyneuritis Cachexia, edema Cardiac failure *Beriberi*	Men: 1.4 mg Women: 1.0 mg Pregnancy: +0.4 mg Lactation: +0.5 mg Infants: 0.3–0.5 mg Children under 11: 0.7–1.2 mg Boys and girls: 1.1–1.5 mg
Riboflavin Vitamin B_2	Milk; organ meats; eggs; green leafy vegetables	Limited body stores, but reserves retained carefully Coenzymes for removal and transfer of hydrogen; flavin mononucleotide (FMN) and flavin adenine dinucleotide (FAD)	Cheilosis (cracks at corners of lips) Scaly desquamation around nose, ears Sore tongue and mouth Burning and itching of eyes Photophobia	Men: 1.6 mg Women: 1.2 mg Pregnancy: +0.3 mg Lactation: +0.5 mg Infants: 0.4–0.6 mg Children under 11: 0.8–1.4 mg Boys and girls: 1.3–1.7 mg
Niacin Nicotinic acid Nicotinamide	Meat, poultry, fish; whole-grain and enriched breads, flours, cereals; nuts, legumes Tryptophan as a precursor	Coenzyme for glycolysis, fat synthesis, tissue respiration. Coenzymes NAD and NADP accept hydrogen and transfer it	Anorexia, glossitis, diarrhea Dermatitis Neurologic degeneration *Pellagra*	Men: 18 mg NE Women: 13 mg NE Pregnancy: +2 mg NE Lactation: +5 mg NE Infants: 6–8 mg NE Children under 11: 9–16 mg NE Boys and girls: 14–19 mg NE
Vitamin B_6 Three active forms: Pyridoxine, Pyridoxal, Pyridoxamine	Meat, poultry, fish; potatoes, sweet potatoes, vegetables	Pyridoxal phosphate is coenzyme for transamination, decarboxylation, transulfuration of amino acids Conversion of tryptophan to niacin; conversion of glycogen to glucose Requirement related to protein intake	Nervous irritability, convulsions Weakness, ataxia, abdominal pain Dermatitis; anemia	Men: 2.2 mg Women: 2.0 mg Pregnancy: +0.6 mg Lactation: +0.5 mg Infants: 0.3–0.6 mg Children under 11: 0.9–1.6 mg Boys and girls: 1.8–2.2 mg
Pantothenic acid	Meat, poultry, fish; whole-grain cereals; legumes Smaller amounts in fruits, vegetables, milk	Constituent of coenzyme A: oxidation of pyruvic acid, α-ketoglutarate, fatty acids; synthesis of fatty acids, sterols, and porphyrin	Deficiency seen only with severe miltiple B-complex deficits; gastrointestinal disturbances, neuritis, burning sensations of feet	Recommended safe and adequate intakes: Adolescents and adults: 4–7 mg Infants: 2–3 mg Children: 3–4 mg

Water Soluble (continued)

NOMENCLATURE	IMPORTANT SOURCES	PSYSIOLOGY AND FUNCTION	EFFECTS OF DEFICIENCY	RECOMMENDED ALLOWANCES
Biotin	Organ meats, egg yolk, nuts, legumes	*Avidin*, a protein in raw egg white, blocks absorption; large amounts of raw eggs must be eaten Coenzyme for deamination, carboxylation, and decarboxylation	Deficiency only when many raw egg whites are consumed for long periods of time Dermatitis, anorexia, hyperesthesia, anemia	Recommended safe and adequate intakes: Adolescents and adults: 100–200 µg Infants: 35–50 µg Children: 65–120 µg
Vitamin B₁₂ Cyanocobalamin Hydroxy-cobalamin	In animal foods only; organ meats, muscle meats, fish, poultry; eggs; milk	Requires intrinsic factor for absorption Biosynthesis of methyl groups Synthesis of DNA and RNA Formation of mature red blood cells	Lack of intrinsic factor leads to deficiency; pernicious anemia, following gastrectomy Macrocytic anemia Neurologic degeneration	Adults: 3 µg Pregnancy: 4 µg Lactation: 4 µg Infants: 0.5–1.5 µg Children: 2–3 µg Boys and girls: 3 µg
Folacin Folic acid Tetrahydrofolic acid	Organ meats, deep-green leafy vegetables; muscle meats, poultry, fish, eggs; whole-grain cereals	Active form is folinic acid; requires ascorbic acid for conversion Coenzyme for transmethylation; synthesis of nucleoproteins; maturation of red blood cells Interrelated with vitamin B₁₂	Megaloblastic anemia of infancy, pregnancy, tropical sprue	Adults: 400 µg Pregnancy: 800 µg Lactation: 500 µg Infants: 30–45 µg Children: 100–300 µg Boys and girls: 400 µg

Fat Soluble

NOMENCLATURE	IMPORTANT SOURCES	PSYSIOLOGY AND FUNCTION	EFFECTS OF DEFICIENCY	RECOMMENDED ALLOWANCES
Vitamin A Retinol Retinal Retinyl ester Retinoic acid Provitamin A Alpha-, beta-, gamma-carotene, cryptoxanthin	*Animal* Fish-liver oils Liver Butter, cream Whole milk Whole-milk cheeses Egg yolk *Plant* Dark-green leafy vegetables Yellow vegetables Yellow fruits Fortified margarines	Bile necessary for absorption Stored in liver Maintains integrity of mucosal epithelium, maintains visual acuity in dim light Large amounts are toxic	Faulty bone and tooth development Night blindness Keratinization of epithelium—mucous membranes and skin *Xerophthalmia*	Children: 400–700 RE (2,000–3,300 IU) Men: 1,000 RE (5,000 IU) Women: 800 RE (4,000 IU) Pregnancy: 1,000 RE (5,000 IU) Lactation: 1,200 RE (6,000 IU)
Vitamin D Vitamin D₂ Ergocalciferol Vitamin D₃ Cholecalciferol Antirachitic factor	Fish-liver oils Fortified milk Activated sterols Exposure to sunlight Very small amounts in butter, liver, egg yolk, salmon, sardines	Synthesized in skin by activity of ultraviolet light Liver synthesizes 25 (OH) D₃ Kidney synthesizes 1,25 (OH)₂ D₃ Functions as steroid hormone to regulate calcium and phosphorus absorption, mobilization and mineralization of bone Large amounts are toxic	*Rickets* in children Soft, fragile bones Enlarged joints Bowed legs Chest, spinal, pelvic bone deformities Delayed dentition *Tetanic* convulsions in infants *Osteomalacia* in adults	Children 0–18 years: 10 µg Adults 19–22 years: 7.5 µg Adults over 22 years: 5 µg Pregnant or lactating women: +5 µg

Fat Soluble (continued)

Table 22–2. **(continued)**

Fat Soluble (continued)

NOMENCLATURE	IMPORTANT SOURCES	PSYSIOLOGY AND FUNCTION	EFFECTS OF DEFICIENCY	RECOMMENDED ALLOWANCES
Vitamin E Alpha-, beta-, gamma-to-copherol Antisterility vitamin	Plant tissues—vegetable oils; wheat germ, rice germ; green leafy vegetables; nuts; legumes Animal foods are poor sources	Not stored in body to any extent Related to action of selenium *Humans:* reduces oxidation of vitamin A, carotenes, and polyunsaturated fatty acids *Animals:* normal reproduction; utilization of sex hormones, cholesterol	*Humans:* hemolysis of red blood cells; mild anemia; deficiency is not likely *Animals:* sterility in male rats; resorption of fetus in female rats; muscular dystrophy; creatinuria; macrocytic anemia	Infants: 3–4 mg α-TE Men: 10 mg α-TE Women: 8 mg α-TE Pregnancy: 10 mg α-TE Lactation: 11 mg α-TE
Vitamin K Phylloquinone (K₁) Menaquinone Menadione	Green leaves such as alfalfa, spinach, cabbage Liver Synthesis in intestine	Bile necessary for absorption Formation of prothrombin and other clotting proteins Sulfa drugs and antibiotics interfere with absorption Large amounts are toxic	Prolonged clotting time Hemorrhagic disease in newborn infants	Estimated safe and adequate intakes Infants: 10–20 μg Adults: 70–140 μg

Source: Corinne H. Robinson and Marilyn R. Lawler: *Normal and Therapeutic Nutrition.* 16 ed. Macmillan, New York, 1982, pp. 204 and 240.

Table 22–3. **Summary of the Minerals**

MINERALS	FUNCTIONS IN THE BODY	METABOLISM	FOOD SOURCES	DAILY ALLOWANCES
Calcium	Hardness of bones, teeth Transmission of nerve impulse Muscle contraction Normal heart rhythm Activate enzymes Increase cell permeability Catalyze thrombin formation	*Absorption:* about 15–40 percent, according to body need; aided by gastric acidity, vitamin D, lactose; excess phosphate, fat, phytate, oxalic acid interfere *Storage:* Trabeculae of bones; easily mobilized *Utilization:* needs parathyroid hormone, vitamin D *Excretion:* 60–85 percent of diet intake in feces; small urinary excretion; high protein intake increases urinary excretion *Deficiency:* retarded bone mineralization; fragile bones; stunted growth; rickets; osteomalacia; osteoporosis	Milk, hard cheese Ice cream, cottage cheese Greens: turnip, collards, kale, mustard, broccoli Oysters, shrimp, salmon, clams	Infants: 360–540 mg Children: 800 mg Teenagers: 1,200 mg Adults: 800 mg Pregnancy: 1,200 mg Lactation: 1,200 mg

MINERALS	FUNCTIONS IN THE BODY	METABOLISM	FOOD SOURCES	DAILY ALLOWANCES
Chlorine	Chief anion of extracellular fluid Constituent of gastric juice Acid-base balance; chloride-bicarbonate shift in red cells	*Absorption:* rapid, almost complete *Excretion:* chiefly in urine; parallels intake *Deficiency:* with prolonged vomiting, drainage from fistula, diarrhea	Table salt	Estimated safe and adequate intake: Infants 275–1,200 mg Children 500–2,775 mg Teenagers 1,400–4,200 mg Adults 1,700–5,100 mg Daily diet contains in excess of need
Chromium	Efficient use of insulin in glucose uptake; glucose oxidation, protein synthesis, stimulation of fat, and cholesterol synthesis Activation of enzymes	Usable form in organic compound; glucose tolerance factor	Liver, meat Cheese Whole-grain cereals	Estimated safe and adequate intake: Infants 0.01–0.06 mg Children 0.02–0.20 mg Teenagers 0.05–0.20 mg Adults 0.05–0.20 mg
Copper	Aids absorption and use of iron in synthesis of hemoglobin Electron transport Melanin formation Myelin sheath of nerves Purine metabolism	*Transport:* chiefly as protein, ceruloplasmin *Storage:* liver, central nervous system *Excretion:* bile into intestine *Deficiency:* rare; occurs in severe malnutrition Abnormal storage in Wilson's disease	Liver, shellfish Meats Nuts, legumes Whole-grain cereals Typical diet provides 1 to 5 mg	Estimated safe and adequate intake: Infants 0.5–1.0 mg Children 1.0–2.5 mg Teenagers 2.0–3.0 mg Adults 2.0–3.0 mg
Fluorine	Increases resistance of teeth to decay; most effective in young children Moderate levels in bone may reduce osteoporosis	*Storage:* bones and teeth *Excretion:* urine Excess leads to mottling of teeth	Fluoridated water: 1 ppm	Estimated safe and adequate intake: Infants 0.1–1.0 mg Children 0.5–2.5 mg Teenagers 1.5–2.5 mg Adults 1.5–4.0 mg
Iodine	Constituent of diiodotyrosine, triiodothyronine, thyroxin, regulate rate of energy metabolism	*Absorption:* controlled by blood level of protein-bound iodine *Storage:* thyroid gland; activity regulated by thyroid-stimulating hormone *Excretion:* in urine *Deficiency:* simple goiter; if severe, cretinism—rarely seen in U.S.	Iodized salt is most reliable source Seafood Foods grown in nongoitrous coastal areas	Infants: 40–50 μg Children: 70–120 μg Teenagers: 150 μg Adults: 150 μg Pregnancy: 175 μg Lactation: 200 μg
Iron	Constituent of hemoglobin, myoglobin, and oxidative enzymes: catalase, cytochrome, xanthine oxidase	*Absorption:* about 3 to 23 percent, depending on food source and body need; aided by gastric acidity, ascorbic acid *Transport:* bound to protein, transferrin *Storage:* as ferritin in liver, bone marrow, spleen	Liver, organ meats Meat, poultry Egg yolk Enriched and whole-grain breads, cereals Dark-green vegetables Legumes Molasses, dark Peaches, apricots, prunes, raisins Diets supply about 6 mg per 1,000 kcal	Infants: 10–15 mg Children: 10–15 mg Teenagers: 18 mg Men: 10 mg Women: 18 mg Pregnancy: 18 + mg Lactation: 18 mg

Table 22–3. (continued)

MINERALS	FUNCTIONS IN THE BODY	METABOLISM	FOOD SOURCES	DAILY ALLOWANCES
Iron (continued)		*Utilization:* chiefly in hemoglobin; daily turnover about 27 to 28 mg; iron used over and over again *Excretion:* men, about 1 mg; women, 1 to 2 mg; in urine, perspiration, menstual flow; fecal excretion is from unabsorbed dietary iron *Deficiency:* anemia; frequent in infants, preschool children, teenage girls, pregnant women		
Magnesium	Constituents of bones, teeth Activates enzymes in carbohydrate metabolism Muscle and nerve irritability	*Absorption:* parallels that of calcium; competes with calcium for carriers *Utilization:* slowly mobilized from bone *Excretion:* chiefly by kidney *Deficiency:* seen in alcoholism, severe renal disease; hypomagnesemia, tremor	Whole-grain cereals Nuts; legumes Meat Milk Green leafy vegetables	Infants: 50–70 mg Children: 150–250 mg Women: 300 mg Men: 350 mg Pregnancy and lactation: 450 mg
Manganese	Activation of many enzymes; oxidation of carbohydrates, urea formation, protein hydrolysis Bone formation	*Absorption:* limited *Excretion:* chiefly in feces *Deficiency:* not known	Legumes, nuts Whole-grain cereals	Estimated safe and adequate intake: Infants 0.5–1.0 mg Children 1.0–3.0 mg Teenagers 2.5–5.0 mg Adults 2.5–5.0 mg
Molybdenum	Cofactor for flavorprotein enzymes; present in xanthine oxidase	Absorbed as molybdate Stored in liver, adrenal, kidney Related to metabolism of copper and sulfur	Organ meats Legumes Whole-grain cereals	Estimated safe and adequate intake: Infants 0.03–0.08 mg Children 0.05–0.31 mg Teenagers 0.15–0.50 mg Adults 0.15–0.50 mg
Phosphorus	Structure of bones, teeth Cell permeability Metabolism of fats and carbohydrates: storage and release of ATP Sugar-phosphate linkage in DNA and RNA Phospholipids in transport of fats Buffer salts in acid-base balance	*Absorption:* about 70 percent; aided by vitamin D *Utilization:* about 85 percent in bones; controlled by vitamin D, parathormone *Excretion:* About one third of diet in feces; metabolic products chiefly in urine *Deficiency:* poor bone mineralization; poor growth; rickets	Milk, cheese Eggs, meat, fish, poultry Legumes, nuts Whole-grain cereals	Infants: 200–400 mg Children: 800 mg Adults: 800 mg Pregnancy: 1,200 mg Lactation: 1,200 mg

MINERALS	FUNCTIONS IN THE BODY	METABOLISM	FOOD SOURCES	DAILY ALLOWANCES
Potassium	Principal cation of intracellular fluid Osmotic pressure; water balance; acid-base balance Nerve irritability and muscle contraction, regular heart rhythm Synthesis of protein	*Absorption:* readily absorbed *Excretion:* chiefly in urine; increased with aldosterone secretion *Deficiency:* following starvation, correction of diabetic acidosis, adrenal tumors; some diuretics; muscle weakness, nausea, tachycardia, glycogen depletion, heart failure	Widely distributed in foods Meat, fish, fowl Cereals Fruits, vegetables	Estimated safe and adequate intake: Infants 350–1,275 mg Children 550–3,000 mg Teenagers 1,525–4,575 mg Adults 1,875–5,625 mg Diet adequate in calories supplies ample amounts
Selenium	Antioxidant Constituent of glutathione oxidase	Stored especially in liver, kidney Spares vitamin E	Meat and seafoods Cereal foods	Estimated safe and adequate intakes Infants: 0.01–0.06 mg Children: 0.02–0.20 mg Teenagers 0.05–0.20 mg Adults 0.05–0.20 mg
Sodium	Principal cation of extracellular fluid Osmotic pressure; water balance Acid-base balance Regulate nerve irritability and muscle contraction "Pump" for active transport such as for glucose	*Absorption:* rapid and almost complete *Excretion:* chiefly in urine; some by skin and in feces; parallels intake; controlled by aldosterone *Deficiency:* rare; occurs with excessive perspiration and poor diet intake; nausea, diarrhea, abdominal cramps, muscle cramps	Table salt Processed foods Milk Meat, fish, poultry	Estimated safe and adequate intake: Infants 115–750 mg Children 325–1,800 mg Teenagers 900–2,700 mg Adults 1,100–3,300 mg Diets supply substantial excess
Sulfur	Constituent of proteins, especially cartilage, hair, nails Constituent of melanin, glutathione, thiamin, biotin, coenzyme A, insulin High-energy sulfur bonds Detoxication reactions	Absorbed chiefly as sulfur-containing amino acids Excreted as inorganic sulfate in urine in proportion to nitrogen loss	Protein foods rich in sulfur-amino acids Eggs Meat, fish, poultry Milk, cheese Nuts	Not established Diet adequate in protein meets need
Zinc	Constituent of enzymes: carbonic anhydrase, carboxypeptidase, lactic dehydrogenase	*Absorption:* limited; competes with calcium for absorption sites *Storage:* liver, muscles, bones, organs *Excretion:* chiefly by intestine *Deficiency:* marginal occurs in U.S.	Seafoods Liver and other organ meats Meats, fish Wheat germ Yeast Plant foods are generally low Usual diet supplies 10 to 15 mg	Infants: 3–5 mg Children: 10 mg Teenagers: 15 mg Adults: 15 mg Pregnancy: 20 mg Lactation: 25 mg

Source: Corinne H. Robinson and Marilyn R. Lawler: *Normal and Therapeutic Nutrition.* 16 ed. Macmillan, New York, 1982, pp. 180–182.

Table 22–4. **Dietary Guidelines for Americans and Suggestions for Food Choices**

1. Eat a variety of foods daily. Include these foods every day: fruits and vegetables; whole-grain and enriched breads and cereals; milk and milk products; meats, fish, poultry, and eggs; dried peas and beans.
2. Maintain ideal weight. Increase physical activity; reduce kcalories by eating fewer fatty foods and sweets and less sugar, and by avoiding too much alcohol; lose weight gradually.
3. Avoid too much fat, saturated fat, and cholesterol. Choose low-fat protein sources such as lean meats, fish, poultry, and dried peas and beans; use eggs and organ meats in moderation; limit intake of fats on and in foods; trim fats from meats; broil, bake, or boil—do not fry; read food labels for fat content.
4. Eat foods with adequate starch and fiber. Substitute starches for fats and sugars; select whole-grain breads and cereal, fruits and vegetables, dried beans and peas, and nuts to increase fiber and starch intake.
5. Avoid too much sugar. Use less sugar, syrup, and honey; reduce concentrated sweets like candy, soft drinks, cookies, etc.; select fresh fruits or fruits canned in light syrup or their own juices; read food labels—sucrose, glucose, dextrose, maltose, lactose, fructose, syrups, and honey are all sugars; eat sugar less often to reduce dental caries.
6. Avoid too much sodium. Reduce salt in cooking; add little or no salt at the table; limit salty foods like potato chips, pretzels, salted nuts, popcorn, condiments, cheese, pickled foods, and cured meats; read food labels—for sodium or salt contents especially in processed and snack foods.
7. If you drink alcohol, do so in moderation. For individuals who drink, limit all alcoholic beverages (including wine, beer, liquors, etc.) to one or two drinks per day. Note: Use of alcoholic beverages during pregnancy can result in the development of birth defects and mental retardation called fetal alcohol syndrome.

Source: USDA, U.S. Department of Health, Education and Welfare, 1979.

Regulation of Nutritional Status

Both internal and external factors affect the ingestion, digestion, and absorption of food. Internal factors are stimulated by events or activities within the body. External factors affecting food intake and nutrition come from the environment.

Internal Regulation of Nutritional Status

In the ideal system, the body's energy needs are met each day, but not exceeded, by the food ingested. Regulation of this entire process is complex and not completely understood. The basal metabolic rate (BMR) is a measure of energy utilization by the body at rest. The energy demands of the body are also reflected by the blood glucose level and cellular metabolic rates. The body regulates the level of blood glucose between 70 and 120 mg/100 ml through the action of insulin and glucagon, which are both secreted from the pancrease. The beta cells of the pancreas secrete insulin in response to a rising blood glucose level following ingestion of carbohydrates. The insulin increases the intake of glucose by the cells, thus lowering the level in the blood to normal. In the cells, the glucose is either converted into energy or stored as glycogen. When the blood glucose level begins to decrease, the alpha cells of the pancreas secrete glucagon which stimulates the conversion of stored glycogen in the liver to glucose, bringing the blood glucose level back up to normal. Stress, either physical or emotional, also stimulates the conversion of glycogen to glucose and raises the blood glucose level. This is accomplished through the release of cortisol from the adrenal cortex and epinephrine from the adrenal medulla. Ingestion of large amounts of sugar causes rapid elevation of blood glucose and release of insulin. Reactive hypoglycemia occurs when the sugar is all absorbed, but insulin production and release remain high. The blood glucose level then drops rapidly.

Much of the actual regulation of digestion and absorption occurs at a local level within the gastrointestinal system. Table 22–5 summarizes some of these local control mechanisms.

What controls the amount and type of food an individual consumes? This remains a partly unanswered question. Eating is a voluntary activity and is, therefore, under the control of the central nervous system and the cerebral cortex. Eating is partially a response to various internal stimuli. The effects of learning are certainly re-

Table 22-5. **Local Control of Digestion and Absorption Within the Gastrointestinal System**

STIMULUS	RESPONSE	EFFECT
Increased acidity in duodenum from stomach contents	Release of hormone secretion which inhibits HCl secretion within the stomach	Reduces acidity in the duodenum to maintain action of digestive enzymes in the duodenum
Distention of small intestines from unabsorbed food	Increases peristalsis within the small intestines; inhibition of peristalsis in stomach	Mixing of digestive enzymes with food to increase digestion and absorption; decreased rate of stomach emptying
Fatty acids or amino acids (proteins) in the duodenum	Release of cholecystokinin from duodenal wall	Inhibits gastric peristalsis; causes gallbladder to contract, releasing bile for fat digestion; causes pancreas to release fat-digesting enzymes
Distention or presence of proteins in the stomach	Release of hormone gastrin which increases HCl secretion by stomach	Digestion of ingested foods
Fatty acids or simple carbohydrates in the small intestine	Release of gastric-inhibitory peptide by cells in small intestine	Inhibits HCl secretion in the stomach
Milk products containing lactose (carbohydrate) in small intestine	Release of lactase by cells in small intestine	Digestion of lactose so absorption is possible

lated to the type and quality of food ingested, but the mechanism within the body that initiates and terminates the desire to eat is unknown. It was believed to be controlled by the hypothalamus, but recent research indicates the hypothalamus within the brain is not the control center for feeding, although it is most likely involved (Vandern et al., 1980). Internal stimuli from the senses, from receptors for blood glucose levels, body temperature, and other areas are also involved in regulating food intake. Obesity is a condition in which this complex regulation process has failed, and excess calories are repeatedly consumed. The obese individual may actually eat less than a person of normal weight but often has a reduced level of activity and, therefore, reduced energy needs. The calories are then stored as fat. "Low levels of activity seem to stimulate eating" (Vander et al., 1980), which is the opposite of what should happen to maintain the body's energy balance.

Hunger indicates a desire for food. When the stomach is empty, peristalsis increases, to cause "hunger pains" or rumblings. This physical discomfort is relieved by eating. A blood glucose below 70 mg/100 ml usually causes hunger. Distention of the stomach decreases the desire to eat and contributes to the internal stimuli causing cessation of eating.

Learned behavior that contributes to food intake involves the individual's culture, religion, recreation patterns, ways of dealing with stress, and family behavior patterns regarding food. Understanding of the body's nutritional needs through education is another learned behavior affecting food consumption.

External Regulation of Nutritional Status

Poverty is one of the major deterrents to adequate nutrition throughout the world. Individuals with low incomes tend to consume inadequate protein which is found in more expensive foods. Some types of foods may not be available to people in some geographic areas because of climate and growing seasons. When foods are transported from distant areas, the price usually increases, making the items too expensive for some people's budgets.

Poverty is the leading cause of *marasmus* and *kwashiorkor*. Marasmus is a state of near starvation because of an inadequate caloric intake. Kwashiorkor is a severe protein deficiency when calorie intake may be adequate. Both diseases are most commonly seen in children living in poverty. After being weaned from the breast milk, the child may be given affordable, cereal-type foods with grossly inadequate protein supplies. The child gradually withers and may die from protein deficiency. Together these and related diseases are called protein-calorie malnutrition or PCM and are the world's leading nutritional problem.

Environmental temperature also plays a role in the amount of food ingested. People in colder climates consume more food than people in warm climates. Table 22-6 presents a summary of various factors that affect the body's nutritional needs. Some factors increase an individual's nutritional needs, and other factors decrease the need.

Table 22–6. **Factors Affecting the Body's Nutritional Needs**

Factors Increasing Nutritional Needs

Periods of rapid growth (infants, toddlers, teenagers, pregnancy)

During times of tissue repair from injury or surgery

Elevated or slightly reduced body temperatures (shivering and heat increase cellular metabolic rate—caloric needs increase by 7 percent for each degree F rise in body temperature [Bodinski, 1982])

Increased muscular actitivity

Sex (men have faster BMR than women)

Tall, thin build (increased heat loss requiring increased metabolism)

Some medication (increases nutrient excretion; decreases nutrient production or absorption within body)

Infection or disease

Stress (increases thyroid hormone and epinephrine released which increases metabolism)

Increased loss of nutrients through body fluid losses (hemorrhage, diarrhea, draining wounds, perspiration, kidney dialysis, lactation, menstruation, burns)

Chronic diseases affecting metabolism, ingestion, digestion, absorption, and elimination (diabetes, hyperthyroidism, cancer, psychosis, kidney or liver disease, respiratory problems)

Factors Decreasing Nutritional Needs

Cessation of growth

Fasting and constant malnutrition (decreases BMR)

Severe hypothermia (decreased cellular metabolism)

Hypothyroidism (decreases BMR)

Sex (women have lower BMR than men)

Sedentary life-style

Immobility or bed rest (decreases caloric needs but increases protein needs)

Short, fat build (conserves body heat and heat calories)

Losing weight (as the individual loses weight, it takes less muscular activity to move the lighter load—accounts for the plateau reached by many dieters who have lost significant amounts of weight and suddenly stop losing while consuming the same amount of calories)

Effect of Unmet Nutritional Needs on Other Basic Needs

When nutritional needs are unmet, the body's ability to meet other basic needs is compromised. Inadequate or excessive nutrition affects all areas, from oxygenation to self-actualization. Table 22–7 presents a summary of the effect of unmet nutritional needs on the individual's ability to satisfy other needs.

Table 22–7. **Effect of Unmet Nutritional Needs on Satisfaction of Other Basic Needs**

Oxygen Needs

Inadequate protein or iron may result in anemia and reduced ability to transport oxygen on the hemoglobin molecule

Inadequate water causes dehydration and reduced blood volume for transport of oxygen to all body cells

Inadequate protein and vitamin K will reduce the blood's ability to clot, resulting in excessive blood loss and reduced ability to transport oxygen

Excessive intake of saturated fatty acids is associated with coronary artery disease, jeopardizing the pumping action of the heart

Deficiency of vitamin B_{12} results in pernicious anemia and decreased ability to transport oxygen

Excessive caloric intake resulting in obesity is associated with hypertension, coronary artery disease

Severe malnutrition leads to wasting of heart muscles

Temperature Maintenance

Inadequate nutrient intake reduces the ability to produce heat

Loss of subcutaneous fat from inadequate intake reduces the body's ability to conserve heat

Consumption of excessive amounts of alcohol increases heat loss and decreases the sensation of being chilled, thus increasing the risk of hypothermia

Elimination Needs

Inadequate fluid and nutrient intake results in hard, difficult-to-pass stool

Inadequate production of insulin by the pancreas results in elevated blood glucose levels; increased excretion of glucose by the kidney draws water from the blood into urine formation; excessive urine production (polyurea)

Rest and Sleep

Inadequate intake may lead to hunger, making it difficult to fall asleep

Obesity is associated with apneic sleep disorder

Pain Avoidance

Inadequate nutrition results in delayed healing and longer periods of pain and discomfort from injured tissues

Nutritional deficiencies may result in pain in the legs when walking

Inability to digest and absorb foods can result in pain in the abdomen from distention and excess formation of gas (flatus)

Sexual Needs and Sexuality

Inadequate nutrition can result in temporary loss of reproductive ability

Obesity is associated with decreased sexual attractiveness in many cultures

Obesity is associated with reduced fertility

Stimulation Needs

Inadequate intake of nutrients results in muscle wasting and weakness, reducing the individual's ability to interact with the environment

Inadequate protein intake interferes with vision by preventing the normal function of the light receptors in the retina which are composed of protein

Vitamin deficiencies can result in loss of position and vibration sense

Inadequate nutrition results in a general lack of interaction with the environment to conserve energy, resulting in lack of sensory and motor stimulation

Safety and Security Needs

Inadequate nutrient intake results in generalized muscle weakness and increased risk of injury from falls

Confusion and loss of consciousness may result from inadequate nutrition and uncontrolled blood glucose levels, resulting in increased risk of injury from falls or accidents

Inability to ingest foods normally may result in anxiety, fear of choking

Love and Belonging Needs

Inadequate or excessive nutrition may result in rejection by family and peers

Esteem Needs

Inability to ingest foods without assistance frequently results in loss of self-esteem

Obesity may lead to rejection by others, causing the individual to dislike self

Nutritional deficiencies can result in altered body features, reducing the individual's personal feelings of attractiveness

Repeated failures to gain or lose weight may lead to self-condemnation

Self-Actualization

Obesity may interfere with ability to obtain desired employment or pursue a chosen career

Inadequate intake of nutrients will reduce the energy the individual has available to pursue desired goals

Factors Associated with Unmet Nutritional Needs

Factors Affecting Ingestion of Food

During the process of ingesting foods, the individual may encounter problems with chewing, tasting, swallowing, and hand/mouth coordination. Large changes in an individual's weight may affect the fit of dentures, making them uncomfortable or too loose for good chewing control. Talk with patients about the fit of their dentures and obtain dental consultations as necessary. Clean the patient's dentures several times each day to refresh the patient's mouth. If the patient is alert and oriented, help the patient to insert the dentures before meals. Dentures that fit poorly can injure the gums and discourage the patient from attempting to eat certain foods.

A stroke (cerebrovascular accident or CVA) often affects the individual's ability to take in food. Loss of dominant hand and arm control can make eating awkward and embarrassing. Food or fluids are often spilled, and eating utensils are difficult to manipulate. The stroke may affect the mouth, leaving one side of the mouth drooping. Control of fluids in the mouth becomes difficult. Drooling may require the wearing of a bib and be associated with loss of self-esteem. Swallowing may be difficult for a patient following a stroke, depending on the area of the brain involved. Choking occurs frequently if the coordination of swallowing has been affected by the CVA.

The patient may be physically unable to bring food to the mouth because of paralysis, as occurs for patients with quadriplegia, and because of casts, amputations, congenital absence of arms, or because of age (infants). These patients will require feeding by another individual which may be viewed as a sign of helplessness by older children and adults. Patients may prefer not to eat or to eat only small amounts of food to limit the embarrassment created by being fed.

Patients may be unwilling to eat. Depression and low self-esteem may lead the individual to ignore internal and external stimuli to eat. Patients who are 10 percent underweight or who have lost large amounts of weight recently are at nutritional risk. Low self-esteem is related to a condition called *anorexia nervosa* in which individuals starve themselves to lose weight and may cause their own death. This disease seems to be unique to teenagers and young women who continually view themselves as overweight, even though they may be grossly underweight. Nutritional intervention, coordinated with family and individual counseling, is needed for individuals with anorexia nervosa. Anorexia nervosa occurs in 1 out of every 200 young, white, Western females, which is a tenfold increase from a decade ago.

Injury or damage to the face, mouth, gums, or esophagus will interfere with the ability to consume food. An individual with a fractured jaw has the jaws wired together (top to bottom) during healing. This prevents the individual from separating the teeth. Foods must be able to pass between the teeth. This results in ingestion of a fluid diet for several weeks. Cancer of the mouth or esophagus may make chewing and swallowing difficult or impossible. Nutrition may have to be introduced directly into the stomach, bypassing the damaged or obstructed area.

Illness and hospitalization put the patient at risk for inadequate intake of nutrients. The patient may experience loss of appetite (*anorexia*) and nausea or vomiting during an illness. Administration of some medications, surgery, or diagnostic tests may also cause anorexia and nausea. This will reduce the individual's normal nutritional intake. The practice of restricting foods and fluids for many hours before diagnostic tests will interfere with good nutrition, especially if testing continues for several days, followed by surgery and further food abstinence. Surgery is associated with termination of food and fluid intake for varying periods of time, depending on the severity of the patient's condition and the type of surgery performed. Maintenance on IV therapy for three or more days without any oral intake of nutrients is associated with a compromised state of nutrition. Approximately 60 percent of the people admitted to the hospital lose an average of 13 lb during their stay. Thirty-seven percent are anemic when admitted, and another 16 percent become anemic during hospitalization (Lichtenstein, 1982). Acute illness increases the body's nutritional needs, especially protein needs, and most patients consume less food and fluids than normal. The increased need, coupled with decreased intake, results in 40 to 65 percent of all hospitalized patients being malnourished (Lichtenstein, 1982).

Manipulation of the gastrointestinal tract and general anesthesia are associated with elimination of normal peristalsis in the tract, with delayed return of function. Peristalsis returns to the stomach and large intestines in 48 to 72 hours after general anesthesia. The small bowel regains peristaltic action in 8 to 12 hours (Patterson and Andrassy, 1983). Ingesting food when peristalsis is absent or greatly reduced results in abdominal distention and discomfort, nausea, and vomiting. Return of bowel sounds is an indication that peristalsis has resumed, and ingestion of small amounts of food and fluid can be attempted. Absence of bowel sounds in all areas of the abdomen is an indication that food and fluids should be withheld. Increasing the patient's activity level is helpful in reestablishing peristalsis in the tract. Passing flatus is another indication that peristalsis has returned, and ingestion of food may begin. Hunger is a sign of returning peristalsis, although it is not as reliable as the other two indicators. The postoperative patient is frequently started on a clear liquid diet and advanced gradually to a regular solid diet over one to several days, if no problems develop. If signs of abdominal distention begin to develop, intake of additional food should be discouraged, and activity such as walking in the halls should be increased, if possible. Medications that decrease peristalsis, such as codeine, should be used only when needed, or other medications should be substituted that have less effect on bowel motility. Medications are changed by the physician.

Clients with restricted activity are at nutritional risk. Immobility and extended periods of bed rest result in breakdown of body proteins faster than they are produced. If nutritional intake remains constant or decreases, as is often the case, inadequate intake of protein can be expected. Reduced activity and bed rest tend to decrease the individual's appetite. Certain positions in bed make eating difficult.

Other conditions associated with inadequate nutritional intake include living and eating alone, low or fixed incomes, alcoholism, and lack of understanding the body's nutritional needs or of what an appropriate daily intake should include. The cause of this lack of knowledge may be cultural, family-based, or a result of reduced cognitive functioning. The mentally retarded individual striving to maintain independence is often inappropriately nourished because of the foods chosen for consumption. Older patients who are experiencing memory and thinking difficulties may alter normal intake of foods in their confusion. They may be unable to buy and prepare foods as they previously did.

Obesity is a problem with regulation of intake. The obese individual is one who is more than 20 percent over ideal weight for height and body build. Obesity is a very serious and complex problem which is often very resistant to treatment. Stated simply, caloric intake exceeds caloric utilization in a continuing pattern. Obese individuals have a mortality rate 50 percent higher than people of normal weight. It is estimated that 15,000,000 Americans are obese to the point that they are severely jeopardizing their health. Obesity is associated with hypertension, diabetes, heart disease, gallbladder problems, and reproductive problems. Factors related to obesity include a sedentary life-style, eating rapidly, eating while doing other things (such as watching TV), aging, skipping meals, and using foods to deal with strong emotions, fatigue, and boredom.

Choking and aspiration of food or fluids into the respiratory system are problems of ingestion. A decreased level of consciousness is most often associated with an inability to coordinate swallowing, which results in choking and possible aspiration. The technique for removing food obstructing the airway is presented in Chapter 20.

Patients are being discharged from the hospital in weakened conditions to settings where little or no help is available with grocery shopping and meal preparation. Patients who live alone are discharged from the hospital and may not have the strength to buy and prepare meals for several days to weeks. Inadequate intake of nutrients is the result, which further reduces healing time and prolongs generalized weakness. Public health nursing referrals are needed for any patient whom the hospital nurse anticipates will have problems providing adequate nutritional intake after discharge. Community services can be used to deliver nutritious meals to the patient's home, one or more times each day, at reasonable costs. Patients might be encouraged to stay with friends or relatives for a few days or to have someone stay with them until they are stronger. They also might choose to remain in the hospital a few more days.

Problems with Digestion and Absorption

Problems with digestion and absorption of nutrients involve disturbances in function of the various parts of the digestive system. There may be obstructive problems interfering with the movement of food through the system. Problems with regulation and secretion of digestive juices may be another area where problems develop, making absorption of nutrients impossible. Trauma or inadequate blood circulation to the digestive tract may result in damage to the cells and loss or partial loss of function. Infection of the digestive tract may result in minimal absorption of nutrients, as in severe diarrhea. Table 22–8 summarizes common problems affecting digestion and absorption of foods from the gastrointestinal tract. These problems are all associated with various forms of inadequate nutrition. Table 22–9 presents classifications of drugs used in treating GI problems.

Patients taking medication, either prescribed or over-the-counter, that may affect ingestion, digestion, absorption, metabolism, or elimination are at nutritional risk. This is especially true if the medications have been used for extended periods of time. Diet pills, very large doses of some vitamins or minerals, and laxatives are some examples of drugs many people use and abuse without medical supervision. Drugs prescribed by the physician may also cause problems with a patient's nutritional status. Some medications are expected to cause some gastrointestinal disturbances or to create nausea or anorexia. Other medications may have these undesirable side effects and need to be changed. Some patients may need to increase or decrease their consumption of certain foods and fluids to avoid nutritional deficits or problems while on some medications.

Table 22–8. **Common Problems Affecting Digestion and Absorption**

PROBLEM	RELATED DATA
Transport Problems	
Vomiting (emesis)	Forceful regurgitation of ingested food from the stomach or duodenum associated with excessive distention, increased intracranial pressure, motion sickness, intense pain, hormone production in pregnancy, chemical irritation of digestive tract; often preceded by sweating, nausea, increased heart rate, and salivation; can be initiated by tactile stimuli to back of throat.
Dumping syndrome	Associated with surgical reduction in stomach size; gastric contents empty into duodenum before adequately digested and liquefied; acidity in duodenum greatly increased, causing fluids to be pulled from blood into gut to dilute acidity; associated with weakness, nausea, cramps, and diarrhea
Hiatus hernia	Stomach displaced upward through diaphragm; reflux of gastric fluids into esophagus, resulting in "heartburn"
Gallstones	Obstructive disease affecting release of bile into small intestine for fat digestion; stones are composed of cholesterol; associated with diarrhea, abdominal pain, nausea and vomiting, and jaundice with elevated levels of serum bilirubin
Injury/Damage Problems	
Peptic ulcers	Lining of stomach or duodenum damaged; affects one in ten people; more common in men; related to life stress, either physical or emotional; pain caused by food, acid, and enzymes coming in contact with damaged stomach cells and unprotected cells below these damaged mucus-secreting cells; bleeding and perforation of wall possible
Inflammatory bowel disease (Crohn's disease in small bowel; also called *regional enteritis*)	Inflammatory lesions in one area of the bowel which may spread to other areas; may result in obstruction of digestive tract and reduced absorption of nutrients; chronic disease of unknown cause; associated with loss of weight, anorexia, diarrhea, fever, and pain
Celiac disease	Lining of small intesting damaged with decreased area for absorption of nutrients; cause unknown
Gastritis	Inflammation of mucosal lining of the stomach; associated with ingestion of irritating substances such as alcohol, medications, caffeine, pepper, and meat extracts
Digestion/Absorption Problems	
Lactose intolerance	Common in all adults except Caucasians of European ancestry (Kloster, 1982); inability to digest milk and milk products because of lack of enzyme lactase required to break down lactose; associated with increased production of gas in intestines, distention, abdominal pain, and diarrhea
Diabetes mellitus	A metabolic rather than a gastrointestinal problem; affects nutritional status by preventing utilization of glucose from the blood at a cellular level, leading to elevated blood glucose levels; inadequate production of effective hormone insulin by beta cells of pancreas

Table 22-9. **Medication Classifications Associated with Nutrition**

Anti-infective Agents

Used to treat bacterial infections in GI tract; long-term use may destroy bacteria in large bowel and eliminate synthesis of vitamin K; use related to decreased appetite, diarrhea, decreased vitamin absorption

Autonomic Drugs

Parasympatholytic agents (anticholinergics) used to decrease motility and muscle spasms in the GI tract; decrease gastric acid secretions

Gastrointestinal Drugs

1. Antacids. Inorganic salts that dissolve in acidic gastric secretions to neutralize part of HCl; used to relieve discomfort of heartburn, indigestion, and peptic ulcer pain
2. Digestants. Replace inadequate secretion of gastric and pancreatic secretions needed for digestion
3. Absorbents. Used as an antidote to ingestion of poisons; absorbs poison, preventing absorption.
4. Emetics and Antiemetics. Emetics are used to induce vomiting in early stage of poison ingestion; antiemetics are used to decrease nausea and vomiting and are usually given parenterally
5. Miscellaneous GI Drugs. Cimetidine: Used in treatment of duodenal ulcers; reduces gastric acidity

Hormones and Synthetic Substitutes

Insulins and antidiabetic agents used to treat diabetes mellitus; used to lower blood glucose level

Thyroid and antithyroid.

Thyroid preparations are used to treat conditions in which thyroid secretion is inadequate; antithyroid drugs are used to decrease thyroid secretion when it is excessive

Vitamins and Mineral Supplements

Used to supplement an inadequate diet; may be toxic in very large doses; essential nutrients for adequate nutrition

Central Nervous System Drugs

Cerebral stimulant
  Amphetamines used to treat depression, and in treatment of obesity to decrease appetite

Assessment of Nutritional Need Satisfaction

During the assessment process, the nurse collects data indicating any of the following problems affecting nutrition:

1. Evidence of inadequate intake of nutrients because of physical, emotional, financial, medical, religious, or cultural reasons

2. Evidence of increased loss of nutrients from the body through loss of body fluids from the skin, the gastrointestinal tract, or the blood

3. Evidence of increased nutritional needs based on an increased metabolic rate from such things as fever, tissue healing, pregnancy, cancer, or growth

4. Evidence of decreased nutritional need compared to food intake from such things as reduced activity or a decreased metabolic rate such as accompanies normal aging

Data Related to Satisfaction of Nutritional Needs

The following data are associated with an appropriately nourished individual.

Objective Data. Satisfaction of nutritional needs can be confirmed by the following observations:

- Shiny hair which does not pull out easily from the scalp when combed or brushed
- Consistent skin color over the face with no evidence of facial swelling
- Clear, bright eyes with white sclera, pink and moist inner lids, and intact skin surrounding the eyes
- Smooth, pink lips with no evidence of swelling
- A pink tongue with bumpy texture from elevated taste buds; no swelling
- Adequate teeth for biting and chewing; few dental caries; intact gum tissue; consistent color of tooth enamel
- Smooth, intact skin with color distribution common to racial group and individual's age over entire body
- Fingernails and toenails that are straight and smooth; ability to grow long nails.
- Bowel sounds heard over abdomen; auscultation of bowel sounds with a stethoscope results in a gurgling or rumbling sound over various areas of the abdomen. The sound is created by normal peristalsis moving the food through the intestine
- Some fat between skin and muscle; triceps skinfold approximately 11 to 12 mm for men and 19 to 22 mm for women; midupper arm circumference approximately 29 to 31 cm for men and 26 to 29 cm for women

The amount of subcutaneous fat is measured using the fat-fold test on the back of the upper arm or by measuring the circumference of the middle of the upper arm. The midpoint between the shoulder and the elbow is located and a nonstretching tape measure is used to measure arm circumference at this point. A device called a caliper is needed to measure the tricep fat fold. At the midpoint of the back of the upper arm, the skin is pinched up between the nurse's fingers without including the underlying muscle tissue. The caliper is placed over the pinched-up tissue, and the tension on the device is allowed to compress the skin between the pinch. The caliper is then read after 3 sec.

- Good muscle tone with normal (2 +) reflexes (see Chapter 28 for assessment of deep tendon stretch reflexes)
- Energy balance (calorie intake approximately equal to total energy expended each day)

Total caloric intake is estimated based on the type and amounts of foods consumed in a 24-hour period. Tables of calorie content in various foods are widely available. Total energy utilization is calculated by the following four steps:

1. First calculate the basal metabolic rate (BMR) for the individual:

    a. Body weight $\times$ 9.9 kcal (women) or 1.0 kcal
       (kg) 1 kg/hr (men) = kcal the individual uses each hour

    b. Kcal used $\times$ 24 hr = Kcal used each day at rest
       each hour (BMR)

2. Next calculate additional energy utilized in voluntary activities in a day:

    BMR $\times$ | 0.2 (sedentary—most patients)
    0.3 (lightly active)
    0.4 (moderately active—most nurses)
    0.5 (extremely active) | = Voluntary energy utilization

3. Next, calculate the additional energy utilized in processing the food consumed:

    (BMR + voluntary energy $\times$ 0.1 = Energy utilized
    utilization) to process food

4. Total energy utilization = BMR + Voluntary energy utilized + Energy used to process food

- Ingestion of approximately 33 kcal/kg of ideal body weight
- Body weight appropriate for height (actual weight close to "ideal weight")

Tables from insurance companies provide data on average weight for height and are used as "ideal weight" guides. Body build affects the amount of weight appropriate for an individual's height. A small

Table 22–10. **Body Build Based on Wrist Measurement**

HEIGHT	WRIST CIRCUMFERENCE	BODY BUILD
4′8″–5′2″	5–5¹/₂″	Small frame
	5¹/₂–5³/₄″	Medium frame
	5³/₄″ or more	Large frame
5′2″–5′5″	5–6″	Small frame
	6–6¹/₄″	Medium frame
	6¹/₄″ or more	Large frame
5′5″ or taller	5–6¹/₄″	Small frame
	6¹/₄–6¹/₂″	Medium frame
	6¹/₂″ or more	Large frame

body build carries less weight than a large body build. Body build is based on the individual's bone structure. An easy way of assessing body build is to measure the smallest circumference of an individual's wrist, distal to the prominent bones at the wrist. Table 22–10 indicates body build based on height and wrist circumference. Table 22–11 presents a height and weight table considering body build.

- Normal heart rate and rhythm (based on age)
- Normal blood pressure (based on age)
- Alert and oriented to time, place, and person
- Laboratory values normal

Serum albumin	3.5–5 gm/100 ml
Hemoglobin	12–16 gm/100 ml (women)
	14–18 gm/100 ml (men)
Hematocrit	37–47% (women)
	42–52% (men)
Total serum protein	6–8 gm/100 ml
Cholesterol	150–300 mg/100 ml
Serum glucose	65–105 mg/100 ml
Blood urea nitrogen	10–20 mg/100 ml
Creatinine (urine)	1.5–2.0 gm/24 hr (men)
	0.8–1.5 gm/24 hr (women)
Urine glucose	negative
Urine ketones	negative

- Soft-formed stools passed regularly with minimal effort
- Normal growth rate for age

Table 22–11. **Height and Weight Standards Based on Body Build**

Men				Women			
HEIGHT	SMALL	MEDIUM	LARGE	HEIGHT	SMALL	MEDIUM	LARGE
5′ 2″	128–134	131–141	138–150	4′10″	102–111	109–121	118–131
5′ 3″	130–136	133–143	140–153	4′11″	103–113	111–123	120–134
5′ 4″	132–138	135–145	142–156	5′ 0″	104–115	113–126	122–137
5′ 5″	134–140	137–148	144–160	5′ 1″	106–118	115–129	125–140
5′ 6″	136–142	139–151	146–164	5′ 2″	108–121	118–132	128–143
5′ 7″	138–145	142–154	149–168	5′ 3″	111–124	121–135	131–147
5′ 8″	140–148	145–157	152–172	5′ 4″	114–127	124–138	134–151
5′ 9″	142–151	148–160	155–176	5′ 5″	117–130	127–141	137–155
5′10″	144–154	151–163	158–180	5′ 6″	120–133	130–144	140–159
5′11″	146–157	154–166	161–184	5′ 7″	123–136	133–147	143–163
6′ 0″	149–160	157–170	164–188	5′ 8″	126–139	136–150	146–167
6′ 1″	152–164	160–174	168–192	5′ 9″	129–142	139–153	149–170
6′ 2″	155–168	164–178	172–197	5′10″	132–145	142–156	152–173
6′ 3″	158–172	167–182	176–202	5′11″	135–148	145–159	155–176
6′ 4″	162–176	171–187	181–207	6′ 0″	138–151	148–162	158–179

Source: 1983 Height and Weight Card. Courtesy of the Metropolitan Life Insurance Company, New York, 1983.

Subjective Data. If nutrition needs have been adequately satisfied, a patient would report the following:

- Ability to walk and run without pain
- Alcohol consumption limited to one or two drinks per day
- Having enough energy for activities
- Consuming appropriate number of servings from the basic food groups each day
- Normal appetite for a variety of foods
- Normal sense of taste and smell
- Maintenance of stable weight over the last several years (adult)

Data Associated with Unmet Nutritional Need

Objective Data. If nutritional needs have not been satisfied, the following observations would be made:

Dull, dry, brittle hair which pulls out during combing or brushing; loss of normal color in sections of hair

Lightened areas of skin on the face or other parts of the body; dry, scaling skin on face or body; facial, abdominal, or general edema

Unusual colored spots on sclera of eyes; dulling of normal eye color; softening of the cornea; cracking of skin around the eyes

Cracked, swollen, or reddened lips

Excessively reddened or pale tongue; smooth appearance of the tongue from atrophied taste buds

Inadequate teeth for chewing; decayed teeth; gums that bleed easily; tenderness

Open areas on the skin; dry, flaking areas; excessive coarseness

Thin, brittle nails; spoon-shaped nails

Inadequate or excessive fat between skin and muscle; triceps fatfold less than ½ inch or more than 1 inch (normally less in men than in women of ideal weight); midarm circumference on upper arm less than 28 cm or more than 34 cm in men, less than 24 cm or more than 34 cm in women

Large, edematous abdomen with thin extremities, especially in children

Ingestion of excessive or inadequate calories in relation to total body energy needs

Absent or diminished bowel sounds, especially with abdominal distention

Loss of deep tendon reflexes

Body weight 10 percent or more above or below "ideal weight" for height

Persistent vomiting

Bruising or petechiae on skin

Tachycardia, enlarged heart, arrhythmia

Irritable, confused, lethargic

Retarded growth for age

Very hard stools passed with much difficulty, diarrhea, change in bowel habits

Recent, unplanned weight losses or gains

Continuous IV solutions for several days with nothing taken orally

Low income

Poorly fitting dentures

Enlarged liver

Softening of bones in skull of children or failure of anterior fontanel to close by two years of age

Legs curved outward at knees in children

Abnormal laboratory values

- Low hemoglobin or hematocrit (inadequate iron intake)
- Elevated blood urea nitrogen (breakdown of body proteins for energy)
- Blood glucose abnormally low or high (high in diabetes mellitus; low in hyperinsulinism)
- Glucose in urine (elevated blood glucose in diabetes)
- Ketones in urine (using protein for energy; inadequate caloric intake)
- Low serum albumin (inadequate protein in diet)
- High or low serum protein (high in dehydration; low in liver disease)
- Elevated cholesterol levels in blood (related to ingestion of too many fats)
- Decreased urine creatinine (reduced body muscle mass, breaking down body protein for energy)

Subjective Data. If nutritional needs have not been met satisfactorily, the patient would report some of the following:

- *Anorexia* (loss of appetite)
- Consumption of three or more alcoholic drinks each day
- Excessive fatigue
- Jitteriness; feeling weak and shaky
- Trouble thinking clearly
- Headaches
- Nausea/vomiting
- Eating sporadically, few regularly planned meals each week
- Eating one or two food types predominantly to the exclusion of foods from other major food groups
- Practicing crash diets; lose-weight-quick diets; abuse of diet pills

- Use of megadoses of vitamins/minerals over several months or longer
- Problems with digestion, "stomach problems"
- Lives and eats alone
- Difficulty chewing and/or swallowing
- Loss of taste and smell
- Feelings of depression much of time
- Pain or tenderness in ankles and calf muscles when walking

Nursing Diagnoses Associated with Unmet Nutritional Needs

Listed below are some general nursing diagnoses associated with excessive or inadequate nutrition.* Following the general diagnoses are some specific ones:

Activity intolerance
Potential obesity
Obesity
Nutritional deficit
Alteration in bowel elimination patterns: constipation or diarrhea
Self-feeding deficit
Body-image disturbance
Self-esteem disturbance
Examples of specific nursing diagnoses:
    Decreased self-esteem related to 35-lb weight gain
    Calorie and protein deficit
    Diarrhea related to initiation of tube feedings (enteral nutrition)
    Obesity related to consumption of food during times of stress

Nursing Interventions to Facilitate Satisfaction of Nutritional Needs

Initial assessment of the patient following admission to any nursing care facility, hospital, or clinic will provide baseline data for evaluating the patient's current and future nutritional status. Inadequate or excessive nutrient intake can be identified by combining the patient's nutritional information with objective observations during the first few days in the facility. Measurements and laboratory data contribute additional data on the body's nutritional status. Any factors associated with unmet nutritional needs identified on admission should serve as a stimulus for a nutritional care plan to prevent problems and improve the patient's nutrition. Patients are placed on daily assessment of intake and output (I & O), daily weights, vital signs, and urine acetone (ketones). A referral to the dietitian is often appropriate as soon as possible. Patients at risk include those grossly (20 percent) overweight or underweight, individuals unable to consume food for several days (if adequately nourished initially), or less if initially poorly nourished. Risk of inadequate nutrition is high in patients with abnormal losses of body fluids and solids, inadequate intake, digestion, or absorption, and increased metabolic rate.

Interventions to Maintain Adequate Nutrition

Therapeutic Diets.   Different types of foods and fluids may be ordered by the physician to improve the pa-

tient's medical condition, to provide adequate nutrition during recovery from treatment, to reduce the risk of potential nutritional problems, or to treat obvious nutri-

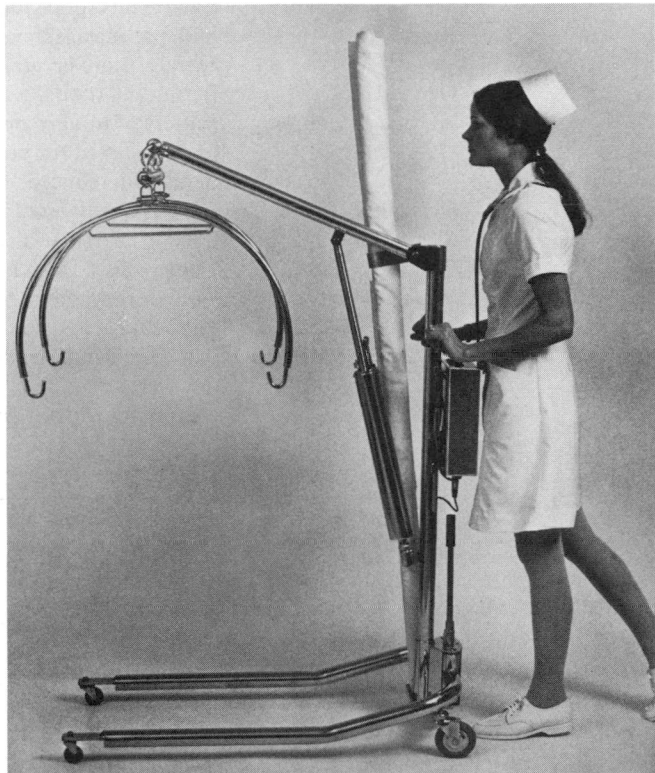

Figure 22–5.   Daily weights for a patient unable to get out of bed can be obtained by using a sling scale which lifts the patient off the bed and indicates the patient's weight. (Photo courtesy of Scale-Tronix, White Plains, NY.)

*National Group for Classification of Nursing Diagnosis: List of Nursing Diagnoses accepted at Fourth National Conference, St. Louis, 1982.

Table 22–12. **Common Therapeutic Diets**

DIET	TYPES OF FOOD/FLUIDS
Clear liquid	Consists of fluids that are liquid at body temperature; nutritionally inadequate in calories and nutrients (400–500 kcal in three meals); frozen clear liquids acceptable; often the first meal after surgery; used to treat diarrhea; used for some diagnostic tests; leaves little residue in bowel.
Full liquid	Consists of any foods and drinks that are liquid at room temperature; may provide adequate caloric intake but minimal residue left in bowel, includes cooked cereals, puddings; diet frequently advanced from clear to full liquids for postoperative patients in the transition to solids; leaves little residue in bowel; nutritionally inadequate.
Surgical soft	Easy-to-digest foods, omits rough grains, nuts, spicy or fatty foods, dried fruits, raw vegetables and fruits, relishes, chocolate, rich desserts; adequate nutrients; 2,000–2,500 kcal; used in transition from full liquid to regular diet.
Mechanical soft	Consistency of food altered; ground meats; little or no chewing needed; for patients with difficulty chewing and swallowing.
Fractured jaw or pureed diet	Consistency of food altered; thick-liquid quality; no food chunks present; baby food; for patients unable to chew or open jaws; nutritionally adequate.
Bland diet	Removal of the following known stomach irritants: caffeine drinks, citrus fruits, foods with meat extracts, raw fruits and vegetables, spices, whole-grain foods; used for patients with peptic ulcers and other GI problems.
Low residue	Used to reduce food in gastrointestinal tract before tests or surgery on tract; limits foods producing residue in large bowel; limits milk and milk products, spicy foods, vegetables and fruits; may include refined cereals, white bread, peeled white potatoes, strained fruit juices.
General diet	Permits all foods.
Six small feedings	Variety of foods from any type of diet divided into six fairly equal portions; used for postoperative patients, anorexia, poor appetite, patients with reduced stomach capacity.
Diets altering fiber	Fiber is not digested and forms the fecal material
High fiber	Used in constipation and noninflammatory diseases of the colon; whole grains, fresh fruits, and vegetables.
Low fiber	Used during acute phase of chronic GI diseases or when inflammation of bowel occurs; contains a minimum of fiber.
Residue restricted	Same as fiber-restricted diet without milk, used in acute phase of GI diseases.
Fiber restricted	Used before and after surgery on the large bowel or rectum, in partial obstructive GI problems, and in acute inflammatory problems in the large bowel.

tional problems. (See Table 22–12.) Some diets are designed to make ingestion of food easier for the patient. Others are designed to reduce the activity in the gastrointestinal tract by providing few indigestible or difficult-to-digest foods. Some diets are designed to exceed the patient's nutritional needs so body weight will be gained. Others are designed to be inadequate in calories so the patient will lose weight.

There are three routes to provide nutrition to the patient using therapeutic diets. One way is through the mouth as the patient ingests and swallows the food and fluids. Another way is by placing a feeding tube into the patient's stomach or small intestine. The tube may enter the body through the nose, mouth, or directly through a surgically created opening in the stomach or small bowel. This method of feeding using a tube is called *enteral nutrition*. The third method of providing nutrition to a patient is through the circulatory system. A tube is inserted into the patient's vein, and nutrient-containing fluids are introduced directly into the blood. This method is called *parenteral nutrition*. An IV infusion is a form of parenteral nutrition, usually providing glucose, water, and minerals. Total parenteral nutrition and hyperalimentation are terms used to describe total replacement of fluids and nutrients using the vascular system. These forms of feeding are used for patients with nonfunctioning digestive tracts as a temporary measure during repair and healing of the tract. Enteral nutrition will be discussed in this chapter, but total parenteral nutrition is beyond the scope of this text.

Assisting Patients with Ingestion. Helping patients eat or feeding them can be awkward for both the nurse and the patient. Most adults are not accustomed to feeding another adult. People tend to feed another person the way they feed themselves. Some people eat all of one food first and then move on to another. Other people prefer a bite of each type of food. Some people drink fluids with their meals and others do not. Each individual may have a certain pattern of activity before, during, and after meals which is associated with a sense of well-being. How is the nurse to know which pattern of food ingestion is comfortable for any particular patient? The answer, of course, must come from the patient or from friends or relatives familiar with the patient's eating pattern.

If patients are able, encourage them to direct the nurse's activity during feeding. Have the patient decide which foods to eat, addition of condiments, and timing of fluid intake during the process of eating or being fed. If the patient is completely unable to bring food to the mouth, talk with the patient before beginning to feed about normal pattern of meal consumption. Try to follow the pattern while you feed that patient and document it in the patient's care plan so every individual feeding the patient does not have to collect the same information. If the patient can partially feed self, do all you can to encourage the effort. Self-feeding not only provides some exercise to the patient's joints and muscles but increases the feelings of independence and progress in recovery. Self-feeding may take patients much more time than if the nurse or another assistant fed them, but learning self-care is important for the patient's eventual physical and emotional recovery. If fatigue becomes a factor in reducing a patient's intake, the nurse may encourage the patient to eat more easily manipulated foods and assist with foods requiring use of utensils. The following suggestions may be helpful when preparing to assist patients with ingestion:

1. Elevate the head of the bed to a sitting position or help the patient sit in a chair or wheelchair before beginning to eat. This uses gravity to encourage the movement of food down the esophagus to the stomach and is a more familiar position for the patient. This position also reduces the risk of aspiration. If patients must remain flat, position them on their side to reduce the risk of aspiration and to permit adequate inspection of the food tray.

2. Reduce the energy expenditure of eating for the weakened patient by opening cartons, cutting meats, buttering breads, and assisting with repositioning.

3. If the patient is unable to see the food tray because of visual problems or position restrictions, describe the food on the tray and take the patient's hand and locate the placement of food and utensils on the tray. Ask the patient what type of assistance is needed for eating.

4. Prepare patients for meals ahead of time by repositioning and offering them a chance to brush their teeth and wash their hands or go to the bathroom. By doing this ahead of time, less time is spent with each patient when the meal trays are delivered, making it more likely that hot food will arrive hot and cold food will still be cold for all patients.

5. If some patients will need assistance with eating, deliver the other patients' trays first. Keep the trays of patients needing help in the oven until personnel are available to assist with feeding. If foods have become cold, use the microwave oven, if available, to reheat them. Do not leave the tray in the patient's room to become cold when feeding help is unavailable. It not only may anger the patient but may increase the patient's sense of helplessness, resulting in loss of appetite, especially if foods are fed to the patient at the wrong temperatures. Talk with volunteer services or nursing services within the institution about getting additional personnel at mealtime if many patients require feeding help.

6. For patients with varying degrees of muscle weakness or paralysis of the mouth and facial muscles, keeping food in the mouth, chewing, and swallowing may be difficult. Liquids are the most difficult for these patients to handle. Semisolid foods and fluids frozen into a slushy consistency are easier for these patients to handle (Hargrave, 1979).

7. Feeding patients too rapidly may tire them and reduce their total intake. Ask the patient if the pace of feeding is too fast or too slow and adjust the rate accordingly.

8. Position the patient to allow the nurse to sit while feeding whenever possible. Avoid bending over to prevent back strain. Sitting with the patient also implies an unhurried pace which may encourage the patient to eat more.

9. Provide the patient with assistive devices to facilitate food ingestion. Straws are often much easier to handle for both hot and cold liquids than attempting to use a spoon or to pick up cups and glasses. Talk with occupational or physical therapy about specialized plates,

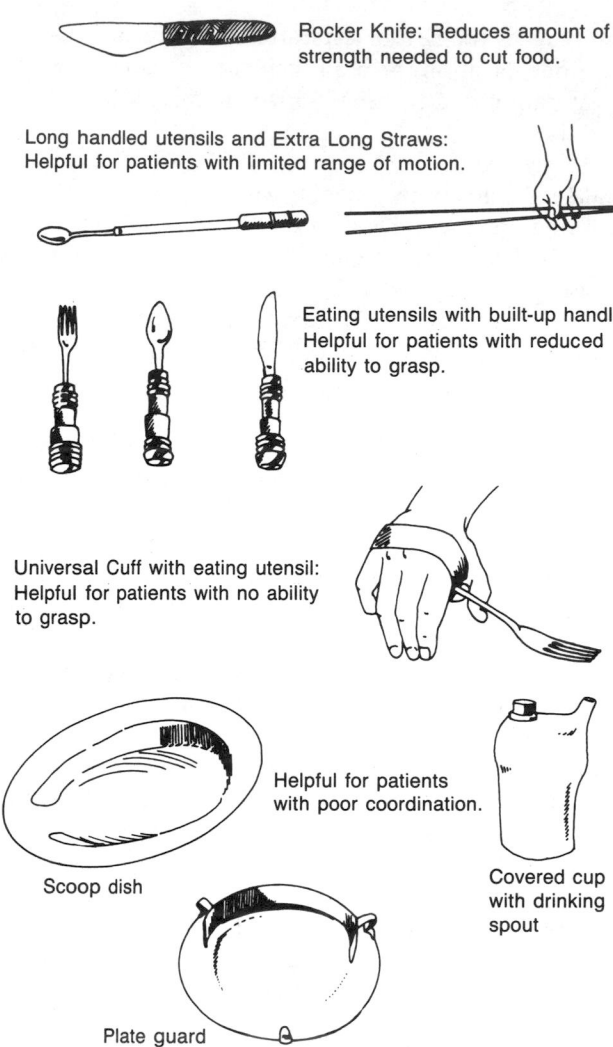

Rocker Knife: Reduces amount of strength needed to cut food.

Long handled utensils and Extra Long Straws: Helpful for patients with limited range of motion.

Eating utensils with built-up handles: Helpful for patients with reduced ability to grasp.

Universal Cuff with eating utensil: Helpful for patients with no ability to grasp.

Helpful for patients with poor coordination.

Scoop dish

Covered cup with drinking spout

Plate guard

Figure 22–6. Assistive eating devices.

cups, and utensils available to assist patients with impaired upper arm mobility to feed themselves. (See Figure 22–6.)

10. Be alert to the risk of choking, vomiting, and aspiration during and after meals. If patients are in locked restraints, the key should be visible in the room so the patient can be quickly unlocked and repositioned to prevent aspiration. Patients with jaws wired shut should have metal clippers visible in the room for the same reason, and every nurse must know which wires to clip to open the jaws should vomiting occur. Patients can be positioned on their side and slightly elevated following meals to reduce the risk of aspiration and vomiting. Limiting activity after meals will also decrease the risk of vomiting, especially in infants.

11. Consider the patient's culture and religious beliefs in regard to food and fluids. Some cultural groups prefer rice as a staple, while others rely more on corn products. When attempting to increase the amount of nutrients a patient ingests, serving favorite, familiar foods may be helpful. Table 22–13 presents some cultural groups and traditional food preferences. The dietitian may be able to provide some of the patient's preferred foods, while family and friends can be encouraged to bring in others.

Increasing a Patient's Food Consumption

There are times when the nutritional goals for patients involve increasing their intake of all nutrients, especially carbohyrdates, protein, and fats, to promote weight gain. Often these patients have reduced appetites, small stomach capacities from long-term reduced intake and feelings of nausea. They may be apathetic about eating. Many people are so accustomed to hearing about the problems of obesity and reduction diets that weight gain does not receive much attention. It is as difficult for patients with inadequate weight to gain as it is for overweight patients to lose. Both patients will have to exert voluntary control over whatever internal stimuli are resulting in undernutrition or overnutrition.

Frequent small meals, high in carbohydrates, are usually tolerated by patients trying to gain weight compared to three large meals. A large plate of food may be so overwhelming to patients with anorexia that they feel defeated before they begin and do not eat anything. Many people feel they should clean their plate and not waste food. By being given small portions more frequently, the individual is more likely to feel capable of eating most of the food on the plate. It is a smaller, more achievable goal, so the patient is more likely to attempt it.

Involving the patient in recording food and calories consumed may also be helpful in increasing the amount of food ingested. If realistic daily intake goals can be set with the patient, that individual may be more internally motivated to eat the food necessary to achieve a certain caloric intake. Setting short- and long-term weight-gain goals with the patient may also motivate increased food consumption.

Keeping the patient adequately warm and moderately active is helpful to facilitate weight gain. A chilled patient is continually using nutrients to produce heat rather than storing them to cause weight gain. A very inactive patient may have a reduced appetite and begin breakdown of body proteins. The goal is to encourage patients to participate in activities without tiring them or jeopardizing a medical condition. Any increase in activity should be discussed with the patient's physician before implementing.

Table 22–13. **Cultural Considerations in Food Preferences***

Black culture	Vegetable foods include greens (mustard and collard), chard, kale, black-eyed peas
	Meat group favors pork; ham, pork, bacon, chitterlings, pig's feet, neck-bones
	Bread group utilizes corn, flour, cornbread, grits, hominy
	Boiling and frying common preparation methods
	Incidence of hypertension and use of high-sodium foods merit assessment
American Indian	Food preferences and rituals involving foods vary among tribes
	Vegetable groups focus on corn, squash, and beans
	Meat traditionally includes wild game and fish
	Bread group utilizes cornmeal
	Abstinence from some foods part of cultural healing
	Low intake of milk and dairy products
Vietnamese	Fish and rice diet mainstays with reduced use of red meat and poultry
	Concept of "hot" and "cold" foods unrelated to temperature; balance between hot and cold in body needed for health; healing involves reestablishing hot/cold balance in body through hot/cold food intake
	Chopsticks used commonly after two years of age
	Diet low in milk; fluids rarely consumed with meals
	Tea and rice wine, and beer common fluids. Seasoning usually high in sodium and merits assessment if patient hypertensive; soy sauce, MSG
Latino culture	Vegetables favor corn and tomatoes; pinto beans used (high in iron)
	Low intake of dairy products
	Corn used in breads, tortillas; rice used commonly
	Low in animal protein
Chinese	View most foods as "hot" or "cold" and idea of balance needed for health and healing
	Milk intake low; tofu and soy milk used
	Variety of foods from food groups used
	Stir frying preferred to raw; preserves vitamins, and nutrients
	Rice, noodles, and steamed buns in bread group; seasonings high in sodium; soy sauce, MSG
Philippine	"Hot" and "cold" food concept; dishes try to combine both for balance
	Rice, fish, and vegetables are staples
	Low milk intake; diets may be low in calcium
	Seasonings high in sodium
	Marinated meats common
Japanese	Consume both raw and cooked vegetables
	Seasonings high in sodium
	Low intake of milk and milk products
	Soybean products common
	Common use of fish
	Tea most common fluid
Jewish	Religious laws affect type of foods consumed and preparation; Kosher food prepared according to Jewish dietary laws (frozen Kosher dinners are available)
	Meats from animals with cloven hooves that chew cuds are the only meats allowed. This includes lamb, beef, venison, and goat; no pork
	Fish with fins and scales permitted (no shellfish, catfish, bullhead or eels)
	Meat and dairy products not permitted at same meal (milk may be consumed before or after the meal following a lapse of three to six hours). Separate utensils required to cook and serve meat and dairy products

*Traditional foods presented in this table should in no way substitute for assessment of an individual's food preferences which may or may not be similar to the foods associated with the individual's culture.

Providing a social atmosphere for meals also increases food ingestion. One study found patients in a nursing home ate more when they were seated in groups of three to five rather than at long tables or large, circular ones (Hargrave, 1979).

Many patients attempting to gain weight will have between-meal snacks ordered for them. Many are high-calorie or high-protein drinks which are to be served cold. Unfortunately, they are often forgotten by nursing personnel and are never delivered to the patient. If these drinks or foods can be left at the patient's bedside in a bucket of ice, they are more likely to be ingested since the patient can sip on them between meals. Between-meal snacks which cannot be left at the patient's bedside for several hours should be scheduled into the nurse's work plan just as any other treatment.

Enteral Nutrition—Tube Feedings

Provision of nutrients through a tube is used for many different types of problems, from the tiny preterm newborn unable to suck and swallow to the elderly adult with a decreased level of consciousness. Tube feedings may also be used to supplement inadequate oral intake. Tube feedings are used when there are obstructions in the esophagus; paralysis, trauma, or inadequate coordination of chewing and swallowing; after radical surgery on the face or neck; or radiation and chemotherapy of the area.

The question whether or not enteral nutriton is an extraordinary means of supporting life during terminal illness is an ethical issue. Since nutrition is such a basic need for survival, withholding foods by not feeding a patient via the enteral route means certain death. The decision to feed or not to feed is often made by the physician, the patient, and the family when a patient is unable to eat normally, and death is a short-term certainty. Nursing is usually not involved in the decision but is responsible for caring for the patient, whether nutrients are to be provided or withheld. The nurse may benefit from talking with the physician, clergy, and other nurses if the decision is in opposition to personal beliefs.

Tube feedings are administered in either a large amount several times each day or as an intermittent or continuous drip The large feedings usually contain up

Table 22–14. **Types of Enteral Feedings**

Bolus Amount	Intermittent Drip	Continuous Drip
250–400 ml/feeding	250–400 ml/feeding	2,000–2,500 ml/day 100–150 ml/hr
Feeding into stomach	Feeding into stomach	Feeding into small bowel or stomach
May be poorly tolerated, causing cramping, nausea, diarrhea, vomiting, aspiration	Generally well tolerated by patients with normal stomach and bowel function or patients not critically ill	Tolerated by critically ill patients or patients with some GI problems
Administered over 5–10 min	Administered over 20–60 min	Administered over 16–24 hr
4–6 feedings/day	4–6 feedings/day	Feedings often continuous
Uses gravity flow	Uses gravity flow	Uses a pump or gravity flow
Tube placement verified before each feeding	Tube placement verified before each feeding	Tube placement verified every 4–8 hr
Feeding given at room temperature (allow to sit out for 1/2 hour before feeding)	Feeding given at room temperature	Ice used to keep feeding cold in reservoir (4–hr portion is maximum to hang each time to reduce risk of bacterial growth)
Patient in Fowler's or sitting position to decrease risk of aspiration	Patient in Fowler's or sitting position	Patient in Fowler's or sitting position or head elevated
Tube flushed with water after feeding	Tube flushed with water after feeding	If feeding interrupted, water given to flush tube

to 400 ml of formula which run into the stomach by gravity over several minutes. Table 22–14 contrasts the feeding methods. Most tube-feeding preparations contain 1 cal in each milliliter of solution. Some formulas provide 2 cal per milliliter for weight-gain goals. Some formulas are designed to be absorbed almost totally, leaving little residue for the large bowel. This results in less frequent stools, perhaps once every five days. A total of 2,000 to 2,500 ml is usually given each day for patients who are unable to take food and fluids by mouth. Some formulas contain mixtures of carbohydrates, fats, proteins, water, vitamins, and minerals to replace normal food intake. This type of formula is used on patients with normally functioning gastrointestinal tracts. Another type of formula provides nutrients in a more elemental form such as amino acids, glucose, and triglycerides which are forms of nutrients after partial breakdown. This formula is used for patients with poorly

functioning gastrointestinal systems and is more expensive for the patient, costing up to $25 per day. Formulas are available for patients with kidney or liver disease to reduce the work load of these organs. Lactose-free formulas are also available.

In adults, the feeding tube is put down the esophagus to the stomach or small intestine through the nose and left in place as long as tube feedings are required. (See Figure 22–7.) Correct placement of the tube is checked before each administration of feeding by attaching a syringe to the feeding tube and aspirating stomach contents. Placement can also be checked by pushing a few cubic centimeters of air from a syringe through the tube and listening for the bubbling sound over the stomach. Nursing Skills 22–1 and 22–2 present insertion of a nasogastric tube and the activities involved in administering a tube feeding. The first few days a tube feeding is given, the formula is usually di-

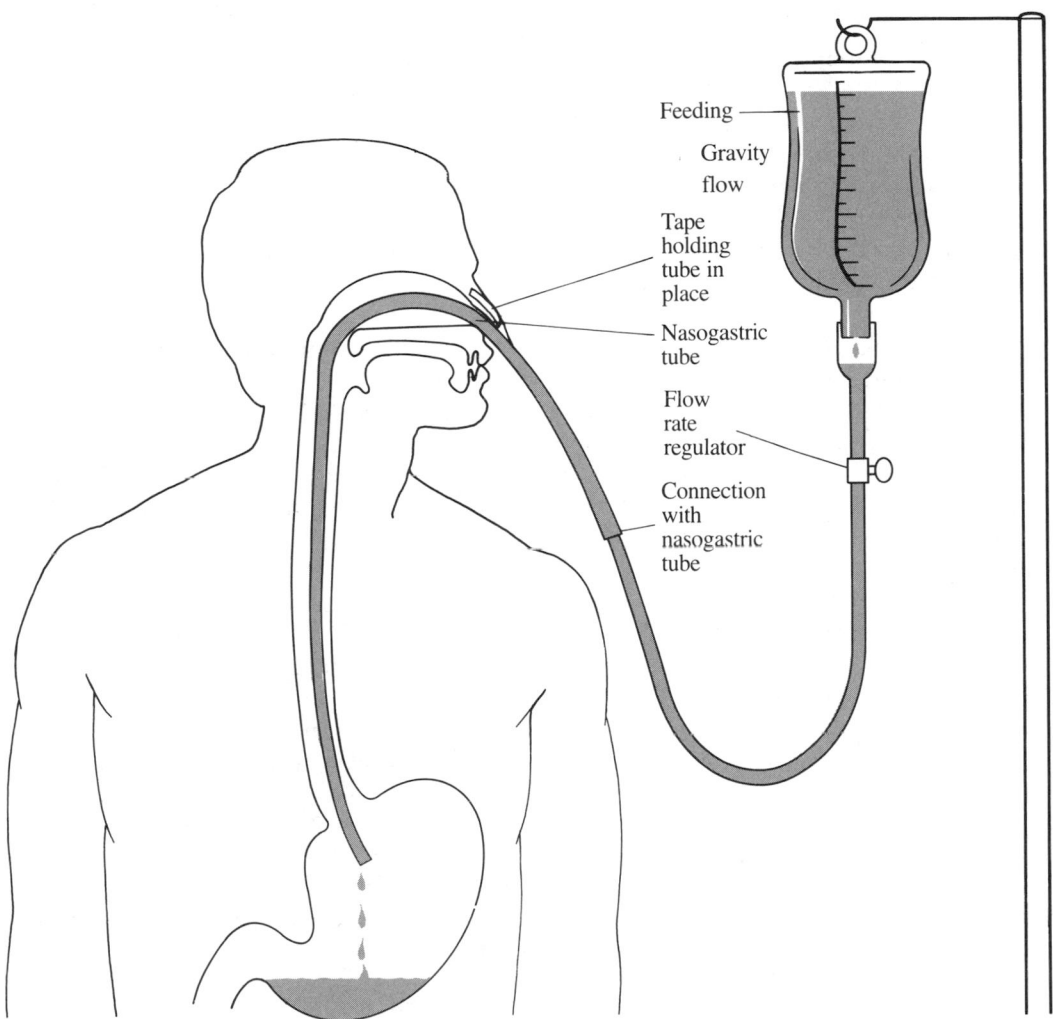

Figure 22–7.   Tube feeding with gravity flow of feeding into the stomach. Clamp on tube regulates flow of feeding into the stomach, and tape on tube secured to patient's nose maintains correct tube placement.

Nursing Skill 22–1   Inserting and Removing Nasogastric Tubes

Preparation

1. Determine need. The patient's physician will order both the insertion and removal of a nasogastric tube. The nasogastric tube is inserted to feed individuals who are unable to swallow. The tube is also used to remove air and secretions from the stomach, to remove ingested medication overdoses or poisons, to empty the stomach before surgery on the digestive tract.
2. Equipment. Nasogastric tube, portable gastric suction machine (intermittent) or wall suction, tape, tissues, stethoscope, glass of water with a straw (if patient able to swallow), water-soluble lubricant, basin, large syringe.
3. Wash hands.
4. Explain procedure to patient.
5. Provide privacy as needed.

Procedure	Explanation
1. Position the patient in high Fowler's position or sitting in a chair.	1. Uses gravity to move the tube down esophagus into stomach.
2. Occlude each side of the nose separately and assess air flow.	2. An obstructed air passage may block movement of the tube.
3. Measure distance from patient's nose to ear and down to tip of xiphoid process. Mark on tube with tape or note distance from markers printed on NG tube.	3. Distance needed to go through nose, down the esophagus to stomach.
4. Lubricate the tube with water-soluble lubricant and insert into nares directing it back toward ear and down.	4. Reduces friction in nose and throat to decrease discomfort and tissue damage.
5. Advance tube until visible in back of patient's throat. Have patient tip head down toward chest and swallow water. Advance tube each time patient swallows. Advance to marker.	5. Avoids curling of tube in mouth. Reduces risk of entering lungs. Lubricates tube, decreasing friction, and occludes trachea; peristalsis in esophagus aids movement of tube to stomach.
6. Use a large syringe to aspirate some stomach contents or inject 5 to 10 cc of air into tube while listening for bubbling over stomach.	6. Assures correct tube placement in stomach and not in respiratory tract.
7. Tape tube to nose; wrap additional tape around tube further down and pin tape to patient's gown in proper position for tube drainage. (Check package label.)	7. Prevents tube from being displaced; if tube is pulled, the tension will pull on patient's gown rather than nose; tube position facilitates drainage.
8. Attach to suction machine or to feeding or cap end of tube.	8. Refers to reason for tube placement; prevents stomach contents from draining on patient and bedding.
9. Reposition patient for comfort.	9. Pain avoidance need.
10. Remove any unneeded equipment from the room.	10. Improves room appearance and provides space for other activities.
11. Document tube insertion (or removal) in care plan and patient's chart.	11. Legal responsibility; communication among health team members.

The tube is removed by disconnecting suction and all tape, having the patient swallow some water to lubricate the tube, and gently pulling the tube out after completion of swallowing.

Nursing Skill 22–2 Giving a Tube Feeding

Preparation

1. Determine need. The physician will order the rate and type of feeding (either continuous drip by IV infusion pump or intermittent drip or bolus dose by gravity flow). In a bolus dose, the amount to be given will be specified.
2. Equipment. Stethoscope, large syringe, feeding bag, IV pole (or infusion pump in continuous drip), glass of water.
3. Wash hands.
4. Explain procedure to patient.
5. Provide privacy as needed.

Procedure	Explanation
1. Position the patient in Fowler's or sitting position.	1. Gravity assists feeding into stomach.
2. Check placement of tube by aspirating gastric contents and reinserting aspirate or by inserting 5 to 10 cc of air into tube and listening for bubbling over stomach.	2. Assures feeding will enter stomach and not respiratory system; repeated removal of gastric contents may lead to electrolyte disturbances; if more than 150 ml left in stomach, hold feeding, and notify physician.
3. Bolus feeding placed in feeding bag and attached to NG tube; given slowly by gravity flow; feeding warmed to room temperature. Intermittent drip is regulated at flow clamp to administer feeding over 10 to 20 minutes or longer. Continuous drip is set by adjusting flow rate to administer 24 hour intake continuously. For example: 24h total = 2000 ml feeding (ordered by physician) $$\frac{2000\ ml}{24h} = 83.3\ ml/hr \text{ or } \frac{83.3\ ml/hr}{60\ min} = 1.4\ ml/min$$	3. Decreases ''cramping'' feeling in stomach.
4. Give several ounces of water through the tube following the feeding for bolus or intermittent drip.	4. Clears tube, preventing obstruction and bacterial growth.
5. Clamp tube. Remove feeding bag and rinse out for next use.	5. Prevents backflow of feeding.
6. Leave patient elevated for $^1/_2$–1 hr following feeding; then reposition for comfort.	6. Uses gravity to keep feeding in stomach, reducing risk of emesis and aspiration.
7. Document feeding and amount and type of gastric aspirate present before feeding.	7. Legal responsibility; communication among health team members.

luted to half or one-third strength and given slowly to allow the gastrointestinal tract time to adjust to the feeding. It is advanced to full strength and more rapid administration over several days' time if no problems with abdominal distention, cramps, or diarrhea develop. Administering the feeding by continuous drip, rather than by bolus doses of several hundred milliliters at one time, usually decreases the incidence of complications. When the feeding is given in a bolus dose, the amount of feeding left in the stomach (*gastric aspirate*) may be measured as an indicator of gastrointestinal function. If a large part of the original feeding still remains in the stomach (150 ml or more) when the next feeding is due, it is an indication that the food is not moving through the tract as it should. If the nurse administers the next feeding in its entire dose, on top of the feeding still remaining in the stomach, the capacity of the stomach may be exceeded. This leads to nausea, vomiting, and possible aspiration. When a large portion of the last feeding remains in the stomach, hold the next feeding and notify the physician. Half the usual feeding amount may be ordered, or a more dilute feeding may be ordered, or one or more feedings may be withheld to allow time for the stomach to empty. Patients receiving tube feedings are assessed daily for intake and output (I & O), weight, vital signs, and urine glucose and ketones (acetone).

The necessity of receiving nutrients through a tube will affect the patient's self-esteem. It may create anxiety and a sense of lost body control. The individual is deprived of the sense of taste and smell, and time is no longer broken up by three meals each day. The patient may feel dependent on the machine regulating the continuous flow of liquid into the stomach. The patient who is unable to eat and drink normally is also experiencing a form of sensory deprivation since a considerable amount of daily activity and stimulation (both physical and social) centers around meals. Offering patients on tube feedings a chance to brush their teeth and rinse their mouth out may increase the patients' comfort. Some patients are allowed to suck hard candy or to chew favorite foods and spit them out. Support, reassurance, education, and other comfort measures are important to the patient and the family adjusting to this altered method of nutritional intake.

Nasogastric Suction

Nasogastric suction is the process of applying continuous or intermittent suction to the contents of a pa-

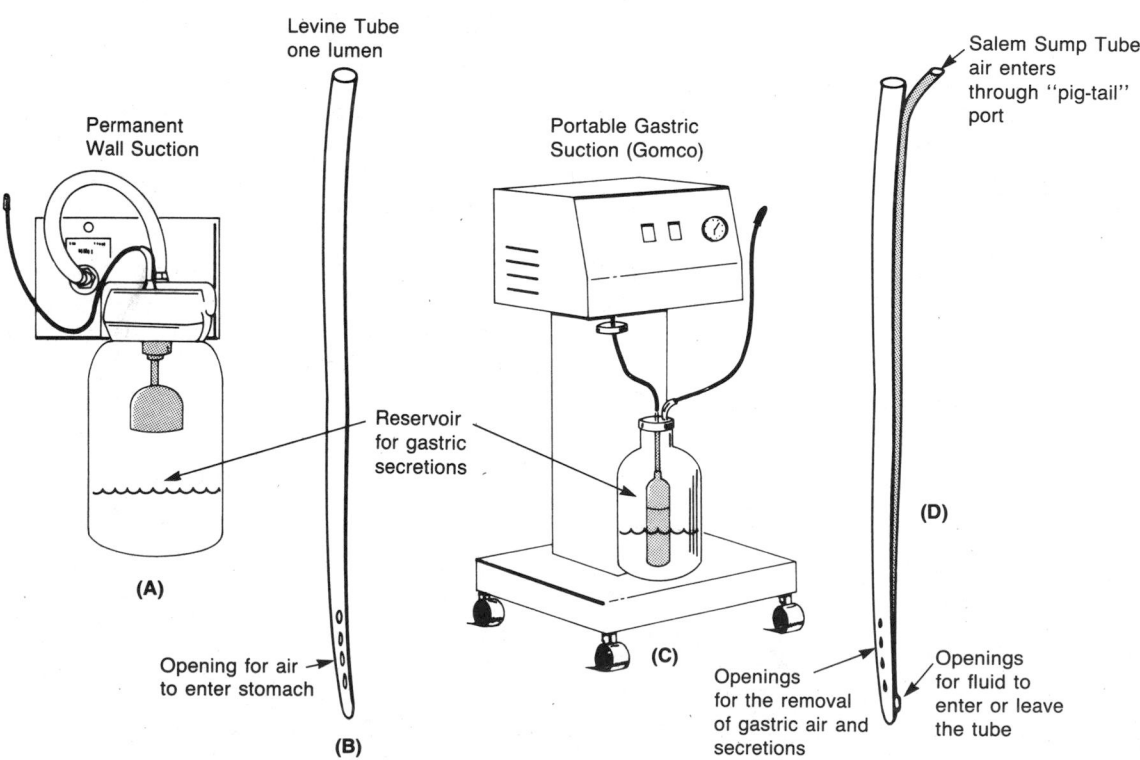

Figure 22-8. Nasogastric tubes. The Levin tube (**B**) has one lumen, while the Salem sump tube (**D**) has a double lumen allowing air to be drawn into the stomach as gastric suction draws air and secretions out through the larger section of the tube. Both tubes can be used with either portable (**C**) or permanent (**A**) suction equipment.

tient's stomach through a tube entering the nose and ending in the stomach. An electrical pump provides suction to one end of the tube. The purpose of the tube and suction is to draw out the air and secretions in the stomach to prevent abdominal distention. Lack of peristalsis in the bowel is usually the reason the suction is needed. The patient is NPO, and the fluid being drawn out of the stomach is usually measured and replaced, volume for volume, with IV fluid.

Two types of tubes are commonly used for gastric suction, one being a Levin tube and the other a Salem sump tube. The first type has one lumen and the Salem tube has two lumens. Both drain air and fluid out of the stomach. The Levin tube exits from the patient's nose and should be positioned downward toward the patient's chest to facilitate drainage. The Salem tube should be draped in a U-shaped curve and pointing up. This prevents gravity from draining stomach secretions out the pigtail port which is designed to allow air to en-ter the stomach and prevent excess suction from damaging the lining of the stomach. (See Figure 22–8.)

If the suction is not draining fluid from the stomach, the tube may have slipped up too far to reach the secretions, or the tube may be obstructed, or the drainage may be too thick to move through the tube. Check the placement of the tube first. If the tube is in place, try irrigating the tube with 10 ml of normal saline for the Levin tube or 10 cc or air through the pigtail port of the Salem sump tube. If the air does not clear the Salem tube, try 10 ml of normal saline. Also check to make sure the suction machine is plugged in and turned on. Repositioning the patient may also improve the drainage of fluid if the tube was lying against the wall of the stomach. In some institutions, a physician's order may be needed to irrigate the tube with normal saline, so check with the nurse in charge before irrigating a blocked tube.

Nursing Care Plan for a Patient with Unmet Nutritional Needs

Assessment

Data: Mr. Hays is an 89-year-old, white male who has been living with his 83-year-old wife in a senior citizen's high-rise apartment in a small town. He is a retired farmer, having sold his farm five years ago. He was admitted to the hospital with mild congestive heart failure and edema in the lower extremities. He was started on digoxin (LANOXIN) for his heart. His height is 5'10", and weight on admission was 120 lb. After several days on LANOXIN, his weight was 110 lb, and much of the edema in his legs was gone. His teeth are badly decayed, and he has never had dentures. His wife is a very thin woman who is reported by relatives to be increasingly confused about people and events. Mr. Hays says his wife fixes mostly potatoes, no meat, and few vegetables. She forgets to cook or serves things undercooked or overcooked and dry. The family reports that their father has lost a lot of weight over the last few months and that, "Mom just cannot seem to prepare meals anymore." The couple refuses to consider moving in with any of the relatives, and they have an adequate financial income. The children all live an hour's drive or more from their parents. Mr. Hays appears pale and very thin. His triceps skinfold on the back of the upper arm is 0.3 inches. He reports having little energy for any activities other than reading. He was surprised to learn how little he weighed after the edema disappeared. Mr. Hays is alert and oriented but is weak and slightly unsteady on his feet. He is to be discharged from the hospital in two days.

Nursing Diagnoses. Nutritional deficit related to inadequate meals available in home setting.

Planning

Goals of Care. Patient's weight to be 112 lb at the end of two weeks.

Planned Actions

1. Contact public health nurse in community about patient's discharge and diagnosis of nutritional deficit.
2. Contact hospital dietitian to plan needed caloric and nutrient intake for weight gain, based on patient's total energy expenditure.

3. Schedule family conference with wife, family, patient, and dietitian about the need for the nutrients in the diet and how inadequate protein intake may be related to Mr. Hays's weakness, edema, heart problems, and muscle wasting. Discuss alternatives for providing the couple with several nutritious meals each day. Discuss long- and short-term weight-gain goals with Mr. Hays and the family. Plan for weekly assessment and support from the visiting community nurse.

4. Assist Mr. Hays with meals in the hospital as needed; discuss a mechanical soft diet with the patient and implement if acceptable.

5. High-protein strawberry milk shake at bedside on ice between meals; alternate with vanilla-flavored shakes.

6. Discuss the possibility of a dental consultation with the patient and the physician.

7. Encourage Mr. Hays to eat with his wife in the patients' dining room.

8. Record intake and output daily.

9. Weigh every morning before breakfast.

10. Assist Mr. Hays to keep track of the food he eats each day and to total the caloric intake; explain his daily caloric goal based on the dietitian's assessment of his total energy utilization and amount of additional calories needed for gaining weight.

Evaluation:

Goal partially met. Visiting nurse reported that patient had gained 1½ lb in eight days following hospital discharge. Patient was using the "Meals-on-Wheels Program," and the family was doing the grocery shopping for high-calorie and high-protein foods that required little or no preparation.

Reassessment. The patient is still experiencing a nutritional deficit. The goal of gaining 1 lb each week may be more realistic for this patient. The visiting nurse will continue to assess the patient's diet and progress in gaining weight during the next month.

Summary

Nutrition is essential to survival. Adequate nutrition is required for new cell growth, maintenance of existing cells, and disposal and replacement of old or damaged cells. Nutrition provides the raw materials for cellular metabolism. Adequate nutrition puts the body in energy balance by providing approximately the same number of kcalories coming in as are being utilized. The kcalories in an adequate diet are divided among the four food groups of milk, meat, fruits and vegetables, and grain products. These four food groups provide the body with nutrients necessary for cellular functioning. These include protein, carbohydrates, fats, vitamins (especially A, C, and B complex), minerals, (especially calcium and iron), and water.

The process of ingestion brings food from the environment into the stomach. Digestion breaks the food down into a fluid consistency called chyme. The complex structures of some nutrients are reduced to simpler structure through the action of peristalsis, enzyme action, and HCl acid. Absorption involves the movement of nutrients from the digestive tract into the blood for delivery to the body cells.

Both internal and external stimuli affect the amount and type of food ingested. The feeding center of the brain initiating and terminating eating behavior is incompletely understood. Learning, environmental temperature, activity level, blood glucose level, amount of food in the stomach, and food availability all affect ingestion. Various factors affect the individual's nutritional needs. Things that increase cellular metabolism, such as fever, periods of growth or stress, also increase the nutritional needs if energy balance is to be maintained. Situations that decrease cellular metabolism, such as reduced activity or severe hypothermia, also decrease nutritional needs. When nutritional needs are unmet, the individual's ability to meet other needs is compromised.

Data related to unmet nutritional needs are diverse,

from retarded body growth to problems with vision. Depending on the nutrients lacking in the diet, various signs and symptoms will appear. PCM (protein-calorie malnutrition) is the world's leading nutritional problem. Other problems relate specifically to digestion, absorption, or metabolism of nutrients. Most nursing problems related to nutrition focus on ingestion of appropri-

ate amounts of nutrients. Enteral nutrition is one way of providing nutrients when a patient is unable to chew and swallow, but when the GI tract is still functioning. Nasogastric suction may be needed to remove air and fluids from the stomach when peristalsis is absent or greatly reduced or when movement of fluids through the tract might cause problems.

Terms for Review

absorption	chyme	ingestion	metabolism	peptic ulcers
anorexia	digestion	ketones	minerals	peristalsis
anorexia nervosa	dumping syndrome	kwashiorkor	nasogastric suction	protein
calorie	emesis	lactose intolerance	nutrient	regional enteritis
carbohydrates	enteral nutrition	lipids	obesity	vitamins
celiac disease	glycogen	marasmus	parenteral nutrition	

Self-Assessment

The following questions help you to do a nutritional self-assessment. Many students find that the stress and time commitments involved in returning to school affect the amount and types of foods they eat. Weight gain over the course of nursing education is common. If you are inappropriately nourished, your ability to learn, work, and play will be compromised.

Comparison of Real Weight with Ideal Weight

Compare your height and body build type to the "ideal weight" suggestions in Table 22-11. Are you more than 10 percent above or below the average weight? More than 20 percent above or below?

Use a table of caloric equivalents to estimate your total calorie intake for three days, and divide this by three to get an average daily calorie intake. Compare this to your total calorie utilization. Is your intake and output fairly balanced? Are you running an excess caloric intake? Are your calories inadequate for your energy expenditures?

If your body weight is not within the "ideal" weight for your height, a "yes" answer to any of the following questions may indicate possible problems with your eating habits.

1. Is your weight above or below the suggested range for your height and body build?
2. Do you frequently have large weight losses or gains?
3. Do you weigh yourself less than several times each month?
4. Do you usually allow yourself as many sweets as you want?
5. Do you eat moderate to large amounts of fats such as butter, oils, and fried foods?
6. Is your alcohol consumption more than one or two drinks each day?
7. Do you use get-thin-quick diets that use only one type of food or starvation?
8. Do you eat foods such as candy, potato chips, cookies, and soft drinks for quick energy, instead of meals, while you study?
9. Do you usually eat quickly, taking less than 20 minutes at the table?
10. Do you eat while you study or do other activities?
11. Do you take more than one portion of foods at a meal?
12. Do you usually skip one or more meals each day rather than eat three times a day?
13. Do you eat when you are bored, angry, or depressed?
14. Do you keep foods in the house for others that you know you should not eat?
15. Do you eat foods off the plates of others when clearing off the table?
16. Do you snack after dinner?

Learning Activities

1. Talk with dietetic services within a hospital or nursing care facility about the type of services they offer patients. Find out how a staff nurse can request the services of a dietitian.

   Discuss the roles of the student nurse, the dietitian and the public health nurse when a patient at risk for unmet nutritional needs is being discharged from the hospital.

2. Practice eating food from a tray when your vision is impaired by a blindfold. Try feeding another student in the laboratory when the other student is unable to move either arm. Have another student feed you.

   How did you feel?

   Could you enjoy the food?

   Which foods were easiest to handle?

   Try eating in various positions in bed.

3. Go to the hospital or school cafeteria and observe the types of food available.

   What types of foods are selected most often?

   Do most people select a well-balanced diet?

4. Maintain a seven-day diary of all the foods and beverages you consume each day.

   Is your kcaloric intake fairly consistent each day?

   Do you eat a wide variety of foods from each of the four food groups each day?

Review Questions

1. Which of the following nutrients is the body's preferred energy source?
   a. Protein
   b. Fats
   c. Minerals
   d. Vitamins
   e. Carbohydrates

2. Where in the gastrointestinal tract are the majority of nutrients absorbed?
   a. Mouth
   b. Stomach
   c. Small bowel
   d. Large bowel

3. A patient with a stroke affecting the muscles of the mouth and face will probably have the least difficulty ingesting which of the following foods?
   a. A glass of water
   b. A popsicle
   c. A slice of roast beef
   d. Chicken bouillon soup

4. Which of the following patients is most at risk for unmet nutritional needs?
   a. A 5'-tall woman weighing 98 lb admitted for knee surgery.
   b. A 5'8''-tall man weighing 130 lb who has been NPO for three days with continuous IVs during testing and is scheduled for back surgery in the morning
   c. An older adult who refuses to eat any fresh fruit because of denture problems
   d. A 5'3''-tall woman with a small body frame who weighs 150 lb and is attempting to lose weight by consuming approximately 1,100 kcal per day.

5. Which of the following patient data do *not* indicate possible nutritional problems?
   a. Weight loss of 20 percent in three months
   b. Absence of bowel sounds 12 hours after surgery
   c. Anemia
   d. Edema
   e. Triceps skinfold of 20 mm for a woman (4/5 inch)

6. For which of the following reasons might a nasogastric tube be inserted?
   a. To stimulate peristalsis in small bowel
   b. To reduce abdominal distention from flatus (gas) in the lower bowel
   c. To remove fluids in the stomach
   d. To open an obstructed nasal passage

7. Which of the following diets has the best balance of nutrients?
   a. Sausages with fried green peppers and onions, mustard, and a glass of beer
   b. Grilled cheese sandwich, mixed green salad with blue-cheese dressing, and skim milk
   c. Yogurt, and glass of tomato juice
   d. Pancakes with butter and syrup, bacon and glass of milk

Answers

1. e
2. c
3. b
4. b
5. e
6. c
7. b

References and Bibliography

Bayer, L,; Bauers, C.; and Kapp, S.: Psychosocial aspects of nutritional support. *Nurs. Clin. North Am.*, **18**:119–28, 1983.

Bayer, L.; Scholl, D.; and Ford, E.: Tube feeding at home. *Am. J. Nurs.*, **83**:1321–25, 1983.

Beal, V.: *Nutrition in the Life Span.* Wiley, New York, 1980.

Bodinski, L.: *The Nurse's Guide to Diet Therapy.* Wiley, New York, 1982.

Cataldo, B., and Smith, L.: *Tube Feedings: Clinical Application.* Ross Laboratories, Columbus, Ohio, 1981.

Corbin, C.: *Nutrition.* Holt, Rinehart and Winston, New York, 1980.

Crocker, K.; Gerber, F.; and Shearer, J.: Metabolism of carbohydrates, protein and fat. *Nurs. Clin. North Am.*, **1**:3–28, 1983.

Grant, A.: *Nutritional Assessment Guidelines*, 2nd ed. Anne Grant, Box 25057, Northgate Station, Seattle, 1979.

Hargrave, M.: *Nutritional Care of the Physically Disabled.* Sister Kenny Institute, Minneapolis, 1979.

Hunt, S.; Groff, J.; and Holbrook, J.: *Nutrition: Principles and Clinical Practice.* Wiley, New York, 1980.

Keithley, J.: Infection and the malnourished patient. *Heart Lung*, **12**:23, Jan., 1983.

Kloster, P.: Nutrition—nurse—dietician teamwork. *Geriatr. Nurs.* **4:**49, Jan.–Feb., 1983.

Kloster Yen, P.: Diet and digestive problems. *Geriatr. Nurs.* **3:**411, Nov.–Dec., 1982.

Konstontinides, N., and Shronts, E.: Tube feeding: Managing the basics. *Am. J. Nurs.*, **83:**1312–18, 1983.

Lichtenstein, V.: Nutritional management. *Geriatr. Nurs.* **3:**386, Nov.–Dec., 1982.

Mangieri, D.: Looking at the tube . . . and we don't mean T.V. *Nursing 83,* **13:**47, Apr. 1983.

Orgue, M., and Bloch, B.: *Ethnic Nursing Care. A Multicultural Approach.* Mosby, St. Louis, 1983.

Patterson, R., and Andrassy, R.: Needle-catheter jejunostomy. *Am. J. Nurs.*, **83:**1325–26, 1983.

Rambo, B., and Wood, L.: *Nursing Skills for Clinical Practice.* 3rd ed. Saunders, Philadelphia, 1982.

Twin Cities District Dietetic Association: *Manual of Clinical Nutrition.* Minneapolis, 1981.

Vander, A.; Sherman, J.; and Luciano, D.: *Human Physiology—The Mechanisms of Body Function*, 3rd ed. McGraw-Hill, New York, 1980.

Whitney, E., and Hamilton, E.: *Understanding Nutrition*, 2nd ed. West, St. Paul, 1981.

THE NEED FOR FLUID

Objectives

1. Describe the use of water within the body.

2. Identify normal, abnormal, and therapeutic sources of water loss and gain for patients.

3. Describe the route of fluid from the mouth to the cells of the body.

4. Describe several basic mechanisms for regulating body fluid balance.

5. Identify factors that affect fluid needs.

6. Describe patient conditions or problems that may interfere with normal fluid balance.

7. Describe the effect of surgery and trauma on body fluid balance.

8. Describe how unmet fluid needs may affect the satisfaction of other basic needs.

9. Identify data related to normal hydration, overhydration, dehydration.

10. Identify groups of patients at risk for unmet fluid needs.

11. Identify nursing interventions to increase fluid intake; to decrease or limit fluid intake.

12. Identify safety considerations during IV therapy; identify complications of IV therapy.

13. Safely perform the following skills:
    Measurement of I & O
    Setting up an IV
    Discontinuing an IV
    Regulating an IV
    Calculating drip rate of an IV based on physician's order
    Changing IV tubing and solution container

Fluid as a Basic Human Need

Water is the most essential nutrient for survival. A water molecule consists of two molecules of hydrogen and one molecule of oxygen (H_2O). Water is required for formation of all body fluids: blood, cerebrospinal fluid, gastric and other digestive secretions, perspiration, urine, hormones, and enzymes. Fluids differ from water because of varying concentrations of additional substances such as minerals, proteins, hormones, and electrolytes. The major component of all body fluids or liquids ingested is water. Metheny and Snively (1983) state, "Water is required for the countless chemical reactions of the body; no major physiological function can proceed without it." The adult is approximately 60 percent fluid, while the newborn is closer to 80 percent fluid.

Body fluids are divided into two components: *cellular fluids* and *extracellular fluids (ECF)*. The fluids within the cells of the body contain approximately three-fourths of the body's total fluid. The extracellular fluid is composed of the *plasma*, which is the liquid part of the blood, the fluid around all body cells (*interstitial fluid*), and other body secretions such as digestive fluid and the cerebrospinal fluid around the brain and spinal cord. Only about one-eighth of the fluids within the body are in the blood. Each body fluid area has its own concentration of electrolytes and water. *Electrolytes* are minerals or molecules which develop an electrical charge when dissolved in water. Table 23-1 shows the common electrolytes found in each body compartment. The body uses 20 percent of its ATP to maintain the electrolyte and water differences between various parts of the body.

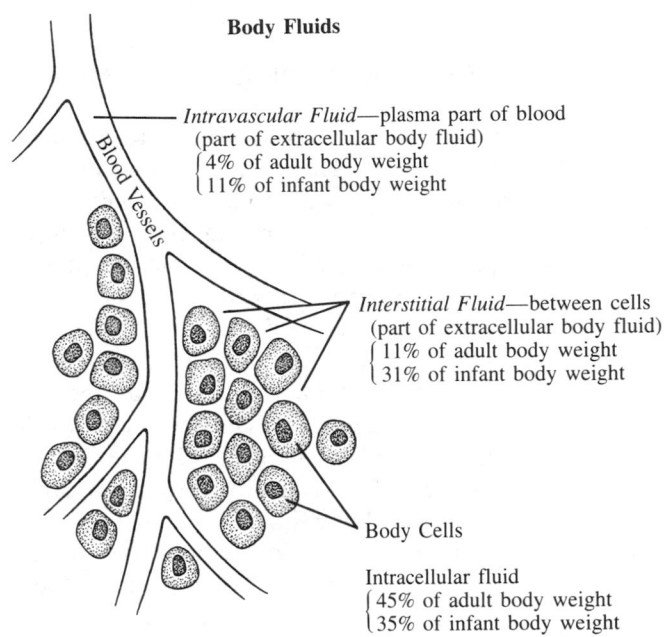

Body Fluids

Intravascular Fluid—plasma part of blood (part of extracellular body fluid)
{ 4% of adult body weight
{ 11% of infant body weight

Interstitial Fluid—between cells (part of extracellular body fluid)
{ 11% of adult body weight
{ 31% of infant body weight

Body Cells

Intracellular fluid
{ 45% of adult body weight
{ 35% of infant body weight

Figure 23-1.   Types of body fluids.

Losses of electrolytes and water will cause problems of varying severity. Loss of 20 percent of the body water is usually fatal (Bodinski, 1982). Loss of 10 percent of total body weight in the form of water is considered severe dehydration (inadequate water in body fluids) which may result in death.

Table 23-1.   **Electrolytes in Body Compartments**

	CATIONS (+ IONS) (CREATE A POSITIVE CHARGE IN WATER)	ANIONS (− IONS) (CREATE A NEGATIVE CHARGE IN WATER)
Plasma (liquid part of blood)	Sodium (Na^+) primary cation	Chloride (Cl^-) primary anion
	Potassium (K^+)	Bicarbonate (HCO_3^-)
	Calcium (Ca^{++})	Sulfate (SO_4^{--})
	Magnesium (Mg^{++})	Phosphate (PO_4^{--})
Interstitial fluid (fluid between cells)	Na^+ (primary cation), K^+, Ca^{++}, Mg^{++}	Cl^- (primary anion), HCO_3^-, SO_4^{--}, PO_4^{--}
Intracellular fluid (fluid within the cells)	K^+ (primary cation), Mg^{++}, Na^+	HPO_4^{----}, SO_4^{--}, HCO_3^-

Normal Means for Meeting Fluid Needs

Water Supply

Water for body fluids normally comes from two sources. One source is in the foods and fluids the individual consumes each day. An average adult fluid intake is approximately 1,300 ml. The water contained in solid foods adds another 1,000 ml of fluid to the body. This fluid is absorbed into the body primarily in the large bowel. The second source of water comes from the chemical reactions occurring within the cells. As the nutrients carbohydrate, protein, and fats are oxidized for use by the cells, carbon dioxide and water are produced as waste products. This adds another 300 ml of water to the body. Total body water intake and production will equal approximately 2,600 ml in the healthy adult under normal circumstances. The fluid lost from the body each day is also approximately 2,600 ml. (See Figure 23-2.) Through urine production, the body excretes an average of 1,500 ml each day. Only 100 to 200 ml are lost each day in the stool. Another 900 ml are excreted through the skin and lungs. This 900 ml is called the *insensible water loss* because the individual is unaware of losing fluid while breathing or through the skin by perspiration, and the nurse cannot measure the loss. The body attempts to maintain the balance between intake and output of fluid. The amount of fluid ingested by the individual is usually very close in amount to the urine output in a 24-hour period. The added fluid from food and cellular metabolism is balanced by the insensible water loss. During hot weather or exercise, more fluid is lost through perspiration, and urine output may be reduced, but fluid ingestion usually increases so water losses equal water gains.

Movement of Water in the Body

Water reaches the cell and enters in several ways. *Osmosis* is the process by which *water* moves from a body compartment with a low concentration of electrolytes, to a body compartment with a higher concentration of electrolytes. Water is able to move freely between the body compartments, but the membranes separating the compartments do not allow free movement of electrolytes. If the blood has more electrolytes than the body cells and interstitial fluid, water moves into the blood to increase volume by the process of osmosis. If the intravascular fluid (blood) has less electrolytes than the interstitial fluid and body cells, water will leave the blood and move into the interstitial area and body cells by os-

blood. *Colloid osmotic pressure* is the force that tends to hold water in the vascular system. It is measured as osmolality of the blood, meaning the concentration of particles in water. High osmolality of the blood occurs when the concentration of particles in blood fluid is elevated, either because of reduced fluid or excessive numbers of particles such as proteins. Particles that cannot move through the walls of the blood vessels because of their large size, such as protein molecules, cause water to move from the cells and interstitial fluid into the blood. Since water follows the movement of proteins and electrolytes because of the higher concentration, mosis. This will decrease the volume of circulating

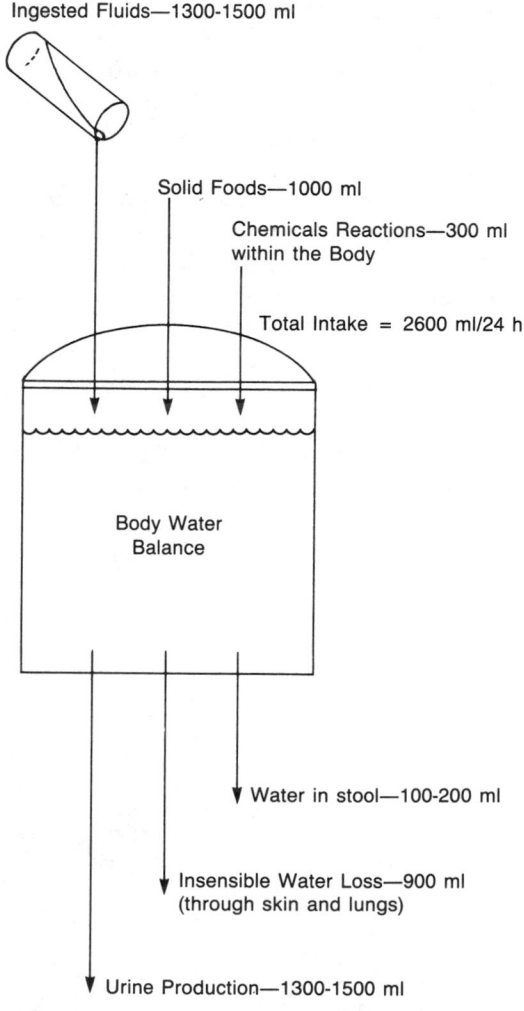

Figure 23-2. Body water balance.

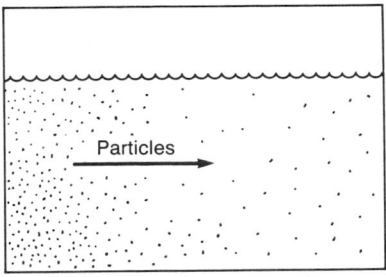

Diffusion—Movement of <u>particles</u> from area of high concentration to area of lower particle concentration

Membrane through which only <u>water</u> may move

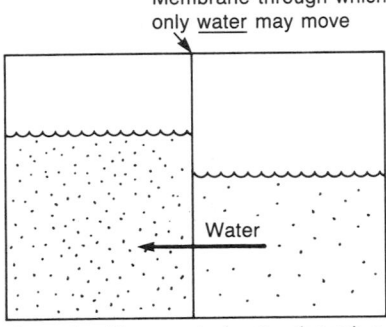

Osmosis—Movement of <u>water</u> through a semi-permeable membrane from area of low particle concentration to an area of higher particle concentration

Figure 23-3.   Diffusion and osmosis. Particles move by diffusion and water moves by osmosis.

water movement is accomplished secondary to movement of electrolytes.

Electrolytes and other particles of nutrients move through the body by *diffusion* and *active transport*. In *diffusion*, the constant random movement of the particles tends to equalize concentrations of the particles in a fluid medium. Figure 23-3 contrasts diffusion and osmosis. The *particles* move from areas of higher concentrations to areas of lower concentrations by diffusion. This is how oxygen and carbon dioxide move in and out of the cells, blood, and lungs. During *active transport*, electrolytes are moved from areas of lower concentrations to areas of higher concentrations, across a body membrane separating the two compartments. This requires energy because it is opposing the process of diffusion. By using active transport, the cells of the body maintain higher internal concentrations of potassium than the interstitial fluid or the blood.

Filtration is a process that moves both water and dissolved molecules from an area of high pressure to an area of low pressure. The pressure differences are created by the pumping action of the heart. The water and molecules tend to be forced out of the blood into the interstitial fluid spaces by this pressure within the vascular system. This pressure is called *hydrostatic pressure*. Hydrostatic pressure is opposed by osmotic pressure, and a balance between the two maintains a normal fluid volume in the vascular and interstitial fluid compartments.

Regulation of Body Fluids

Hormonal Regulation

The kidney is the primary regulator of body fluid. When excess fluid is ingested, the kidney increases excretion of water in the urine, making the urine more dilute. When fluid intake is inadequate, the kidney conserves water by reabsorbing it, making urine more concentrated. The hypothalamus in the brain produces *antidiuretic hormone* (ADH). This hormone is stored in the posterior pituitary and is released into the blood when the concentration of osmotically active particles (particles that will cause water to be drawn to them) in the blood increases. This increase in serum osmolality reflects less water than normal in comparison to the concentration of electrolytes, proteins, and other cells within the blood. It is related to inadequate fluid intake, reduced blood volume, or excessive amounts of electrolytes. ADH stimulates the kidney to conserve water by reabsorbing both sodium and water. *Aldosterone* is a

hormone secreted by the adrenal cortex located above the kidney. Aldosterone causes retention of sodium by the kidney. As sodium is reabsorbed, water is reabsorbed by osmosis. When the osmolality of the blood decreases because there is more fluid within the blood than normal, the release of ADH and aldosterone is inhibited, and the kidney excretes more sodium and water to reestablish the balance between fluids and osmotic particles within the blood. As blood osmolality increases, aldosterone and ADH are released in increasing amounts, and the kidney reabsorbs water.

Thirst

Intake of fluids is controlled by the sensation of thirst. As plasma osmolality increases, the thirst center in the hypothalamus is stimulated, and the individual becomes increasingly thirsty. The individual will drink

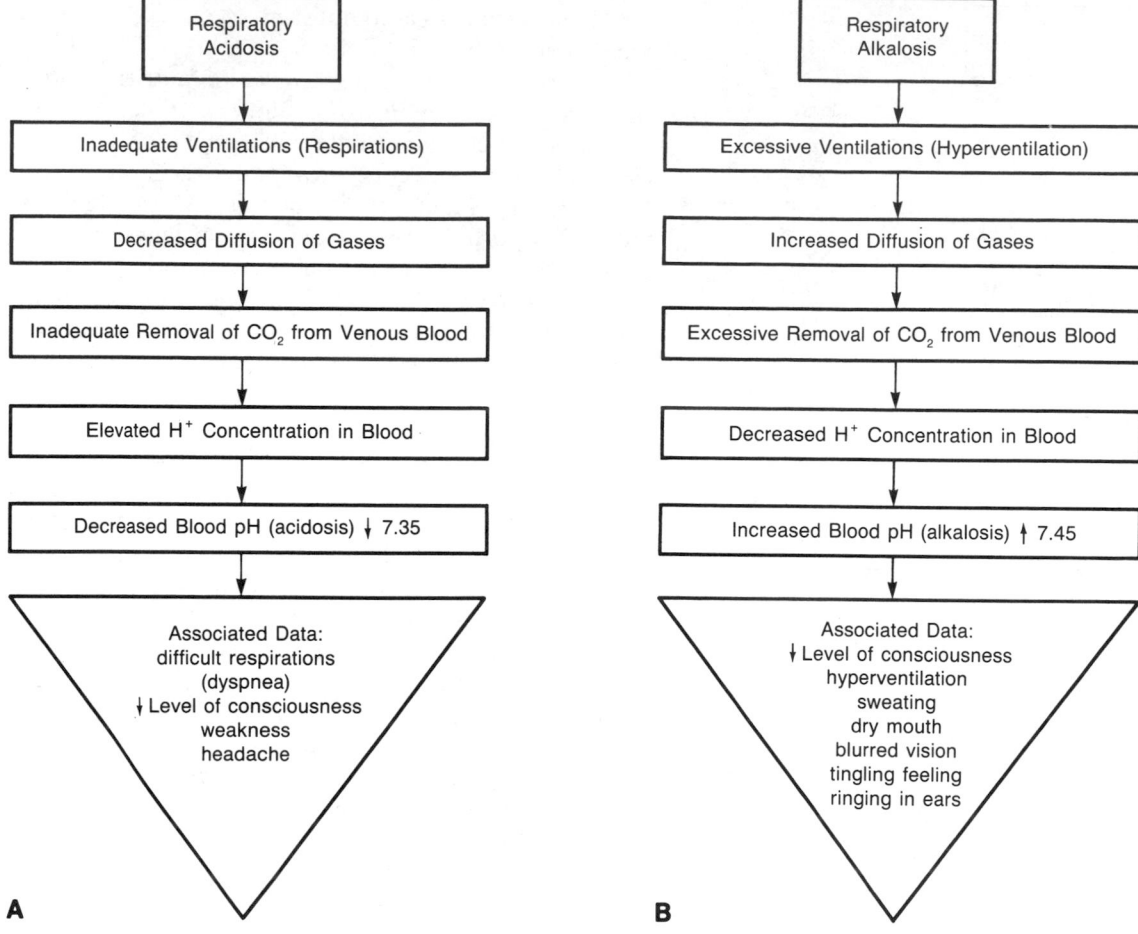

Figure 23–4.   A. Respiratory Acidosis. **B**. Respiratory alkalosis.

Table 23–2. **Regulation of Fluid and Electrolyte Balance**

Lungs	Regulate acid-base balance in extracellular fluid by rate of CO_2 excretion
	Increased CO_2 decreases blood pH and stimulates respirations to blow off more CO_2 to reduce blood acidity
	Low CO_2 levels in the blood depress respirations, causing retention of CO_2 and a decrease in blood pH
	Insensible water loss through respirations
Hypothalamus and pituitary	Antidiuretic hormone (ADH) produced in hypothalamus and stored in pituitary causes the kidney to reabsorb water
	Thirst center in hypothalamus stimulated by increased blood osmolality
Adrenal cortex	Produces and releases aldosterone into the blood to cause the kidney to reabsorb sodium chloride and water and excrete potassium
Parathyroid	Regulates the concentration of calcium in the extracellular fluid
	Without this electrolyte, muscle tetany will result
Skin	Insensible water loss through perspiration
Kidneys	Selectively reabsorb electrolytes and water based on body's needs for fluid and electrolyte balance
	Help to maintain acid-base balance in extracellular fluid through secretion of hydrogen ions with ammonia and other buffers

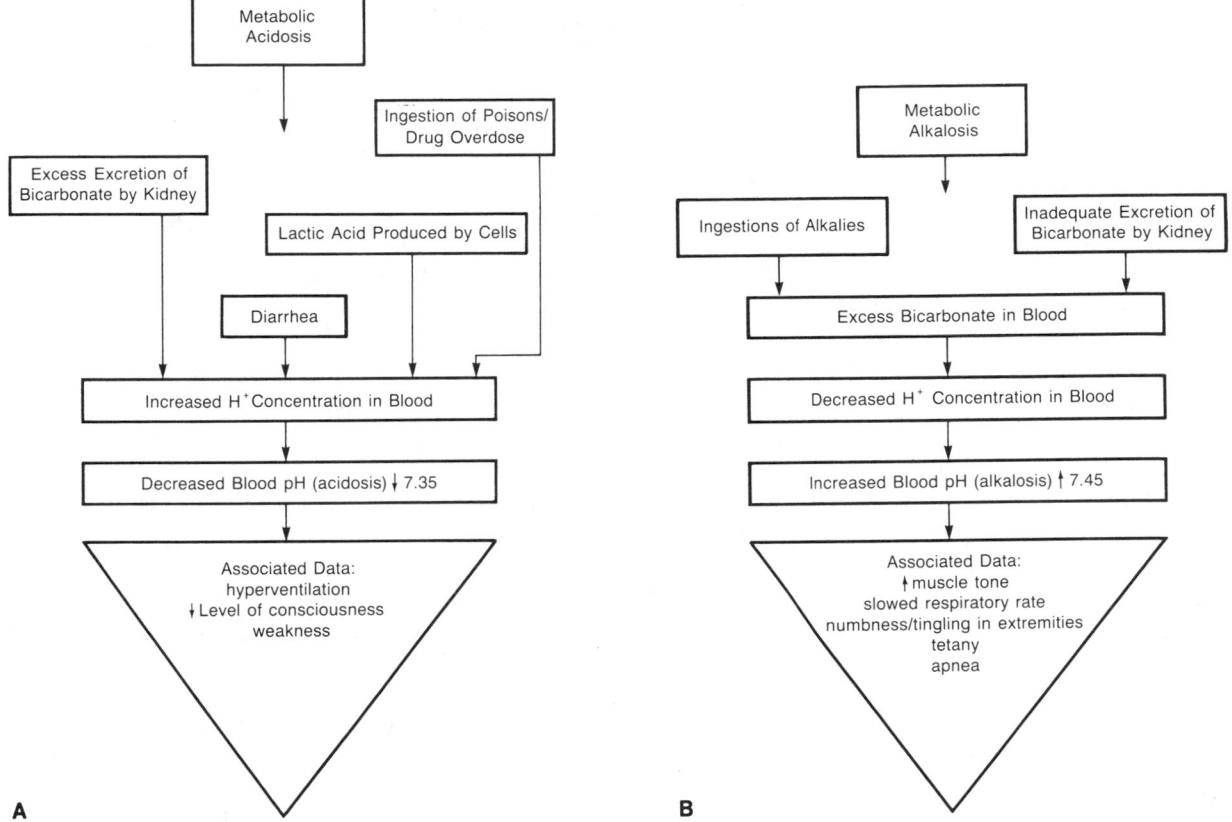

Figure 23-5. **A**. Metabolic acidosis. **B**. Metabolic alkalosis.

enough fluids to reestablish the balance within the blood, but the mechanism monitoring the fluid ingested is not understood at this time. The individual will stop drinking and thirst will be satisfied before the fluid is absorbed from the digestive system to return blood osmolality to normal values. Dryness of the mouth will also cause the sensation of thirst, but this type of thirst can be relieved by rinsing the mouth out with water or sucking on ice, if the blood osmolality is normal. Learning or habits also affect ingestion of fluids in the absence of thirst. Some people associate social events with drinking certain beverages such as coffee, punch, or alcoholic beverages. The body often does not need these extra fluids, and they will be excreted by the healthy kidney through increased urine production.

Acid-Base Balance and Electrolytes

Electrolytes within the body fluids are critically important in regulating the acid-base balance within the blood and other types of fluids. Some electrolytes are capable of combining with hydrogen ions to form a base, thus reducing the acidity created by free hydrogen ions. Electrolytes are also capable of combining with each other to form a salt. Retained CO_2 in the blood results in the formation of carbonic acid. Carbonic acid will result in free hydrogen ions and increased acidity of the blood, resulting in acidosis. The lungs can increase the excretion of CO_2 which will decrease the acidity of the blood. The kidneys can increase or decrease the acidity of the blood by the rate of excretion of bicarbonate ions. If the lungs are unable to remove CO_2 adequately, a respiratory acidosis will develop. (See Figure 23-4.) If the lungs remove too much CO_2, a respiratory alkalosis (carbon dioxide deficit) will occur. If the kidney excretes too much bicarbonate, metabolic acidosis (bicarbonate ion deficit) occurs. (See Figure 23-5.) If the kidney is unable to excrete enough bicarbonate, metabolic alkalosis results (excess bicarbonate ions). The kidneys also remove hydrogen ions from the blood through the production of ammonia (NH_3) which will pick up an additional hydrogen ion (NH_4) and be excreted into the urine. Table 23-2 summarizes primary fluid-regulating systems in the body.

Factors Affecting Fluid Needs

The following factors may increase or decrease an individual's need for water:

1. Age. The younger the individual, the greater proportion of the body weight that is composed of water and the greater the water needs for every pound of body weight. This does not mean that an infant must consume more fluid than an adult to meet fluid needs. It means the infant requires more fluid for each pound of body weight to meet fluid needs compared to an adult. If an adult's fluid needs per pound of body weight were the same as an infant's, the average-size man would have to consume over 10,000 ml or approximately 45 cups of water daily. Adults require 55 ml per kilogram body weight and infants require 150 ml per kilogram.

2. Sex. Men have 17 percent more body fluids compared to women, as young adults. This decreases to only 5 percent more fluid by their senior years.

3. Amount of body fat. Thin people have a greater percentage of their total weight composed of water compared to an overweight individual. Approximately 50 percent of an obese person's weight is fluid compared to 75 percent of a very trim individual's weight.

4. Body temperature. An elevated body temperature increases the need for water. For every degree Fahrenheit rise in body temperature, the individual needs 50 to 75 ml more fluid per day. An individual with a temperature of 103° F needs at least 250 ml of additional fluid to meet fluid needs. If sweating occurs, more fluid will be required to replace the increased loss of water from the body.

5. Increased loss of fluids from body. Abnormal losses of body fluids from draining wounds, hemorrhage, vomiting, diarrhea, gastric suction (removal of stomach secretions through a tube), or hyperventilation will increase the body's daily fluid needs.

6. Increased metabolic states. As the metabolic rate increases, the need for fluids increases. Hyperthyroidism, stress, and fear are examples of conditions that increase fluid needs.

7. Kidney failure. If the body is unable to form urine, fluid will be lost from the body at a greatly reduced rate, resulting in decreased fluid needs.

8. Environmental temperature. As the temperature rises, the body increases heat loss through perspiration. The more a person perspires, the more fluid is needed to balance the increased loss.

9. Physical activity. Body temperature and cellular metabolism are increased by physical activity, especially heavy, sustained exercise. There is an increased fluid loss which must be replaced as perspiration and respirations increase. The increased metabolism in the cells also increases the fluid needs.

Factors that May Interfere with fluid Need Satisfaction

Intake of Fluids

Anything that interferes with an individual's ability to bring fluids to the mouth and swallow will interfere with adequate hydration. When inadequate fluids enter the body, dehydration results. *Dehydration* is a reduction in total body water. It affects the body cells, the blood volume, and the interstitial fluid volume. The following problems affect the individual's ability to ingest fluids and, therefore, are likely to interfere with meeting fluid needs: paralysis of arms or immobility, stroke, injury to the mouth or throat, obstructions of the esophagus from swelling or tumor growth, depressed level of consciousness, restraints, absence of fluids in the immediate environment, some diagnostic tests, surgery.

Transport and Absorption of Fluids

Transport of fluids to the cells will be affected by the hydrostatic pressure and osmotic pressure in the vascular system. Inadequate nutritional intake will result in reduced body proteins and electrolytes within the blood, reducing the osmotic pressure and leading to fluid moving into the interstitial areas causing edema. A weakly pumping heart will decrease hydrostatic pressure and reduce perfusion of the kidney and decrease water excretion through urine. Fluid will also tend to remain in the circulation increasing blood pressure and decreasing fluid movement into the cells of the body. Gastrointestinal problems will reduce the transport of water from the GI tract into the blood. Very rapid peristalsis decreases the absorption time in the large bowel, resulting in excess fluid being lost through the feces as diarrhea. Obstructions or inflammation of the GI tract can result in reduced absorption and failure of fluids to move into the lower bowel for absorption. Nausea and vomiting reduce fluid intake and increase loss of previously ingested fluids and electrolytes.

Regulation of Fluid Balance

Problems with regulation of water balance in the body may leave fluid needs unmet. Problems of regulation may result in excess hydration or dehydration depending on the specific problem. Excess ADH production can result in overhydration with excess fluid in the blood, cells, and interstitial areas. Inadequate ADH production may result in excess water losses as the kidney produces large amounts of dilute urine. The same is true with inadequate or excessive production of aldosterone. Without production of aldosterone, death will occur within several days to weeks from excessive loss of sodium and water (Guyton, 1981). Diabetes insipidus is a disease with inadequate and ineffective ADH production. Tumors of the hypothalamus, pituitary, or adrenal cortex may alter production and release of these hormones. Kidney failure is another problem which can result in excess fluid losses or inadequate excretion of body water by an inability to respond to normal body control mechanisms. Electrolyte imbalances in the blood can result in excess or inadequate excretion of water by the kidneys, leading to dehydration or overhydration.

Increased Loss of Fluids

Any condition of a patient which results in an increased loss of fluid from the body will increase the risk of dehydration and electrolyte imbalances. Draining wounds such as burns, pressure sores, incisional sites, and surgically placed drains, all increase fluid loss from the body. Vomiting, diarrhea, and gastric suction are possible ways of losing fluids from the GI tract before absorption has occurred. Bleeding disorders or actual hemorrhage can cause rapid loss of fluids from the vascular system. Rapid respiration during exercise or resulting from trauma or disease of the medulla will increase water loss through rapid respirations and increased evaporation from the airways. Excessive perspiration from fevers, heavy work, and hot environmental temperatures will increase the loss of body water through the skin.

Therapies Disrupting Fluid Balance

Some medical and nursing treatments may disturb the patient's fluid balance. Excessive fluid gains without comparable fluid loss will result in overhydration. Loss of electrolytes with body fluids and replacement with

Table 23-3. **Potential Routes for Gaining and Losing Body Water**

Water Gains	Water Losses
Drinking fluids	Ventilations
Water in foods	Tears
Tube feedings	Vomiting
IV fluids	Hemorrhage
Cellular metabolism	Diarrhea
Enemas (water absorbed by lower bowel)	Urine
Irrigation of tubes	Perspiration
	Feces
	Wound drainage
	Respiratory secretions
	Gastric suction
	Menstruation
	Lactation (breastfeeding)

water alone will also disturb fluid balance. Tube feedings with inadequate water content can result in dehydration. Intravenous fluid therapy may lead to overhydration if not carefully monitored and ordered based on a patient's current fluid needs. Table 23-3 presents therapeutic and body-regulated ways of gaining and losing fluid.

Surgery

Surgery results in a shifting of body water into the interstitial fluid spaces because of the stress reaction. During the first 48 to 72 postoperative hours, the capillaries become more permeable to large particles in the blood, and proteins leak out into the interstitial fluid. Water then follows by osmosis. This decreases the blood volume, which, in turn, decreases the urine output because of poor perfusion of the kidney. During this period of time, intake exceeds output. As the body recovers from the stress of surgery, the water in the interstitial fluid is reabsorbed as capillary permeability returns to normal and osmotic pressure draws the water back into the vascular system. This increases the circulating blood volume, resulting in increased perfusion of the kidney and decreased blood osmolality. Urine production is increased to reestablish fluid balance. During this period of time, output exceeds intake until total body water content is reestablished. Then fluid intake will again equal fluid output.

Effect of Unmet Fluid Needs on Other Basic Needs

Because of the interrelated nature of human needs, problems meeting one need can affect the satisfaction of some or all other needs to varying degrees. Since the body cannot survive long without water, altered satisfaction of this need can seriously affect all survival needs. There are some positive outcomes of dehydra-

Table 23–4. **Possible Effects of Unmet Fluid Needs on Other Basic Needs**

Oxygen

Electrolyte imbalances will affect the heart and may result in irregular contractions or cardiac arrest

Hypotension may result from dehydration and decreased plasma volume

Hypertension may result from overhydration and electrolyte imbalances

Overhydration may result in pulmonary edema which will interfere with the exchange of gases in the alveoli

Dehydration increases the viscosity of respiratory secretions and decreases the volume of secretions

Severe dehydration may reduce the circulating blood volume to the point that body cells are not being adequately supplied with oxygen

Overhydration may result in cerebral edema and a decreased heart and respiratory rate with an increasing pulse rate because of inadequate central nervous system (CNS) control

Temperature Maintenance

Inadequate fluid intake reduces the body's ability to lose heat through perspiration

Sodium excess from too much water being lost may raise the temperature

Nutritional Needs

Electrolyte imbalances and dehydration may cause nausea and loss of appetite

Dehydration results in a dry mouth and tongue and decreased saliva production which all interfere with chewing and swallowing food

Consumption of high-calorie fluids (beer, pop) may lead to excess weight gains

Elimination Needs

Inadequate fluid intake results in decreased urine production

Inadequate fluid intake leads to constipation

Inadequate fluid intake results in more concentrated urine with a specific gravity above 1.030 and increased risk of urinary infections

Pain Avoidance

Electrolyte imbalances are associated with muscle cramps, bone pain, and headache

Severe dehydration causes reduced level of consciousness which decreases the sensation of pain; dying patients are dehydrated without IV therapy and feel less discomfort because of this reduced level of consciousness (reduced level of alertness and orientation to time, place, and person)

Stimulation Needs

Blurred vision may result from excess water intake

Electrolyte imbalances may result in unusual sensations such as warm skin, increased sensitivity to sound, and numbness

Ringing in the ears is associated with acid-base imbalances

Reduced muscle coordination and reduced level of consciousness are associated with dehydration

Excess water in the body is associated with muscle cramps and twitching, decreased coordination, and seizures as intracranial pressure increases; hemiplegia can also result from water excess and cerebral edema

Safety/Security

Fluid and electrolyte imbalances are associated with an altered level of consciousness, increasing the risk of injury from poor judgment

Inadequate fluid in circulatory system results in feelings of apprehension and confusion

Hypovolemia from inadequate fluid in blood causes dizziness and increased risk of falls when attempting to stand

Love/Belonging Needs

The parental-infant bond may be affected in a negative way when an infant is unable to meet fluid/nutritional needs through sucking and swallowing or has problems with colic, vomiting, or breastfeeding; parents may feel anger, frustration, and guilt when feeding problems persist

Partaking of food/fluids has social, cultural, and religious components which may alienate the individual who is unable to drink or eat certain things because of medical problems

Self-Esteem

Intervention in an individual's normal pattern of food/fluid ingestion because of medical conditions may affect the individual's self-concept in a negative way, making the individual feel different and defective

Loss of control over fluid consumption (as in alcoholism, fluid restrictions) may decrease self-esteem

Self-Actualization

When fluid needs are unmet, the body and mind are not functioning optimally and may prevent an individual from developing potentials

---

tion. As a normal process of dying Zerwekh (1983) states, "After three years as a hospice nurse, I now believe we should not routinely give fluids to all patients." She feels the benefits of rehydrating or maintaining hydration in a dying patient through IV or tube-feeding therapy must outweigh the detrimental effects. Increased respiratory secretions, breathing difficulty and the need for suctioning, increased level of conscious-

ness, and increased perception of discomfort and pain are all possible effects of hydrating the dying patient. She feels that for some patients, dehydration is a natural part of dying and should not be treated because fluid replacement increases patient discomfort and other problems. Table 23–4 presents possible effects of unmet fluid needs on other basic needs.

Assessment of Fluid Need Satisfaction

When assessing a patient's hydration, look for any data that would indicate an excess intake of fluids, an inadequate intake of fluids, an excess loss of fluids, or an inability to lose fluids through normal means. Any of these areas may result in unmet fluid needs through overhydration or underhydration. The following data are related to adequate hydration:

Adequate Hydration

Objective Data. Certain objective observations can identify the patient who has adequate hydration.

Maintenance of body weight over time
Moist mucous membranes
Intact skin with good turgor

When assessing skin turgor, the skin is pinched up between two fingers and released. Skin tissue with adequate water content will quickly return to shape. Dehydrated tissue will remain pinched or wrinkled for a

much longer time. Older people lose skin elasticity as they age, making the assessment for tissue turgor a more reliable test for dehydration on the younger and middle-aged adult.

Normal pulse rate for age
Normal blood pressure for age
Normal temperature
Normal respiratory rate for age
Normal breath sounds
Routine passage of well-formed, soft stools
Urine output of approximately 1,500 ml per day
Fluid intake of approximately 1,500 ml per day
Adequate nutritional intake of foods from all four food groups
Alert and oriented
Urine specific gravity approximately 1.012 to 1.025 (may be as low as 1.003 or as high as 1.030 in health) (Metheny and Snively, 1983)
Normal blood values for hematocrit, serum protein, sodium, BUN, creatinine, osmolality

Subjective Data. Subjective data associated with satisfaction of fluid needs are obtained when the patient reports:

- No difficulty swallowing fluids
- Consuming a variety of fluids, approximately 6 or 7 cups a day (more if active or in warm weather)
- Drinking two alcoholic beverages a day or less as an average consumption
- No unusual sensations or muscle problems

Excessive Hydration

Associated Data. The following observations are indicative of excessive hydration (overhydration or water intoxication):

Weight gain from fluid over the last few days or weeks (gain of 2.2 lb = 1 liter of retained fluid). Weight gains of:
    2–5% = mild overhydration
    5–8% = moderate overhydration
    above 8–10% = severe overhydration
Bounding pulse
Distention of the jugular veins in the neck
Difficulty breathing (dyspnea); shortness of breath (SOB)
Increased respiratory rate
Auscultation of rales in the lungs (pulmonary edema)
Edema in dependent (lowermost) body parts

Edema is an abnormal collection of fluid in the interstitial fluid compartment of the body. *Pitting edema* is evaluated on a four-point scale from +1 to +4. In slight edema of an area, there is a small depression left after pressing a finger firmly into the tissue and removing it. This is caused by forcing fluid out of the interstitial space and into adjacent areas. In severe pitting edema, a deep 1-inch pit is left in the tissue which disappears slowly over several minutes.

Increased blood pressure and pulse
Increased urine output (if kidney function is normal)

Fluid Deficit

Associated Data. The following observations are indicative of fluid deficit (underhydration or dehydration):

Weight loss of fluid over last few days or weeks
  Weight loss of:
    2–5% = mild dehydration
    5–8% = moderate dehydration
    8–10% or greater = severe dehydration
Dry, sticky mucous membranes
Depressed anterior fontanel in infant; newborn
Reduced tearing , salivation
Eyes appear sunken
Longitudinal furrows in tongue
Dry, cracked lips; speech may be difficult with dryness of lips and mouth
Increased pulse and respiratory rate; weak, thready pulse
Lowered blood pressure
Decreased urine output with increased specific gravity (above 1.030)
Output may exceed intake of fluids
Respiratory secretions become thick (viscous) and difficult to remove; reduced in amount
Dry skin with poor skin turgor
Hard, difficult-to-pass stools
Vomiting
Elevated temperature
Slow filling of veins

When the patient's hand is resting on a firm surface, compress the distal end of one of the veins and stroke the vein toward the patient's heart with the other hand. After the vein empties, release the pressure on the vessel and watch how long it takes for the vein to refill with blood. It should refill instantly. Any delay in refilling is another indication of dehydration.

- Agitation or confusion; reduced level of consciousness
- Patient may report dizziness, especially when standing up, anorexia, nausea, and especially thirst

Nursing Diagnoses Associated with Unmet Fluid Needs

Following are some general and specific examples of nursing diagnoses:

Fluid volume, alteration in: Excess or deficit (related to a specific patient condition)
Fluid volume deficit, potential

Self-feeding deficit: unable to manipulate fluid containers to mouth related to severe arthritis (or any other feeding problem)
Potential fluid deficit related to repeated vomiting (or any other abnormal loss of fluid)
Dehydration related to diarrhea

Nursing Interventions to Facilitate Satisfaction of Fluid Needs

Anticipating Problems—Preventive Nursing Care

Whenever a patient is admitted to a nursing care facility or hospital or is seen in a clinic setting, assessment of fluid status is done. Patients known to be at high risk for unmet fluid needs include:

1. Patients about to have surgery
2. Patients with inadequate fluid intake for their age and body build, or for their activity level, or the environmental conditions (as activity and environmental temperature increase, so should fluid intake)
3. Patients with physical problems affecting the intake of fluids and food
4. Patients with excess loss of body fluids: bleeding, wound drainage, diarrhea, gastric suction, perspiration
5. Patients with inadequate loss of body fluids because of kidney disease
6. Patients with large amounts of fluids entering the body through oral, intravenous, or rectal routes
7. Patients who are very old or very young are also more likely to have problems maintaining fluid balance during illness or treatments than younger adult patients

Monitoring Intake and Output

High-risk patients or patients already having difficulty with meeting fluid needs are started on intake and output recordings and daily weights to monitor their progress. These measurements should be done with as much accuracy as possible. Weights are done at the same time each day, using the same scale, with the patient dressed in the same type of clothing. Intake recordings include measurement of all fluids that are liquid at body temperature, including frozen fluids. Because some institutions include cooked hot cereal as a full liquid, it is necessary to check hospital procedure. The amount of each fluid consumed is also recorded. Estimate how much of the total was consumed and record this amount on the intake sheet. (See Figure 23–6.) Each beverage container should have a "full" measurement in milliliters readily available to the nurse recording intake. For example, if the coffee pitcher, when full, contains 300 ml and the patient drank three-fourths of the coffee in the pitcher, the nurse would record 225 ml as an estimate. If ice-cream servings in a hospital are 100

ml and the patient ate almost all of the ice cream, the nurse would record 90 ml on the intake record.

Other things recorded as intake include:

1. Any tube feedings. Record total amount taken.
2. Any water used to clear the tube before or after a tube feeding. First measure out some water and then flush the tube for accurate fluid intake.
3. Any fluid introduced into a tube that was not completely withdrawn. If the nurse irrigated a patient's NG tube because it was obstructed and injected 10 ml of normal saline into the tube but was only able to retrieve 3 ml, the patient would be credited with an intake of 7 ml.
4. Any fluid the patient consumes as part of oral hygiene.
5. Intravenous fluid is considered intake but may be recorded on a separate sheet in the patient's chart and added to the 24-hour total intake on one shift or on each shift.
6. Any water consumed from the patient's bedside water pitcher. Measure the total volume in the pitcher and record. When fresh water is given, record how much of the total the patient has consumed over the last several hours. Ice counts for one-half the same volume of water (1 cup of ice is equal to ½ cup of water). For example, if the water pitcher contains 600 ml, and when fresh water is passed out, the pitcher is half empty, the nurse records 300 ml water on the patient's intake sheet.

Output may be only a measure of urine if no other fluid losses are obvious. If intake and output are to be as accurate as possible, other fluid losses must be measured or estimated and recorded. One way to obtain an accurate measurement of the amount of fluid lost is to weigh the fluid-soaked dressings and subtract the weight of identical clean dressings. The difference is the weight of fluid lost and can be recorded in milliliters. A gram scale is used to weigh dressings. Each gram is equal to 1 ml of body fluid. For example, if a patient was bleeding heavily on admission to the emergency room, the nurse weighs the sterile dressings applied to the wound at 35 gm. When those dressings are removed, the nurse reweighs the dressing at 138 gm. The weight gain in grams is considered to be the blood loss in milliliters. In this example, the blood loss would be 103 ml.

If a patient is on any type of suction device which is withdrawing body fluids such as wound drains or gastric suction, the actual amount of drainage is poured out of the container and measured. This is usually done once a shift or once a day, depending on the amount of fluid leaving the body and the severity of the patient's condition.

Diarrhea stools and vomited material are also

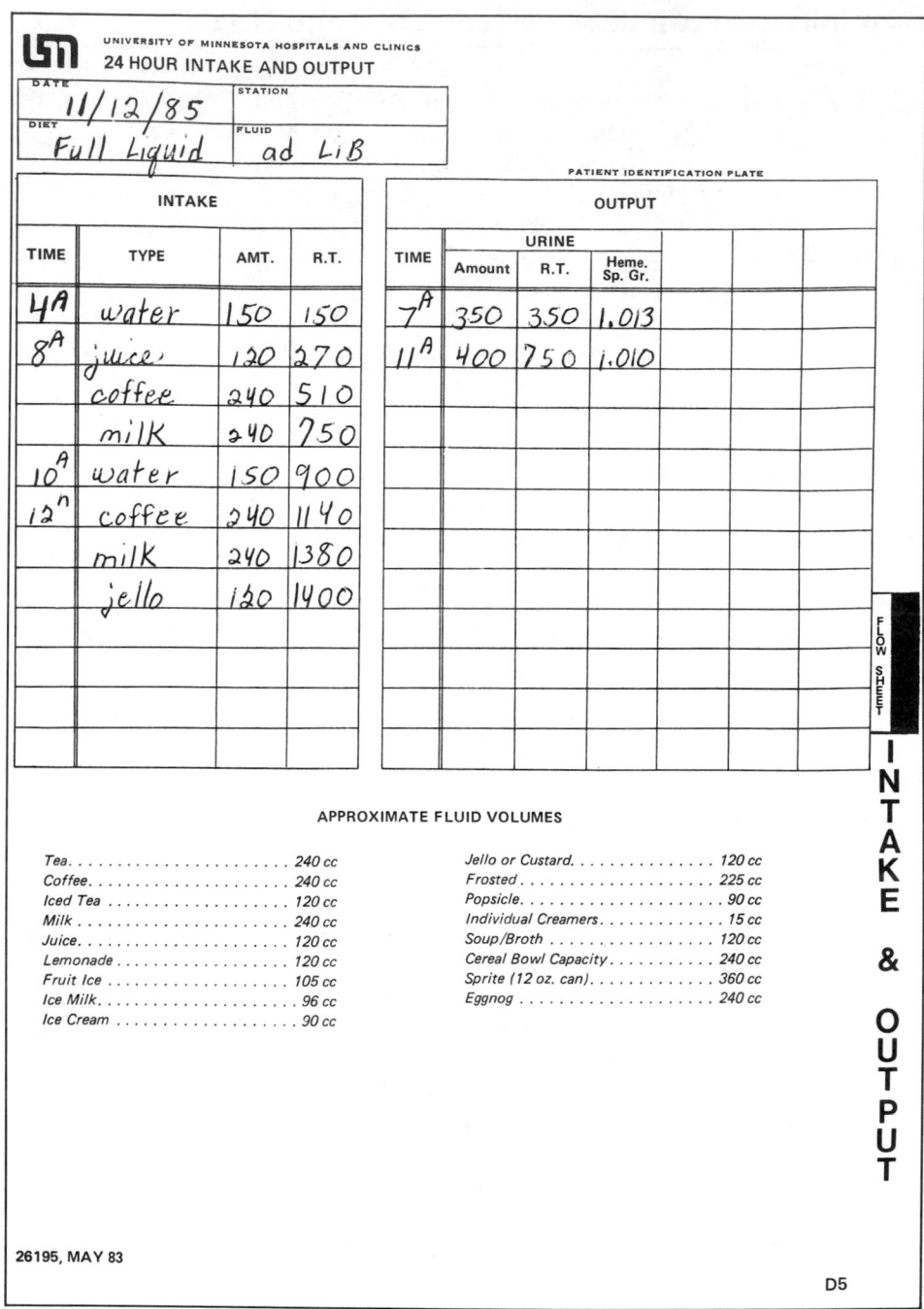

Figure 23–6. Intake and output (I & O) recordings. (Forms courtesy of the University of Minnesota Hospitals and Clinics, Minneapolis, MN.)

weighed, measured, or estimated, and added to the output tally.

Increasing Fluid Intake

Other nursing interventions helpful in maintaining or restoring a patient's fluid balance include giving patients help at meals, offering fluids between each meal and before bedtime, and serving fluids during breaks from other treatments such as in physical therapy or during education classes. Helping the patient assume an upright position whenever possible makes drinking easier and safer. Assistive devices are available for drinking to enable the patient to consume fluids independently or to make it easier for the patient to get the fluids from the container into the mouth. Some cups have spouts on them to reduce spilling. Spoons can be used to feed fluids if the patient is unable to drink or sip through a straw.

Frequent oral hygiene may also improve fluid intake by leaving a more pleasant taste in the patient's mouth and by reducing dryness. If a patient is on a fluid-restricted diet, frequent oral hygiene may reduce thirst, especially if the patient holds water in the mouth for several seconds before spitting it out.

The physician or another nurse may write "force fluids" as an order for a patient's care. Ethically and legally, the nurse may not "force" a patient to do anything. A "force fluid" order means the nurse is to encourage the patient to drink as much fluid as that patient is willing to drink. Explaining to the patient and family the reason more fluids are needed by the individual is helpful. If patients refuse to drink, that is their choice. Force or threats are inappropriate, being both unethical and a violation of the patient's rights.

The nurse seeks information from the patient and relatives about fluid preferences and the temperatures at which the individual prefers beverages to be served. Some cultures may prefer fluids of only one temperature as a traditional healing technique. If the nurse does not seek this information, any fluid that does not comply with cultural or religious guidelines will be untouched, and fluid intake will be less than it could have been. Providing the patient with small glasses of fluids several times during the day is usually more effective in increasing fluid intake than offering one or two large glasses of fluid. Having the names of patients at risk of inadequate fluid intake on the nourishment/juice cart is another way of making staff aware of individual patient's fluid needs.

Goals for fluid intake may be written as specific amounts for a 24-hour period, such as 3,000 ml/24h. Most adults sleep at night, so this is a time of reduced fluid intake if sleep is to be undisturbed. Encouraging the patient to drink most of the desired fluid intake during the waking hours is usually more successful in meeting a fluid-intake goal than dividing the amount of fluid to consume equally over the three nursing shifts.

Fluid Restrictions

When a patient is on restricted fluids, the cause of the problem is usually inadequate kidney function. To limit a patient's intake of fluids, the following suggestions may be helpful:

1. Make sure the patient and family understand why fluid is being restricted and how much fluid is allowed each day. Discuss this treatment with the patient before limiting fluids.

2. Divide the total amount of fluid the patient is permitted over a 24-hour period into three sections: one for each shift of nurses. Without doing this, the night nurse may be left with almost no fluid allowed to that patient for the entire eight hours.

3. Each shift should maintain an intake-and-output record and not exceed the amount for that shift.

4. Subtract fluid not eaten or drunk from premeasured containers so the patient receives all the fluid allowed.

5. Frequent oral hygiene is used to reduce feelings of dry mouth and thirst.

6. Plan with the patient how fluids should be served: some with the meal, none with the meal and all between, only certain fluids such as coffee with the meal and all other fluids between meals.

7. Remove water pitchers and other visual stimuli associated with drinking from the patient's room.

8. Patients who will be discharged on fluid restrictions may find it helpful to pour all fluid permitted (in a 24-hour period) into one pitcher. Every time they drink something, they are to pour an equal amount of liquid out of the large container. This provides a visual monitor of how much fluid is left for consumption. The patient will be able to see if too much fluid is being consumed and decrease the rate of drinking to provide fluids for later in the day.

9. The use of hard candies and lemon and glycerine swabs actually increase thirst by drawing water from the tissues into the mouth by osmosis because of the greater concentration of glucose and other electrolytes. Rinsing the mouth out with water and mouthwash is more effective in relieving thirst than the above-mentioned techniques.

Diets Regulating Electrolytes

Patients may be placed on diets to increase fluid intake or limit fluid intake based on their fluid needs. Diets may also be devised to rebalance the electrolytes within the patient's body, such as with low or high sodium, potassium, or calcium. Some medications, especially diuretics, will increase the loss of some electrolytes from the body, and dietary supplement may be necessary to maintain a normal balance. Low potassium is especially at risk when a patient is on diuretic therapy. Refer to Chapter 22 regarding foods high in sodium, potassium, calcium, and magnesium.

Parenteral Fluids

When fluid needs are unmet or in risk of being unmet, *parenteral fluid supplement* (IV therapy) is frequently used. The sterile fluid is introduced directly into the vein (*intravenous*) and the rate of infusion and the type of solution are matched to individual patient's fluid needs. Parenteral fluid can totally replace ingestion of fluids, but it bypasses normal body regulatory mechanisms. The patient may experience no thirst when permitted no food or fluid by mouth (NPO) if IV fluid supplement is adequate. The risk of overhydration exists with parenteral fluid therapy, and the nurse should be alert for the signs and symptoms, especially if kidney function is questionable. The physician orders IV fluid administration and specifies rate and type of solution. Like any other medication, the nurse does several checks to make sure the correct type of solution is being administered. The physician or specially trained nurses or technicians will start the IV infusion. The skill of venipuncture is one that requires repeated practice and is beyond the expertise of the beginning nursing student. Table 23-5 presents the various types of commonly used IV fluid.

Intravenous fluids may be started to maintain normal fluid intake, to replace fluids lost during surgery, trauma, or hemorrhage, to administer medications, and as a precautionary measure to provide rapid access to the circulatory system should problems arise during a treatment or procedure. Most patients have an IV infusion begun before surgery. The patient returns from surgery with the IV infusion still in place. It is left infusing until the patient is alert and able to take adequate fluids orally. The patient may be NPO for a period of time after surgery to give the GI tract time to reestablish peristaltic action. Once bowel sounds return indicating peristalsis, fluids are usually begun.

Safety Considerations in IV Therapy. There are both risks and benefits to intravenous therapy. Bacterial contamination of the needles, tubing, or solution will increase the patient's risks of infection. (See Figure 23-7.) Underhydration and overhydration are also risks if flow rate is not correctly calculated and maintained. Administration of the incorrect IV solution could also have disastrous results for the patient. Whenever providing IV therapy to a patient, consider the following points:

1. Maintain sterile technique when working with an IV infusion. Begin by washing your hands. If the protective caps are off the ends of the tubing when a package of tubing is opened, assume the tubing is contami-

Table 23-5. **Common IV Solutions**

1. Isotonic Solutions

Same osmotic pressure as blood; no water movement occurs into or out of vascular system from interstitial fluid or cells

D_5W (5% dextrose in water) contains no electrolytes; provides 170 kcal in 1,000 ml (approximately 5.4 kcal/oz); main benefit is in maintaining or replacing water; considered isotonic; not to be used with blood

Normal saline (0.9% sodium chloride in water) considered isotonic; contains no other electrolytes besides sodium and chloride; used to reestablish or maintain sodium balance and to replace lost extracellular fluid volume; used to begin and end blood administration; supplies no calories

Ringers solution contains sodium, chloride, potassium, and calcium; used to supplement inadequate fluid intake or when water losses from body are excessive; considered isotonic

Lactated Ringer's—same as Ringer's solution but contains lactate; considered isotonic; used to treat dehydration and shift of fluid from vascular system to interstitial space; also used to treat mild acidosis from diarrhea and kidney disease

2. Hypertonic Solutions

Higher osmotic pressure than blood; interstitial fluid drawn into blood; used to replace electrolytes and fluid deficits

5% dextrose in 0.9% normal saline
5% dextrose in lactated Ringer's
10% dextrose in water ($D_{10}W$)
20% dextrose in water ($D_{20}W$)

3. Hypotonic Solutions

Lower osmotic pressure than blood; used to move water into interstitial fluid from blood
0.45% normal saline

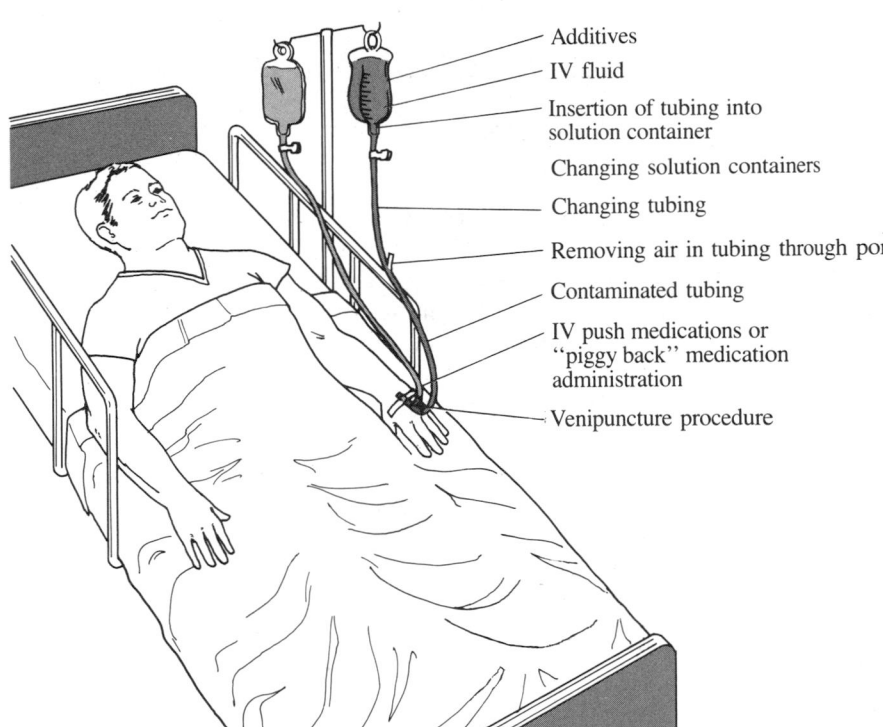

- Additives
- IV fluid
- Insertion of tubing into solution container
- Changing solution containers
- Changing tubing
- Removing air in tubing through port
- Contaminated tubing
- IV push medications or "piggy back" medication administration
- Venipuncture procedure

Figure 23–7. Sites for potential contamination during initiation and maintenance of an intravenous infusion.

nated and get new tubing. The tubing should not be disconnected unless absolutely necessary, as this practice increases the risk of bacterial contamination. To remove a patient's gown, slide the tubing and the IV bottle/bag through the armhole of the gown. (See Figure 23–8.) Put a clean gown on the patient by first slipping the IV bottle/bag through the armhole of the gown in the same direction that the patient's arm will go through

it. A better solution to the problem is to have the hospital or nursing home investigate buying or making gowns with openings at each shoulder for easy gown removal during IV therapy. IV tubing may be changed routinely every 24 to 48 hours for patients on IV therapy to reduce the incidence of bacterial growth within the tube. This policy should be checked at each institution in which you are giving nursing care.

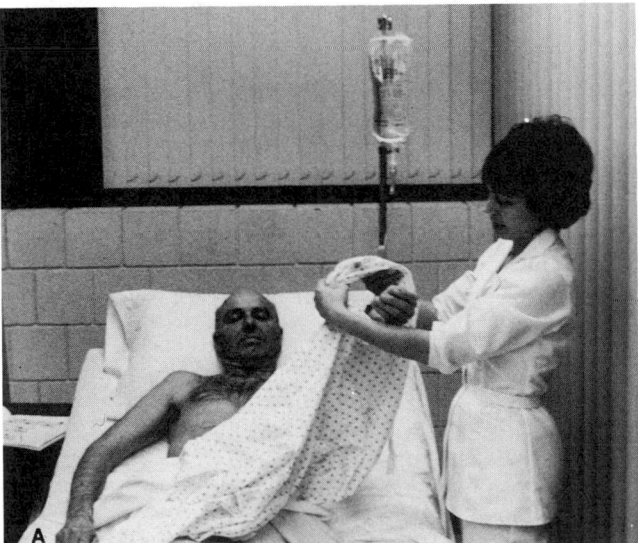
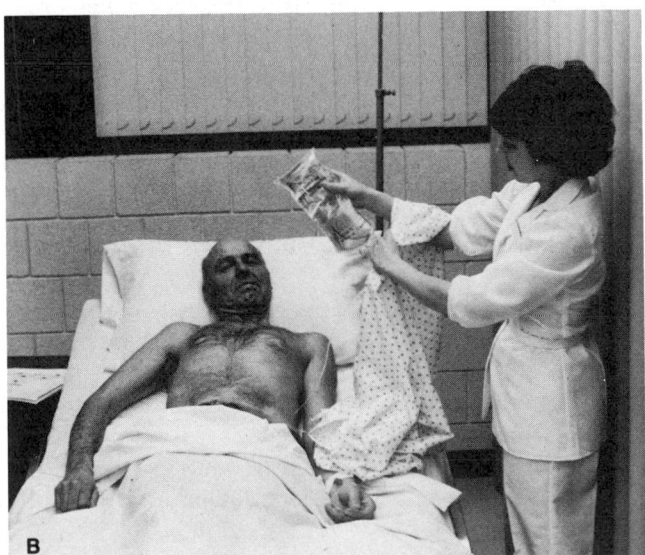

Figure 23–8. Getting a patient's gown on and off during an intravenous infusion. Tubing and solution container passed through sleeve of gown to maintain uninterrupted infusion and prevent possible contamination from disconnecting the tubing.

Nursing Skill 23–1   Calculating and Regulating IV Infusion Drip Rates

Preparation

1. Determine need. Any IV infusion will require regulation if the correct amount of fluid is to be given to the patient. The flow rate is calculated and regulated initially and should be rechecked every two hours, or more often if there are any problems maintaining the correct rate of flow. The physician will order a specific flow rate, as 150 ml/hr, or a specific volume of fluid to infuse over a given time period, as 1,000 ml q8h.
2. Calculate the flow rate before entering the patient's room. Information needed:
   a. Number of drops from drip chamber that equal 1 ml (varies with manufacturer, from 10 to 60 drops; read label on box of tubing or call hospital pharmacy)
   b. Volume of fluid to infuse (physician's order)
   c. Time over which volume is to be infused (physician's order)

Calculations

$$\frac{\text{Drops from drip chamber equal to 1 ml}}{60\ \text{min}} \times \frac{\text{Total volume of fluid}}{\text{Total time in hours}} = \frac{\text{Number of drops}}{\text{to infuse each minute}}$$

Example: Physician orders 1,000 ml q8h
　　　　Drip chamber = 10 drops (gtt) in 1 ml

$$\frac{10\ \text{gtt}}{60\ \text{min}} \times \frac{1,000}{8\ \text{hr}} = \frac{10,000}{480} = 20.8\ \text{gtt/min or 21 gtt}$$

If ordered as 125 ml/hr

$$\frac{10\ \text{gtt}}{60\ \text{min}} \times \frac{125\ \text{ml}}{1\ \text{hr}} = \frac{1,250}{60} = 20.8\ \text{gtt/min or 21 gtt}$$

3. Equipment needed: a watch or clock with a second counter.
4. Explain what you are doing to the patient.
5. Wash hands.
6. Mark off IV solution container in one-hour increments for future assessment of volume of solution infused compared to desired volume.

Procedure	Explanation
1. Check the patient's name band.	1. To get correct solution and flow as ordered for each patient.
2. Divide number of drops per minute by four.	2. Gives drops each 15 sec for more rapid regulation of flow.
3. Count the number of drops falling in 15 sec	3. To assess current rate of flow.
4. If too many drops were released, tighten the clamp lightly and recount; if too few drops were released, loosen the clamp slightly and recount.	4. To adjust current flow rate to ordered flow rate.
5. Continue step #4 until correct number of drops falls every 15 sec.	5. To adjust current flow rate to ordered flow rate.
6. Recheck rate in 10 to 15 min and again every 2 hr or as needed to maintain flow rate.	6. Patient movement, vein irritation, a clot in the needle, BP, and positioning can all affect rate of flow.

Nursing Skill 23-2   Setting Up an IV and Changing Solutions or Tubing

Preparation

1. Determine need. A physician may order an IV to be started or may start one. The container of solution, tubing, needles, and tape must all be prepared ahead of time. Once the venipuncture is performed and the needle is in place in the vein, the solution must be at the end of the tubing ready to attach to the hub of the needle. Flow is initiated as soon as the connection is made to prevent clotting of the needle. The needle and tubing are then secured in place with tape to the patient's skin. In a life-threatening emergency, the nurse can anticipate a patient's need for an IV and set up all equipment for the responsible physician or start the IV without the physician, if the nurse has been trained in venipuncture. Institutions usually have prewritten orders (standing orders) to guide a nurse in such an emergency as to what fluid to start, a rate of flow, and under what circumstances venipuncture may be done.

2. Equipment needed: ordered IV solution (bag or bottle), tubing, tape, assortment of needles, alcohol wipes, Band-Aids, tourniquet, IV pole (many hospitals have an IV tray containing most of these items), filters (check hospital policy for use of IV filters)

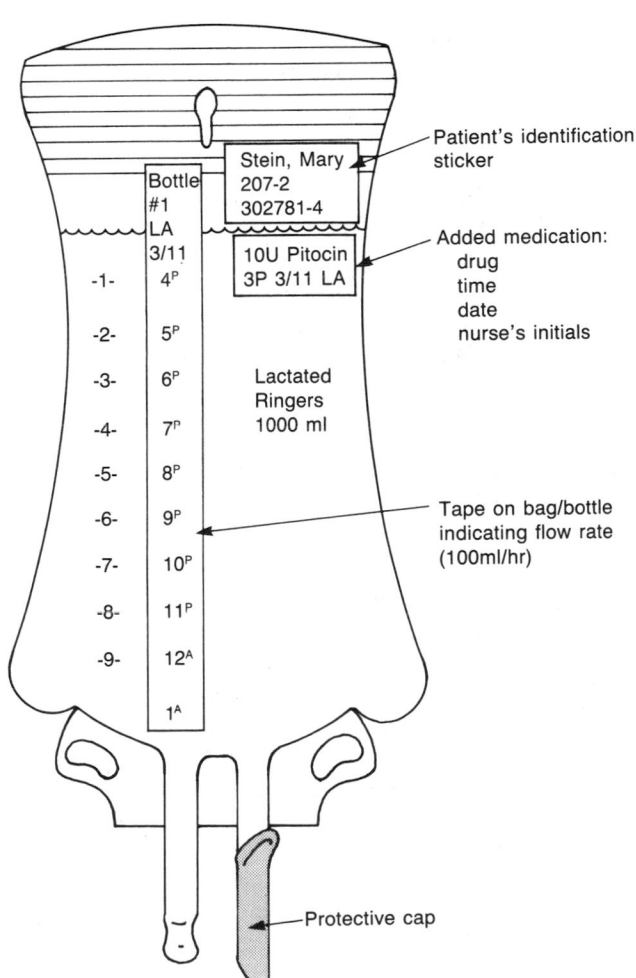

Figure 23-9. Labeling intravenous solution container. The bottle or bag of IV solution is labeled with the rate of flow per hour, name and amount of any added medication, time initiated, patient's name, and initials of nurse who prepares the solution for administration and hangs the container.

3. Wash hands.
4. Check the patient's name band.
5. Explain to the patient when and why the physician wants an IV infustion started.
6. Open box of tubing; for glass bottles, remove metal lid from top of bottle.
7. Label bottle with date, time, patient's name, number (1st bottle, 2nd bottle, etc.) with a piece of tape. Any medications added to the bottle should be labeled on the bottle (medication, dose, date, time, initials of nurse). (See Figure 23–9.)

Procedure	Explanation
1. Remove latex cover from top of IV bottle by pulling at edge; sound of air rushing into bottle must be present when latex cover removed. For the bag, two flaps are pulled back to reveal the insertion site for the drip chamber.	1. Opens site for tubing insertion. Guarantee of sterile solution; vacuum in bottle indicates no air leaks; discard any bottle having no vacuum to prevent infusing possibly contaminated solution.
2. Remove cover from plastic tip above drip chamber on tubing.	2. Protects sterility until ready for inserting into IV solution container.
3. Insert plastic tip into largest hole in IV solution container while compressing drip chamber (bags have only one entrance, but bottles have an additional smaller hole which is an air vent). (See Figure 23–10.)	3. Prevents air from entering drip chamber.
4. Tighten clamp on tubing completely and invert IV solution container and hang on pole.	4. Prevents solution from runing out other end of tubing causing possible contamination.
5. Fill one-half the drip chamber by squeezing it and releasing.	5. Prevents air from entering tubing or entire drip chamber from filling with fluid preventing nurse from counting drops.
6. Remove cap on other end of tubing and hold above a container such as a cup or basin. (See Figure 23–11.) Release the clamp until fluid is dripping rapidly through the drip chamber and fills the tubing completely.	6. Clears tubing of air; prevents contamination of sterile tip if not touched by hands or to cup or basin.
7. Tighten clamp completely.	7. Prevents fluid from running out end of tube.
8. Replace cap on end of tubing and drape over IV pole.	8. Protects sterility of tubing tip.

To change solution containers (done before old container completely empty to prevent air from entering drip chamber and tubing):

1. Wash hands.	1. Reduce microorganism transfer.
2. Check patient's name band.	2. Assures correct solution for each patient.
3. Open new bottle.	3. Preparation of bottle increases speed in changing containers, reducing time for clot formation in needle.
4. Clamp off flow rate.	4. Prevents fluid from running on patient and bedding when disconnected.
5. Take old solution container down from IV pole, invert and pull out plastic tip.	5. Prevents fluid from running on patient and bedding when disconnected.
6. Insert plastic tip in new solution container, invert and hang on pole.	6. To establish new flow.
7. Open clamp and readjust flow rate.	7. To reestablish ordered drip rate.
8. Document in chart.	8. Legal responsibility; communication among health team members.

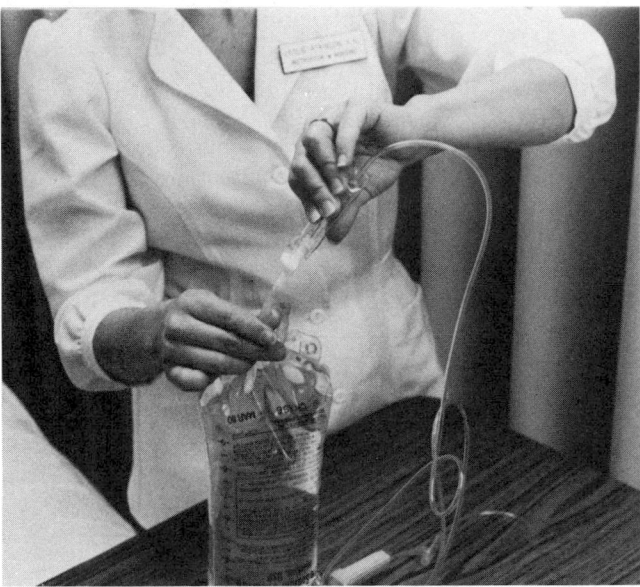

Figure 23-10. Inserting tubing into intravenous solution bag. Drip chamber is squeezed when it is inserted.

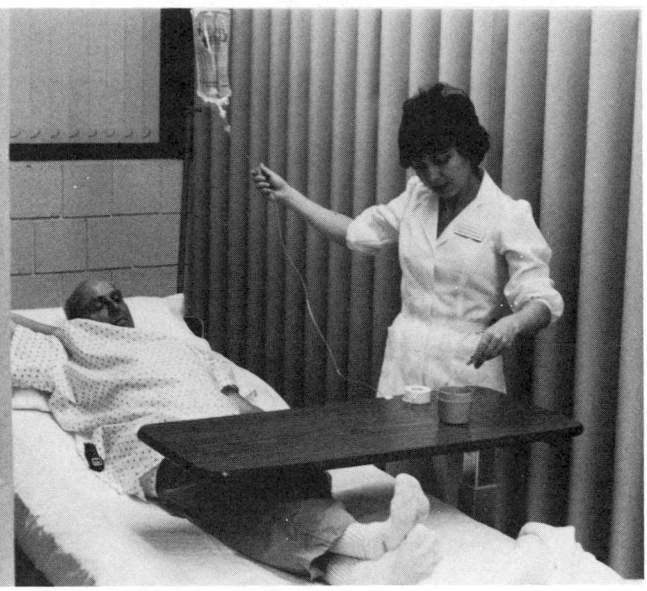

Figure 23-11. Clearing the IV tubing of air before starting infusion. Tip of tubing held several inches above container; when all air is removed, the flow clamp is tightened so no solution drips out.

To change solution container and tubing:

1. Wash hands.
2. Obtain new container of IV solution and fill new tubing with fluid to remove air.
3. Remove tape holding old tubing to hub of needle.
4. Clamp off old tubing and remove from needle hub; insert new tubing into hub (remove cap from end of new tube and hold in third and fourth fingers as thumb and first finger of same hand used to remove old tubing from needle hub). (See Figure 23-12.)

1. Reduce microorganism transfer.
2. Reduces time that IV flow is interrupted; prevents air from entering vein.
3. To remove old tubing.
4. Prevents fluid from running on patient and bedding; allows rapid insertion of new tubing and IV flow, reducing risk of clotting in the needle.

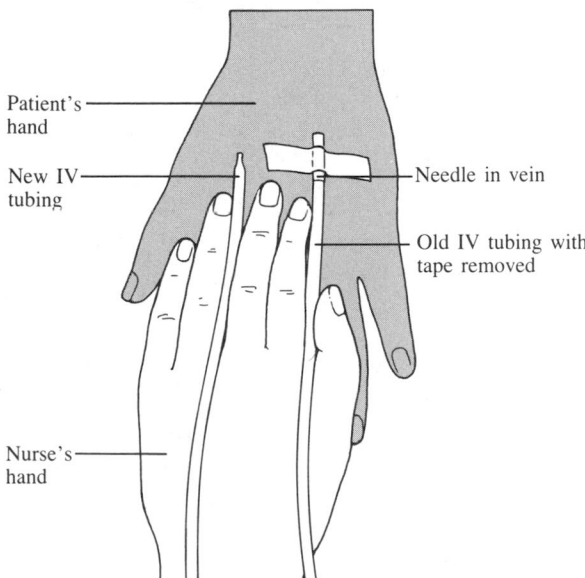

Patient's hand

New IV tubing

Needle in vein

Old IV tubing with tape removed

Nurse's hand

Figure 23-12. Changing tubing during an IV infusion. Care must be taken not to contaminate new tubing while removing old tubing from needle hub.

Procedure	Explanation
5. Loosen clamp on new tubing to establish drip pattern.	5. Reduces risk of needle clotting.
6. Tape new tubing in place to needle hub and skin.	6. To prevent tubing from separating from needle hub; prevents pull on needle with patient movement.
7. Regulate drip rate.	7. Reestablish ordered flow rate.
8. Document in patient's chart.	8. Legal responsibility; communication among health team members.

2. Treat the IV solution as a medication and do the appropriate checks to assure the correct medication, the correct patient, and the correct time and dose (rate of flow). Review Chapter 19 on medication administration.

3. Check the IV solution container for any signs of leaks or particles in the solution. There should be no visible particles in any IV solution. If there are visible particles, do not use the solution, but notify pharmacy and obtain another bottle or bag for the patient.

4. Check the IV site several times each shift for any signs of redness, pain, edema, or leaking around the needle insertion site. If any of these conditions are present, the IV may need to be restarted or repaired. Have a more experienced nurse check your findings, and never discontinue the IV without the direction of the responsible nurse or your nursing instructor.

5. Do not shut off the infusion without consulting the staff nurse or your nursing instructor as this will result in very rapid clot formation in the needle. See Nursing Skills 23-1, 23-2, and 23-3 for correct techniques in handling IV infusions.

6. Do not lower or raise the level of the IV container for more than a few moments without readjusting the flow rate. Raising the height of the container will make the solution run into the vein at a faster rate. Lowering the container will slow or stop the rate of flow.

7. If air gets into the tubing, do not let it run into the patient's vein. Even though small sections of air in the tubing will not cause physical harm to the patient, it may be very upsetting to a patient who thinks death will result from an air embolism. It is estimated that 70 cc of air are needed to cause death from an air embolism in an adult, but very rapid injection of lesser amounts of air may also cause death, as may lesser amounts in very ill patients (Metheny and Snively, 1983). It is also poor technique. Do not disconnect the tubing to remove the air as this leads to contamination. If there are only a few air bubbles in the tube, pull the tube taut and straight down from the solution container and flick the tubing

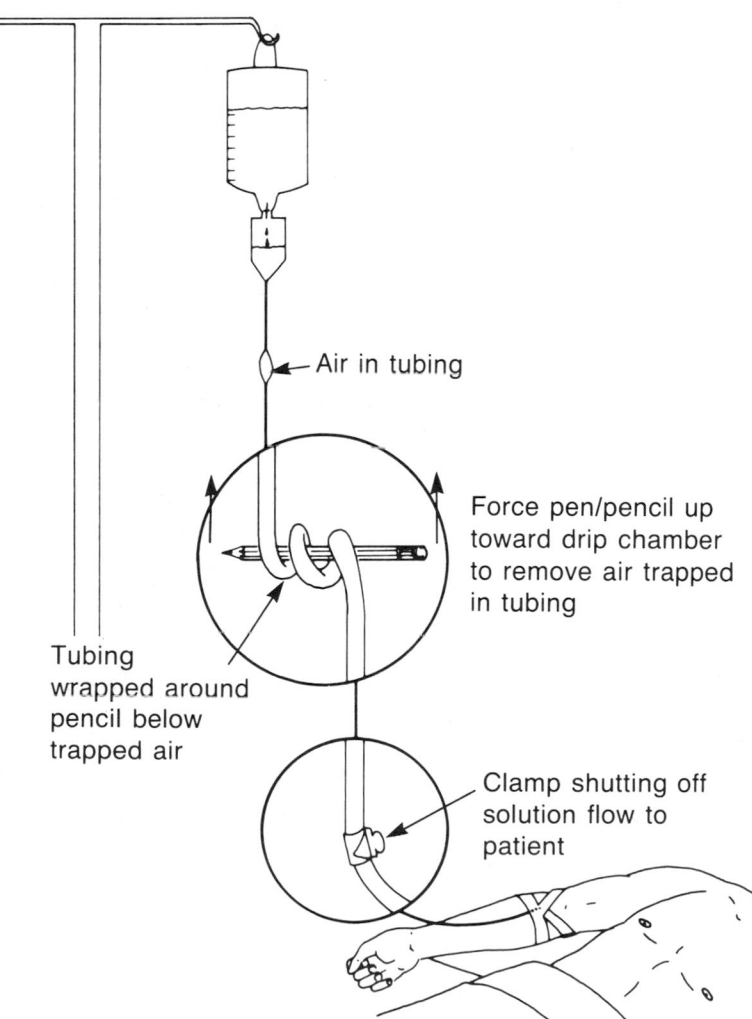

Air in tubing

Force pen/pencil up toward drip chamber to remove air trapped in tubing

Tubing wrapped around pencil below trapped air

Clamp shutting off solution flow to patient

Figure 23-13. Removing air trapped in tubing during an IV infusion. The air is between the patient and the drip chamber with the flow clamp below the trapped air. The clamp is tightened to shut off the flow of solution to the patient and to prevent blood from being drawn up into the tubing as the nurse compresses the tubing with a pencil, forcing out the trapped air.

Nursing Skill 23–3   Discontinuing an IV Infusion

Preparation

1. Determine need. As a student, never discontinue an IV without consulting the responsible staff nurse or your nursing instructor. An IV infusion may be discontinued by the nurse for the following reasons:
   a. Physician's order to discontinue IV
   b. Occlusion of needle by blood clot (fluid will not flow through needle, and it is not possible to aspirate blood back with a syringe injected at port nearest the needle)
   c. Redness, tenderness, swelling, and warmth of area around needle indicate irritated vessel which may result in phlebitis; it is better to restart the IV in another site than continue to irritate an inflammed vessel
   d. Infiltration. Needle is no longer in vein; fluid being infused into interstitial space, causing edema, tenderness; no blood return when aspirated with syringe at nearest port

   If the patient has very fragile vessels that are difficult for IV needle insertion, such as the old or very young patient, seek assistance from the nurse with the most IV experience before discontinuing in case the current IV can be maintained.
2. Equipment needed: sterile 2 × 2s or alcohol wipes; Band-Aids.
3. Wash hands.
4. Check patient's name band.
5. Explain procedure to patient.
6. Provide privacy as needed.

Procedure	Explanation
1. Remove the armboard, if used.	1. Removal of armboards and tape allows straight backward pull on needle or catheter for removal.
2. Shut off IV flow by tightening clamp on tubing. Shut off any IV pump or machine used to regulate flow.	2. Prevents fluid from infusing into interstitial tissue or on skin or bedding.
3. Remove the tape holding the IV tubing and needle to the patient's skin; use a quick pull if taped over hairy area.	3. Removal of armboards and tape allows straight backward pull on needle or catheter for removal.
4. Place alcohol wipes or sterile gauze over and in front of needle insertion site and pull straight back on needle.	4. In readiness to apply pressure after removal of needle; pressure during removal may damage vein or break catheter.
5. Apply pressure over site for 1 min after entire needle out of vein.	5. Prevents formation of hematoma (collection of blood in tissues).
6. Examine needle or catheter to make sure it is unbroken.	6. Broken tip of catheter could lodge in smaller vessels of body as embolism; medical emergency.
7. Apply Band-Aid to injection site after all bleeding has stopped.	7. To absorb any further bleeding and protect site from bacteria.
8. Document discontinuation of IV, amount of IV fluid infused and amount of fluid remaining, if any; identify reason for discontinuation and any patient data indicating problems.	8. Legal responsibility; communication to other health team members.

with your finger or a pen. The bubbles will be dislodged from the tubing and rise up into the drop chamber. If there is a large amount of air in the tube, clamp the tube between the patient and the air and quickly wrap the tubing around a pencil several times below the air. Then force the pencil up toward the drip chamber, and the air should be pushed into the drip chamber. Turn the flow back on and regulate the rate. (See Figure 23–13.) If that technique did not work, slow the drip rate and obtain a syringe and alcohol wipe. Cleanse the IV tubing at a port below the air by wiping it with alcohol. Insert the sterile needle into the cleansed port and clamp off the IV tubing between the patient and the port. Pull back on the syringe (aspirate), and the IV solution and the trapped air will come up into the syringe. Remove the syringe and open the clamp to reestablish the flow. Regulate the rate.

8. Record administration of IV fluid by including the type of solution, the amount the patient received, the amount remaining in the container, any problems with the infusion, and any reasons why an infusion was discontinued or initiated. Always include times and dates and sign your name when documenting IV therapy. (See Figure 23–14.)

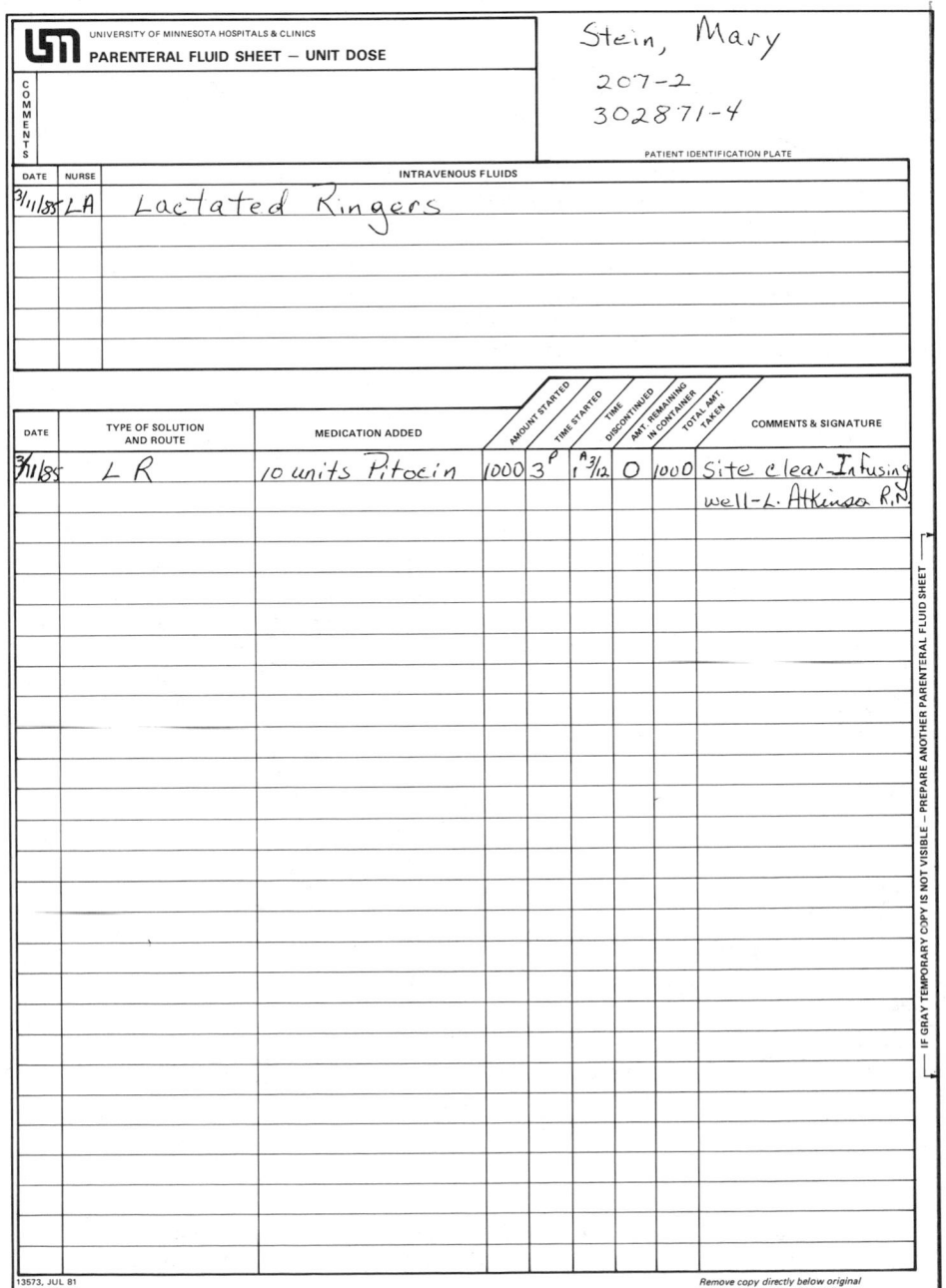

Figure 23–14. Recording intravenous infusions. (Forms courtesy of the University of Minnesota Hospitals and Clinics, Minneapolis, MN.)

Table 23–6. **Complications of IV Therapy**

Infiltration	Needle out of vein and in subcutaneous tissue; tissue edema, painful, IV infusion slowed; IV must be discontinued; warm packs and elevation of arm helpful in reducing discomfort.
Hematoma	Bleeding into the subcutaneous tissue from the vein; discoloration and swelling around needle insertion site; failure to apply adequate pressure while discontinuing an IV may result in hematoma, as may pushing needle through other side of vein when attempting to start infusion; pressure dressing and elevation of affected area are helpful.
Phlebitis	Inflammation of a vein resulting in tenderness/pain along vein, discoloration of skin near needle, swelling of tissue, increased local and/or body temperature; IV is discontinued, warm packs at site and elevation used to relieve discomfort. Bed rest and anticoagulant therapy may be started. Inflammation may be from bacterial action, chemical, or physical irritation of the vein.
Local infection	Caused by poor aseptic technique; results in fever, pain at site, inflammation, discoloration, and drainage; IV discontinued, site cultured, and antibiotic ointment and sterile dressing applied to site; systemic antibiotic may be used.
Nerve damage	Excessive pressure from restraints, unpadded armboards, and tape may interfere with circulation in the area and damage the local nerves, resulting in numbness or tingling in the extremity.
General infection	Caused by poor aseptic technique; results in blood infection, causing elevated temperature, chills, backache, vomiting, discomfort.
Embolism	A section of the catheter may break loose and lodge in another part of the body, causing obstructed blood flow; air may enter vein when solution container runs dry, but generally, in a gravity flow system, the patient's blood pressure will cause the solution to stop running before the air reaches the vein and the needle clots.

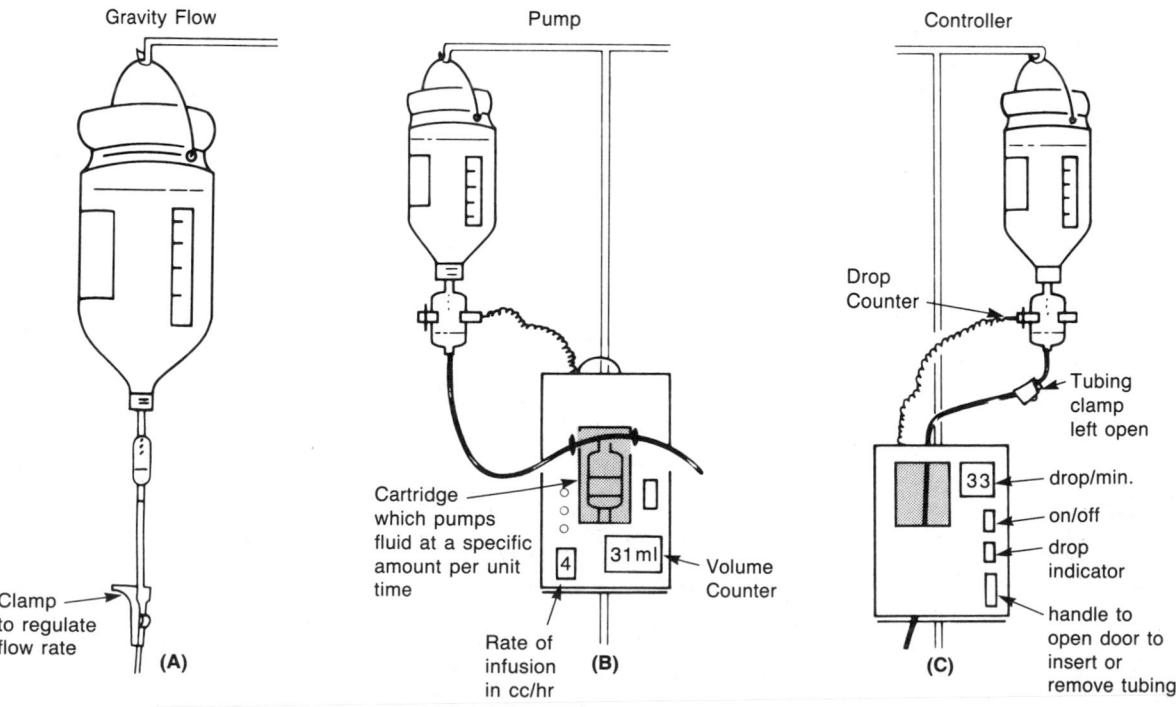

Figure 23–15. Three methods for administering intravenous fluids. **A.** Gravity flow using tube clamp to regulate flow. **B.** Infusion pump using a syringe device to measure volume of fluid infused. **C.** Controller using a drop counter around the drip chamber to regulate flow in drops per minute.

Table 23-6 presents some complications of IV therapy.

Mechanical Regulation of IV Rates. There are three basic ways of regulating an IV infusion. (See Figure 23-15.) The first method involves the use of *gravity flow* from the solution container above the patient. The height of the container and the diameter of the tubing regulate the flow. A clamp control valve is adjusted to constrict the tubing in varying degrees until the desired flow rate is obtained. This method is the most unreliable since patient movement, changing levels of the infusion site (as when the patient sits or stands), and viscosity of the fluid can all alter the rate of flow without the nurse's knowledge. Continuous administration of very small amounts of fluid by gravity flow is extremely difficult to regulate.

The second method of administering IV solution is by using a mechanical *controller*. (See Figure 23-16.) This involves one of various machines designed to regulate flow by monitoring the number of drops given each minute. An electronic counter is placed around the drip chamber and as each drop falls, it breaks the light beam sent through the chamber by the electronic counter, and the machine counts a drop. If the drop rate decreases because of an occlusion (blockage such as a blood clot) in the needle or in the tube, an alarm will sound, alerting the nurse to a decreased flow rate. The machine will not allow an accelerated rate of flow to occur. A guide on the side of the machine allows the nurse to find the correct drop rate to achieve an ordered infusion rate. This conversion is based on the number of drops needed to equal 1 ml, which varies from 10 to 60 drops, depending on the type of drop chamber and manufacturer. The machine is then set to advance that many drops per minute. This system is also affected by gravity and can be slowed by patient position changes but will sound an alarm if altered rates occur.

The third method involves the use of a *pump* to administer IV solutions instead of gravity. The pumps come in various shapes and sizes but are most appropriately used when very small amounts of solution are to be administered. The constant pressure on the fluid in the

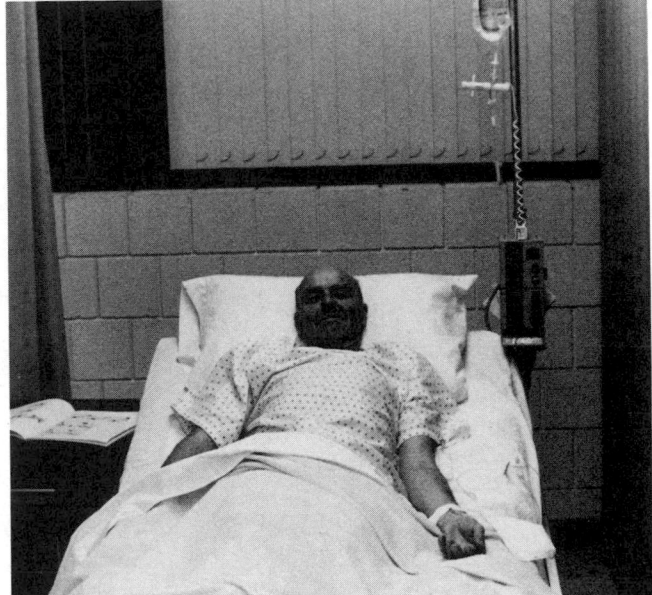

Figure 23-16. An intravenous infusion using a controller to monitor drip rate.

tubing from the pump keeps the needle open, where it often clots with either of the other systems. When volume accuracy is critical, the pump is also the best choice since a specific volume of fluid is infused continuously over time. The pump is also the best choice for more viscous fluids since thick fluids tend to run slowly by gravity alone and the needle is more likely to clot. The pumps may have alarms to warn the nurse of problems, and the newer models will have a visual printout of the probable problem, such as "empty solution container" or "occlusion." A significant problem with the pump is that it will continue to infuse solution into the patient even if the needle comes out of the vein into the tissue. This solution, pumped into the subcutaneous tissue, causes painful edema, and, if strong medication is in the solution, tissue damage and cellular death may occur. In contrast, using a gravity system, the pressure caused by fluid within the tissue is enough to greatly slow or stop the flow of solution and the dislodged needle clots over.

Nursing Care Plan for a Patient with Unmet Fluid Needs

Assessment

Data. Mrs. Johnson was admitted on 9/18 for gallbladder surgery the following day. She was 42 years old and moderately overweight. She had three children at home, ranging in age from 8 to 20 years. She reported being nauseated and having repeated bouts of vomiting over the last week. She reported that she has been able to eat very little all week and has been eating only Jell-O, tea, and juice. She reports that her current weight of 148 lb is 10 lb less than her normal. Her urine output for the 11 P.M. to 7 A.M. shift was 150 ml of dark urine with a specific gravity of 1.032. She returned from surgery with an IV of D₅W infusing at a rate of 150 ml/hr. She was to be NPO for 24 hours and then to begin clear liquids and advance as tolerated. She was ordered to be on daily weights and I & O recordings by her physician. She was to sit at the bedside on the day of surgery and begin ambulating the first postoperative day. The IV was to be maintained at 125 ml/hr until she was taking adequate fluids, and then it could be discontinued. She had a urinary catheter in place which was to be discontinued on the first postoperative day. She began taking fluids well on the first postoperative day but by noon was feeling slightly nauseated and had considerable abdominal distention. Her IV had been discontinued at 10 A.M. after she had taken 500 ml of fluid with no apparent problem. No bowel sounds were heard over the abdomen by the nursing student assigned her care.

Nursing Diagnoses

1. Abdominal distention related to fluid ingestion and inadequate persistalsis.
2. Potential fluid deficit.

Planning

Goals (Short Term)

1. Abdominal distention to be lessened by 3 P.M.
2. Total fluid intake (IV + PO) to be 1,800 ml or more for 24 hours on 1st POD (postoperative day).

Planned Actions (Interventions)

For Goal 1

1. Reduce fluid intake to sips of water until peristalsis returns.
2. Ambulate every two hours as much as tolerated.
3. Turn and reposition in bed between ambulations.
4. Assess bowel sounds q2h (every 2 hours).

For Goal 2

1. Measure total fluid taken by "sips" and record.
2. Begin clear fluid intake when bowel sounds return and when patient begins to pass flatus.
3. If nausea persists and bowel sounds do not return by 4 P.M., contact patient's physician regarding restarting IV infusion.
4. If urine output falls below 30 ml/hr, notify physician for order to restart IV infusion.

Evaluation

Goal 1 met; abdominal distention greatly reduced by 3 P.M. with fairly good bowel sounds heard.
Goal 2 met; patient began to take fluids slowly at 3 P.M. with no problems. Ate clear liquid supper with no increase in abdominal distention or reappearance of nausea. 24-hour total 1,875 ml and output 1,700 ml.

Reassessment

Problem 1 still exists since patient still experiencing some abdominal distention. Alter goal to: "Abdominal distention resolved within next 24 hours." Change planned actions to: "Ambulate q2h while awake, auscultate bowel sounds q4h, encourage patient to turn in bed ad lib."
Problem 2 no longer a realistic concern; no fluid deficit probable now that patient taking fluids with little problem.

Summary

Fluids is essential for all physiological functions in the body. Without fluid intake, death is a certainty within a matter of days. Fluid balance is maintained in the body by the ingestion of foods and fluids and metabolically created water remaining equal to fluid losses through respirations, perspiration, and urine production. The effects of thirst, body hormones, and electrolytes work together to maintain a balance between fluid intake and fluid losses. Various factors affect fluid needs such as age, activity, health status, body build, and sex. Anything that increases loss of fluids from the body, reduces normal loss of fluid from the body, increases fluid entering the body, or decreases fluid entering the body has the potential for interfering with satisfaction of body fluid needs.

Data indicating normal hydration, dehydration, and overhydration were presented. Nursing interventions helpful in increasing or limiting an individual's fluid intake were discussed. Administration of parenteral fluids is one way of increasing or maintaining hydration when a patient is unable to consume food and fluids orally. Safety considerations and complications of IV therapy were presented, along with the skills of calculating IV rate, discontinuing an IV infusion, changing bottles (bags) and tubing during an infusion, and setting up an infusion.

Terms for Review

active transport	diffusion	hypertonic solution	isotonic solution
air embolism	edema	hypotonic solution	osmosis
aldosterone	electrolyte	infiltration (related to IV therapy)	parenteral fluid
antidiuretic hormone	extracellular fluids	insensible water loss	phlebitis
colloid osmotic pressure	filtration	interstitial fluid	pitting edema
dehydration	hydrostatic pressure	intracellular fluids	plasma

Self-Assessment

Answer the following questions to assess your own ability to meet your fluid needs:

	T	F
1. My skin turgor is good.		
2. I usually have no edema in my legs.		
3. My blood pressure is less than 140/90.		
4. I eat a well-balanced diet.		
5. I usually do not eat a lot of salty foods.		
6. I usually consume 2 oz or less of 70-proof alcohol per day (or its equivalent).		
7. I usually void five to six times a day in fairly large amounts.		
8. I drink about 6 to 10 cups of fluids each day.		
9. I am not usually troubled by constipation.		
10. I am not taking diuretics.		

"False" answers are associated with possible problems with fluid and electrolyte balance within the body fluid compartments.

Self-assessment related to ethical/legal problems in nursing are presented for your consideration. A patient's wishes may be in conflict with ordered medical treatments the nurse or student is expected to carry out. The nurse may attempt to persuade the patient that a treatment should be accepted but may not use force or threats. Think about how you might respond to the following situations based on your personal ethical beliefs. Consider if you might be risking the patient's health, a legal complaint of professional negligence, or violation of the nurse's Code of Ethics by your response.

1. I believe all patients should receive adequate hydration by IV therapy even if they are dying and near death.
2. A patient on a fluid-restricted diet could probably talk me into giving extra fluid and not recording it, if the individual was thirsty.
3. I feel a patient who refuses to drink adequate amounts of fluids should have an IV started whether the individual wants it or not.
4. I think I & O recordings are usually very inaccurate and not worth doing.
5. I think patients are usually competent and honest enough to record their own intake accurately, after being shown how it is done.

6. I feel the nurse is better able to get a patient to drink than a patient's friends or family.
7. I feel a dying patient does not have the right to refuse fluids and become severely dehydrated.
8. I am so afraid of IVs and of doing something wrong that I usually don't even look at them when I am with a patient on IV therapy.

Learning Activities

1. Accompany a nurse who specializes in venipuncture and IV therapy on a clinical site.

   How is sterility maintained?

   What common problems occur and how are they remedied?

   What type of special training did this individual nurse receive to become an IV specialist in the hospital?

   What does the IV nurse do if a patient refuses venipuncture?
2. Visit physical therapy departments or rehabilitation centers and talk with nurses about specialized equipment and techniques for helping patients ingest fluids. Attempt to drink a glass of water using one of these devices.
3. Visit a hospice and talk with the nursing supervisor about their policy on maintaining hydration using IV therapy for dying patients. Discuss your feelings about such policies with classmates, clergy.

Review Questions

1. Which individual has a greater percentage of body weight composed of fluid?
   a. An 85-year-old man who is very thin
   b. A 9-lb newborn
   c. An overweight teenage girl
   d. A 36-year-old marathon runner
2. Mr. Johnson has a pituitary tumor which is severely reducing the amount of ADH released into the blood. How would Mr. Johnson's problem affect urine production?
   a. Urine production would be greatly increased and specific gravity would be above 1.030.
   b. Urine produced would be more concentrated than normal.
   c. Urine production would be reduced, but concentration of waste products would be increased.
   d. Urine production would be greatly increased and more dilute than normal.
3. During the first 24 to 48 hours after surgery, how is fluid balance affected?
   a. Fluid moves into the vascular system from the interstitial fluid.
   b. Fluid osmotic pressure of the blood increases.
   c. Output of fluid usually exceeds intake.
   d. The kidney produces large amounts of dilute urine.
   e. Fluid moves into the interstitial fluid from the blood by osmosis.

4. Which of the following dominant electrolytes is appropriately matched to the body fluid compartment?
   a. Plasma—sodium dominant cation
   b. Cell—sodium dominant cation
   c. Interstitial fluid—calcium dominant cation
   d. Plasma—potassium dominant cation
5. How does a fever affect fluid needs?
   a. Fluid needs decrease during a fever unless the patient is perspiring, at which point they increase.
   b. Body fluid needs increase with each degree Fahrenheit rise in temperature in the absence of obvious perspiration.
   c. Body temperature does not affect fluid needs.
6. Which of the following is considered a normal amount of insensible fluid loss in a 24-hour period?
   a. 100 ml
   b. 200 ml
   c. 500 ml
   d. 900 ml
   e. 1,500 ml
7. Risks of IV fluid therapy include all of the following *except*:
   a. Infiltration
   b. Embolism
   c. Phlebitis
   d. Abdominal distention from flatus (gas) in the intestines
   e. Overhydration
8. Which of the following nursing interventions is helpful in limiting a patient's fluid intake?
   a. Explaining the reasons for fluid restriction to the patient
   b. Providing 2,000 to 3,000 ml of IV fluid in 24 hours so the patient is not thirsty
   c. Providing as many ice chips or popsicles as the patient desires
   d. Letting the patient drink as much as desired until the fluid allotment for the day is consumed and then having the patient remain NPO
9. *True or False*
   _____ When discontinuing an IV, apply firm pressure over the vein while pulling the needle (catheter) out.
   _____ An IV flow can be shut off safely for several minutes to remove air from the tubing without risking clot formation in the needle.
   _____ The most serious complication of IV therapy is tissue edema near the needle site.
   _____ When the IV flow rate is being maintained by a pump, the risk of tissue edema and necrosis from vein perforation is reduced.
   _____ If a patient has an IV in the hand, the IV flow rate will tend to slow when the patient ambulates.

Answers

1. b
2. d

3. e
4. a
5. b
6. d
7. d
8. a
9. F, F, F, F, T

References and Bibliography

Aspinall, M.: A simplified guide to managing patients with hyponatremia. *Nursing 78*, **8**:32–35, Dec., 1978.

Baylan, A., and Marbach, B.: Dehydration: Subtle, sinister . . . preventable. *RN*, **42**:37–41, Aug., 1979.

Bodinski, L.: *The Nurse's Guide to Diet Therapy*. Wiley, New York, 1982.

Ellis, J.; Nowlis, E.; and Bentz, P.: *Modules for Basic Nursing Skills*, Vol. 2. Houghton Mifflin, Boston, 1984.

Guyton, A.: *Textbook of Medical Physiology*. Saunders, Philadelphia, 1981.

Hunt, S.; Groff, J.; and Holbrook, J.: *Nutrition: Principles and Clinical Practice*. Wiley, New York, 1980.

Keithley, J., and Fraulini, K.: What's behind that IV line? *Nursing 82*, **12**:33–42, Mar., 1982.

Kurdi, W.: *Modern Intravenous Therapy Procedures*. Medical Education Consultants, Los Angeles, 1978.

Menzel, L.: Clinical problems of fluid balance. *Nurs. Clin. North Am.*, **15**:549–58, Sept., 1980.

Metheny, N., and Snively, W. D.: *Nurse's Handbook of Fluid Balance*, 4th ed. Lippincott, Philadelphia, 1983.

Monitoring Fluid and Electrolytes Precisely. Intermed Communications, Horsham, Pa., 1978.

Rambo, B., and Wood. L.: *Nursing Skills for Clinical Practice*. Saunders, Philadelphia, 1982.

Roberts, A.: The posterior pituitary and water homeostasis. *Nurs. Times*, **76** (Feb. 7), Center Section, 1980.

Robinson, C., and Lawler, M.: *Normal and Therapeutic Nutrition*, 16th ed. Macmillan, New York, 1982.

Suitor, C., and Hunter, M.: *Nutrition: Principles and Application in Health Promotion*. Lippincott, Philadelphia, 1980.

Urrows, S.: Physiology of body fluids. *Nurs. Clin. North Am*, **15**:537–47, Sept., 1980.

Vander, A.; Sherman, J.; and Luciano, D.: *Human Physiology: The Mechanisms of Body Function*. McGraw-Hill, New York, 1980.

Zerwekh, J.: The dehydration question. *Nursing 83*, **13**:47–51, Jan., 1983.

CHAPTER 24

THE NEED FOR ELIMINATION*

Objectives

1. Explain the physiological need for elimination.
2. Describe the process of urine formation and excretion.
3. Describe the process of formation and excretion of feces.
4. Indicate factors that influence amount and pattern of waste elimination.
5. Explain how elimination is related to satisfaction of each of the other basic needs.
6. Describe briefly these common elimination problems: oliguria, constipation, fecal impaction, diarrhea, flatulence, obstruction, infection, incontinence, urinary retention, dysuria, hemorrhoids, and ostomies.
7. Identify data associated with normal urinary elimination.
8. Identify data related to normal intestinal elimination.

*Written by Mary E. Schuler Richards, R.N., M.S., an instructor in nursing at Normandale Community College, Bloomington, Minnesota, where she teaches various levels of the Associate Degree Nursing Program.

9. List data indicating urinary retention, constipation, diarrhea, fecal impaction, and intestinal distention.
10. State nursing interventions to promote normal elimination.
11. Describe nursing interventions for the relief of urinary retention.
12. Describe management of the indwelling catheter.
13. Present nursing measures for the treatment and prevention of constipation.
14. State indications for the use of laxatives, suppositories, and enemas.
14. Compare these enemas in regard to use, type of solution, and volume: cleansing, oil retention, carminative, return flow, and medicated.
16. Describe nursing interventions to assist in diarrhea, intestinal distention, incontinence, and hemorrhoids.
17. Describe the following nursing measures: collection of urine and stool specimens, assisting with a bedpan or urinal, catheter and bladder irrigation, digital removal of fecal impaction, insertion of a rectal tube, bowel and bladder retraining, and application of a condom catheter.
18. Explain nursing interventions to prevent elimination problems related to diagnostic tests, surgery, activity restrictions, and medications.
19. Demonstrate safe performance of these nursing techniques: obtaining a urine specimen from an indwelling catheter, measuring urinary output, measuring specific gravity, palpating the bladder, percussing the abdomen for distention, auscultating the abdomen for bowel sounds, inserting an indwelling catheter, irrigating an indwelling catheter, administering an enema, emptying an ostomy pouch.

Elimination as a Basic Human Need

The process of elimination provides for the body's need to get rid of surplus and undesirable substances. Some of these substances are ingested in amounts greater than needed by the body; others are produced in the body as the result of cell metabolism. If allowed to accumulate, these substances interfere with cell function and survival. Although the skin and lungs play a part in the removal of unnecessary substances, the main organs of elimination are the urinary and intestinal tracts. Most of the body's liquid wastes, consisting of water, end products of metabolism, and excess inorganic salts, are eliminated through the urinary tract. The intestinal tract, while excreting small amounts of end products and some water, primarily eliminates solid wastes, made up of bacteria and ingested materials not digested or absorbed by the body. Problems with elimination interfere with daily living and, in some cases, threaten life.

Normal Means for Meeting Urinary Elimination Needs

Under normal conditions, the amount of water lost from the body each day equals the water gained. Water occurs in the body as the result of its ingestion in foods and liquids and of metabolic processes of oxidation. Some water is lost from the body through the lungs, skin, and intestinal tract. Most excess water, however, is excreted through the urinary tract. The kidneys provide the main mechanism for maintaining fluid balance by eliminating or retaining water in accordance with the body's need. When large amounts of water are ingested, the kidneys excrete large amounts in the urine. When little water is taken in, or large amounts are lost through heavy sweating, heavy breathing, vomiting, or diarrhea, the kidneys produce a small amount of concentrated urine. The amount of urine excreted each day can vary from as much as 25 liters (about 26 qt), when water intake is extremely high, to as little as 400 ml (about 1⅔ cup) when there is a need to conserve water (Vander *et al.*, 1980).

Structure of the Urinary Tract

The urinary tract consists of the kidneys, ureters, bladder, and urethra. (See Figure 24–1.) Urine is formed in the kidneys and passes through the ureters into the bladder. It is stored in the bladder until, at intervals, it is eliminated from the body through the urethra.

The two kidneys are located at the back of the abdominal cavity on either side of the spinal column, just above the waistline. They are bean-shaped, about 4 inches long, and held in place by fat and connective tis-

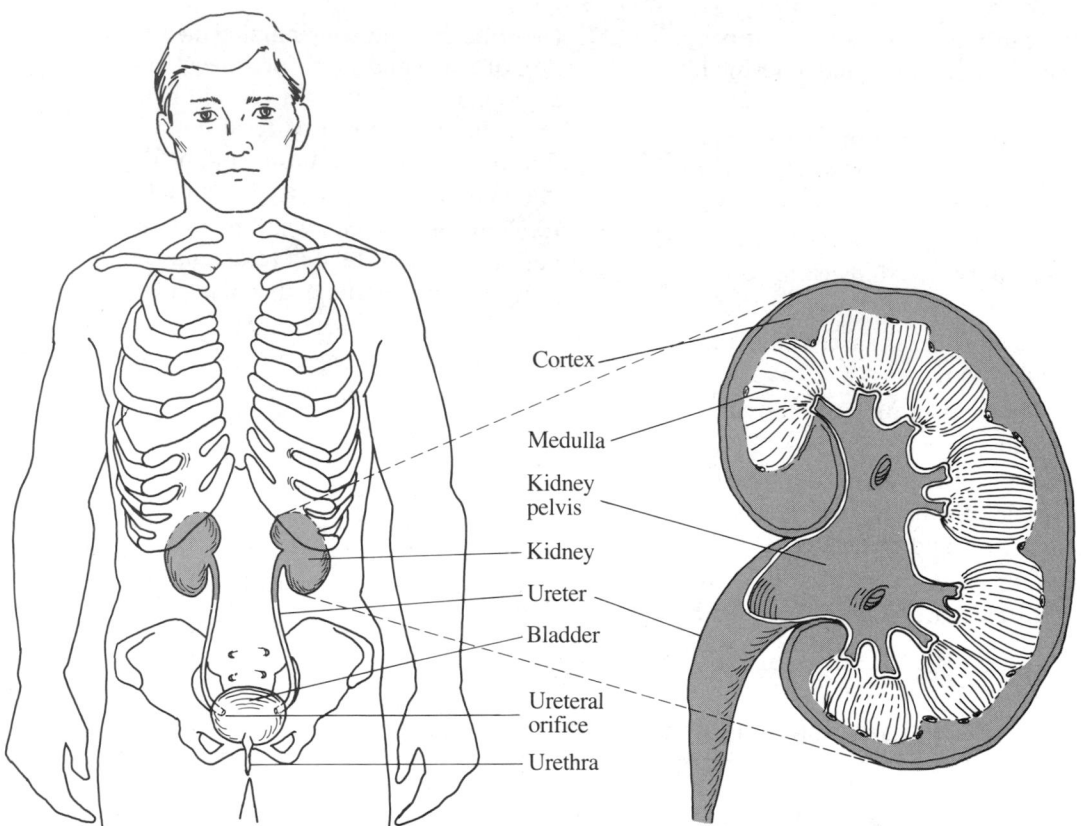

Cortex

Medulla

Kidney pelvis

Kidney

Ureter

Bladder

Ureteral orifice

Urethra

Figure 24–1. Structures of the urinary system. (Adapted from F. Strand: *Physiology: A Regulatory Systems Approach*. Macmillan, New York, 1978, p. 274.)

sue. Each kidney has an outer portion called the *cortex*, an inner portion, the *medulla*, and a central collection area, the *pelvis*.

The functional units of the kidneys are known as *nephrons*. Each of the one million nephrons in each kidney consists of a cluster of capillaries (the *glomerulus*) and a tubule (see Figure 24–2). The tubule originates as a sac (Bowman's capsule) encasing the capillary cluster. It winds through the kidney tissue and ends in the collecting tubule, which empties into the kidney pelvis. The nephrons are situated in the kidney so that the cortex contains the glomeruli, while the medulla is made up of the collecting tubules.

Continuous with the kidney pelves are the ureters, tubes of smooth muscle 25 to 30 cm (10 to 12 inches) in length. The two ureters enter the back of the bladder on either side. The bladder, a distensible sac of smooth muscle, can expand to hold as much as 2 liters (about 2 qt) or more, although its usual capacity is 200 to 500 ml (about 1 to 2 cups). At its lower end, the bladder connects to the urethra, a narrow tube leading to the exterior of the body. In the adult female, the urethra is 3 to 5 cm (1½ to 2 inches) in length; in the male, it is about 20 cm (8 inches). The opening of the urethra to the outside of the body is called the *meatus*.

Muscle fibers at the juncture of the bladder and urethra form the internal urethral sphincter, which remains tightly closed to hold urine in the bladder. A second sphincter, the external urethral sphincter, reinforces this function. It is located in the urethra, just below the prostate gland in males (see Figure 24–3) and at approximately midurethra in females.

Formation of Urine

Approximately 1,700 liters of blood enter the kidneys each day. This blood is channeled through the glomeruli, where 125 ml per minute are filtered into Bowman's capsules. The fluid filtered from the blood (*glomerular filtrate*) has the same composition as blood plasma, except that it contains almost no protein. The plasma proteins are, for the most part, too large to pass through the pores of the glomerular capillaries and remain in the blood vessels.

As the glomerular filtrate flows through the twisting tubules, its composition is continuously altered. Substances needed by the body are reabsorbed into the blood. These include water, sodium chloride and other electrolytes, glucose, urea, creatinine, and amino acids.

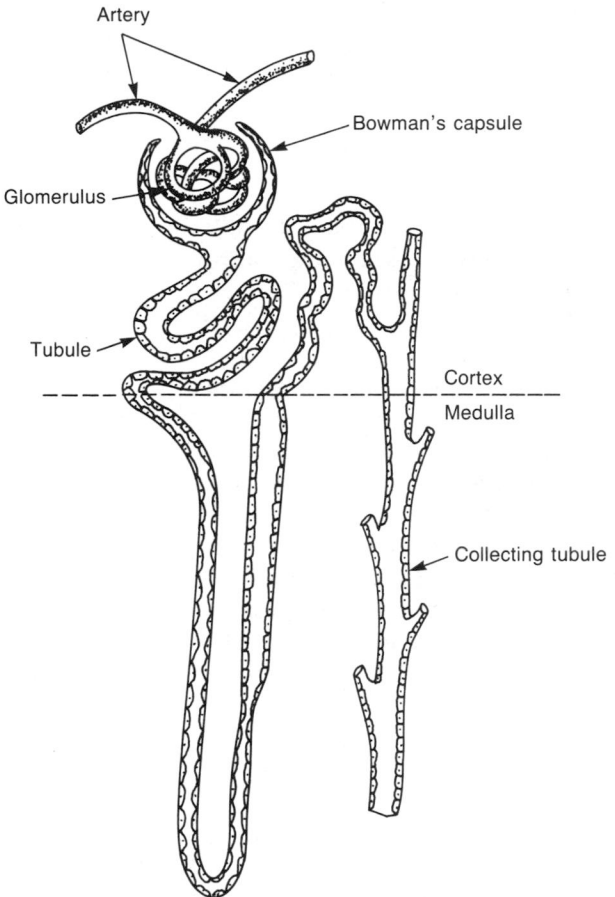

Figure 24-2. The nephron. (Adapted from F. Strand: *Physiology: A Regulatory Systems Approach.* Macmillan, New York, 1978, p. 275.)

In addition, substances in excess supply in the body are secreted from the blood into the tubules for excretion. Secreted substances include potassium, hydrogen ions, ammonia, and foreign substances such as drugs and poisons. By the time the filtrate reaches the collecting tubules, about 99 percent of the water has been reabsorbed. Thus, from a total filtered volume of about 180 liters per day, there remains only about 1½ liters each day which reaches the kidney pelvis to be excreted as urine.

Transport and Storage of Urine

From the kidney pelvis, urine flows through the ureters into the bladder, propelled by wavelike contractions of the ureteral walls. The frequency of these waves is increased by parasympathetic stimulation and decreased by sympathetic stimulation. A fold of membrane forms a valve at each ureter's entrance to the bladder. These valves prevent the backflow (*reflux*) of urine into the ureters during contraction of the bladder. The urine collects in the bladder and is stored there until, at intervals, it is discharged from the body through the urethra.

Normal Micturition

Micturition means the process of emptying the urinary bladder. Other terms for this process are *urination* and *voiding*. Slang terms referring to this process abound and may need to be used if the patient is to un-

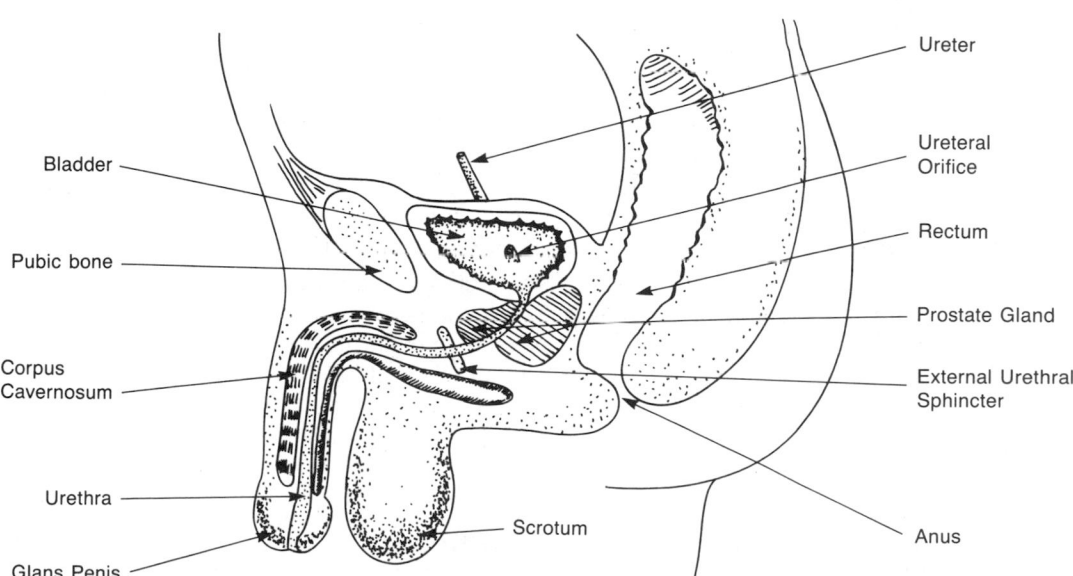

Figure 24-3. The male bladder, urethra, and surrounding structures. (Adapted from F. Strand: *Physiology: A Regulatory Systems Approach.* Macmillan, New York, 1978, p. 512.)

derstand the nurse's communication related to the need to void. Parents often invent terms to use with their children. These terms should be documented in the care plan to facilitate communication about this process with the pediatric patient.

The bladder muscle is supplied with parasympathetic nerves, stimulation of which causes the bladder to contract. When there is little urine in the bladder, these nerves are inactive, allowing the bladder muscle to remain relaxed. When relaxed, the lower portion of the bladder, which forms the internal urethral sphincter, remains closed, preventing the escape of urine. Meanwhile, muscles of the external urethral sphincter are maintained in a state of contraction, causing this sphincter to remain closed also. As urine accumulates to a volume of about 200 to 500 ml in the adult, stretch receptors (nerve endings sensitive to stretch) in the bladder wall are stimulated. They send impulses to the spinal cord which activate the micturition reflex. This reflex, if permitted its course, results in urination. It produces parasympathetic stimulation which contracts the bladder. Contraction changes the shape of the bladder, pulling open the internal sphincter, and permitting urine to enter the urethra. The presence of urine in the urethra stimulates the external sphincter to relax and voiding occurs.

The micturition reflex can be suppressed by the person who has learned to control voiding. At the same time that the stretch receptors transmit impulses to the spinal cord, signals are sent to the higher centers in the brain. The person recognizes the urge to void, but can consciously contract the external sphincter to delay urination. When a micturition reflex is suppressed, the bladder contractions die out. With continued filling of the bladder, however, the micturition reflex returns again and again, and each time the urge to void is more powerful. When the time for urination becomes appropriate, the person can consciously initiate a micturition reflex by relaxing the external sphincter.

Regulation of Urinary Elimination

Fluid and Dietary Intake.   The major determinant of the amount of urine produced and the frequency of urination is the amount and frequency of fluid intake. Some fluids, such as coffee, tea, and alcoholic beverages, have a *diuretic* effect, that is, they increase the amount of urine produced in excess of the amount taken in. Salty fluids and foods may decrease urine production because their osmotic effect tends to hold fluids in the body. A high dietary intake of protein may increase the amount of urine eliminated since the end products of protein metabolism require plentiful amounts of water for their excretion.

Neural Influences.   Neural influences on urine production include those related to the control of blood volume and pressure and to stress. Changes in blood volume and blood pressure stimulate nerve endings sensitive to stretch (baroreceptors) in the walls of the heart and blood vessels. Impulses are transmitted to the medulla in the brain. The medulla transmits messages through the sympathetic nervous system to the kidneys. When blood volume and pressure are high, the kidneys increase the amount of fluid excreted in the urine. Conversely, when blood volume and pressure are low, the kidneys retain fluids. Stimulation of the sympathetic nervous system in states of stress or anxiety may increase urine production as a result of the increased blood pressure and rate of circulation through the nephrons.

Hormonal Influences.   Antidiuretic hormone (ADH) prevents *diuresis*, the rapid excretion of abnormally large amounts of urine. It does this by increasing the amount of water reabsorbed into the blood from the kidney tubules. ADH is secreted by the posterior pituitary gland in response to a low blood volume or to an increased concentration of solutes in the body fluids (increased osmolality). When blood volume gets low, or body fluids become too concentrated, volume receptors in the heart and vessels or osmoreceptors in the hypothalamus stimulate the posterior pituitary to produce more ADH. This ADH, in turn, stimulates the kidney tubules to reabsorb more water, thereby returning the blood volume and concentration to normal. On the other hand, when blood volume is increased or body fluids are diluted, little ADH is produced, and more water is excreted in the urine.

Aldosterone is another hormone that affects urine production. Produced in the adrenal cortex, aldosterone stimulates the reabsorption of sodium by the kidney. Sodium excreted in the urine carries water with it. By retaining sodium, the body is also able to retain enough water to meet its fluid needs. The more aldosterone secreted, the smaller the amount of urine eliminated, and vice versa.

Normal Means for Meeting Intestinal Elimination Needs

Solid wastes are eliminated from the body through the lower part of the intestinal tract. This portion of the tract is called the large intestine, the large *bowel*, or the *colon*.

Structure of the Large Intestine

The large intestine is a tube about 5 ft long and 2½ inches in diameter. Its walls are made up of two layers of smooth muscle, lined with mucosa, and well supplied with nerves. It begins at the *ileum* (last and major portion of the small intestine) and ends in the *anus* (the opening to the outside of the body). The large bowel consists of the cecum, ascending colon, transverse colon, descending colon, rectum, and anus. (See Figure 24-4.) The *ileocecal*, or *ileocolic*, valve is a fold of membrane between the ileum and the colon which controls the passage of chyme.

The last part of the colon, the *rectum*, is approximately 13 cm (5 inches) long in the adult. Its end (distal) portion, about 2.5 cm (1 inch), is the *anal canal*, which terminates at the anus. Two sphincters control the exit from the body. The internal sphincter, consisting of smooth, involuntary muscle, is located within the anal canal. The external sphincter, made up of voluntary muscle, is at the anus.

Formation of Feces

The function of the colon is to concentrate the chyme into a more solid mass and to store it until it is expelled from the body. About 750 ml of chyme each day enter the colon from the ileum. By the time the chyme reaches the colon, most of the nutrients have already been digested and absorbed. The colon absorbs most of the remaining water, sodium, and chlorides. This absorption is facilitated by churning movements which gradually expose all of the waste material to the colon surface. Periodic propulsive movements of the colon advance the waste through the tract. By the time it reaches the descending colon, all but about 150 to 200 ml of the chyme have been reabsorbed. The material is now semisolid and is called *feces* or *stool*.

Contained in the feces are undigested food residue, bacteria, debris sloughed from the intestinal lining, dried constituents of digestive juices, bile pigments, and a small amount of salts. The characteristic odor is the result of gases produced by bacterial fermentation of the food residue. Approximately 400 to 700 cc of gas are produced in the colon and expelled from the anus each day.

Transport and Storage of Solid Wastes

The ileocecal valve is normally closed, slowing or blocking the flow of chyme into the colon. This extends the time available for the absorption of nutrients in the small intestine. After a meal, food moving from the stomach into the duodenum stimulates increased peristalsis throughout the small intestine. With each peristaltic wave of the ileum, the ileocecal valve relaxes, and chyme is pushed into the colon. Backflow from the cecum to the ileum is prevented by the structure of the valve.

Transport of chyme through the colon is accomplished by periodic propulsive movements called *mass movements*. In mass movements, colon contents are moved one-third to three-fourths the length of the colon in a few seconds' time (Vander *et al.*, 1980). These movements result from the *gastrocolic* reflex (nervous stimulation of colonic movements initiated by the emptying of gastric contents into the duodenum).

Mass movements occur three or four times a day, primarily after meals, or on arising from sleep. They usually last for 10 to 30 minutes. With mass movements, stool is advanced into the lower portion of the descending colon, the *sigmoid* colon, where it is stored until another mass movement propels it into the rectum for excretion from the body. Movement of stool through the colon is facilitated by the secretion of mucus which lubricates the fecal mass. Fecal material passes through the colon in about eight hours to several days. Transit time varies with the individual's bowel habits and with the amount and type of foods eaten. The longer feces remain in the colon, the more water is absorbed. This can eventually lead to the formation of hard, dry stools which are difficult to pass, a condition known as *constipation*.

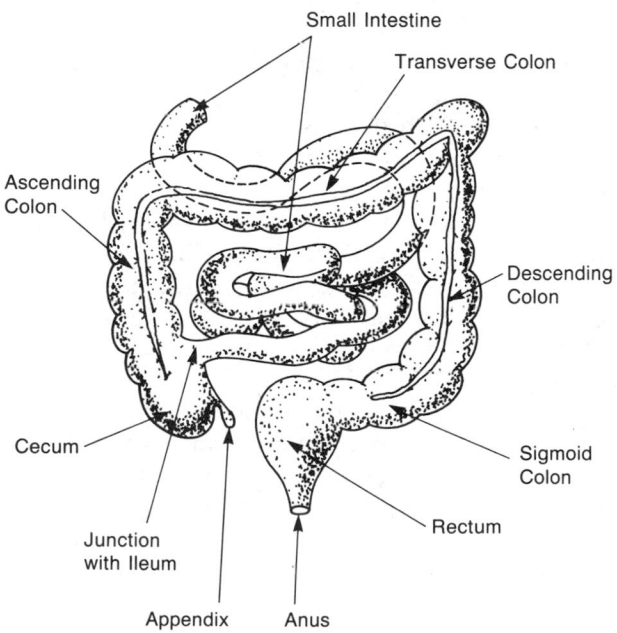

Figure 24-4. The large intestine. (Adapted from F. Strand: *Physiology: A Regulatory Systems Approach.* Macmillan, New York, 1978, p. 333.)

Normal Defecation

The rectum is usually empty until just before *defecation* (the process of expelling feces from the body). Feces propelled into the rectum by a mass movement distend the rectum, activating stretch receptors in the rectal walls. Nerve impulses are transmitted to the spinal cord and to motor nerves in the colon walls, activating the *defecation reflex*. This reflex causes contraction of the rectum, relaxation of the internal sphincter, and further contractions of the descending colon. If the external sphincter is concurrently relaxed, the feces are propelled through the anus and out of the body. Defecation is usually assisted by voluntary closure of the glottis following a deep breath and contraction of the diaphragm and abdominal muscles. This increases the pressure on the colon contents, facilitating expulsion. In addition, contraction of the levator ani muscle of the perineum lifts the pelvic floor upward over the feces, assisting in its elimination.

Since the external sphincter is under voluntary control, defecation can be consciously inhibited. At the same time that nerve impulses are being transmitted from the distended rectum to the colon walls and spinal cord, impulses are also sent to the brain. The person recognizes the urge to defecate, but can choose to delay defecation by contracting the external sphincter. If defecation does not proceed, the defecation reflex gradually subsides. It does not recur until another mass movement propels more feces into the rectum, once again stimulating the stretch receptors.

Regulation of Intestinal Elimination

Nervous control of the intestines is supplied by the myenteric plexus, a network of nerve fibers within the muscular layers of the intestine, as well as by the sympathetic and parasympathetic nervous systems. The myenteric plexus transmits peristaltic waves along the tract and is responsible for transmitting the gastrocolic reflex. In general, stimulation of the sympathetic nervous system inhibits intestinal motility, causing a slowdown of peristalsis and less frequent elimination. Parasympathetic stimulation, on the other hand, increases intestinal motility, its excessive stimulation leading to frequent, watery stools (*diarrhea*).

Relationship of Other Basic Needs to Elimination

Fluid Need

When the body's fluid balance is low, blood flow through the kidneys is reduced, decreasing the filtration of water and wastes into the nephrons; therefore, the kidneys are less effective in removing wastes from the body. The kidneys' ability to function is also diminished by the decreased blood flow to the kidney tissue. An additional effect of low fluid intake on urinary elimination is infrequent emptying of the bladder. This increases the incidence of urinary tract infections in susceptible individuals since stagnant urine provides a medium for bacterial growth. Intestinal elimination is also compromised by a low fluid intake. In dehydration, the body attempts to compensate for the low fluid level by reabsorbing more water from the feces in the colon. Although this improves the internal fluid balance, it has the disadvantage of producing hard, dry stools which are difficult to pass.

Individuals experiencing incontinence or painful urination tend to restrict fluid intake in an attempt to limit the frequency of urination. The feeling of fullness accompanying constipation may deter a person from drinking adequate amounts of fluid.

Nutrition Need

Intestinal elimination is closely related to food intake. Lack of fiber in the diet results in less bulk of the waste materials, therefore, slower passage through the intestinal tract and a greater tendency for constipation. An irregular meal schedule also increases the probability of constipation since it hinders the development of a regular pattern of mass movements of the colon. Malnutrition leads to poor muscle tone, which reduces the individual's ability to efficiently expel urine and feces, and to poor nervous control, which reduces the individual's command of sphincter muscles. Additionally, malnutrition reduces resistance to urinary and intestinal infections.

Appetite is decreased in the presence of elimination problems such as infection, pain, constipation, and gaseous distention (*flatulence*). Distention and inflammation interfere with the digestion of food. Persons with diarrhea may be reluctant to eat since the ingestion of food stimulates peristalsis, increasing the frequency of defecation. The individual with diarrhea may be temporarily restricted to clear liquids only or nothing by mouth to reduce the number of stools.

Oxygenation Need

A lack of oxygen to the kidneys and intestine, depending upon the degree, can lead to diminished function or destruction of tissue. Complete kidney failure is a frequent consequence of severe shock. Kidney failure can also result from prolonged hypertension. Individuals who are short of breath from whatever cause may delay or limit trips to the bathroom because of fatigue with even minimal exertion. This disruption of normal elimination patterns may lead to increases in retention of urine, infection, and constipation. Use of the Valsalva maneuver in attempts to expel hard stool can precipitate a stroke or heart attack in the susceptible individual.

Temperature Maintenance

Elimination is affected in the person who has a fever. Although more fluid is produced in the body during fever as a result of the increased metabolic rate, the urinary output tends to be low because excessive water is lost as exhaled water vapor, insensible evaporation from the skin, and perspiration. The potential for constipation increases in fever due to anorexia, general muscle weakness, and the decrease in body fluids.

Sleep

An irregular sleep schedule prohibits regular times for meals and elimination. Persons whose work requires frequent changes between day and night shifts often find it difficult to maintain elimination patterns. Sleep and rest may be disturbed by frequent urination at night (*nocturia*), the inability to control urination or defecation (*incontinence*), or diarrhea.

Pain Avoidance

Pain interferes with the maintenance of regular elimination. It is difficult for the individual in pain to eat a balanced diet, to get the exercise necessary for maintaining good muscle tone, and to relax the sphincters involved in defecation or urination. Energy and strength are sapped by pain, diminishing that available to walk to the bathroom or to expel stool. Walking to the bathroom or trying to use a bedpan or urinal may aggravate existing pain, leading the individual to delay voiding and defecation urges as long as possible. Pain associated with the passage of urine or stool leads to infrequent elimination and possibly to urinary retention or consti-

pation. The person who has pain from abdominal surgery will hesitate to contract the abdominal muscles to assist in defecation. Perineal pain may inhibit the ability to relax the external sphincters. Some medications used to decrease pain also reduce intestinal motility, thus increasing the potential for constipation and abdominal distention.

Exercise

Physical activity promotes muscle strength and stimulates peristalsis. Weak muscles of the diaphragm, abdomen, and pelvis are less effective than well-toned muscles in applying pressure to the abdominal contents to aid in defecation or in providing sphincter control. The sluggish peristalsis associated with inadequate exercise contributes to constipation. Lack of exercise also reduces blood flow to the kidneys, so urinary wastes are not as efficiently eliminated. The extreme activity limitations of bed rest prohibit the normal positions for defecation and voiding. Drainage of urine from the kidneys to the bladder is slowed, increasing the potential for infection and kidney stone formation.

Bowel and bladder problems often interfere with satisfaction of the need for exercise. Activity is avoided when it stimulates diarrhea or urinary or fecal incontinence. Exercise may also be avoided for fear of dislodging tubes, bags, or pads for the collection of urine or feces.

Psychosocial Needs

Emotional states affect elimination patterns. Much importance is attached by society to having privacy for elimination. This requirement is learned from early childhood, and situations where the sights, sounds, and odors of elimination are apparent to others are embarrassing for the individual. Hospitalized persons may experience embarrassment and difficulty in relaxing sphincters when a curtain around the bed is the only provision for privacy. A patient who needs assistance may void less frequently or delay defecation because of embarrassment in asking for assistance. At times, a person may delay elimination because of reluctance to draw attention to the reason for leaving a group or activity.

The control of bowel and bladder function is a highly valued skill, and loss of competence is this area leads to a decrease in self-esteem. Elimination problems are often accompanied by soiled clothing, odors, and interrupted activities. Individuals who experience these difficulties tend to reduce the potential for embarrassment by avoiding other people. This severely limits social interactions, sexual activity, and the feeling of being loved and accepted.

Stress may increase or decrease the frequency of both urination and defecation, depending upon individual response. In some individuals, the heightened awareness associated with the stress response intensifies sensitivity to the urge to void, increasing the frequency of urination. In others, the generalized muscle tension inhibits relaxation of the sphincters, hindering urination. Stress increases peristalsis in some individuals, decreases it in others.

Stress may cause children who were previously toilet trained to revert to urinary and bowel incontinence. This behavior is an attempt to gain additional support from others while trying to cope with the stressful situation. Incontinence of urine may occur with fear in some individuals, especially children. Depression, which slows peristalsis along with other body processes, predisposes to constipation.

Common Urinary and Intestinal Problems

Problems with Formation of Wastes

Anuria is the absence of urine production by the kidneys. The term is applied when urine production is less than 100 ml per day. Normal daily production is about 1,500 ml. Anuria is the result of kidney failure, or renal shutdown, the causes of which include kidney disease, urinary tract obstructions, and any conditions that severely decrease blood flow to the kidneys, such as hemorrhage or shock. Renal shutdown can be fatal if untreated.

Oliguria refers to the production of diminished amounts of urine, about 100 to 500 ml per day. It may progress to anuria and stems from the same causes.

Polyuria, also referred to as diuresis, is the production and elimination of excessive amounts of urine. It is the result of kidney disease, systemic diseases such as diabetes mellitus, or hormonal imbalances, such as occur after childbirth or with inadequate ADH production. Polyuria may be accompanied by dehydration and excessive thirst.

Problems with Transport and Storage of Wastes

Constipation. In constipation, stools are very hard and difficult to pass. The consistency of the stool rather than the frequency of defecation is the main determinant of constipation, since some individuals have only one or two bowel movements a week, but have stools that are soft and passed with ease. Although the retention of stool may be accompanied by headache, anorexia, and a feeling of fullness, it does not result in the reabsorption of harmful toxins and has been known to continue for long periods without causing illness.

Common causes of constipation, in addition to the lack of fluids, fiber, and exercise previously mentioned, are irregular defecation habits, overuse of laxatives, and neuromuscular effects of aging, injury, or disease. When the urge to defecate is consistently ignored, perhaps because of inconvenience or discomfort, the nerve endings in the rectum become less responsive to the presence of stool. Defecation reflexes become progressively weaker and less frequent and eventually cease to occur.

The overuse of laxatives or enemas leads to the development of chronic constipation in many people. Laxatives and enemas empty the colon more completely than a normal bowel movement, so after their use, a longer than normal period of time is required for feces to again reach the rectum. With this delay in the next bowel movement, the individual, fearing a recurrence of constipation, repeats the laxative or enema. Thus begins a cycle in which normal defecation reflexes do not occur since distention of the rectum is never permitted. Constipation occurs in the elderly and in individuals with neuromuscular disorders because their weakened muscles are less effective in expelling stool, and deterioration of nervous stimulation to the bowel slows peristalsis.

Continued constipation leads to the accumulation of hardened feces in the rectum. The mass continues to lose water and becomes increasingly hard. Fecal material collects behind it until, ultimately, the mass becomes too hard and too large to pass through the anal canal. This condition is called *fecal impaction*. The chief indicator of fecal impaction is the passage of watery stools from the rectum in the absence of any normal stools. The fecal mass blocks the exit of formed stool, and only the liquid is able to seep past the obstruction.

Diarrhea. Diarrhea is the frequent passage of liquid or unformed stool. It results primarily from the passage of wastes through the intestinal tract too rapidly for the absorption of the normal amounts of water. It is usually accompanied by cramping pain in the abdomen and by difficulty in controlling the urge to defecate.

Diarrhea may be caused by infections, in which irritation of the intestinal mucosa stimulates the increase of both motility and secretions. This mechanism serves to protect the body by flushing out the offending agent. Traveler's diarrhea results from exposure to microorganisms to which the individual has not developed an immunity. Irritation of the mucosa also results from some foods, beverages, and medications. Stress causes diarrhea in some individuals. Prolonged diarrhea results in fatigue, weakness, weight loss, and dehydration. The large loss of water and electrolytes can be extremely dangerous, especially to the very young and the very old.

Flatulence.   An excessive amount of gas in the stomach or intestines is known as flatulence. Gas in the gastrointestinal tract, *flatus*, normally occurs as the result of swallowed air or bacterial decomposition of food. Most of the swallowed air is expelled from the stomach by belching (*eructation*). The rest passes along the intestinal tract where, along with the gas produced in the tract, it is either absorbed or expelled through the anus.

Increased swallowing of air may occur with eating rapidly, chewing gum, drinking through a straw, or hyperventilating due to pain or anxiety. Increased gas production occurs with the ingestion of foods whose decomposition produces large amounts of gas, for example, beans, onions, and cabbage, or when foods are not thoroughly digested as in diarrhea or individual food intolerances.

Interferences with gas absorption or movement lead to accumulation within the bowel. With increasing accumulation, the intestinal lumen fills with gas and expands, creating a condition called *intestinal distention* or *abdominal distention*. The abdomen becomes swollen, firm, and uncomfortable. Interferences with peristalsis and gas movement most commonly result from abdominal surgery, certain medications, or decreased activity.

Obstruction.   Obstruction, which can occur in either the urinary or intestinal tract, is a blockage that prevents passage of the waste materials. Tumors are a frequent cause of obstruction. They may block a tube by growing within the lumen or by pressing on the tube from the outside. Tubes may also be blocked by swelling due to inflammation or trauma, or by tight bands of scar tissue (*adhesions*). Partial obstructions may be caused by *strictures*, which are constricted or narrowed areas of a tube. Strictures are due to congenital malformations, infections, trauma, or scarring. Stone formation (*lithiasis*) causes obstruction of the urinary tract when the stones (*calculi*) become lodged in the kidney pelvis, ureter, or urethra. In men over the age of 50, ure-

thral obstruction frequently occurs as the result of *prostatic hypertrophy*. In this condition, the prostate gland, which surrounds the male urethra at its exit from the bladder (See Figure 24-3), becomes enlarged, pressing inward on the urethral lumen and obstructing the flow of urine.

Functional obstruction may occur in either the urinary or intestinal tract. In this condition, there is no mechanical blockage but rather a failure of the nerves to stimulate the muscle contractions necessary to move waste materials along the tract. Functional obstruction results from irritation or trauma to the nerves, as from toxins or manipulation during surgery, which causes temporary cessation of peristalsis. It may also be present in neurological disorders.

Obstructions produce distention of the tube above the blockage, as wastes, secretions, and gases collect and swelling develops. The area becomes prone to infection. Pressure on the blood vessels in the walls of the system leads to impaired circulation and possibly ischemia and necrosis. Pain is usually severe. In urinary tract obstructions, the prolonged pressure of the backed-up urine permanently damages the kidney. Also, the pool of stagnant urine increases the potential for infection and for stone formation. In the intestinal tract, obstruction may lead to rupture of the wall, resulting in leakage of fecal material into the sterile abdominal cavity. Life-threatening infection results.

Problems with Infections and Inflammations

Urinary Infections and Inflammations.   Except at the lower end of the urethra, the urinary tract is normally free of microorganisms. Bacteria that ascend into the bladder are flushed out with urination or are destroyed, apparently by antibacterial characteristics of the bladder lining and the urine. An infection arises when pathogens overcome the body's resistance. Urinary infections may result from pathogens carried through the blood or lymph vessels, but are most commonly caused by organisms ascending through the urethra. Causative organisms for urinary tract infections are generally those found in the colon. They are part of the normal flora in the colon, but cause infection in the sterile urinary tract.

Urinary infections are named for the portion of the tract in which they occur. Infection of the urethra is called *urethritis*, of the bladder, *cystitis*, and of the kidney pelvis, *pyelonephritis*. An infection of any part is likely to spread to the others, traveling along the continuous mucous membrane which lines the entire tract. Women are more likely than men to contract urinary tract infections. This is mainly due to the short female urethra and the nearness of the meatus to the anus.

Complete or partial obstructions to the flow of urine, for example, strictures, stones, or pregnancy, increase the potential for *urinary tract infection (UTI)*. Urine remaining in the bladder becomes more alkaline, providing a better growth medium for bacteria than more recently produced urine with a more acid pH. Pressure of the retained urine on the bladder walls restricts blood flow, increasing their susceptibility to infection.

Inflammations of the urinary tract occur along with infections, but may also result from trauma, bacterial toxins, chemicals, or obstructions. Glomerulonephritis and nephrosis are examples of kidney inflammations. Both infections and inflammations, if not treated, can lead to permanent kidney damage and renal failure. Symptoms of cystitis and urethritis may include burning on urination, a frequent and urgent need to void, and small amounts of blood in the urine. Kidney infections and inflammations may be accompanied by anorexia, fatigue, fever, edema, flank pain, and cloudy urine.

Intestinal Infections and Inflammations. Infection of the bowel generally results from ingestion of the offending organism. It is accompanied by pain, fever, and diarrhea, which may progress to dehydration and electrolyte imbalance as bowel function is compromised. Typhoid fever and dysentery are examples of intestinal infections. Antibiotic therapy may destroy the normal bacteria in the bowel, leaving it more susceptible to infection from other organisms.

Inflammation of the colon may be due to infection, trauma, obstruction, or disease processes. Ulcerative colitis and Crohn's disease are types of bowel inflammation. Symptoms, in addition to those of infection, include colicky pain and possibly the passage of blood and large amounts of mucus. Inflammation can lead to malabsorption, weakness, hemorrhage, abscesses, and *fistulas* (abnormal openings between two body organs or surfaces).

Problems with Excretion

Incontinence. Incontinence is the inability to control urination or defecation. It usually results from weakened or damaged sphincters, disorders of the nervous system, or altered awareness of the elimination urges. In the elderly, a common cause is fecal impaction. Incontinence may be a chronic problem or occur temporarily in infections or emotional states such as acute fear or anger.

Urinary incontinence takes many forms. In *reflex incontinence*, which occurs in some neurological disorders, the bladder empties automatically when it fills to a certain point, or when other stimuli produce a micturition reflex. In *overflow incontinence*, or *retention with overflow*, the bladder retains relatively large amounts of urine at all times. As more urine enters the bladder, the pressure is increased to the point where it forces a small amount of urine out through the external sphincter. The amount is just enough (usually less than 50 ml) to reduce the pressure within the bladder to its previous level, at which point the sphincter is again able to remain closed. Causes of overflow incontinence include urethral obstruction or impaired nervous control of the bladder and sphincters.

Stress incontinence is that which occurs with an increase in intra-abdominal pressure. Coughing, sneezing, laughing, or lifting may cause this type of incontinence in the person with weakened sphincters. It is most prevalent in women who have had several pregnancies, or men who have had prostate surgery. *Urge incontinence* occurs when the desire to void is so urgent that micturition results before the individual can reach the toilet. Frequent causes are bladder spasms or infections of the bladder or urethra.

Enuresis is a general term meaning involuntary urination, but it is frequently used more specifically to refer to urinary incontinence while sleeping (bedwetting). It may result from urethral or bladder irritation, excessive fluid intake, neurological conditions, emotional disturbances, or very deep sleep patterns. It may occur in the elderly as an effect of decreased muscle tone which reduces sphincter control.

In fecal incontinence, stool is evacuated with each defecation reflex. As with normal defecation, incontinent stools are most likely to occur after meals, at the time of mass movements of the colon. They also occur irregularly, especially with activity or position changes. The incidence of fecal incontinence is higher when stools are very loose.

Retention. In urinary retention, urine is produced normally by the kidneys but is not excreted from the bladder. As urine accumulates, the bladder becomes distended and can be felt as a firm, rounded protuberance of the lower abdomen. Temporary retention occurs when trauma and its resultant swelling obstruct the urethra. This kind of retention sometimes follows childbirth or surgery to the lower abdomen, bladder, urethra, or perineum. Obstructions that, without treatment, may lead to permanent retention are tumors, strictures, scarring, some urinary stones, and prostatic hypertrophy. Long-term retention is also produced when the micturition reflex is blocked by spinal cord injuries or other nervous disorders.

In some cases of retention, the amount and frequency of voiding appear normal, but the bladder fails to empty completely. Urine remaining in the bladder immediately after voiding is called *residual urine*. Normally, this amount is less than 3 ml, but in urinary retention, amounts can be several hundred milliliters or more. Extreme distention may rupture the bladder.

Discomfort and Difficulty. Painful or difficult urination is called *dysuria*. A burning sensation often accompanies voiding in infections or lesions of the bladder or urethra. Difficulty voiding, with or without discomfort, may result from partial obstruction of the urethra or neurological impairment. *Hesitancy* is the term that refers to a delay or difficulty in initiating urination. Hesitancy often accompanies infections or enlargement of the prostate gland. Straining or forceful contraction of the abdominal muscles may sometimes be necessary to expel urine from the bladder or hard stool from the rectum. Pain with defecation most commonly accompanies constipation or hemorrhoids, which are discussed below.

Hemorrhoids. Hemorrhoids are distended, tortuous veins (varicose veins) of the rectum or anus. They result from increased pressure in the veins, such as occurs with prolonged sitting, the passage of hard stools, or pregnancy and childbirth. Hemorrhoids may be internal or external. Internally, they appear within the rectum where they are usually painless, but may bleed with the passage of stool. External hemorrhoids appear as swollen protrusions of tissue in or around the anus. Because

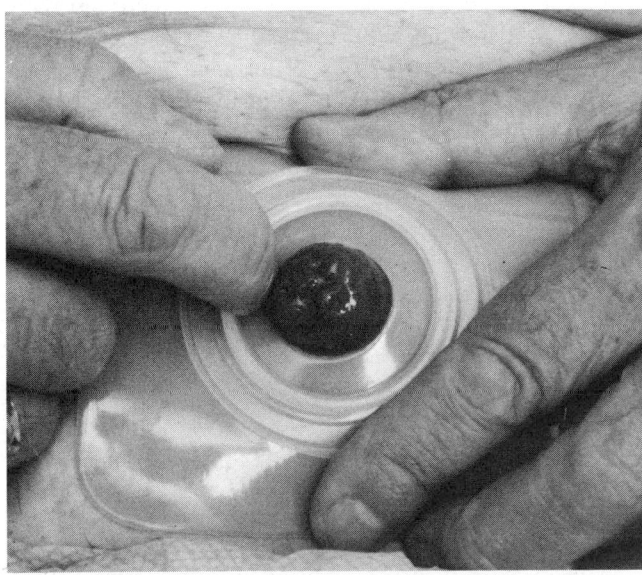

Figure 24-5. A colostomy stoma. A collecton pouch is being applied to this colostomy by the patient. (Photograph courtesy of the Sur-Fit System, Convatec; E. R. Squibb and Son, Inc. Princeton, N.J.)

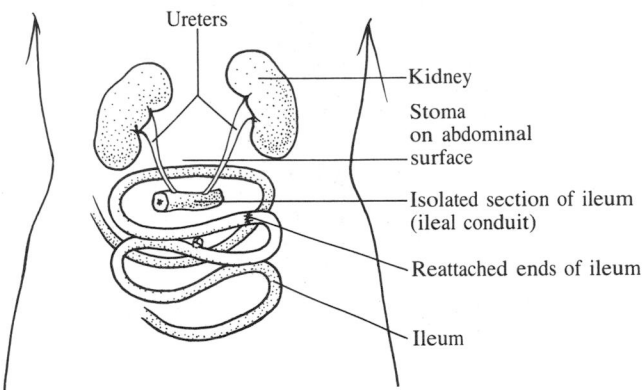

Figure 24-6. Diagram of an ileal conduit.

the anus is more plentifully supplied with nerves than the rectum, external hemorrhoids tend to produce itching and pain, sometimes of a severe nature. External hemorrhoids may obscure the opening of the anus making it difficult for the nurse to identify the site for insertion of a thermometer, rectal tube, or suppository. These procedures may also be extremely painful for the patient.

Alternate Routes of Excretion. In some individuals, wastes are not excreted through the urinary meatus or the anus, but are diverted through a surgically created outlet called an *ostomy*. An ostomy is created by suturing a part of the urinary or intestinal tract to the abdominal wall and creating an opening to the outside of the body. The opening itself is referred to as a *stoma*. The stoma may appear simply as a slit in the skin. Usually, however, it is surrounded by a circle of mucosa which has been turned back and sutured to the skin, forming a smooth, reddish doughnut-shaped protuberance. (See Figure 24-5.)

An opening from the ileum is called an *ileostomy*, from the colon, a *colostomy*. An ostomy which drains urine is a *urostomy*. The most common type of urostomy is the *ileal conduit*, in which urine drains from the ureters into a surgically created pouch of ileal tissue and out of the body through an abdominal stoma. (See Figure 26-6.)

Ostomies may be located in various areas of the abdomen, depending upon the section of the intestine involved. (See Figure 24-7.) Ostomies may be temporary or permanent. They are constructed temporarily to allow a lower portion of the tract to heal after surgery, injury, or inflammatory disease. Permanent ostomies are created when a lower portion of the tract is removed or permanently damaged.

Since the stoma has no sphincter, elimination through an ostomy in most cases cannot be controlled.

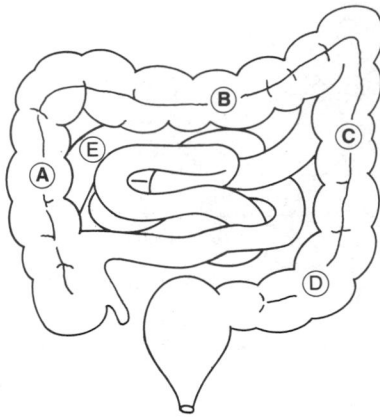

Figure 24-7. Examples of stoma placement for (**A**) ascending colostomy, (**B**) transverse colostomy, (**C**) descending colostomy, (**D**) sigmoid colostomy, (**E**) ileostomy. (Adapted from F. Strand: *Physiology: A Regulatory Systems Approach*. Macmillan, New York, 1978, p. 394.)

Drainage is collected in a plastic pouch attached to the skin with adhesive. Surgical techniques that create an internal pouch have succeeded in giving control to selected individuals with ileostomies and urinary stomas. The internal pouch is periodically emptied by insertion of a *catheter* (tube) which permits drainage of the urine or liquid fecal material.

Control of colostomies is related to the consistency of the drainage. A colostomy in the ascending colon yields liquid drainage and cannot be regulated. By the time the fecal material reaches the sigmoid colon, it has attained the consistency of stool normally excreted through the anus. A sigmoid colostomy, therefore, can often be managed so that, as with normal bowel movements, emptying occurs at a regular time each day. Some individuals with transverse or higher descending colostomies irrigate the colostomy daily in order to gain control over the time of emptying. A colostomy irrigation is similar to an enema, except the water is inserted through the stoma. Freedom from wearing a pouch is achieved by the individuals for whom these methods of bowel regulation are successful. Ostomies create the potential for skin irritation, odor, obstruction, diarrhea, fluid and electrolyte imbalance, and urinary tract infections. They also alter body-image and may affect self-esteem.

Assessment of Elimination Need Satisfaction

In assessing elimination, the nurse considers the influencing factors including diet, fluid intake, exercise, medications, disease, and the patient's knowledge and feelings about any problems and their treatment. Also examined are specific data related to elimination patterns and characteristics of urine and feces.

Data Associated with Urinary Elimination

Voiding Patterns. When urinary elimination is proceeding satisfactorily, approximately 1,500 ml of urine are excreted every 24 hours. The frequency of urination varies among individuals according to personal habits and the amount of fluid intake. Most individuals void four to six times a day, excreting about 250 to 400 ml each time. In the absence of a large fluid intake, most people do not awaken from sleep to urinate, but void before going to bed and again upon arising. Urination is under the voluntary control of the individual and is accomplished without difficulty or pain.

Characteristics of Urine. Urine normally ranges in color from pale yellow when dilute to amber when more concentrated. When first voided, it is clear and has a characteristic aromatic odor. After standing, it may become cloudy due to the precipitation of some of its constituents and may develop an ammonia odor as decomposition occurs. The pH of urine is usually about 6, slightly acid. It varies, from 4.5 to 7.5, with changes in activity and dietary intake. The normal specific gravity or urine ranges from 1.003 to 1.030 (Metheny and Snively, 1983). *Specific gravity* is a measure of the concentration of dissolved solids in the urine. It indicates the kidneys' ability to concentrate or dilute urine according to the body's need to conserve or excrete fluids. Constituents of normal urine include water, nitrogenous wastes, diluted toxins, mineral salts, pigments, and hormones. Occasionally, traces of protein or glucose are also present. Table 24-1 summarizes normal urinary data, as well as data associated with possible urinary problems.

Nursing Procedures for Assessing Urinary Elimination

The nursing measures most commonly used in the assessment of urinary elimination are collecting specimens, measuring urinary output, measuring urine specific gravity, testing for abnormal constituents, palpat-

Table 24-1. **Urinary elimination**

POSSIBLE PROBLEMS	DATA ASSOCIATED WITH NORMAL ELIMINATION	DATA INDICATING POSSIBLE PROBLEMS
Frequency	4–6 times daily	Less than 3 times or more than 8 times/day
Amount	250–400 ml/voiding	Less than 150 or more than 500 ml/voiding
	1,500 ml/day; at least 30 ml/hr	Less than 500 or more than 3000 ml/day; less than 30 ml/hr
Nocturia	Absent	More than once/night
Control	Voluntary control of micturition	Incontinence; retention (distended bladder, hesitancy, straining, voiding very small amounts frequently, absence of urination for 6–8 hr)
Comfort	Absence of discomfort	Burning on urination, pressure, sharp cramping pain, aching flank pain
Characteristics of Urine		
Color	Yellow to amber	Red, brown, or smoky due to bleeding or disease; various colors due to medications
Clarity	Clear	Cloudiness due to presence of blood cells, pus, or mucus
Odor	Characteristic aroma	Strong odor due to concentration; foul odor due to infection
pH	6	Less than 4.5, more than 7.5
Specific gravity	1.003–1.030	Less than 1.003, more than 1.030, or remains constant despite hydration changes
Constituents	Water, nitrogenous wastes, diluted toxins, mineral salts, pigments, hormones	Blood (*hematuria*), protein (*proteinuria*), glucose (*glucosuria*), ketones (*ketonuria*), pus (*pyuria*), increased mucus or epithelial cells, casts, red and white blood cells

ing for bladder distention, and assessment of residual urine.

Collecting Specimens. The nurse is responsible for collecting urine samples to be analyzed. In some cases, the nurse provides the equipment and instructions to the patient who then collects the specimen. Laboratory instructions are followed regarding the type of container to be used and any special care the specimen is to receive, such as refrigeration or immediate transport to the laboratory. The specimen is labeled with the patient's name and identification number. The nurse records in the patient's record the type of specimen and the time it was collected.

ROUTINE URINALYSIS. Because it economically provides valuable data about body functions, urinalysis is commonly performed routinely for each patient on ad-

mission to the hospital or on the initial visit to a clinic or physician's office. The first morning voiding is sometimes preferred for this test since its concentration increases the likelihood that certain abnormal contituents will be identified. Five to 10 milliliters of urine are usually sufficient for analysis.

TIMED URINE SPECIMENS. For certain tests, urine is collected at precisely spaced intervals. The intervals vary according to the type of constituent sought. The nurse collects the specimens as directed by laboratory personnel, or the procedure manual, and labels them with the exact times at which they were obtained. The 24-hour specimen is a common type of timed specimen. At the beginning of the collection period, the patient voids, the urine is discarded, and the time is noted. All urine voided during the next 24 hours is collected. The last specimen is obtained exactly 24 hours after the test was begun. Decomposition of the urine is delayed by adding a preservative to the container and/or refrigerating the urine.

URINE SPECIMEN FOR CULTURE.   Urine is cultured to determine the presence of microorganisms in the urinary tract. For accurate results, the urine must not be contaminated with organisms from the urinary meatus or other parts of the body. Specimens for culture are therefore obtained by inserting a sterile tube into the bladder or by the clean-catch midstream technique. The latter method is preferred since catheterization carries the risk of introducing infection into the bladder. When a catheter is already in place, a specimen for culture can be withdrawn from the catheter or tubing. This technique is described later in the chapter.

The clean-catch midstream urine specimen is collected in a sterile container after careful cleansing of the urinary meatus. Cleansing is carried out in the same manner as for catheterization. Refer to Nursing Skill 24–1, Steps 12 to 14, for the female; Nursing Skill 24–2, Steps 11 to 13, for the male. The first urine voided is not collected since it contains organisms and cells flushed from the urethra and meatus. The sample is drawn instead from the middle of the stream. The patient voids approximately 30 ml of urine into the toilet. Then, without stopping the flow, the specimen container is passed under the stream to collect several milliliters of urine. The container is pulled away before voiding stops, and the patient finishes voiding into the toilet. Care is taken throughout the procedure to avoid touching and con-

taminating the inside of the container or its lid. The patient, if able, carries out the procedure unassisted after receiving instructions from the nurse. When the patient is weak, confused, or bedridden, the nurse collects the specimen. In obtaining a specimen from a female on a bedpan, the nurse asks the patient to void forcibly so that urine can be collected that has not drained across the perineum.

OBTAINING A SPECIMEN FROM AN INDWELLING CATHETER.   A urine specimen is obtained from an indwelling catheter by inserting a sterile needle into the sampling port on the catheter tubing or into the catheter itself. Sterile technique is used to avoid introducing pathogens into the bladder. Urine from the drainage bag is not used since it is not fresh and may yield inaccurate results. The catheter is not disconnected from the tubing since opening the system would provide an entry for microorganisms.

The nurse wipes the sampling port with an antiseptic swab, inserts a 21- or 22-gauge needle attached to a 3-ml syringe, and withdraws about 3 ml of urine. When the tubing has no sampling port, and when the catheter is made of a self-sealing material, the needle can be inserted directly into the distal portion of the catheter. The needle is inserted at a 45-degree angle to promote resealing, and caution is used to avoid puncturing the channel which leads to the balloon that holds the catheter in the bladder. Figure 24–8 illustrates these methods of obtaining a specimen. When the tubing contains too little urine to permit aspiration, the tubing may be

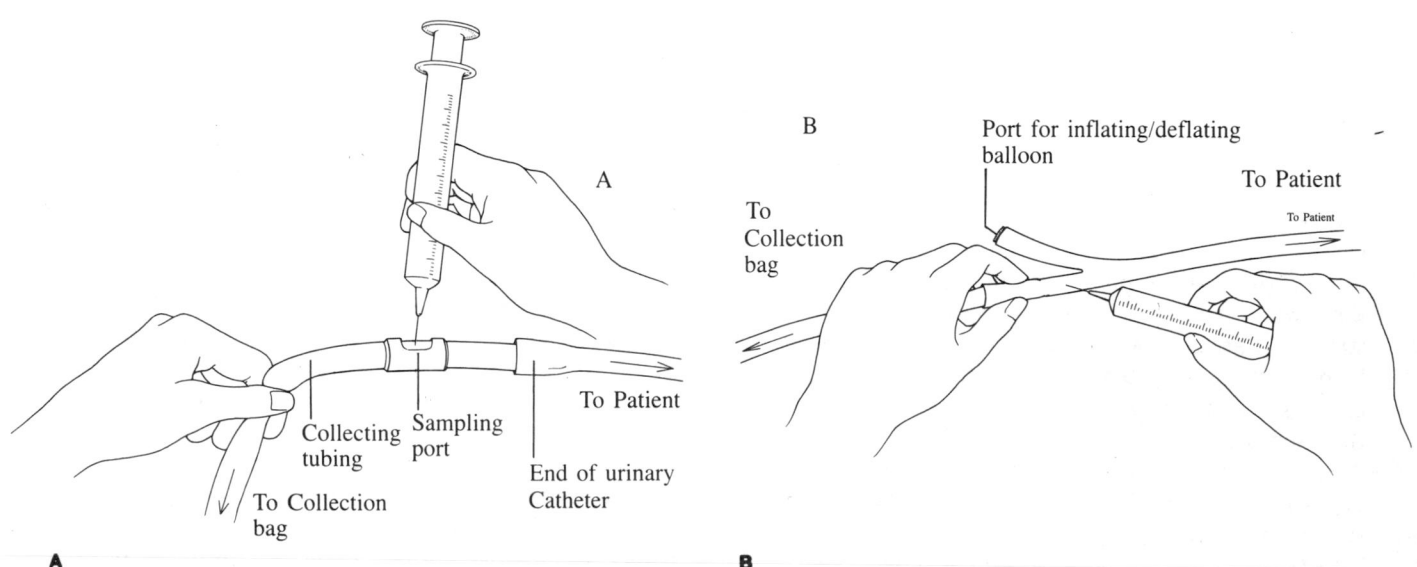

Figure 24–8.   Obtaining a urine specimen from an indwelling catheter by inserting a needle into (**A**) a sampling port and (**B**) a self-sealing catheter.

clamped just below the port or the catheter for several minutes to allow urine to collect. The clamp is removed promptly following specimen collection.

SERIAL URINE SAMPLES. Samples of consecutive voidings are sometimes collected to distinguish progressive changes in the color or clarity of urine, as may occur with bleeding or purulent infections. A small amount of urine from each voiding is saved in a separate clear container. Three or four containers are lined up with the oldest specimen on the right, the most recent specimen on the left. With successive voidings, the oldest specimen is discarded, the remaining cups are moved one place to the right, and the newest specimen is added on the left. With this technique, gradual changes are readily apparent.

Measuring Urinary Output. Urinary output is measured, along with fluid intake, to provide data related to the patient's fluid balance. The patient is informed that all urine is to be saved. The urine is voided into a collecting container positioned under the toilet seat, a bedpan, or a urinal. It is poured into a graduated container for measuring and then discarded. The time and the amount are noted on the individual's intake and output record, which is typically kept in the patient's room. Some patients are able to take the responsibility of measuring and recording their own output. Others are instructed to save the urine voided and notify the nurse, who then measures it. If the patient is occasionally incontinent, or if a voiding is accidentally discarded, it may be possible to estimate the approximate amount voided.

Output is commonly totaled at the end of each eight-hour period and again at the end of the 24-hour period. These totals are entered in the patient's permanent record. For patients with indwelling catheters, the drainage bag is emptied every eight hours, or as needed, and the amount included in that period's total. The output for critically ill patients is totaled as often as every one or two hours. Vomitus, liquid feces, and drainage from wounds are included, in addition to urine, in the total output.

Measuring Specific Gravity. The specific gravity of urine is measured with an instrument called a *hydrometer,* or *urinometer.* The urinometer is a sealed glass cylinder with a calibrated stem and a weighted bottom. The gradations range from 1.000, the specific gravity of distilled water, to 1.060. The urinometer is placed in a tube filled three-fourths full with fresh urine. (See Figure 24–9.) It is given a slight spin to prevent its adherence to the sides of the tube. The measurement, taken at eye level, is read where the lower line of the meniscus crosses the scale on the urinometer: the more concen-

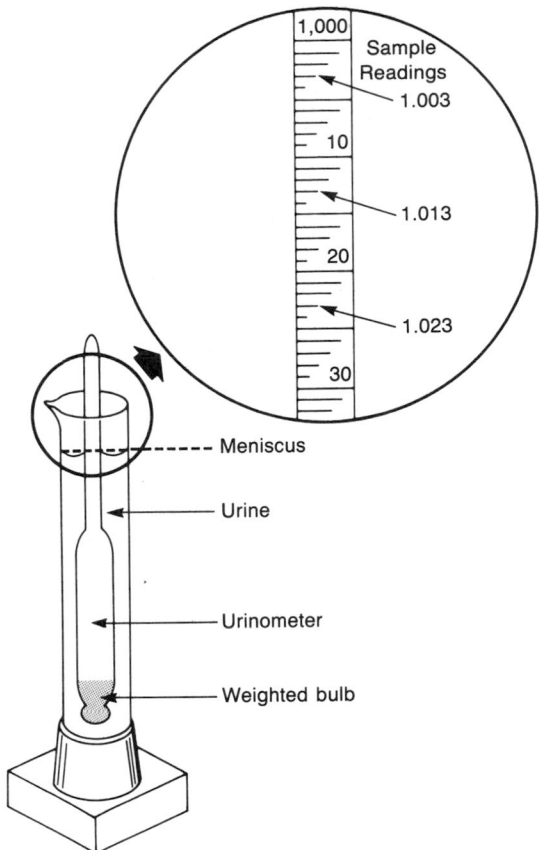

Figure 24–9. Urinometer for measuring specific gravity. The value is read at the lower level of the meniscus.

trated the urine, the higher the instrument floats, and the higher the specific gravity reading.

Testing for Abnormal Constituents. In some situations, the nurse performs tests to detect in the urine abnormal substances such as glucose, acetone, protein, bilirubin, or blood. Commercially prepared diagnostic kits are available for the specific substances. The tests are generally done by dipping chemically treated strips or tapes into the urine and noting color changes. The color of the strip or tape is compared with an accompanying chart that describes the significance of the given color. The manufacturer's directions are followed precisely to ensure accurate results.

Palpating for Bladder Distention. When the bladder fills to about 200 ml, it begins to extend above the pubic bone and can be felt as a firm, rounded mass in the lower abdomen. Palpation is done to assess the degree of bladder retention in patients having difficulty voiding. To palpate, the fingers of both hands are placed on the lower abdomen below the umbilicus and pressed gently inward and down toward the pubic bone. (See

Here

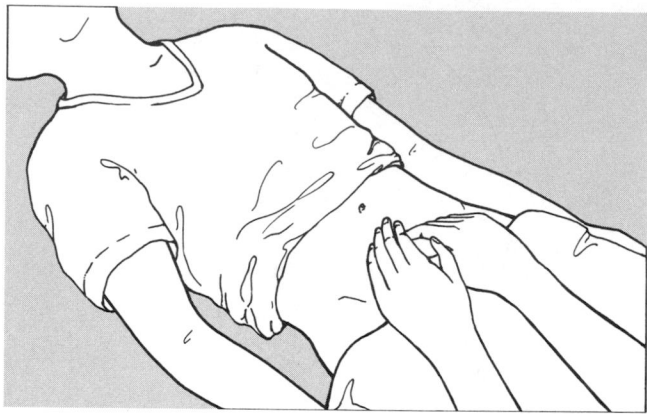

Figure 24–10.   Hand placement for palpation of the bladder.

Figure 24–10.) The upper border of the bladder is located, and its distance below the umbilicus, or above the public bone, is noted in centimeters. A distended bladder may extend as far upward as the umbilicus. (You may practice this skill by delaying the urge to void and palpating your own full bladder.)

Assessing Residual Urine.   In some persons, the bladder fails to empty completely with each voiding, continually leaving some urine residing in the bladder. When this type of retention is suspected, as, for example, in repeated bladder infections, a catheter is inserted into the bladder immediately following voiding. The amount of urine returned, the *residual urine*, is noted and recorded. Normally, residual urine is less than 3 ml. Larger amounts indicate some degree of urinary retention.

Nursing Diagnoses Related to Inappropriate Urinary Elimination

Several examples of general nursing diagnoses are provided below. Under each are listed examples of specific diagnoses related to that general category.

Altered urinary elimination pattern
  Potential for urinary tract infection related to indwelling catheter
  Painful urination related to urethritis
Impairment of urinary elimination: Incontinence
  Stress incontinence related to weakened perineal muscles
  Intermittent incontinence related to bladder spasms
Impairment of urinary elimination: Retention
  Inability to void related to urethral trauma
  Anxiety related to difficulty in initiating urination

Data Associated with Intestinal Elimination

Characteristics of Feces.   Normal stool is medium brown in color, its color resulting from bile pigments and bacterial decomposition of food. The color, along with the distinctive odor, varies somewhat with the types of food eaten. Normal stool is formed and soft in consistency. It is composed of undigested food residue, bacteria, intestinal debris, bile pigments, and small amounts of salts. Occasionally, threads of mucus or particles of partially digested food may be observed in the stool. Table 24–2 presents data that indicate normal or abnormal feces.

Defecation Patterns.   The frequency of defecation varies normally among individuals, from three or four times a day to once or twice a week. The amount of stool produced varies directly with the amount of undigestible fiber in the food ingested. The average amount of stool excreted daily by an adult is about 200 ml. Approximately 75 percent of this is water; the rest is fiber and intestinal debris. The amount of stool is usually described by the nurse as small, moderate, or large. When stools are liquid, they may be measured and the amount expressed in milliliters. Defecation is controlled by the individual and is not accompanied by pain or discomfort.

Table 24–2. **Characteristics of Feces**

	NORMAL DATA	ABNORMAL DATA
Color	Brown	Red or black in bleeding; clay colored when bile absent; green in some infections; varied colors caused by some foods, medications, or diseases
Odor	Characteristic odor due to bacterial decomposition	Foul odor due to digestive disorders or intestinal infection
Consistency	Formed, soft	Watery or hard
Constituents	Occasional shreds of mucus or particles of undigested food	Excessive fat or mucus, blood, pus, pathogens, or parasites

Table 24–3. **Altered Bowel Elimination Patterns**

	CONSTIPATION	FECAL IMPACTION	DIARRHEA	ABDOMINAL DISTENTION
Consistency of stool	Excessively hard	Seepage of liquid fecal material; hard stool felt in rectum	Liquid, unformed	————
Frequency of stools	Less often than usual for the individual	No stool passed	More than 3 liquid stools per day	No stool passed
Passage	Difficult, requires increased muscular effort; may be painful	Unable to pass	Difficult to control defecation	No gas passed through rectum; no bowel sounds (since no movement of gas)
Associated data	Rectal pressure, headache, anorexia; hemorrhoids may result	Abdominal and rectal discomfort, anorexia, abdominal distention	Cramping in abdomen, anorexia, irritation of skin around the anus; dehydration may occur	Progressive swelling and discomfort in abdomen, "drumlike" sound of abdomen on percussion, shortness of breath, cramping

Defecation patterns are altered in constipation, fecal impaction, diarrhea, and abdominal distention. These problems affect the consistency and frequency of stools, the ease of passage, and patient comfort. Data related to these conditions are listed in Table 24–3.

Nursing Procedures for Assessing Intestinal Elimination

Abdominal Percussion.   Percussion of the abdomen is done to determine the presence of excess gas in the gastrointestinal tract. The middle finger of one hand is placed on the abdomen. The finger is then tapped sharply, several times in quick succession, just below the nail, with the middle finger of the other hand. (See Figure 24–11.) A dull sound is heard in the absence of distention; a hollow, "drumlike" sound (*tympanites*) is heard when gaseous distention is present. Bowel sounds are assessed by listening to the abdomen through a stethoscope (auscultation). Active peristalsis is accompanied by frequent gurgling or bubbling sounds as fluids and gas move through the tract. Absence of sounds indicates an interference with peristalsis.

Collecting Stool Specimens.   Stool specimens are analyzed for blood, fat, bile, pathogenic bacteria, viruses, and parasites or their ova (eggs). The stool is collected in a clean or, in some cases, sterile bedpan or collecting container placed beneath the toilet seat. The patient first voids in the toilet or other receptacle to prevent contamination of the specimen with urine. One or two tongue blades are used to transfer the necessary amount of stool, typically about ½ oz, into the specimen container. Smaller amounts are required for cultures, while tests for fat or bile may require the entire stool. The container is then capped, labeled, and sent to the laboratory. Care is taken to avoid contamination of the outside of the container with stool, and the hands are washed thoroughly after the specimen is collected.

To ensure accurate test results, the nurse follows the specific instructions provided by the laboratory for each

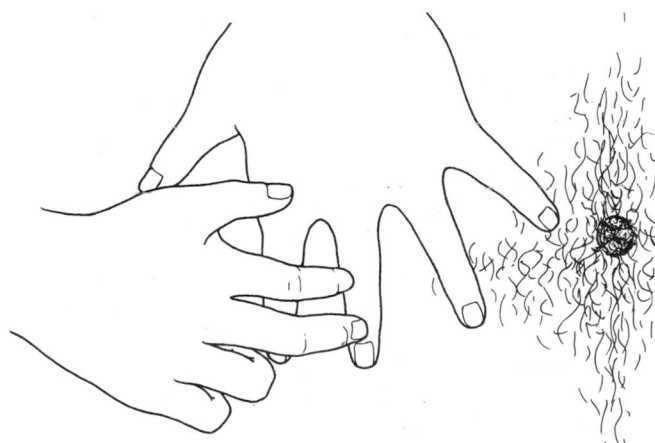

Figure 24–11.   Finger placement for percussion of the abdomen.

type of test. For example, a specimen to be analyzed for parasites and ova is sent to the laboratory immediately since it must be examined while warm and the parasites still alive.

Specimens for pinworms or their ova are collected by pressing the adhesive side of clear cellephane tape to the anal region. The tape is immediately pressed onto a glass slide and sent to the laboratory for microscopic examination. Since pinworms emerge from the rectum and deposit their eggs in the perianal area while the patient is sleeping, the specimen is collected in the early morning before the patient bathes or wipes the anus.

Testing for Occult Blood.   Nurses frequently test the stool for blood which is not apparent on visual examination (*occult blood*). Various methods, including commercially prepared packets, are used. Directions for the particular method are followed. Typically, a small amount of stool is spread thinly onto guaiac-impregnated filter paper. A chemical reagent is then applied, producing a color change in the presence of blood. These tests are useful in screening for colon and rectal cancers, which usually produce intermittent bleeding. They are more accurate when the patient has followed a meat-free, high-roughage diet for three days preceding the test.

Nursing Diagnoses Related to Intestinal Elimination Problems

Several examples of general and specific nursing diagnoses are presented below.

Alteration in bowel elimination
  Painful defecation related to hemorrhoids
  Flatulence related to food intolerances
Alteration in bowel elimination: Constipation
  Constipation related to inadequate fluid and fiber intake
  Lack of information regarding constipation prevention
Alteration in bowel elimination: Diarrhea
  Excoriation of perianal skin related to frequent stools
  Potential for dehydration related to diarrhea
Alteration in bowel elimination: Incontinence
  Potential for skin irritation related to incontinence
  Decreased self-esteem related to bowel incontinence

Nursing Interventions to Facilitate Satisfaction of Elimination Needs

Nursing interventions that facilitate elimination are directed toward promoting normal habits, intervening in elimination problems, and preventing treatment-related problems.

Promoting Normal Habits

Individuals often find it difficult to maintain normal elimination when admitted to the hospital. Diet, mealtimes, convenience of obtaining preferred fluids, exercise level, sleep schedule, and opportunity and privacy for elimination are all changed. In addition, the level of stress is generally increased. Nursing interventions to minimize these changes include:

- Arrange for special dietary needs (such as daily bran cereal or prunes).
- Provide a pitcher of fresh water at the bedside, iced or at room temperature as the patient prefers.
- Determine the preferred beverages and provide them to approximate the patient's usual schedule.

- Offer fluids hourly to patients who lack the ability or motivation to take fluids by themsleves.
- Encourage and assist the person to be out of bed and/or as active as possible. Schedule regular exercises for patients whose mobility is limited.
- Place the call light within easy reach for patients who need help with elimination.
- Maintain a matter-of-fact attitude about elimination that does not deter patients from requesting needed help.
- Provide privacy to the degree possible—close the door, pull the curtains, ask visitors to step out of the room.
- Provide instruction about factors that influence elimination. Many individuals are aware of the need for fiber in the diet, but not the need for fluids and exercise.
- Provide information related to the method of elimination expected or required while the person is hospitilized. Patients need to know whether ambulation to the bathroom is expected or permitted, or whether a bedpan, commode, or urinal is to be used. Do not assume patients know how to use these special receptacles; provide instruction.

Assisting with Normal Elimination

The hospitalized patient may need assistance to the bathroom or to use the bedpan, urinal, or commode. Assistance should be offered at regular times throughout the day, especially when the patient awakens in the morning, before and after meals, before bathing, and at bedtime. The offered assistance indicates the nurse's acceptance of elimination as a normal and expected function and facilitates the process for patients who are reluctant to ask for help. Privacy is provided, and the call light and toilet tissue left within reach. If continued assistance is necessary, the nurse remains with the patient. After elimination, any required assistance is provided with cleansing the perineal area and with handwashing. In cleansing the female, the perineum is wiped from front to back to prevent transferring organisms from the rectum to the urethra or vagina. The date of each bowel movement is usually noted on the patients's record to facilitate early recognition of constipation.

Assisting with a Bedpan.   Bedpans are used by males for defecation and by females for both defecation and urination. A typical bedpan and a fracture pan are shown in Figure 24–12. The smaller, flatter fracture pan is easier to slide under a patient who is immobilized by fractures or cannot be turned. It is also more comfortable for the individual who must remain flat. Bedpans are made of plastic or metal. Metal pans are rinsed with warm water before use since the cold surface may interfere with sphincter relaxation and is uncomfortable for the patient. A bedpan for each patient's personal use is typically kept in the bedside stand or bathroom rack.

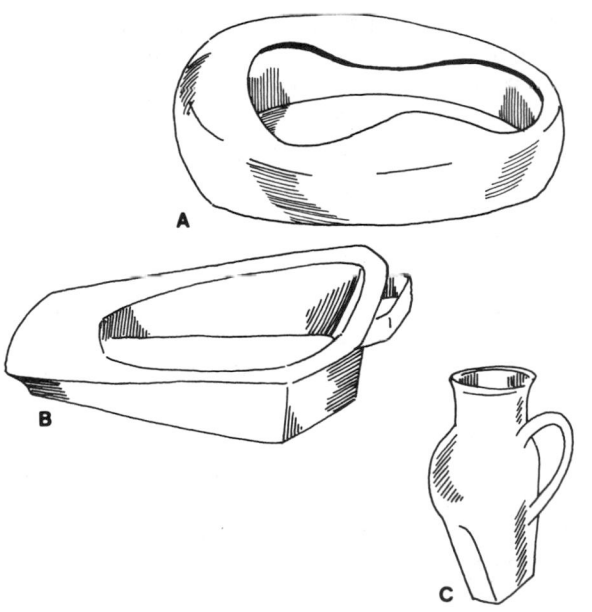

Figure 24–12. Bedpans and urinal: **(A)** adult bedpan, **(B)** fracture pan, **(C)** male urinal.

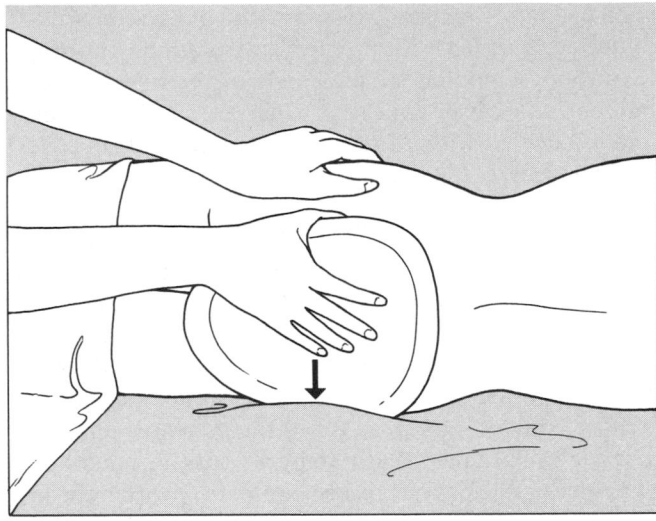

Figure 24–13. Assisting the patient onto a bedpan from the side-lying position.

When assisting a patient with a bedpan, the nurse raises the bed to working height and pulls the curtains around the bed. Bed linens are folded back diagonally to the patient's knees; the gown covers the genital area but is lifted as necessary to check proper placement of the pan. The patient lies on the back with knees flexed and feet flat on the bed. Pushing with the feet, the patient raises the buttocks off the bed. At the same time, the nurse places one arm under the lower back to assist in raising the buttocks and, with the opposite hand, slides the bedpan under the patient. Powder may be used on the pan to ease its placement and decrease skin irritation. The patient who is unable to assist by raising the buttocks is positioned on the side. The nurse stands at the patient's back and places the bedpan against the buttocks. One of the nurse's hands presses on the top edge of the pan, pushing it downward and toward the patient. The other hand, at the same time, pulls on the upper hip, rolling the patient onto the pan. (See Figure 24–13.)

Correct placement of the pan is checked. The flattened rim should be under the sacrum, the upper edge of the opening just above the anus. Unless contraindicated, the head of the bed is raised to a comfortable degree, and the patient's knees are bent. The bed linens are replaced, and the upper side rails raised. Unless constant attendance is required, the nurse leaves the room to provide privacy. A patient should not be left on the bedpan for more than 30 minutes at a time, since the pressure of the pan interferes with circulation, and the position may cause back discomfort.

The pan is removed in the same manner it was placed. To avoid spilling, the pan is stabilized with one hand while the patient is lifted or turned with the other.

The bedpan is emptied, rinsed with cold water, and, if required, cleaned with a detergent solution. Thorough cleansing, including the underside of the rim, alleviates odor. If there is no toilet in the patient's room, the bedpan is covered with a square of material (bedpan cover) during transfer to the utility room.

Assisting with a Urinal. Urinals are used by male patients for voiding. A male urinal is illustrated in Figure 24–12. If at all possible, the urinal is used with the patient standing at the bedside because the upright position facilitates complete emptying of the bladder. In bed, the patient lies on the side or back, or sits with the head of the bed elevated. When the patient is unable to use the urinal unassisted, the nurse positions and holds it in place. The penis is placed completely within the urinal so it does not slip out when urination begins. The bed linen can be pulled up over the urinal to provide privacy while it is being used. After use, the urinal is rinsed with cold water and stored in the bedside stand.

Female urinals are also available. They have a large, oval cup-shaped top which is held firmly against the perineum. Since leakage is difficult to control except in a standing position, they are infrequently used.

Use of a Commode. A commode is a portable toilet, usually on wheels, that can be brought to the bedside. It has a receptacle which slides under the toilet seat and can be removed for emptying. Figure 24–14 illustrates one type of commode. Some commodes can be rolled into the bathroom and, with the receptacle removed, positioned directly over the toilet. Many have a cushioned cover which can be closed over the toilet seat giving the commode, between uses, the appearance of a chair. The individual is provided with robe and slippers and a blanket over the knees if needed for warmth. After elimination, assistance is provided with cleansing and returning to bed. The receptacle is removed from the commode, emptied into the toilet, and rinsed with cold water. If the commode is shared with other patients, it is cleaned according to institutional policy and returned to the storage area.

Intervening in Elimination Problems

Urinary Retention. When the patient is unable to void, noninvasive techniques are first employed in attempts to stimulate urination. If these are not successful, a catheter is inserted to empty the bladder. Overfilling of the bladder is not allowed since this damages the bladder walls, interferes with reflex contractions, and results in backflow into the ureters and kidney pelves, all of which predispose to infection.

NONINVASIVE MEAURES. Noninvasive measures to stimulate voiding include:

1. Decrease discomfort and anxiety. Offer ordered medications to relieve pain. Project a calm, unhurried attitude. Allow adequate time for voiding. Refrain from overemphasizing the fact that the patient is not voiding.

2. Provide a generous fluid intake. Filling of the bladder assists in stimulating micturition.

3. Respond promptly to requests for assistance with voiding. If urination must be delayed, the urge will die out.

4. Suggest urination even though the patient does not initiate a request. Offer assistance at times consistent with the patient's previous voiding patterns or at regular intervals.

5. Provide privacy.

6. Position the patient as near normally as possible. Unless contraindicated, assist the male patient to stand at the bedside; help the female to a commode or to sit on a bedpan on the edge of the bed, feet resting on a stool. If bed rest is essential, elevate the head of the bed and flex the patient's knees.

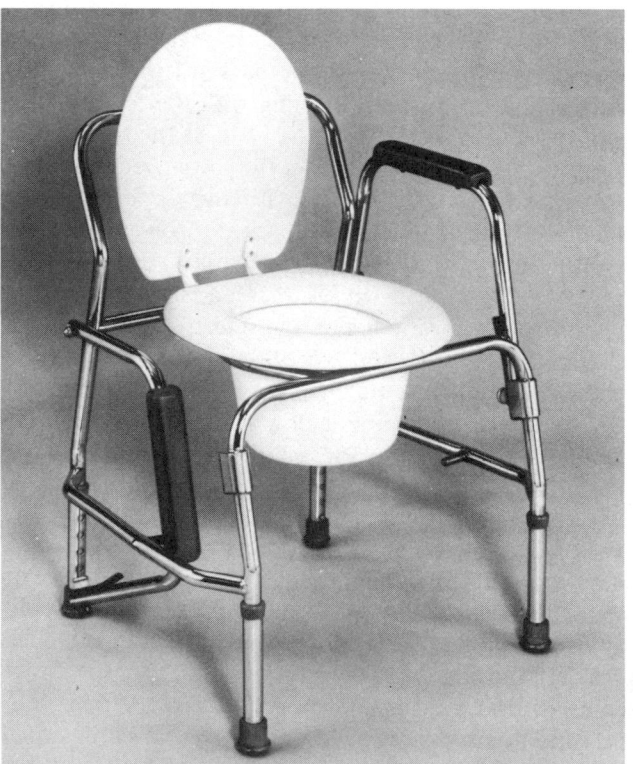

Figure 24–14. A type of commode. Note that the armrest folds down to facilitate patient transfer from bed to commode. Many models have wheels for moving the patient into the bathroom following the transfer from the bed. The wheels must be locked during the transfer onto and off the commode. (Photograph courtesy of Lumex, Bayshore, NY.)

7. Introduce stimuli suggestive of voiding. Let water run within the patient's hearing; dangle the patient's fingers in warm water; or pour warm water over the genitalia.

8. Assist muscle relaxation with a warm shower, bath, or sitz bath. Encourage the patient to void during the shower or bath, if able. The shower or tub can be easily cleaned, and this method is highly preferrable to catheter insertion.

9. Apply warm packs to the lower abdomen to promote muscle and sphincter relaxation.

10. Instruct the patient to contract the abdominal muscles. The added pressure on the bladder may stimulate a micturition reflex.

11. Stimulate areas that trigger urination. In some patients with neurological dysfunction, the micturition reflex may be stimulated by tapping over the bladder, stroking the inner thigh, or pulling the pubic hair.

12. Give medication prescribed to stimulate bladder contraction (see Table 24-4).

13. Apply manual pressure over the bladder, in special cases, to force urine out. This technique, the Crede method, is used with caution since excessive force may damage the bladder and sphincters.

Table 24-4. **Medications Associated with Elimination Needs**

TYPE OF DRUG	ACTION	EXAMPLES
Laxatives	Promote evacuation of the bowel	
Bulk-forming laxatives	Absorb water, leading to large, soft stools which stimulate peristalsis through increased bulk	Psyllium hydrophilic muciloid (METAMUCIL, HYDROCIL)
Saline or osmotic laxatives	Provide an osmotic effect which draws fluid into the intestine, softening the feces and providing bulk	Magnesium hydroxide (milk of magnesia), lactulose (CHRONULAC)
Lubricants	Lubricate the stools for easier passage; coat the fecal material, preventing reabsorption of water from the stool	Mineral oil
Stool softeners	Facilitate the mixing of water with fecal contents by a wetting or detergent action	Dioctyl sodium sulfosuccinate (COLACE), dioctyl calcium sulfosuccinate (SURFAK)
Stimulant laxatives	Stimulate peristalsis by irritating the colonic mucosa; inhibit water reabsorption from the colon	Bisacodyl (DULCOLAX), castor oil, phenolphthalein (PHENOLAX), senna (SENOKOT)
Antidiarrhea Agents	Reduce the frequency and liquidity of stools; two or more types are often combined	
Opiates and related derivatives	Reduce peristalsis	Paregoric, diphenoxylate (LOMOTIL), loperamide (IMODIUM)
Anticholinergics	Reduce peristalsis and decrease intestinal secretions; seldom used because of unacceptable side effects	Atropine sulfate, isopropamide (DARBID), mepenzolate (CANTIL)
Adsorbents	Believed to bind toxins, bacteria, and irritants to their surface for excretion	Bismuth salts (PEPTO-BISMOL); other drugs used but not proven effective include kaolin, pectin, and activated charcoal (Clark *et al.*, 1982)

Table 24–4. (*Continued*)

TYPE OF DRUG	ACTION	EXAMPLES
Bacterial cultures	Believed to reestablish normal intestinal flora in diarrheas resulting from antibiotic-induced disruption	Lactobacillus acidophilus and bulgaricus (Lactinex)
Bulk-forming laxatives	Absorb excess fecal fluid, producing soft, rather than liquid, stools	Psyllium hyrophilic muciloid (METAMUCIL)
Antispasmodics and Anticholinergics	Relieve hypermotility and spasms of the ureters, bladder, and intestine; may cause constipation and urinary retention	Dicyclomine hydrochloride (BENTYL, DYSPAS), propantheline bromide (PRO-BANTHINE)
Cholinergic Agents	Increase tone and motility of the bladder and intestine; used to treat nonobstructive urinary retention and intestinal distention	Bethanechol (URECHOLINE), neostigmine (PROSTIGMIN)
Urinary Antiseptics	Provide antibacterial activity in the urine with little systemic effect; used in kidney and bladder infections	Trimethoprim-sulfamethoxazole (BACTRIM, SEPTRA), nalidixic acid (NEGGRAM)
Antibiotics	Destroy or inhibit the growth of susceptible infecting microorganisms	Cephalexin (KEFLEX), sulfasalazine (AZULFIDINE)
Glucocorticoids	Reduce inflammation; may be used to treat kidney and bowel inflammations	Dexamethasone (DECADRON, HEXADROL), prednisone (METICORTEN), methylprednisolone (MEDROL)
Antiflatulents	Claimed to relieve flatulence with a defoaming action that disperses gas trapped in the gastrointestinal tract and facilitates its elimination by belching or passing flatus	Simethicone (MYLICON, SILAIN)
Diuretics	Increase the volume of urine produced; most act by inhibiting sodium and water reabsorption in the kidney tubules; useful in the treatment of hypertension and edema; some may be used to increase urine production in decreased kidney function	Hydrochlorothiazide (HydroDIURIL), spironolactone (ALDACTONE), furosemide (LASIX)

INVASIVE MEASURES—CATHETERIZATION. Urinary catheterization is the insertion of a tube (catheter) through the urethra into the bladder to drain urine or to instill medication or fluid. Catheterization is performed only when absolutely necessary since it carries a high risk of introducing infection into the bladder.

Depending upon their purpose, catheters may be inserted briefly and removed (*straight* catheters), or left in

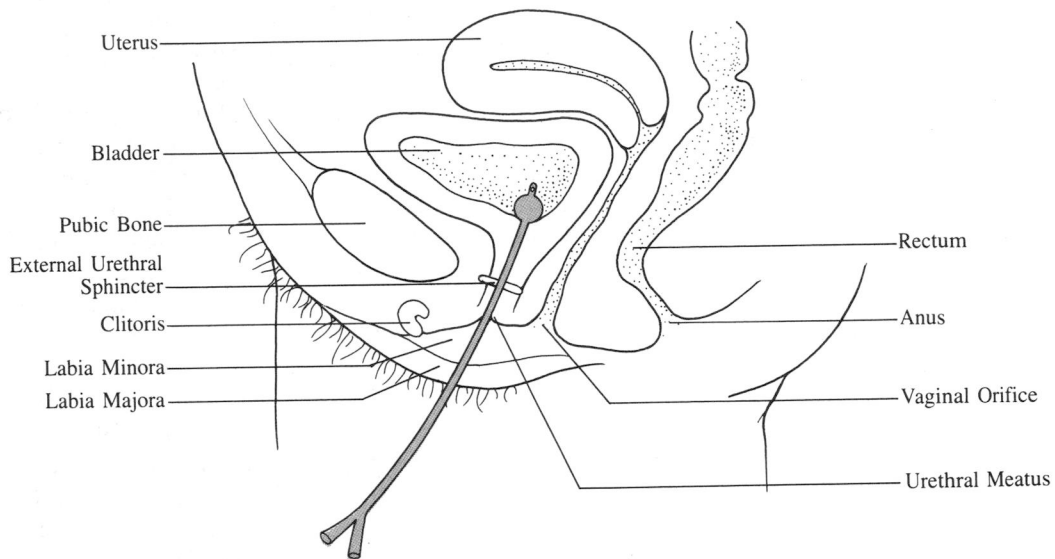

Figure 24-15. Indwelling catheter in place in a female. (Adapted from F. Strand: *Physiology: A Regulatory Systems Approach*. Macmillan, New York, 1978, p. 568.)

place for several days or more (*indwelling, retention*, or *Foley* catheters). Straight catheters are inserted to:

Drain a distended bladder
Obtain a sterile urine specimen
Measure residual urine
Empty the bladder prior to surgery on adjoining structures

Indwelling catheters are used to:

Provide continuous or intermittent bladder drainage
Permit repeated instillation of medications or irrigating fluids
Monitor urine production in critically ill patients
Manage incontinence

An indwelling catheter is connected to drainage tubing and a bag for collecting the urine. Figure 24-15 illustrates an indwelling catheter in the bladder of a female.

Sizes and Types of Catheters. Urinary catheters are rubber or plastic tubes, about 16 inches long. They are sized according to the French scale, which refers to the circumference measured in millimeters. A size 8 or 10 is generally used for children, 14 or 16 for women, and 16 or 18 for men. Too large a catheter interferes with the drainage of urethral secretions and causes pressure on the urethra. There is no evidence that a larger catheter is more resistant to obstruction than a smaller one, except, perhaps, in the presence of large blood clots.

Straight catheters are single-lumen tubes. Indwelling, or retention, catheters have a double lumen. One

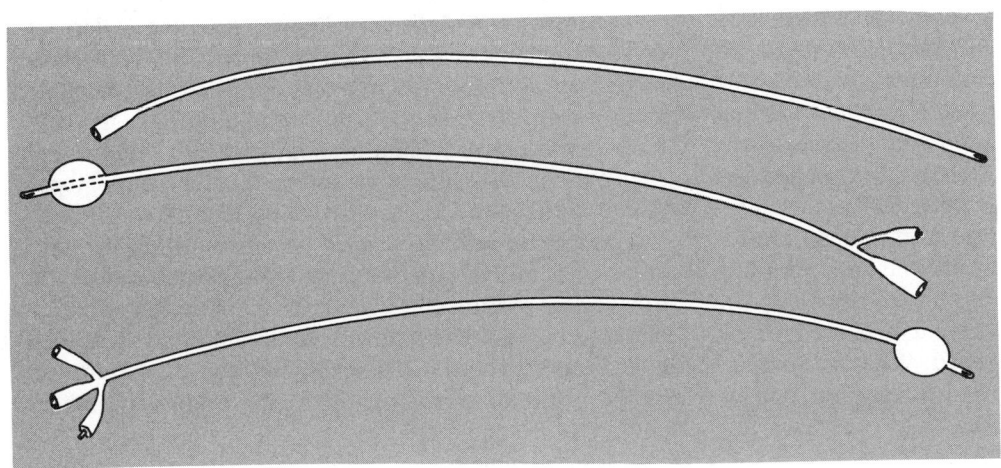

Figure 24-16. Types of catheters: **(A)** straight catheter, **(B)** indwelling catheter with balloon inflated, **(C)** triple-lumen catheter with balloon deflated.

lumen drains the urine; the other provides for inflation of a small balloon near the tip of the catheter. The balloon, inflated with 5 to 30 ml of sterile water or saline, holds the catheter in the bladder. A triple-lumen catheter (three-way Foley) is also available. The third lumen serves as a channel for introducing irrigation fluid. These three types of catheters are shown in Figure 24–16.

Techniques of Catheter Insertion. The techniques for inserting indwelling catheters in females and males are described in Nursing Skills 24–1 and 24–2. The technique for inserting straight catheters is identical, except there is no need for balloon inflation or attachment of a collection bag. The straight catheter is withdrawn slowly as urine flow begins to subside, so the tip of the catheter moves slowly through, and drains, any urine remaining in the base of the bladder.

Management of the Indwelling Catheter.

PREVENTING INFECTION. The indwelling catheter, the tubing, and the collection bag form a closed sterile system. Because of the danger of introducing organisms, the catheter and tubing are not separated unless absolutely necessary. The nurse's hands are washed before and after handling the bag or tubing, and the bag is kept off the floor at all times. The perineum is cleansed with soap and water daily, rinsed well, and dried. Any dried secretions at the catheter-meatal junction are gently removed. Care is taken to avoid pulling on the catheter as this exposes a part of the catheter that has been in the urethra. When tension is released, this part of the catheter again recedes into the sterile urethra, carrying organisms with it. It was formerly the policy in some institutions to cleanse the perineum and catheter twice daily with soap and water or antiseptic solution and to apply antiseptic ointment to the meatus. This was believed to remove or destroy bacteria which would otherwise ascend along the catheter into the bladder. Recent evidence indicates, however, that these procedures are associated with a higher, rather than lower, incidence of bladder infection, possibly due to the increased handling of the catheter (McGill, 1982).

Maintaining Drainage. Urine flows through the catheter into the drainage bag by gravity. This method of drainage is called *straight drainage*, as opposed to other types of fluid drainage which employ suction devices. For effective drainage, the collection bag must remain lower than the bladder, and the catheter and tubing must remain free of obstruction. The collection bag is hung on the bed frame. (See Figure 24–18.) It is not attached to the side rail since this could raise it above the bladder when the side rail is elevated. When the patient is up, it is carried, pinned to the robe or gown, or attached to a lower portion of the chair or wheelchair. If it

becomes necessary during position changes or transfers to raise the bag above bladder level, the tubing is pinched to prevent backflow of urine into the bladder. Excess tubing, which allows for patient movement, is coiled on the bed. This prevents its hanging down below the level of the collection bag and forcing the urine to overcome gravity to reach the bag. For the patient who remains in bed, the coil of tubing is held on the bed by fastening it to the bottom sheet. Some systems have attached clips for this purpose. With other systems, a piece of tape or an elastic band is looped around the tubing and then pinned to the sheet. The tubing may be placed either over or under the patient's thigh. When placed over the thigh, urine has to overcome gravity to reach the drainage bag. When placed under the thigh, the tubing may be compressed by the weight of the leg. A small pillow or pad may be used to lift the leg slightly off the bed, reducing compression of the tubing. The nurse decides which position is most effective for the individual patient. As the patient is repositioned, the tubing is adjusted for maximal drainage. Instructions in handling and ambulating with the catheter and bag are provided to the patient.

The catheter is checked at least every four hours to see that it remains patent (unobstructed). A high-fluid intake contributes to catheter patency by providing a continuous flushing of the lumen. Intake and output are monitored, and if output decreases in relation to intake, or ceases entirely, the patient is assessed for other signs of urinary retention. An obstructed catheter must be irrigated or replaced. Catheter irrigation is discussed later in the chapter.

Once in place, a catheter is usually not changed unless it becomes obstructed, its lumen begins to fill with gritty sediment, odor cannot be controlled, or an infection occurs. Catheters are left in place for two to four weeks, and even longer in individuals who are permanently dependent upon catheter drainage, up to two or three months. The tubing and drainage bags are changed as needed to control odor, leakage, or infection, usually once a week.

Emptying the Collection Bag. The urine collection bag is emptied every eight hours, more often if the output is large. A container is taken to the bedside to collect the urine as it is drained through a small tube in the bottom of the bag. A separate container is provided for each patient since infections spread readily from one patient's catheter to another. Aseptic technique is used. The nurse's hands are washed before handling the bag, and care is taken to avoid touching the open end of the tube. Some institutions require the end of the drainage outlet to be wiped with an antiseptic solution before and after draining the urine. The amount and characteristics of the urine are noted on the intake and output sheet and on the patient's record.

Nursing Skill 24-1   Female Catheterization: Indwelling Catheter

Preparation

1. Determine need. Catheterization is carried out only with a physician's order. An order is frequently written, however, to "catheterize as necessary for urinary retention." Data that lead to the decision to catheterize in this case include the absence of urination in the past six to eight hours despite normal intake, discomfort in the bladder area, restlessness, diaphoresis, and palpable bladder distention.
2. Gather equipment:
   a. Sterile catheterization tray containing catheter, collection container, gloves, antiseptic solution and cotton balls (or antiseptic-soaked swabs), forceps, water-soluble lubricant, waterproof absorbent drapes, specimen container, syringe with solution for balloon inflation
   b. Sterile drainage bag and tubing
   c. Flashlight or lamp
   d. Bath blanket
3. Identify the patient.
4. Explain the procedure to the patient. Include the fact that catheterization is not painful unless inflammation or abnormalities are present.
5. Place sterile tray on the overbed table.
6. Provide privacy by closing the door and pulling the curtain around the bed.
7. Position the patient on her back with hips and knees flexed, knees spread apart. If this position is difficult to maintain, the legs may be left flat on the bed, widely abducted at the hips; or the patient may be placed on her side with the upper leg flexed at the hip and knee.
8. Drape with a bath blanket placed diagonally, one corner on the chest, the opposite corner between the legs.
9. Arrange lighting as necessary.
10. Wash hands.

Procedure	Explanation
1. Remove the drainage bag and tubing from the package and set to one side; leave the sterile cover on the tip of the tubing.	1. Provides availability when needed; maintains necessary sterility.
2. Fold back the lower corner of the bath blanket to expose the patient's perineum.	2. Provides privacy until exposure is necessary.
3. Open the sterile tray touching only the outer corners of the wrap.	3. Preserves sterility of the inner surface of the wrap, providing a sterile work area.
4. Remove the first waterproof drape from the tray; touching only the two upper corners, place it, plastic side down, on the bed between the patient's legs, tucking the upper edge under the patient's buttocks.	4. Keeps the bed dry; maintains sterility of the center of the drape.
5. Don the sterile gloves.	5. Maintains sterility of the items handled.
6. Pick up the fenestrated drape (the one with a hole in the center) and either	6.
a. open it and place it over the genital area, maintaining sterility of the gloves, or,	a. Enlarges the sterile field, for those experienced in its use.
b. drop it aside.	b. Slips out of place easily, contaminating the area and equipment, when placed over the perineum. It can be dropped to one side of the sterile field to later receive the used cotton balls or swabs.

Procedure

7. Pour antiseptic solution over the cotton balls, or open the package of antiseptic-soaked swabs.
8. If collecting a specimen, set the container to one side, within easy reach, with the lid placed loosely on top.
9. Lubricate 2.5 to 5 cm (1 to 2 inches) of the catheter tip.
10. Place the lubricated catheter in the collection container.
11. Move the sterile tray with prepared equipment onto the bed between the patient's legs, touching only sterile parts of the tray and wraps.
12. With the fingers of one hand, separate and pull gently upward on the labia minora.
13. Maintain separation of the labia with this hand until the catheter has been inserted.

14. Cleanse the meatal area with antiseptic-soaked cotton balls or swabs:
    a. Hold the cotton balls with the forceps; swabs are on a stick so forceps is not necessary.
    b. Use each cotton ball or swab for only one stroke.
    c. Discard each cotton ball or swab, as it is used, on an edge of the package wrapper or drape, being careful not to reach across the sterile field.

Explanation

7. Prepares them for use when needed.

8. Facilitates opening the container later when only one hand is free.

9. Reduces friction and possible irritation as catheter is inserted.
10. Places it aside and maintains sterility until it is needed.
11. Places all equipment within easy reach; maintains sterility of equipment.

12. Exposes the meatus. (Figure 24–17 illustrates exposure of the meatus for catheterization.)
13. Prevents labia from closing over the meatus and contaminating it after cleansing; contaminates this hand so it can no longer be used to handle sterile items.
14. Reduces the probability of introducing organisms from the meatus into the bladder.
    a. Prevents contamination of the sterile glove.

    b. Removes organisms rather than redistributing them.
    c. Prevents contaminated solution from dropping onto sterile field.

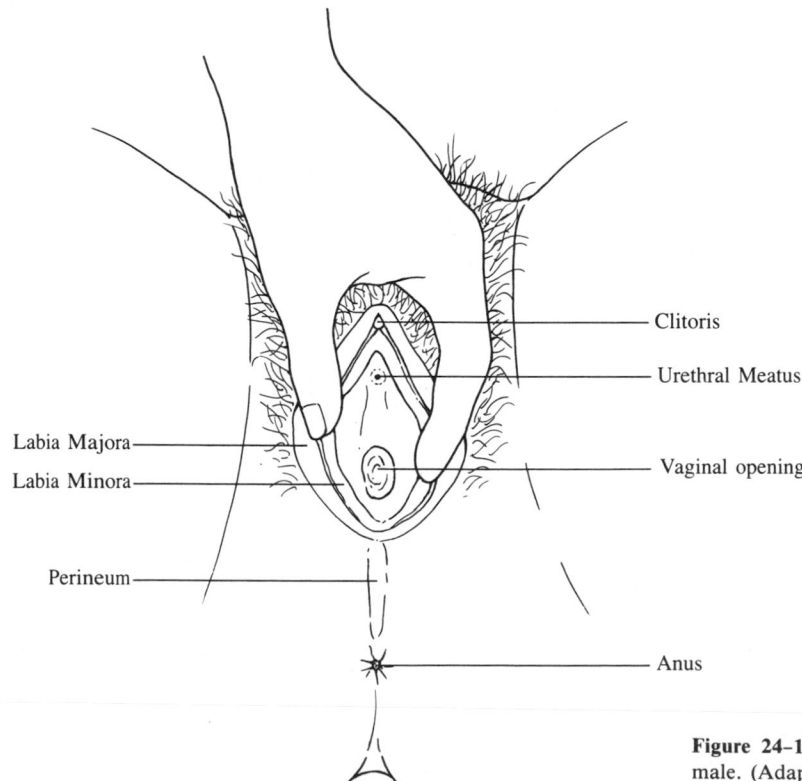

Figure 24–17. Exposure of the meatus for catheterization of a female. (Adapted from F. Strand: *Physiology: A Regulatory Systems Approach.* Macmillan, New York, 1978, p. 521.)

d. Wipe from front to back, from above meatus toward the anus.

e. Use three cleansing strokes, wiping along one side of the meatus, then along the other side, and finally, directly across the meatus.

15. Pick up the catheter with the sterile gloved hand, holding it about 8 cm (3 inches) from the tip.

16. Position the drainage end of the catheter in the collection container.

17. Ask the patient to take a slow, deep breath just as the catheter is inserted.

18. Gently insert the catheter 5 to 7.5 cm (2 to 3 inches); when urine starts to flow, insert 2.5 cm (1 inch) more to ensure placement of the balloon entirely within the bladder.

    a. Do not force insertion against resistance.

    b. If the catheter is contaminated at any point prior to insertion, a new catheter is obtained and the procedure begun again.

19. Release the labia and hold the catheter securely in place with the hand that formerly held the labia; maintain grasp until the balloon is inflated.

20. Collect a specimen if required:

    a. Pinch the catheter.

    b. Remove the specimen container lid and set it, top down, on the overbed table.

    c. Set the specimen container beside the collection container.

    d. Place the drainage end of the catheter in the specimen container and collect about 30 ml of urine.

    e. Replace the end of the catheter in the collection container and allow the urine to drain from the bladder.

    f. Set the specimen container on the overbed table and replace the lid with one hand.

21. Allow urine to flow into the collection container until the bladder is empty, or until the amount reaches 1,000 ml.

22. Inflate the balloon:

    a. Bring the inflation valve to the hand holding the catheter in the bladder.

    b. Stabilize the valve with two fingers of this hand, while continuing to maintain the position of the catheter.

    c. With the other hand, attach the syringe of solution to the inflation valve and inject 5 to 10 ml of solution. (The amount varies with agency policy.)

    d. Pull gently on the catheter to determine that the balloon is inflated.

23. Attach the catheter to the drainage tubing and bag.

24. Wipe excess antiseptic from meatal area; wash and dry the area, and remove the drape(s).

d. Moves organisms away from the meatus

e. Removes microorganisms from the catheter insertion area.

15. Provides control of the catheter tip; allows for full insertion with minimal finger movement.

16. Prevents drainage of urine onto the bed.

17. Relaxes the urinary sphincters for easier passage of the catheter.

18. The female urethra is 3 to 5 cm (1½ to 2 inches) long; inflation of the balloon in the urethra causes pain and tissue damage.

    a. Traumatizes tissues.

    b. Protects the patient from the introduction of organisms by contaminated equipment.

19. Prevents the catheter from slipping out of position.

20.

    a. Stops urine flow.

    b. Maintains sterility of the inside of the lid.

    f. Allows other hand to continue maintaining the position of the catheter.

21. It is believed that rapid emptying of large amounts of urine may cause shock as a result of the sudden movement of blood into the formerly constricted abdominal vessels.

22. Holds the catheter in the bladder.

23. Establishes closed urinary drainage system.

24. Prevents tissue irritation from prolonged contact with the antiseptic.

Procedure	Explanation
25. Assist the patient to a comfortable position.	25. Provides physical comfort.
26. Tape the catheter to the thigh, allowing some slack (See Figure 24–18).	26. Prevents pressure on the meatus and possible mucosal erosion.
27. Hang the drainage bag at the side of the bed; coil the excess tubing on the bed—do not let it hang down below the drainage bag (See Figure 24–18).	27. Keeps the bag away from microorganisms on the floor; allows the bladder to be drained freely by gravity. If the tubing hangs below the level of the drainage bag, urine has to overcome gravity to reach the bag.
28. Dispose of the equipment properly.	28. Prevents contamination of the environment.
29. Instruct the patient on management of the catheter (see the section on management of an indwelling catheter which follows.)	29. Decreases anxiety, promotes adequate drainage, reduces potential for complications.
30. Wash hands.	30. Prevents the transmission of microorganisms to the nurse and other patients.
31. Record the reason for catheterization, the type and size of catheter inserted, the amount and appearance of urine removed, and the patient's response to the procedure.	31. Makes the information available to other health team members; provides official documentation of care given.

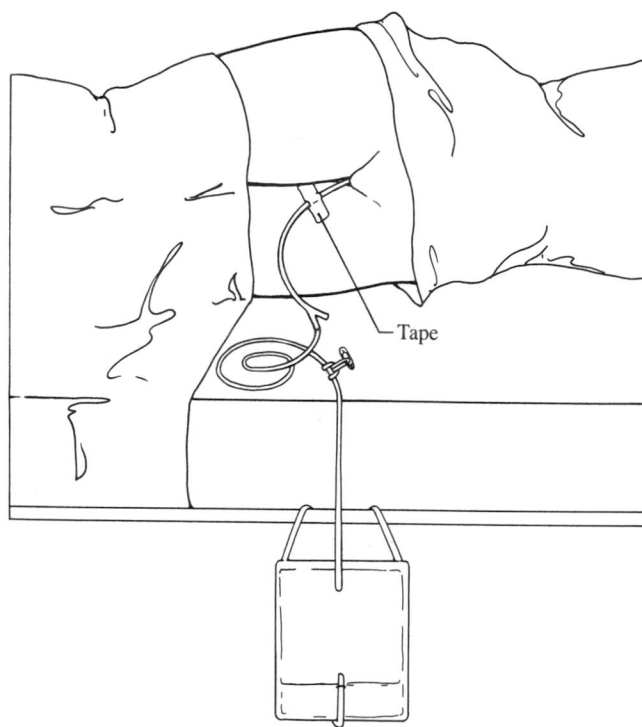

—Tape

Figure 24–18. Position of drainage bag and tubing for an indwelling catheter.

Nursing Skill 24–2   Male Catheterization: Indwelling Catheter

Preparation

The preparation for catheterization of the male is the same as for the female, except that extra lighting is seldom needed, and the positioning and draping are different. The patient is positioned on his back with legs together. A bath blanket is placed across the upper body, while the legs are covered with the bed linen.

Procedure	Explanation
1. Remove the drainage bag and tubing from its package and set it to one side; leave the sterile cover on the tip of the tubing.	1. Provides availability when needed; maintains necessary sterility in the interim.
2. Open the sterile tray touching only the outer corners of the wrap.	2. Preserves sterility of the inner surface of the wrap, providing a sterile work area.
3. Remove the first sterile drape from the tray; touching only the two upper corners, unfold and place it, plastic side down, across the patient's legs and under the penis.	3. Provides a sterile field.
4. Don the sterile gloves.	4. Maintains sterility of the items handled.
5. Unfold the fenestrated drape and position it so the penis protrudes through the hole, or place the drape, folded in half, across the lower abdomen just above the penis. Take care to maintain sterility of gloves.	5. Increases the sterile area.
6. Pour antiseptic solution over cotton balls, or open package of antiseptic-soaked swabs.	6. Prepares them for use when needed.
7. If collecting a specimen, set the container to one side, within easy reach, with the lid placed loosely on top.	7. Facilitates opening the container later when only one hand is free.
8. Lubricate 10 to 13 cm (4 to 5 inches) of the catheter tip.	8. Reduces friction and possible irritation as the catheter is inserted.
9. Place the lubricated catheter in the collection container.	9. Places it aside and maintains sterility until it is needed.
10. Move the sterile tray with the prepared equipment onto the patient's legs or onto the bed beside his hips, touching only sterile parts of the tray and wrap.	10. Places all equipment within easy reach; maintains sterility.
11. Grasp the penis firmly behind the glans, retract the foreskin of an uncircumcised patient, and spread the meatus open. (See Figure 24–19).	11. Exposes the meatus and glans for effective cleansing.
12. Maintain the hand in this position, retracting the foreskin and spreading the meatus, until the catheter is inserted.	12. Prevents the foreskin from carrying organisms back over the glans after cleansing; prevents this hand, which is now contaminated, from handling sterile equipment.
13. Cleanse the meatus and glans with antiseptic-soaked cotton balls or swabs: a. Hold the cotton balls with a forceps. b. Starting at the meatus, wipe in a circular motion over the meatus and down toward the base of the glans; repeat this step twice more, using a new cotton ball or swab each time.	13. Reduces the probability of introducing organisms from the meatus into the bladder. a. Prevents contamination of the sterile glove. b. Prevents the transfer of organisms from the glans to the meatus; moves organisms away from the meatus.

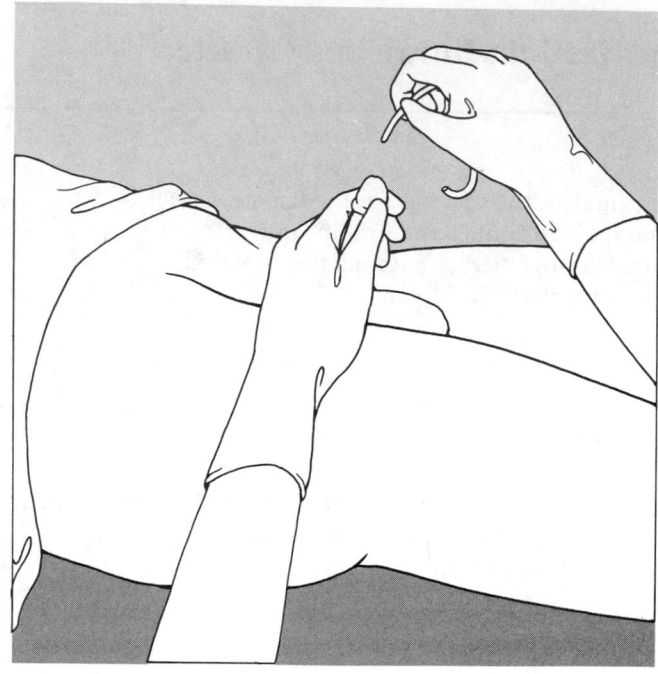

Figure 24–19.   Position of the penis for catheterization.

Procedure

14. Pick up the catheter with the thumb and forefinger of the sterile gloved hand, holding it about 7.5 cm (3 inches) from the tip. With the last three fingers, hold the drainage end of the catheter in the palm of the hand.

15. Gently pull the penis upward with the fingers around the shaft.

16. Gently insert the catheter 17.5 to 20 cm (7 to 8 inches); when urine starts to flow, insert 2.5 cm (1 inch) more to ensure that the balloon is entirely within the bladder.

17. If resistance is felt, do not force insertion:
   a. Wait a few seconds.

   b. Have the patient take a deep breath or bear down as if to force urination.
   c. Change the angle of the penis.

18. Position the drainage end of the catheter in the collection container and lower the penis.

19. Continue holding the catheter securely in place until the balloon is inflated.

Explanation

14. Provides control of the catheter.

15. Helps to straighten the urethra.

16. The male urethra is about 20 cm (8 inches) in length; inflation of the balloon in the urethra causes pain and tissue damage.

17. Injures urethral lining.
   a. Allows time for a temporary sphincter spasm to subside.
   b. Helps to relax the sphincters.

   c. Straightens the urethra; facilitates passage of the catheter past the prostate gland.

18. Prevents drainage of urine onto the bed; lowers urethra so urine can flow from the bladder.

19. Prevents catheter from slipping out of position.

Continue the procedure as described in Nursing Skill 24–1, Female Catheterization: Indwelling Catheter, Steps 20 through 31.

In some institutions the catheter is taped, not to the thigh as suggested in Step 26, but to the lower abdomen. This position of the penis is thought to reduce pressure on the urethra at the junction of the penis and scrotum, thus reducing the potential for tissue necrosis. This factor is especially important when catheters are in place for prolonged periods, as in spinal cord injury. Figure 24-20 illustrates the two methods of anchoring the catheter for a male.

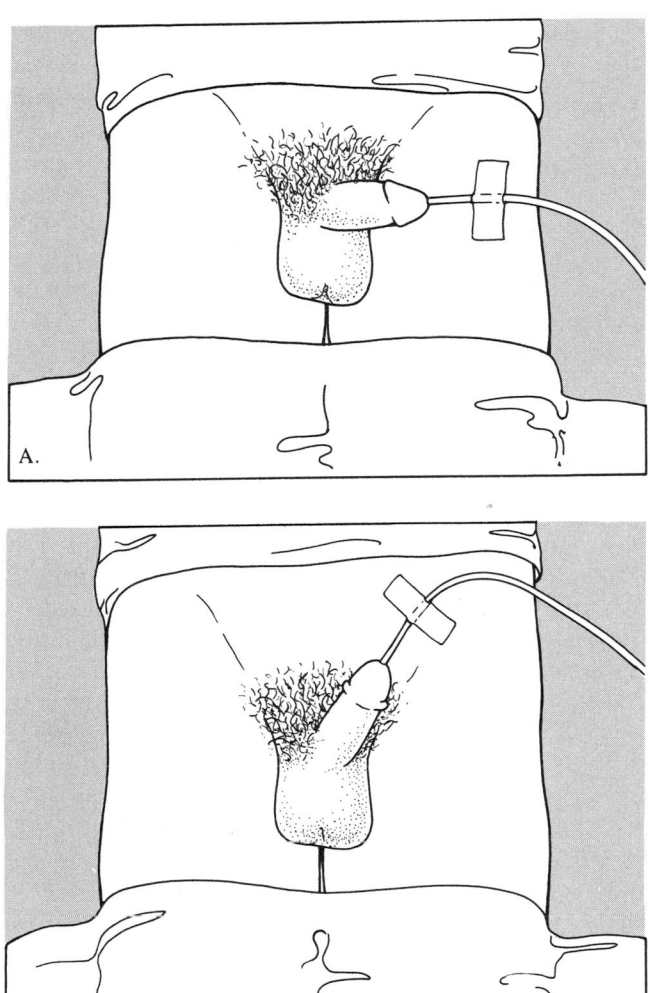

Figure 24-20. Stabilization of the catheter in a male by taping it to **(A)** the thigh, **(B)** the abdomen.

CATHETER AND BLADDER IRRIGATIONS. Irrigation is the flushing or washing out of a tube or body area with solution. Catheter and bladder irrigations are done to flush out blood clots, mineral precipitates, pus, or debris that are obstructing, or have the potential to obstruct, the catheter. Sterile normal saline is the solution commonly used. It is usually introduced at room temperature. Refrigerated solution can be warmed by immersing the solution bottle in warm water. Cold solution may cause bladder spasms. A total amount of 120 to 200 ml is usually used for adult catheter irrigation, 1,000 ml (or the amount specifically ordered) for adult bladder irrigation. Since the goal of bladder irrigation is to flush out the bladder, more fluid is needed than for catheter irrigation which simply flushes the catheter lumen. Catheter and bladder irrigations are carried out in one of three ways—the open method, the needle method, or the closed method. Sterile technique is observed in each method; once opened, a bottle of irrigating solution is used for no longer than 24 hours.

Open Method. In the open method, the drainage system is opened by temporarily disconnecting the tubing from the catheter, and the irrigation solution is introduced into the catheter with a syringe. (See Figure 24–21.) Catheters were routinely irrigated by this method in the past before it was learned that opening the system leads to bladder infections. Current practice is to use this method only when irrigation is definitely required, the needle method is not effective, and a closed system is not in place. The technique for open catheter irrigation is presented in Nursing Skill 24–3. A new sterile irrigation set is used each time the catheter is irrigated.

Needle Method. The needle method of irrigation is similar to the open method, except the solution is inserted through a needle, alleviating the need to open the system. A needle attached to a large syringe is inserted into the catheter lumen or the port on the tubing, using the aseptic technique described earlier for collecting a sterile specimen from a catheter. During instillation, the tubing below the needle insertion site is pinched off to ensure solution flow toward the bladder, rather than down the tubing. When the syringe is refilled, it is separated from the needle rather than the needle being withdrawn from the catheter, thus reducing the opportunity for introduction of organisms with repeated needle insertions. Care is taken to maintain sterility of the syringe tip and needle hub. Since the size of the fluid stream from the needle is smaller than that from an irrigating syringe, the rate and strength of flow are dissipated as the stream enters the larger catheter lumen. For this reason, the needle method of irrigation may be less effective than the open method in dislodging debris from the catheter lumen.

Closed Method. The closed method of catheter and bladder irrigation permits the introduction of solution without opening the system to the entry of microorganisms. This method, which utilizes a triple-lumen catheter, is especially desirable when repeated irrigations are required. A bag or bottle of irrigating solution is hung on an IV pole and connected by tubing to the irrigation lumen of the catheter. Solution flow is controlled by a clamp on the tubing. A closed irrigation system is illustrated in Figure 24–22. With this system, irrigation can be continuous or intermittent. In continuous irrigation, the clamp is adjusted to permit a slow, steady flow of solution into the bladder. There is a corresponding steady outflow from the bladder, through the drainage lumen of the catheter, into the collection bag. Patency of the catheter is checked frequently to prevent overdistention of the bladder. In intermittent irrigation, the tubing from the irrigation bottle is clamped until the time specified for the irrigation. The clamp is then opened and the ordered amount of solution allowed to flush the bladder and catheter. Because the system remains closed, the danger of infection is significantly reduced. The nurse replaces the solution container and empties the drainage bag as required. When urinary output is being measured, the amount of irrigating solution is subtracted from the fluid in the collection bag to arrive at the amount of urine produced.

BLADDER INSTILLATION. In bladder instillations, medicated solutions are introduced into the bladder and retained for a specified length of time. Medications may be instilled for their ability to reduce precipitates in the urine or for their antiseptic or anticancer effects on the bladder mucosa. Medicated solutions are introduced in the same way as irrigating solutions—by the open, closed, or needle methods. In instillations, however, the drainage tubing is clamped just prior to introduction of the solution and remains clamped until the medication has been in the bladder for the specified period. The patient is asked to turn from side to side to allow contact of the medication with all bladder surfaces.

CATHETER REMOVAL. When catheter removal is ordered, the tape anchoring the catheter to the thigh or abdomen is removed. A syringe is inserted into the balloon deflation valve, and the fluid inflating the balloon is withdrawn. The catheter is then gently pulled out and placed in a towel or basin. The amount and appearance of urine in the collection bag are recorded, along with the time of catheter removal.

After catheter removal, the nurse monitors intake and output for 24 hours and checks for any difficulty with voiding. The patient may temporarily experience burning on urination, difficulty voiding, frequency, or dribbling. These problems are related to the urethral irritation, loss of bladder tone, reduced bladder capacity,

Nursing Skill 24–3   Catheter or Bladder Irrigation: Open Method

Preparation

1. Determine need. A physician's order is usually required for catheter and bladder irrigation, although agency policies may permit it without an order in certain situations. Becuase of the high risk of introducing infection, the open method of irrigation should be used only when the needle method does not produce adequate results. When repeated irrigations are required, the insertion of a triple-lumen catheter connected to a closed system is preferred. The need for catheter irrigation is demonstrated by a stoppage or reduction in urine flow despite adequate fluid intake and by the other signs of urinary retention discussed previously.
2. Gather equipment:
   a. Sterile irrigation set composed of solution container, 60-ml irrigation syringe, antiseptic swab, linen protector, collection basin, cover for tip of drainage tube and, in some institutions, sterile gloves.
   b. Ordered irrigation solution—about 200 ml for catheter irrigation, 1,000 ml (or amount ordered) for bladder irrigation.
3. Identify the patient and explain the procedure.
4. Provide privacy.
5. Wash hands.
6. Place solution and irrigation set on the overbed table.

Procedure	Explanation
1. Fold back the bed linen to expose the catheter at its junction with the drainage tubing.	1. Minimizes patient exposure while providing for nurse's visualization of the area.
2. Remove the tape anchoring the catheter to the thigh.	2. Facilitates manipulation of the catheter.
3. Open the sterile irrigation set using aseptic technique. Parts of the equipment that must remain sterile are the solution, the lip of the solution bottle, the inside of the solution container, the inside of the syringe and as much of the outside of the syringe as is allowed to contact the solution in the container, open ends of the drainage tubing and catheter.	3. Reduces potential for introducing microorganisms into the bladder.
4. Pour the required amount of solution into the sterile container, and replace the cap on the solution bottle.	4. Preserves sterility of irrigating solution.
5. Place the linen protector under the catheter.	5. Provides a sterile field; protects the linen from moisture.
6. Position the collection basin on the bed next to the patient's hips, or between the thighs.	6. Provides receptacle for return flow of solution.
7. Wipe the juncture of catheter and tubing with the antiseptic swab.	7. Removes microorganisms.
8. Disconnect the drainage tubing from the catheter with a twisting and pulling motion. Avoid touching either open end or the part of the tubing that will be reinserted into the catheter.	8. Twisting helps loosen the tight-fitting junction; touching introduces organisms to the sterile area.
9. Position the open end of the catheter securely in the sterile collection basin.	9. Frees the nurse's hands; maintains sterility of the catheter.

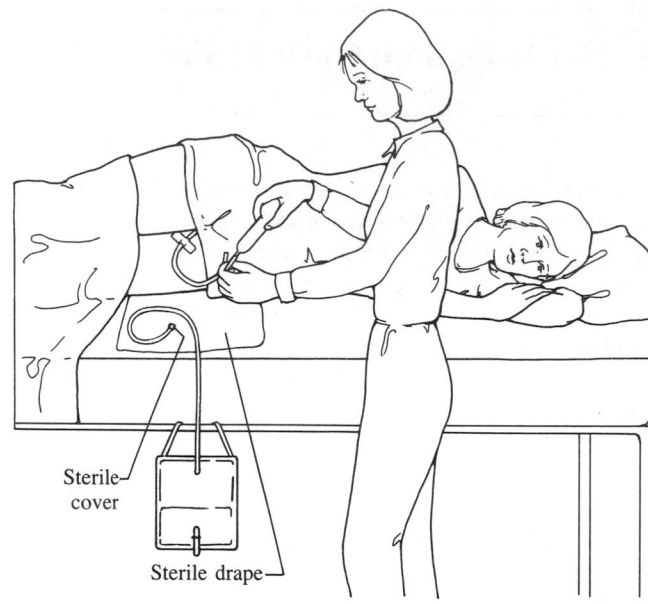

Sterile cover

Sterile drape

Figure 24–21. The open method of catheter irrigation.

<table>
<tr><td align="center">Procedure</td><td align="center">Explanation</td></tr>
</table>

Procedure	Explanation
10. Cover the open end of the drainage tubing with the sterile tube cover, and coil the tubing on the bed securely so that it will not slip to the floor.	**10.** Maintains sterility and cleanliness of the drainage tubing.
11. Draw 30 to 60 ml of irrigation solution into the syringe.	**11.** Provides an amount sufficient to fill the catheter lumen, and is well within the limits of bladder capacity.
12. Insert the syringe tip into the catheter and gradually instill the solution (Figure 24–21); do not instill air.	**12.** Gradual instillation provides for patient's comfort and reduces incidence of bladder spasm; air is thought to cause bladder spasms.
13. For *catheter* irrigation:	**13.**
a. Instill about 30 ml at a time.	a. Provides sufficient fluid to fill and flush the catheter lumen.
b. Withdraw the syringe, lower the catheter, and let the solution drain into the collection basin.	b. Lowering the catheter allows the solution to flow by gravity.
c. Repeat the instillation and drainage three more times, or until the drainage is clear.	c. Provides for adequate flushing of the catheter.
d. If the solution does not return after 60 ml have been introduced, do not instill more until this has been removed.	d. Prevents overdistention of the bladder.
14. For *bladder* irrigation:	**14.**
a. Withdraw the syringe and, without allowing drainage, repeat instillation until the ordered amount has been introduced, usually 60 or more ml.	a. Delivers sufficient fluid to flush out the bladder as well as the catheter.
b. Lower the catheter and let the solution drain into the collection basin.	b. Provides for gravity flow.
c. Repeat steps a and b as ordered, or until the drainage is clear.	c. Provides for adequate flushing of the bladder.

15. If the solution does not return from either type of irrigation:
    a. Change the patient's position—turn from side to side or raise the head of the bed.
    b. Pinch and rotate the catheter between thumb and fingers.
    c. Reinsert the syringe and withdraw the solution with gentle suction.
16. Reconnect the catheter and tubing, maintaining the sterility of both ends.
17. Retape the catheter to the thigh.
18. Remove the linen protector and assist the patient to a comfortable position.
19. Coil the drainage tubing on the bed.

20. Dispose of equipment properly and wash hands.

21. Record on the intake and output sheet the difference between the amount of fluid instilled and fluid returned.

15.
   a. Changes position of catheter tip and urine in the bladder, increasing the likelihood of flow.
   b. Helps dislodge any debris that may be present.

   c. Strong suction may pull mucosa into the catheter and cause tissue damage.
16. Reestablishes the closed, sterile system.

17. Prevents pressure and erosion at meatus.
18. Provides patient comfort.

19. Prevents tubing from hanging below the level of the drainage bag, which would require urine to overcome gravity to reach the bag.
20. Prevents contamination of the environment; prevents the transmission of microorganisms to the nurse and other patients.
21. Provides for an accurate account of urine output.

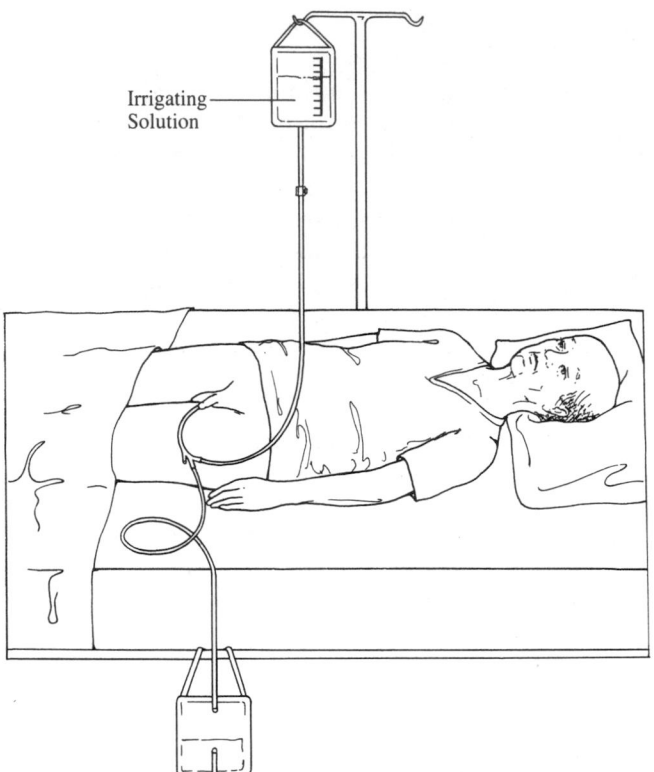

Irrigating Solution

Figure 24–22. Closed system for catheter of bladder irrigation, or bladder instillation.

and interference with sphincter closure caused by the catheter. They may be aggravated by the patient's anxiety. A high-fluid intake is encouraged to dilute the urine and to increase bladder tone and capacity. Sphincter control is improved by perineal exercises which are discussed later. Bladder tone and capacity may be reinstated before catheter removal by clamping the catheter for about three hours, allowing it to drain for 5 to 10 minutes, and then reclamping. This cycle is repeated at least three times. If the catheter has been in place for more than a week, it may be clamped for shorter periods initially and the time progressively increased to gradually stretch the bladder to its former capacity.

Constipation. The treatment for constipation requires a plan for its prevention in the future. The nurse and the patient together develop a plan that will be effective and acceptable to the patient. The plan provides for an adequate fluid intake (2,000 ml or more daily), a high-fiber diet (generous amounts of fruits, vegetables, and whole grains), physical activity including exercises to strengthen the abdominal and perineal muscles, withdrawal from laxatives if being used inappropriately, a regular time set aside each day for defecation, prompt response to the defecation urge, privacy, and measures to promote comfort and relaxation. Before the patient is

ready to discuss prevention, however, the immediate problem must be relieved. Laxatives, suppositories, and enemas are used in the treatment of constipation.

LAXATIVES. Laxatives and cathartics are medications that promote defecation. The term *laxative* usually denotes a gentle-acting drug, while a *cathartic* produces a stronger effect. Types of laxatives and their modes of action are presented in Table 24–4. In addition to treating constipation, laxatives are used to empty the colon before surgery or examination, and in situations where straining at stool would be dangerous or painful, for example, perineal incisions, heart conditions, or hemorrhoids. In the treatment of constipation, laxatives are used only as a temporary measure until changes in habits can bring about more normal evacuation.

SUPPOSITORIES. Rectal suppositories stimulate bowel emptying by chemical irritation or mechanical distention of the rectum. Medication is gradually released as the suppository melts, bringing about defecation in about 10 to 30 minutes. Suppositories are usually administered to produce defecation at the patient's usual time, such as after breakfast. They are frequently used in bowel retraining to establish a regular defecation pattern. The technique of suppository insertion is described in Chapter 19.

ENEMAS. An enema is the introduction of a solution into the rectum and sigmoid colon. Enemas are most frequently given to cleanse the bowel, but are also used to soften hardened feces, promote the expulsion of flatus, or instill medication.

Cleansing Enemas. Cleansing enemas are administered to empty the rectum and colon to (1) relieve constipation, (2) promote visualization during x-rays and instrument examinations, or (3) prevent contamination during childbirth or surgery. Cleansing enemas soften the feces and stimulate peristalsis by distending and irritating the rectum and colon.

Solutions commonly used for cleansing enemas are tap water, normal saline, and soapsuds. Although all of these soften the feces and distend the bowel, soapsuds have the additional effect of combining more rapidly with the feces and irritating the intestinal mucosa. The safety of their use is questioned since the irritation sometimes progresses to rectal inflammation and colitis. To avoid excessive irritation, only soap solutions made with castile soap, 5 ml or less per 1,000 ml of water or saline, should be used. Tap-water enemas are not used for infants, nor for repeated enemas in adults. The hypotonicity of tap water can lead to dangerous fluid shifts as water is drawn from the bowel into the body tissues by osmosis.

The amount of solution instilled for adults is 500 to 1,000 ml. The lesser amount is given to empty the lower colon; the larger amount to remove feces higher in the colon. Proportionately less solution is used for children—250 to 350 ml for preschoolers. The temperature of the emema solution is 105° F. This is sufficiently warm to stimulate peristalsis, but not hot enough to damage the bowel lining. Cold solutions cause discomfort and increase the potential for cramping. Nursing Skill 24-4 describes the technique for administering a cleansing enema.

Hypertonic solutions are used for low-volume cleansing enemas. These solutions, commercially prepared, typically contain 120 ml of a sodium phosphate solution packaged in a soft plastic container with a prelubricated tip. These enemas are used for their convenience, as well as for patients who cannot tolerate a large volume of fluid. They are generally administered at room temperature, but can be warmed by immersing the container in warm water. Hypertonic solutions stimulate peristalsis by irritating the mucosa and by drawing water into the bowel from the blood and surrounding tissues by osmosis. Distention of the bowel gradually increases over a period of 5 to 10 minutes until defecation is stimulated. Since some sodium may be absorbed from the enema solution, hypertonic enemas are not given to persons whose sodium intake is restricted. They are also withheld from dehydrated patients and children, who are prone to serious fluid imbalance from the increased loss of water through the bowel.

Oil Retention Enemas. Oil retention enemas are given to treat constipation or fecal impaction. The oil softens the feces and lubricates the rectum for easier passage of the stool. About 180 ml of vegetable or mineral oil are instilled. These enemas are available commercially in plastic squeeze bottles with prelubricated tips. Alternately, the oil is administered through a small funnel and rectal tube. Since retention for one to three hours is desired, the oil is warmed to body temperature and introduced slowly with a small rectal tube to reduce the potential for stimulating a defecation reflex before the oil has had an effect.

Carminative Enemas. Carminative enemas promote the expulsion of excessive flatus. They consist of combinations of ingredients that release gas, thus further distending the colon and stimulating peristalsis. Amounts range from about 200 to 350 ml, depending upon the ingredients used.

Return Flow Enemas. The return flow enema, or Harris flush, is also used to expel flatus. In this procedure, solution is repeatedly introduced into, and drained from, the colon. About 200 to 300 ml of solution are instilled. The solution container is then lowered so the fluid flows back out into the container. The passage of gas is noted as it bubbles up through the liquid. The process is repeated four or five times, or until the alternate filling and emptying of the bowel stimulate

peristalsis and relieve the distention. As the solution becomes thick with feces, it is emptied into the bedpan and replaced with clean solution. A total of 1,000 ml is usually used.

Medicated Enemas. Enemas containing medication are intended to be retained in the bowel for an extended period. Amounts are small to prevent stimulation of defecation. Medications include those used to destroy intestinal parasites, to reduce bacteria in the bowel, to reduce bowel inflammation, or to bind and remove excess electrolytes in renal failure. Dextrose solutions or other nutrients are occasionally administered by enema.

Positioning for Enemas. Patients are typically positioned on the left side for enemas. In this position, the flow of fluid from the rectum to the sigmoid colon is assisted by gravity. This is believed to introduce more solution into the colon, rather than permitting it to distend the rectum and stimulate early defecation. When distribution of the solution throughout the entire colon is desired, the patient may begin the procedure on the left side, then turn to the back, and finally to the right side, promoting flow of the solution to the transverse and ascending colon. This type of positioning is useful for carminative and medicated enemas, or for cleansing enemas where complete emptying of the colon is desired. The knee-chest position is also effective in delivering solution to the colon, but it is awkward and often uncomfortable for the patient. Good results can be obtained from enema administration in most positions as long as the solution is administered slowly. The supine position is used when the individual is unable to retain the solution. The patient is placed on a bedpan and the head of the bed elevated about 30 degrees. The nurse wears a glove on the hand used to hold the enema tube in place, as feces and solution drain from the rectum throughout the procedure.

DIGITAL REMOVAL OF FECAL IMPACTION. Fecal impaction is usually treated with an oil retention enema followed by cleansing enemas. When this approach is unsuccessful, digital removal becomes necessary. The patient is positioned on the side with a pad under the buttocks. The nurse inserts into the rectum a gloved finger, generously lubricated. The fecal mass is gently manipulated and small pieces broken loose. The pieces are worked down through the anus, wiped on toilet tissue, and/or deposited in a bedpan. Caution is required to avoid injuring the bowel mucosa. The procedure is painful for the patient, as well as embarrassing, requiring considerable emotional support. Removal of the mass may need to be done in stages, allowing the patient time to rest. A second oil retention enema can be administered to further soften the partially broken mass and facilitate its complete removal.

Nursing Skill 24–4   **Administering a Cleansing Enema**

Preparation

1. Determine need. Enemas are ordered by the physician. The order is frequently written in response to data provided by the nurse which indicate constipation. Cleansing enemas are also given as part of established protocols to prepare the bowel for diagnostic and surgical procedures.
2. Gather equipment. Ordered solution at 105° F, fluid container (can, bucket, or plastic bag), rectal tube and tubing to connect it to the fluid container (may be constructed in one piece), clamp to control flow, lubricant, waterproof absorbent pad, tissues, robe and slippers if appropriate, bedpan or commode if patient cannot walk to bathroom, IV pole or overbed table.
3. Wash hands.
4. Identify the patient.
5. Discuss the procedure with the patient:
   a. Explain the reason for the enema.
   b. Determine the patient's prior experience with enemas.
   c. Explain the desirability of retaining the solution for 10 to 15 minutes.
   d. Determine whether the patient will use the bedpan, commode, or toilet.
6. Provide privacy.
7. Elevate the bed to working height.

Procedure

1. Position the patient on the left side with the right hip and knee flexed. (see Figure 24–23).
2. Place waterproof pad under the patient's buttocks.
3. Cover the patient, exposing only the anal area.

Explanation

1. Permits gravity to assist flow of solution to the colon; facilitates visualization of the anus.
2. Protects the bed linen from water and soiling.
3. Provides warmth and privacy.

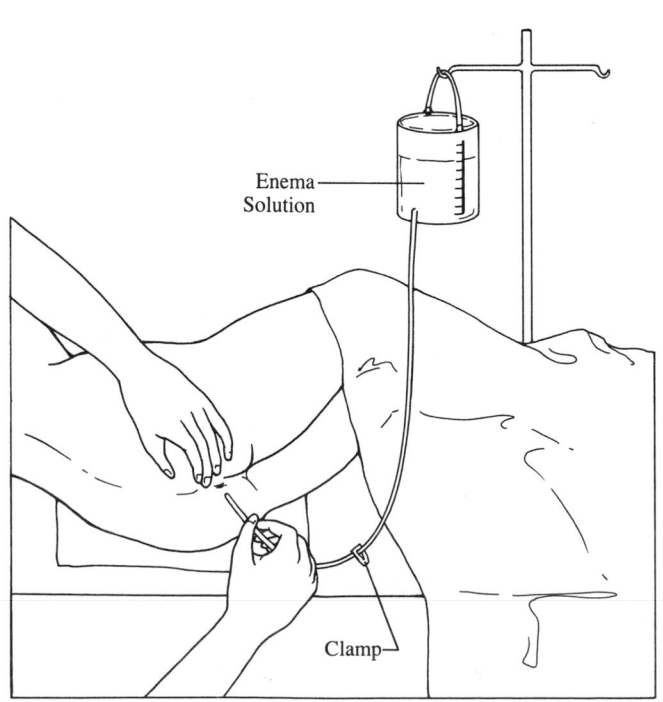

Enema Solution

Clamp

Figure 24–23. Enema administration.

4. Set the container of solution on the overbed table or hang it on the IV pole. Adjust the height of the pole so the fluid level is 12 to 18 inches above the rectum.
5. Open the clamp allowing solution to fill the tubing; close clamp.
6. Lubricate the last 5 to 8 cm (2 to 3 inches) of the rectal tube.
7. Separate buttocks to clearly expose the anus.

8. Begin to insert the rectal tube into the anus, wait a few seconds, then continue to insert 7.5 to 10 cm (3 to 4 inches) for an adult, 5 to 7.5 cm (2 to 3 inches) for a child.
   If resistance is felt, withdraw the tube slightly and allow a small amount of solution to flow. Ask the patient to take a deep breath, and continue insertion during exhalation.
9. Raise the solution container, or check the height of the IV pole, so the fluid level is 12 to 18 inches above the rectum.
10. Open the clamp and run the solution in slowly, over 5 to 10 minutes for 1,000 ml, less time for smaller amounts.

11. Hold the rectal tube in place throughout the procedure.
12. If cramping occurs, or if the urge to defecate occurs before most of the solution has run in, pinch the tubing or lower the container to slow or stop the flow temporarily. Ask the patient to take several slow, deep breaths or to pant. When cramping subsides, resume slow administration.
13. Clamp the tubing after all the solution has run in, or when the patient can no longer retain it.
14. Apply firm pressure over the anus with tissues as the rectal tube is withdrawn.
15. Encourage retention of the enema for 10 to 15 minutes, or until the urge to defecate becomes strong.
16. Assist the patient into a sitting position on the bedpan, commode, or toilet to expel the enema.
17. If the enema is expelled in the toilet, ask the patient to avoid flushing until the nurse has noted the returns.
18. If the enema solution is not expelled, an attempt may be made to remove it by siphoning:
    a. Position the patient on the right side.

    b. Pour 150 to 200 ml of warm water into the enema solution container.
    c. Expel air from the tubing and reclamp.
    d. Insert the rectal tube.
    e. Open the clamp and allow a small amount of water to flow into the rectum.

4. Frees the nurse's hands; this height allows gravity flow but prevents tissue damage from excessive force.

5. Expels air and warms the tubing.

6. Decreases friction for ease of insertion and reduced risk of tissue injury.
7. Provides for comfort and safety of insertion; facilitates identification of the anus if partially obscured by hemorrhoids.
8. Allows time for initial contraction of the external sphincter to subside; positions the end of the tube beyond the anal sphincter.

   Warm fluid and deep exhalation facilitate relaxation of the internal sphincter; forced insertion damages the tissues.

9. Allows gravity to move fluid into the rectum; prevents tissue damage from excessive force.

10. Prevents stimulation of a defecation reflex until sufficient fluid is introduced to promote thorough cleansing. Lowering the container reduces the rate of flow.
11. Prevents its slipping out or being expelled by bowel contractions.
12. Allows time for colon contractions to subside; distracts attention from defecation urge.

13. Indicates an adequate amount of solution has probably been administered.
14. Assists retention of fluid.

15. Produces sufficiently strong muscle contractions to adequately empty the bowel.
16. Protects safety of patients who are weak or in a hurry; provides normal position for defecation.
17. Permits the nurse's observation of the amount and character of the feces expelled.

18. Increases the patient's comfort; decreases the potential for fluid and electrolyte imbalance.
    a. Allows gravity to assist initiation of return flow from the sigmoid colon.

Procedure	Explanation
f. Before any air enters the tubing, lower the rectal tube below the level of the rectum and allow the water to drain into the bedpan.	f. Creates a siphon effect, or negative pressure, which draws fluid out of the colon.
g. Steps b through f may be repeated several times.	
19. Assist the patient to clean the rectal area, wash hands, and return to a comfortable position.	
20. Dispose of equipment properly and wash hands.	20. Prevents contamination of the environment by fecal material; prevents transmission of organisms.
21. Record on the patient's record the amount and appearance of stool and fluid returned, the amount of gas expelled, and the patient's tolerance of the procedure.	21. Provides for continuity of care; provides necessary documentation of care given.

Intestinal Distention. Flatulence and intestinal distention are relieved by limiting the amount of air swallowed, reducing gas formation, and promoting the evacuation of gas. Patients who swallow large amounts of air while anxious or in pain are taught relaxation techniques or offered pain-relieving medication. Avoiding the use of drinking straws, chewing gum, and carbonated beverages also reduces the gas swallowed. Gas production in the colon is limited by restricting gas-forming foods. Since individual tolerances vary, the patient is asked to identify foods that are particularly troublesome.

Peristalsis is stimulated in several ways, the most effective of which is exercise. Ambulation is encouraged as appropriate. When the patient must remain in bed, assistance is provided with frequent turning and activity. A high-fiber diet is provided when foods are not restricted. When peristalsis is severely reduced, as after abdominal surgery, food and fluids are withheld until bowel sounds are present, and flatus is being expelled from the rectum. Unless contraindicated, a warm heating pad may be applied to the abdomen.

RECTAL TUBES. When the above methods are not successful in removing flatus, a rectal tube may be inserted. The rectal tube stimulates peristalsis and facilitates passage of flatus through the sphincters. The tube is lubricated and inserted 15 to 20 cm (4 to 6 inches) into the rectum. It is usually held in place by taping to the buttocks. To collect any fecal seepage, a pad is placed under the buttocks, and the end of the rectal tube placed in a rolled absorbent pad or small waterproof container. The patient may change positions to facilitate passage of the gas, or may remain in a side-lying, prone, or knee-chest position. The tube is left in place for 20 minutes. After this time, nerve endings cease to respond to the stimulation and peristalsis decreases. Prolonged use also reduces sphincter control and irritates the tissues. Insertion may be repeated every two to three hours. The nurse records the procedure, noting the amount of flatus expelled and any changes in the patient's comfort level.

Diarrhea. Goals in the treatment of diarrhea are to decrease peristalsis and to maintain fluid and electrolyte balance, nutrition, skin integrity, and patient morale.

PERISTALSIS. Peristalsis is decreased by removing the cause of the diarrhea, if possible. This may mean providing medication for an intestinal infection, discontinuing medications that cause diarrhea, restricting food or fluids not tolerated by the individual, or reducing stress. Food and possibly fluids may be temporarily withheld and activity restricted to avoid peristaltic stimulation. Peristalsis may also be reduced by giving antidiarrhea medications, types of which are summarized in

Table 24-4. Although the physician is responsible for ordering and discontinuing medications, the data collected in the nursing assessment help to identify the types of medication changes required.

NUTRITION AND FLUIDS. The patient with diarrhea is reluctant to eat since the ingestion of food provides the stimulus for additional stools. Intake and output are measured and fluids provided to replace the water lost in the stools. Fluid replacement is especially important in infants because they can develop dehydration and electrolyte imbalance within hours. In severe infant diarrhea, regular formulas are replaced with water and electrolyte solutions for 24 hours or more, then reintroduced gradually over a period of several days. In patients of all ages, fluids are given intravenously if not tolerated orally. Foods and fluids are less likely to stimulate peristalsis when served at lukewarm, rather than very hot or very cold, temperatures, and when taken in small amounts. Greasy, spicy, and high-fiber foods are avoided. Full liquid and soft, bland diets are better tolerated and are better absorbed during the rapid passage of food through the intestine. Yogurt or medications containing lactobacillus may be given in diarrhea resulting from antibiotic therapy to replace the normal intestinal bacteria.

SKIN INTEGRITY. Diarrhea stools are highly irritating to the skin and mucosa because of their acid and enzyme content. To prevent skin breakdown, the anal area is washed with warm water and mild soap promptly after each defecation. The area is gently dried and a protective coating of petroleum jelly or zinc oxide cream applied. Cotton balls and a nonirritating lotion are sometimes used for greater comfort in cleansing.

EMOTIONAL SUPPORT. Diarrhea is embarrassing for the patient. The increased frequency, sounds, and odors of defecation greatly limit privacy. The urgency associated with diarrhea creates the fear of soiling, and patients find it humiliating to require clean-up help from others. The patient's emotional comfort is advanced by providing rapid access to the bathroom, commode, or bedpan. The call light is answered promptly. The patient may want to keep the bedpan in the bed, out of sight under the linen. Most feel more secure with a waterproof pad on the bed. The bedpan or commode is emptied immediately after use, the patient washed, and any soiled clothing or bed linen promptly changed. Room deodorizers are used, and room ventilation is provided as available.

Incontinence. The loss of bladder or bowel control may be humiliating for the individual. The importance attached by society to being clean and odor free heightens the person's distress. An accepting and understanding attitude on the part of the nurse is essential in helping the patient to cope with the problem. Meticulous skin care is required to prevent skin irritation and breakdown, as well as to provide physical and psychological comfort to the patient. The skin is washed with mild soap and water and dried gently, but thoroughly, after each bowel or bladder evacuation. Disposable bedpads or waterproof absorbent undergarments are used to keep bed linen and outer clothing clean and dry and to reduce the patient's embarrassment from soiling. Dependence on the pads and undergarments is not allowed to develop, however; a regular toileting schedule is maintained even with their use. Female patients with stress incontinence may wear sanitary napkins to absorb the relatively small amounts of urine expelled with physical stress.

BOWEL AND BLADDER RETRAINING.   In many situations, a period of retraining can restore normal functioning to the incontinent individual. Incontinence can be reduced by these nursing measures:

1. Involve mentally capable patients in development of the plan.

2. Get the patient out of bed and into daytime clothing. This tends to decrease dependency and to increase the motivation to remain continent.

3. Provide easy access to the bathroom, commode, or bedpan. Answer the call light promptly.

4. Provide clothing that is easy for the patient to manage.

5. Establish a regular schedule for voiding and defecation. Defecation is planned for the same time every day, 15 to 30 minutes after a meal to take advantage of the gastrocolic reflex. Urination is encouraged according to the observed pattern of the individual, at least every two to three hours, to empty the bladder before an uncontrollable micturition reflex occurs.

6. Encourage fluid intake of 2,000 to 3,000 ml each day. Patients may be hesitant to drink because it increases the frequency of urinary incontinence. The large intake, however, promotes normal filling of the bladder, which is necessary to stimulate the micturition reflex and establish a voiding pattern. Fluids are offered 20 to 30 minutes before the planned voiding time; they are withheld after the evening meal to reduce nocturia.

7. Prevent constipation.

8. Teach perineal exercises to improve sphincter tone. Perineal exercises are performed by contracting the perineal muscles as though to prevent defecation and to stop the urinary stream. A workable schedule is to perform four contractions each hour of the day, over a period of several weeks or months.

9. Have the patient hold the urine in the bladder a little longer with each urge to void to gradually increase bladder capacity.

10. Administer suppositories and laxatives in the initial phase to establish a defecation pattern.

11. Insert a urinary catheter as a last resort. A catheter may be chosen when the skin is irritated to prevent breakdown, or by the active person whose incontinence cannot be controlled by other methods. Intermittent catheterization produces less irritation and fewer infections than an indwelling catheter. Individuals with certain types of neurological dysfunction have remained infection-free using a clean, rather than sterile, catheterization technique to empty their own bladders intermittently.

THE CONDOM CATHETER.   Incontinent males may wear a condom catheter to collect urinary drainage. This device consists of a condom (a thin, flexible rubber or plastic sheath worn over the penis) connected to tubing which drains into a collection bag. When the individual is ambulatory, a leg bag collects the urine; when in bed, an indwelling catheter collection bag is used. The bags are washed daily with soap and water. Vinegar soaks may be used to alleviate odor and bacterial growth. Figure 24–24 illustrates a condom catheter connected to a leg bag. The condom is attached to the penis with skin adhesive and elastic tape. The penis is washed

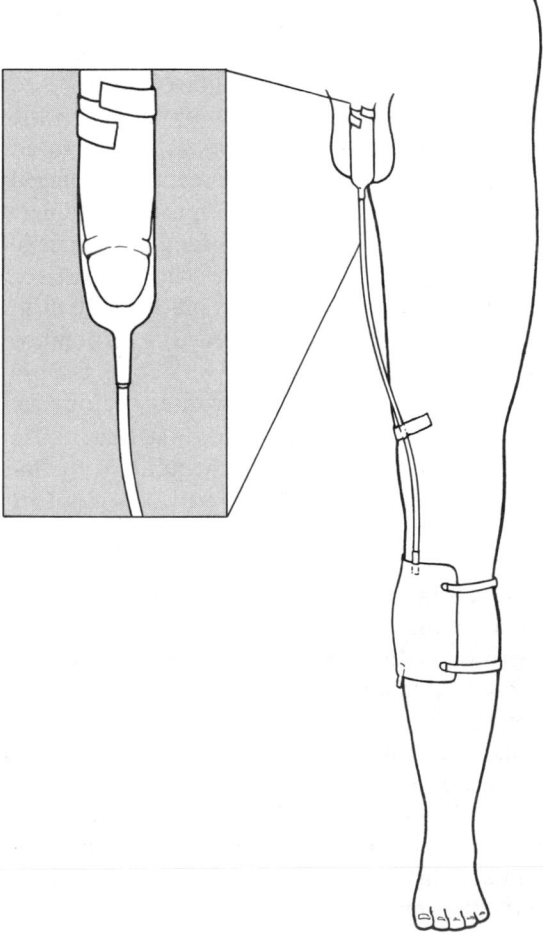

Figure 24–24.   Condom catheter attached to a leg bag.

and dried, and the adhesive applied around the top. The condom is rolled up over the penis, leaving ½ to 1 inch extending beyond the tip of the penis, preventing irritation of the tip of the penis by the end of the condom. A strip of elastic adhesive tape is then applied spirally around the top of the condom and penis. The penis is not completely encircled since this could compromise circulation with erection or swelling. The tape is applied snugly enough to prevent leakage, but not so tight as to interfere with circulation. Since this is difficult to accomplish, damage to the penis is not uncommon. The condom is left on for one to two days if the patient's skin remains free of irritation. The condom, because it is flexible, tends to twist around itself at the tip of the penis. The nurse checks periodically to be sure that urine flow and blood circulation is not obstructed.

Hemorrhoids.   Nursing interventions are instituted to decrease constipation and discomfort. Relieving constipation decreases pressure on the swollen veins, allowing inflammation and swelling to subside. Pain is relieved by the application of heat, as in sitz baths, and with medications. Stool softeners reduce the pain of defecation. Ointments are used to anesthetize the area, especially prior to defecation, and to shrink swollen tissues. Severe hemorrhoids are treated surgically.

Altered Routes of Elimination.   Nursing care of patients with colostomies, ileostomies, and urinary diversions involves emptying and changing pouches, maintaining integrity of the surrounding skin, teaching the patient, and providing psychological support. Emptying the pouch (also called a bag or appliance) will be described here. The other measures are beyond the scope of this book and can be found in medical-surgical nursing textbooks. Several types of bags are pictured in Figure 24-25.

The bag for a urinary diversion is emptied much the same as the collection bag for an indwelling catheter. A cap or spigot at the bottom of the pouch is opened, allowing the urine to drain into a graduate or other receptacle. When the patient is able, the bag is emptied directly into the toilet. Aseptic technique is used to prevent the entrance of pathogens into the opened end of the tube or spigot. At night, or when in bed, the patient's urinary pouch is connected to a catheter collection bag to remove the need for getting up at night to empty the pouch.

Pouches for ileostomies and colostomies are washed out with each emptying to remove odor. Clean technique is used since the intestine is not sterile. A waterproof pad is placed across the patient's abdomen, under the pouch, to prevent soiling of the patient or bed. The bottom of the pouch is opened by removing a clamp and unfolding the bottom of the pouch. The lightweight,

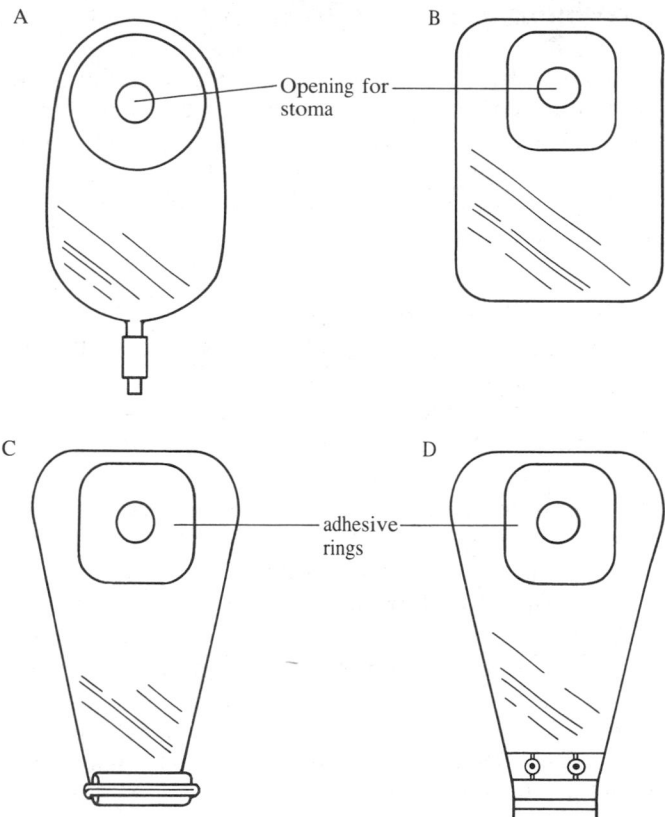

Figure 24-25. Ostomy pouches: **(A)** urostomy bag with push-pull drainage valve, **(B)** closed colostomy bag which is discarded rather than emptied, **(C)** drainable colostomy or ileostomy bag closed by folds and a clamp, **(D)** drainable colostomy or ileostomy bag with zip lock and snap closure.

clear pouches applied in surgery may be closed with an elastic band. The contents of the pouch are emptied into a graduate or small basin. A solution of warm water and mild detergent is poured into the pouch and swished around while the open end of the pouch is held closed. The solution is then drained into a basin or container. The introduction and drainage of solution are repeated until all the fecal material has been washed out. The pouch is then rinsed with clear water. The open end is dried thoroughly, inside and out, refolded, and closed as before. Thorough drying of the folded end is essential for odor control. Any remaining liquid prevents a tight seal and provides a pathway for the escape of feces and gas. Containers and equipment are promptly removed from the room, and the patient left clean and dry. The patient's psychological comfort is enhanced when the nurse performs the procedure efficiently and without soiling skin, bed linen, or clothing. When the patient's strength permits, the procedure can be done in the bathroom. The patient sits far back on the toilet seat or on a chair facing the toilet. The feces and cleansing solution can then be drained directly into the toilet.

Preventing Treatment-Related Problems

Diagnostic tests, surgery, activity restrictions, and medications all carry the potential for interfering with elimination. In these situations, nursing actions for promoting normal habits are continued within the prescribed limitations, and additional measures related to the specific problem are instituted.

Problems Related to Diagnostic Tests. The radiopaque substance (barium) given orally or rectally for gastrointestinal x-rays causes constipation and fecal impaction unless thoroughly evacuated. Following its administration, the nurse monitors the appearance and frequency of stools until the barium is expelled, and provides ordered laxatives or cleansing enemas as necessary.

Tests in which instruments are inserted through the urethra cause irritation and swelling, and may lead to infection or urinary retention. The nurse observes for data indicating these conditions, monitors intake and output, and encourages a large fluid intake. Fluids dilute the urine, decreasing tissue irritation, swelling, and discomfort. They also flush out bacteria that may have been introduced during the procedure.

Problems Related to Surgery. Following many types of surgery, patients are prone to develop urinary retention, abdominal distention, and constipation. These problems result from the antiperistaltic effects of anesthetics, narcotics, sedatives, irritation of tissues during surgery, anxiety, pain, inactivity, and food and oral fluid restrictions. Nursing measures include frequent assessment for early recognition of developing problems, and the institution of specific interventions, within surgery-related limitations, presented earlier in the chapter.

After surgery, urine production is reduced for several days, apparently due to a stress-related increase in the production of ADH. A bowel movement is usually expected by about the third postoperative day. The enemas or laxatives often given prior to surgery and the withholding of food during the surgical period delay the accumulation of sufficient residue to stimulate the defecation reflex.

Problems Related to Activity Restrictions. Restricted mobility interferes with elimination by contributing to muscle weakness, prohibiting body positions conducive to elimination, predisposing to urinary stone formation, and decreasing appetite. Nursing measures to minimize these interferences are a high fluid intake, a schedule of regular exercise within the patient's limitations, position changes every one to two hours to promote urine drainage from the kidneys, and establishment of a bowel and bladder evacuation schedule.

Problems Related to Medications. Medications prescribed for other purposes may coincidentally predispose the patient to elimination problems. Constipation or urinary retention are likely to result from drugs that decrease the frequency and strength of muscle contractions in the urinary and intestinal tracts. These include many pain relievers, sedatives, and tranquilizers, as well as drugs used to treat nausea, spasms of the urinary and intestinal tracts, and psychosis. Iron supplements cause constipation in some people, diarrhea in others. Certain antacids cause constipation, others cause diarrhea. Diarrhea also results from drugs that irritate the intestinal mucosa, from antibiotics that alter the normal colon bacteria, and from the overuse of laxatives. Urinary tract inflammation occurs when drugs eliminated through the kidneys form crystals and/or irritate the tract lining. The nurse observes the patient for data indicative of these side effects, informs the patient of symptoms to be noted and reported, and provides nursing care specific to the constipation, diarrhea, retention, or inflammation.

Nursing Care Plan for a Patient with Unmet Elimination Needs

Assessment

Data. Mrs. Meadows was admitted to the hospital on 10/18 for the treatment of lower back pain which began after she rearranged her living-room furniture. She is a 59-year-old widow who lives alone. She works 30 hours a week as a secretary. Her treatment in the hospital consists of pain control, physical therapy for her back, and instruction in exercises to strengthen her abdominal and back muscles. She is allowed to be up and about at will, but is reluctant to move because of the pain in her back.

On 10/20, her third hospital day, she complains of the urge to defecate but inability to expel the stool. She has had no bowel movement since admission and believes her last bowel movement occurred the day before she entered the hospital. Mrs. Meadows states that her bowels usually move every two or three days. She often feels the urge to defecate after breakfast, but doesn't usually have time before she leaves for work. Sometimes bowel movements occur after lunch, sometimes after the evening meal. About once a month she becomes constipated and takes a laxative which she buys without a prescription at her neighborhood pharmacy. Her diet includes foods from the basic four food groups, but she eats only white bread. Most fruits and vegetables are canned or frozen because of the convenience of preparation. Her fluid intake consists of about four cups of coffee each day; she doesn't like to drink water. Her hobbies include reading, knitting, and gardening. She occasionally takes walks, of about three or four blocks, on the weekends. The pain medications she is taking while in the hospital have minimal potential for causing constipation.

Nursing Diagnoses

1. Constipation related to immobility and irregular defecation habits
2. Potential for recurring constipation related to irregular defecation habits and lack of exercise

Planning

Goals

1. Bowel movement within the next 24 hours
2. Knowledge of methods to prevent constipation

Planned Actions (Interventions)
For Goal 1

1. Fluid intake of at least 2,000 ml today.
2. Assist to walk at least 20 ft four times today; give medication for pain one hour before walking.
3. Send a dietary request for whole-grain bread and raw fruits or vegetables with each meal.
4. Give prune juice at bedtime.
5. Assist to the bathroom 15 minutes after breakfast 10/21.
6. Provide privacy and an uninterrupted time for defecation.

For Goal 2

1. Explore with the patient ways to consistently include more fluid and fiber in her daily diet.
2. Explain the value of responding promptly to the urge to defecate.
3. Explore the possibility of establishing a regular time each day for defecation.
4. Establish a plan for increasing daily exercise.

Evaluation

Goal 1 not met; no bowel movement on 10/21.
Goal 2 partially met; patient has identified a plan for getting up one-half hour earlier in the morning to allow time for a bowel movement before going to work.

Reassessment
Diagnosis 1 is retained since the problem has not been resolved. The goal and the planned actions are continued with the addition of a new intervention, "Obtain physician's order for a laxative."
Diagnosis 2 continues to be relevant. The actions are modified to reinforce the patient's decisions to date and to continue working on the rest of the plan.

Summary

Elimination of waste products from the body is essential for continued cell function. The urinary tract removes most of the liquid wastes and end products of metabolism, while the intestinal tract removes primarily the solid wastes. Elimination is influenced by neural and hormonal mechanisms as well as by activity level, fluid and dietary intake, cultural patterns, environmental factors, and the degree of satisfaction of other basic needs. Common problems of elimination are related to waste formation, transport, and storage, and to infection and inflammation.

Assessment of elimination involves the collection of data regarding factors that influence elimination, voiding and defecation patterns, waste characteristics, control, and comfort. Nursing techniques for assessing elimination are presented. Interventions are described for assisting with normal elimination, intervening in elimination problems, and preventing treatment-related problems. The procedures for carrying out female and male catheterization, catheter irrigation, specimen collection, and enema administration are presented in a step-by-step format.

Terms for Review

abdominal distention	diuretic	ileostomy	pyuria
adhesions	dysuria	ileum	rectum
anal canal	enema	incontinence	reflex incontinence
anuria	enuresis	intestinal distention	reflux
anus	eructation	ketonuria	residual urine
bowel	fecal impaction	kidney pelvis	retention with overflow
calculi	feces	laxative	sigmoid
cathartic	fistula	lithiasis	specific gravity
catheter	flatulence	meatus	stoma
Foley catheter	flatus	micturition	stool
indwelling catheter	functional obstruction	nephron	stress incontinence
retention catheter	glomerular filtrate	nocturia	strictures
straight catheter	glomerulus	occult blood	tympanites
colon	glucosuria	oliguria	urethritis
colostomy	hematuria	ostomy	urination
commode	hemorrhoids	overflow incontinence	urinometer
constipation	hesitancy	polyuria	urge incontinence
cystitis	hydrometer	prostatic hypertrophy	urostomy
defecation	ileal conduit	proteinuria	UTI
defecation reflex	ileocecal valve	pyelonephritis	voiding
diarrhea	ileocolic valve		

Self-Assessment

Individual Elimination Habits

1. I have soft, formed bowel movements of a regular schedule. Yes/No
2. If not, what changes can I make to establish a normal consistency and regular pattern?
   Diet

Fluid intake
Exercise
Meal schedule
Responding to the urge
Allowing time
Reducing stress

3. Do I frequently delay the urge to void? If so, what problems do I have an increased risk of developing?
4. Are my elimination habits working for me now, but such that I may develop problems as I get older?

Attitudes Toward Elimination

1. Will I be embarrassed to assist a patient with urinary or bowel elimination? If so, in what ways may this affect my nursing care?
2. What behaviors on my part will decrease any embarrassment the patient may feel?
3. When explaining to a patient the method for collecting a clean-catch specimen, how can I determine that the patient understands my directions?
4. When a patient does not understand my terms for elimination or associated body parts, what other terms will I use?
5. Do I feel that genital care or catheterization is best performed by a care-giver of the same sex as the patient? What is my rationale?
6. Do I feel that catheterization should be performed by a specially trained and experienced "Catheterization Team," or by the nurse primarily responsible for the patient's care? What are the benefits of each to the patient? What are the advantages of each for the health care institution?
7. Do I feel that waterproof undergarments decrease patients' self-esteem by making them feel like babies, or help to increase self-esteem by controlling soiling? How can I verify my opinion?
8. Under what circumstances can I justify the insertion of an indwelling catheter for the purpose of controlling incontinence, considering the risk of infection to the patient?

Learning Activities

1. Observe a staff nurse or member of a hospital "Catheterization Team" insert one or more indwelling catheters. Note the precautions for maintaining sterility of the catheter, provisions for the patient's self-esteem, and any patient education related to catheter management.
2. Visit a nursing home or extended care facility. Investigate the methods used to monitor and evaluate the adequacy of the residents' elimination. What provisions are made for ensuring appropriate fluid intake? How is constipation prevented and treated? How are urinary and fecal incontinence managed? Are bowel and bladder retraining programs in progress? Are residents taken to the toilet at regular times? Are diapers and incontinent pads in evidence? Is the facility free of odor?

Review Questions

1. A micturition reflex is stimulated when the normal bladder contains approximately how much urine?
   a. 150 ml
   b. 350 ml
   c. 750 ml
   d. 1,500 ml
2. Mass movements of the colon, which frequently result in defecation, usually occur
   a. Before meals
   b. Continuously throughout the day
   c. For 30 to 60 minutes at a time
   d. Three or four times a day
3. Normal urine contains significant amounts of
   a. White blood cells
   b. Glucose
   c. Nitrogenous substances
   d. Protein
4. Mr. Artz's care plan includes a nursing diagnosis of "Urinary retention related to partial obstruction of the urethra." Which set of data supports this diagnosis?
   a. Voiding 100 ml at a time, burning immediately following urination, loss of small amounts of urine with heavy lifting
   b. A feeling of extreme urgency accompanying the need to urinate, voiding 700 ml at a time, pale-yellow urine
   c. Voiding every six hours, sharp pain in the lower abdomen immediately preceding urination, cloudy urine
   d. Voiding 50 ml every hour, palpable bladder distention, difficulty in initiating urination
5. A high fluid intake is beneficial for persons with
   a. Diarrhea
   b. Urinary incontinence
   c. Constipation
   d. Indwelling catheters
   e. All of the above
6. Which method is most appropriate *initially* in assisting the person who has difficulty voiding?
   a. Applying manual pressure over the bladder
   b. Administering prescribed medications to stimulate bladder contraction
   c. Running water within the patient's hearing
   d. Inserting a catheter
7. A straight catheter is inserted approximately _____ inches in a women, _____ inches in a man.
   a. 3, 8
   b. 1, 5
   c. 6, 12
   d. 5, 6
8. While a catheter is being inserted, it is most important that which equipment remains sterile?
   a. Gloves
   b. Cotton balls
   c. Specimen container
   d. Insertion end of catheter
9. Which statement related to catheter irrigation is true?
   a. Irrigation fluid is instilled at refrigerator temperature to reduce the potential for infection.
   b. With the open method of irrigation, the bladder contains no more than 30 to 60 ml of irrigating solution at a time.
   c. Of the three methods of catheter irrigation, the needle method carries the least risk of infection.
   d. The continuous closed method of irrigation is the least effective in removing debris from the catheter lumen.

10. Which statement accurately represents one of the steps in administering a cleansing enema that is not of the hypertonic type?
    a. The amount of solution instilled is 500 to 1,000 ml.
    b. The solution container is held 24 inches above the rectum.
    c. Temperature of the solution is 115° F.
    d. Soapsuds solution is used for its soothing effect.
11. The nursing intervention most useful in alleviating intestinal distention is
    a. Withhold all pain medications.
    b. Apply an ice bag to the abdomen.
    c. Assist the patient to exercise.
    d. Give all fluids through a straw.
12. When used to reduce intestinal distention, the rectal tube
    a. Stimulates peristalsis and facilitates passage of gas through the anal sphincters.
    b. Is kept in position by instructing the patient to lie very still.
    c. Provides the best effect when kept in place for one to two hours at a time.
    d. Is inserted 2 to 3 inches.
13. Which technique is most beneficial in reestablishing bowel and bladder control?
    a. Have the patient wear pajamas for ease in toileting.
    b. Limit fluid intake to reduce incontinence.
    c. Avoid the use of suppositories.
    d. Offer help with urination every two to three hours.
14. Which foods are least likely to stimulate peristalsis?
    a. Soft, bland
    b. Very hot
    d. Very cold
    d. Large servings
15. Treatment for hemorrhoids includes all except:
    a. Prevention of constipation
    b. Anesthetic ointments
    c. Stimulant laxatives
    d. Sitz baths
    e. Stool softeners

Answers

1. b
2. d
3. c
4. d
5. e
6. c
7. a
8. d
9. b
10. a
11. c
12. a
13. d
14. a
15. c

References and Bibliography

Aman, R.: Treating the patient, not the constipation. *Am. J. Nurs.,* **80:**1634–35, 1980.

Burns, K., and Johnson, P.: *Heatlh Assessment in Clinical Practice.* Prentice-Hall, Englewood Cliffs, N.J. 1980.

Butts, P.: Assessing urinary incontinence in women. *Nursing 79,* **9:**72–74, Mar., 1979.

Campbell, C.: *Nursing Diagnosis and Intervention in Nursing Practice.* Wiley, New York, 1978.

Clark, J.; Queener, S.; and Karb, V.: *Pharmocological Basis of Nursing Practice.* Mosby, St. Louis, 1982.

Gordon, M.: *Manual of Nursing Diagnosis.* McGraw-Hill, New York, 1982.

Guyton, A.: *Textbook of Medical Physiology,* 6th ed. Saunders, Philadelphia, 1981.

Hargiss, C. and Larson, E.: Infection control: Guidelines for prevention of hospital acquired infections. *Am. J. Nurs.,* **81:**2175–83, 1981.

Hargiss, C., and Larson, E.: Infection control: How to collect specimens and evaluate results. *Am. J. Nurs.,* **81:**2166–74, 1981.

Hogstel, M.: How to give a safe and successful cleansing enema. *Am. J. Nurs.,* **77:**816–17, 1977.

Introduction to Bowel and Bladder Care. Sister Kenny Institute, Minneapolis, 1975.

Killion, A.: Reducing the risk of infection from indwelling urethral catheters. *Nursing 82,* **12:**84–88, May, 1982.

Luckmann, J., and Sorensen, K.: *Medical-Surgical Nursing: A Psychophysiologic Approach,* 2nd ed. Saunders, Philadelphia, 1980.

Malseed, R.: *Pharmacology: Drug Therapy and Nursing Considerations.* Lippincott, Philadelphia, 1982.

McConnell, E.: Urinalysis: A common test but never routine. *Nursing 82,* **12:**108–11, Feb., 1982.

McGill, S.: Catheter management: It's the size that's important. *Nurs. Mirror,* **155:**48–49. Apr. 7, 1982.

Metheny, N., and Snively, W. D.: *Nurses' Handbook of Fluid Balance,* 4th ed. Lippincott, Philadelphia, 1983.

Perston, Y.: Urinary incontinence: Ways to help solve a sensitive problem *Nurs. Mirror,* **154:**38–42, Oct. 21, 1981.

Porth, C.: *Pathophysiology: Concepts of Altered Health States.* Lippincott, Philadelphia, 1982.

Promoting urine control in older adults. *Geriatr. Nurs.,* v.1 236–76, Nov./Dec., 1980.

Strand, F.: *Physiology: A Regulatory Systems Approach.* Macmillan, New York, 1978.

Vander, A.; Sherman, J.; and Luciano, D.: *Human Physiology: The Mechanisms of Body Function,* 3rd ed. Mc-Graw-Hill, New York, 1980.

The Verdict is in on clean cath. *Am. J. Nurs.* **83:**1644, 1983.

Whaley, L., and Wong, D.: *Nursing Care of Infants and Children.* Mosby, St. Louis, 1979.

CHAPTER **25**

THE NEED FOR REST AND SLEEP*

Rest and Sleep as Basic Human Needs

Sleep Architecture: What Happens When We Sleep

Individual Sleep Needs

Sleep Deprivation: What Happens When We Don't Sleep

Factors that Influence Sleep
Age
Environment
Nutrition
Exercise
Stress
Drugs

Sleep Disorders
The Insomnias—Disorders of Initiating and Maintaining Sleep (DIMS)
Disorders of Excessive Somnolence (DOES)
The Parasomnias: Disorders of Arousal

Assessment of Rest and Sleep Need Satisfaction
The Sleep History
Nursing Diagnosis Related to Rest and Sleep

Nursing Interventions to Promote Rest and Sleep

Objectives

1. Identify the two types of sleep and the associated stages.
2. List three recordings that are used to measure activity in a polysomnograph recording.
3. Name five factors that influence sleep.
4. Identify three of the most common sleep disorders.
5. Name three foods that contain L-tryptophan.
6. List five questions that are important when taking a nursing history for rest and sleep.

7. Discuss three nursing interventions to promote rest and sleep.
8. Name three factors that interfere with rest and sleep in the hospital.
9. Name three psychosocial problems of a patient who suffers from sleep apnea.
10. Discribe four symptoms of a patient with the diagnosis of narcolepsy.
11. List two of the most common drugs that alter the sleep/wake cycle.

Rest and Sleep as Basic Human Needs

Shakespeare's plays abound with dissertations on sleep, the lack of sleep, the quest for sleep, and the mystery of sleep. Hundreds of years later, scientists and researchers are still searching for the answers. The question is, why? How much sleep do we need? What happens when we sleep? What happens when we don't sleep?

The need for rest and sleep is a basic human need.

*Written by Jan Davis Schluter, a registered nurse specializing in sleep disorders at the Minnesota Regional Sleep Disorders Center, Hennepin County Medical Center, Minneapolis, Minnesota. She has given seminars on various topics related to sleep disorders and nursing care to health professionals and nursing students. She has worked in neurology in both in-patient and out-patient settings. She is currently head nurse of the opthomology, otolaryngology and neurology ambulatory care clinics.

Rest may be defined as a state of well-being, free from feelings of anxiety or fear. The body and mind need to wind down, to take time to rejuvenate, to be free from physical and mental stresses. If one is not rested, the body and mind do not function to the optimal level. Feelings of tiredness, irritability, depression, or loss of control develop if one is not rested.

Sleep is one of the things we can do to feel rested. Sleep is a regeneration of the body's processes. Mental and physical activities of the day deplete the body of energy. *Sleep* is defined as "a period of rest for the body and mind, during which volition and consciousness are in partial or complete abeyance and the bodily functions partially suspended" (*Dorland's*, 1981). When a person is deprived of sleep, energy diminishes, concentration wanes, activity slows, judgment dulls, and the body will have increased sensitivity to pain and discomfort.

The inability to sleep and feel rested is a common complaint during hospitalization. The patient is subjected to a new and unfamiliar environment, pain and discomfort, loss of independence, and feelings of loss of self-control. An important aspect of the nurse's role is to recognize the patient's needs for rest and provide measures to promote sleep.

Sleep Architecture: What Happens When We Sleep

Sleep is measured by recording the brain's electrical activity from an electroencephalogram (EEG), muscular activity from an electromyogram (EMG), and eye movements by an electro-oculogram (EOG). These recordings are used to determine the stages and cycles of sleep. Other recordings may include an electrocardiogram (ECG), respiration, leg movements, and O_2 (oxygen) saturations by ear oximetry. These sophisticated all-night recordings are called *polysomnograms* (Figure 25–1).

There are two types of sleep: *rapid eye movement*, called *REM*, when twitching of the closed eyelids occurs from eye movements underneath, and *nonrapid eye movement*, called *nonREM (NREM)* which has four stages. Stage I of NREM is the transition between full wakefulness and sleep. The person may be aware of surroundings, but thoughts begin to drift, and short dreaming may develop. Stage I may last approximately one-half minute to seven minutes.

Stages II and III of NREM sleep consist of short, fragmented thoughts, then progress into deeper sleep. The person may be unaware of surroundings, but awakens easily.

Stage IV of NREM sleep is called delta sleep or slow-wave sleep. Most young adults enter delta sleep within 30 to 45 minutes after falling asleep. The body is relaxed, and arousal is difficult. There are slow or rolling eye movements. The heart rate is decreased, and blood pressure lowers. Respiratory rate decreases, as does body temperature and metabolic rate. Stage IV restores the body physically.

After about 70 to 90 minutes of sleep, the first REM period of the night occurs and lasts about five minutes. The second REM period occurs about three hours after falling asleep. Following the second REM period until awakening, REM sleep occurs in 90-minute cycles. During REM sleep, most dreaming occurs (Hauri, 1982). Muscle tone is relaxed, but twitching of the eyelids (REM) can be observed. The pulse is irregular, heart rate is increased, and blood pressure is higher. Cerebral blood flow and brain temperature increase. Respiratory rate and gastric secretions increase. Men experience penile erections, and women have increased vaginal blood flow (Hauri, 1982).

The sleep/wake cycle is an example of a *circadian rhythm* (from the Latin word *circa*, about, and *dian*, day). The cycle completes in about a day or 24 to 26 hours. The body has high and low levels of functioning dictated by an internal clock. Human beings function best during daylight hours, and sleep during darkness. However, there are those who prefer the reverse, the "owls" of the world are examples. Human biological clocks correspond to the 24-hour rotation of the earth. It may be that the 90-minute cycles that occur during sleep also occur during the day, and this might explain mood changes, temperature changes, and other biological changes during the waking hours.

The most beneficial sleep occurs during the low period of the circadian rhythm. If individuals sleep at

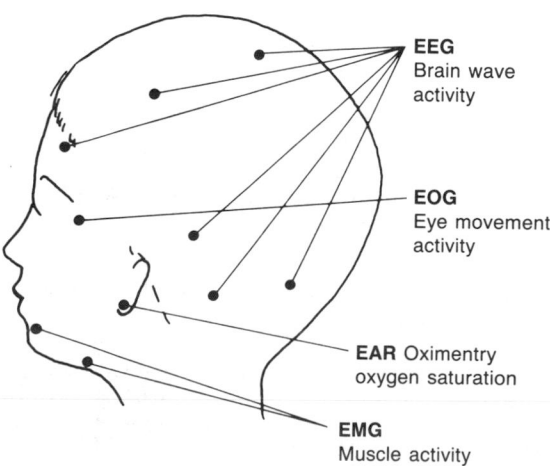

Figure 25–1. Polysomnogram.

EEG
Brain wave
activity

EOG
Eye movement
activity

EAR Oximentry
oxygen saturation

EMG
Muscle activity

other times during the day, they become desynchronized. Some examples are jet-lag syndrome (crossing time zones) and shift workers. Because hospitals provide 24-hour services, nurses are obliged to rotate between shifts. The most common complaint is chronic fatigue, disturbed sleep, lowered performance (the incidence of work errors is much higher in the early morning hours, 3 to 5 A.M., than at any other time). Gastrointestinal symptoms, plus increased stress on social and family life, are common.

The psychological basis for sleep is that the process of sleep restores. Sleep is necessary for maintaining mental health. Sleep is the time for gathering the day's information, selecting and processing that information, then putting it aside. Dreaming is the key mechanism to sorting information. Most dreams are about daily concerns. Everybody dreams, but we do not always remember those dreams. Dreaming helps us review problems of the day and enables us to cope with pain and discomfort.

Individual Sleep Needs

The range of individual sleep requirements is wide. Eight hours of sleep is not the magic number. Some individuals can sleep three to five hours and feel refreshed, while those who sleep ten to twelve hours per night awaken feeling tired.

Studies have shown that adults who sleep seven to eight hours a night have lower mortality rates than those that sleep more (Kripke et al., 1979) and are likely to be artistic and creative. Hartmen el at. (1973) claims that long sleepers appear to be worriers and nonconformists, while short sleepers appeared to be successful, outgoing, energetic, ambitious, and confident.

Sleep alterations, stress, and illness create special sleep needs. During the first trimester of pregnancy, the patient will experience excessive sleepiness, and during the last trimester, the patient may complain of insomnia due to increased fetal movements, failure to find a comfortable position for sleep, and the increased need to urinate. Hormonal changes during menopause alter the patient's sleep pattern. Night sweats, hot flashes, insomnia, and daytime sleepiness reduce the ability to fall asleep.

Chronic diseases play a role in sleep patterns. Nocturnal angina (chest pain at night) occurs during REM sleep. Arthritis causes awakenings during sleep as inactivity causes joint pain and stiffness. Patients with peptic and duodenal ulcers have increased gastric secretions at night, and those with COPD (chronic obstructive pulmonary disease) complain of shortness of breath at night.

Sleep Deprivation: What Happens When We Don't Sleep?

Most researchers agree that an occasional night of poor sleep has no ill effects, however, chronic sleeplessness causes lowered performance, irritability, inability to concentrate, listlessness, and increased fatigue. Sleep deprivation decreases the patient's ability to cope with pain. Patients in intensive care units for more than three to five days may experience a syndrome known as intensive care delirium, characterized by hallucinations, irritability, and confusion caused by excessive stimulation and unmet rest and sleep needs. Patients with epilepsy may have an increase in seizure activity when sleep needs are unmet, and patients with psychiatric disorders report an increase in depression if sleep deprived.

Factors that Influence Sleep

Age

Age is the most important factor affecting rest and sleep needs. Infants sleep most of the time, and sleep needs decrease with age. The elderly require longer to fall asleep and awaken earlier in the morning. Sleep disturbances also increase with age. (See Figure 25-2.)

Environment

Environment alters or enhances an individual's ability to sleep. The patient tries to adjust to new surroundings, temperature changes, sleeping alone if previously used to sleeping with a bed partner. Too many or not enough blankets, sensory overload from hospital paging

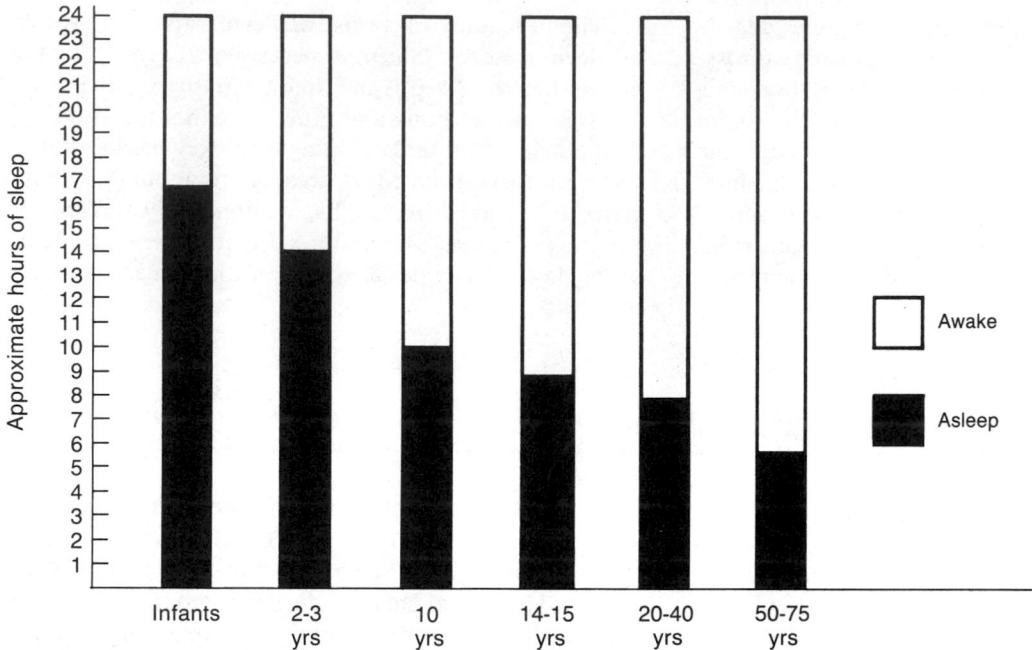

Figure 25–2. Sleep changes with age.

systems, lights, a snoring roommate and disruption of the normal bedtime ritual are some of the things the nurse must consider if promoting the patient's ability to sleep.

Nutrition

Weight gain is associated with long and uninterrupted sleep; weight loss with short and fragmented sleep. Insomnia is a common symptom in anorexia nervosa (Hauri, 1982). Foods high in protein induce sleep. Foods that contain L-*tryptophan* (an amino acid) found in milk, cottage cheese, tuna fish, chicken, turkey, and cashews are natural hypnotics that promote sleep. Grandma's advice to drink a glass of warm milk before bedtime had a scientific basis.

Although milk may induce sleep, coffee, chocolate, and cola drinks with their high caffeine content disrupt sleep. A small amount of alcohol (1 oz) may help sleep, but more than that produces sleep that is fitful and fragmented. The two most common drugs responsible for patients' complaints of poor sleep are coffee (caffeine), a stimulant, and alcohol, a depressant.

Exercise

There is evidence that routine physical exercise promotes sleep. It must be regular exercise, limited to hours in the afternoon, not just before bedtime.

Stress

Life-style changes influence sleep. A change in occupation, marital status, depression, loss of a loved one, anxiety about parenting, financial concerns, attending college, in addition to an illness are some of the stressors a patient might be experiencing that interfere with ability to sleep.

Drugs

Drugs alter the sleep/wake cycle. Over 100 million people in the United States have complaints relating to sleep/wake functions. There is evidence that the largest single use of over-the-counter medications, such as hypnotics, tranquilizers, and alcohol is for the treatment of sleep complaints (Dement, 1974).

Sleep Disorders

The Association of Sleep Disorders Centers has classified over 35 sleep and arousal disorders. Sleep research and assessment of sleep/wake disorders has necessitated a new field of medicine. Sleep disorders centers are usually located at major medical centers. The staff consists of a multidisciplinary team: an expert in sleep disorders (somnologist); sleep laboratory technologists; physicians from the disciplines of neurology, otolaryngology, psychiatry, cardiology, urology, pulmonary medicine, child psychiatry, pediatric neurology; social services, and nursing.

The sleep disorders center may diagnose, evaluate, and manage patients with the following disorders: sleep apnea, narcolepsy, insomnia, excessive daytime sleepiness, nocturnal myoclonus, restless leg syndrome, nocturnal seizures, night terrors, somnambulism, circadian rhythm disturbances, hypoventilation in infants and children, sleep-related cardiovascular symptoms, and impotence. Treatment may include medication, supervised drug withdrawal, counseling, psychotherapy, and tracheostomy.

The Insomnias—Disorders of Initiating and Maintaining Sleep

The most common sleep complaint is, "I can't sleep" or "I don't get enough sleep." A *disorder of initiating and maintaining sleep (DIMS)* is the inability to fall asleep or the complaint of too little sleep. *Insomnia*, a form of DIMS, is characterized by failure to fall asleep within 30 minutes after going to bed, reduced amount of total sleep time, awakening for an hour or more each night, and feeling tired during the day. A sleep log is used in sleep centers to determine the quality of sleep and the patient's perception of sleep time. Treatment for insomnia may include improving the sleep through a regimen of sleep hygiene, hypnosis, self-hypnosis, hypnotics, and drug withdrawal.

Causes of insomnia may include drug abuse, alcoholism, psychiatric and personality disorders, *nocturnal myoclonus* (jerking of the leg muscles while asleep), and *restless leg syndrome* (complaints of sensation of "crawling" or "creeping" inside the calf while awake). Insomnia can result from sensory deprivation or excess sensory stimulation, pain and discomfort, depression, fear, and anxiety.

Disorders of Excessive Somnolence (DOES)

Our society does not condone sleepiness which is basically what *disorders of excessive somnolence (DOES)* are. We are expected to be awake, productive individuals. If you sleep too much, you are labeled as "lazy" or "no good" and subject to ridicule. We are expected to rise at 6 A.M., jog for one-half hour, spend eight hours at our occupation, arrive home, eat the evening meal, then pursue community activities, or engage in hobbies for the remaining hours before bedtime. Patients with excessive daytime sleepiness rarely complain about their disorder for fear of not being taken seriously. The medical profession's standard answers were, "You need more sleep." "You're depressed." "You need to get out more." "You could stay awake if you really wanted to." With increased awareness of sleep disorders, patients with DOES are being treated in sleep centers throughout the world. At the sleep center, a physician does a physical, psychosocial, medical, and detailed sleep history. Because many of the patients with DOES are not aware of how sleepy they are, information from family, bed partners, or friends is useful. The most common disorders of excessive somnolence are narcolepsy and sleep apnea.

Narcolepsy. The narcolepsy syndrome is manifested by four symptoms called the narcolepsy tetrad: excessive daytime sleepiness, cataplexy, sleep paralysis, and hypnagogic hallucinations. Not all four of these symptoms are present in all narcoleptic patients. The most debilitating of the symptoms is excessive daytime sleepiness, sometimes first noticed in the teens. Narcoleptics complain of being too tired to get up for school, sleepiness during classes, failing grades, and inattentiveness (one wonders if some children labeled as behavior problems might be suffering from narcolepsy).

Patients with narcolepsy experience many daytime naps, some lasting 10 to 30 minutes, they awake feeling refreshed, then fall asleep again. Narcoleptics state that

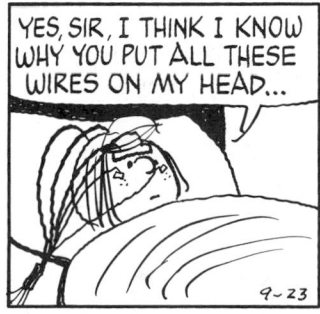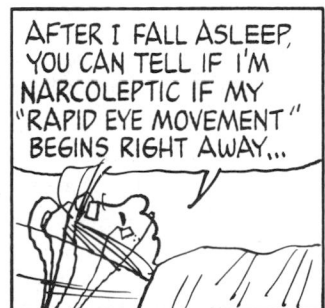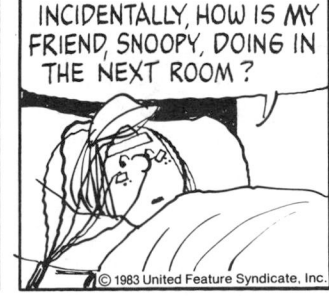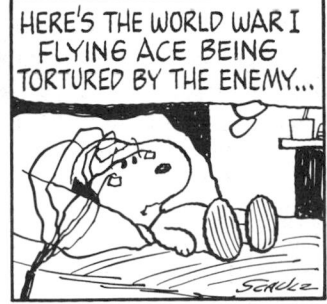

Figure 25–3. Peanut's cartoon. Taking a laboratory sleep test to assess narcolepsy. (Reproduced with permission of United Feature Syndicate, New York, 1983. © 1983 United Feature Syndicate, Inc.)

even though they get a normal amount of sleep at night, they constantly feel sleep deprived.

Cataplexy, one of the four symptoms of narcolepsy, is a brief episode of loss of muscle tone. It can be a slight drooping of the facial muscles or complete collapse. Cataplexy is usually precipitated by an emotion such as anger, humor, or surprise. During cataplexy, patients remain aware of their surroundings. Many narcoleptics become isolated, choosing not to interact with others because of the fear of the debilitating cataplectic attacks.

Hypnagogic hallucinations, another symptom of narcolepsy, are very vivid, frightening dreams that appear at sleep onset. Many patients decline to describe these dreams for fear of being labeled "crazy."

Sleep paralysis occurring with narcolepsy is the inability to move, and it occurs at sleep onset or upon awakening in the morning. At times, sleep paralysis occurs in conjunction with hypnagogic hallucinations, leaving the patient feeling frightened and helpless.

An important documentation for the diagnosis of narcolepsy is the multiple sleep latency test (MSLT). The patient is asked to sleep all night in the sleep laboratory, then asked to nap five to six times during the day. Normal subjects take 20 to 25 minutes to fall asleep during naps, however, patients with narcolepsy fall asleep within five minutes and begin REM sleep immediately.

Narcolepsy is a lifelong condition afflicting more than 250,000 Americans. There is a tendency toward the disease if another family member has narcolepsy. The psychosocial problems are profound. People with narcolepsy have difficulty learning and reading, therefore, education is a struggle. Marital problems, occupational stress, and decreased social interactions isolate the patient with narcolepsy. It is interesting to note that the same syndrome has been identified in dogs. Doberman pinchers are especially susceptible to the disease.

Treatment consists of medications to increase wakefulness, drugs that act as REM suppressants, and support groups to help the narcoleptic cope with daily living.

Sleep Apnea.   Sleep apnea is a life-threatening illness, characterized by excessive daytime sleepiness and cessation of breathing at night. Apnea during sleep may be caused by obstruction of the upper airway [obstructive sleep apnea (OSA)] or loss of nervous stimulation to breathe (central apnea) or a combination of the two, called mixed apnea. The most common is obstructive sleep apnea. The patient may have as many as 300 to 600 obstructions and awakenings every night. The cause is not known, but some physicians feel that the muscles of the tongue and upper airway collapse during sleep. The patient is usually male, obese, middle-aged, and has a short, thick neck. He may complain of loud snoring, night sweats, morning headaches, and have hypertension and right-sided heart failure. The patient is studied in the sleep laboratory by monitoring sleep stages, heart rate, respirations, and oxygen saturations. Normal hemoglobin oxygen saturation is 92 to 94 percent. Apnea patients may have O_2 saturations of 0 to 50 percent (Hauri, 1982).

Treatment for obstructive sleep apnea depends on the degree of disability during daytime hours, severity of other medical symptoms (heart failure), and degree of oxygen deprivation. The treatment that guarantees a cure is a tracheostomy. The surgeon creates a new airway, and the obstruction is bypassed. The larynx is not damaged. The patient can speak when the tracheostomy is plugged during the day. The plug is removed at night, thereby letting the patient sleep normally with unobstructed breathing.

A new surgical procedure, the uvulopalatopharyngoplasty or UPP, has been performed without or in addition to the tracheostomy. It involves a "face lift" of the upper airway and removing redundant laryngeal tissue.

Patients with sleep apnea have many psychosocial problems caused by excessive daytime sleepiness. They may have marital problems (the wife may move out of the bedroom because loud snoring interrupts her sleep).

Table 25-1.   **Affect of Sleep Apnea on Other Basic Needs**

  I. Physiological needs
Decreased oxygen to body
Fluid overload (congestive heart failure)
Obesity—increased food intake, eats to stay awake
Impotence

 II. Safety and security
Unsafe due to need to sleep during the day. May fall asleep while driving a car. Potential for accidents on the job.

III. Love and belonging
Behavior is not acceptable, falls asleep at family gatherings and social interactions. Falls asleep at work.

IV. Self-esteem
Loses respect of co-workers and is an embarrassment to family because of excessive sleepiness. Feels rejected by family and friends. Feels nonproductive.

 V. Self-actualization
Unable to become self-actualized because they can't meet other needs. Too sleepy to appreciate and enjoy beauty, unable to be creative.

She assumes financial, household, and family responsibilities because the patient is too tired. Many patients have lost their jobs and turn to drugs or alcohol. Their quality of life is drastically altered. They can't drive safely or take part in recreational activities. They are shunned by their family and don't take part in family activities because they are too tired. (See Table 25–1.)

The Parasomnias: Disorders of Arousal

Parasomnias are events that occur exclusively during sleep or are exaggerated by sleep (Hauri, 1982). They occur most often in children. They usually occur about an hour after sleep onset. Parasomnias usually occur during stage IV or delta sleep, and patients rarely remember the events. Some of the events of the parasomnias are *somnambulism* (sleepwalking), *enuresis* (bedwetting), which is more common to boys and can be very distressing to both parent and child, and *pavor nocturnus* or sleep terror (a very frightening dream). People experiencing sleep terror start with screaming and are difficult to console. Sleep terrors usually disappear in adolescence. Other parasomnias include *jactatio capitis nocturna* (head banging or rhythmic body movements before or during sleep), and *bruxism* (teeth grinding). If the habit persists, mouth guards may be worn to prevent dental problems.

Drugs used to treat some sleep disorders are presented in Table 25–2.

Table 25–2. **Drugs Used for Sleep Disorders**

DRUG	PHARMACOLOGIC ACTIONS	USES	SIDE EFFECTS	DOSAGE
Methylphenidate (RITALIN)	Similar to amphetamines and includes central nervous system and respiratory stimulants	Treatment of narcolepsy	Nervousness, insomnia, anorexia, nausea, dizziness, tachycardia, lowers convulsive threshold among others	Tablets (U.S.P.), 5 mg, 10 mg, 20 mg. Dosage must be carefully adjusted according to individual requirements
Pemoline (CYLERT)	Similar to those of amphetamines and methylphenidate and includes central nervous system and respiratory stimulation	Treatment of narcolepsy	Insomnia, anorexia, stomachache, irritability, skin rash, nausea, dizziness, headache	Tablets, 18.75 mg, 37.5 mg, 75 mg scored. Dosage must be carefully adjusted according to individual requirements
Protriptyline (VIVACTYL)	Tricyclic antidepresant	Treatment of sleep apnea, cataplexy, and sleep paralysis	Dry mouth, blurred vision, constipation, urinary retention, nausea, vomiting, anorexia	Tablets (N.F.), 5 mg, 10 mg. Dosage must be carefully adjusted according to individual requirements
Imipramine hydrochloride (TOFRANIL)	Tricyclic antidepressant	Treatment of disorders of arousal, enuresis, in children	As above	Treatment of enuresis: 25 mg 1 hr before bedtime. Tablets, 10 mg, 25 mg, 50 mg
Clonazepam (CLONOPIN)	Anticonvulsant. Pharmacologically related to diazepam (VALIUM) and other benzodiazepines	Petit mal seizures, psychomotor seizures, infantile spasms, and may be used for restless leg syndrome	Drowsiness, ataxia, irritability, gastritis, nausea	Tablets, 0.5 mg, 1 mg, 2 mg scored.
Flurazepam (DALMANE)	Hypnotic	Short-term management of insomnia	Drowsiness, dizziness, ataxia, falls	Capsules, 15 mg, 30 mg

Assessment of Rest and Sleep Need Satisfaction

The Sleep History

The nurse who is aware of sleep disorders and sleep-related problems will be able to gather data and form a plan of care using a sleep history. Most initial history forms in health care settings have few questions relating to rest and sleep. The usual questions is, "How many hours do you sleep at night?" and no further discussion follows. The observant nurse not only will collect data pertaining to sleep-related problems and normal hours of sleep but will include information on the individual's presleep activities, medications used for sleep, and fears or anxieties that might preclude sleep. Table 25–3 presents some questions that are helpful to include when assessing a patient's ability to rest and sleep.

Nursing Diagnoses Related to Rest and Sleep

Listed below are some general and specific examples of nursing diagnoses associated with unmet rest and sleep needs.

Sleep pattern disturbance
  Impaired ability to sleep at night
  Impaired ability to stay awake during the day
Alteration in thought processes related to lack of sleep.

Table 25–3. **A Nursing History for Rest and Sleep**

1. Whether or not excessive sleepiness during the day is a problem.
2. Does the patient snore or have unusual breathing problems at night?
3. How long does it take the patient to fall asleep after retiring?
4. Does the patient have unusual leg movements at night?
5. What medications are used, if any?
6. Amount of coffee, alcohol, or caffine containing cola consumed during the day?
7. The time of retiring and arising.
8. The number of naps during the day.
9. Does the patient sleep alone or have a bed partner?
10. Methods used for relaxation: watching TV, reading, etc.
11. Number of awakenings at night; reason for awakening.
12. What environmental factors contribute to the ability to sleep, such as tolerance of noise, light, temperature?
13. The patient's conception of the adequacy of personal sleep pattern.
14. Affect of any previous hospitalization on ability to meet rest and sleep needs.

Social isolation related to constant daytime sleepiness.
Potential for ineffective breathing pattern related to sleep apnea.

Nursing Interventions to Promote Rest and Sleep

The hospital is a noise-producing environment. Hospital paging systems, delivery systems, monitoring machinery, cleaning equipment, and inappropriate staff discussions all contribute to heightened noise level. You've all heard the complaint, "I just got to sleep then the nurse woke me up to give me a sleeping pill." Schedules are necessary, but are they for the nurse's benefit or the patient's? The nurse who uses good judgment and common sense will be able to provide rest and promote sleep for the patient.

Environmental Management.   Provide an environment that is conducive to sleep. Draw the drapes to minimize light, close the door to the patient's room to minimize sound. Check to see if the patient is too warm or cold. Offer blankets if too cold. Discourage unnecessary talking or laughter near the patient's room. Change room assignments if a roommate is disruptive. Offer a light

snack before bedtime. Know and understand the effects of sleep medications. If possible, schedule treatments, activities, and vital signs at a time when the patient will not be disturbed.

Fears and Concerns.   Offer to discuss patient's fears and concerns. The fear of pain or the fear of dying is a common concern. The absence of loved ones, feelings of loneliness, loss of independence, and loss of self-control are common to the hospitalized patient.

Observation.   Learn to observe the sleeping patient. Is sleep restless? Are there many leg movements? Does breathing stop many times during the night? Are there an unusual number of awakenings? If so, why? These observations will determine whether or not the patient has had a "good" night's sleep.

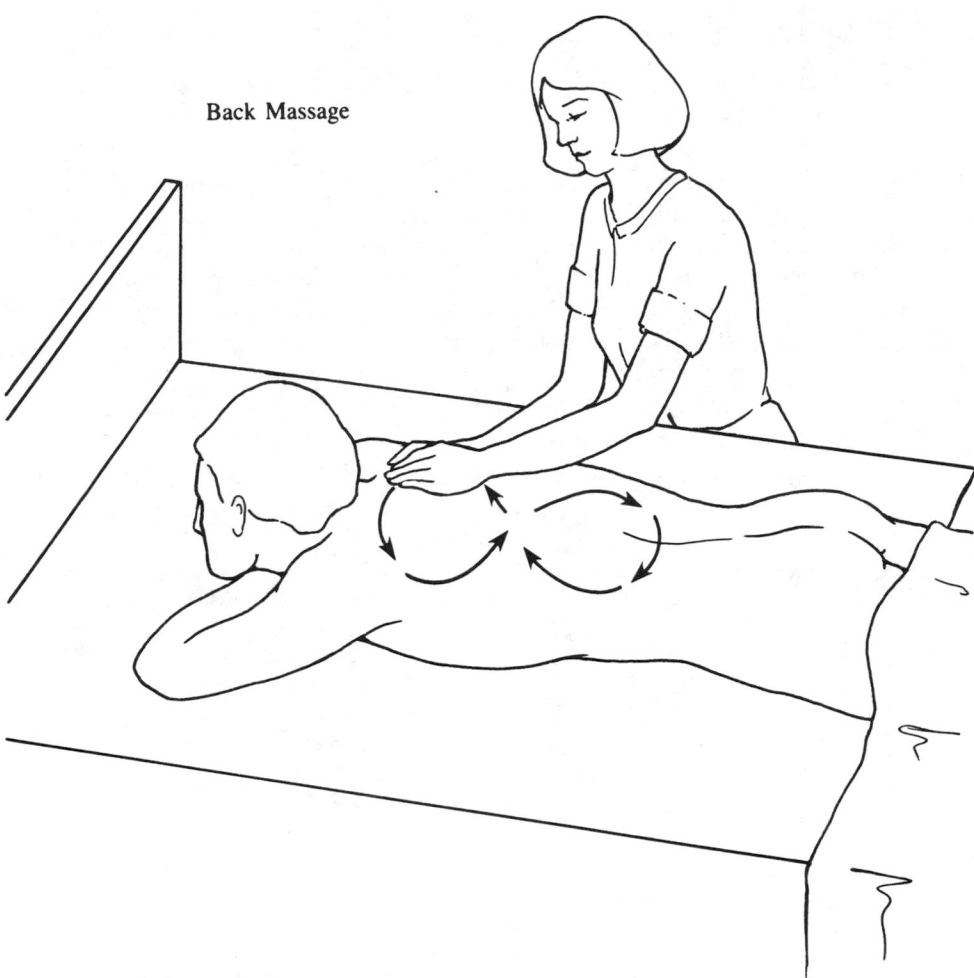

Back Massage

Figure 25-4.   Back massage.

Offer a Back Rub.   The back massage promotes feelings of relaxation and acts as an aid to sleep. It can serve two purposes: relaxation and time for the nurse to explain procedures and answer questions the patient might have (Figure 25-4). During the back rub is an excellent time to discuss some of the patient's concerns to help relax the patient psychologically in addition to physical muscle relaxation.

The following are suggested steps for a back massage:

1. Provide privacy.
2. Wash hands.
3. Adjust bed to working height so nurse may use good body mechanics.
4. Position patient, usually prone position, with pillow under head as comfortable.
5. Drape patient with bath blanket so back, shoulders, and buttocks are exposed.
6. Warm lubricant (lotion) under warm water and rub between hands.
7. Inform patient as you begin that it might feel cold.
8. Apply lubricated hands to lower back. Stroke from the buttocks, up to the shoulders, over arms, and back down to the buttocks.
9. Use long, slow, stroking motions with continuous contact of hands.
10. Using a kneeling motion and working down, begin at the muscles of the neck at the hairline; include the shoulders. Work down to the sacral area. A figure 8 massage pattern over the buttock may be included.
11. Assess patient's level of relaxation and condition of skin.
12. Wipe extra lotion from back with bath towel.
13. Put away equipment. Wash hands.
14. Document procedure in chart.

Nursing Care Plan for a Patient with Unmet Rest and Sleep Needs

Subjective data: Mrs. C. is a 32-year-old, recently divorced woman with three children, ages 7, 9, and 12, admitted to the hospital from home with complaints of "I haven't slept for a week and I'm so tired during the day. My husband is gone and I'm afraid to sleep alone, so I sit on the couch all night." She states a concern regarding family finances and ability to pay for hospitalization.

Objective data: Thin, pale, anxious woman, hair uncombed, wringing her hands, crying, and asking for sleeping pills. Blood pressure 130/88, respiration 20, pulse 94, weight 108, height, 5'4". Alert and oriented to time, person, and place but refuses to answer questions about sleep patterns or nutritional status.

The following format is a common way of documenting a patient's care plan on the Kardex.

No.	Problem	Goals and/or Expected Outcome	Intervention	Evaluation
1.	Insomnia related to life-style changes	Improve nighttime sleep to at least 6 h/night	1. a. Obtain sleep history b. Encourage good sleep hygiene: Going to bed and arising at same time Encourage activity during the day Limit coffee and cola during the day Limit cigarette smoking Offer a light snack before bedtime c. Offer back rub d. Minimize environmental factors: light, sound, etc.	1. Slept 6–7 hours 2nd hospital night
2.	Excessive daytime sleepiness related to inability to sleep at night	Decrease daytime sleepiness to no more than a 1 hr nap/day	2. Same as #1 interventions	2. Took ½ h nap on 3rd hospital day and reports feeling rested
3.	Anxiety related to financial worries and increased responsibilities	Decrease anxiety prior to hospital discharge.	3. a. Encourage to express fears and concerns regarding financial and parenting worries b. Contact social service for financial aid and information	3. States less anxiety after talking with social service and getting financial aid.
4.	Potential for drug dependency related to inability to sleep at night	Knowledge of medications used for sleep and consequences of abuse	4. a. Offer medication as ordered b. Teach alternative methods for relaxation c. Inform of possible physiological changes from medication	4. Stated correct dose and use of sleep medication before discharge

Summary

The nurse who understands the need for rest and sleep as a basic human need and is knowledgeable about individual sleep needs and factors that influence sleep will be able to provide for rest and promote sleep for the patient.

Knowing what foods promote sleep, the importance of taking a nursing history for sleep, the ability to observe a sleeping patient and identify abnormal behavior during sleep, the importance of establishing a routine or practicing good sleep hygiene—all will give the nurse a basis for teaching the patient.

Knowledge about sleep disorders and the availability of sleep disorders centers can provide the nurse and the patient with resources that before were unavailable.

Providing an environment that is conducive to sleep, understanding the effects of medications used for sleep, offering a back rub, or taking the time to listen to a patient's fears about hospitalization are some of the nursing interventions that will help the nurse develop a plan of care.

Terms for Review

bruxism	hypnagogic hallucinations	parasomnia	sleep apnea
cataplexy	insomnia	polysomnograph	sleep hygiene
circadian rhythm	narcolepsy	REM sleep	sleep paralysis
DIMS	nocturnal myoclonus	rest	somnambulism
DOES	NREM sleep	sleep	L-tryptophan
enuresis			

Self-Assessment

The nurse not only provides for the patient's rest and sleep, but takes responsibility for personal rest and sleep needs as well by practicing proper sleep hygiene and knowing individual sleep needs.

The student is especially vulnerable to unmet sleep needs. Late night studying, cramming for finals, and increased stress (I wonder if I flunked my chemistry test?) are a few examples of behavior that interferes with rest and sleep. The student who skips meals and exists on coffee or cola drinks is subjected to fragmented sleep at night, irritability, and gastrointestinal symptoms during the day.

Practicing proper *sleep hygiene* is the most effective aid to a good night's sleep. Ask yourself if you practice the components of sleep hygiene that are designed to maximize your ability to sleep.

Do you?

	Yes	No
1. Go to bed and get up at the same time every day?	____	____
2. Have a comfortable mattress, large enough for turning and stretching?	____	____
3. Fall asleep with the television or radio on? (Light and sound may help some people to fall asleep, but can be a detriment to others.)	____	____
4. Keep your bedroom temperature comfortable?	____	____
5. Use your bedroom as a place for other activities (studying, craftwork, ironing clothes)? Except for sexual activity, the bedroom is a place for sleeping.	____	____
6. Consume large amounts of coffee, cola, or alcohol during the day? (More than two cups of coffee can alter sleep.)	____	____
7. Nap during the day?	____	____
8. Smoke cigarettes? Nicotine is a stimulant. Do you wake up at night to have a cigarette?	____	____
9. Study just before bedtime? Use the hour before bedtime to relax. Take a warm bath, listen to music, minimize anxiety.	____	____
10. Take drugs to keep you awake or consume more than an ounce of alcohol in the evening?	____	____

A "Yes" answer to questions 3, 5, 6, 7, 8, 9, and 10 may indicate a violation of one or more components of sleep hygiene. If you feel tired and poorly rested or do have trouble falling asleep, consider altering your behavior so you can answer "yes" to questions 1, 2, 4, and "No" to the rest.

Learning Activities

1. Visit a sleep disorders center in your area. Ask to observe a polysomnograph recording and have the technologist explain the stages of sleep.
2. Interview two nurses who work the night shift. Ask about the quantity and quality of their sleep.
3. Using Maslow's hierarchy-of-needs model, list five needs that a patient with sleep apnea has difficulty in satisfying.
4. Take a sleep history from five nursing students. Discuss answers that you feel constitute sleep abuse.
5. Interview an elderly person (over 70 years of age) and a young adult (under 20 years). Compare and contrast sleep needs, methods used for promoting sleep, and reasons needs are not met.
6. Read the *Dr. Seuss Sleep Book* to a young child. Encourage a discussion about sleep. Listen to the fears and anxieties relating to bedtime or sleep.

Review Questions

1. Mrs. A. has been evaluated at a sleep disorders center for excessive daytime sleepiness. Mrs. A. was instructed to come to the sleep laboratory for an all-night recording. This recording is which of the following?
   a. Cardiac stress test
   b. Basal metabolic rate
   c. A polysomnograph
   d. ECG
2. Mrs. A.'s physician told her that she had narcolepsy. Mrs. A. probably had all the following symptoms, except:
   a. Enuresis
   b. Cataplexy
   c. Hypnagogic hallucinations
   d. Excessive daytime sleepiness
3. Mrs. A.'s physician prescribed a stimulant to help her stay awake. Which of the following drugs is a stimulant?
   a. L-Tryptophan
   b. DALMANE
   c. Wine
   d. RITALIN
4. Mr. B. is a 60-year-old, 385-lb male admitted to the hospital. His wife states he has hypertension (180/100), he snores, and he stops breathing many times during the night. Mr. B's symptoms are most characteristic of which of the following problems?
   a. Insomnia
   b. Alcoholism
   c. Narcolepsy
   d. Sleep apnea
5. L-Tryptophan, an amino acid that promotes sleep, is found in which of the following foods?
   a. Milk
   b. Tuna fish
   c. Cashews
   d. Chicken
   e. All of the above
6. Mr. D. is considering a surgical procedure for sleep apnea. He would choose which of the following?
   a. A colostomy
   b. A tracheostomy
   c. A laryngectomy
   d. A hemorrhoidectomy
7. Mrs. M. complains that her son, Bobby, age 2, bangs his head against the mattress before he goes to sleep. This behavior is which of the following?
   a. Pavor nocturnus
   c. Somnambulism
   c. Enuresis
   d. Jactatio capitis nocturna
8. Nursing interventions to provide rest and promote sleep would include
   a. Offer a light snack
   b. Offer a back massage
   c. Minimize sound and light
   d. All of the above
9. Everybody needs eight hours of sleep at night.
   a. True
   b. False

Answers

1. c
2. a
3. d
4. d
5. e
6. b
7. d
8. d
9. b

References and Bibliography

American Society of Hospital Pharmacists: American Hospital Formulary Service, 1983. Drug Information, Bethesda, Md.

Armstrong, Ester, C. A., and Hawkins, L. H.: Day for night, circadian rhythms in the elderly. *Nurs. Times,* **78**:No. 30, p. 1263–65, July 28, 1983.

Association of Sleep Disorders Centers: Diagnostic classification of sleep and arousal disorders. *Sleep,* **2**:17–19, 1979.

Dement, William C.: *Some Must Watch While Some Must Sleep.* Norton, New York, 1974.

Dorland's Illustrated Medical Dictionary, 26th ed. Sauders, Philadelphia, 1981.

Fernsebner, B.: *Sleep deprivation in patients. AORN J.,* Jan. 1983. **37**:35–42

Franceschi, M., *et al.* Excessive daytime sleepiness: A one year study in an unselected inpatient population. *Sleep,* **5**:239–47, 1982.

Fujita, S., *et al*.: Surgical correction of anatomic abnormalities in obstructive sleep apnea syndrome: uvulopalatopharyngoplasty. *Otolaryngol. Head Neck Surg.* **89**:923–34, 1981.

Guilleminault, C. (ed.): *Sleeping and Waking Disorders: Indications and Techniques*. Addison-Wesley, Reading, Mass., 1982.

Hartman, E.: Sleep requirement: long sleepers, short sleepers, variable sleepers and insomniacs. *Psychomatics,* **14**:95–103, 1973.

Hauri, Peter: *Current Concepts, The Sleep Disorders*, 2nd ed. Upjohn Kalamazoo, Mich., 1982.

Iber, Conrad: Sleep-disordered breathing: Differential diagnosis and treatment. *Respiratory Medicine for Pulmonary Care Physicians Journal*. Academic Press, New York, 1982.

Jenkinson, V.: Nurse education: Night duty and the nurse. *Nurs. Mirror*, May, **152** (May):25–30, 1981.

Karacan, I.: Managing marital conflicts: Association with sleep disorders. *Med. Aspects Human Sexuality*, **16**:No. 3, p. 71–94, 1983.

Kripke, D. F.; Simons, R. N.; Garfinkel; *et al.*: Short and long sleep and sleeping pills. Is increased mortality associated? *Archives Gen. Psychiatry*, **36**:103–116, 1979.

Lehmann, Phyllis: I didn't sleep at all last night. *The American Legion Journal*, Mar., 1983.

Lerner, R.: Sleep loss in the aged: Implications for nursing practice. *J. Gerontol. Nurs.* **8** (June):323–26, June, 1982.

Lindsay, M: The problem of staying awake. *Nurs. Times*, **78** (Mar.):379–381, 1982.

Orr, W. C.,: Allshuler, K. Z.; and Stahl, M. L: *Managing Sleep Complaints*. Year Book Medical Publishers, Chicago, 1982.

Roth, T.; Zorik, F.; Sicklesteel, J.; and Stepanski, E.: Effects of benzodiazepines on sleep and wakefulness. *B. J. Clin. Pharmacol.,* **5**:28–45, 1982.

Torbjorn, A., *et al.*: Sleepiness and shift work: Field studies.*Sleep,* **5**:595, 1982.

Walsh, J. K.; Bertelson, A. D.; and Schweitzer P. K.: Clinical aspects of sleep disorders. Proceedings of a Symposium. Deaconess Hospital, St. Louis, Mo., 1983.

Walsleben, J.: Sleep Disorders. *Am. J. Nurs.*, **82**(June):936–40, 1982.

THE NEED FOR PAIN AVOIDANCE*

Objectives

1. Discuss pain avoidance as a basic human need.

2. Explain the differences between acute and chronic pain.

3. Discuss factors that affect the initiation of pain impulses, the perception of pain, and the response to pain.

4. Discuss adaptation of physiological and behavioral responses occurring in chronic pain.

5. Recognize attitudes that hamper health professionals' accurate assessment and treatment of pain.

6. Identify the patient's verbal description and nonverbal behavior that indicate pain.

7. Discuss nursing interventions that assist patients in avoiding or reducing pain, alleviating pain, and coping with pain.

8. Explain the gate control theory as a framework for pain relief from cutaneous stimulation or relaxation with guided imagery.

Introduction

Avoidance of pain is a basic human need. Although a person can survive with pain, its continual presence interferes with an individual's well-being. Pain that is unrelieved becomes the focal point of a person's life, thereby disrupting the ability to eat, sleep, or exercise.

Pain is one of the most common circumstances that cause a person to seek health care assistance. As a result, all nurses inevitably will work with patients experiencing pain. As the health care team member who spends the most time with the patients, the nurse can make a significant difference in how patients perceive pain, react to pain, and the degree of relief obtained.

Pain is a complex phenomenon which, in most cases, acts as a protective mechanism to warn a person of actual or impending tissue damage. One definition identifies *pain* as a concept which involves "a personal, private sensation of hurt; a harmful stimulus which signals current or impending tissue damage; a pattern of responses which operate to protect the organism from harm" (Sternback, 1968). This definition points out the

*Written by Alexandra Wright, R.N., M.S., who works on an oncology unit with patients in pain. She writes and gives workshops on pain control for nurses and for people experiencing pain.

important components of pain which involve not only a stimulus and a sensation of hurt but also the responses of the person experiencing pain. These responses are individual and are influenced by the physiological, psychological, cultural, and spiritual makeup of the person in pain.

McCaffery (1972), a nationally known nursing expert in the field of pain management, defines pain as "whatever the experiencing person says it is, existing whenever he says it does." Inherent in this definition is the attitude that the person with pain is believed. This attitude is basic to working effectively with a patient in pain.

Neurophysiological Mechanisms for Pain

Although the exact basis for the transmission and perception of pain is not known, neurophysiological, psychological, and sociological research has helped in the formation of pain theories. These theories serve as the framework for specific pain-relieving actions.

Although several theories exist, the *gate control theory* proposed in 1965 by Melzak and Wall currently provides the most comprehensive explanation of pain (Jacox, 1977). It not only proposes that pain is a neurophysiological phenomenon based on the transmission of a stimulus which produces pain sensation but also suggests that thoughts, past experiences, and emotions influence the perception of pain and the response to pain, thereby establishing that the pain experience involves the mind and the body. Also, it provides a conceptual framework for understanding and developing measures that will help control a patient's pain. These specific nursing measures will be presented later in the chapter.

According to the gate control theory, a mechanism in the spinal cord acts as a gate that permits or prevents the transmission of pain impulses to the brain. It is believed that the site for the gate is an area within the spinal cord called the *substantia gelatinosa*. If the gate is open, then the impulses are permitted through to transmission cells (T cells); they then ascend the spinal cord to the brain where pain is perceived. If the gate within the substantia gelatinosa is closed, the transmission of pain impulses to T cells and to the brain is blocked, and pain is not realized.

Activity involving three specific areas within the nervous system influences the opening and closing of the gate. These areas are the large and small nerve fibers in the spinal cord, the brainstem, and the cerebral cortex and thalamus.

Stimulation of Small and Large Nerve Fibers

Small-diameter nerve fibers transmit pain signals to the spinal cord, through the open gate, and to the brain. Activation of the large-diameter nerves on the skin surface, by rubbing for instance, closes the gate and blocks or decreases the transmission of pain impulses (Figure

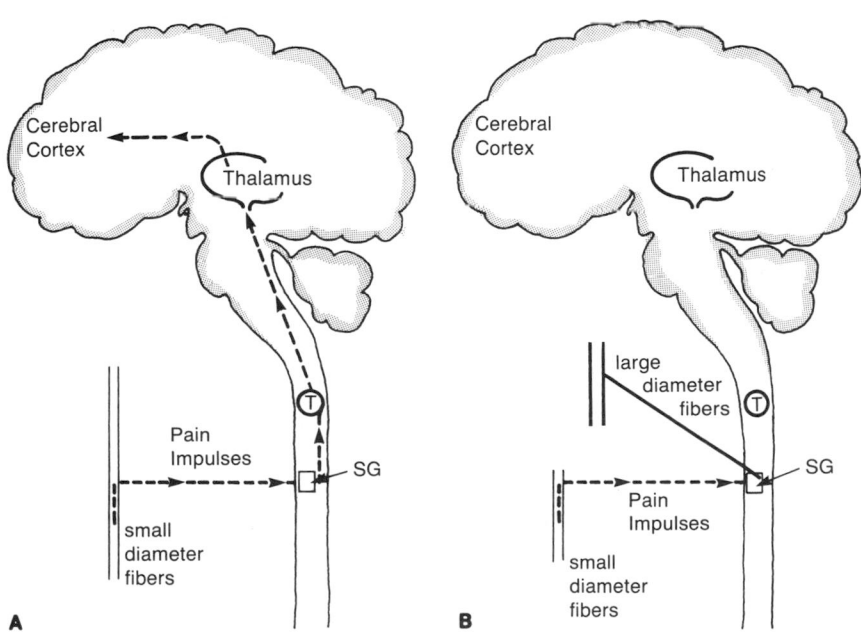

Figure 26–1. Diagram illustrating key concepts from the gate control theory. *SG* stands for substantia gelatinosa; *T* stands for transmission cells. **A.** Open gate location. **B.** Closed gate location. (From P. Burkhalter and D. Donley: *Dynamics of Oncology Nursing.* McGraw-Hill, New York, 1978. Reprinted with permission.)

26–1). Therefore, the sensation of pain is not felt or is reduced.

Impulses from the Brainstem

The core of the brainstem is composed of fibers and nerve cells which make up the reticular formation. The reticular formation monitors sensory input. If enough sensory input is received, through distraction techniques, for example, the brainstem transmits impulses that close the gate which blocks pain sensation. Monotony or minimal sensory input instead can facilitate pain by opening the gate.

Impulses from the Cerebral Cortex

Other factors in opening or closing the gate are thoughts, emotions, and memories processed in the cerebral cortex and thalamus. Therefore, an individual's fears and past negative experiences with pain can facilitate opening the gate and allow pain perception. On the other hand, measures to reduce anxiety through accurate information or positive relationships with health care professionals who relieve a patient's pain can result in inhibitory signals from the cortex and thalamus, resulting in pain alleviation.

Endorphins

Additional pain research has identified portions of the outer surface of specific nerve cells that attract and hold narcotics, called narcotic (opiate) receptor sites. In 1975, the body's own internally secreted, narcoticlike substances that hooked onto these receptors were identified. These naturally occurring narcoticlike substances called *endorphins* (a combination of the words "endogenous" and "morphine") tend to occur in the same locations as the narcotic receptor sites (Jacox and Rogers, 1981). These locations include the spinal cord, brainstem, and cerebral cortex. It is believed that endorphins block the transmission of a pain signal between nerve cells. Normally, a pain impulse (signal) is transmitted across the space between two nerve cells and ascends toward the brain. The release of endorphins is triggered by a descending impulse from the brain; it locks into the narcotic receptors and blocks the transmission of the pain impulse, thereby preventing the impulse from reaching the brain (West, 1981).

Gaps in knowledge about the gate control theory and the release of endorphins persist, however. Continued research will provide a better understanding of pain mechanisms, perception, and response, establishing the framework on which interventions for pain relief will be based.

Acute Pain and Chronic Pain

An important process for the nurse is to differentiate between acute and chronic pain. These differences have implications for assessment and treatment of pain.

Acute pain is usually described as pain of short duration that lasts from seconds to weeks. The pain may result from injury, such as missing a nailhead with a hammer and hitting the finger. It may result from surgical trauma, such as an abdominal incision for an appendectomy, or it may be the result of a disease, such as arteriosclerosis of the coronary artery which could result in the pain of myocardial infarction. Generally, however, acute pain decreases and eventually disappears with healing of the injury, surgical trauma, or disease.

Chronic pain, in contrast, is described as lasting for months, years, or a lifetime. There may be intermittent occurrences of chronic pain characterized by periods of pain interspersed with intervals that are pain free. This pattern may be repeated continuously over the years. Examples of intermittent chronic pain include migraine headaches, sickle cell anemia, or back pain that flares up several times a year.

Chronic pain can also be constant, persist, and grow progressively worse despite treatment. Arthritis and advanced cancer are diseases in which continuous chronic pain may occur.

Three terms that are used as descriptors of a specific type of pain are referred pain, phantom pain, and intractable pain. Pain that is perceived in one area of the body when the actual stimulus is in another area is *referred pain*. For example, pain from a myocardial infarction may be described as pain in the left shoulder extending down the left arm. For referred pain, the nerve fibers carrying pain impulses from the viscera (or internal organs) join with other fibers in the spinal cord. If the pain stimulus is intense, the sensation spreads over into areas that normally receive stimuli only from the skin. Thus, the person perceives the pain sensation as originating in the skin instead of from its actual source. Many patterns of referred pain occur and are useful for diagnostic purposes.

Phantom pain is pain that a person feels from a body part that is no longer present. An example is the pain that a patient feels in a calf after the leg has been amputated. Although not clearly understood, phantom pain is thought to be the persistence of "pain memory" after the cause for the pain has been removed.

Intractable pain reflects the inability to control or relieve pain despite various treatment regimens. In some cases, this term "may be as much a reflection of the health care providers' inability to find an effective treatment as it is a characteristic of the pain itself" (Jacox and Rogers, 1981).

Factors that Influence the Pain Experience

Components of the pain experience involve the initiation of the pain impulse, perception of the pain, and response to the pain. Each component affects the other, and these components, in turn, influence the patient's pain experience. Therefore, all three are vital factors which the nurse considers when working with a patient with pain.

Initiation of the Pain Impulse

A number of different stimuli—chemical, mechanical, and thermal, for instance—may initiate a pain impulse. Chemical stimuli include external irritants, such as acid in contact with the skin, and internal irritants released by specific cells. It is thought that damaged tissue cells release chemical substances, such as histamine and bradykinin, that excite pain nerve receptors.

Mechanical stimuli result from a physical force, such as a door slamming closed on a person's finger. Pain is thought to be caused by pressure on the nerve endings and the chemical substances released by the damaged cells.

Stretching or distention of tissue, another form of mechanical stimuli, can result in pain. For example, distention of an organ such as the stomach or esophagus by a tumor can exert pressure on the nerve endings and occlude the small blood vessels.

Mechanical stimuli can also include muscle spasms. The contraction that occurs exerts mechanical pressure on pain fibers and constricts small blood vessels, which prevents metabolic cellular waste products from being carried away. The buildup of these products is chemically irritating to the sensory nerve endings, thereby causing pain.

Extremes of hot or cold substances in contact with the skin are examples of thermal stimuli that initiate pain impulses. A burn caused by excessive heat to a body part is thought to cause pain by the destruction of tissue and the release of irritating chemical substances from the injured cells. Extreme cold constricts the blood vessels and may completely cut off the blood supply, allowing the buildup of acidic waste products of cellular metabolism.

Tissue ischemia is another cause of pain. When the blood supply to a part is not sufficient to carry away the acidic waste products of cell metabolism, the accumulation results in the irritating effect of these substances on nerve endings. The loss of blood supply to tissue cells can result in the death of these cells, thereby releasing irritating chemical substances that would contribute to pain. An example of pain from tissue ischemia is myocardial infarction or the continued presence of an inflated blood pressure cuff on the arm.

Perception of Pain

The *pain perception threshold* is the point at which the intensity of noxious stimulation results in the person's reporting pain. This point varies from person to person and may not be consistent within the same individual at different times because of the influence of physical and psychosocial factors.

The perception of a pain stimulus may be altered because of an interruption in the mechanism for receiving, transmitting, and interpreting the pain impulse. For example, a tumor or injury to the spinal cord can prevent transmission of pain stimuli so that a person does not feel pain in the affected area. The patient must then be protected from harmful stimuli. For example, a paraplegic is taught to inspect the area of skin that lacks sensory perception and to change position frequently to prevent decubitus ulcers.

Fatigue or persistent unrelieved pain can influence a person's perception of pain. A person who has had little sleep may react more readily to painful stimuli than a well-rested patient. It may be tempting, therefore, to conclude that the more pain a patient experiences, the more immune that person will become to it. However, the opposite usually occurs. As the pain persists, the patient perceives the pain more readily and, therefore, fearfully anticipates its increasing intensity.

The underlying cause of pain can also influence a person's pain perception. For instance, a person may perceive the pain of delivering a baby as different from the pain that results from advancing cancer.

Response to Pain

Response to pain includes both physiological and behavioral manifestations.

Physiological Responses. These include a voluntary reflexive action and an involuntary or autonomic response. The voluntary action involves a withdrawal reflex in which local muscles are triggered to remove the involved part from the pain stimulus. For example, touching a hot stove triggers a reflex reaction in which the person immediately withdraws the hand.

The autonomic or visceral response involves the internal organs and glands. This response is protective in nature and prepares the body for "fight or flight" by increasing the body's alertness to pain. The autonomic response involves pupil dilation, muscle tension, perspiration, and an increase in blood pressure, pulse, and respirations.

Behavioral Responses. The responses to pain vary from individual to individual. The person's emotional state, cultural background, childhood training, and past experience with pain are just some of the factors that will influence how a person responds to pain. The individual may have grown up in a culture that values "suffering in silence," or in one in which loud groaning and screaming are approved responses to pain. Phrases such as "It is not grown up to cry" or "Be brave" reinforce stoic pain behavior in a child. These values are instilled in childhood and influence the response to pain throughout life.

Much of the written material on cultural responses to pain tends to identify specific characteristics according to a certain sociocultural group. This can mislead health care providers to assume that members of cultural groups will automatically have certain pain responses. Avoid stereotyping any individual's response to pain; instead, try to establish each person's individual response to pain and understand the reason for the response. This will result in effective nursing assessment and management of a patient's pain.

The nurse brings personal cultural background, childhood teachings, and attitudes to the patient's situation. If nurses value a "suffer in silence" attitude, they may find themselves reacting negatively to a patient who is openly verbal about pain. The nurses' reaction is normal and reflects personal social values which, in this instance, are different from the patient's. If these differ-

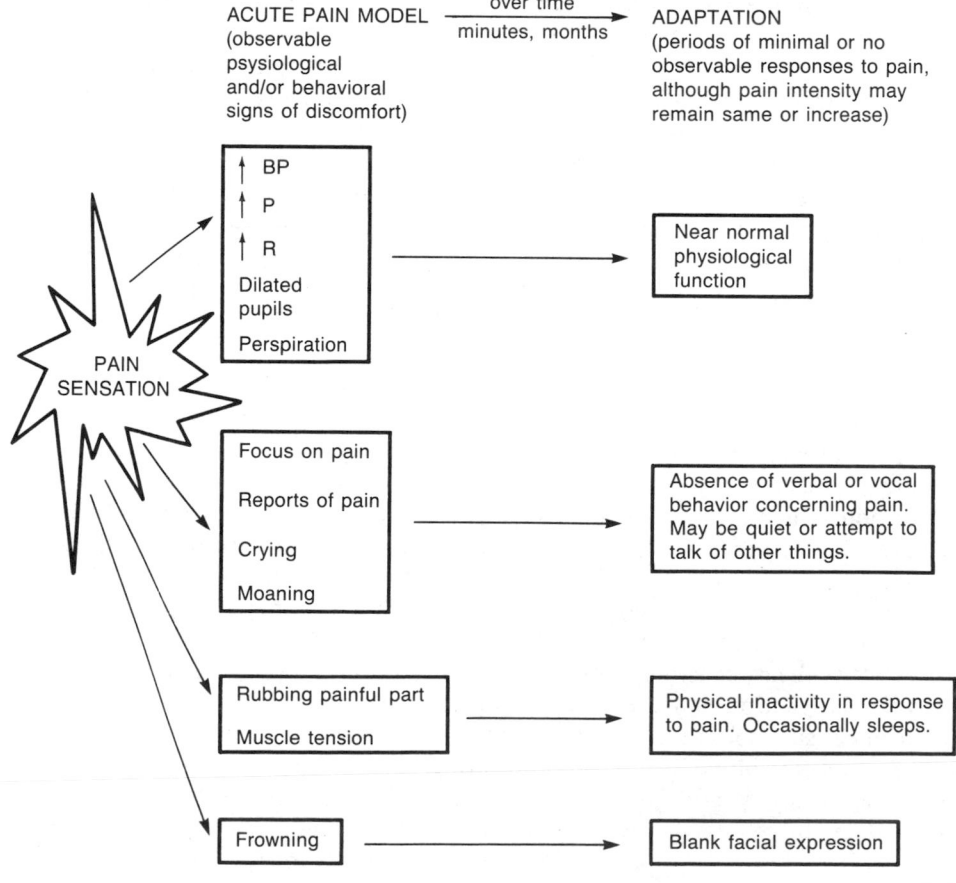

Figure 26–2. Differences between acute pain and the adaptation that occurs with chronic pain. (From M. McCaffery: The person experiencing pain. In L. Brunner and D. S. Suddarth: *Textbook of Medical-Surgical Nursing*, 4th ed. Lippincott, Philadelphia, 1980. Reprinted with permission.)

ences are recognized and accepted, nurses will be able to give effective patient care without letting the differences hamper their ability to assess and manage a patient's pain.

Anxiety, fear, and exhaustion, as mentioned earlier, not only influence pain perception but aggravate a patient's reaction to pain. A patient who has experienced a great deal of pain will probably increase fearful anticipation of the pain. For example, a patient who has had continuous painful debridement of a wound may become tense and fearful anticipating the next debridement.

Adaptation of Responses.   An adaptation of both physiological and behavioral responses occurs with chronic pain. Responses to pain of long duration (chronic) are very different from the body's responses to the sudden onset of acute pain (see Figure 26–2). The body is unable to maintain the autonomic response of increased blood pressure, pulse, and respirations over a period of months or years. Therefore, adaptation occurs, and there may be no detectable physiological changes.

One of the behavioral responses to persistent pain is a blank facial expression. Continuous pain may leave a person too exhausted to frown, moan, or groan. Patients may appear relaxed and involved in watching television or talking with friends because they have become expert at distracting themselves from the constant pain. Therefore, the nurse who does not understand the differences between acute pain and the adaptation that occurs with chronic pain may erroneously assume that lack of pain expression means lack of pain. For example, a patient with advanced cancer of the breast with pain from tumor invasion of the vertebra in her spine may calmly and with no facial expression state that she has back pain. A nurse's or physician's reaction may be that she does not look or act as though she is in pain. This attitude could hamper assessment of the intensity of her pain and therefore interfere with the initiation of pain-relieving measures.

As illustrated, cancer pain, a type of chronic pain, will not elicit the same pain behaviors or physiological signs as those of a patient who has just had surgery. The nurse's awareness of these differences is vital to the ability to work effectively with patients in pain.

Effect of Pain on Other Needs

As mentioned earlier in the chapter, persistent, unrelieved pain can become the focal point of a person's life. Pain can disrupt sleep and decrease appetite, thereby affecting a person's basic need for rest and nutrition. Persistent pain retards recovery and produces a disabling condition which leads to a lack of activity, the end result of which is weakness and muscle atrophy. This lack of activity can compound already existing disturbances in sleep and appetite.

The progressive interference of pain with these basic physiological needs will, in turn, affect a person's need for love, belonging, and self-esteem. Increasing disability can interfere with a person's ability to hold a job or maintain a role within the family; decreased self-esteem is the result. Persistent pain can alter interpersonal relationships and lead to decreased social contacts and eventually isolation. Thus, it becomes evident that pain can affect both physiological and psychological human needs.

Assessment of Pain

Assessment is the first step in solving any nursing problem. In order to alleviate a patient's pain, the nurse gathers information helpful in understanding what the pain is like for the patient and its effect. The data gathered guide the nurse in planning and evaluating nursing interventions. Assessment of a patient with pain is not a one-time process but rather is continual and ongoing and, in some instances, may be warranted every two hours or every day, week, or month.

Attitudes that Can Hamper Assessment

The individual's attitudes about a topic or subject are important to consider, as these attitudes influence behavior toward that subject (Freedman *et al.*, 1974). Therefore, nurses' attitudes about pain will influence their behavior toward patients in pain and can hamper their ability to assess and manage a patient's pain.

1. Health care professionals decide whether pain ex-

ists and the degree of intensity. This erroneously assigns authority about the pain experience to the nurse or physician. Pain is subjective; however, the experiencer is the only one who really knows what it is like. This is a vital premise for the nurse's assessment of any patient with pain.

2. The patient's statement of pain is not believed unless a physical cause is found. Physical causes for pain cannot always be identified. Authorities in the management of pain no longer argue with the patient about whether or not pain exists; the patient's own statement of pain is believed.

3. All pain can be verified by the same behavioral and physiological responses. As discussed earlier in the chapter, this attitude erroneously assumes that the person who does not exhibit these signs is not in pain. If the nurse assumes lack of pain based only on a blank facial expression and no change in vital signs, then appropriate assessment and pain alleviation is seriously hampered.

4. Health professionals tend to praise a patient for exhibiting a high pain tolerance and become judgmental if the patient exhibits a low pain tolerance. Patients may be labeled "good" patients if they put up with the pain and seldom ask for pain relief. However, a patient who reacts to any stimulus as pain and who constantly requests relief may be judged as a "problem" patient who has "little tolerance" for pain. *Pain tolerance* is defined as "that duration or intensity of pain the patient is *willing* to endure" (McCaffery, 1979). Because pain tolerance is based on what the patient is willing to endure, and because each patient's perception of and reaction to pain are unique, it is inappropriate to make a value judgment about a patient's pain tolerance. "It is well to remember," McCaffery (1979) writes, "that the patient's tolerance for pain is not a matter of good or bad, bravery or cowardice. The patient's tolerance for pain is his own *unique response to pain to which he is entitled*."

The purpose of the discussion on attitudes toward pain is to increase the nurse's awareness of them. Awareness of these attitudes is often enough to prevent them from interfering with the nurse's effectively working with a patient with pain.

Data for the Assessment Process

The patient's verbal description of the pain and accompanying nonverbal behavior provide information needed for planning and evaluating nursing intervention. McGuire's assessment tool provides the nurse with a short, systematic way to gather this important information (see Figure 26–3).

Location. Ask the patient to point to or trace the painful area. The location of pain assists the physician in diagnosing the condition and the nurse in planning appropriate care. Do not *assume* the location of pain, even though it may appear obvious. For instance, a patient three days postoperative for gallbladder surgery asks the nurse for pain medication. It is tempting to assume that the pain is caused by the incision and administer pain medicine before assessing the patient. In this case, the nurse asks the exact location of the pain. The patient points to the lower abdomen, nowhere near the incision, and states that the pain is different from the "surgery pain" because it "rolls around." The nurse, aware of the effect of anesthesia on the intestines, establishes that it is probably gas pains. The nurse suggests that the patient first increase activity. If this is not helpful, then a rectal suppository is provided to help expel the gas. In this instance, careful questioning as to the location of pain prevented the inappropriate use of pain medicine.

Quality. How does the patient describe the pain? What does it feel like? Words and phrases such as burning, aching, "like something is twisting my insides," "like a knife cutting through me" are examples of descriptions of pain. In documenting or reporting the quality of pain, the nurse uses the patient's exact words. Determining the quality of pain helps the physician to discover its cause and also helps with the choice of appropriate pain medicine. For instance, a muscle relaxant is more appropriate for muscle spasms than a narcotic analgesic.

Intensity. Ask the patient to rate the intensity of the pain on a scale of 0 to 10 (0 means no pain; 10 is the worst pain imaginable). Using this scale, the nurse gains a clear understanding of the patient's pain, a consistent method for documentation, and a concrete method for evaluating the effectiveness of interventions. A rating of 8 provides a more consistent interpretation than a patient's statement of "a lot of pain." The nurse is able to demonstrate the effectiveness of an intervention if it lowers the patient's original rating of pain from 8 to 4.

Onset and Duration. When does the pain occur? How long does it last? Is it a continuous pain that never goes away or an intermittent pain that recurrs? With this data, the nurse and the patient can plan interventions to prevent the pain or control the pain before it becomes severe.

Precipitating Factors. What makes the pain better? What makes the pain worse? What has helped control pain in the past? For instance, pain may be brought on by exertion in some cardiac patients. Therefore, it is im-

---

PAIN ASSESSMENT

Name_____ Room_____

Age_____ Diagnosis_____

Primary nurse_____ Doctor_____

Date first seen_____

Medications for pain_____

Location

Have patient point to or trace the area of pain._____
_____

Quality

Have patient describe pain in his words._____

Intensity

Rate pain on a 0 to 10 scale: At present_____

1 hour after medication_____

Worst it gets_____

Best it gets_____

Onset

When did the pain start? _____

What time of day does it occur?_____

How often does it appear? _____

How long does it last? _____

Patient's view of pain

What makes the pain better? _____

What makes the pain worse?_____

Any associated symptoms? _____

What has helped control pain in the past? _____

What is the pain preventing the patient from doing that he'd like to do?
_____

Plan:

_____
_____
_____
_____
_____

Figure 26–3. This pain assessment tool was developed by Lora McGuire, R.N., M.S., Nursing Pain Consultant, Joliet, Ill. (Reprinted with permission from the March issue of *Nursing '81*. Copyright © 1983, Springhouse Corporation. All rights reserved.)

portant to know how much activity a patient can tolerate when planning the care. A heating pad may control a patient's pain at home, but in the hospital the patient may not think about using one. Eliciting what has helped the patient in the past can be useful in planning present pain control measures.

Nonverbal Behavior. The very young, the aphasic, or confused or disoriented patient may be unable to communicate verbally about pain. Therefore, the nurse may have to rely on several varieties of nonverbal behavior. The patient's family member can be a vital resource for the nurse in detecting and interpreting certain responses. A variety of facial expressions may be an indication of pain. These may include a frown, facial grimace, or clenched teeth. Other nonverbal indications could in-

clude groaning or crying out, holding or rubbing a part of the body, restlessness, or lying rigidly still.

This is not an all-inclusive list, but rather a sampling of possible nonverbal behaviors that communicate pain. Pain assessment includes the patient's *verbal* and *nonverbal* communication. However, as discussed earlier, the nurse cannot assume lack of pain in patients with chronic pain based only on the absence of nonverbal behavior.

Nursing Diagnoses Related to Pain

A nursing diagnosis describes signs and symptoms that indicate an actual or potential health problem the nurse can help to resolve through interventions (Dossey and Guzzetta, 1981; Atkinson and Murray, 1983). The

National Group of Classification of Nursing Diagnoses continues to identify accepted nursing diagnoses.

For a patient who has a problem with pain, the following nursing diagnosis is made: Comfort, alteration in: Pain.

The patient's problem and its probable cause form the diagnostic statement that is documented on the patient's care plan. For example, a patient with a fractured right hip from a fall complains of hip pain. A nursing diagnoses for this particular problem is: Comfort, alteration: Right hip pain related to fracture of right hip as the result of a fall.

A patient with breast cancer states she has pain in her left and right anterior ribs. A recent bone scan shows metastasis of the cancer to these ribs. One of the nursing diagnoses on her care plan reads: Comfort, alteration in: Left anterior rib pain related to tumor involvement.

After the nursing diagnosis is made, measurable objectives are set, and nursing interventions are planned accordingly. Additional nursing diagnoses as related to a specific patient's pain are shown in the nursing care plan (see pages 670–71).

Nursing Interventions to Facilitate Pain Relief

Nursing interventions for pain relief involve assisting patients in avoiding or reducing the stimuli causing the pain, in alleviating the pain, and in coping with the pain.

The approach of the nurse is basic to working effectively with any patient in pain. The nurse who conveys to the patient that the statement of pain is believed, that the nurse cares about helping obtain pain control, may be able to enhance the effectiveness of other pain-relief measures.

Measures to Avoid or Reduce Painful Stimuli

In some instances, pain can be avoided once the cause is known. The nurse's primary role in this case is patient teaching. The patient with a heart condition, for instance, notices that exertion brings on pain. The nurse helps the patient learn which activities are responsible for the pain and how to moderate them to prevent further discomfort. A patient with chronic low-back pain that has resulted from many years of heavy lifting learns correct posture and body mechanics from the nurse in order to prevent further damage to the back muscles.

Assisting the patient to meet other basic physiological needs can eliminate sources of pain. The discomfort of a distended bladder or constipation can be relieved by specific nursing interventions (see Chapter 24).

In some instances, painful stimuli cannot be avoided. However, the nurse can play an important role in reducing or minimizing a patient's pain. For example, the postoperative patient must ambulate, breathe deeply, and cough immediately after surgery to prevent respiratory complications. The nurse can reduce the pain by instructing the patient to support the incision with the hands or with a pillow while coughing or deep breathing.

A patient with cancer that involves the ribs and lower back finds any movement to be painful. The nurse can minimize the patient's pain by requesting several team members to help support as much of the patient's body as possible during a move. The use of a draw sheet (positioned directly under the patient and on top of the bottom sheet) to turn or move the patient can prevent painful handling and pulling of the patient.

Helping a patient change position frequently prevents pressure on a particular body area which can lead to a breakdown of the tissue. Maintaining good body alignment by careful positioning can help minimize painful muscular contractures.

Assisting Patients to Alleviate Pain

Nursing measures to alleviate pain include giving medications and using noninvasive techniques.

Medications. The use of pain medications is one of the most effective ways to control pain. An important differentiation is between anesthetic and analgesic medications. General anesthetic drugs prevent pain by suppressing consciousness; they are limited mostly to use in surgery. The most common pharmacological means of controlling pain is with analgesic (pain-relieving) medications. Unlike anesthetic drugs, the goal in the use of analgesic drugs is to achieve relief from or control of pain without the loss of sensation or consciousness.

The analgesic drugs that will be discussed here are narcotics and nonnarcotics. In this chapter, it is not possible to present the numerous important concepts related to the pharmacological control of pain. (For an in-depth coverage of this subject, the nurse is encouraged to read the references by McCaffery cited at the end of this chapter.)

Narcotics, also called opiates, include natural drugs such as morphine and codeine, and synthetic agents such as meperidine (DEMEROL), propoxyphene (DARVON), and methadone (DOLOPHINE). The exact nature of pain relief by narcotics is not known, but the mechanism is the same as described earlier for endorphins. The narcotic attaches to the opiate receptor site and inhibits or modifies the pain impulses, thereby preventing their transmission to the brain for pain preception. The discovery of receptor sites in the cerebral cortex to which the narcotic combines supports the hypothesis that narcotics alter the perception of pain (West, 1981). The person is aware of the pain, but it is not bothersome.

Nonnarcotic analgesics include such drugs as aspirin, acetaminophen, ibuprofen, and naproxen. These drugs have both anti-inflammatory and antipyretic properties. Their precise analgesic activity is also unknown; however, it is thought that they work at the peripheral level of the nervous system to inhibit prostaglandins (a hormonelike substance present in all tissues of the body) which irritate pain nerve endings.

The nursing considerations important to the effective use of medications for relief of pain are presented below.

A PREVENTATIVE APPROACH. By encouraging a patient to take pain medicine before the pain becomes unbearable, the nurse assists the patient to achieve relief or effective control of the pain. If the patient "toughs it out" or delays taking the pain medicine, it often takes a higher dose to relieve the intensity of pain as opposed to the dose needed to relieve milder pain. Therefore, the nurse can encourage the fresh postoperative patient to ask for pain medicine when the pain first begins. Activity can be scheduled during the peak action of the medicine, generally, 30 minutes after IM pain medicine, one hour after PO medicine, and 15 minutes after IV medication.

If the patient's pain occurs repeatedly throughout the day, suggest to the physician that pain medication be ordered on an around-the-clock schedule at regular intervals instead of on a prn schedule. The regular schedule prevents the pain from becoming severe, and it erases the memory of pain and the fearful anticipation of its recurrence. The around-the-clock schedule is a particularly appropriate treatment for chronic cancer pain.

If the patient experiences pain upon wakening in the morning, then the nurse awakens that patient during the night to take pain medication. The patient continues this practice at home by setting an alarm clock. Continuous pain relief or control is obtained because consistent levels of pain medicine remain in the bloodstream.

Some physicians hesitate to order and some nurses hesitate to give regularly scheduled dosages of narcotics because of a belief that this will enhance the patient's chances of addiction. The facts demonstrate that this is a misconception which, unfortunately, is the basis for inadequate pharmacological treatment of patients with pain (Marks and Sachar, 1973). In a recent study, 39,946 hospitalized patients where monitored for narcotic addiction. Of the 11,882 patients who received a narcotic, only *four patients* showed well-documented cases of addiction (Porter and Jick, 1980).

Addiction is defined as a behavioral pattern of overwhelming involvement with obtaining and using a drug, coupled with a high tendency to return to this behavior after stopping the drug (Jaffe,1980). When pain is relieved, most patients stop taking narcotic medication. The scheduling of medicine to provide a patient with adequate pain relief does not of itself result in addiction. The nurse cannot allow this misconception to prevent good pharmacological control of the patient's pain.

INDIVIDUALIZED ROUTE, DOSAGE, AND INTERVAL. The route, dosage, and interval of pain medicine are adjusted according to the individual patient's need and response. The oral route of medication is used whenever possible because the patient is not dependent on someone else to administer the drug, and levels of analgesia are longer lasting than with the intramuscular or intravenous route. However, the patient's condition may necessitate a parenteral injection of pain medication, as in the immediate postoperative patient or in the patient who is vomiting or unable to swallow.

Dosages of pain medicine will vary according to the varying intensity of a patient's pain or the different rates of metabolism and absorption of a drug from one patient to another. Unfortunately, a set dosage and an inflexible interval may be ordered on one patient after another, regardless of any factors individual to that patient. If the patient states the medicine is not relieving the pain, the nurse cannot complacently continue to administer the dose because "it is what is usually ordered." An appropriate nursing action is to talk with the physician about increasing the dosage for more effective analgesia. A helpful practice for the nurse is viewing dosages of pain medicine not in terms of a large or small dose but in terms of whether it is relieving or controlling a patient's pain. For example, a patient may be labeled as "liking shots too much" when stating that DEMEROL, 75 mg IM, just barely relieves the pain for one to two hours. It is well documented that DEMEROL's duration of analgesia is only two hours in some patients. Therefore, DEMEROL, 75 mg IM, every four hours may be an appropriate dosage and interval for some patients but are ineffective for this particular patient.

DRUG COMBINATIONS. When narcotics are indicated, combining a nonnarcotic analgesic (acetaminophen, aspirin) with a narcotic analgesic (morphine, dolophine) can result in more effective analgesia than with the narcotic alone. For instance, aspirin is believed to act at the level of the peripheral nervous system. If it is given concurrently with morphine, which is believed to act in the central nervous system, the combination produces better analgesia than administering the morphine alone (Houde *et al.*, 1960).

If anxiety is part of the patient's pain, the patient may complain of feeling "tense inside" and "unable to relax." The nurse may notice rigid posture or continual clenched fists. Hydroxyzine may be given with the pain medication to ease the patient's anxiety which, in turn, can help relieve pain. Hydroxyzine has its own analgesic and antinausea properties which can be helpful for a patient with pain.

Because many patients with chronic pain are depressed, an antidepressant medicine (doxepin, amitriptyline) is often given. It has also been discovered that these medicines have an analgesic effect, along with a sedative effect, which can help the sleep disturbances that can occur with persistent pain.

MYTH ABOUT PLACEBOS.   For the purpose of this discussion, a *placebo* is an inert substance given as medication. A placebo in the form of a saline shot or a sugar pill may be given to the patient who continuously complains of pain despite pain medication and no documented cause for the pain. If the patient obtains relief from the placebo, the health care team will conclude that the patient does not have real pain. This is an erroneous conclusion which can result in a patient's pain being ignored (McCaffery, 1979). Fact: 35 to 40 percent of patients suffering from acute postoperative pain or chronic pain from cancer demonstrate pain relief following a placebo (Lasagna *et al.*, 1954). Certainly, it cannot be concluded that these patients do not have pain. The only accurate conclusion about a patient who responds to a placebo is that the patient *trusts* care-givers to help obtain pain relief and is confident that "the medicine" administered will relieve the pain.

A typical physician's order may read: Administer a placebo of 1 ml normal saline IM every three hours prn pain. Do not tell the patient that this is a placebo. A vital component in any nurse-patient relationship is mutual trust. This trust is destroyed when the nurse deceives a patient by administering a placebo in this manner. Once trust is lost, the nurse can be of little help to the patient with pain.

It is important that the nurse is aware of personal feelings about these issues, the administration of a placebo to diagnose "real" pain, and the effect this has on the nurse-patient relationship. The nurse perpetuates the myth about placebos by erroneously concluding that the patient who obtains relief from a saline injection is not in real pain. If the nurse believes that administering a placebo would damage the nurse-patient relationship, then the nurse has the right and responsibility to refuse to administer it. Ultimately, nurses must decide as individuals how they feel about these issues.

Noninvasive Pain-Relief Techniques.   Medications are not the only method of pain relief; instead, there are many noninvasive nursing techniques that can help patients with pain. For brief pain lasting only seconds to minutes, a noninvasive technique may be all that is needed. However, for pain of longer duration—hours or days—the use of these techniques along with medication may provide the most effective relief of a patient's pain.

Three types of noninvasive techniques will be discussed: distraction, cutaneous stimulation, and relaxation techniques. The following discussion is not intended to provide the nurse with the complete skills needed to use these techniques effectively. For acquiring more complete knowledge and skills the nurse is referred to McCaffery's book (1979) and Donovan's article (1981) listed at the end of the chapter. Before beginning with a patient, the nurse is encouraged to practice one or two techniques with friends and co-workers to become comfortable with them and to be skilled in their use.

DISTRACTION.   Distraction involves focusing a patient's attention away from the pain sensation, thereby sacrificing attention to pain in favor of attention to other stimuli (McCaffery, 1979). Specific distraction methods include listening to music, talking on the phone, using slow, rhythmic breathing techniques. The gate control theory provides the framework to understand the effectiveness of these techniques (Exhibit 26-1). In each of these method, the brainstem is flooded with sensory stimuli which results in the closing of the gate. Pain impulses do not pass through to the higher centers of the brain, and pain is not perceived, or the awareness of pain is lessened. For example, slow rhythmic breathing may be helpful to divert a patient's attention from a painful dressing change. The nurse encourages the patient to look fixedly at an object and deeply breathe in and out while slowly counting out loud "In 1, 2—out 1, 2."

In another situation, the patient states a worry about the pain recurring just after taking a pain medication. The patient has previously stated an enjoyment of listening to classical music. The nurse then might suggest listening to music as a specific pain-relieving technique right after taking the pain medicine or whenever the patient feels anxiety increasing the pain.

CUTANEOUS STIMULATION.   According to the gate control theory, stimulation of the large-diameter nerve

Exhibit 26–1. Gate Control Theory

Major Contributions

1. An integrated conceptual model for appreciating the many factors that contribute to individual differences in the experience of pain.
2. Conceptualization of categories of activity that may form a theoretical base for developing various pain-relief measures.

Nature of the Gate

The transmission of potentially painful impulses to the level of conscious awareness may be affected by a gating mechanism, possibly located at the spinal cord level of the CNS.

STRUCTURES INVOLVED	NO PAIN OR DECREASED INTENSITY OF PAIN	PAIN
Spinal cord (?)	Results from CLOSING THE GATE by:	Results from OPENING THE GATE by:
Nerve fibers	1. Activity in the *large-diameter nerve fibers,* e.g., caused by skin stimulation,	1. Activity in the *small-diameter nerve fibers,* e.g., caused by tissue damage,
Brainstem	2. Inhibitory impulses from the *brainstem,* e.g., caused by sufficient or maximum sensory input arriving through distraction or guided imagery, or	2. Facilitory impulses from the *brainstem,* e.g., caused by insufficient input from a monotonous environment, or
Cerebral cortex and thalamus	3. Inhibitory impulses from the *cerebral cortex* and *thalamus,* e.g., caused by anxiety reduction based on learning when the pain will end and how to relieve it.	3. Facilitory impulses from the *cerebral cortex* and thalamus, e.g., caused by fear that the intensity of pain will escalate and will be associated with death.

Source: McCaffery, M.: *Nursing Management of the Patient with Pain,* 2nd ed, Lippincott, Philadelphia, 1979. Reprinted with permission.

fibers in the skin closes the gate, thereby inhibiting pain impulses on the small fibers from ascending to the brain for pain perception (Exhibit 26–1). Stimulation of the skin involves the use of massage, pressure, heat, cold, menthol ointment, or *transcutaneous electric nerve stimulation (TENS).* Some of these measures require a physician's order; others are contraindicated for specific disease processes. Therefore, the nurse is responsible for checking first on the appropriateness of these techniques before planning on their use.

In many cases, the type, location, duration, and intensity of stimulation involve the use of common sense and a trial-and-error approach.

Generally, the application of heat is effective in the relief of muscular pains. Cold decreases peripheral circulation and can be helpful to reduce swelling and the resulting pressure on nerve endings. A back rub or massage to a patient's back can relieve the muscular tension or pain resulting from maintaining one position or posture too long. The immediate effect of warmth from a menthol ointment can be very soothing for muscle and joint pain.

The use of TENS, by doctor's prescription, can be an effective pain-relief measure for acute or chronic pain. Originally, it was thought that TENS blocked pain by the gate control theory. Data now suggest that TENS stimulates the release of endorphins in the thalamus which bind to the receptor site and prevent pain impulses from traveling to the cerebral cortex (Jacox and Rogers, 1981).

TENS is delivered by a battery-operated unit that transmits a buzzing sensation through electrodes that are applied to the skin in the area of the pain. The TENS unit can be worn all day to deliver continuous cutaneous stimulation.

In some instances, stimulation of the skin can be located right over or near the painful site. If direct stimulation to the area is too painful or simply not possible, then the skin in an opposite area can be used for pain relief. This is contralateral stimulation. For example, a patient with a superficial burn on the left forearm might obtain significant pain relief from an ice pack placed in the same location on the right forearm.

RELAXATION TECHNIQUE. Both anxiety and muscular tension can intensify a patient's reaction to pain. A relaxation technique reduces anxiety and tension by combining slow rhythmic breathing with a progressive relaxing of muscle groups throughout the body. This technique can be used alone or in combination with medications or other noninvasive measures for pain relief.

A patient may already know a relaxation technique which the nurse can suggest using when the pain begins or before it becomes severe. It is important that the patient understand that relaxation is a skill that takes practice and should not be given up after only a few times.

Initially, the nurse may coach the patient through the relaxation technique while the patient lies or sits in a comfortable position. With slow, rhythmic breathing, the patient concentrates on relaxing the muscles throughout the entire body beginning with hands, then arms, until progression to the toes. The nurse may then encourage the patient to imagine a favorite place as vividly as possible and to enjoy this image for a few minutes (this is called guided imagery).

A relaxation technique can be as short as a few minutes or last as long as 15 minutes, depending on the individual needs of the patient. For an in-depth look at a script for a relaxation technique, refer to Donovan's article (1980) listed at the end of the chapter.

Assisting Patients to Cope with Pain

As discussed earlier, the pain experience involves not only the physical sensation, but also psychosocial components. Therefore, effective relief or control of a patient's pain requires interventions not only for physical support but also for psychological support. Discussing with patients what the pain prevents them from doing may help the nurse understand the effect the pain has on patients' lives and goals. The nurse may discover that, although patients talk about pain all the time, what really frightens them is the implication of the pain. Is the pain caused by an incurable condition? Does this condition mean premature death? Once nurses are aware of these underlying fears, they can alert the physician and other appropriate health team members to the patient's fears and unanswered questions. A chaplain, psychologist, or counselor might be appropriate resources for the patient.

For some patients, knowing what to expect during a procedure in terms of discomfort or pain can be helpful. This can reduce some of the anxiety or fear of the unknown that can increase a patient's perception of pain.

Helping patients maintain as much control over the situation as possible can help to minimize their response to the pain. The noninvasive techniques discussed earlier restore some of the patients' control over pain by allowing them to decide when and how frequently they will use these techniques to alter pain perception.

Special facilities are available to help specific populations of patients cope with pain. Using a multidisciplinary approach to control chronic pain, pain clinics help a patient deal with pain by the use of biofeedback, group therapy, hypnosis, physical therapy, nerve blocks, or medications.

Nationwide hospices have been developed to provide symptomatic relief and emotional support to dying patients and their families.

Nursing Care Plan for a Patient Experiencing Pain

Mrs. Rogers is 50 years old with breast cancer with metastasis to her cervical and thoracic spine. She is bedridden due to the bone destruction in her spine. She is tearful and states the pain is at 8 or 9 on a 0 to 10 scale (0 is no pain, 10 is the worst pain imaginable). Because of the pain, she has been unable to sleep for the past week. The physician has just ordered an increase in pain medicine.

The following format is a common way of documenting a patient's care plan on a Kardex.

Date	Nursing Diagnosis	Goal	Nursing Approach or Intervention	Evaluation
3/20	Comfort, alteration in: Back pain related to metastasis from breast cancer	The patient will state that her pain is below 4 on 0–10 scale during hospitalization.	1. Monitor and document pain control using 0–10 scale every 1 hour during first 4 hours of new pain medication regimen. Then monitor and document every 4 hours for 24 hours. Then monitor and document at least once each shift. 2. Ask once each shift if pain relief lasts for the full 4-hour interval between pain medication. 3. Notify physician for change in pain medicine if pain is above 4 at any time during hospitalization or if pain is not controlled for full 4-hour interval.	3/20 Patient rates pain at 2. 3/22 Patient states that pain returned 1 hour before dose of medicine is due. Physician notified, interval changed to every 3 hours.

3/20	Sleep-pattern disturbance related to unrelieved pain	The patient will state that she is able to sleep throughout the night	1. Assist patient into a comfortable position for sleep. 2. Encourage patient to use the relaxation technique that she uses during the day to relax her muscles right before sleep. 3. Administer gentle back rub right after 10:00 P.M. pain medication to help patient relax before sleep	3/21 Patient states she slept throughout the night.
3/20	Self-bathing–hygiene deficit related to intolerance of pain	The patient will participate in bath as much as condition allows.	1. The nurse or aide will assist patient with parts of bath she cannot complete during first week. 2. By second week (4/3), nurse will encourage patient to bath herself.	3/22 Presently needing complete bath except for face and hands. 3/26 Patient now able to complete own bath from her waist up.
3/20	Potential for impairment of skin integrity due to bed rest related to progression of the disease and pain	Patient's skin will not become reddened or break down.	1. Check and document skin integrity, especially over bony prominences once each shift. 2. Water mattress on bed. 3. Have patient shift position twice each shift. She is most comfortable on back with knees elevated. 4. Reinforce to family members importance of shifting her position and massaging skin to prevent breakdown.	3/25 No reddened area or skin breakdown 3/21 In place 3/22 Too painful for patient to turn on left or right side, so just shift her weight to the side by placing pillows at back. 3/26 Husband and daughter stated that they were doing this at home.

Summary

Pain is one of the most common causes of discomfort, and its avoidance is a basic human need. Pain involves not only a stimulus and a sensation of hurt but also the various responses of the person experiencing pain. These responses are individual and are influenced by the physiological, psychological, cultural, and spiritual makeup of the person in pain.

Persistant pain becomes the focal point of a person's life, affecting both physiological and psychological human needs.

The gate control theory proposes that thought, past experiences, and emotions interact with neurophysiological activities in the perception of and reaction to pain.

The discovery of endorphins, the body's own internally secreted narcotic-like substances, adds more to understanding mechanisms for pain relief.

The differences between acute and chronic pain suggest implications for assessment and treatment. The nurse who does not understand these differences may erroneously assume that lack of pain expression means lack of pain.

Components of the pain experience involve the initiation of the pain impulse, perception of the pain, and response to the pain. Each component affects the other, and all three, in turn, influence the patient's pain experience.

Pain is subjective; the experiencer is the only one who knows whether it is present and the degree of its intensity. Therefore, the patient's verbal description and nonverbal behavior provide the data for pain assessment.

Nursing interventions for pain relief involve assisting patients in avoiding or reducing the stimuli causing pain, in alleviating the pain, and in coping with the pain. These interventions consist of the administration of narcotics, nonnarcotics, and/or the use of distraction techniques, cutaneous stimulation, and relaxation techniques.

Discussion on attitudes toward pain increases the nurses' awareness of them. Awareness of these attitudes is often enough to prevent them from hampering the nurse's effective assessment and treatment of a patient with pain.

As the health care team member who spends the most time with the patient, the nurse can make a significant difference in how a patient perceives pain, reacts to pain, and the degree of relief obtained.

Terms for Review

acute pain	gate control theory	pain perception threshold	placebo
addiction	intractable pain	pain tolerance	referred pain
chronic pain	pain	phantom pain	TENS
endorphins			

Self-Assessment

The purpose of the following questions is to help the nurse focus on experiences of personal pain and on attitudes about pain expression and treatment that will influence interactions with patients in pain. It may be helpful for the student to discuss personal responses to these questions with a fellow student in order to gain perspective on the various individual differences involved.

1. Think back on how you reacted to painful stimulus as a child. When you cried, were you told to "Be brave" or "You're to old to cry"?
2. Was there anyone in your family in continuous pain as you were growing up? Did they talk openly about it—cry or moan? Or were they silent about the pain, and did they try not to show it?
3. How much personal experience have you had with pain? Think back on the most recent time that you were in pain. How did you act? Did you want someone with you or did you want to be alone? Did you moan or cry out or did you not make a sound? Did you take medicine for the pain or did you just "tough it out"? If you did take pain medicine, was it before the pain got bad or did you take it only when you could not stand the pain anymore?
4. What are your feelings about administering a narcotic for pain relief in the following instances: to a dying cancer patient, to a patient with acute pancreatitis secondary to alcoholism?
5. The doctor's order states: "1 ml saline IM every 3 hours prn pain. Do not tell patient that this is a placebo. If Mrs. Smith asks, tell her that this is medicine for pain." What are your feelings about giving this to the patient? Do you think you have a choice to give it or not? You decide to give the placebo and the patient discovers what you have given her. She accuses you of deceiving her and tells you not to come near her again. What are your feelings?
6. What are your feelings about causing pain in patients in the following instances: venipuncture for blood studies, wound care to a patient with second-degree burns, turning a patient with bone metastasis from advanced cancer.

Review Questions

Circle all the appropriate answers *or* place T for true or F for false beside questions 7 through 12.

1. For the most effective control of chronic pain with analgesics, the following statement(s) apply:
   a. Pain medication is given on a prn basis.
   b. The patient wakes at night to take the pain medicine.
   c. The oral route of medication is used as long as the patient can take oral medication and is comfortable.
   d. Narcotics should be avoided as long as possible because of the problem of addiction with most patients.
   e. Pain medication is given on an around-the-clock schedule.
2. The gate control theory proposes that which part(s) of the nervous system are involved in facilitating or inhibiting the transmission of pain impulses?
   a. Small nerve fibers
   b. Cerebral cortex
   c. Large nerve fibers
   d. Brainstem
   e. All of the above
3. Acute pain is described as
   a. Long in duration
   b. Specific to patients with cancer
   c. Generally decreasing and eventually disappearing as the tissue heals
   d. Short in duration
4. A person's perception of pain can be influenced by
   a. An injury to the spinal cord
   b. Fatigue
   c. A nurse who communicates belief in the patient's statement of pain
   d. The underlying cause of the pain
   e. None of these
   f. All of these
5. The following statement(s) apply to listening to music as a pain-relief measure:
   a. It is the most effective measure for long-term chronic pain.
   b. It is a form of distraction and therefore a noninvasive method of pain control.
   c. It is thought to "close the gate" by increasing sensory input, thereby inhibiting pain impulses from the brainstem to the cortex.
   d. It is not an appropriate measure to use in combination with pain medication.
6. A placebo given to test whether or not a patient's pain is real
   a. Is an appropriate use of a placebo.
   b. Is the only test which tells health professionals whether or not a patient is having pain.
   c. Is an inappropriate use of a placebo.
   d. Says nothing about the presence or absence of pain.

7. _____ Unrelieved pain has little effect on other basic human needs such as activity, nutrition, and sleep.

8. _____ It is correct to conclude that if a physical cause for the pain cannot be found, then the patient is not having pain.

9. _____ Assessment of the intensity of a patient's pain is based mostly on the patient's nonverbal communication about his pain (i.e., body position, facial expression).

10. _____ Fear and anxiety from past experiences with pain can facilitate impulses from the cerebral cortex, causing "the gate to open" and allowing transmission of pain.

11. _____ The physiological and behavioral responses of a patient with acute pain are similar to those of a patient with chronic pain.

12. _____ Assessment of a patient's pain is a frequent, ongoing process that includes the patient's verbal and nonverbal communications.

Answers

1. b, c, and e
2. e
3. c, d
4. f
5. b, c
6. c, d
7. F
8. F
9. F
10. T
11. F
12. T

Suggested Readings

Donovan, M.I.: Relaxation with guided imagery: A useful technique, *Cancer Nurs.* 3(1):27–32, 1980.

McCaffery, M.: Understanding your patient's pain. *Nursing '80,* 10(9):26–31, Sept., 1980.

_____: Patients shouldn't have to suffer—Relieve their pain with injectable narcotics. *Nursing '80,* 10(10):34–39, Oct. 1980.

_____: Relieve your patient's pain fast and effectively with oral analgesics. *Nursing '80,* 10(11):58–64,Nov. 1980.

_____: Relieving pain with noninvasive techniques. *Nursing '80,* 10(12):55–57, Dec. 1980.

References and Bibliography

Atkinson, L., and Murray, M.: *Understanding the Nursing Process.* 3rd ed. Macmillan, New York, 1983.

Dossey, B., and Guzzetta, C.: Nursing diagnosis. *Nursing '81,* 11:34–38, 1981.

Freedman, J. L.; Carlsmith, J. M.; and Sears, D. O.: *Social Psychology.* Prentice-Hall, Englewood Cliffs, N.J., 1974.

Houde, R.; Wallenstein, S.; and Rogers, A.: Cinical pharmocology of analgesics. *Clin. Pharmacol. Ther.,* 1:163–74, 1960.

Jacox, A.: Sociocultural and psychological aspects of pain. In Jacox, A. (ed.): *Pain: A Source Book for Nurses and Other Health Professionals.* Little, Brown, Boston, 1977.

Jacox, A., and Rogers, A.: The nursing management of pain. In Marino, L.: *Cancer Nursing.* Mosby, St. Louis, 1981.

Jaffee, J. H.: Drug addiction and drug abuse. In Goodman, L. S., and Gilman A. (eds.): *A Pharmacological Basis of Therapeutics,* 6th ed. Macmillan, New York, 1980, pp. 535–44.

Lasagna, H.; Mosteller, F.; VonFelsinger, J.; and Beecher, H.: A study of the placebo response. *Am. J. Med.* 16:770–79, 1954.

Marks, R. N., and Sachar, E. J.: Undertreatment of medical inpatients with narcotic analgesics. *Ann. Intern. Med.* 78:173–81, 1973.

McCaffery M.: *Nursing management of the Patient with Pain.* Lippincott, Philadelphia, 1972.

_____ *Nursing Management of the Patient with Pain,* 2nd ed. Lippincott, Philadelphia, 1979.

National Group for Classification of Nursing Diagnoses: List of Nursing Diagnoses accepted at Fourth National Conference, St. Louis, 1982.

Porter, J., and Jick, H.: Addiction rare in patients with narcotics. *N. Engl. J. Med.,* 302:123, 1980.

Sternback, R. A.: *Pain: A Psychophysiological Analysis.* Academic Press, New York, 1968.

West, B. A.: Understanding endorphins: our natural pain relief system. *Nursing '81,* 11 (2):50–53, Feb., 1981.

CHAPTER **27**

THE NEED FOR SEX AND SEXUALITY

Objectives

1. Contrast the concepts of sex, reproduction, and sexuality.

2. Describe the phases of the sexual response cycle and physical changes associated with each phase.

3. Describe hormonal factors controlling reproduction and sex drive.

4. Describe various methods of fertility control.

5. Describe various types of sexual stimulation.

6. Identify factors affecting sexual expression.

7. Describe characteristics associated with satisfaction of sexual needs.

8. Describe the nurse's role related to patient's sexual needs.

9. Write a nursing diagnosis based on a data base from a patient with unmet sexual needs.

10. Identify interventions for assisting patients with sexual concerns or problems.

11. Identify possible ways of dealing with the patient who is seductive or sexually aggressive toward the nurse.

Sexual Needs and Sexuality

Sexual needs are similar to and different from other basic needs. Labby (1975) states, "Our sexuality is a critical component of our expressive life, necessary to general well-being and devastating in its loss." In terms of an individual's survival, sex is not an essential need in the sense of fluid, nutrition, or oxygen. In terms of survival of the human race, sex is a survival need. In this chapter, the term *sex* will be used to refer to the behaviors of the individual that are likely to result in orgasm. *Gender* is used to denote male or female. *Reproduction* is closely associated with sexual activity and is the basis for species survival. The term *sexuality* is a broader term

referring to the individual's integration of biological drives and physiology with the self-concept and sexual expression. Sexuality is affected by social, cultural, and religious factors, in addition to physical structure, functioning, and appearance. Sexuality is integrally involved in the way people relate to one another. DeLora *et al.* (1981) view sexuality as one's sexual behavior and all of the attitudes the individual holds related to sexual matters. Mann and Katsuranis (1975) view sexuality as a combination of:

1. Male or female gender identity as part of the self-concept. This is established by the age of two or three

years and is most often dependent on body structure and hormonal influences during development.

2. Sex role. The sex role appropriate for men or women within a society will change over time and among different cultures, religions, and families. The school-age child develops a sense of the range of appropriate male/female behavior, which is then incorporated into the self-concept. (In some cultures or groups, there may be little or no distinction between male/female roles. Roles are negotiated within families based on individual interest and talents. In other groups, rigidly defined sex roles are enforced.)

3. Sexual object choice. This is the type of person who becomes acceptable to the individual as a sexual partner. It involves the choice of same-sex or opposite-sex partners on a continuum from exclusively heterosexual to exclusively homosexual.

4. Preferred sexual activity. This is a combination of unique sensitivity of body parts and learned behavior related to ways of showing love, releasing sexual tension, and causing sexual arousal.

Satisfaction of individual sexual needs may serve some or all of the following functions (Mann and Katsuranis, 1975):

1. Reproduction
2. Source of immediate and ongoing pleasure
3. Relief of sexual tension and other forms of tension
4. Increase in self-esteem through positive sexual experiences with another person (the opposite is also true of negative sexual relationships)
5. Satisfaction of love and belonging needs
6. Clarification of relationship that exists between two people (lovers versus friends)

This chapter presents sexual needs of patients as an aspect of total nursing care. People's needs will vary from total lack of concern to a preoccupation with sexual ability and functioning. The nurse's role in this area is to assess the individual's needs and provide interventions to assist the patient resolve or reduce sexual concerns. Many health problems and treatments will affect a patient's sexuality and sexual abilities, either temporarily or permanently. The patient should not leave the health care setting worried about sexual concerns, afraid or too embarrassed to ask for information or help. Just as the patient is taught how to do a dressing change before discharge from the hospital, patients recovering from a heart attack, spinal cord injury, or mastectomy should be given the opportunity to talk with an informed nurse about the impact of their health problems on their sexuality and sexual functioning.

Normal Means of Meeting Sexual Needs

Sexual Response Cycle

There are many avenues of sexual expression available to individuals based on their knowledge, experiences, and willingness to experiment with ways of giving one another sexual pleasure. Common to all forms of sexual activity is the human sexual response as explained by Masters and Johnson in their 12-year research on human sexual activity (1966). They divided the sexual response into four stages: excitement, plateau, orgasm, and resolution. All individuals do not always move through all stages during sexual activity. Some individuals may only rarely or may never reach the stage of orgasm, yet be very comfortable and satisfied with their individual sexual adjustment. Exhibit 27-1 presents these four stages of sexual response and associated physiological changes.

Control of Sexual Functioning

Control of the sexual response and sexual drive (libido) is a result of the integrated functioning of the cerebral cortex, hypothalamus, anterior pituitary gland, and the gonads (male or female reproductive organs). The gonads release the sex hormones and the egg or sperm for reproduction. The anterior pituitary, under the direction of the hypothalamus, releases follicle-stimulating hormone (FSH) and lutenizing hormone (LH) in both men and women. In men, these hormones are released at a fairly fixed rate during health, but in women, the release of these hormones varies within the menstrual cycle. (See Figure 27-1.) Both hormones affect the gonads. In men, FSH and LH stimulate the testes to release the male sex hormone, *testosterone*, responsible for sex drive and secondary sexual characteristics. FSH and LH also stimulate the testes to produce sperm cells (spermatogenesis). In women, FSH and LH result in the production and release of a mature egg cell and in the production of the female sex hormones, *estrogen* and *progesterone*. These horomones are primarily concerned with preparing the uterus for implantation of a fertilized egg and maintaining secondary sexual characteristics. A woman's sexual drive is more dependent on the release of testosterone from her adrenal gland than on estrogen or progesterone.

Exhibit 27-1 Human Sexual Response

Excitement Phase

The excitement phase is the first stage of sexual response to arousing physical or mental stimulation. If the arousing stimulation continues, the individual will move into the second phase of the sexual response. If the stimulus is stopped or becomes unpleasant, the excitement phase will end, and any physical changes will quickly reverse. The major physical changes involve engorgement of the genital tissues with blood, called *vasocongestion*, and increased muscle tension throughout the body. These two changes occur in both men and women. In men, the vasocongestion results in an erection of the penis. Men may have an erection and lose part or all of it several times during the excitement phase because of conflicting environmental stimuli or changes in sexual stimulation. In the woman, the labia enlarge and partially separate, making the vaginal opening less obstructed. The vasocongestion in the vagina results in rapid lubrication as cells along the entire vagina release a fluid coating. The clitoris also enlarges and is especially sensitive to physical stimulation. Erection of the nipples occurs in women and in 60 percent of men (McCary, 1979). Women with inverted nipples may have no erection. Heart rate, respiratory rate, and blood pressure increase from normal levels.

Plateau Phase

Sexual tension continues to increase. Vasocongestion and muscle tone continue to increase. The testes increase in size, up to 50 percent, and fluid containing a small amount of sperm may be secreted onto the end of the penis. The breasts in women who have not breastfed a child also increase in size by 20 to 25 percent; women who have breastfed do not experience this change. Rapid, irregular uterine contractions occur in the woman; this is not a reason to abstain from sexual intercourse during pregnancy since it is not related to premature labor in the normal pregnancy. Rapid pelvic thrusts occur in both sexes from voluntary and involuntary muscle contractions and general muscle tension. The heart rate may increase to double its normal rate in both sexes, and hyperventilation occurs. Blood pressure also rises 20 to 80 mm Hg systolic and 10 to 40 mm Hg diastolic above the normal range for individuals. Average length of time in this stage is 30 seconds to 3 minutes (Siemens and Brandzel, 1982).

Orgasmic Phase

During this period, sexual tension peaks. Involuntary contractions occur in the vagina at the rate of every 0.8 second. The involuntary contractions of the urethra and muscles at the base of the penis result in ejaculation of seminal fluid in the male. The urethral opening may dilate in women with the release of small amounts of urine or an urge to void. The uterus continues to contract irregularly. Involuntary rhythmic contractions of the rectal sphincter may occur in both sexes but are more common in the male. The orgasmic phase lasts from 3 to 15 seconds (Siemens and Brandzel, 1982). Heart rate increases to 110 to 180 beats per minute. Orgasms from masturbation increase heart rate more than intercourse (Siemens and Brandzel, 1982). Respiratory rate may increase to 40 breaths each minute. Blood pressure increases by 30 to 100 mm Hg systolic and 20 to 50 mm Hg diastolic above normal values for individuals. In hypertensive patients, blood pressures as high as 260/150 mm Hg have been reported during intercourse (Labby, 1975). Periods of maximum stress on the heart are estimated to be 10 to 15 seconds in most people.

Resolution Phase

During this phase, the changes which peaked during the orgasmic phase return to normal states. If stimulation continues, the woman is capable of repeated orgasms, but the man is unable to reach orgasm again until after a refractory period. The penis quickly loses 50 percent of its size (10 to 15 seconds) and then returns to normal size more slowly. If orgasm does not occur, vasocongestion dissipates more slowly. In the woman, most of the changes are reversed and back to normal in 5 to 15 minutes. Continued stimulation of the man is usually unsuccessful in maintaining an erection. Erection of the penis is again possible in most men within several minutes to several hours. Many people experience a sudden release of perspiration during the early resolution phase. Blood pressure, pulse, and respirations go back to normal values. Total energy expenditure during the sexual response cycle in married people is comparable to climbing two flights of stairs (Thompson, 1980).

The central nervous system controls the physical changes associated with the sexual response through reflex activity and through the interaction of conscious thought with physical stimulation of the senses. Skin receptors in the genital tissues of men and women are triggered by pressure and touch. This stimulation results in parasympathetic nervous system activity and inhibition of the sympathetic system, leading to physical changes identified in the sexual response cycle.

Reproduction and Fertility Control

In both men and women, the gonads produce egg or sperm cells which have half the normal number of chromosomes as are present in all other body cells. The union of the male and female cells results in one complete cell with 46 chromosomes, which is then capable of duplicating itself and developing into a unique individual. Over eight million different combinations are possible

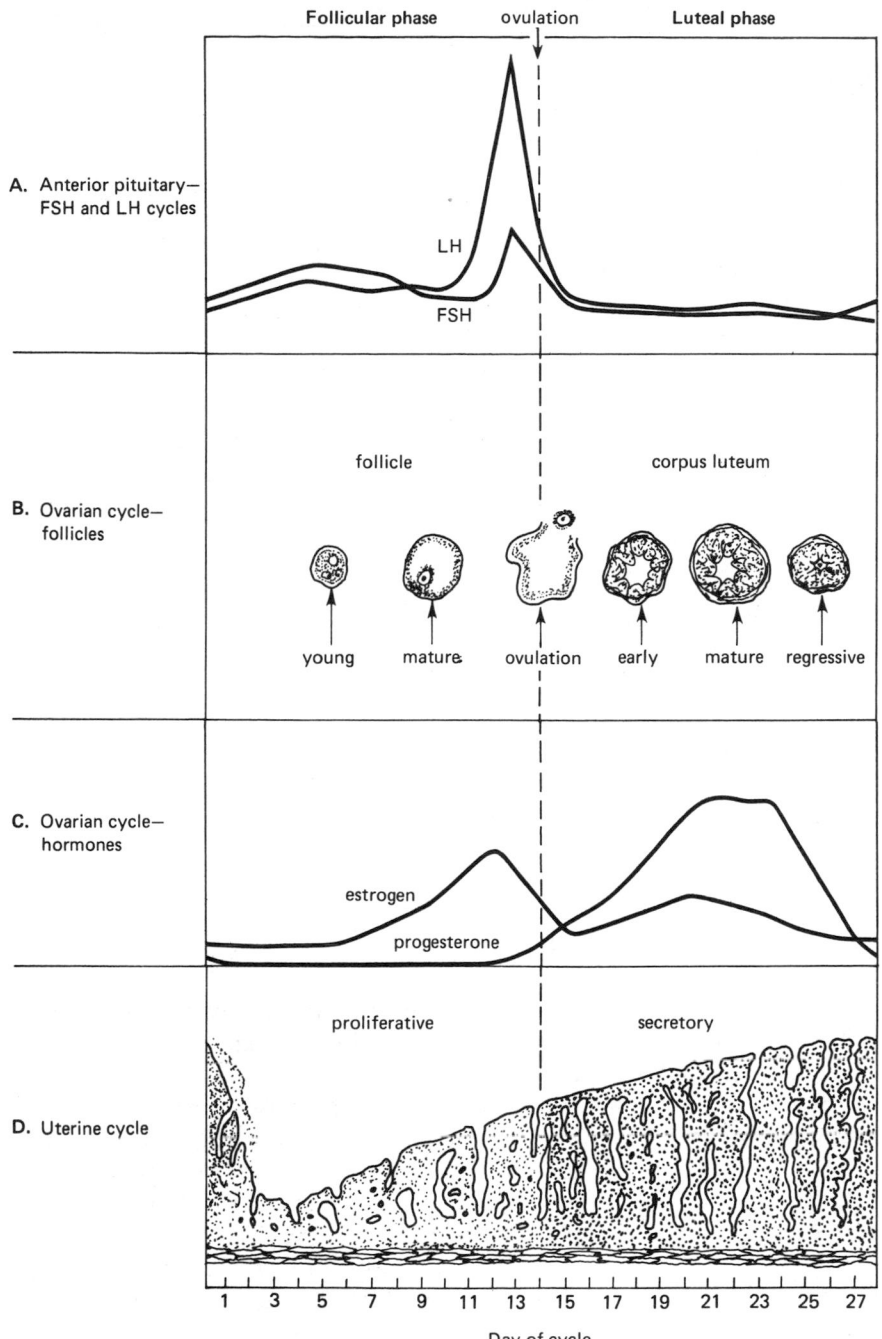

Figure 27-1. Hormonal changes during a normal menstrual cycle. (From M. Griffiths: *Introduction to Human Physiology*, 2nd ed. Macmillan, New York, 1981, p. 450.)

from the process of meiosis (formation of egg/sperm cells) and fertilization. During ejaculation, the man releases approximately 3 ml of fluid containing an average of 300 million sperm. A healthy man may produce an average of several hundred million sperm each day which are stored in the testes until ejaculation occurs.

A woman is born with all the egg cells she will ever have, which is estimated to be one million. After men-

struation begins, one egg cell matures and is released each month. An egg cell released when a woman is 14 years old is also 14 years old. An egg cell released when she is 45 years old is also 45 years old. The increasing incidence of some birth defects in older women is thought to be related to aging eggs. This is not true in men since new sperm are constantly being produced throughout life. In a normal lifetime, a woman will probably release

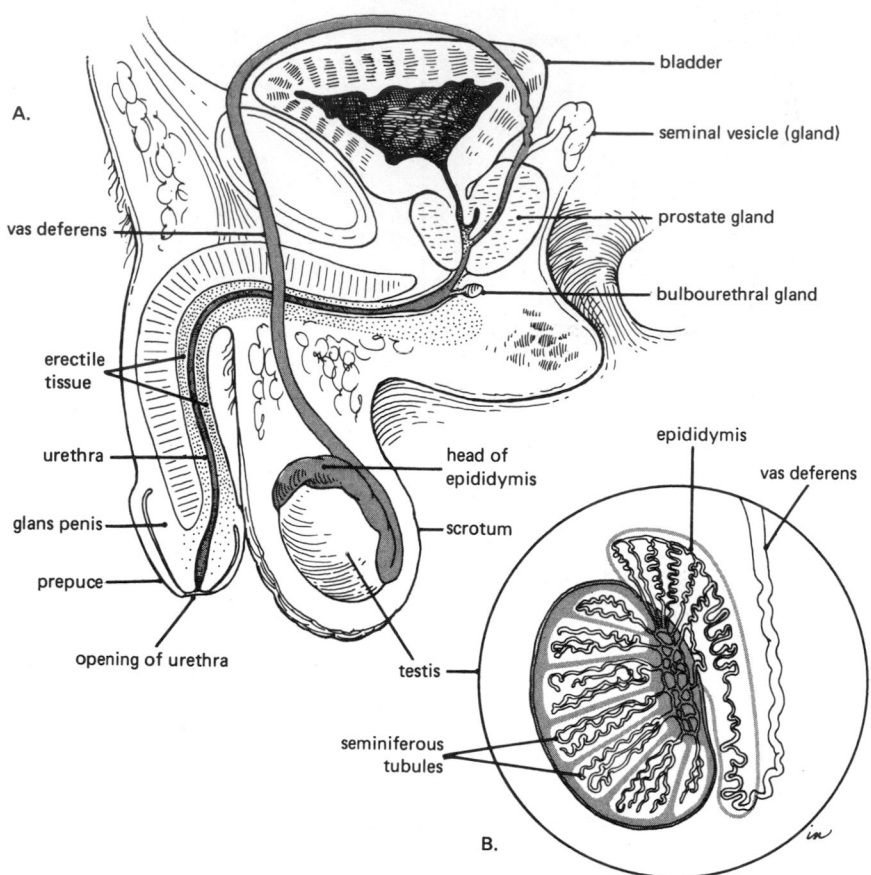

Figure 27-2. Male reproductive structures. (From M. Griffiths: *Introduction to Human Physiology*, 2nd ed. Macmillan, New York, 1981, p. 435.)

400 eggs for possible fertilization. The rest of the eggs in the ovary will degenerate so that few, if any, are left by the time the woman reaches menopause. Ovulation in the woman is triggered by a rapid but short-lasting release of LH from the anterior pituitary which occurs on approximately day 14 in a 28-day menstrual cycle. The first day of the cycle is marked by the beginning of the menstrual flow. Fertilization is most likely to occur within 48 hours of ovulation since, after this time, the egg cell begins to deteriorate. Fertilization usually takes place in the woman's fallopian tubes, and the fertilized egg then moves into the uterus and implants in the wall approximately seven days after ovulation. The sperm is able to travel the distance to the egg within the fallopian tube in 30 minutes following intercourse.

Fertility control is the ability to prevent or achieve a pregnancy based on a conscious decision. Birth control is aimed at preventing pregnancy by interrupting the normal cycle of hormone release in the woman, at killing the sperm before fertilization occurs, at obstructing sperm passage into the uterus or fallopian tubes, at preventing fertilization or at preventing implantation of the fertilized egg in the uterine wall. Figure 27-4 presents the current methods available for preventing pregnancy.

Sex Roles

Based on studies in 1948, Kinsey developed a seven-point scale for describing a range of sexual behavior, from exclusively heterosexual to exclusively homosexual. The term *homosexual* is used medically to refer to people of either gender who seek out sexual partners or are sexually attracted to people of the same sex. *Heterosexual* people are attracted to and involved sexually with people of the opposite sex. (See Table 27-1.) Only a very small percentage of people rate themselves as having exclusively homosexual interests and experiences. Between 20 to 50 percent of people have had some homosexual responses or experiences, with men having a higher percentage than women. Approximately 50 to 80 percent of people are exclusively heterosexual, with women having a higher percentage than men (Brodoff, 1980).

The term *lesbian* is used to refer to homosexual women. *Transexuals* are people who want to change their anatomy to that of the opposite sex because their self-identity is closer to the opposite sex than to their own physical sexual characteristics. Someone who is *bisexual* is equally divided between heterosexual and homosexual interests. *Asexual* means someone is lacking

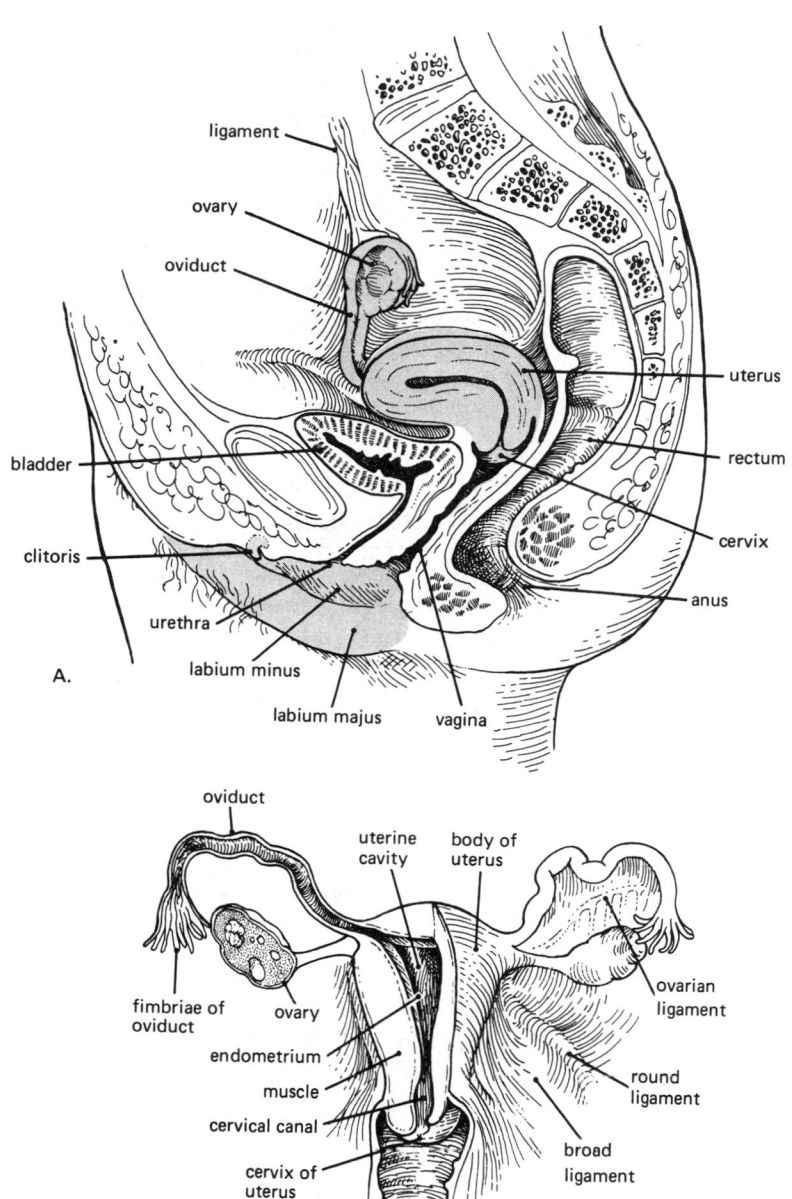

A.

B.

Figure 27-3. Female reproductive structures. (From M. Griffiths: *Introduction to Human Physiology*, 2nd ed. Macmillan, New York, 1981, p. 443.)

Table 27-1. **Kinsey's Scale of Sexual Behavior**

Scale		
0	Exclusively heterosexual (50% men, 70–80% women)	
1	Predominantly heterosexual, only incidentally homosexual	
2	Predominantly heterosexual, occasionally homosexual	20–30%
3	Equally heterosexual and homosexual (bisexual)	women,
4	Predominantly homosexual, occasionally heterosexual	46% men
5	Predominantly homosexual; only incidentally heterosexual	
6	Exclusively homosexual (4% men; 1–2% women)	

Source: Kinsey, A. *et al.*: *Sexual Behavior of the Human Male*, 1948; *Sexual Behavior of the Human Female*, 1953, Saunders, Philadelphia.

Oral Contraceptives "The pill"

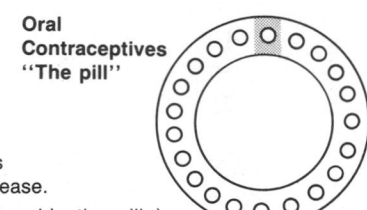

Prevents Ovulation
if taken every day for 21 days
by suppressing FSH & LH release.
Estrogen and Progesterone (combination pills)
Progesterone only ("minipills")—prevents fertilization and implantation by altering cervical mucus and lining of uterus.
Most reliable method 99.7%.
Risk of thromboembolism 3/100,000 (in young nonsmokers)
Prescribed by physician
Reduced menstrual flow

Intrauterine Device

Prevents implantation or alters transport in fallopian tube to prevent pregnancy.
May contain copper or progesterone which are gradually released.
Prescribed, inserted and removed by physician/midwife.
Effective for 1-3 years depending on type.
97% effective
Increased menstrual flow; cramping as side effects
Strings checked periodically to assure correct placement

Diaphragm

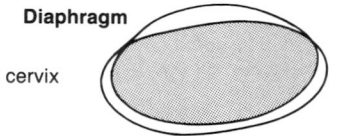

Prevents sperm from entering cervix by blocking entrance.
87% effective with cream
Inserted up to 1 hour before intercourse
Left in place 6-8 hours after intercourse
Fitted by physician/midwife
Diaphragm refitted after 2 years or after 10 pound weight gain or loss or following childbirth

Contraceptive Cream

Condom

Reservoir for evaculate
Prevents pregnancy by containing sperm.
Protects against STD
90% effective
Put on over erect penis
"Over the Counter"

Vaginal Sponge

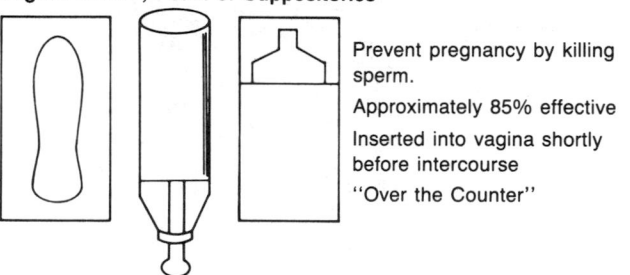

Prevents pregnancy by killing sperm and obstructing cervical opening.
Activated by putting 2 T. of water in depression and squeezing before insertion into vagina
Effective for 24 hours after insertion; "over the counter" 85-95% effective

string for removal

Vaginal Cream, Foam or Suppositories

Prevent pregnancy by killing sperm.
Approximately 85% effective
Inserted into vagina shortly before intercourse
"Over the Counter"

Coitus Interuptus—No sperm released into vagina 85% effective
Abstinence—100% effective
Rhythm—based on basal body temperature, dates or cervical mucous changes—70-90% effective—prevents introduction of sperm to viable egg cell

Surgical Sterilization:

Vasectomy (male)—No sperm released in ejaculate
Tubal Ligation (female)—Egg unable to reach sperm } essentially 100% effective

---

functioning sexual organs or is without sex, as when people feel they have lost their femininity or masculinity. *Transvestites* are usually heterosexual individuals who occasionally or consistently wear clothing of the opposite sex for sexual excitement. They are usually not interested in changing their gender.

A word of warning about the use of labels may be appropriate at this point. Labels are helpful in describing one or several characteristics about an individual, but they in no way reflect the total person. Sexual orien-

tation is not the only important facet of an individual's personality or health needs. Just as it is dehumanizing to consistently refer to an individual with a spinal cord injury as a quadriplegic, it is equally inappropriate to refer to patients as lesbians or homosexuals. People with homosexual orientations are found in both sexes and in every social class and occupation. Less than 15 percent of males who consider themselves homosexual have feminine qualities and behavior (Brodoff, 1980).

Factors Affecting Sexual Needs and Behavior

Many things can affect an individual's sexual behavior and ability to satisfy personal sexual needs. Table 27–2 describes various forms of sexual stimulation. Illness and injury or chronic diseases will affect an individ-

ual's ability to meet sexual needs. Labby (1975) states, "During illness, the loss of a sense of intactness, especially as related to body image, can cause great anxiety about the capacity to function sexually; feelings of self-

Table 27-2. **Forms of Sexual Stimulation**

Tactile stimulation—touching any body area can be a form of sexual stimulation for an individual.

Masturbation—sexual stimulation (especially of genital area) by self usually with the hand; common in men and women, infants and children.

Sexual fantasies may occur anytime during work, relaxation, or sexual activities.

Kissing may involve mouth-to-mouth touching of lips, teeth, and tongues or licking, sucking, or kissing other body areas of sexual partner.

Breast stimulation—tactile stimulation of nipples and breasts may be sexually arousing in both men and women; more often arousing in women who may reach orgasm during this form of stimulation.

Genital stimulation—sexual arousal to the point of orgasm can occur in both sexes; genital area usually stimulated by hand or mouth of partner.

　Cunnilingus—stimulation of the female by sexual partner's tongue and mouth (against the law in some states).

　Fellatio—stimulation of male genitals by sexual partner's tongue and mouth (against law in some states).

　Coitus (sexual intercourse)
　　Face to face, man-above postion
　　Face to face, woman-above position
　　Face to face, side-lying position
　　Front to back, rear-entry position (woman in crawling position or prone)
　　Face to face, sitting on partner's lap
　　Anal intercourse—penis in anus of sexual partner, more common among male homosexuals

havior are learned as the child matures into adulthood. Knowledge about sex and sexual behavior is gained through family teaching and practices, personal sexual experiences, talking with others about sexual matters, peer-group practices, religion, health education, and through the media. These methods may provide the individual with a very sound base for a satisfying sex life, or they may leave the individual uninformed or misinformed. When sexual concerns arise because of other health problems or as a major health problem, the less accurate information the individual possesses about sexual functioning and sexuality, the less likely it is that the individual can handle the problem without professional help.

An individual's body-image and self-concept will affect sexual behavior and ability to satisfy sexual needs. People who feel attractive to themselves and have confidence in who they are are more likely to be able to attract desirable sexual partners. People who feel unattractive and insecure may choose to isolate themselves physically or emotionally from other people rather than risk rejection. Confinement to a wheelchair, because of lower body paralysis, may isolate someone physically by making mobility to and from social events more difficult. Other people may be uncomfortable interacting sexually with a handicapped person, especially if they are unfamiliar with the handicap or the adaptations that might be needed for intimate relations. Handicapped individuals may be unsure about the safety of intercourse or their ability to function, especially if this topic was never discussed as part of their rehabilitation. As a result, self-condemnation, frustration, and abstinence from sexual relationships may result.

Priority of other needs will affect sexual behavior. The basic survival needs of oxygen, temperature, nutrition, fluids, and pain avoidance must usually be met to some degree before sexual needs begin to be a concern. Individuals who are intensely involved in a particular focus, such as school or a work-related project, may find their sexual drive is reduced, and sexual activity decreases until the preoccupation with one concern lessens. Stress from any number of sources not only will reduce sexual drive but will interfere with sexual functioning. Menstruation may cease temporarily in a woman because of excessive physical or mental stress. A man may be unable to achieve and maintain an erection during times of stress.

worth and attractivness to others are threatened at a time when need for intimacy is greatest." Hospitalization usually results in "sexual deprivation" according to this author because of the lack of privacy, opportunity, and attention to other needs and health problems.

Children are guided by their specific culture into acceptable behavior with same- and opposite-sexed individuals. What is acceptable in one culture may be quite unacceptable in another. Most cultures in some way discourage sexual relationships between close relatives or forced sexual relationships, such as rape. Kissing is a learned behavior in our culture, but in some cultures this practice is completely unknown. One culture may be very tolerant of premarital sex while another is not. The range of behavior and the acceptability of that be-

Common Sexual Problems Affecting Need Satisfaction

Sexual problems can be grouped into two broad categories: primary dysfunction and secondary dysfunction (Levitt, 1975). In *primary dysfunction*, the sexual

problems have existed during the major part of the individual's adult life. When the nurse encounrters this type of sexual problem with any patient, the best recommendation is to refer the patient to a professional trained in sexual counseling and therapy. With *secondary sexual dysfunction*, the sexual problems are recent in origin and may appear suddenly. They may be directly or indirectly related to other health problems or treatment. An example of this is the patient who reports an alarming inability to achieve an erection several weeks after beginning to take a medication for high blood pressure control. Another example is the woman who reports painful intercourse and inadequate vaginal lubrication several months after giving birth. The fact that breast-feeding her infant reduces vaginal lubrication was never discussed with her by the nurse prior to her hospital discharge. These secondary sexual problems are the primary focus for nursing interventions. Table 27-3 presents common sexual problems and concerns which the nurse may encounter or prevent by appropriate interventions.

Table 27-3. **Common Sexual Problems and Concerns**

Dyspareunia	Pain that occurs during or just after sexual intercourse; may be related to inadequate vaginal lubrication, injury or scarring of the vagina, vaginal infections, allergic reactions to contraceptives, tumors of the pelvic area, damage to the ligaments supporting the uterus, thinning of the vaginal walls with aging or anxiety. The man may also experience painful intercourse from infection under the foreskin, inability of foreskin to retract (phimosis), and allergic reactions to contraceptives. Prostate problems may produce pain during ejaculation.
Impotence	Inability to achieve an erection or maintain one; may be related to anxiety, stress, fatigue, alcohol consumption, medications, loss of interest in partner, pain in other body parts, illness, fear of hurting partner or of worsening own medical condition; conditions especially associated with impotence involve cardiac problems, diabetes mellitus, low spinal cord damage, and alcoholism.
Premature ejaculation	Excessively short period of orgasm, resulting in ejaculation shortly after or before entering the vagina; related to psychological factors or rarely to degeneration of nervous tissue, as in multiple sclerosis.
Anorgasmia	Inability of woman to achieve orgasm; may be related to premature ejaculation by partner, inadequate foreplay, a particular partner, form of sexual stimulation used, illness, fatigue, depression.
Sexually transmitted diseases (venereal diseases)	Approximately 25 diseases are transmitted through sexual activity (Siemens and Brandzel, 1982); some examples are syphilis, gonorrhea, pelvic inflammatory disease, herpes, and infections by Trichomonas, Candida, and Chlamydia; antibiotic treatment and use of condoms is needed to prevent spread.
Fertility control	Fertility control is the ability of a woman or couple to prevent or initiate a pregnancy; birth control measures are designed to prevent unwanted pregnancies by preventing fertilization, ovulation, or implantation. *Infertility* is the inability to conceive after a year of unprotected intercourse and affects 15 to 20 percent of married couples. Without any form of fertility control, it is estimated that 60 to 80 women out of 100 will become pregnant within one year.
Surgically altered body form	Surgical procedures such as hysterectomy, mastectomy, breast reconstructive surgery, or augmentation and creation of ostomies (for removal of urine and feces when disease prevents normal elimination patterns)—all have the potential for interfering with sexual need satisfaction and making the individual feel less sexually attractive and desirable; any disfiguring injury or treatment involving nonsexual parts of the body has the same potential.
Decreased sexual desire	Decreased sexual interest may be viewed by the individual as normal and even desirable, but if the patient identifies it as a problem, regardless of age or physical health, it should receive attention from qualified professionals; it may be related to fatigue, preoccupation

	with other needs or concerns, medications, weakness, hormonal disorders, stress and fear, cultural learning and expectations, decreased interest in partner, and boredom with consistent sexual techniques.
Sexual abuse	Includes rape, sexual relations with children, and using force or fear as a means of getting another person to perform sexual activities; reportable crimes.
Homosexuality	Same-sex sexual preference was classified as an illness by the American Psychiatric Association until 1973. At that time, it was declassified as an illness and viewed as a sexual orientation which had the potential for a lasting and satisfying intimate relationship with another human being. Sexual preference, as an isolated trait, does not make a person unhealthy or mentally unstable. The cause of homosexuality is unknown but is not determined by an occasional sexual experimental encounter during adolescence. It is determined internally and is separate from the sense of gender identification. Homosexuality has been recognized throughout history and in many different cultures. Homosexual experiences during adolescence are common, especially among boys, and are a part of the general experimentation occurring among this age group. These isolated experiences have little or no relationship to later adult sexual preference, although it may be stressful to the adolescent and his family at the time.

Assessment of Sexual Need Satisfaction

Data indicating sexual need satisfaction or lack of satisfaction are not as obvious as the data associated with other unmet physical needs. Even the obvious state of being pregnant may or may not indicate satisfaction of sexual needs, depending on whether the pregnancy was desired by the man and woman involved. Maddock (1975) has identified several factors associated with sexually healthy individuals which will be presented as the basis for assessing sexual needs.

The student in nursing is not an expert in sexual counseling. As a new student, the idea of assessing an individual's sexual needs may seem very inappropriate or an invasion of privacy. Also, the fear of embarrassment or lack of knowledge in this area may prevent many students and graduate nurses from assessing patients' sexual needs. If the medical community does not address sexual needs and provide the patient with answers to questions related to sexual functioning, who will? Commonly, patients' questions will focus on ability to function sexually, when sex can safely be resumed, and any adaptations that altered health status may require for sex and feelings of sexuality.

During assessment, the nurse presents the topic for the patient's consideration. When the nurse presents the topic of sexual functioning and sexuality, the nurse gives the patient permission to discuss concerns and ask questions. Without presenting the topic for the patient,

the individual patient may be too embarrassed to ask about concerns or may feel the topic is inappropriate and that the nurse may think the patient is being sexually aggressive or seductive. The young adolescent with a spinal cord injury may believe sexual intercourse is just as impossible as moving his paralyzed legs, when, in fact, intercourse and reproduction are possible for both men and women with spinal cord injuries. The patient may wonder if sex is safe following a heart attack and abstain from sexual activity for fear of another attack. Does the woman who has recently given birth understand that breastfeeding is an unreliable method of birth control, or is she to be allowed to discover this fact through an unwanted pregnancy because her nurse was uncomfortable talking about sexual concerns?

Data Associated with Sexually Satisfied Individuals

1. The individual has accurate information about sexual functioning, sexuality, and reproduction. For example, the patient who understands how a particular method of birth control actually prevents pregnancy is more likely to be able to use that method correctly to meet sexual needs. One young adolescent the author worked with believed that a woman was most fertile just

before and just after her menstrual period. Because of this incorrect information she used the rhythm method of birth control to time intercourse in the center of her cycle not realizing this was her most fertile time and was very surprised to find herself pregnant in a short time. This was not an unintelligent person, only misinformed. The number of misconceptions related to sexual issues is surprisingly large, even in supposedly educated people, because of the lack of open, factual discussions in the family, churches, schools, and health care facilities. The lack of information is especially acute when physical problems are superimposed on sexual functioning and feelings of sexuality. People who are most at risk for having inaccurate or inadequate information are those who are experiencing major changes in their life which are either temporary or permanent in nature. Any type of surgery that alters an individual's outward physical form or ability to function has implications for sexual need satisfaction. Common patient questions may include: "How will a mastectomy affect my ability to relate sexually to a man?" "What will happen with my colostomy if I have sexual relations?" "Can I have an erection with a spinal cord injury?" "Can I have sex during pregnancy or will it hurt the baby?"

2. The individual has an understanding of personal sexual attitudes and is comfortable with gender identity, sexual role, and behavior. This concept is very important to the success of some activities that may have sexual connotations. These include such things as breast-feeding an infant, control of fertility, and willingness to experiment sexually to provide optimum satisfaction for both partners when previous modes of sexual expression are blocked or altered because of physical problems. Some people may view the handicapped person as asexual. The thought of having sex with someone in a wheelchair or without a breast may be offensive or not even considered as potentially healthy and satisfying, depending on how the individuals feel about themselves and appropriate sexual behavior. This applies to both the handicapped individual and an unaffected person. For example, a woman who is uncomfortable with touching her own body is going to have a hard time breastfeeding or inserting a diaphragm, suppository, or sponge into the vagina for birth control.

3. The individual has a value system that supports decisions and behavior related to sexuality so behavior is not in conflict with beliefs and values. The individual who is unable to seek professional help related to sexual concerns because of a personal belief system may be in a constant state of conflict. Problems can be anticipated when an individual's belief system is in conflict with current sexual behavior or sexual abilities, as when a woman continues to feel sexually attracted to men well into her later years, even though such behavior is viewed by her as inappropriate.

4. An individual experiencing sexual well-being is able to relate effectively to both sexes in a variety of relationships, including potential relationships leading to long-term commitment and intimacy. Fear of rejection or lack of information about ability to function sexually may block people with physical handicaps or medical problems from attempting close intimate relationships. Some patients may be sexually aggressive or seductive toward the nurse as a reaction to forced dependence and be unable to behave in an appropriate manner. Patients may make repeated sexually suggestive statements to the nurse or touch the nurse in sexually suggestive ways. Often, the patient is experiencing decreased feelings of sexual attractiveness. The patient may be questioning ability to function and attempting to elicit responses in the nurse that reinforce the fact that the individual is still a sexually attractive being rather than repulsive or asexual. This situation is also difficult for the nurse since sexual interaction with the patient is unethical and not considered professional. It also makes most nurses quite uncomfortable; they tend to avoid the patient, and inadequate patient care results. Dealing with the seductive or sexually aggressive patient is discussed later in this chapter.

The Nurse's Role in Assisting Patients with Sexual Need Satisfaction

Health care providers should be informed about sexual matters, especially if it is the patient's primary reason for seeking medical assistance, but also as a part of any patient's recovery or rehabilitation from other health problems or injuries. The nurse accepts the patient's sexual orientation and sexual concerns without judging "right/wrong," "good/bad." This is necessary if an effective helping relationship is to develop between the nurse and the patient. At times, acceptance of the patient's sexual needs may be incompatible with the nurse's personal value system. At this point, the best course of action is to admit and recognize personal beliefs and bias and refer the patient to another nurse who is capable of providing the needed care.

The role of the nurse in helping patients with sexual needs focuses on:

1. Becoming aware of personal beliefs and values related to sexual issues
2. Providing information on sexual issues
3. Communication skills for assessing and discussing patients' concerns
4. Making referrals to more experienced health professionals based on specific patient needs

The self-assessment section of this chapter is designed to help the student begin to recognize beliefs and values related to sexual issues and how these may affect the ability to give nursing care. Sexual concerns of patients are a neglected area because many nurses are uncomfortable with the topic and have inadequate knowledge to plan helpful interventions.

Understanding of sexual functioning includes: knowledge of normal growth and development, of gender identification, and sexual activity of the growing child. It includes information on physical changes in puberty, pregnancy, and menopause. Sexual knowledge of the nurse includes the stages of the sexual response cycle, ranges of normal sexual functioning and expression, and adaptations that make sexual functioning possible for the patient with a variety of physical handicaps or health problems.

Nurses should begin with the assumption that if they do not present requested information about sexual issues to the patient or refer the patient to someone more knowledgeable, no one else will. The patient's health concerns related to sexual activity can be discussed with the physician for clarification and for any contraindicated activity. The nurse assesses the patient's current knowledge level regarding sexual activity to correct misconceptions and provide appropriate information. Providing a dissertation on sexual function to a patient who has no interest in such information is as inappropriate as discharging a patient from the hospital who has many unasked, unanswered questions. The nurse should know how disease, injury, treatments, and medications may affect sexual functioning and offer to discuss these problems with each patient. The nurse makes the offer to provide the patient with information. It is up to the patient to accept or reject the offer based on personal needs at the time. If the patient is not currently concerned about sexual needs, but later finds that concerns are developing as recovery progresses, the fact that the nurse offered the information earlier will make it more likely that the patient will request the information as needs arise.

Skills in communication are necessary if patients are to feel accepted and comfortable discussing sexual issues. Good listening skills and clarification of patient's actual concerns are needed if problems are to be identified. Confronting patients with their verbal and nonverbal behavior that may indicate sexual concerns will help a patient recognize problems or fears, if they exist.

The nurse must be able to understand the words the patient is using to explain sexual concerns, just as the patient must be able to understand the words the nurse uses to provide information or make suggestions for reducing problems. There may be a large gap between professional medical terminology and slang expressions. It is more appropriate for the nurse to try to bridge this communication gap by altering the words used to communicate than it is for the patient to attempt this. Many professionals need to be desensitized to words before they are able to use them comfortably. One way of doing this is to repeatedly write or verbalize words related to sex and sexuality. After a time, the words lose their impact for creating discomfort in the health care provider. Using technical words that the patient does not understand is not professional. It is a failure to communicate.

Some of a nurse's communication skills involve making verbal or written referrals to people who will be more likely to assist the patient with sexual problems. The referrals may be to clergy, physicians, support groups of people with similar problems and concerns, another nurse, or a family planning service, to name a few.

Self-awareness of personal values and beliefs about sexual matters will prevent the nurse from unconsciously imposing personal values and behavior patterns on patients. The patient's fear of how the nurse may react to sexual concerns may be sufficient to prevent a patient from mentioning the topic. If the patient mentions the topic and feels a lack of acceptance or rejection and discomfort from the nurse, the topic may be dropped by the patient for the nurses's sake, leaving the patient with unmet sexual needs.

Nursing Diagnoses Associated with Unmet Sexual Needs

A listing of some common nursing diagnoses follows but is in no way an all-inclusive list. The diagnosis of a sexual problem for each patient will be individualized based on physical, cognitive, social, religious, family, and behavioral factors.

Rape trauma syndrome
Sexual dysfunction
Feelings of emasculinization/loss of femininity related to illness or altered body-image
Inadequate/incorrect information related to sexual activity or functioning
Infertility
Fear of sexual dysfunction
Grief related to lost reproductive function
Grief related to altered body-image and feelings of lost sexuality
Inappropriate sexual behavior (with health care providers, other patients)
Fear of rejection by sexual partner
Unwanted pregnancy

Nursing Interventions to Facilitate Satisfaction of Sexual Needs

Some general suggestions will be presented related to sexual need satisfaction.

Consider the following when dealing with patients' sexual concerns:

1. Consider resumption of sexual activity as part of every patient's total rehabilitation or recovery program.

2. Use language the patient understands.

3. Start with general questions and move toward specific questions based on the individual patient's needs. For example, the nurse may ask, "You will be going home in a few days to your family, and I am wondering if anyone has talked with you about resuming sexual activity?" This opens the topic for the patient who may reply that no one has, but that no concerns or questions exist. The patient may also begin an outpouring of questions and fears related to resumption of sexual activity. Finding out exactly what the patient is worried about will make interventions more effective in meeting a particular patient's needs.

4. Consider sexual assessment and counseling as another form of teaching.

5. The nurse may begin discussing sexual needs by presenting some common misconceptions related to a patient's health status to assess if the patient has inaccurate information. For example, the nurse may begin by saying to a patient recovering from an MI, "Many patients are afraid of having another heart attack if they resume sexual activity, when actually the strain on the heart during intercourse is similar to that from climbing two flights of stairs and is safe for many patients after six to eight weeks. Do you have any concerns about resuming sexual activity once other forms of exercise are approved by your physician?" Some common misconceptions related to sexual functioning are presented in Table 27–4.

6. Give the patient time to ask and answer questions. Finding the words for self-expression may be difficult for patients who are not used to talking about sexual topics.

7. Discuss the importance of open, honest communication between sexual partners in resuming sexual activity. The partner may be fearful of hurting the patient to the point of lost sexual interest or function. Previous forms of sexual stimulation may feel differently and be less desirable than others, and this can be communicated between partners.

8. Discuss physiological responses to sexual stimulation and how a patient's current level of health may affect responses. For example, a breastfeeding woman should understand that her milk may let down with orgasm.

Table 27–4. **Myths Associated with Sexual Functioning and Sexuality**

Paralyzed men are unable to have intercourse or father children.
Quadriplegic women are unable to conceive or carry a pregnancy.
Intercourse with a catheter in place is impossible.
Letting your partner know what feels good to you in a sexual relationship will make your partner feel inadequate and reject you.
Intercourse with the man on top of the woman provides both people with the best sexual stimulation during intercourse.
Sex during pregnancy is dangerous.
Women lose all interest in sex while they are pregnant or breastfeeding.
Orgasm is reached only when a man has intercourse with a woman.
Handicapped people usually lose most of their ability to function sexually.
A woman with an ostomy cannot carry a pregnancy or have a normal delivery.
A breast cannot be reconstructed surgically for a woman following a mastectomy.
A woman who has had her breast size increased (augmentation mammoplasty) cannot breastfeed any future children.
Following a hysterectomy, a woman will need hormone replacement therapy for the rest of her life.
A hysterectomy decreases the size of the vagina, making it too short for the full length of the erect penis, and causes discomfort for both the man and the woman.
Infertility is usually caused by failure of the woman to reach orgasm.
Infertility is a rare problem for couples who really want children.
Most teenage pregnancies are planned.
Young girls who become pregnant usually have less physical complications than older women.
Impotence is to be expected as a man ages.
Sexual activity among older people is unusual and may endanger their health.
After a heart attack, most people should abstain from sexual intercourse because of the risk of a repeat attack.
Sexual abuse of children is more rare than physical abuse of children.
Most rapes are reported.
Most rapes are unplanned.
Rape is most often committed by a stranger to the victim.

9. Identify activities that other patients with similar health problems have used to ease the resumption of sexual activity. Describe any preparation that may be helpful prior to sexual intercourse to prevent undesirable interruptions from other body needs. For example, some patients may choose to remove a urinary catheter

or to tape it out of the way prior to beginning sexual activity. Other patients may find that some form of vaginal lubrication is helpful before intercourse. They may insert some water-soluble lubricant, such as K-Y jelly, into and around the vaginal opening or on the penis before or during the exictement phase.

10. Identify a time range for the patient in which people with similar health problems have resumed sexual activity.

11. Identify activities or positioning that may facilitate intercourse as requested by the patient. For example, late in pregnancy, the woman being in a superior position is more comfortable for many women. For the recovering cardiac patient, having the woman in a superior position initiating rocking movements during intercourse puts less strain on the man's heart than when the man is in a superior position doing the thrusting. How might a person in a wheelchair engage in intercourse? What is to be done with any tubes, dressings, or prostheses during sexual activity? These are questions for the nurse to consider and investigate in preparation for sexual counseling of patients and their families.

12. Describe any physical signs the patient may experience during intercourse indicating danger to physical health. Indicate appropriate actions to take, such as terminating sexual activity and notifying the physician. What if the recovering cardiac patient begins to have chest pains during sexual activity? What if the woman experiences pain when beginning to have intercourse following childbirth? What if breathing becomes difficult for the patient with COPD?

13. Consider all patients as sexual beings and consider the possibility and implications of pregnancy for the patient's total health. Offer to discuss control of fertility and use of specific methods compatible with the patient's beliefs and physical abilities. One patient, with whom the author worked, had severe diabetes and was blinded from the disease, had experienced renal failure, and had a kidney transplant. Previous sexual counseling of this 30-year-old patient involved telling her she was infertile because of the extent of her diabetes. She confided that for three months she had been aware of the increasing size of her abdomen but had been afraid to go to the doctor because she was sure she had a cancerous tumor. When she finally sought medical assistance, she was diagnosed as being six and a half months pregnant! This infertile patient gave birth to a healthy baby boy, but the risk to her transplanted kidney and diabetes was great.

14. Consider the effect of prescribed medication on sex drive and sexual functioning, and if potentially problematic, discuss it with the patient. (See Table 27–5.)

15. Consideration for sexual need satisfaction is the responsibility of the nursing staff in a long-term care facility. The nurse can expect to assist patients or residents by discussing sexual concerns, providing information, providing privacy, preventing interruptions, creating an accepting environment for sexual activity between two adults desiring intimacy, and assisting with physical needs prior to sexual activity.

Table 27–5. **Drugs/Medications Related to Sexual Functioning**

Nicotine	Long-term impairment of sexual function because of association with chronic lung and malignant diseases. As a vasoconstricting drug, it may interfere with erection in the male and lubrication and separation of the labia in the female. During pregnancy, it reduces the circulation of blood to the placenta.
Alcohol	Light to moderate consumption will reduce fears and anxiety which may block normal sexual functioning. Abuse of alcohol in the man leads to loss of fertility, inability to achieve an erection, and reduced testosterone production. Consumption of alcohol by the pregnant woman is associated with fetal alcohol syndrome in the newborn; the more the woman drinks, the greater the risk of FAS to the fetus.
Steroids	Used to reduce inflammation in arthritis and other chronic diseases; tends to reduce sexual drive by decreasing amount of testosterone in the body of both men and women.
Antihypertensives	Used to control high blood pressure and are related to problems with erection, lubrication, and decreased sex drive.
Oral contraceptives	Birth control pills are one of the most effective methods of preventing pregnancy by preventing ovulation. The estrogen and progesterone in the pills may reduce sexual drive, but this effect may be balanced by the reduced concern over unwanted pregnancy.

Dealing with Sexually Aggressive or Seductive Patients

Sexual harassment or aggression by patients may be experienced during your learning activities as a student in nursing and later as a graduate nurse. Watson (1982) felt nursing students are more likely to receive sexual harassment from patients because they are viewed by patients as less experienced, uncertain of how to respond, having less authority, younger, and more likely to feel at fault for eliciting sexual behavior in a patient. Some people are unaware of the implications of their behavior and appearance in a clinical setting where close and intimate physical care of others is expected. Makeup, jewelry, and a social relationship may be inappropriate while caring for a patient. The nursing student's appearance or behavior may make the patient uncomfortable sexually or may make the patient or other health care-givers feel that the student nurse is trying to attract their attentions on a social level. This does not mean that a nurse or student should play down natural good looks. It does mean that students in nursing should examine their intentional and incidental behavior and general appearance, in addition to their attitudes, when providing patient care.

For example, the inexperienced nursing student may take more time manipulating a male patient's condom catheter while attempting to change it than an experienced nurse. This added stimulation may cause the patient to have an erection and be interpreted by the patient as sexual stimulation.

If a patient makes suggestive statements or physical advances to you as a student, talk with your instructor about the incident. A professional interpretation of the patient's behavior and your own behavior is needed to validate your own interpretation. Examine your verbal and nonverbal behavior. Could your behavior have been interpreted as seductive by the patient? Assey and Herbert (1983) suggest two techniques for dealing with patients who are exhibiting unacceptable sexual behavior toward the nurse. First the nurse examines personal behavior to determine if it could have legitimately been interpreted by the patient as seductive or socially inviting. If the nurses's behavior was not the stimulus for the patient's sexual behavior, the suggestion is to confront a patient with the unacceptable behavior and express your negative reactions to such behavior and how it affects your ability to provide competent nursing care. This approach is directed at stopping the behavior, while opening up the area of sexual concerns. The nurse might begin by looking at the patient and saying, ''Mr. Anderson, don't touch me like that. It really makes me uncomfortable, and I find myself avoiding some of your care. Other patients don't act that way with me so I'm wondering if something is bothering you?'' Another approach involves setting limits on the patient's behavior by identifying the unacceptable behavior and telling the patient the consequences of continuance of the behavior. For example the nurse may say, ''Ms. Gess, whenever I am your nurse, I find you are exposing your breasts while I am giving you care. The other nurses report you do not do this with them. If you continue to expose yourself to me, I am going to assign your care to another nurse.'' Bear in mind that a sense of anxiety and dependence that many patients experience in the hospital may result in aggressive or seductive behavior. Patients may be trying to assure themselves that they are still attractive or still a ''man'' or ''woman'' when altered body-image is involved. This does not mean the nurse or student should allow the patient to continue to be sexually aggressive or seductive toward them. But the behavior may be less personally related to the nurse as an individual and more related to the patient's sexual needs at the time.

Nursing Care Plan for a Patient with Unmet Sex/Sexuality Needs

Data.   Jim North was admitted to the rehabilitation unit of the hospital as a transfer patient from the neurosurgery station of the hospital. He had experienced a fracture of his spine one month ago with damage to the spinal cord resulting in permanent paraplegia. He was 22 years old, single, and had lived with a roommate prior to the accident in which he had injured his spinal cord. He had a Foley catheter in place, was on a regular diet, and had a lack of all feeling and muscle control below the area of his waist. After one week in the rehabilitation area, he began to make sexual comments to the nurses. While his genital area was being cleansed, he stated to one nurse, ''I bet you wish that [referring to his penis] was working.'' Another nurse reported that Jim had touched her breasts, but she wasn't sure whether it was accidental or done on purpose. A nursing student reported to her instructor that, upon entering the room of Mr. North, she had found him completely exposed and had been told that she had made him ''hot.'' Another nursing student reported that Jim had been found masturbating and, when interrupted by the student, had said, "It doesn't matter anyway. The damn thing is as dead as my legs. I might as well be forgetting about getting it on with anyone from now on." At the suggestion of the nursing instructor and head nurse, a care conference was held concerning Jim's problems and nursing care. Several of the nurses expressed anger, embarrassment, or fear concerning Jim's sexual behavior which had previously been unreported and admitted avoiding him. The following care plan emerged from the conference.

Nursing Diagnoses
1. Altered body-image from lower body paralysis
2. Fear of lost sexual functioning
3. Inappropriate sexual behavior with nursing staff

Planning

Goals of Care
1. Jim to discuss concerns and feelings about his paralysis and how he sees it affecting him as a person and his life in general, within one week of conference.
2. Jim to discuss feelings related to sex and his sexuality with nurse within one week of conference.
3. Jim will stop making seductive statements and touching female nurses' body parts within one week of conference.

Nursing Actions (Interventions)
Goals 1, 2, and 3 are all in one plan.

1. Assign the same nurses each shift to Jim's care who feel capable of discussing sexual concerns and behavior with him.
2. Present Jim with his currently unacceptable behavior. Emphasize that the behavior is unacceptable but not Jim as a person.
3. Stay with Jim when he makes remarks about sexual functioning; offer opportunity for Jim to discuss the effect of paralysis on his sexuality and ability to function sexually.
4. Set limits for Jim's behavior by indicating nurses will not be able to care for him if he repeats any seductive or sexually aggressive behavior toward them. Explain to Jim that his behavior is making nurses uncomfortable and interfering with his nursing care.
5. Assess knowledge regarding future sexual functioning.
6. Correct inadequate information or incorrect information.
7. Encourage Jim to participate in weekly support groups for spinal cord–injured patients.
8. Offer to provide Jim with printed information from various sources on abilities and management techniques for paraplegic people who are independent.
9. Offer to involve Jim's sexual partner in discussions about sexual functioning and adaptations during intercourse for spinal cord–injured patients.

Evaluation

Goal 1 met. Jim discussed how he no longer feels capable of being a man because of lost sexual attractiveness and functioning. He views himself in a dependent role, relying on others for almost all his needs for the rest of his life. This is in conflict with his image of maleness which involves being independent, strong, and sexually active.
Goal 2 partially met. Jim began to talk about his feelings but feels the nurses are incapable of understanding how a man feels. He equates sexual functioning with sexual attractiveness and feels convinced he will be unable to perform sexually, thus, is undesirable and asexual.
Goal 3 met. Jim has stopped making sexual advances toward the nurses. He apologized for his behavior but felt such a strong need to be viewed as a sexual person that he tried to get sexual responses from the nurses.

Reassessment

Jim's identified problems are not resolved, with the possible exception of his inappropriate behavior toward the nurses. Continued data collection and opportunities to ventilate feelings and find alternative ways of sexual expression will be required to assess and assist Jim's overall adjustment to life and to himself. Try assigning a male nurse to Jim's case to facilitate continued discussion of sexual concerns (since he feels female nurses do not understand his feelings).

Summary

This chapter presents reproduction as a survival need for the human species and sexuality as an integral part of an individual's self-concept. Sexuality is an integration of gender, sex roles and behavior, sex drive, and prefered sexual activity. Sexual need satisfaction may serve the functions of reproduction, pleasurable stimulation, relief of tensions, increased self-esteem, satisfaction of love/belonging needs, and clarification of the relationship between two individuals. The sexual response cycle involves the phases of excitement, plateau, orgasm, and resolution with individuals experiencing some or all of the stages during various forms of sexual stimulation.

Control of sex drive, reproduction, and fertility were presented, as were the range of sex roles and behaviors common to our culture. Some factors affecting sexual behavior involve learning, growth and development, culture, religion, health, body-image, and stress. The nurse's role in assessment and intervention in patient's sexual concerns was discussed. Dealing with sexually aggressive or seductive patients involves self-assessment, setting limits, and confrontation.

Terms for Review

asexual	gender	lesbian	progesterone	sexuality
bisexual	heterosexual	masturbation	reproduction	testosterone
estrogen	homosexual	orgasmic phase	resolution phase	transsexual
excitement phase	impotence	plateau phase	sex	transvestite
fertility control	infertility			

Self-Assessment

Consider the following situations related to sexual behavior as one way of beginning your own assessment of feelings and beliefs and how these values may affect your nursing care. How comfortable would you feel in each situation? Do you feel the need to change the patient's beliefs or sexual behavior? Could you give emotional and physical care to these patients without compromising your own values, or would it be better for you to have the patient assigned to another nurse?

1. A 14-year-old pregnant girl admitted to labor and delivery with her 16-year-old boyfriend
2. A teenager being treated for the third time in one year for a sexually transmitted disease
3. A quadriplegic resident of a nursing home who asked for assistance inserting a vaginal sponge for contraception because her boyfriend was coming shortly to take her for an outing
4. Unmarried teenagers and adults coming to you for birth control information and devices
5. Walking in on a patient of any age who was masturbating
6. Providing sexual counseling for a person who identifies herself as homosexual
7. Providing physical care, including bathing, for a patient known to be a homosexual
8. Handling a woman's breasts as you assist her with breast-feeding
9. Walking in on two residents of a nursing home during your evening rounds who are engaged in mutual sexual stimulation or intercourse
10. A fellow nursing student who complains to you that her male patients often try to "come on to her" sexually. She wears a lot of makeup, earrings, necklaces, and bracelets, and uniforms that are quite tight and too short.

Learning Activities

1. Talk with nurses or others who lead support groups, such as RESOLVE, for infertile couples. Attend a group session, if possible, in your community. What concerns are common to both sexes? Do the men's concerns differ from the women's concerns? What types of communication techniques are used by the group leaders to encourage couples to verbalize their feelings/concerns?

2. Visit a community family planning clinic and talk with the nurses or midwives about how they help clients select birth control measures to match their life-style and sexual activity. Do most adolescents inform their parents that they are sexually active and using birth control? What type of conflicts arise between values of clients/families and taking responsibility for sexual activity and fertility?

3. Visit a rehabilitation center for physically or mentally handicapped people. Are sexual needs and fertility control discussed as part of the overall rehabilitation plan? What type of obstacles do many handicapped people encounter related to meeting their sexual needs?

Review Questions

1. Sexuality is most related to an individual's
   a. Ability to reproduce
   b. Ability to reach orgasm
   c. Self-concept
   d. Physical structure

2. The excitement and plateau phases of the human sexual responses involve two major types of physical changes in both men and women. These changes are
   a. Relaxation of voluntary muscles and reduced blood pressure
   b. Vasocongestion and increased muscle tension
   c. Hypotension and release of FSH
   d. Release of LH and FSH by anterior pituitary

3. Sexual drive or libido is most dependent on which of the following hormones?
   a. Estrogen in the female
   b. Progesterone in the male
   c. Testosterone in both sexes
   d. Testosterone in the male only
   e. FSH and LH

4. When the nurse experiences unwanted sexual advances from a patient, the best course of action is to
   a. Report it to the physician
   b. Apologize for being sexually attractive to the patient
   c. Explain to the patient that the particular behavior is unacceptable and interferes with ability to provide care
   d. Assign all care of that patient to a nursing assistant of the same sex

5. When bringing up the topic of sexual needs and concerns with patients, which intervention is most likely to meet individual needs?
   a. The nurse consistently explains all forms of birth control to each patient prior to hospital discharge.

b. The nurse begins discussion of the topic by taking a detailed sexual history of each patient.
   c. The nurse opens the topic for discussion with each patient as part of the rehabilitation or recovery phase of health care.
   d. The nurse does not pry into a patient's sexual life but waits until the patient asks specific questions.

True or False

6. _____ The blood pressure reaches maximum elevation during orgasm.
7. _____ Hyperventilation often occurs in women but rarely in men during intercourse.
8. _____ Orgasm can be achieved through masturbation.
9. _____ Homosexuals are genetically different from heterosexuals.
10. _____ The pulse rate may increase to twice the normal value during sexual stimulation.

Answers

1. c
2. b
3. c
4. c
5. c
6. T
7. F
8. T
9. F
10. T

References and Bibliography

Altchuler, K., and Kessler, D.: Dealing with seductive behavior. *Patient Care*, pp. 78–79, Sept. 15, 1980.

Assey, J., and Herbert, J.: Who is the seductive patient? *Am. J. Nurs.*, **83**:531–32, 1983.

Bregman, S.: *Sexuality and the Spinal Cord Injured Woman*. Sister Kenny Institute, Minneapolis, 1975.

Brodoff, A.: Who is homosexual? A working definition. *Patient Care*, **14**:22–86, Sept. 15, 1980.

Cole, C.; Levin, E.; Whitley, J.; and Young, S.: Brief sexual counseling during cardiac rehabilitation. *Heart Lung*, **8**:124–29, Jan.–Feb., 1979.

DeLora, J.; Warren, C.; and Ellison, C.: *Understanding Sexual Interaction*, 2nd ed. Houghton Mifflin, Boston, 1981.

Frank, D.: You don't have to be an expert to give sexual counseling to a mastectomy patient. *Nursing 81*, **11**:64–67, Jan., 1981.

Gondek, M.: Post—MI sex: Those unspoken fears. *RN*, **46**:61–63, May, 1983.

Hyde, J.: *Understanding Human Sexualtiy*. McGraw-Hill, New York, 1979.

Kinsey, A.; Pomeroy, W.; Martin, C.; and Gebhard, P.: *Sexual Behavior in the Human Female*. Saunders, Philadelphia, 1953.

Kinsey, A.; Pomeroy, W.; Martin, C.: *Sexual Behavior in the Human Male.* Saunders, Philadelphia, 1948.

Labby, D.: Sexual concomitants of disease and illness. *Postgrad. Med.*, **57**:103–11, July, 1975.

Levitt, E.: Sexual counseling. *Postgrad. Med.*, **57**:91–97, July, 1975.

Ludlow, E.,and Baqwell, M.: Faculty and students confront sexuality. *J. Nurs. Educ.*, **22**:161–64, Apr., 1983.

Maddock, J.: Sexual health and health care. *Postgrad. Med.*, **57**:52–58, July, 1975.

Mann, J., and Katsuranis, J.: The dynamics and problems of sexual relationships. *Postgrad. Med.*, **57**:79–86, July, 1975.

Masters, W., Johnson, V.: *Human Sexual Response.* Little Brown, Boston, 1966.

McCary, J.: *Human Sexuality*, 2nd ed. Van Nostrand, New York, 1979.

Siemens, S., and Brandzel, R.: *Sexuality: Nursing Assessment and Intervention.* Lippincott, Philadelphia, 1982.

Stockard, S. Caring for sexually aggressive patient. *Nursing 81*, **11**:114–16, Nov., 1981.

Thompson, D.: Sexual activity following acute myocardial infarction in the male. *Nurs. Times*, **76**:1965–67, Nov. 6, 1980.

Vander, A.; Sherman, J.; and Luciano, D.: *Human Physiology. The Mechanisms of Body Function.* McGraw-Hill, New York 1980.

Watson, C.: Ordeal by harassment. *Nurs. Mirror*, **155**:38, Aug. 18, 1982.

THE NEED FOR STIMULATION: SENSORY/MOTOR

Objectives

1. Describe the interactions among muscles, bones, joints, and nerves to achieve movement.

2. Describe the effect of immobility on other basic needs.

3. Describe normal sensory input to the central nervous system.

4. Describe the effects of inadequate or excess sensory stimulation on human functioning.

5. Identify factors affecting reception and interpretation of environmental stimuli.

6. Identify patient data associated with unmet stimulation needs.

7. Describe nursing interventions to maintain muscle and joint functioning.

8. Explain the goals of therapeutic positioning.

9. Identify principles and techniques for moving and lifting patients that reduce the nurse's risk of back injury and muscle strain.

10. Describe safety considerations when ambulating a patient.

11. Explain the following types of gaits for patients using assistive devices: four-point gait, two-point gait, three-point gait, partial weight-bearing gait, cane-supported gait.

12. Describe nursing interventions to assist patients meet their needs following loss of vision or hearing.

13. Describe the appropriate use of restraints to help a patient meet safety needs.

14. Identify causes and recommended nursing interventions in the prevention and treatment of pressure sores.

15. Safely perform the following skills:
    Moving and positioning patients in supine, prone, lateral, and Fowler's positions
    Transfer of patient from bed to chair or bed to cart
    Ambulating a patient
    Range-of-motion exercises
    Crutch or cane gaits

Stimulation as a Basic Human Need

This chapter discusses stimulation as a basic human need for health and normal functioning. The stimulation needs considered in this chapter involve the senses of vision, hearing, taste, smell, touch, the vestibular sense of position and balance, and the need for muscular activity and body movement. These forms of stimulation involve a person's interaction with the environment. The stimuli originate in the environment or by movement through the environment. The various internal forms of stimulation occurring between areas of the body and the peripheral and central nervous system are also critically important to normal body functioning but are often below the level of conscious awareness.

The human body seems to be designed following the concept of "use it or lose it." Unless the sensory and motor systems of the body are used continually, their structure and their ability to function effectively begin to deteriorate and may be permanently impaired. The brain receives constant information in the form of coded electrical messages from the nerves serving the muscles, joints, and senses within the body. A specific amount of input from the senses is required for normal brain functioning. When stimulation to the brain from the senses and muscles of the body is inadequate, cognitive, affective, and motor behavior is negatively affected. Experimental studies on restricted sensory environments (exposure to environment without sensory or social stimuli for several hours to days) show that people react to inadequate sensory input by developing a reduced ability to think and reason, decreased coordination, decreased spontaneous movement, decreased mental alertness, and disorientation. The person who has reduced physical movement because of immobility will experience gradual deterioration in the size and strength of the muscles. Hallucinations, both visual and auditory, may develop because of immobility, and people often become anxious and restless.

If one sense is lost or lessened in acuity, the body attempts to compensate through the other senses, which become more acute. This provides the constant stimulation needed by the central nervous system to interpret and interact with the environment. The common example of the blinded person developing increased auditory and tactile abilities is an adaptation made by the nervous system to compensate for decreased information from the visual system. A nursing student or graduate nurse beginning work on the labor and delivery unit will initially have great difficulty in doing an accurate assessment of cervical dilation on the laboring woman. One reason for this is that sighted people rely on vision for information on size and shape of objects much more than on touch. In assessing the cervix, the sense of vision is useless, and the tactile sense must be developed. This takes time and practice as the brain learns to focus on tactile sensory input and give meaning to the messages from the nurse's fingers.

Normal development of the senses and of motor ability requires use during all stages of life but especially during the first few years as the brain and nervous system develop and mature. For example, if stimulation to the brain from one eye is inadequate because of a structural or muscle problem in that eye, the vision center within the brain will not develop normally. Correction with lenses or muscle surgery later in life may be ineffective in restoring normal vision, since the interpreting area in the brain did not develop completely. Muscle requires activity to maintain or increase its size. With total disuse, muscle decreases in size by 50 percent within one month. (See Figure 28-1.) An infant in an environment with inadequate stimulation will not develop normally and will become physically, mentally, and socially retarded compared to other infants. Infants may actually completely withdraw from a nonstimulating physical and social environment until they wither and die.

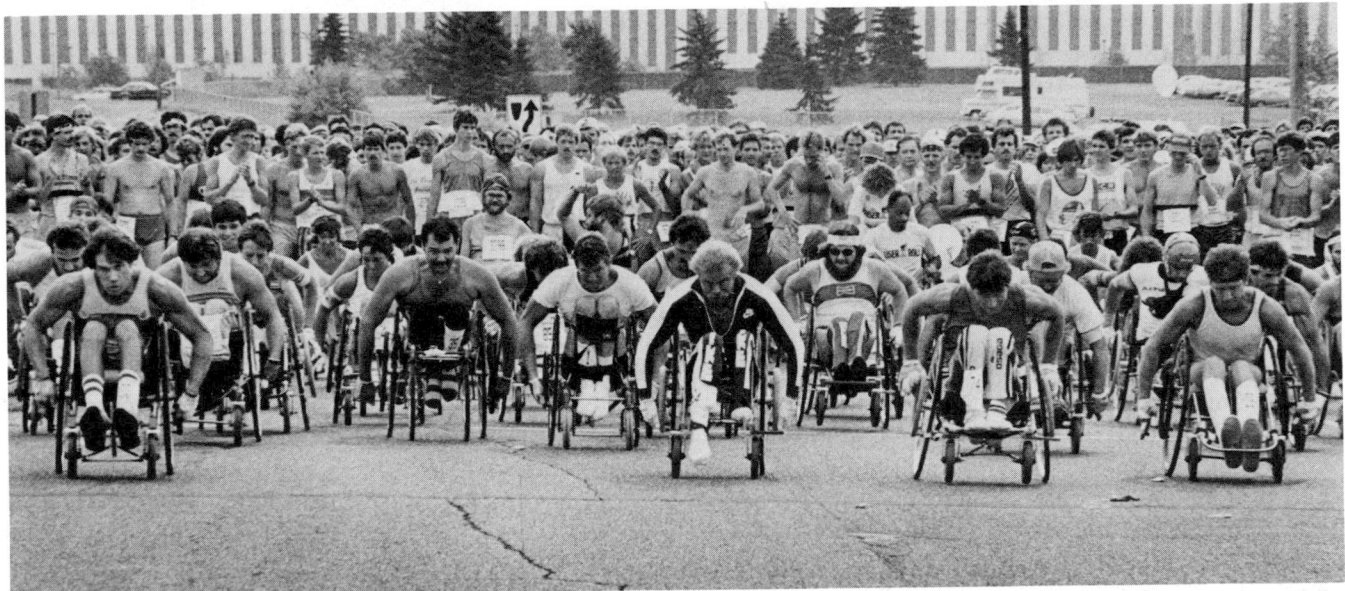

Figure 28-1.   The Kaiser Roll Marathon Race (Minnesota, 1983). Note the upper arm muscle development in the racers in wheelchairs compared to the muscle atrophy in their legs. (Photograph by Steve Downer, *Current* newspaper, Bloomington, MN.)

Normal Means of Meeting Stimulation Needs—Mobility

Mobility is the ability to contract and relax muscle groups to enable the individual to move about purposefully in the environment. Normal mobility is tied very closely to the concept of health for most individuals and is often taken for granted. Mobility is necessary if people are to meet their other needs since it affects not only the ability to interact with others and earn a living but also the internal workings of the body.

Mobility depends on the coordinated functioning of muscles, joints, and bones. This coordination is achieved through the *afferent nerves* (going toward the nerve cell body) and *efferent nerves* (going away from the nerve cell body). These pathways lead to the spinal cord and central nervous system and then back to the muscle, exiting from the spinal cord. (See Figure 28-2.) Normal muscle tissue is maintained in a state of slight contrac-

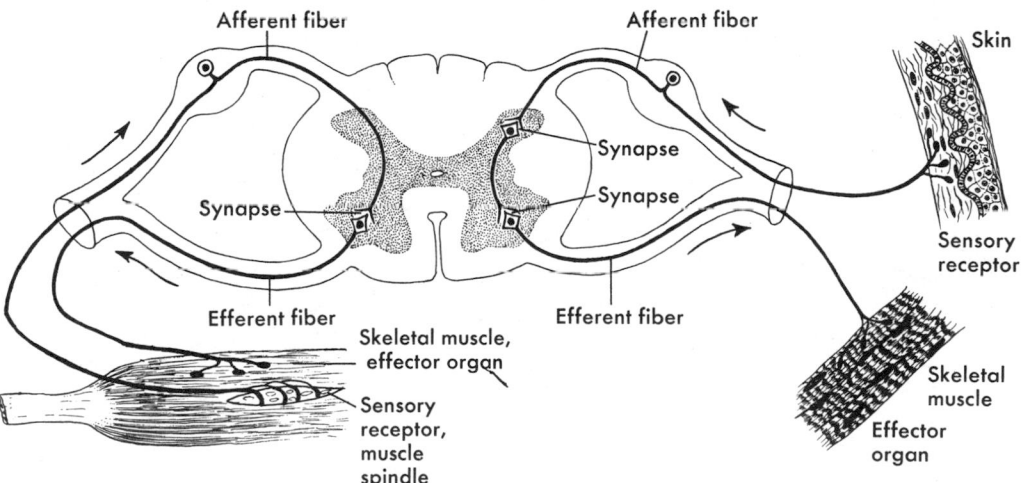

Figure 28-2.   Afferent and efferent nerve fibers. The left side of the diagram shows a monosynaptic reflex involving two nerve cells. On the right, a polysynaptic reflex is illustrated involving three or more nerve cells. (From M. Miller *et al.*: *Kimber-Gray-Stackpole's Anatomy and Physiology*, 17th ed. Macmillan, New York, 1977, p. 212.)

tion called *muscle tone*. This is accomplished by reflexes originating within the muscle. Muscle tone is maintained by a reflex arc, triggered by the degree of stretch present in the muscle and by impulses from the spinal cord and brain. Often there are intermediary neural connections within the spinal cord so three or more neurons are involved in regulating the degree of stretch on the muscle fibers they innervate.

The Motor Unit

One neuron from the spinal cord innervates many individual muscle fibers at one time. The finer the movement performed by the muscle, the fewer the number of muscle fibers innervated by a single neuron. On the average, one neuron innervates 150 muscle fibers. The eye, for example, has only about 13 muscle fibers innervated by one neuron, while the large calf muscles may have as many as 1,700 fibers innervated by one neuron. The neuron and the muscle fibers it innervates are called a *motor unit*. It is the coordinated workings of the innumerable motor units throughout the body that give individuals the ability to move in a purposeful manner. Motor units throughout the body are triggered

to contract in a continuously alternating pattern to prevent jerky, spastic movements. Posture and mobility are maintained through the action of different motor units contracting at slightly different times. This produces one continuous contraction in a muscle group, such as the biceps in the arm, to maintain function without fatiguing individual muscle fibers.

ATP for Muscular Contractions

The maximum amount of contraction possible in an individual muscle fiber is based not only on the rate of neural stimulation causing contraction of the muscle fiber, but also on the ability of the muscle fiber to produce adenosine triphosphate (ATP). As long as the ATP supply lasts, the muscle fiber can maintain a continuous contraction. There are three pathways for ATP production within the muscle. (See Figure 28–3.) The first pathway involves the formation of *creatine phosphate* which stores ATP and is utilized at the onset of muscle fiber contraction. The amount of ATP stored in creatine phosphate is quite small and is rapidly utilized during the first few seconds of a strong contraction.

The second pathway involves a process called *oxida-*

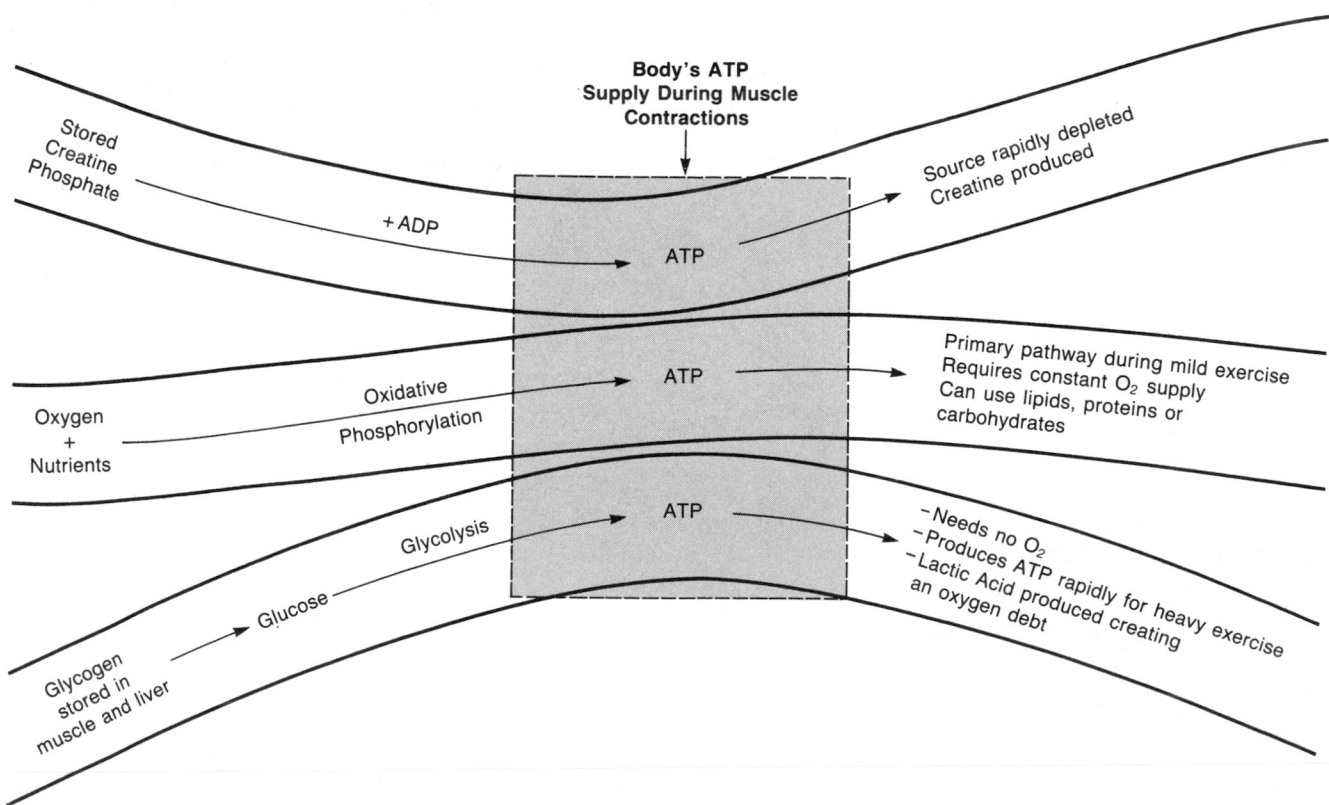

Figure 28–3.   Three pathways for ATP production.

tive phosphorylation. In this process, oxygen and other nutrients, such as fatty acids, amino acids, or glucose, are converted into ATP. This pathway for ATP production is sufficient during mild exercise, when muscle fibers have adequate blood circulation for oxygen supply and time to convert oxygen and nutrients into ATP. Oxidative phosphorylation is an energy-efficient process in which 36 molecules of ATP can be produced from one glucose molecule. This process occurs within the mitochondria of the muscle fibers.

The third pathway, which is called into play during vigorous physical activity, is *glycolysis*. This is an energy-wasting process since only two molecules of ATP are produced from one glucose molecule. The advantage of glycolysis is that it can occur very rapidly and it does not require oxygen. The limiting factor in glycolysis is the supply of glucose to the muscle. As the glycogen stores within the muscle are converted to glucose and used up in the production of ATP by very active muscles, the muscle fibers begin to fatigue. The fatigue is caused by a decreasing supply of ATP when oxidative phosphorylation and glycolysis are inadequate for meeting the muscle fibers' need for energy. The force of the individual fiber's contraction begins to decrease as the ATP supply drops off, and the contraction will eventually cease as the ATP supply is exhausted. During heavy physical activity, when glycolysis is used to produce ATP, lactic acid is formed as a by-product. Lactic acid contains over 70 percent of the energy from the glucose molecule. It must be oxidized to CO_2 and H_2O or reconverted to glucose to retrieve this stored energy and also to prevent the blood from becoming too acidic. The lactic acid diffuses into the circulating blood and can interfere with normal functioning. People continue to breathe heavily after exercise has stopped because they are repaying the oxygen debt created by glycolysis in the muscle fibers. Oxygen is used to convert the lactic acid to CO_2 and H_2O after heavy exercise. ATP produced by oxidative phosphorylation can also convert the lactic acid back to glucose so the glycogen stores in the muscle can be ressteablished.

Isometric and Isotonic Contractions

There are two different types of muscle fibers within muscle tissue. One type is called low oxidative because the fibers utilize ATP rapidly, but produce ATP through oxidation slowly. The other type of fiber is called high oxidative, since these fibers rely more on the production of ATP through oxidation. *Isometric contractions*, in which muscle tension develops but no shortening of the fibers occurs, tend to utilize low-oxidative fibers. Straining to pass a fecal mass and pushing against a footboard are examples. One nurse trying to lift a 190-lb patient, unassisted, is another example of an isometric exercise, which tends to produce more of an oxygen debt than isotonic exercises. *Isotonic* contractions involve shortening muscles to move a load, whether it be bones of the body or books on a table. Walking and all forms of active movement are isotonic and tend to utilize high-oxidative fibers. Isotonic exercises help to maintain the blood flow through the muscles by the pumping action created by contraction, relaxation, contraction. Constant tension is not maintained in isotonic contractions as it is in isometric contractions because the length of the muscle changes. The constant unrelieved tension in an isometric contraction is harder on the muscle fiber because it maintains a constant pressure on the capillaries, partially occluding them and decreasing the blood supply. Isometric exercises also tend to raise the blood pressure and increase the cardiac output while creating local muscle tissue hypoxia.

Muscle Strength

Muscle strength is determined by the diameter and length of the muscle fibers. In skeletal muscle, the total amount of shortening that can occur during a maximum contraction is approximately 30 percent more than the resting muscle length, which is already in some state of contraction or tone. Cardiac muscle, which is not attached to bone, has a much greater ability to contract. There are some 600 different skeletal muscles within the body involved in various movements. The large muscles of the body contain several hundred thousand muscle fibers, while smaller muscles, responsible for more detailed movement, contain a few hundred muscle fibers. "The transmission of force from muscle to bone is like a number of people pulling on a rope, each one corresponding to a single muscle fiber and the rope to the connective tissue and tendons" (Vander, 1980).

The strength that a muscle can exert on a load depends on the number of muscle fibers actively contracting at one particular time and also on the amount of tension or force developed within each fiber. This is controlled by the nervous input into the muscle fibers from the efferent neurons. *Tetanus* is the term given to a maximum sustained contraction when the muscle fibers are contracting to their limit. The tetanic contraction can be maintained until the ATP supply begins to decrease. Then the contraction will begin to lessen, corresponding to the dropping ATP levels within the muscle fibers.

It is interesting to note that ATP is also needed for relaxation of the muscle fibers. The living cell, supplied by blood, continuously replaces the ATP supply for muscle relaxation and contraction. Without ATP, the fibers will remain in a contracted state until death of the cell. This is what happens in rigor mortis when total body death precedes death of individual muscle cells. The muscle cells receive no nutrients or oxygen after cessation of the heartbeat and are thus unable to produce ATP. They remain contracted in the position the patient is allowed to assume after death. The muscle fibers gradually deteriorate, and the proteins of the fibers break down, releasing the contraction some 15 to 72 hours after total body death.

Joints, Bones, and Muscles—The Body's Lever System

Joints are areas where two or more bones meet and make movement in different directions possible. The joint is held together by tough connective tissue. The connective tissue is kept flexible by repeated stretching as the joint moves through its complete range of motion during activity. When a joint is immobilized or not moved through its total range of motion, the connective tissue gradually becomes stiff and fibrotic. This process may begin in as few as five days and progresses until the connective tissue holds the joint immobile.

Muscles and bones work together to form a system of levers within the body. It is through movement of these levers at the joints that mobility is possible. As a

muscle contracts, a force is exerted on the bone called *tension*. The bone exerts a counterforce on the muscle called *load*. When the force of the contraction exceeds the load, movement occurs. (See Figure 28–4.) The total load on the muscle that must be overcome is equal to:

> The weight of the load + The distance of the weight from the joint + The distance of the muscle from the joint.

The muscle is attached to the bone by ligaments and tendons above and below the joints. The farther from the joint that the attachment of the tendon is located, the greater is the load for the muscle moving that joint. The farther the object to be moved is from the joint, the greater the total load the muscle must overcome if movement is to occur. When the total load equals or exceeds the maximum muscle tension of which a muscle is capable, isotonic contractions become isometric because the muscle is unable to shorten and lift the load. Very large, strong muscles are actually capable of tearing the tendons from their attachment on the bone or breaking a bone in an effort to overcome the resistance from a heavy load.

A single muscle group exerts only pulling force against a load, so many muscles are grouped in pairs called *antagonists*. One muscle group moves the load in a direction opposite to that of its antagonist muscle group. *Flexion*, which is bending at a joint, is caused by the contraction of one muscle group, while *extension*, or

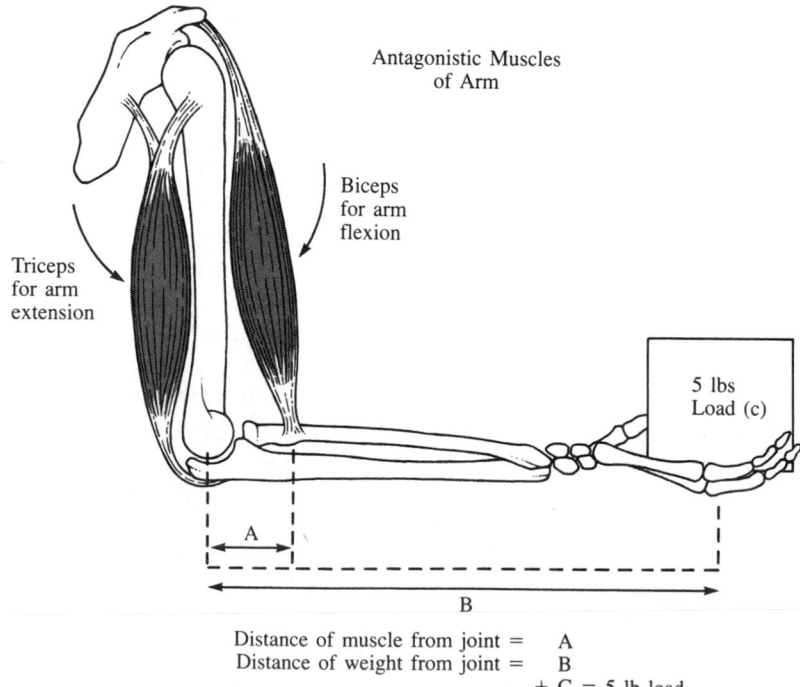

Distance of muscle from joint =   A
Distance of weight from joint =   B
                               + C = 5 lb load
                               ─────────────
                               Total Load

Figure 28–4. Muscles and bones of the arm lifting a load in the hand. Antagonist muscle groups flex (biceps) or extend (triceps) the lower arm. The total load the biceps must overcome to move the load is equal to **A + B + C.**

straightening of that joint, is caused by contraction of the antagonist muscle group, usually located on the opposite side of the bones around a joint.

Normal Posture

Normal posture is maintained while sitting and standing by the repeated and asynchronous contractions of the muscles of the back, legs, abdomen, and neck. The back normally has four separate curves, one in the cervical region, one in the thoracic region, one in the lumbar region, and one in the sacral region. (See Figure 28-5.) The center of gravity is approximately at the level of the pelvic crest or umbilicus in the adult. For optimum balance, the center of gravity should be over a line drawn between the base of support (the feet). The feet point forward and at right angles to the legs. The knees are slightly relaxed in a standing position, as are the elbows. The head is straight, maintaining a slight curve in the cervical vertebrae. The abdominal muscles are contracted slightly to hold the abdomen securely. The hands are at the sides, with palms facing the body, the fingers are slightly flexed. The shoulders are straight and pulled back to maintain a slight curve in the thoracic vertebrae and give maximum height. The buttocks are slightly contracted and tucked under to maintain a slight curve to the lumbar vertebrae.

Muscle and Nerve Growth

All muscles present in the adult body are formed during prenatal life and are found in the full-term newborn. After birth, the muscles grow in length and diameter but not in number. If a muscle cell is damaged after birth, it cannot reproduce itself. Instead, adjacent muscles will increase in size and diameter to compensate as much as possible for the distroyed muscle fibers.

If the nerve cell innervating a group of muscle fibers is destroyed, it cannot reproduce itself, and the muscle will be temporarily paralyzed. The adjacent nerve endings will gradually grow new branches to reach closely located muscle fibers to restore the ability to contract. However, the precision of movement will be slightly reduced since one neuron may now be stimulating several thousand muscle fibers at once, instead of two neurons each stimulating a thousand muscle fibers. If the nerve cell body is intact but the branch of the nerve cell reaching to the muscle is destroyed, the cell body is capable of regenerating the branch to the muscle fiber. The rate of nerve growth is very slow, approximately 1 to 2 mm each day (Porth, 1982). At this rate, it may take weeks or months for a crushed or severed axon to grow back to the muscle fibers it originally innervated.

If the axon does not follow exactly the same path to reach the muscle fibers, it is likely that the entire neuron will degenerate and die. Crushing injuries have a better chance for nerve regeneration than injuries that sever the nerve. The crushed nerve has an intact pathway to follow as it regenerates. It is much more likely to reach the original muscle fibers than a nerve that has been severed and must be realigned with the cut section. The paralyzed muscle fibers will deteriorate rapidly and will be almost completely obliterated by fat and connective tissue after two years without nervous stimulation. External application of electrical stimulation to the muscle fibers will cause them to contract and help preserve structure and function as a temporary measure while the nerve branch regenerates.

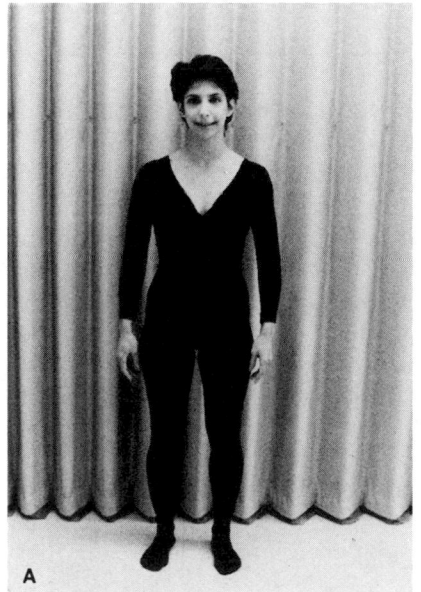
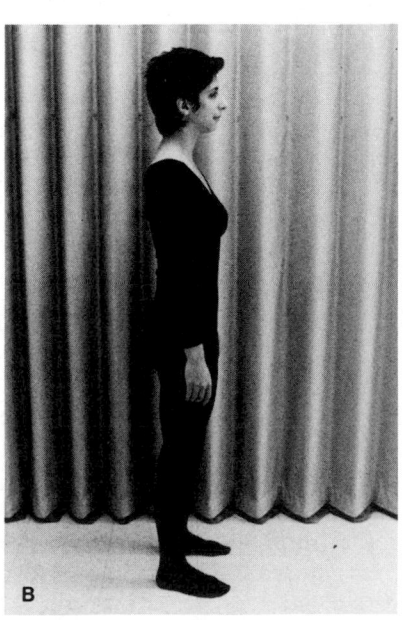

Figure 28-5. Normal posture. **A.** Dorsal (front) view. **B.** Lateral (side) view.

Exercise and Physical Activity—Benefits and Risks

Physical activity, essential as it is for normal body functioning, can be viewed as both a benefit and a hazard. Physical activity is a stressor to the body in the sense that it produces changes and utilizes energy. Physical activity decreases the risks of sensory deficits and social isolation. It prevents the loss of motion that occurs with disuse of muscles and joints. It is a form of nonverbal communication in which strong emotions can be dissipated. The idea of doing something to keep the mind and body busy is associated with increased energy levels and a more positive outlook on the world in general and on the self in particular. People who are physically active often feel better about themselves and have more endurance than people with limited activity.

Regular exercise has the benefits of decreasing blood pressure, heart rate, and serum lipid levels, while increasing cardiac stroke volume and tissue oxygenation. Exercise also promotes relaxation and sleep. These benefits decrease the individual's risk of heart attacks, heart disease, and atherosclerotic changes in the arteries. These benefits are gained when exercise is regularly part of the person's life and high-oxidative fibers are used in isotonic contractions. The term *aerobic exercise* is currently used to indicate the type of exercise that provides these benefits. The stress on the bones, arteries, and muscles helps to delay many of the changes associated with aging, such as bone loss (osteoporosis), loss of muscle mass, and narrowing of the arteries from the deposition of lipid material within the walls (atherosclerosis). Habitual exercise increases the concentration of high-density lipoproteins, which further protects against atherosclerotic changes. The nurse in good physical shape from regular exercise is also less likely to experience personal injury in performing the many muscular activities involved in providing care to patients.

During vigorous physical activity, the cardiac output can go from 5 liters per minute at rest to 30 liters per minute in a trained athlete. The majority of the increase in cardiac output occurs because the pulse rate increases dramatically from a baseline of 70 beats per minute, for example, to a rate of 190 beats per minute. The systolic blood pressure rises the most dramatically, going from a normal value of 120 mm Hg to 200 mm Hg during heavy exercise. The alveolar ventilation within the lungs may increase 20-fold during heavy exercise. The diastolic pressure changes much less, showing approximately a 10- to 15-point rise. The temperature will also rise during heavy exercise and may be several degrees above normal immediately after vigorous sustained activity.

There are some risks to exercise, including muscle strains, sprains of the ligaments and joints, pain from sore muscles, and broken bones. The changes in pulse and blood pressure may lead to serious complications in people with heart disease or respiratory problems. Life-threatening hazards exist for the individual who is unaccustomed to heavy exercise and suddenly begins exercising beyond the point of fatigue. Heart attacks caused by snow shoveling affect a number of people each year. Falls, especially in the elderly, can be life threatening where bone loss and changes of aging make bones more likely to break and slow to heal. Activities such as swimming, diving, and rock climbing can be very dangerous activities if the individual is careless, inexperienced, or out of physical condition.

Regulation of Motor Activity

The control of muscle movement is partially understood. The central nervous system receives information about the degree of tension or stretch on the muscle through the afferent pathways leading from the muscles and joints through the spinal cord. Information is sent to the muscles through the efferent pathways leading away from the spinal cord. The deep tendon reflexes or *stretch reflexes*, such as the knee jerk, contain only two neurons, located in the spinal cord, one afferent and one efferent. All other reflexes and reactions involve at least three or more nervous cells. The skeletal muscles on one side of the body are controlled by motor neurons on the opposite side of the brain. The motor cortex of the brain, located in the posterior part of the frontal lobe, has areas corresponding to different muscle groups throughout the body. Stimulation of the motor cortex in the area associated with the foot will cause contractions of muscle fibers in the foot. The cerebellum plays a role in coordination and achievement of smooth motion and detailed movement. Damage in this area of the brain causes problems with balance and walking. *Intention tremors* are also common in problems with cerebellar function. The person becomes shaky and muscle tremors develop when activity is attempted. The basal ganglia of the brain also plays a role in motor activity. Damage to this area results in tremors, muscle rigidity, and a delay in the person's ability to perform intentional motion. Parkinson's disease affects areas of the basal ganglia. One result is a gradual elimination of the spontaneity people have in their movement, speech, and facial expressions. People with this disease must concentrate very hard to start and stop movement which most people take for granted.

The part of movement and physical activity which is not understood at this time is the origination of the impulses to begin and end activity, the conscious intention to perform some activity. The decisions people make everyday to walk, exercise, and engage in the thousands of activities requiring some degree of physical motion occur in a yet-undiscovered area of the brain.

Effect of Immobility on Other Needs

Immobility of the total body affects all other basic needs. There are both positive and negative effects of bed rest and decreased muscular activity. For the most part, the negative effects outweigh the positive effects, and a great deal of nursing care is directed toward the prevention of complications associated with muscular disuse. Table 28-1 summarizes these effects.

Table 28-1. **Effect of Immobility on Other Needs—The Disuse Syndrome**

Oxygen Needs

INCREASED WORK LOAD ON THE HEART

Elevated pulse rate
Elevated blood pressure
Loss of muscular pumping action in legs to assist venous return to the heart
Occurrence of Valsalva maneuver while moving in bed or straining to have a bowel movement
Decreased filling time for heart

DECREASED ABILITY TO TRANSPORT BLOOD

Decreased vasomotor tone, resulting in vasodilation
Orthostatic hypotension in the vertical position with inadequate venous blood return to the heart, dizziness, and decreased blood
    pressure
Tendency toward venous stasis (pooling of blood in the veins) because of decreased muscular activity and vasodilation
Edema in the tissues from venous stasis
Tendency toward thrombus (clot) formation from venous stasis, external pressure on the veins from body positions, casts, trac-
    tion, pillows, and positional aids
Hypercoagulability of blood occurring during extended periods of immobility increases risk of thrombus formation; increased
    risk of pulmonary embolism

REDUCED VENTILATION VOLUMES

Counterpressure of the bed to respirations decreases lung expansion
Tendency toward atelectasis, infections, and increased secretions from shallow breathing
Weakening of muscles of respiration; reduced ability to cough forcefully

REDUCED OXYGEN NEED

This is one of the benefits of bed rest if a person is having trouble meeting oxygen needs; inactivity reduces oxygen utilization by
    the muscle fibers

Stimulation Needs

Muscular strength decreases rapidly during the first week or two of bed rest or immobility of a muscle group
Immobility tends to increase the risk of sensory deficit
Social interaction, a form of stimulation, is generally reduced with immobility, leading to feelings of isolation
Muscles tend to shorten in disuse, reducing movement
Fibrosis of joints may begin after five days of immobility and limit future range of motion in the joint
Joints may stiffen and muscles may shorten forming abnormal joint positions (*contractures*) which may require surgical interven-
    tion to correct

Table 28–1. **(Continued)**

Stimulation Needs (Continued)

Osteoporosis develops during immobility when the bone does not bear weight; begins after several days of disuse
There is potential for efferent and afferent nerve damage to skin and muscle from ischemia with improper body positioning in bed
Pressure sores caused by local tissue ischemia and resulting cell damage may develop, affecting skin, subcutaneous tissue, muscle, and bone; may affect muscle function and nervous innervation; very slow to heal and an added stressor for the patient; skin areas most at risk for pressure sores are those covering bony prominences.

Elimination Needs

Optimum position for urine to drain from kidneys down the ureters is in the upright position; urine tends to pool in the kidney when the patient is lying down; pooling of urine in the kidney can cause cellular damage and increase the risk of kidney infections
Complete emptying of the bladder is difficult in bed; incomplete emptying of the bladder increases the risk of urinary infections in the bladder
Increased incidence of urinary stones due to increased excretion of calcium in the urine as the bones of the body develop osteoporosis; affects 13 to 30 percent of immobilized patients; pain and obstruction of urine flow may result
Embarrassment and difficult positioning may inhibit defecation, leading to constipation and fecal impaction
Weakened muscles reduce ability to assist with bowel evacuation

Nutritional Needs

Increase in catabolic (breakdown) activity; the muscle cells are broken down faster than they are replaced, leading to muscle loss
Caloric needs are decreased in the immobilized patient compared to needs during activity; protein needs are increased
Appetite is often decreased, leading to reduced intake
Intake may be reduced because food and fluids are out of reach or not available
Decreased peristalsis and mixing of food in stomach may lead to gastritis
Stress of immobility related to peptic ulcer formation

Temperature Needs

Inactivity leads to reduced heat production and a risk of hypothermia if added insulation is not provided to conserve body heat
Loss of muscle mass leads to reduced ability to generate heat through activity and shivering
Inadequate fluid intake may compromise ability to lose heat through perspiration

Rest and Sleep Needs

Inactivity often leads to frequent naps during the day and inability to obtain normal depth and length of sleep at night; the patient feels poorly rested and isolated at night while others sleep

Pain Avoidance

More sensitive to the perception of pain because of the lack of other interesting stimuli in the environment to occupy conscious thought
Inadequate rest and sleep will increase sensations of discomfort
Weakened muscles will make movement in bed more difficult and possibly more painful
Stiffness in muscles and joints increases with the duration of immobilization, adding to other discomforts

Sexual Needs

Immobility frequently alters fertility; women often will not menstruate during the stress of immobility
Sexual closeness and intimacy are often impossible because of a lack of privacy, hospital policies regarding overnight guests, and physical obstacles such as casts, traction, paralysis, and general weakness

Safety Needs

Physical safety can be severely compromised if an immobilized patient becomes disoriented because of sensory deprivation and tries to get out of bed unassisted
Sensory deprivation can lead to hallucinations which are frightening to the patient; these hallucinations may seem very real, or the patient may know it is imagination and fear loss of mental faculties; impaired judgment increases risk of injury
Immobilization usually requires confinement in an unfamiliar place with unfamiliar people which is a stress in itself, regardless of the reason for the limited movement

Love and Belonging Needs

Close friends and family are often encouraged to visit, but the patient may not feel part of the family unit or receive the psycho-
logical and physical attention needed to feel loved and needed by others
Loss of interaction with one's work colleagues increases feelings of isolation
Anger and frustration due to immobility may be taken out on family and friends, causing further isolation

Self-Esteem

Impaired cognitive functioning occurs during extended immobility and may decrease self-esteem
Self-esteem usually decreases during prolonged immobility as feelings of uselessness develop
Inability to attend to personal grooming habits may make the individual feel unattractive and undesirable
Concern for long-term effects of the original problem requiring immobilization can affect body-image if loss of function or alter-
ation of physical appearance is a possible outcome
Depression is common, as are feelings of anger, fear, and guilt

Self-Actualization

Immobility will interfere with the goals of the individual, at least temporarily; personal goals may need to be totally revised if major changes in abilities will result from the original problem
Some patients may find the time to assess their life and where it is headed and make positive decisions to improve their lives; immobility gives a new value to abilities commonly taken for granted and may be enough of a stimulus to make people change
poor health practices in order to avoid future problems

Normal Means of Meeting Stimulation Needs—Sensory

Vision

Sighted people rely a great deal on the sense of vision for information about the environment and themselves. The eye is capable of responding to various amounts and frequencies of light. The clarity of vision is partly due to the structure of the eye and partly due to the functioning of the nervous system and visual cortex area of the brain which receives signals from the receptor cells in the eye.

The Path of Light.   Light can be traced from the environment to the eye and eventually to the brain where impulses are decoded into visual perception. (See Figure 28-6.) As the light enters the eye, it is bent by moving from air through the denser cornea. The cornea redirects the path of light rays more than does the lens of the eye. When the light reaches the lens, it is focused on a specific area of the retina called the *fovea* for optimal visual acuity. It is the lens of the eye that is capable of altering shape through the contraction or relaxation of the muscles holding it in place. This gives the eye the ability to focus light reflected from close, intermediate, and distant objects for near and far vision.

Receptor Cells and Nervous Transmission.   The light on the retina stimulates receptor cells which are of two types: *rods* and *cones*. Cones are capable of communicating light of different wavelengths to the brain by dif-ferent chemical changes. Some cones respond maximally to green, others respond maximally to yellow, and still others respond maximally to blue. From the various chemical responses to light occurring within these three types of cones comes our interpretation of color.

Approximately 10 percent of men and 1 percent of women have some degree of color perception deficit or "color blindness." Actually, most people lack only the yellow or green type of cones and are deficient in this color, while other vision is normal. Color deficit for red is caused by a lack of yellow cones. The gene for color-sensitive cones is on the chromosome determining an individual's sex, the X chromosome. It is recessive, meaning women rarely exhibit a color deficit because they have two X chromosomes, and normal genes are usually present on one or the other. A man has only one X chromosome, therefore, the deficit will develop because there is no normal gene to overcome the recessive trait.

The rods are more sensitive to light than the cones and provide most of the vision in dim lighting and at night. Many more rods connect to one afferent neuron in comparison to cones, so the acuity of vision in the rod is much less than in the cones. The cones provide more precise vision but require much greater illumination than do rods. Rods are capable of summation as many rods provide input to the afferent neuron. Cones, on the other hand, have more of a direct line to the afferent neuron so each cone must receive more light to trigger the response carried by the nerve to the brain.

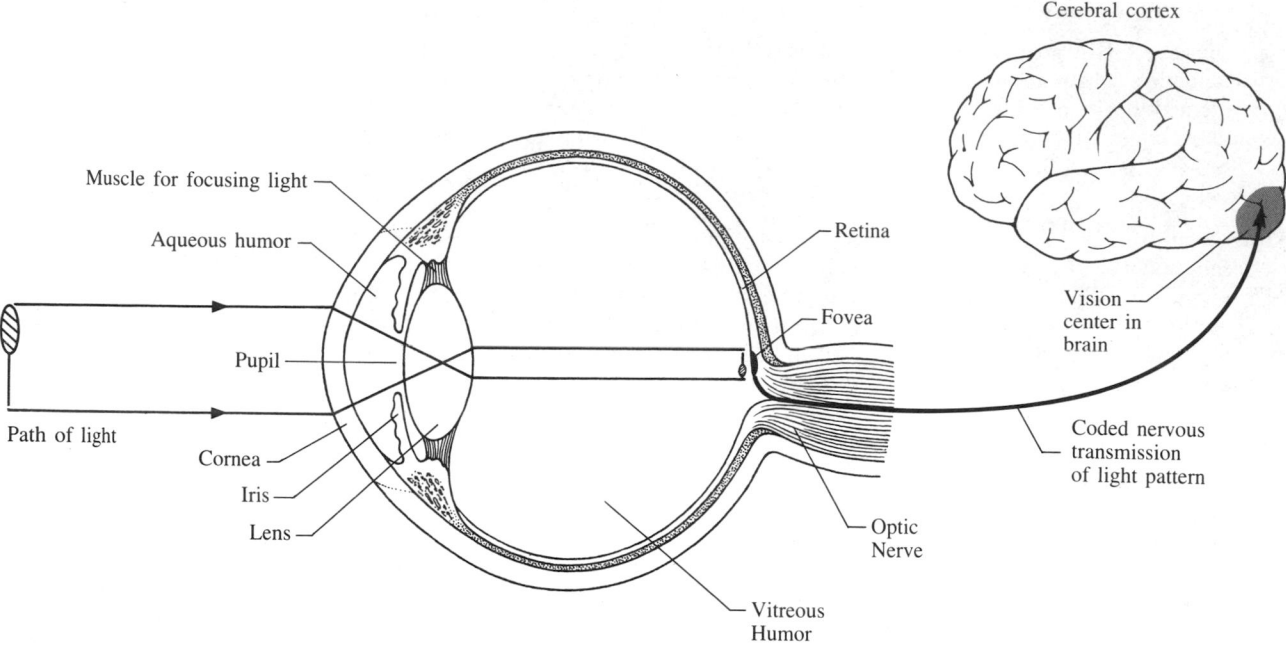

Figure 28-6. Path of light through the eye to the vision center of the brain.

The image focused on the lens is inverted and reversed, but the brain interprets this message so the object being viewed is seen upright with right and left in the correct place. When words are focused on the retina as they appear on paper, as is the case when writing is viewed through a mirror, the message is difficult to interpret because the brain reverses the image so it is seen upside down and backward. Writing words backward on a piece of paper and viewing them through a mirror show how the eye reverses the letters from right to left.

The coded message from the rods and cones is carried on afferent nerves which form the optic nerve. Some of the messages from each eye cross over to the opposite side of the brain. The message reaches the thalamus within the brain where there is a partial processing of the information. From there it goes to the primary visual cortex at the back of the brain in the occipital lobe. Each half of the brain in the visual cortex area receives input from both eyes. In the visual cortex, the impulses from the afferent nerves are further processed, and another coded electrical statement is sent to the visual association area of the brain's cortex about pattern, contrast, movement, and color of the original light stimulus. It is in the visual association cortex that meaning is given to the coded light message, and a particular light reflection pattern is recognized as a close friend, a speed limit sign, or a sunset.

Measuring Visual Acuity. Normal visual acuity in the adult is described as 20/20 vision. This means that an individual is able to read a particular line on an eye chart

at a distance of 20 feet in both eyes. The eye chart commonly used for visual acuity testing is the Snellen eye chart. (See Figure 28-7.) A person with 20/60 vision can read certain letters at 20 feet when most people can read

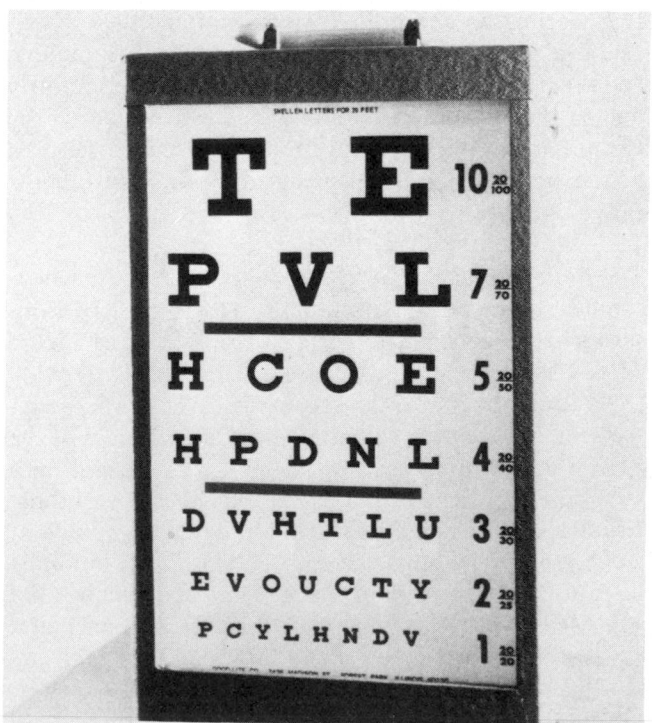

Figure 28-7. Snellen vision chart. This chart is commonly used to test the visual acuity of persons able to identify letters. (Photograph courtesy of Good-Lite Co., Forest Park, IL.)

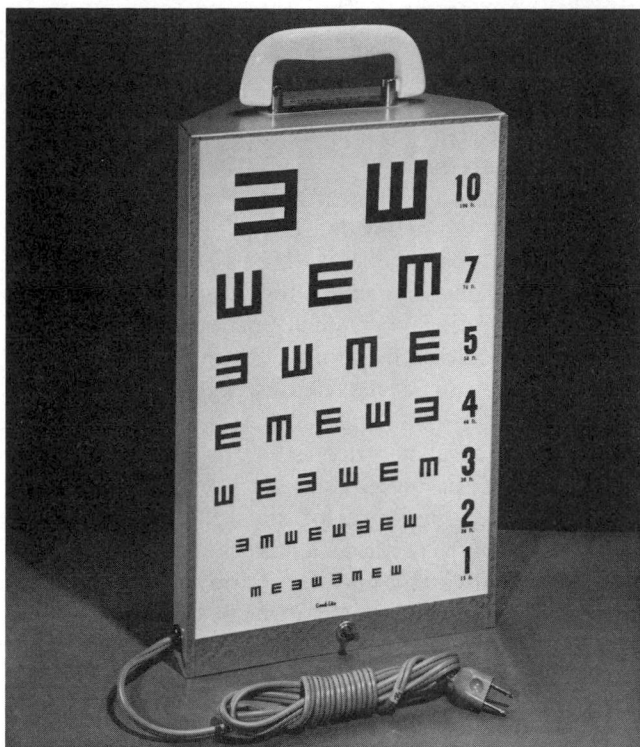

Figure 28-8.   Modified Snellen eye chart (the "E" chart). This chart is used to test visual acuity in individuals who are unable to speak or identify letters. Persons being tested use their hand to indicate which direction the legs of the "E" on the chart are pointing. (Courtesy of the Good-Lite Co., Forest Park, IL.)

those same letters at a distance of 60 feet. 20/15 vision means that an individual can read letters at a distance of 20 feet which most people can only read when they are 15 feet away, so vision is better than "normal acuity." Each eye is assigned a number set since vision in one eye is not always the same as vision in the other eye. Visual acuity in children is usually less than 20/20 until the age of eight or nine years, averaging around 20/30 in both eyes. There are modified Snellen eye charts for people who do not recognize letters, as in Figure 28-8.

Hearing

Sound is transmitted to the ears in the form of sound waves, consisting of areas of molecular compression, alternated with areas of lesser than normal molecular density in the air (rarefaction). When something vibrates such as a bell, a tuning fork, or the human vocal folds, the vibration rearranges the molecules in the air into waves of alternating density which are eventually perceived as sound. There must be both air and vibration for sound. There is no sound in a vacuum.

As the sound waves reach the ear, they enter the ear canal and cause the eardrum (tympanic membrane) to vibrate in and out. This vibration moves bones within the middle ear behind the tympanic membrane. The function of these bones (the malleus, the incus, and the stapes) is to amplify the vibrations from the tympanic membrane. These bones of the middle ear are attached to the oval window within the inner ear and cause it to move in and out in response to vibrations. This movement by the oval window moves fluid within the inner ear which, in turn, stimulates the auditory receptor cells in the organ of Corti. The auditory receptor cells are hairlike structures which are stimulated by the physical force of the fluid moving them back and forth. (See Figure 28-9.)

The afferent neurons leading from the ear's receptor cells form the auditory nerve which synapses with the auditory cortex area of the brain. Location, intensity, and pitch of the sound are interpreted in the auditory

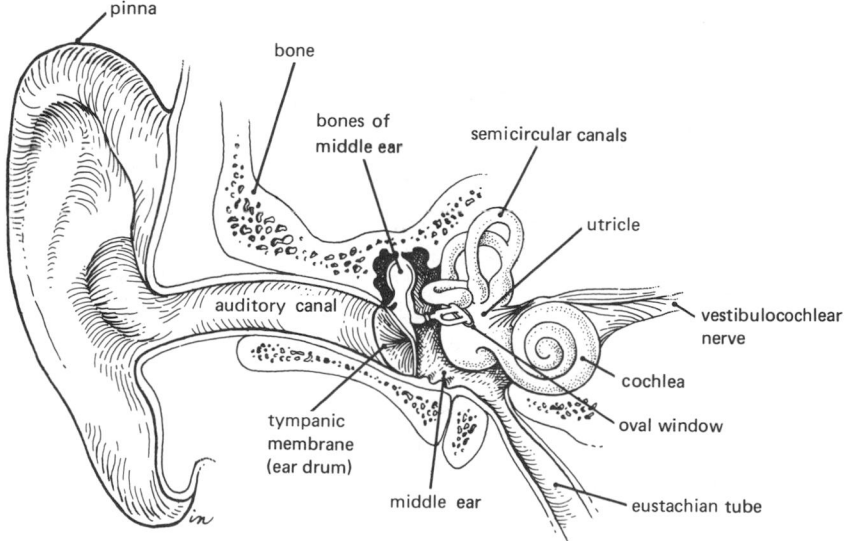

Figure 28-9.   Structures of the ear. (From M. Griffiths: *Introduction to Human Physiology*, 2nd ed. Macmillan, New York, 1981, p. 394.)

cortex by the messages from the receptor cells. The ear closer to a sound is stimulated sooner and more intensely than the opposite ear, and this difference helps the brain localize sound. Pitch and intensity are determined by the rate and number of receptors responding to the vibration.

Hearing can be checked grossly be standing 15 ft away from someone and whispering several words. A person with normal hearing and brain functioning should be able to repeat the words. Make sure the person is not lipreading but actually hearing the sound. The audiometer is a more sophisticated testing method for hearing and is capable of emitting pure tones of various frequencies into each ear.

Smell

The senses of smell and taste are closely related and very important to nutrition. Without the sense of smell, people have minimal tasting sensation, as when people have colds and lose their sense of taste with nasal congestion. Smell enhances the ability to differentiate flavors of foods. Tasting and smelling foods encourage eating, while loss of taste and smell will often reduce normal nutritional intake.

Smell is the least understood sense. It occurs during inspiration as the receptors in the upper part of the nasal cavity are stimulated. The receptors are actually the afferent nerve fibers rather than separate specialized cells, as in other senses. The other end of the neuron in the nasal cavity joins with other nerves to form the olfactory nerve leading into the brain. The molecules carrying odors dissolve in the mucous lining covering the receptor cells in the nose and cause nervous stimulation through chemical changes. How people are able to discriminate so many different odors is a mystery. Discrimination of odors is probably related to the firing pattern of the afferent neuron receptors, level of alertness, and the quality and quantity of the nasal mucus, since excessive mucus decreases the sense of smell. The sense of smell is more acute when the individual is hungry and less acute after smoking. Women tend to have more awareness of odors than men.

Taste

Taste begins with stimulation of the receptor cells in the taste buds on the tongue, roof of the mouth, in the pharynx, and in the larynx. There are approximately 10,000 taste buds involved in creating the sense of taste in the adult. Classically, the taste buds have been said to respond to sweet, sour, bitter, or salty substances, but actual differences in the structure and function of the taste buds cannot be found. Each receptor cell responds to many different tastes by chemical changes which then stimulate the afferent nerve fibers. It is more likely that the receptor cells for taste have different firing patterns to different substances.

The temperature and texture of substances are transmitted to the brain through different receptors in the mouth and throat and contribute to identification of foods and the development of food preferences. Taste is a less sensitive sense than smell since smaller concentrations of molecules will stimulate the sense of smell. The senses of taste and smell decrease in acuity with age, and the actual number of taste buds begins to diminish as a person ages. Diabetes decreases the ability to sense sweet, salty, and bitter. Cancer and pregnancy are known to alter the senses of smell and taste in some way. Radiation to the head and neck area will decrease the flow of saliva and may lessen the sense of taste because fewer molecules are dissolved in solution.

Touch

The sense of touch or tactile sensations are elicited by stimulation of receptors in the skin and subcutaneous tissues. The most sensitive areas to tactile stimulation are those with the greatest density of receptor cells. These areas are located in the fingertips and thumb, the lips, the nose, and cheeks. Each area of the body has a representative area on the cerebral cortex of the brain just behind the division between the frontal and occipital lobes. Receptors on the right side of the body cross over to eventually synapse with the left brain's sensory cortex area. The left-sided sensations are perceived by the right half of the brain. The more intense the tactile stimulations, the greater the rate of firing of the individual receptors, and the more receptors that are stimulated. The ability to locate a stimulus without vision is normally possible on both sides of the body. Discrimination related to sharpness or dullness of a stimulus is present when tactile sensation is normal.

Vestibular Sense

The vestibular sense gives the individual information about motion and position of the head. It is often called the sense of balance. However, damage to this area will not prevent someone from maintaining balance since many other sensations contribute to the ability to walk and maintain an upright posture. The vestibular structures are located within the temporal bone of the skull and work on the principle of inertia. The vestibular structures consist of three semicircular canals positioned at right angles to each other. They are filled with fluid contained in a sac. The sac puts pressure on the hairlike receptor cells when there is a change in motion. The canals move with the bone in which they are embedded, but the fluid-filled sac is free to move and tends to resist the movement of the head. In so doing, it puts pressure on the hair receptors and bends them in the direction opposite to the head movement. Motion at constant speed does not stimulate the receptors. Only changes in direction and speed of movement trigger these receptors. The other components of the vestibular sense are the structures called the utricle and saccule which give the brain information about the position of the head in relationship to gravity. These structures also give information on linear acceleration and deceleration, as when a car speeds up or slows down. The vestibular senses have reflex control of upright posture and of the eye muscles so an individual's gaze can remain focused on an object even though the head is turning.

Factors Affecting Sensory Stimulation and Mobility

The type and quantity of sensory and motor input to the central nervous system can be affected by many aspects of the environment and the individual. The interpretation of the sensory input will depend on genetic characteristics, learning, and the state of functioning of the brain's processing centers.

Degree of Environmental Control

The individual may have a very active role in selecting the amount and type of stimulation received to best meet personal stimulation needs. A person may also be completely helpless in altering the environment and be constantly exposed to sounds, smells, sights, and touching that are excessive or unfamiliar and fairly meaningless, as when a child or adult is hospitalized in critical medical condition. Lack of ability to control the environment puts the individual at risk for both inadequate and excessive amounts of stimulation.

Level of Growth and Development

The individual's level of growth and development affects the type of input and the interpretation of that input. The infant, for example, may be exposed to one taste, hear the sound of the parent's voice primarily, and be wrapped fairly securely in a blanket to prevent gross body movement. The sense of sight is immature, and only very close objects can be brought into some degree of focus. Inadequate stimulation in the infant's environment, in the form of minimal handling, infrequent communication, few toys, and restricted movement in the form of confinement in a playpen, puts the infant at risk for unmet stimulation needs since the baby is fairly helpless to change the environment. Compare this to the active school-age child who chooses to be outside running, jumping, climbing, and balancing, making full use of all senses and mobility. The older child can make choices about the kinds of stimulation to receive, whether it be ten hours of television or constant physical activity and social interaction. Children can select which foods of those served they will eat. They can select the volume on the record player, radio, or television. In health, most children and adults play a very large role in selecting the type and amount of stimulation they receive.

With some of the changes related to aging, there is a decrease in the acuity of many of the senses and, if left uncorrected, the messages reaching the brain are less precise and more likely to be misinterpreted. Many aged people intentionally restrict their movement, and thereby their environment, for fear of falling. Poor sensory input jeopardizes their ability to safely and enjoyably interact with the environment.

Level of Consciousness

The individual's level of consciousness will affect central nervous system processing and interpretation of the stimuli from the body's receptors. Alcohol consumption, drugs, medications, anesthesia, and analgesia will all decrease the ability of the brain to interpret and respond to incoming sensory information. Many people consciously choose to alter their level of consciousness through alcohol and drug abuse. Other people may have an altered level of consciousness because of medical treatment or disease processes. Inadequate nutrients and oxygen to the brain will also rapidly decrease the level of consciousness and ability to interpret the environment.

Culture and Learning

The type and variety of stimuli to which the developing individual is exposed and the interpersonal relationships encountered affect perception of stimuli and response to it. Figure 28–10 shows one example of different perceptions. The fact is that both lines are equally long. People who have been raised in cultures with square corners tend to see line *A* as longer because of the square-corner orientation and learned relationship to depth. People who were raised in cultures with few if any square corners perceive both lines as equal in length. Homes that are round teach the brain to interpret space, line, and depth differently than homes that are square. Pleasant sound in one culture or subculture may be almost painful noise to another subculture. People raised in cultures where touching is common will interpret this stimulus differently than a person who is unfamiliar with frequent touching.

People are able to train their senses by focusing conscious thought on the incoming sensations. They are able to train their muscular responses to stimuli by coordinating tactile, visual, and muscular elements into incredibly precise movement. The detailed muscular coordination needed to crochet a delicate lace or reattach severed arteries in an injured arm is learned and maintained by constant use.

The hospital with its sights and sounds and smells can be considered a subculture that is often foreign to the patients who are served by it. The people and their behavior may seem strange and inappropriate to the inexperienced patient who can frequently misinterpret the barrage of new incoming data from the body's receptors. The reassuring beeping of the cardiac monitor, the clicking of the machine regulating the intravenous infusion rate, and the paging of various hospital personnel may be reassuring to the nurse and incredibly frightening to the patient. This fear can result in muscular tension, increased alertness and perception, and inability to rest or sleep.

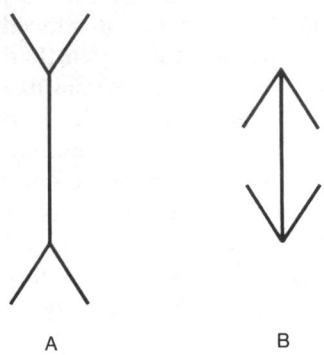

Figure 28–10. Which line is longer? The fact is that they are both equal in length, but to many people line **A** appears longer because of prior perceptual learning in an environment with square corners. In cultures without square corners in their buildings and homes, the lines appear equal in length.

Adaptation to Stimuli

The nervous system is able to "tune in" or "tune out" various forms of stimulation. Receptors in the body will respond differently to a constant stimulus over time, generally decreasing the amount of input sent along the afferent nerve fibers as accommodation takes place. *Accommodation* is a form of adaptation to stimulation over time, with the end result usually being reduced awareness and response to the original stimulus. The sense of smell adapts very rapidly, and even strong odors are difficult to detect after several minutes of constant exposure. People accommodate to sound and may not even hear it after a time. The body seems to respond most to *changes* in the environment. Constant factors in the environment, whether they be sights, sounds, smells, tastes, movement, or interpersonal interaction will become less consciously attended to over time.

Common Problems Related to Stimulation Needs

Sensory deprivation is a problem of inadequate incoming stimulation to the central nervous system from the senses. All sensory stimuli may be reduced to a minimum, as when the person closes the eyes, refrains from or is unable to move, and the room is quiet. This state is desirable for sleep, but even in normal sleep the person moves about frequently, receiving information on position, skin sensation, and muscle tone. True sensory deprivation is rare unless there is a sudden loss of a previously working sense, as in temporary blindness, extensive paralysis, or sudden loss of hearing. The suddenness of the loss is important to the problem. Other receptors and the central nervous system need time to

adapt to the change and compensate for the loss by increasing awareness of other sensory input systems.

Sensory monotony is much more common for patients requiring medical and nursing care. This occurs when environmental stimulation is repetitive and accommodation takes place. The individual does not attend to the environment but rather seems unresponsive. Restricted movement, an unchanging environment, and reduced social interactions are common to many patients in hospitals and other nursing care facilities and lead to sensory monotony. Private rooms, inability to see out windows or windowless rooms, and constant television watching will also contribute to sensory monotony. Without changes in the environment, attentiveness to constant stimuli decreases over time. Hospitals can easily cause sensory overload or deprivation. It seems the more critically ill the patient, the more likely that patient is to experience sensory overload because of the machines, treatments, and variety of health professionals involved in the patient's care. The stable patient or immobile patient in an extended care facility is especially at risk for sensory deprivation or monotony. The patient who is on isolation precautions because of infection is also greatly at risk for sensory monotony and deprivation.

Perceptual deprivation or restriction involves the inability or reduced ability to interpret stimuli from the senses. Damage to the brain as occurs in strokes, tumor growth, or ischemia will decrease the ability of the brain to give meaning to sensory stimulation. The person may be able to hear, but not understand; see, but not recognize.

Sensory and perceptual overload is a result of excessive stimuli reaching the central nervous system to the point that other sensations are blocked or awareness of them is decreased. A state of sensory confusion can result, where the individual is unable to respond to the dominating stimuli, and normal thought patterns are blocked. This may be beneficial, as when tactile stimulation from a transcutaneous electrical stimulator blocks out pain perception. Very loud music may temporarily block out pain and other thoughts so the individual is aware of little else than the music. Sensory overload more often creates problems. If the individual is bombarded by new, intense sensations, thought patterns are disturbed, and the ability to respond appropriately to any one stimulus may be lost or compromised. The person is unable to focus on any one thing and becomes ineffective in dealing with the environment and tends to withdraw from it. Prior learning or lack of learning will affect perception. This is one of the reasons for preoperative or preprocedure teaching. The patient is familiarized with the sights and sounds and feelings associated with surgery or a particular treatment or procedure so accurate interpretation of sensory information is possible during the actual event. This decreases the risk of perceptual overload since more of the sensations will have meaning after effective learning has occurred.

Problems related to stimulation can be grouped into three categories:

1. Problems related to sensory input
2. Problems related to transmission and interpretation of sensory input
3. Problems related to responding to sensory input

Problems of Sensory Input

Trauma to the skin and underlying structures will affect the tactile sense and the perception of pain and pressure. Slight burns, as when the skin is sunburned, will increase sensitivity. Severe burns, which destroy the receptors and afferent nerve endings, will eliminate all tactile sensory input. The structure and function of the sense organs and receptor cells will determine quantity and quality of input into the nervous system. Removal of hearing aids or corrective lenses will affect the type of input from the receptor cells by decreasing intensity and precision of the message sent along the afferent pathways.

Major problems affecting vision include injury, infection, aging, cataracts, and glaucoma. Approximately

Table 28-2. **First Aid for Eye Emergencies**

INJURY	TREATMENT	DO NOT
Specks in eye	Do lift upper eyelid outward and down over lower lid. Do let tears wash out speck. If it doesn't wash out, bandage lightly and see doctor.	Do not rub the eye.
Blows to the eye	Do apply cold compress immediately for 15 min and hourly as needed to reduce swelling and pain. See a physician.	Do not apply heat.
Cuts and punctures of the eye or eyelid	Do bandage lightly. See a physician, immediately.	Do not wash out eye with water. Do not try to remove an object stuck in eye.
Chemical burn	Do flood eye with water immediately and continue for at least 15 min. Do have someone contact physican for further instructions.	Do not bandage eye or use an eyecup.

Source: Minnesota Society for the Prevention of Blindness and the Preservation of Hearing, 1983. Reproduced with permission.

Table 28-3. **Classification of Pressure Sores (Decubitus Ulcers)**

GRADES	DATA
Preulcer	Reddened skin (hyperemia) which disappears within 15 min following relief of pressure
Grade 1	Skin abraded; limited to superficial skin layers
Grade 2	Ulcer extends through skin layers to subcutaneous tissue
Grade 3	Ulcer extends through skin and subcutaneous tissue to involve muscle tissue
Grade 4	Ulcer extends through skin, subcutaneous tissue, and muscle to involve the bones and joints

Source: Adapted from Arnell, 1983.

6.5 million Americans will develop a chronic eye disorder each year; 1.3 million Americans will suffer eye injury each year, with 40,000 injuries resulting in permanent visual impairment. Every 11 minutes, one American goes blind, and the majority of the problems leading to blindness are preventable by appropriate first aid and routine eye testing for acuity and glaucoma (Minnesota Society for Prevention of Blindness and Preservation of Hearing, 1983). Table 28-2 gives first-aid guidelines for eye emergencies. Many states have eye tests which people can use in their home. If they have problems with visual acuity or are at high risk for glaucoma, they are referred to a physician.

Problems of Transmission and Interpretation

Problems of transmission or interpretation involve the functioning of the nerves, spinal cord, and brain. Any trauma or disease of nerves or the brain can affect transmission and interpretation of sensory messages. Decreased level of consciousness is another factor already mentioned that reduces ability to interpret sensory data.

Aphasia is an inability to interpret a verbal message or respond to it and is common in the stroke patient. *Receptive aphasia* is used to describe an inability to understand spoken words, and *expressive aphasia* de-

Table 28-4. **Assessment for Risk of Pressure-Sore Development**

Mental State

0	Alert and oriented
1	Confused
2	Apathetic
3	Stuporous

Nutrition Level

0	Adequately nourished; eating well
1	Occasionally refuses to eat or leaves most of food; encouragement needed to take fluids
2	Poor nutritional intake, inadequate fluid intake, dehydrated
3	No oral intake, IV supplementation

Skin Sensation

0	Normal tactile sensations
1	Decreased sensations
2	Anesthesia in extremities
3	Absence of response to tactile stimulation

Skin Integrity

0	Intact, normal color
1	Reddened areas
2	Broken epidermal/dermal skin layers
3	Pitting edema; skin broken down involving subcutaneous tissue

Activity Level

0	Ambulatory
2	Walks with help
4	Moves to chair with help
6	Bedfast

Mobility

0	Full
2	Slightly limited
4	Very limited; some paralysis of legs
6	Immobile

Elimination Control

0	Complete control
2	Occasional voiding incontinence
4	Bladder incontinence; bowel control
6	Bowel and bladder incontinence

Total score of 12 or greater places the patient at risk for the development of pressure sores.

Source: Adapted from Norton, 1975; Arnell, 1983.

scribes a person who understands but cannot respond appropriately using speech. The person may be unable to utter any words or choose the wrong words to convey a message. Some people will have mixed aphasia after a stroke, with elements of both receptive and expressive aphasia. The frustration patients must experience when they are capable of logical thought but suddenly affected by some form of aphasia is incomprehensible, and the effort patients make to regain this ability is truly remarkable.

A problem with transmission of sensory input frequently occurs in spinal cord injuries. The input coming into the spinal cord below the level of the injury will be lost either temporarily or permanently since nerve cell bodies will not regenerate if they are destroyed. The person may have absolutely no sensation below the nipple line in a high cervical fracture or may have total upper body sensation but no lower body sensation. The loss of sensation in a spinal cord injury runs across the body and affects the right and left sides equally. Injury to areas of the brain may affect the right side, while the left side remains normal, because of the crossover of nerve fibers to the right and left cortex of the brain. *Hemiparesthesia* is loss of sensation from either the right or left side of the body.

Problems Related to Responding to Sensory Input

Stroke.   The stroke patient also has trouble responding to sensory input. Involvement of the motor cortex or speech center results in a reduced ability to move and coordinate muscular activity. The affected muscles are usually flaccid at first and begin to develop spasticity with time. "If spasticity has not begun within six weeks to three months, function will probably not return to that extremity" (Porth, 1982).

Paralysis.   The patient with a spinal cord injury will be able to transmit the messages for appropriate responses from the brain down the cord to the level of the injury. Any nerves leaving the spinal cord below the level of the

Table 28-5. **Conditions Associated with Formation of Pressure Sores**

Poor nutritional status
Less than normal weight for height
Muscular atrophy
Reduced mobility (the greater the reduction, the greater the risk)
Elevated temperatures
Reduced peripheral circulation, peripheral vasoconstriction (shock, hypothermia, excessive
    smoking, reduced blood volume, low arterial blood oxygen content)
Reduced tactile sensations (decrease spontaneous movements)
Paralysis
Sedatives, analgesics (decrease spontaneous movement)
Friction on skin surfaces; tendency to slide forward in a sitting position (stretches skin and
    subcutaneous layers which decreases the cushion between bones and surface on which patient is sitting; interferes with blood flow by stretching and compressing area bearing patient's weight)
Excessive use of soap; failure to remove soap during bathing (soap breaks down normal skin
    protection from bacteria by increasing the pH, making the skin more alkaline instead of slightly acidic)
Repeated injections of medications in an area of tissue (causes tissue trauma and interferes
    with normal capillary circulation and normal sensation)
Anesthesia (decreased spontaneous movement + chilling and vasoconstriction + lowered
    BP)
Use of restraints (increased friction and immobility)
Decreased level of consciousness (may have increased or decreased movement in bed)
Anemia (tissue hypoxia and cells more easily harmed by reduced blood flow during pressure)
Depression or reluctance to cooperate with care
Spasticity (difficult to reposition and increased friction)
Elderly patients (reduced muscle mass, reduced capillary blood flow to skin)
Incontinence (skin becomes macerated and more easily damaged)
Damaged skin on admission
Radiation treatments
Skin-grafted areas
Pain on movement (patient moves less to avoid pain)
Diabetes (poor peripheral circulation)

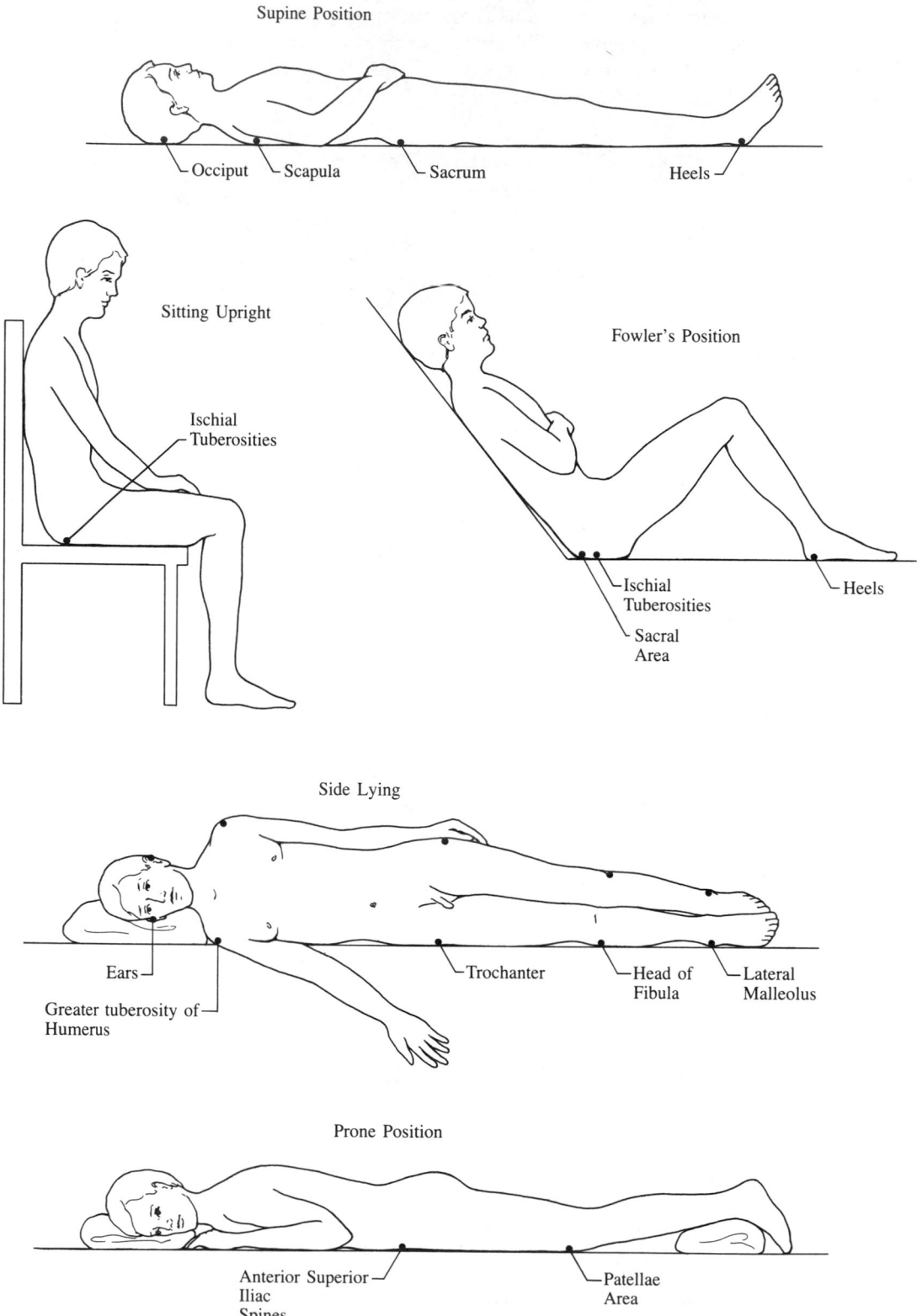

Figure 28–11.   High-risk areas for pressure-sore formation.

injury will not receive the message for action. There are some 250,000 people in the United States with spinal cord injuries. *Quadriplegia* is paralysis of all four extremities and results from damage to the cervical or upper thoracic part of the spinal cord. It may involve the muscles of respiration to reduce ventilation volumes. Posture control is also a common problem for the quadriplegic patient. There may be a return of reflexes for bowel and bladder control after several months. Muscle responses to deep tendon reflexes are increased, and there is often some spasticity and increased tone in the extensor muscles. *Paraplegia* is paralysis of the legs or lower half of the body and involves injury to the lower thoracic, lumbar, or sacral sections of the spinal cord.

Treatments.   Medical treatments will sometimes limit ability to respond. Casts, traction, bed rest, and fear of pain are all effective in reducing muscular activity, even when there is no problem with nervous transmission to the muscle.

Pressure Sores.   An ever-present, potential problem related to immobility is pressure sores (decubitus ulcers or bed sores). The typical high-risk patient is unable to respond effectively to pressure sensations in the skin by changing position. Pressure sores are caused by unrelieved pressure over the skin, muscle, and bone, usually from the weight of the patient's body. Table 28–3 presents various stages of severity in pressure-sore development. Treatment is discussed in the intervention section of this chapter.

The development of pressure sores in patients with reduced mobility or immobility is a serious problem which can develop very rapidly. Once tissue damage occurs and a sore develops, it takes much time and attention to heal. Identifying patients at risk of developing pressure sores allows initiation of a preventive program to eliminate the problems associated with pressure sores, such as infection, permanent muscle-nerve damage, and delayed recovery time. Table 28–4 presents a

rating scale for identification of patients at risk for developing pressure sores: the higher the score, the greater the individual's risk of developing pressure sores. A score above 12 represents a high risk. Table 28–5 indicates conditions associated with the development of pressure sores as an additional discriminator for high-risk patients.

Repeatedly assessing high-risk patients for development of pressure sores will help the nurse evaluate the effectiveness of the preventive therapy or identify the need for additional interventions. Observation of the skin area for any signs of redness (hyperemia) is done during bathing and repositioning. *Hyperemia* is the first sign of a potential pressure sore. Circulatory changes have occurred in response to unrelieved pressure, but not tissue damage. Hyperemia may take up to half an hour to disappear after pressure is relieved so a repeat assessment for redness is appropriate one-half hour after repositioning high-risk patients. Black skin will show a change in color from the rest of the skin in the area, either lighter or darker, if circulatory changes have occurred from excessive pressure on an area.

If the assessment reveals skin areas that look abraded or like they are peeling, tissue damage has already occurred. Another sign of underlying tissue damage is redness and edema that does not disappear within 15 minutes of pressure relief. Blisters may gradually form or the skin may die (necrose), forming an open sore on the skin (ulcer). If pressure to the area continues, further damage may involve not only the skin, but the subcutaneous tissue, muscle, nerves, blood vessels, and bone, resulting in a very deep ulcer. Areas especially prone to developing pressure sores include any skin area over a bony prominence as shown in Figure 28–11. Any area receiving constant friction, such as skin around a cast or prosthesis, is also susceptible. The side-lying position most frequently results in pressure sores in the area of the trochanter. An upright, sitting position predisposes to ulcer formation around the center fold area of the buttocks. A semireclined position puts the sacral area at risk.

Assessment of Stimulation Need Satisfaction

Data Associated with Satisfied Stimulation Needs

Objective Data.   The following objective data are associated with individuals whose stimulation needs are being adequately met:

- Developmental level is appropriate to chronological age

- Joints have full range of motion (see Figure 28–15)
- Weight and muscle mass appropriate for age and height
- Skin intact, no evidence of pressure sores (decubitus ulcers)
- Coordinated muscle movements
- Normal posture and balance when sitting or standing

- Walks about in the environment at will (fully ambulatory)
- Near and far visual acuity in the normal or near normal range (20/20)
- Hears a whisper from approximately 15 ft and understands the message
- Able to taste and smell
- Able to manipulate environmental stimuli to meet personal preferences
- Gives meaning or identifies various forms of stimuli in environment
- Normal pupil response to light stimuli; pupils equal and react to light; opposite pupil constricts when light shone in one eye (tested using a flashlight by moving light in from side of face)
- Muscle strength equal, bilaterally
- Normal level of consciousness (LOC)—The *level of consciousness* represents the person's alertness and ability to respond to environmental stimuli. The Glasgow coma scale is presented in Table 28–6 as a guide for assessing level of consciousness. Assessment of LOC includes a person's sensory, motor, and mental responses to stimuli provided by the nurse during the assessment.
- Perceives and identifies tactile stimulation by location on body and as sharp or dull

Normally, a person is able to identify the location on the body of stimulation without the use of vision. People can discriminate between two simultaneously applied stimuli on slightly different body areas. Normal tactile sensation allows the person to identify an object placed in the hand in terms of size, shape, and weight, even if the object is unfamiliar to the individual. Discrimination between heat and cold is also expected when the tactile sense is functioning adequately. People should also be able to identify the position of their joints. Movement of a patient's joints by the nurse through ten degrees or more should be recognized when the patient has normal sensory input from the joints and muscles. The big toe or index finger is frequently used to test a patient's ability to recognize joint movement and position sense by moving the extremity up, down, and sideways while the patient's eyes are closed. Ability to identify position is then assessed. Sensations are evaluated in the same area on both sides of the body for consistency. A patient's ability to discriminate sharp and dull can be tested using a safety pin. The pointed end, gently touched to the skin, will create a sharp sensation, and the curled end will create a dull sensation. As the tactile sense is evaluated, ask the patient to identify where the touch is occurring and to identify any areas

Table 28–6. The Glasgow Coma Scale for Evaluating Level of Consciousness*

Eye Response

4	Opens eyes spontaneously
3	Opens eyes to verbal stimulation
2	Opens eyes to painful stimulation
1	Does not open eyes to any stimulation

Verbal Response

5	Identifies correct time, place, and person when asked
4	Confused about time, place, or person when asked
3	Verbal response to questions is not appropriate; unrealistic; unrelated to question; repeats words, phrases; profanity
2	Verbal response is not comprehensible; does not complete words; groans or mumbles response to questions or spontaneously
1	No verbal response to questions or spontaneously

Motor Response

5	Correctly follows directions
4	Withdraws or tries to remove painful stimuli
3	Flexes arms at elbows to painful stimuli
2	Extends arms at elbow to painful stimuli
1	No response to painful stimuli

The lower the total score, the more depressed the level of consciousness.

*The assumption is made that the patient is able to hear the verbal stimuli, so make sure hearing aids are in place and functioning before making any assessment.

where the touch feels different. Occasionally, ask the patient to identify location and sharp or dull stimuli without actually touching the skin. This seems like a deception of the patient, but periodically people will be guessing about the stimuli, and this technique will usually point out this problem.

On occasion, the patient will be unresponsive to all forms of tactile stimulation except deep pain. Squeezing the Achilles tendon will elicit deep pain for the purpose of this assessment in a nonresponsive patient. At times, the level of consciousness may be so depressed that the person does not even respond to painful stimuli.

- Normal muscle tone and stretch reflexes of 2 (+ +)

  The *deep tendon reflexes* or *stretch reflexes* are elicited by a sudden, quick blow to the skin over a tendon attached to a relaxed muscle group. The blow causes the muscle to be rapidly stretched, and the reflex, transmitted through the spinal cord, results in quick muscle contraction. A

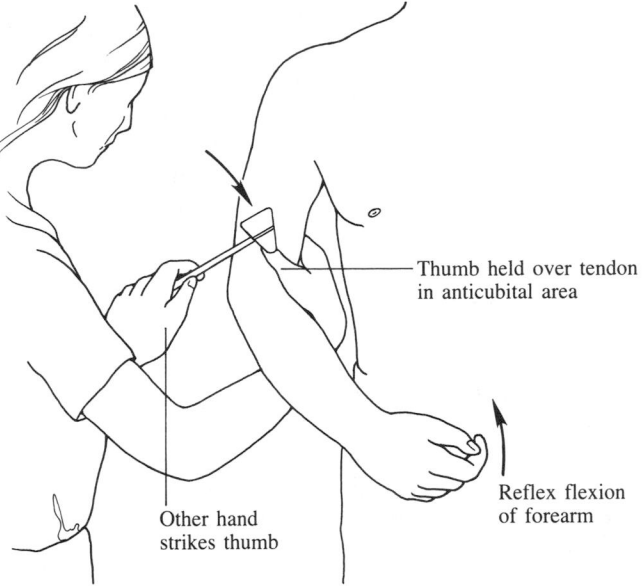

Figure 28–12.   Biceps reflex.

stretch reflex is involuntary. The amount of movement of the body part is evaluated when assessing a patient's reflexes. Reflexes are normally of equal intensity on both sides of the body. An exaggerated reflex or a depressed reflex may indicate a developing problem with muscle-nerve coordination. Some medications will depress the stretch reflexes. This may serve as a warning of a developing overdose with the potential for respiratory and cardiac arrest if increasing amounts of medication are administered.

The following stretch reflexes are commonly assessed as a guide to neuromuscular integrity:

1. *Biceps Reflex.* (See Figure 28–12.) The arm is bent at the elbow (flexion), with the palm up (supination). The nurse supports the length of the arm by holding it or resting it on a flat surface. The nurse's thumb is placed on the antecubital area of the patient's arm. The nurse then strikes the positioned thumb with a reflex

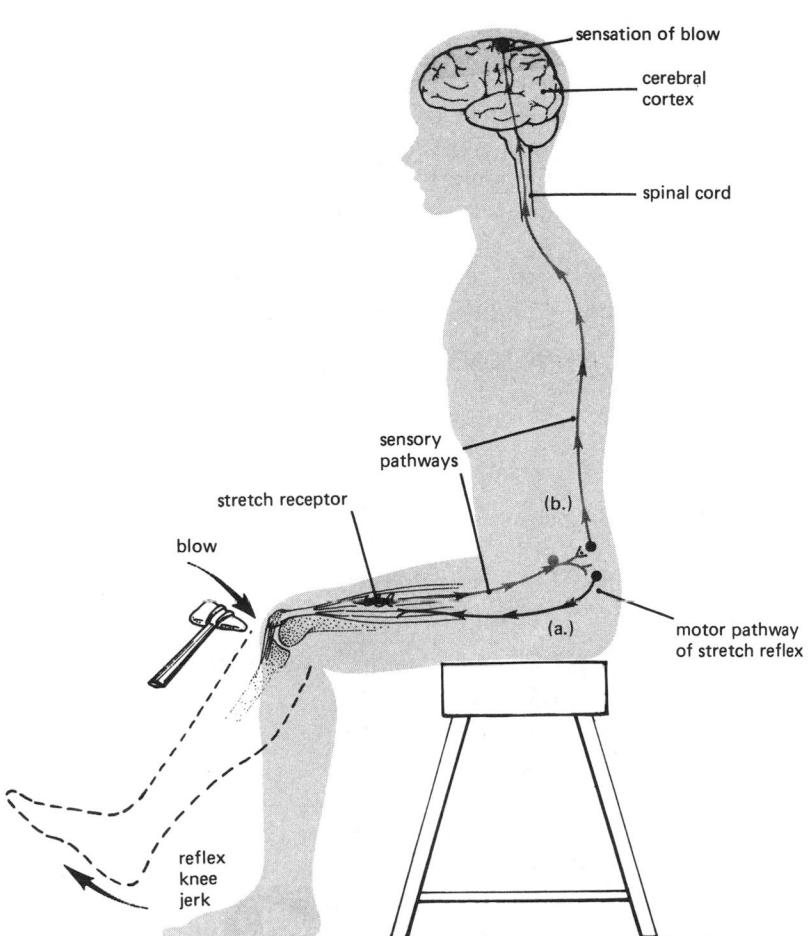

Figure 28–13.   Patellar reflex (knee jerk). (From M. Griffiths: *Introduction to Human Physiology*, 2nd ed. Macmillan, New York, 1981, p. 363.

hammer, thereby stretching the underlying tendon. The muscle contracts reflexively, flexing the forearm.

2. *Knee or Patellar Reflex.* (See Figure 28–13.) The knee is partially reflexed and hanging freely, forming a right angle behind the knee. The area just below the knee is struck with a reflex hammer, stretching the quadriceps tendon. The muscles reflexively contract, and the lower leg is pulled up in a slight kicking motion.

3. *Ankle Jerk or Achilles Tendon Reflex.* (See Figure 28–14.) The ankle is supported in a relaxed position with the nurse pressing up slightly on the ball of the foot to form a right angle between the top of the leg and the top of the foot (dorsiflexion). The nurse then strikes the Achilles tendon located at the back of the foot, level with the ankle and slightly inside (medial) on the big toe side of the foot. The muscles will contract, causing the foot to push against the nurse's hand in a toe-pointing jerk (plantar flexion).

A condition known as clonus may be discovered when the reflexes are assessed. *Clonus* is a hyperactive neuromuscular state in which a muscle group alternately contracts and relaxes rapidly following sudden stretching. A blow with the reflex hammer or sudden dorsiflexion of the relaxed foot will trigger clonus if there is in-

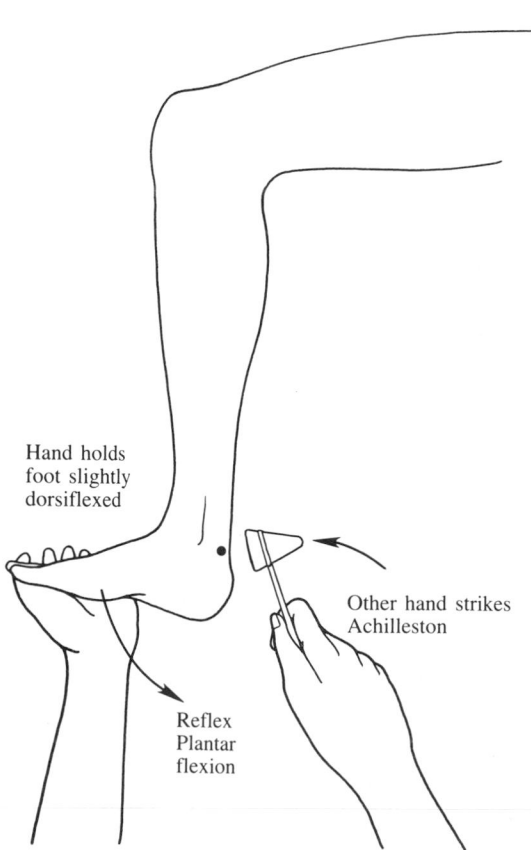

Figure 28–14. Achilles tendon reflex (ankle jerk).

Hand holds
foot slightly
dorsiflexed

Other hand strikes
Achilleston

Reflex
Plantar
flexion

Table 28-7. Evaluation of Deep Tendon Stretch Reflexes

0	No muscle contraction
1 (+)	Slow or diminished muscle contraction
2 (+ +)	Normal, active muscle contraction
3 (+ + +)	Slightly increased muscle contraction
4 (+ + + +)	Brisk contraction with some clonus
5 (+ + + + +)	Very brisk contraction with sustained clonus

creased nervous stimulation to the muscles. Table 28–7 shows the range of scores given to responses during stretch reflex assessment. When taking over the care of a patient whose reflexes are being assessed, have the nurse who has been assessing reflexes initiate the reflex and score it in your presence. This ensures reliability in assessment between nurses in a somewhat subjective scoring system.

Subjective Data. A person whose stimulation needs have been adequately met will report the following subjective data:

Reports no problems with dizziness
Reports no unusual visual or auditory perceptions
Reports no unusual tactile sensations (paresthesia)
Reports no loss in muscular strength or reduction in joint mobility

Data Associated with Unmet Stimulation Needs—Sensory, Motor, or Both

Objective Data. The patient with unmet stimulation needs would be identified by the following observations:

- Retarded developmental level for age; consistently below norms in motor coordination, intellectual functionings, or social interaction
- Joints have decreased range of motion, measured in degrees; assess degree or angle at which resistance or pain is encountered and move the joint no further (for example, wrist dorsiflexion met resistance at 30°)
- Weight is low for height (loss of muscle mass or weight)
- Strength is less than average for individual of that age, or strength is less than in previous assessment
- Uncoordinated muscular movements; difficulty starting and stopping movement
- Body out of alignment when sitting, lying, standing

- Spastic or flaccid muscle tone
- Exaggerated or depressed stretch reflexes (ratings of 0, 1, 3, 4, or 5)
- Altered level of consciousness (disoriented, confused)
- Restlessness, irritability
- Varying degrees of mobility impairment (casts, paraplegia, quadriplegia, hemiplegia, traction, ordered bed rest, unable to bear own weight)
- Reduced visual acuity, accommodation, or peripheral vision
- Corrective lenses not being used as prescribed
- Hearing losses leading to auditory distortion or absence of auditory sensations
- Hearing aids not being used as prescribed
- Altered sensations to touch such as *analgesia* (absence of normal pain perception), *anesthesia* (absence of all sensation), *paresthesia* (abnormal sensations with no observable stimuli), reduced sensations, inability to localize or identify stimuli as sharp or dull, differences in perception of stimuli on right and left sides
- Decreased spontaneous movement
- Difficulty maintaining balance in upright position without assistance
- Decreased or absent sensations of taste and smell
- Unable to manipulate stimuli in environment because of physical, mental, or financial problems; others control sounds, lighting, temperature, foods, odors, visual stimuli, interpersonal interaction, activity, (for example, intensive care units, hospitals, nursing homes, or infants, dependent elderly, and immobile patients)
- Confused about meaning or identity of environmental stimuli for such reasons as lack of knowledge, impaired cognitive functioning, sedation, culture, level of growth and development
- Unable to resolve simple problems or make decisions
- Abnormal pupil responses to light (no response, unequal response, excessive dilation or constriction)
- Muscle weakness or atrophy, generally or in one or more extremities
- Sudden loss of one or more senses, either permanently or temporarily from such things as trauma, surgery, bandages, spinal cord or nerve damage, infection
- Apathy, decreased mental alertness
- Skin shows evidence of damage from unrelieved pressure (pressure-sore formation)

Subjective Data. Patients whose stimulation needs have not been met report that they experience the following symptoms:

> Weakness
> Inability to sleep
> Dizziness
> Hallucinations, both auditory and visual
> Feelings of depression, anger, anxiety
> Changes in sensory input not accounted for by environmental stimulation
> Feelings of fatigue
> Difficulty thinking
> Stiffness in joints or pain

Nursing Diagnoses Associated with Unmet Stimulation Needs

The following general nursing diagnoses are related to various forms of inadequate stimulation, either sensory or motor or both.*

> Social isolation
> Problems (or potential with problems) related to activities of daily living (ADLs)
> Deficit in diversional activities
> Potential for cognitive impairment
> Uncompensated sensory deficit
> Sensory deprivation
> Sensory overload
> Potential for injury related to
>   Use of restraints
>   Sensory deficit
>   Altered level of consciousness
> Potential joint contractures
> Impaired physical mobility
> Potential for skin breakdown (pressure-sore formation)
> Decubitus ulcer
> Impaired muscle strength
> Powerlessness
> Alterations in family processes
> Body-image disturbance
> Self-esteem disturbance
> Self-care deficit

The following are some specific nursing diagnoses for individual patients:

> Potential sensory overload related to intensive care setting and altered level of consciousness

*National Group for Classification of Nursing Diagnoses: List of Nursing Diagnoses from Fourth National Conference, 1982.

Disturbance in body-image related to spinal cord injury and paraplegia

Impaired right-sided muscle strength related to stroke

Social isolation related to protective isolation environment for leukemia

Sensory deprivation related to immobility and loss of sensation below nipple line following spinal cord injury

Potential for cognitive, physical, social retardation related to lack of parental responsiveness to infant's needs and confinement in playpen

Inability to feed self following casting of arms

Potential for pressure-sore development related to unwillingness to change positions while on bed rest

Nursing Interventions to Facilitate Satisfaction of Stimulation Needs

Initial assessment of patients will provide baseline information from which the effectiveness of preventive nursing care can be evaluated. Patients at risk for unmet stimulation needs are identified during the assessment process, and appropriate nursing interventions are chosen, implemented, and evaluated.

Any patient who experiences a loss or restriction in ability to move about in the environment is at risk for problems with unmet mobility needs. Any patient who experiences the loss of one or more senses or the ability to interpret and control environmental stimuli is at risk for problems with appropriate satisfaction of stimulation needs. To preserve a patient's ability to meet stimulation needs, the following nursing interventions are used:

1. Active and passive range-of-motion exercises
2. Exercises to maintain or increase muscle strength
3. Therapeutic positioning
4. Ambulation
5. Interpretation and management of the environment
6. Assistance with satisfaction of other needs

Active and Passive Exercises

Range-of-Motion Exercise. The primary role of the nurse in assisting patients with range-of-motion exercises is to maintain their current level of joint mobility and muscle strength. However, movement also provides sensory, motor, and social stimulation for the patient. The physical therapy department is utilized to help restore function in muscles and joints, while nursing focuses on preservation. This means that range-of-motion exercises will be slightly different for each patient, based on individual joint and muscle functioning at the time preventive nursing treatment is initiated. A patient's maximum range of motion is reached at the point of re-

sistance or pain. The nurse is not to force joints past the point of pain or resistance because of the risk of causing trauma or pain. This is why accurate assessment and documentation of each patient's current capabilities in joint movement are important as a baseline guide for evaluating later range of joint motion. Without some form of range-of-motion exercises, joints begin to stiffen in several days of disuse and may be permanently impaired. Deformities of the bones and joints with loss of movement (*contractures*) are the result.

During *active range-of-motion exercises*, the patient moves various body joints through all possible movement. In *passive exercises*, the nurse or another person moves the patient's joints through their range of motion. Active exercises are preferred whenever possible because the patient is actively involved, both physically and mentally, in preserving healthy joint and muscle function. Only when the patient is unable to participate are exercises of joints performed completely by another person. Encourage the patient to move the joints as much as possible, and assist with complete range as needed. *Active assisted exercises* are joint-motion exercises done by the patient with the help of some assistive device, such as using a normally functioning strong arm to exercise a weakened, partially paralyzed arm following a stroke.

Before assisting with range-of-motion exercises, the nurse considers any medical contraindications for each patient. Any type of joint problem, edema, cardiac problem, or other conditions that may be aggravated by energy expenditure or joint movement indicates a need to discuss range-of-motion exercises with the patient's physician. The type and amount of exercises are then approved by the physician and often by physical therapy.

To perform range-of-motion exercises, move each joint through its range of motion smoothly and slowly with three repetitions of the complete range. In passive exercises, the patient's body part being moved is supported, using maximum surface area under the part. For example, the arm is cradled from underneath, being supported by the nurse's hand and forearm rather than gripping the arm from above. The joint being exercised is held with one hand for support, while the nurse's other hand moves the attached body part to exercise the joint. Rapid, jerky movements may trigger muscle contractions in the form of spasticity or clonus. If the patient begins to develop spastic muscle contractions during range-of-motion exercises, the movement of the affected part is stopped, and continuous gentle pressure is placed on the muscle group until it relaxes. Exercises are then restarted, using slower, steady movement. As with all treatments, the exercises are explained to the patient, as is the reason for doing them. The bed is raised to the nurse's hip level for passive or active assisted exercises to reduce the nurse's back strain while moving and lifting the patient's arms and legs. Figure 28–15 demonstrates the full range of motion possible for each joint in the body. Table 28–8 offers suggestions for handling patient's body parts. A suggestion for children capable of active range of motion would be to adapt the game of "Simon Says" to provide range of motion to all joints.

Some patients may require complete passive range-of-motion exercises several times a day if motion in the joint is to be preserved. This is especially true for the totally immobile patient. A patient who is able to move in bed may be able to maintain joint motion with specific exercises only once a day. Some patients may adequately exercise all upper body joints during normal daily activity but require assistance in exercising lower body joints. Each patient's needs will vary, based on abilities, activity level, prognosis, and willingness to cooperate with suggested exercises. Some patients may refuse to exercise alone. They may want the nurse there to remind and encourage them. Other patients may benefit from group exercise classes, which add support and competition with other patients and also serve a social function.

Group exercise sessions for the elderly held three times each week for 30-minute sessions can result in increased strength and joint mobility, especially in the shoulders (Bassett *et al.*, 1982.)

Exercises to Maintain or Increase Muscle Strength.   In addition to range-of-motion exercises, some patients are able to do isometric exercises to maintain and improve muscle strength for future ambulation. Patients in casts or following procedures such as surgery, whose joints are not to be moved but whose muscle strength is to be preserved, are examples of patients commonly encouraged to do isometric exercises. Consult with the physician before initiating any isometric exercises since they are known to raise the blood pressure and pulse and temporarily obstruct some of the blood flow around the tensed muscle. The patient's medical condition may be a

Table 28–8. **Suggestions for Performing Passive Range-of-Motion Exercises**

Joint	Patient and Nurse Position
Shoulder joint	Patient may be lying supine or sitting; if lying, prone position needed for full shoulder hyperextension. Support elbow with one hand and hold patient's hand to move arm. (See Figures 28–16, 28–17, and 28–18.)
Elbow	Grasp patient's wrist with palm of hand, and encircle with fingers; support elbow with other hand.
Forearm	Hold patient's hand as in a handshake, and turn palm up and down to cause forearm (not shoulder) movement. (See Figure 28–19.)
Wrist	Support wrist with one hand, and hold patient's other hand palm to palm. (See Figure 28–20.)
Fingers and thumb	Nurse's fingers are placed over the top of the patient's fingers and alternately curled and straightened; patient's wrist is supported in a straight position with other hand; fingers are held together for thumb motion. (See Figure 28–21.)
Hip	With patient in supine position, hold leg under ankle with one hand and along length of leg with other hand and arm; knee may be bent to increase movement in hip as it is moved toward patient's chest; lift leg slightly off bed to avoid dragging across bedding and creating friction; internal and external rotation is accomplished by rolling the leg, exerting force at the ankle and knee; prone or side-lying position for hyperextension. (See Figures 28–22 and 28–23.)
Knee	Support under knee with one hand and under ankle with other. Move patient's heel toward thigh to flex knee.
Ankle	Stabilize the leg just above the ankle with one hand, and move the foot by grasping the ball of foot with palm of other hand. (90° angle at foot and leg needed for standing and slightly greater angle needed for normal walking.) (See Figure 28–24.)
Toes	Stabilize lower leg with one hand and move toes all at once by placing other hand over toes and curling and straightening them.

Functional Description of Joint Motions

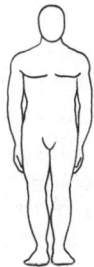

All the motions described are begun from the neutral position; that is, the person is standing or lying straight, arms at the side, palms toward the body, and heels together.

1. Head and neck

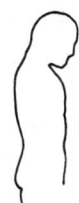   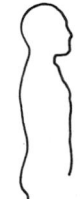   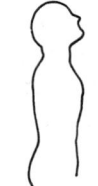

Bending head forward:
flexion

Holding head straight:
extension

Bending head backward:
hyperextension

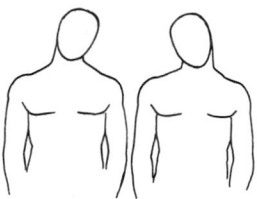   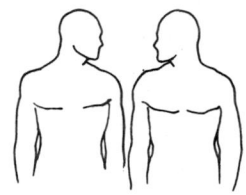

Bending head to either side,
ear toward shoulder:
lateral flexion

Turning head to either side to
look over shoulder:
rotation

Note: These motions of the head and neck are active exercises. They are seldom done passively.

2. Trunk

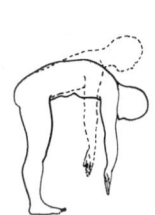   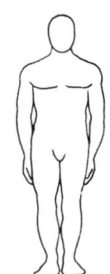   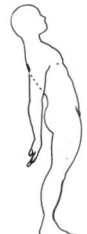   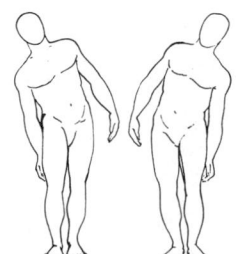

Bending forward from waist:
flexion

Standing or sitting with trunk
straight:
extension

Bending backward from waist:
hyperextension

Bending sideways from waist to
left or right side:
lateral flexion

Figure 28–15.   Range of motion for joints of the body. (Reproduced with permission from *Range of Motion Exercise: Key to Joint Mobility* by Patricia Toohey, R.N., B.S., and Corrine W. Larson, R.P.T., M.S., copyright 1977, Sister Kenny Institute, Minneapolis, MN, pp. 3–6.)

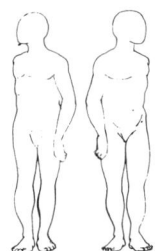

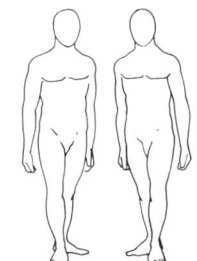

Turning shoulders to either side.
keeping hips in place:
rotation

Turning hips to either side.
keeping shoulders in place:
rotation

3. Shoulder

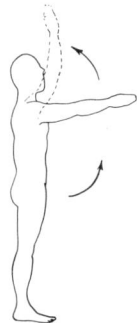

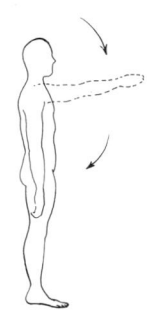

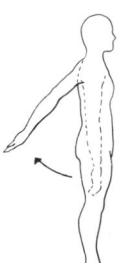

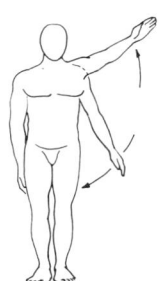

Bringing arm forward and raising
it above head:
flexion

Returning arm to side:
extension

Bringing arm backward:
hyperextension

Moving arm away from side and
above head:
abduction
Returning arm to side:
adduction

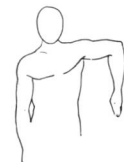

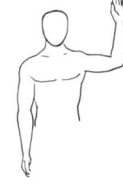

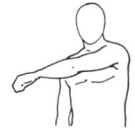

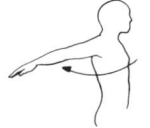

With arm out to side at shoulder
level and elbow bent to right angle,
bringing arm forward so that palm
faces backward:
internal rotation

Using same position, taking arm
back toward head so that palm
faces forward:
external rotation

With arm out to side at shoulder
level, moving it backward (keeping
elbow straight):
horizontal abduction

With arm out to side at shoulder
level, moving it across chest
toward opposite shoulder (keeping
elbow straight):
horizontal adduction

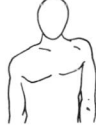

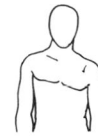

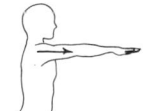

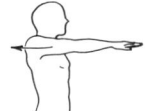

Lifting shoulder toward ear:
elevation

Lowering shoulder toward hip:
depression

With arm at shoulder level (keeping elbow straight), reaching forward as far as possible:
protraction

Using same position, drawing arm
and shoulder back as far as possible:
retraction

Figure 28–15.   (*Continued*)

4. Elbow

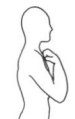 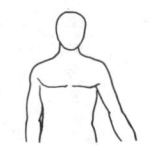

Bending elbow, hand toward shoulder: flexion

Straightening elbow: extension

5. Forearm

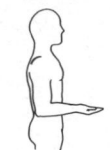 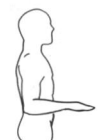

Turning palm upward: supination

Turning palm downward: pronation

6. Wrist

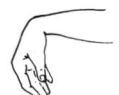 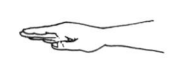 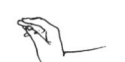

Bending wrist forward: palmar flexion

Returning wrist to neutral position: extension

Bending wrist backward: dorsiflexion

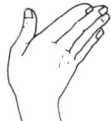 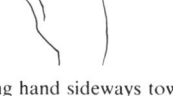

Moving hand sideways toward little finger: ulnar deviation

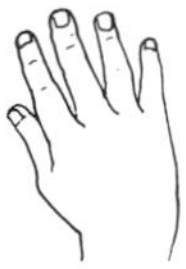

Moving hand sideways toward thumb: radial deviation

7. Finger

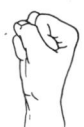 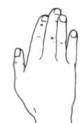 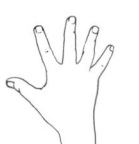 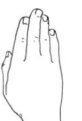

Bending fingers at all three joints (making a fist): flexion

Straightening fingers: extension

Spreading fingers apart (including thumb): abduction

Bringing fingers together (including thumb): adduction

8. Thumb

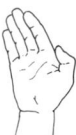 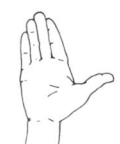 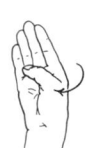

Bending thumb at two outer joints: flexion

Straightening thumb: extension

Moving thumb out and around toward little finger: opposition

Figure 28–15.   *(Continued)*

9. Hip

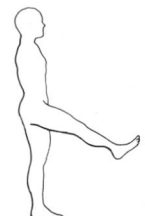

Bringing leg forward by bending hip:
flexion

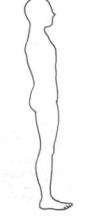

Returning hip to straight position:
extension

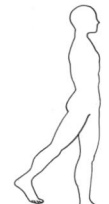

Moving leg backward:
hyperextension

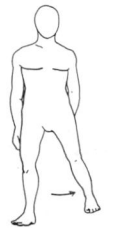

Moving leg out to side:
abduction

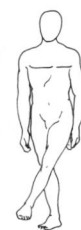

Returning leg to middle and crossing over other leg:
adduction

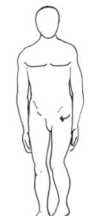

Rolling leg toward middle (knee pointing toward other leg):
internal rotation

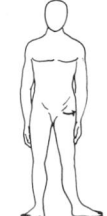

Rolling leg away from middle:
external rotation

10. Knee

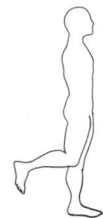

Bending knee:
flexion

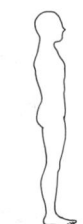

Straightening knee:
extension

11. Ankle

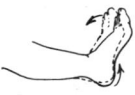

Bending foot up:
dorsiflexion

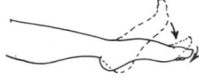

Bending foot down:
plantar flexion

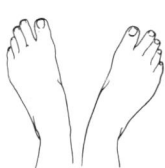

Bringing foot outward:
eversion

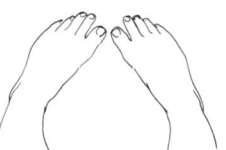

Bringing entire foot inward:
inversion

12. Toe

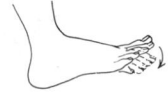

Bending toes down:
flexion

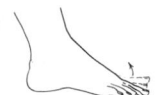

Bending toes back:
extension

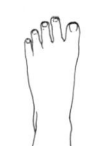

Moving toes apart:
abduction

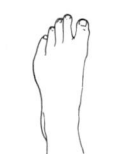

Bringing toes together:
adduction

Figure 28–15.   (*Continued*)

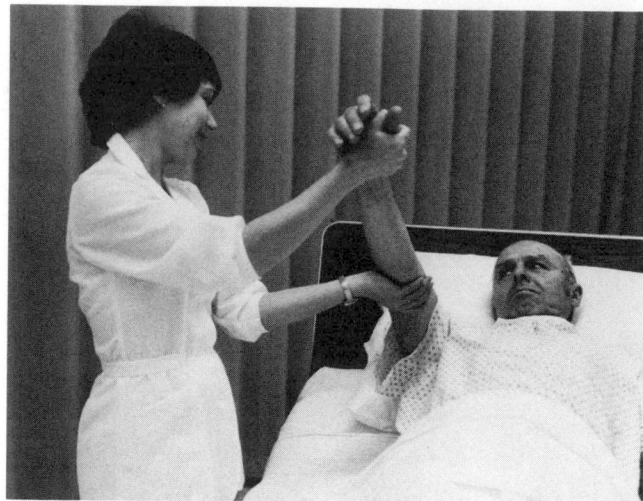

Figure 28–16. Supporting the hand and elbow while flexing shoulder joint.

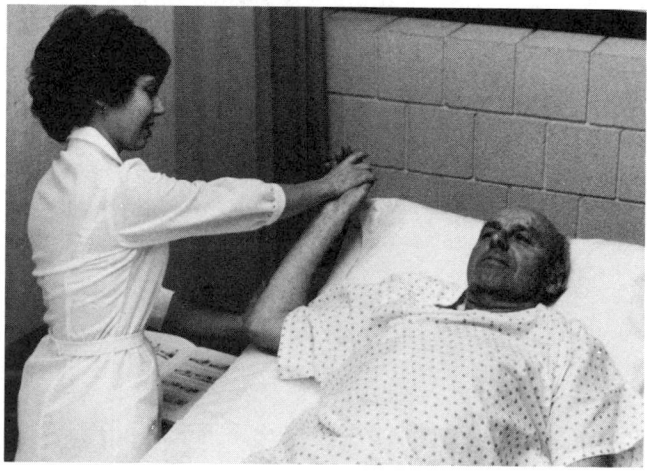

Figure 28–17. Supporting the hand and elbow while moving shoulder joint into external rotation.

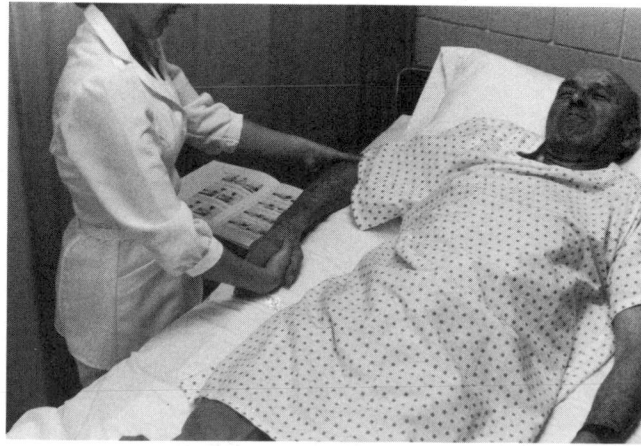

Figure 28–18. Internal rotation of shoulder joint with arm supported.

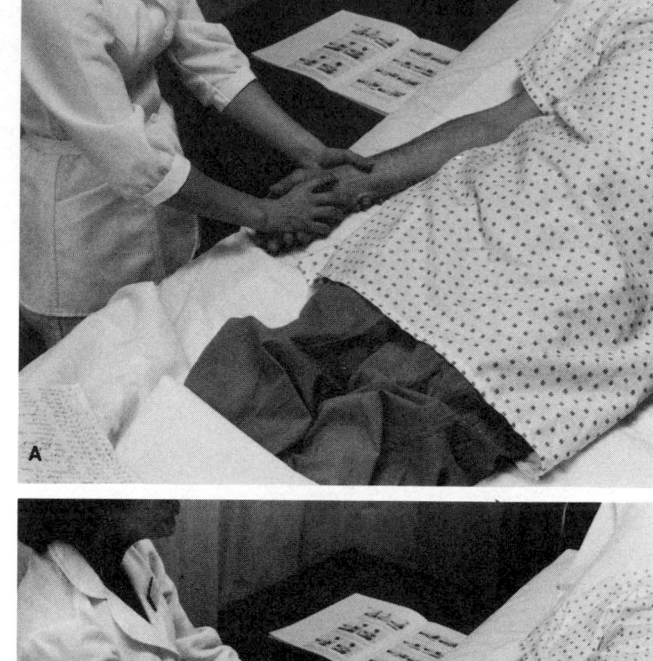

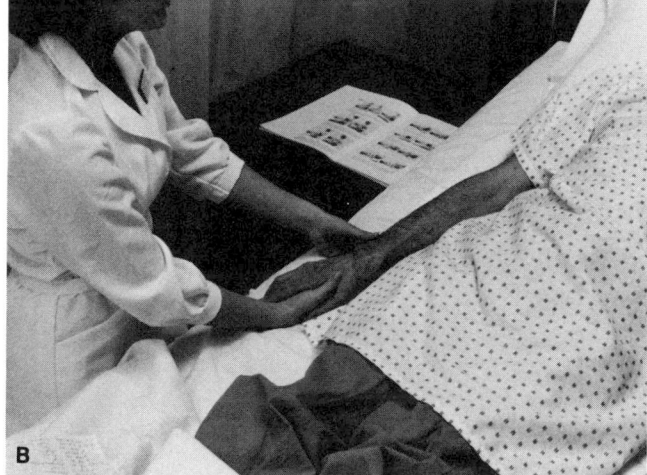

Figure 28–19. Providing range of motion to forearm. **A.** Supination. **B.** Pronation.

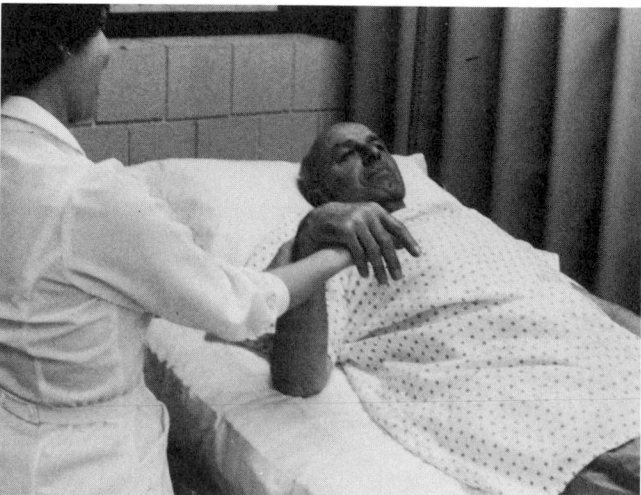

Figure 28–20. Range of moton to wrist (palmar flexion).

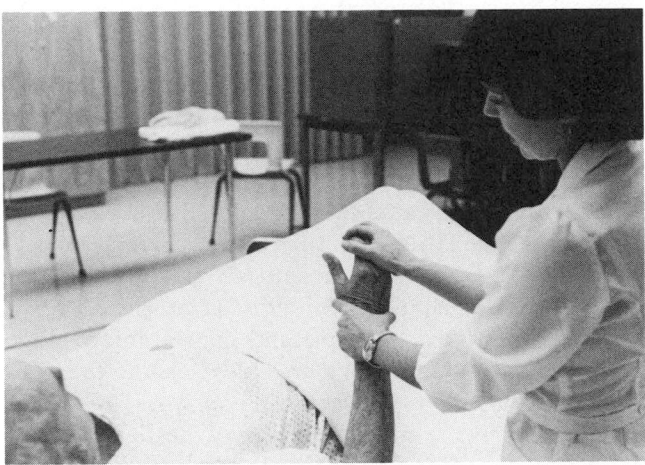

Figure 28-21. Flexion of fingers during range-of-motion exercises.

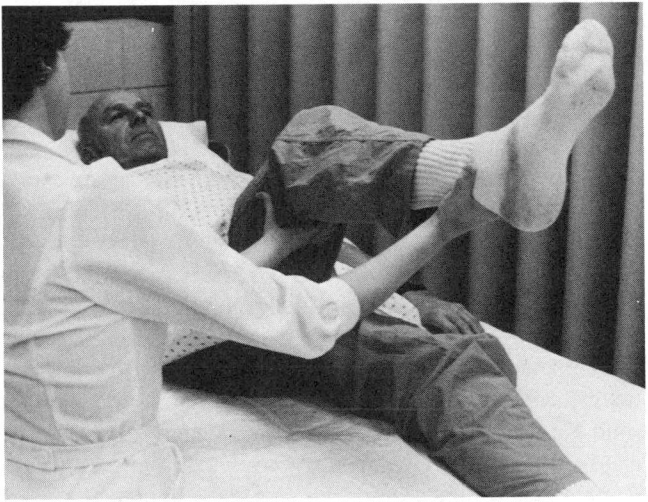

Figure 28-22. Support of the leg during hip and knee flexion.

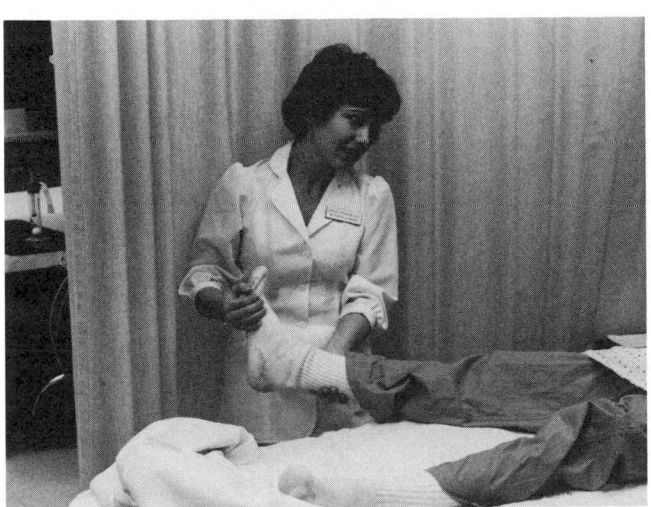

Figure 28-23. Abduction of hip.

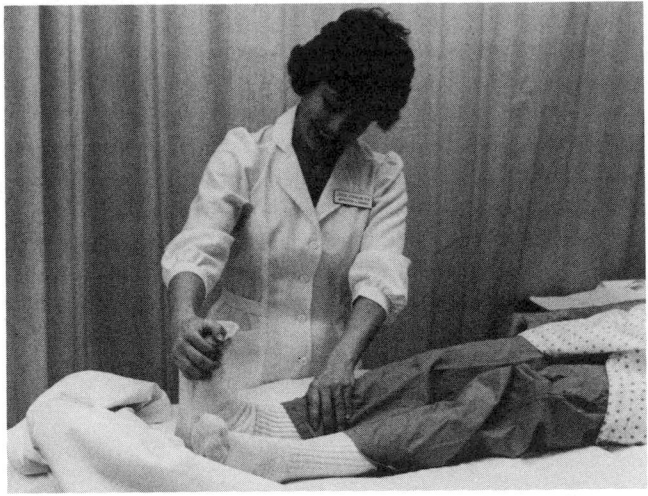

Figure 28-24. Dorsiflexion of ankle.

contraindication for isometric or isotonic exercises. Isometric exercises are also known as muscle-setting exercises. Isometric exercises performed for short periods several times each day are more effective in maintaining muscle strength than one extended exercise session (Lentz, 1981). The muscle groups used for walking—the quadriceps femoris, abdominal, and gluteal muscles—should be exercised isometrically four times each day until the patient is ambulatory. The muscle group is tightly contracted for 8 seconds and then completely relaxed for several seconds. This is repeated ten times for each muscle group at each exercise session.

Pushing against the footboard will put stress on the long muscles of the leg and the bone to help reduce bone demineralization and foot contractures from plantar flexion (footdrop). (See Figure 28-25.) These exercises

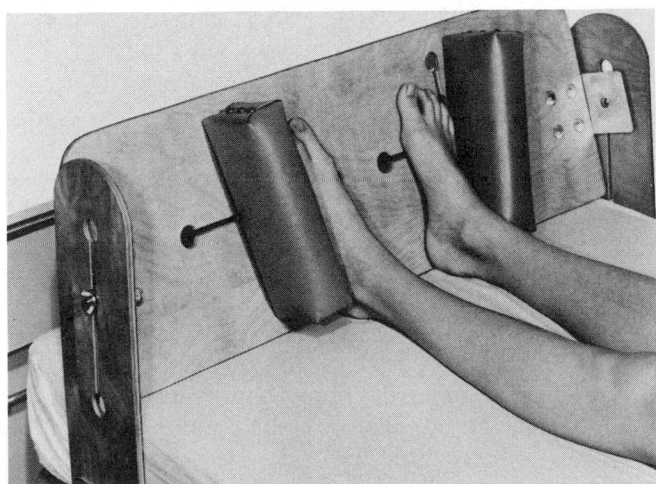

Figure 28-25. A footboard for preventing plantar flexion of the foot and external rotation of the hip. (Photograph courtesy of J. T. Posey Co., Arcadia, CA.)

should also be done several times each day with ten repetitions at each session. Encouraging the patient to perform plantar and dorsiflexion of the ankle and circumduction in an hourly exercise session will increase muscle activity in the leg and thereby promote venous blood return to the heart.

Therapeutic Positioning

Patients with limited mobility will require assistance in changing their positions. The goals of therapeutic positioning are:

1. Even distribution of body weight on supporting surface
2. Maintaining normal body alignment
3. Maintaining unrestricted circulation
4. Use of good body mechanics by lifters
5. Sensory, motor, and cognitive stimulation of patient

Normally, people shift positions slightly every few minutes, even during sleep. Therapeutic positioning is designed to maintain patient comfort, prevent complications, and maintain function of the muscles, joints, and senses of the body. Therapeutic positioning helps to prevent deformities from developing, especially in infants and children whose bones and muscles are growing and may take on the shape of objects pressing against them. Frequent position changes also improve the patient's comfort by relieving pressure on skin, tissues, and bones and reestablishing normal circulation to the area. Some positions are helpful in reducing the intensity of muscle spasticity, which is a sudden continuous muscle contraction occurring in patients with central nervous system damage, as with strokes or spinal cord injuries. Frequent position changes will also help reduce the incidence of other problems associated with immobility.

Assessment of each patient is important to identify their needs related to position changes. Some patients may require repositioning every half hour to avoid the development of pressure sores, while other patients may tolerate position changes every two hours without developing problems. The more risk factors patients have associated with pressure-sore formation, the more frequently they will require repositioning. If no signs of hyperemia develop over pressure areas after turning, the patient may be advanced one-half hour in a turning schedule. For example, instead of turning every hour, the patient is turned every one and a half hour. If no hyperemia develops on this schedule, the patient is advanced to every two-hour turns, but not beyond. At

night, frequent turning will interfere with a patient's rest and sleep. The patient is gradually advanced in a turning schedule at night so a favorite position is maintained up to seven hours, as long as no new risk factors for pressure sores develop. The patient is left in the same position one-half hour longer every week. By the eleventh week, the patient will be tolerating one position all night (Feustel, 1982). If signs of hyperemia or new risk factors develop, the patient is returned to a two-hour turning schedule and gradually advanced again over several months. Some patients may be able to move without difficulty in bed and are able to change their position without help. These people may not need any therapeutic positioning. They may need education about the need to assume positions they normally do not assume in bed in order to achieve good body alignment and maintain joint mobility.

Basic Postions

SUPINE POSITION. In the supine position, the patient is flat on the back with body parts positioned as though the patient were standing with good posture. Pressure point areas over bony prominences, such as the heels, will be at high risk for formation of pressure sores, as will the spine and shoulder blades. The heels are positioned in the space between the mattress and the footboard whenever possible. The feet are supported against a firm surface at a 90-degree angle to the lower leg. Footboards or shoes are often used to achieve this position. The legs will have a tendency to roll outward (external rotation). This is prevented by tucking a small pillow under each hip or by using a trochanter roll. This is a folded towel placed slightly under one hip to secure it and then rolled under against the patient's buttocks and thigh. This causes the leg to return to good alignment at the hip joint. A trochanter roll is placed under each hip. A small pillow supports the head. Arms are

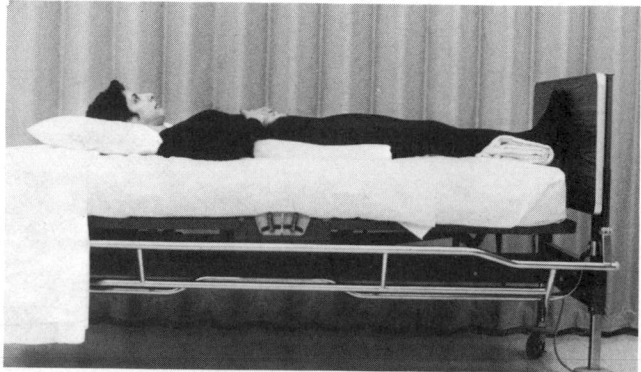

Figure 28–26. The supine position. Note the position of the feet with heels off the bed to prevent any pressure on this area. Trochanter rolls at the hips prevent external rotation.

positioned only if the patient is unable to move them, otherwise active movement in the arms is encouraged. The arms may be positioned in external or internal rotation at the shoulder joint, supported by a pillow. The arms may also be positioned straight down at the sides, slightly abducted from the shoulder, with the forearm in supination. The hands are maintained in position by a hand roll or cone device held in the patient's hand so the fingers are slightly flexed with thumb and fingers in opposition. (See Figure 28-26.) A small pillow under the back supports the lumbar curve.

PRONE POSITION. In the prone position, the patient is lying flat on the stomach with feet off the end of the mattress when possible. No pillow or only a very flat pillow or folded blanket is used under the head. The face is turned to either side. The arms and hands are positioned as in the supine position. Small towels are folded and placed under the shoulders to keep them from protracting. A patient with a large abdomen or large breasts may be uncomfortable in the prone position unless pillows are used to create a space for the prominent body part. Assess the patient after positioning in the prone position for any problems with respirations or discomfort. (See Figure 28-27.)

SIDE-LYING, LATERAL, OR SIMS. In the side-lying position, the patient is positioned on the right or left side with a pillow under the head to keep the neck straight. The back is supported with pillows if the patient tends to roll onto the back. The top leg is flexed at the knee and supported on pillows in front of the bottom leg. The back leg is slightly flexed at the knee with the hip pulled back to stabilize the patient on one side. The top arm is supported by pillows at shoulder height and flexed at the elbow. The lower arm is flexed with the hand up to the level of the face. Make sure the weight of the body is not obstructing blood flow in the lower arm by checking for the presence of a pulse and later check-

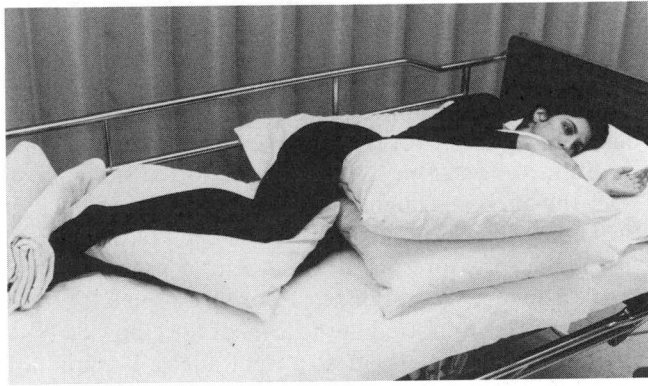

Figure 28-28. The side-lying position. The top arm is supported at the level of the shoulder, keeping the line of vision and breathing unobstructed. The top leg is supported at hip level and slightly in front of the bottom leg for stability. There is slight flexion of the hip and knee. Plantar flexion is prevented by supporting foot.

ing skin color and temperature for similarity with the top arm. A patient with one weak side is positioned more frequently on the strong side rather than the weak side to avoid pressure on affected muscles and nerves. A foot support such as a sandbag may be used to help hold the feet in correct alignment with the leg. Hands are positioned with fingers slightly flexed. (See Figure 28-28.)

FOWLER'S POSITION. In the Fowler's position, the patient is in a semisitting position in bed. The head of the bed is raised to varying degrees for patient comfort or activity, but the knees are straight. In the semi-Fowler's position, the knees are flexed. Common angles of head elevation in the Fowler's position are between 45 and 60 degrees. The patient's heels are supported off the bed by pillows or padding under the lower leg. Trochanter rolls may be needed to prevent abduction at the hips. The elbows are protected from rubbing on the bedding by pillows under the forearms. For patients assessed as very high risk for pressure-sore formation, positioning

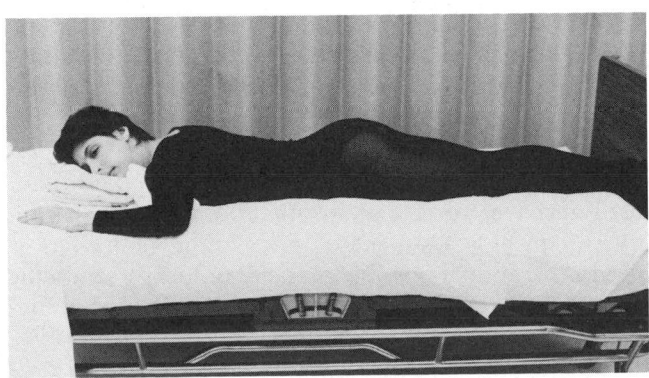

Figure 28-27. The prone position. Feet are flat against a footboard, with the feet positioned in the gap between the mattress and the footboard. Towels under each shoulder prevent protraction of the shoulder in this position.

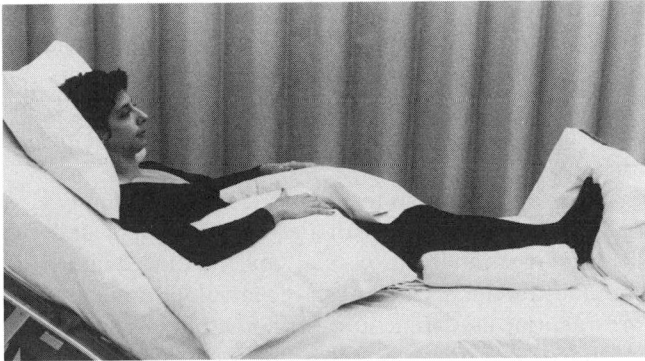

Figure 28-29. Fowler's position. The head of the bed is elevated approximately 45 degrees. The heels are held off the bed by padding under the lower legs. Trochanter rolls may be needed if external rotation at the hip occurs.

in the Fowler's position should be limited to 30 minutes because of the shearing force (force created as the patient slips down in bed and skin stretches away from buttocks). This position is often saved for mealtime to make eating easier for the patient. (See Figure 28–29.)

SITTING POSITION.   In a well-supported sitting position, the back is straight and resting against the back of the chair. The chair ends before the bend in the knee so there is no pressure on the area behind knee (popliteal area). The feet are flat on the floor or flat on a footrest. The arms are supported at the level of the elbow on both sides. The knees are bent at a right angle. If chairs are too high or large, patients will tend to slide forward and slump. This is corrected by placing pillows or blankets behind the patient's back so the knees are allowed to bend freely. A support, which is large enough to position the feet at right angles to the legs, is placed under the feet. If chairs are too small, the knees will be bent to form less than a 90-degree angle in the popliteal area. The hips will also be more flexed. This tends to force the patient backward in the chair with excess weight on the sacral area. This position can be corrected by placing padding under the patient's buttocks to elevate the hips until the feet are flat on the floor and knees are at a 90-degree angle. Added pillows or supports may then be needed for the arms if the armrests have become too low. If the chair is too wide, the patient will tend to lean to one side in poor alignment. This can be corrected by supporting the patient with pillows on both sides of the chair around the hips and waist area so the patient is stable in the middle of the chair.

Positioning to Reduce Spasticity.   Spastic posturing is casued by damage to the central nervous system resulting in the predominance of certain muscle groups. Most spastic posturing results in flexion of the elbows, wrists, and fingers with the arms close to the sides and internal rotation at the shoulder. The legs are straight with internal rotation and adduction at the hips. The toes are pointed down in plantar flexion and turned in. (See Figure 28–30.) Positioning to reduce this spastic muscle activity involves placement in positions opposite to the spastic posturing. The limbs are moved slowly and gradually into position and never forced, since forcing increases spasticity.

In a supine position, the spastic upper extremity is in an abducted position with the elbow straight and the forearm in supination. A small towel is placed under the shoulder by the neck to push the shoulder up into slight protraction, as if reaching for something. The wrist is extended. A soft hand roll is not used since it tends to increase spasticity in the fingers, resulting in excessive flexion. A hard hand cone may be used to hold the fingers in a slightly flexed position. The legs are slightly abducted with the knees in light flexion from a soft pillow

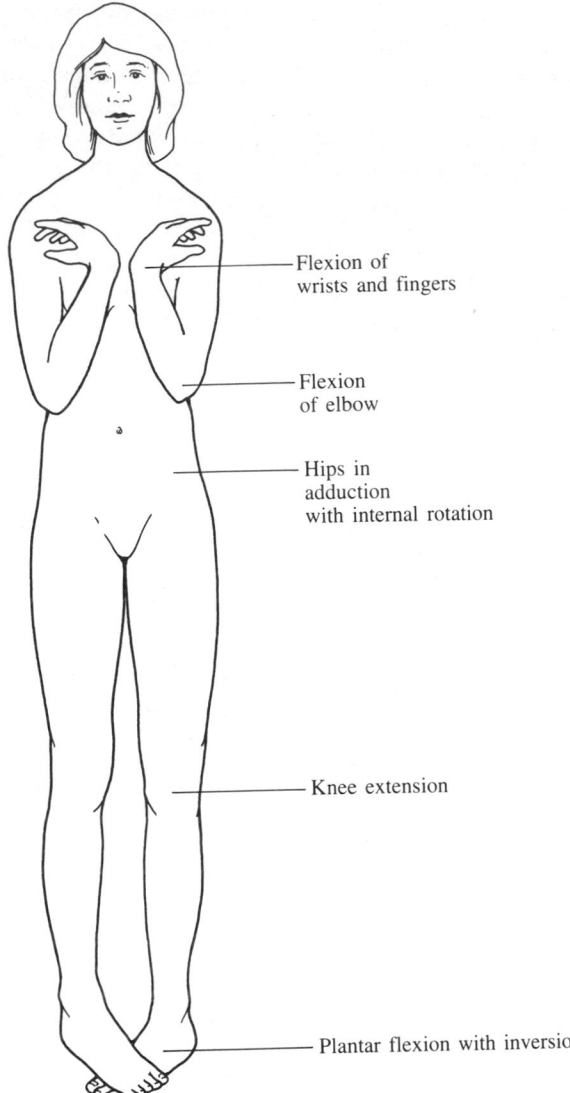

Flexion of wrists and fingers

Flexion of elbow

Hips in adduction with internal rotation

Knee extension

Plantar flexion with inversio

Figure 28–30.   Spastic posturing. Commonly seen to some degree after a CVA or spinal cord injury.

under the knee and lower leg. This also flexes the hip slightly, which is in opposition to the spastic posturing tending to extend the hip. A folded towel is placed under the spastic hips, causing slight protraction of the pelvis. A pillow placed between the legs may help prevent excessive adduction at the hips. A footboard is not used since the pressure against the foot increases spasticity. Frequent assessment of circulation in the feet is needed because of possible pressure on the vessels in the popliteal area from the pillow under the knee. (See Figure 28–31.)

In a side-lying position, spasticity is reduced by pulling the upper arm forward and supporting it on several pillows with the elbow in pronation and wrist extended. The hip is slightly flexed, as are both knees, with the upper leg supported on several pillows at the level of the

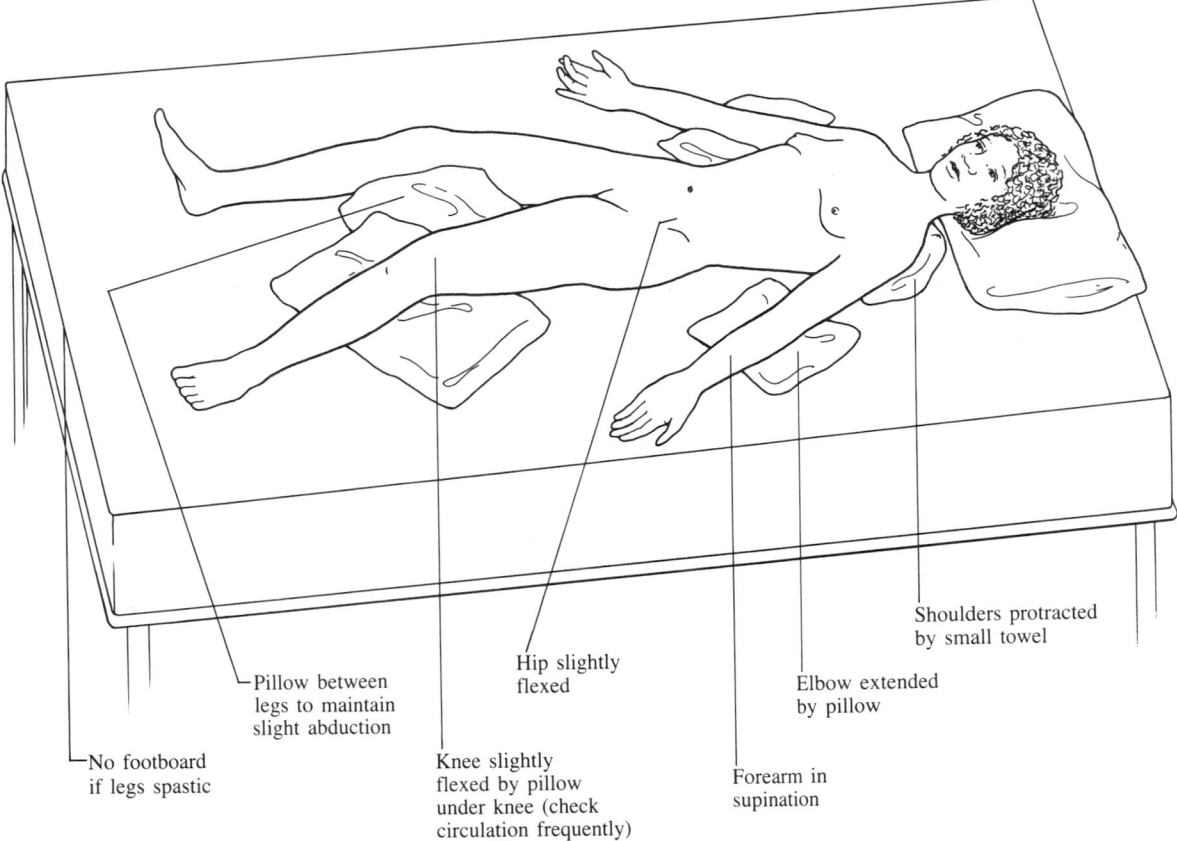

Shoulders protracted
by small towel

Hip slightly
flexed

Elbow extended
by pillow

Pillow between
legs to maintain
slight abduction

Knee slightly
flexed by pillow
under knee (check
circulation frequently)

Forearm in
supination

No footboard
if legs spastic

Figure 28–31.   Positioning to reduce spasticity in the supine position.

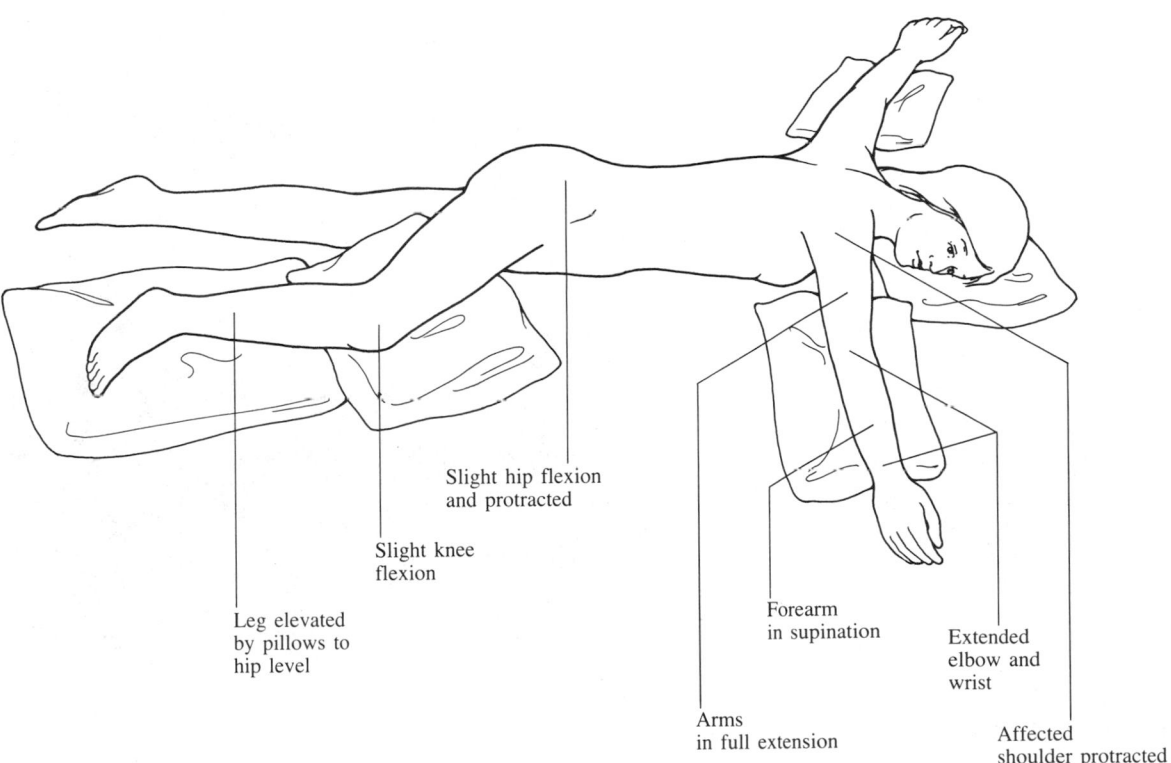

Slight hip flexion
and protracted

Slight knee
flexion

Forearm
in supination

Extended
elbow and
wrist

Leg elevated
by pillows to
hip level

Arms
in full extension

Affected
shoulder protracted

Figure 28–32.   Positioning to reduce spasticity in the side-lying position.

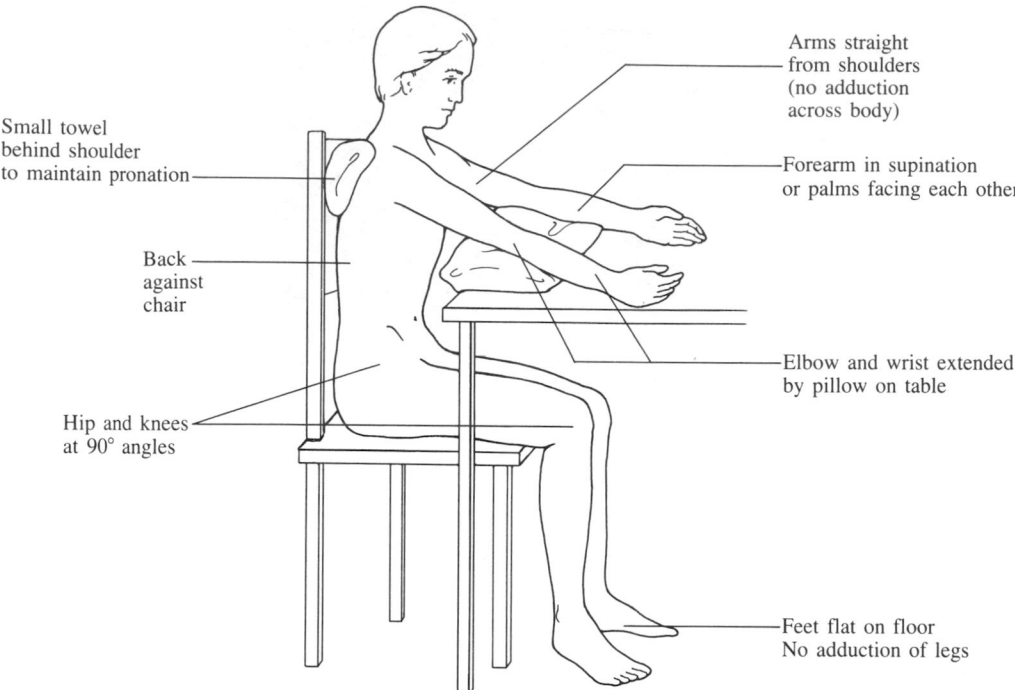

Small towel
behind shoulder
to maintain pronation

Back
against
chair

Hip and knees
at 90° angles

Arms straight
from shoulders
(no adduction
across body)

Forearm in supination
or palms facing each other

Elbow and wrist extended
by pillow on table

Feet flat on floor
No adduction of legs

Figure 28–33. Positioning to reduce spasticity in the sitting position.

upper hip. If the spastic side is in the down position, the arm is still pulled forward with the elbow and wrist extended. The elbow position is in supination. The lower spastic leg is also pulled forward and slightly bent at the knee. (See Figure 28–32.)

In a sitting position, the adaptations for the spastic body parts involve pulling the arms forward at the shoulders (protraction) and supporting them with a

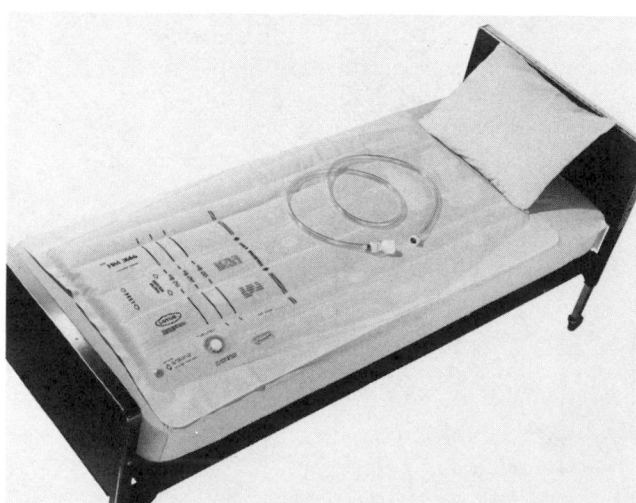

Figure 28–34. A water mattress to reduce pressure to body areas at risk for pressure-sore formation. (Photograph courtesy of the Lotus Health Care Products, CT.)

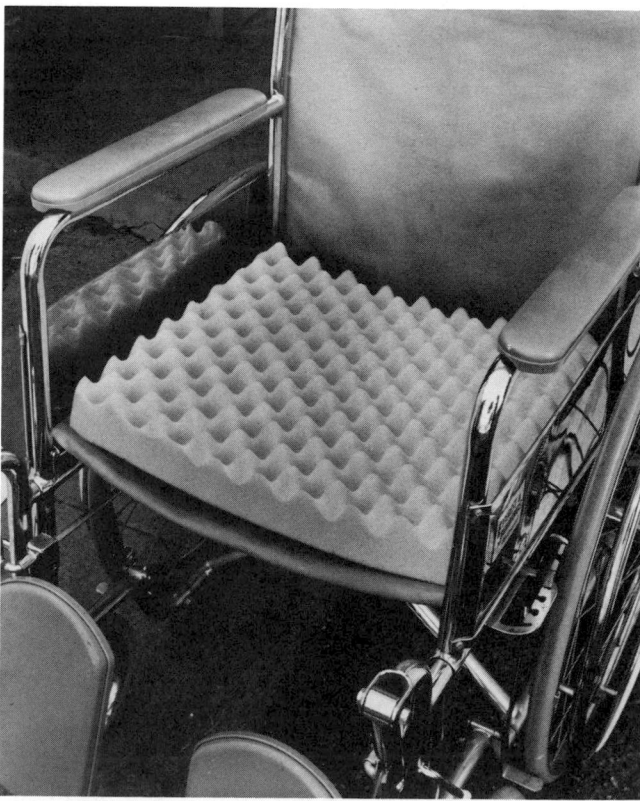

Figure 28–35. Wheelchair cushion ("egg-crate") to reduce pressure on bony prominences (over ischial tuberosities) as a way of preventing pressure-sore formation. Also available for beds. (Courtesy of J. T. Posey Co., Arcadia, CA.)

newer, air-fluidized bed uses a system of round, extremely small beads with air circulating among the beads. The patient's body is supported equally, with no area receiving more pressure than other areas. Other mattresses continuously and gradually lose air to support the patient on a cushion of air. Foam-rubber "egg-crate" mattresses are another adaptation to reduce the pressure on all bony prominences or on specific problem small towel between the shoulders and the back of the chair. The elbows and wrist are extended with the elbow in supination. The elbows are not pronated, nor are the shoulders adducted across the body, since this facilitates spastic posturing. (See Figure 28–33.)

Special Beds and Cushions.   Beds, mattresses, and cushioning equipment are designed to distribute the body weight evenly on the supporting surface, reducing the development of deformities and preventing pressure sores in patients with impaired mobility. Patients who are assessed as being at high risk for pressure-sore formation begin using these devices before any pressure damage is done. Water beds or mattresses are available for incubators, cribs, and full-size hospital beds. (See Figure 28–34.) The warmth of these beds will also cause vasodilation in the skin, improving circulation. The alternating-pressure mattress uses a pump to keep columns in the mattress full of air. At frequent inter-

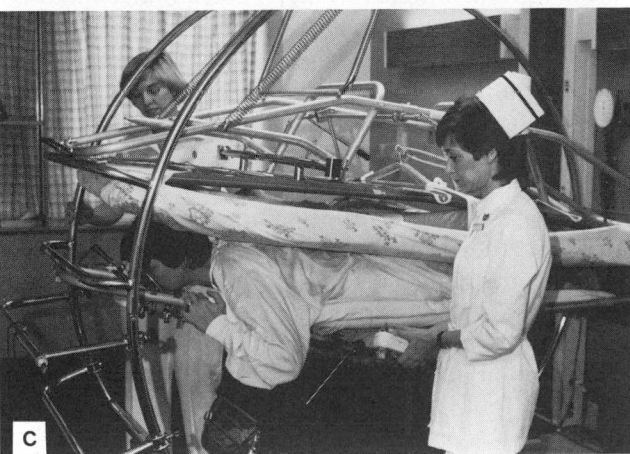

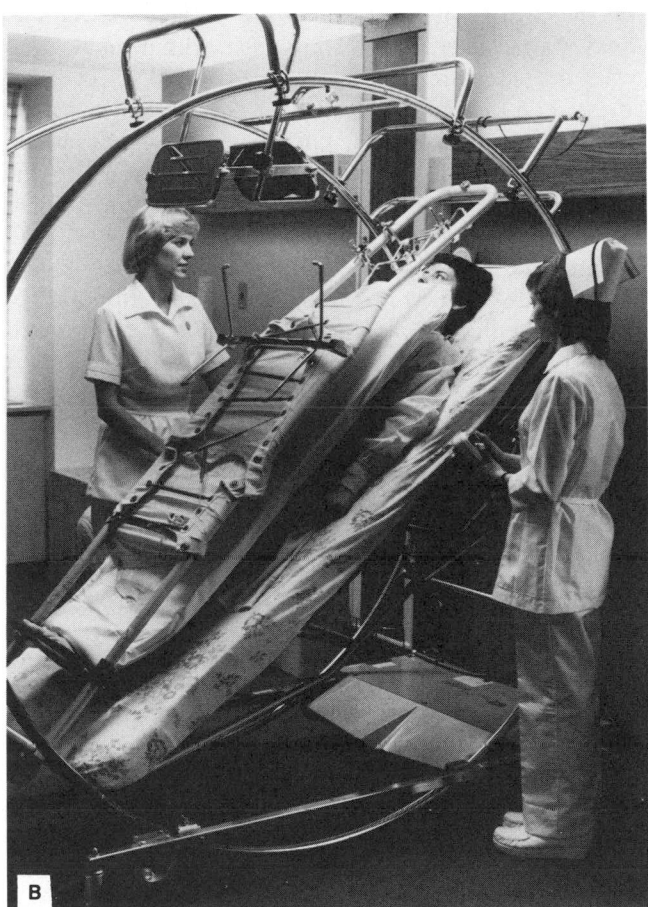

Figure 28–36.   A circle bed. This bed is frequently used to allow turning and repositioning of patients who must maintain perfect alignment of the spinal column following a spinal cord injury. **A.** Supine position. Mirrors allow view of activity in the room. **B.** Patient being turned from a supine to a prone position by rotation of the bed's circular frame. **C.** Patient in prone position at completion of turn. Bedding on top is then flipped up and off patient.

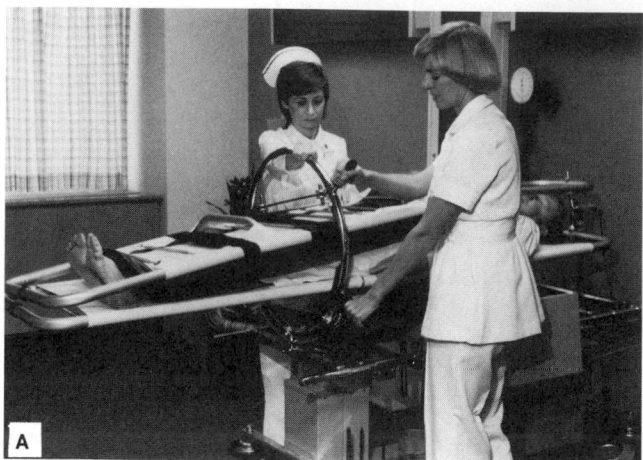 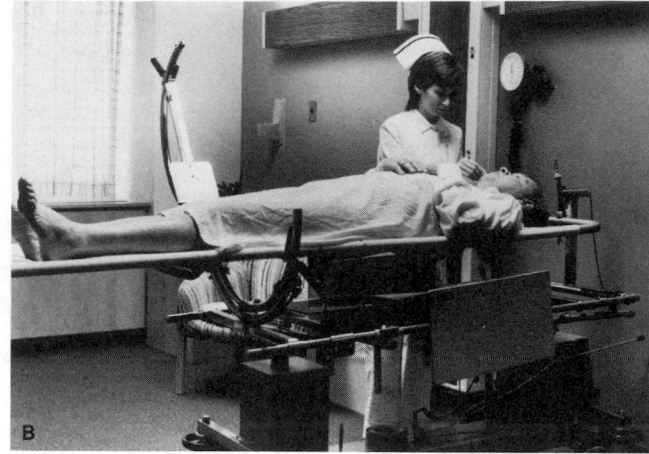

Figure 28–37. A turning frame (Stryker frame). This bed allows the patient to be turned to either a supine or prone position. **A.** Patient supported between two stretchers for turn. **B.** Extra stretcher removed following turn.

vals, some columns deflate, while others inflate, changing the area of tissue bearing the patient's weight. A areas. (See Figure 28–35.) Pads filled with a gel-like material or water are used to reduce the risk of pressure sores while the patient is sitting. There are also special turning beds for immobile patients who must be kept in straight alignment because of possible damage to the spinal cord. One type, the circle bed, turns the patient 180 degrees from supine, to vertical, to prone without moving the patient's position on the bed. (See Figure 28–36.) Another form turns the patient from supine, to prone, and back by flipping the patient over, sandwiched between two stretchers. (See Figure 28–37.) A

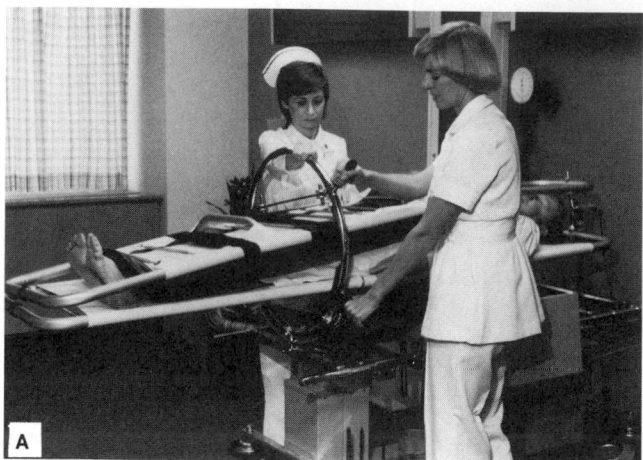

Figure 28–38. The net suspension bed (MECABED). The patient's position can be changed by rotating the cranks on either side of the end of the bed. The patient's weight is evenly distributed and aired, reducing the risk of pressure-sore formation. (Photograph courtesy of Mecanaids Ltd., Gloucester, England.)

net suspension bed distributes the patient's weight, provides air circulation, and allows repositioning by changing the level of the sides of the bed. (See Figure 28–38.) Even with the use of special beds, the patient is turned and responsitioned every two hours at a minimum, and more frequently if signs of excess pressure on body tissue develop or joints begin to stiffen.

Changing a Patient's Position. When moving, lifting, or helping patients change position, the nurse uses good body mechanics to avoid muscle strain and back problems. Good body mechanics involve maintaining a wide base of support with the center of gravity over the base. The large, strong muscles of the legs and arms create the force rather than the weaker muscles of the back. The spine is kept as straight as possible, with little bending or twisting. Body weight is used whenever possible to reduce the muscle force needed to lift or slide the load. Many states have maximum weight-lifting recommendations for men and women for safe working conditions. A nurse is almost always lifting more than these recommended weights while turning, repositioning, and transferring patients in and out of bed. Back problems affect large numbers of nurses, especially if the back muscles are used in lifting rather than the arms, legs, and body weight. Back pain from moving and lifting patients occurs in one out of every three nurses (Chapman, 1981). Each situation requiring muscle work by the nurse in giving patient care has the potential for causing muscle and back strain if incorrect techniques are used. The basic principles and techniques for moving and lifting patients are adapted to each patient's needs and abilities. The equipment and techniques used are also based on the nurse's accurate assessment of personal strength and leverage. Table 28–9 presents some principles and techniques of moving and lifting.

Table 28–9. **Principles and Techniques of Moving and Lifting**

1. More force is required to lift an object than to pull or push it.
   Use roller boards to pull patients onto another surface. (Roller boards have circular rods that revolve under a cover of material. The roller board is positioned partly under the patient, bridging the gap between a cart and bed or any two flat surfaces. The patient is pulled across the board onto the bed. This board and the tubes revolve to move the patient with minimal friction and force needed.)
   Use transfer boards to slide the patient from bed to chair, bed to bed.
   (Transfer boards are flat pieces of solid material, often plastic, which bridge the gap between two surfaces, allowing the patient to slide into the new position gradually rather than being lifted, which requires more work.)
   Creation of friction on patient's skin may cause damage
2. Objects close to the lifter's center of gravity require less force to lift.
   Patient moved close to nurse before lifting
   Nurse's arms flexed rather than extended when lifting
   Reaching while lifting is avoided
   Kneel, squat, and widen base of support to bring load closer to center of gravity
3. A wide base of support gives stability to the body.
   Feet apart approximately 1½ ft
   Feet flat on floor
   (Parallel foot position with one foot forward and one back pulls nurse up onto toes and ball of one foot as weight is shifted, leading to instability.)
   Angled foot position of approximately 60 to 90 degrees, with one foot forward and one back, keeps both feet flat on floor improving stability. (See Figure 28–39.)
4. If the center of gravity moves outside the base of support, the body becomes unstable.
   Position feet so center of gravity in pelvis is over feet. (See Figure 28–40.)
   Bend knees to move down to lift load rather than bending over at waist.
   Knees bend, not back.
5. A twisting motion when moving or lifting a load places strain on the back muscles.
   Back kept straight.
   Weight shifted from front foot to back foot to move load.
   Face direction opposite of movement.
6. When load exceeds the force, no movement will occur.
   Get other lifters to help move heavy or immobile patients.
   Use mechanical lifters.
   Have the patient lift as much of own weight as possible.
   Provide patient's bed with trapeze bar as appropriate to reduce nurse's load.
   Use body weight as a counterbalance to patient's weight to reduce force needed to move load.
7. Muscles of the thighs are ten times as strong as muscles of the back.
   Use the thighs in lifting and moving, not the back.
   Flex knees rather than bending back.
   Tighten abdominal muscles when lifting with thighs for maximum force.
8. Healthy, active muscles are stronger than infrequently used muscles.
   Keep abdominal, thigh, and biceps muscles in good shape.
   Perform regular exercise to strengthen lifting muscles and reduce injury.

Before each position change, the nurse performs the following activities:

1. Determination of a need for the patient to be moved. Some patients will require turning every half hour to two hours throughout the 24-hour day. Other patients may ask to be moved in order to engage in some activity. A patient may slip down in bed or move enough to be in poor body alignment. A patient may be uncomfortable in one position or be having difficulty breathing.

2. Assessment of the amount of force needed to reposition a patient based on ability of the patient to assist the nurse and the nurse's physical strength and leverage. If another lifter will be needed, the nurse explains the new position and the procedures for lifting to the helper; mechanical lifting aids are obtained as needed.

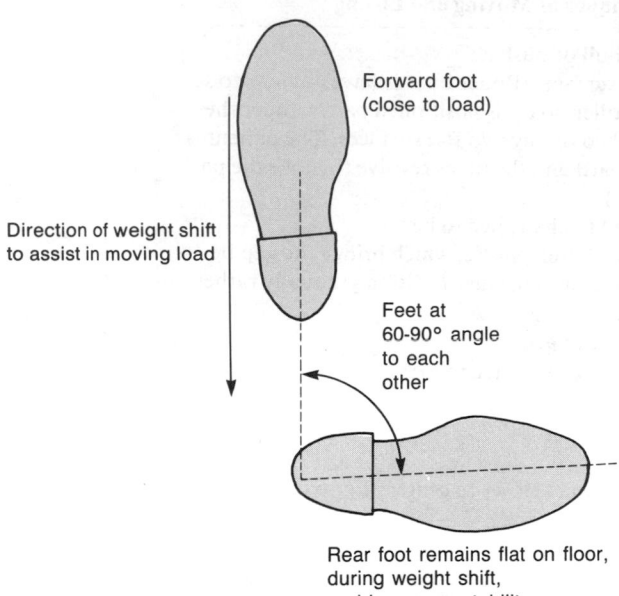

Figure 28–39. Foot position for maximum stability when moving and lifting a load. Rear foot remains in contact with floor when weight shifted backward to move load. Parallel foot positions, with one forward and one back, tend to bring nurse onto toes, decreasing the base of support.

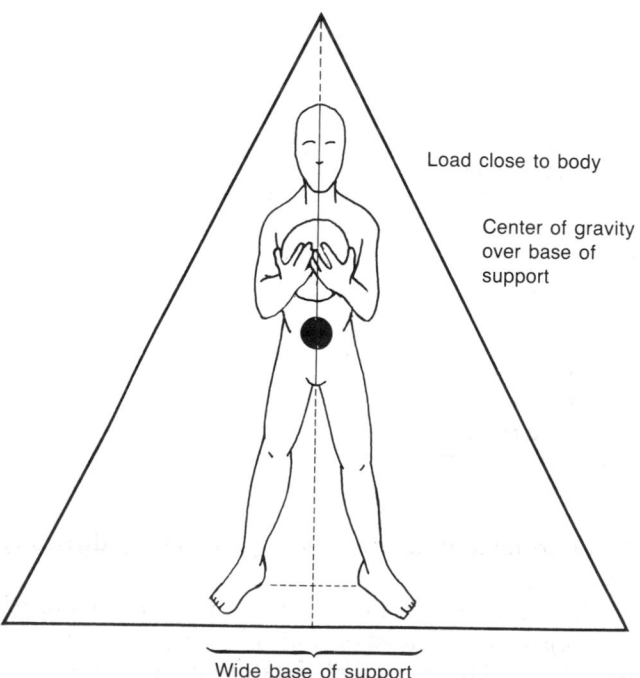

Figure 28–40. Optimum balance and stability. Load is close to body, center of gravity centered over base of support, wide base of support.

3. Lifters wash their hands prior to handling patients.

4. Explanation of the move to the patient and how the patient can help, if able.

5. Provision of privacy during the repositioning.

6. Locking wheels on beds and wheelchairs. This is done to prevent falls. The bed will tend to move away from the direction of the force. Any furniture that may interfere with the move is also moved out of the way.

7. Elevation of bed, when possible, to the nurse' hip level. This prevents bending of the back and use of back muscles. The bed is lowered after the move.

8. Obtaining positioning aids such as pillows, towels, or blankets. These will be needed to support the patient in good body alignment following the move and are brought into the room before beginning.

9. Flatten the bed. This is done before beginning the move so the nurse and patient are not working against the force of gravity.

MOVING PATIENTS UP IN BED. There are several ways of moving patients up in bed, depending on their ability to assist the nurse. Some patients may need little or no help if their bed is equipped with an overhead trapeze. The patient can then lift the major part of body weight, while the nurse assists with the legs. (See Figure 28–41.) The nurse may need to offer slightly more assistance as the patient uses the trapeze bar by bending the patient's legs and placing one arm under the patient's shoulders and the other under the patient's thighs. The nurse faces the opposite direction of movement with the foot farthest from the bed pointing toward the bottom of the bed and the near foot at a 60- to 90-degree angle toward the side of the bed. The feet are wide apart. The knees are flexed so the thighs provide some of the force in moving, along with the biceps and the nurse's weight shift. As the patient lifts, the nurse shifts weight from the front leg to the back leg to move the patient up in bed. If the patient is able to push with the legs, this also reduces the force needed to move. The patient may be able to assist the nurse by pulling on the headboard if a trapeze is not available.

If the patient is able to use the upper body and arms, the shoulder lift (Australian lift) is suggested as the lift placing the least stress on the nurse's back (Scholey, 1982). (See Nursing Skill 28–1.) Most other moves involve some degree of twisting at the waist as the nurse shifts weight while supporting the patient. If the patient is unable to assist with the move, two lifters are recommended, unless the patient is an infant or small child. (See Nursing Skill 28–2.)

A turning sheet, which is a strong piece of material extending from the patient's shoulders to the thighs, is used to move patients up or down in bed. It may also be

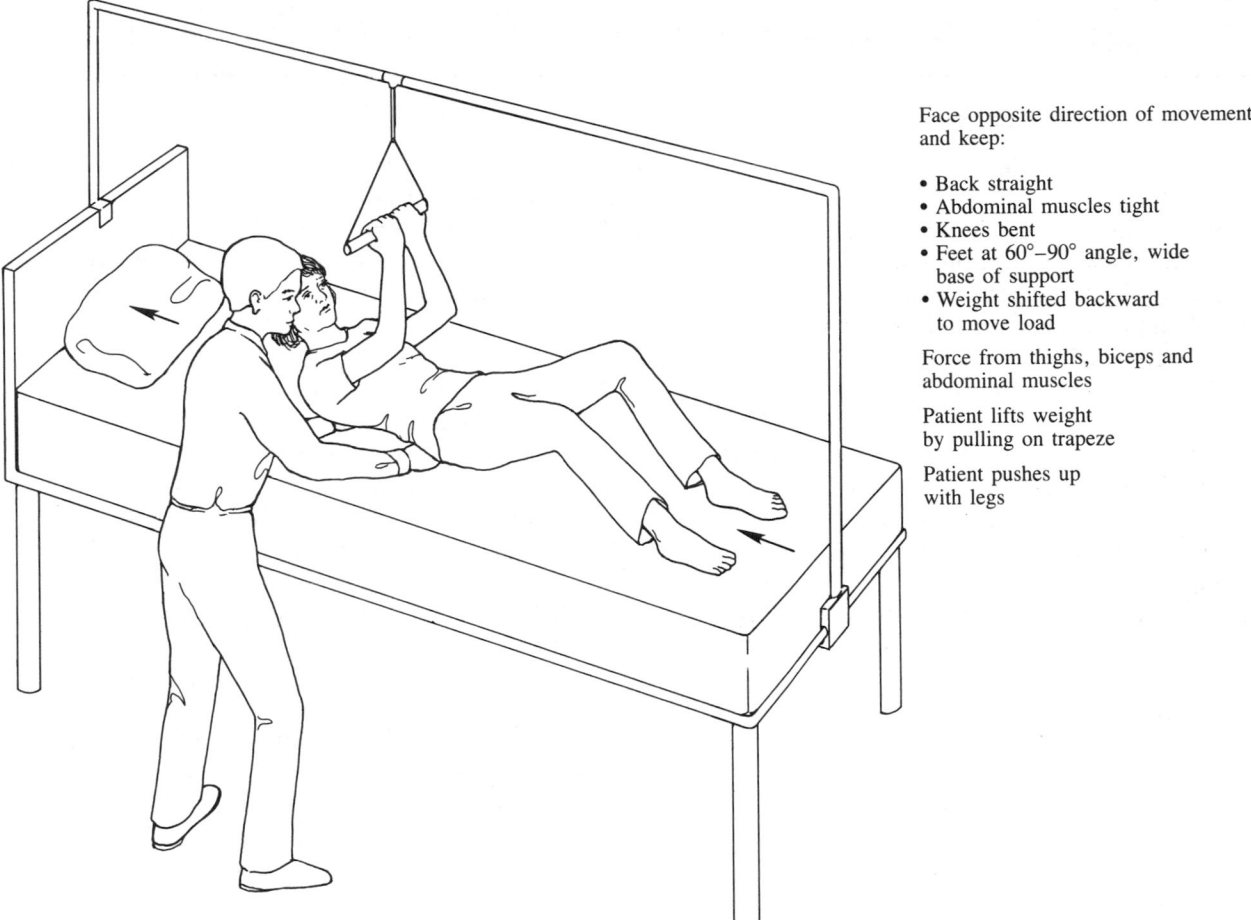

Face opposite direction of movement and keep:

- Back straight
- Abdominal muscles tight
- Knees bent
- Feet at 60°–90° angle, wide base of support
- Weight shifted backward to move load

Force from thighs, biceps and abdominal muscles

Patient lifts weight by pulling on trapeze

Patient pushes up with legs

Figure 28–41.   Moving patient up or down in bed with aid of bed trapeze.

used to move the patient to the side of the bed. Two nurses are needed, with one on each side of the bed. The turning sheet is gripped near the upper and lower sections and rolled in the nurses' hands. When the sheet is bunched and held close to the patient, both nurses pull with their biceps, while shifting their weight backward in the direction of the move. The patient assists by lifting the head during the move, when possible. When moving patients up in bed, it is common to place a pillow against the headboard to protect the patient's head in case the move goes too far.

Whenever the patient is moved up in bed, the supine position is used, unless the Australian lift is possible.

MOVING A PATIENT DOWN IN BED.   The same moving techniques are used to move a patient down in bed with the exclusion of the Australian lift. The nurses face the opposite direction of the move, support the patient with the turning sheet, or under the shoulders and thighs, and transfer their weight backward toward the foot of the bed. The patient's knees are flexed for the move to reduce drag on the bedding, just as when being moved up in bed. (See Figure 28–47.)

MOVING A PATIENT TO THE SIDE OF THE BED.   The patient may be moved to the side of the bed in preparation for sitting on the edge of the bed or for getting out of bed. Patients are also moved to the side of the bed before turning to a prone position so they are not up against the bed rails. One or two nurses may be involved in the move. Again, the nurse's body weight is used as a counterforce to the weight of the patient, as each nurse shifts weight backward with one knee braced against the bed. With two nurses, the entire patient is moved to the side in one motion. With one nurse, the patient is moved toward the side in sections, leaving the patient tempo-

Nursing Skill 28-1   Shoulder Lift (Australian Lift)—Two-Person Lift

Procedure	Explanation
1. The patient is assisted into a sitting position with knees flexed.	1. Reduces friction by having smaller surface area in contact with the bedding.
2. Bed is in low position. Each nurse faces the head of the bed. The nurse's knee near the bed is placed on the bed next to the patient's hips. The nurse's far arm and hand gripping the headboard and near arm under patient's thighs. (See Figure 28-42.)	2. If the headboard can be reached, pulling with the arms creates the least back strain and no twisting. Strong muscles of biceps and thigh used for lifting.
or	
Each nurse faces the head of the bed with feet wide apart and knees braced against bed; the arm nearest the head of the bed is placed perpendicular to the mattress and behind the patient's buttocks; the hand is placed palm down on the mattress (60 to 90° angle foot position). (See Figure 28-43.)	When headboard cannot be reached, wide base of support gives stability, and arm on mattress will act as pivot point for shifting body weight to move patient without twisting back.
3. The other arm is placed under the patient's thighs.	3. Added force of nurse's biceps to move patient weight.
4. The patient's arms are positioned on the nurse's shoulders and down their backs.	4. Pushing force distributed along large area of nurse's body.
5. On the count of three, the patient pushes down as the nurses pull against the headboard and push up with the thigh muscles in the leg on the bed.	5. Counting coordinates efforts by all three people; body weight used to reduce force needed from muscles to move patient weight; patient actively lifting some of own weight to reduce nurses' load; uses largest and strongest body muscles.
or	
On the count of three, the patient pushes down on the nurses' backs, and the nurses push down on the mattress and transfer their weight over the pivot arm to move the patient.	

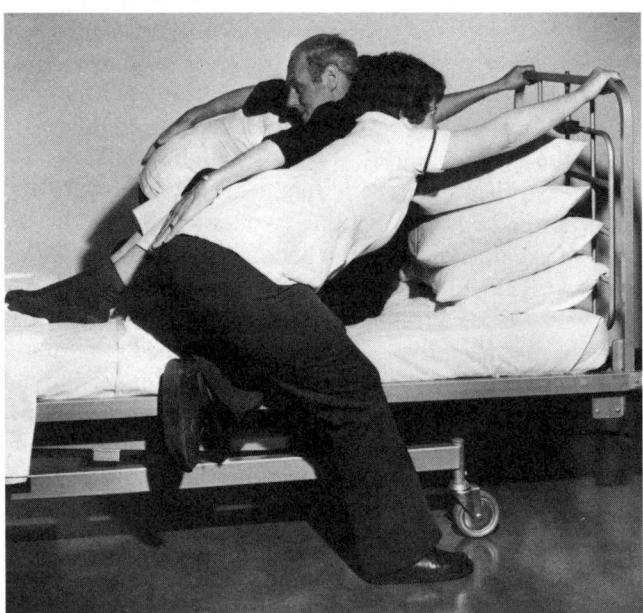

Figure 28-42. Shoulder lift using headboard. Minimal back strain for nurses. (Photograph courtesy of Margaret Scholey and *Nursing Times*.)

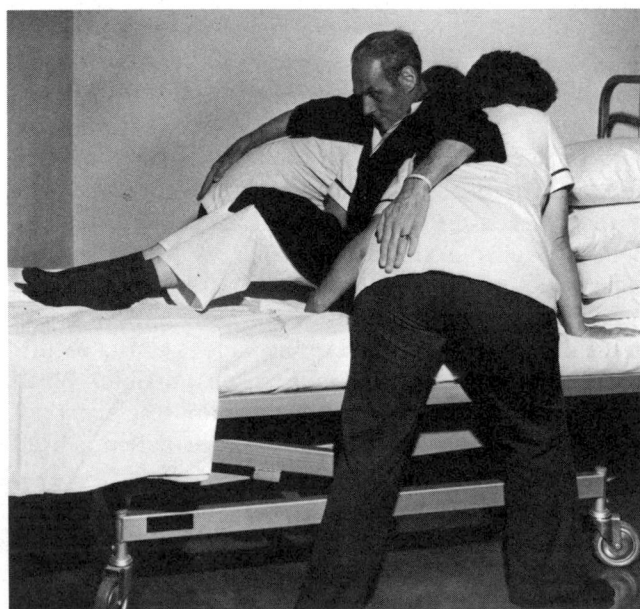

Figure 28-43. Shoulder lift when unable to reach the headboard. Nurses pivot weight over arm braced on mattress. (Photograph courtesy of Margaret Scholey and *Nursing Times*.)

Nursing Skill 28–2   Moving Patient Up or Down in Bed (No Patient Assistance)—Two Lifters

Procedure	Explanation
1. Face opposite direction of movement.*	1. Allows use of pulling force in biceps and thighs, as body weight shifted.
2. One nurse on each side of the bed.	2. Maintains patient in middle of bed so each nurse has minimum reach.
3. Foot close to bed is back, and far foot is forward 1½ ft. Front foot is parallel to bed; rear foot points toward side of bed at a 60 to 90° angle to other foot. (See Figure 28–44*A*.)	3. Wide base of support and feet flat on floor increase stability.
4. Patient's knees are flexed.	4. Reduces friction of legs on bedding.
5. Each nurse places arms under patient's shoulder and thigh.	5. Balanced load.
6. Nurses' knees are flexed; backs straight.	6. Uses thigh muscles rather than back.
7. On count of three, both nurses shift their weight to the back leg. (See Figure 28–44*B*.)	7. Coordinates movement; weight shift reduces force needed to move load.
8. Patient repositioned in good alignment.	8. Preservation of function during impaired mobility or bed rest; prevention of pressure sores.

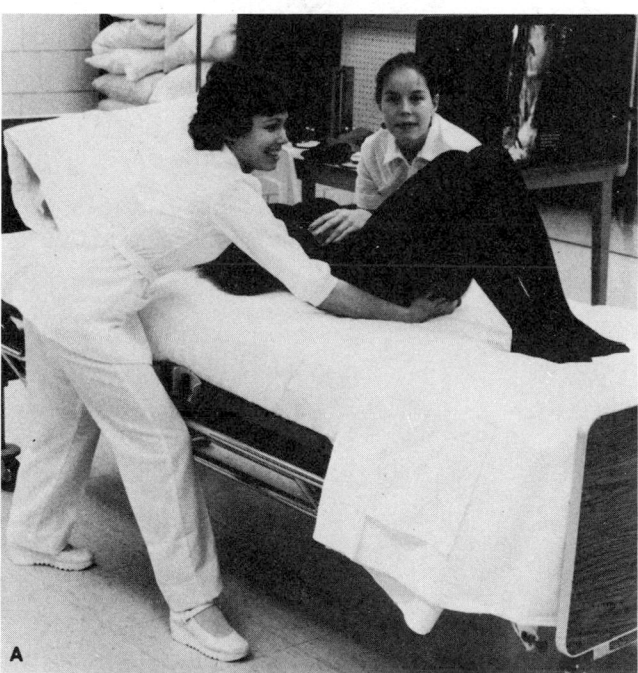 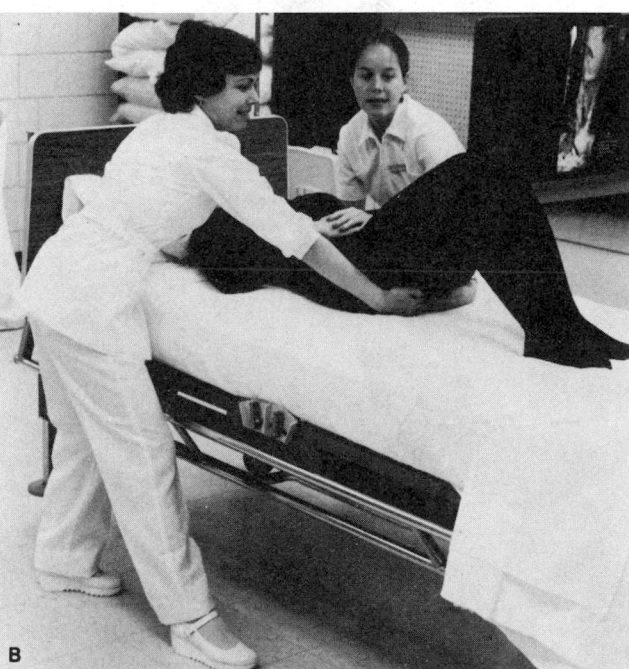

Figure 28–44.   Moving patient up in bed. **A**. Initial position. **B**. Position at completion of move.

---

*If the patient is large and the nurse's arm span is small, the nurses may be unable to support both the shoulders and thighs of the patient. In this case, both nurses would position themselves on the same side of the bed, and one nurse would support the upper body area, while the other nurse supports the lower body area. Both would face away from the direction of movement and proceed as above.

In addition, nurses with shorter arm spans may be reaching too far over their center of gravity to move a patient in the middle of the bed. The smaller nurses would first move the patient to the side of the bed, and then move the patient up or down. Following this, they would put the side rail up, go to the opposite side of the bed, and move the patient back into the middle of the bed.

Nursing Skill 28–3   **Moving Patient to Side of Bed in Supine or Prone Position—One Person**

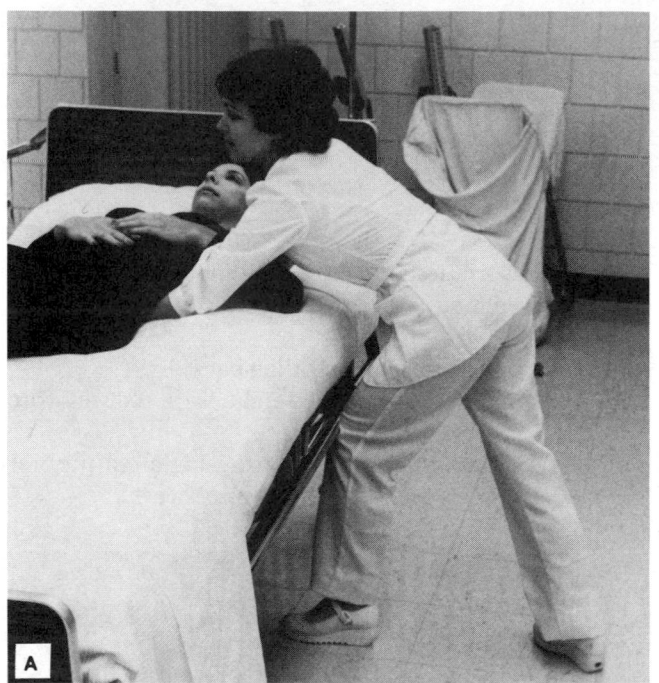

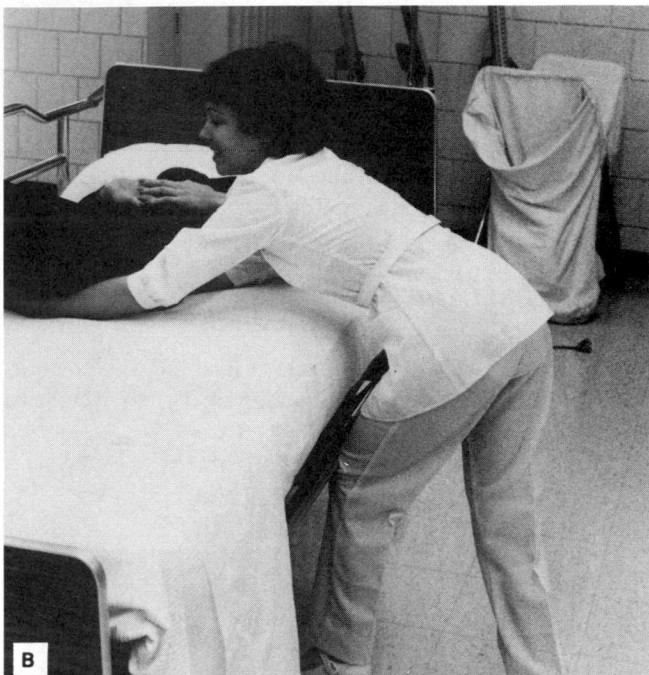

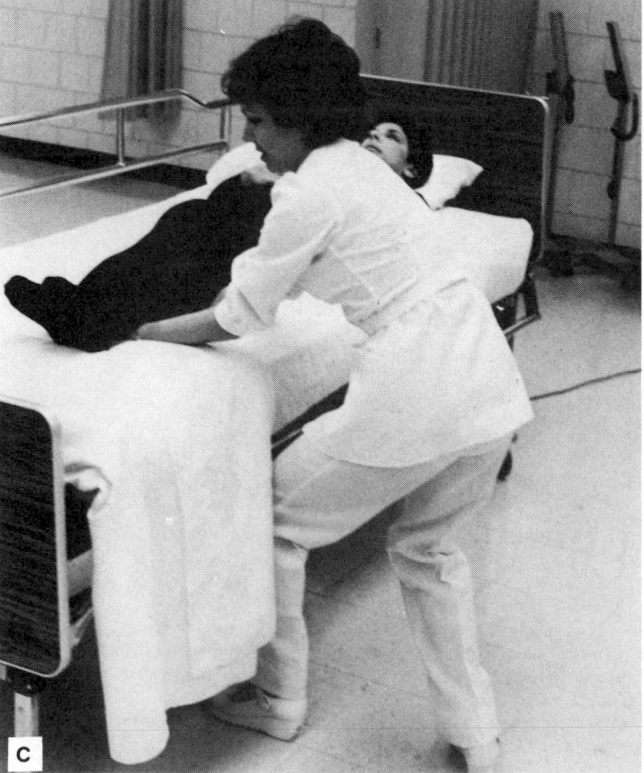

Figure 28–45. One person moving patient to side of bed. **A.** Head and shoulders moved first. **B.** Patient's midsection and hips moved next. **C.** Legs moved last, bringing patient back into alignment.

Procedure	Explanation
1. Lower bed rail on side to which patient will be moved.	1. Reaching over rail causes strain on back; moves center of gravity outside base of support.
2. Face side of bed and brace one knee against bed.	2. Knee will act as a fulcrum when weight is transferred.
3. Place feet approximately 1½ ft apart with forward foot pointing toward side of bed and back foot at a 60 to 90° angle to front foot.	3. Wide base of support for stability; keeps rear foot flat on floor when knees flexed for greater stability.
4. Reach under patient to hold head and shoulder area in one arm, lower chest area in other arm.	4. Moving approximately one-third of patient or 40 to 60 lb so force is greater than load.
5. Flex knees and shift weight to back leg while pulling with biceps and pushing against bed with knee to move patient's upper body to side of bed. (See Figure 28–45.)	5. Body weight of nurse used to help move patient to side of bed; thigh muscles and biceps create force.
6. Reach under patient to hold waist and thigh area and repeat Step 5.	6. Same as 4.
7. Reach under patient's legs and repeat Step 5.	7. Same as 4.

Two nurses may perform this move by each taking half of the patient load and proceeding as above. (See Figure 28–46.) One nurse would hold the patient's head and shoulders with one hand and upper chest with the other. The second nurse would hold the patient's waist area and thighs. On the count of three, both would shift weight and pull patient to side of bed. The lower legs would be moved as a second step if needed. With a small or light patient, one nurse may be able to move half the patient at a time, making the move in two steps.

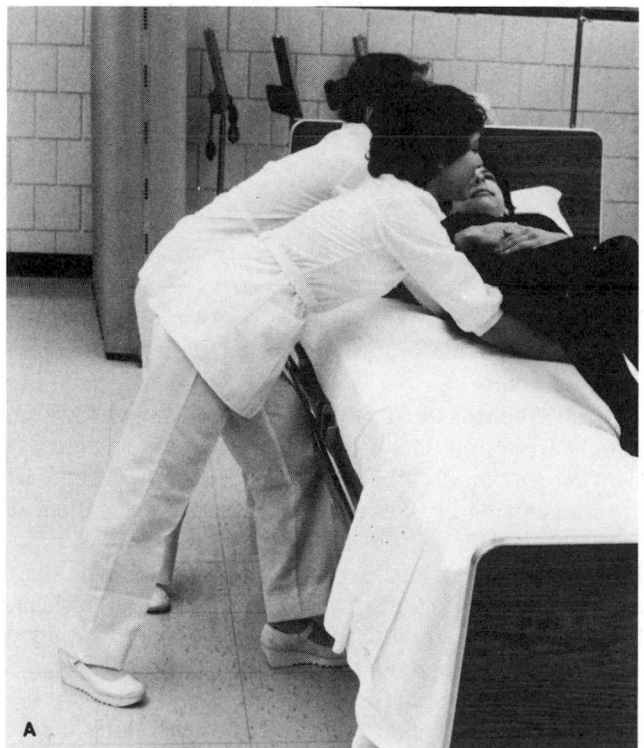
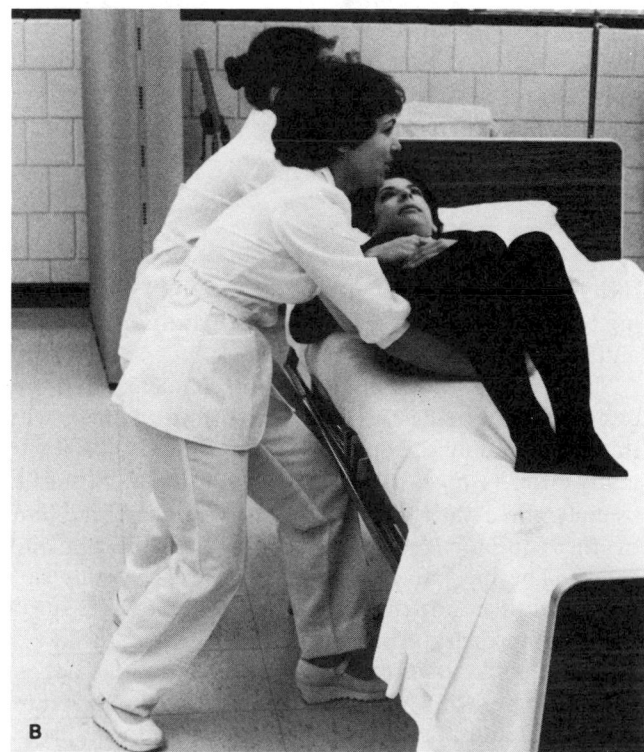

Figure 28–46.   Two people moving patient to side of bed. **A.** Nurses' weight on front legs. **B.** Weight shifted to back legs as patient moved to side of bed.

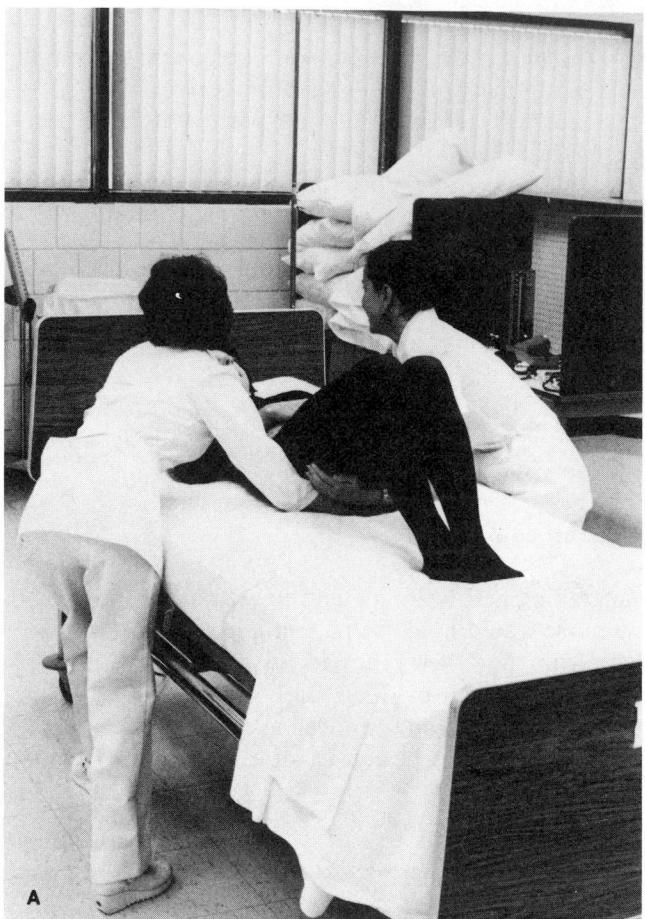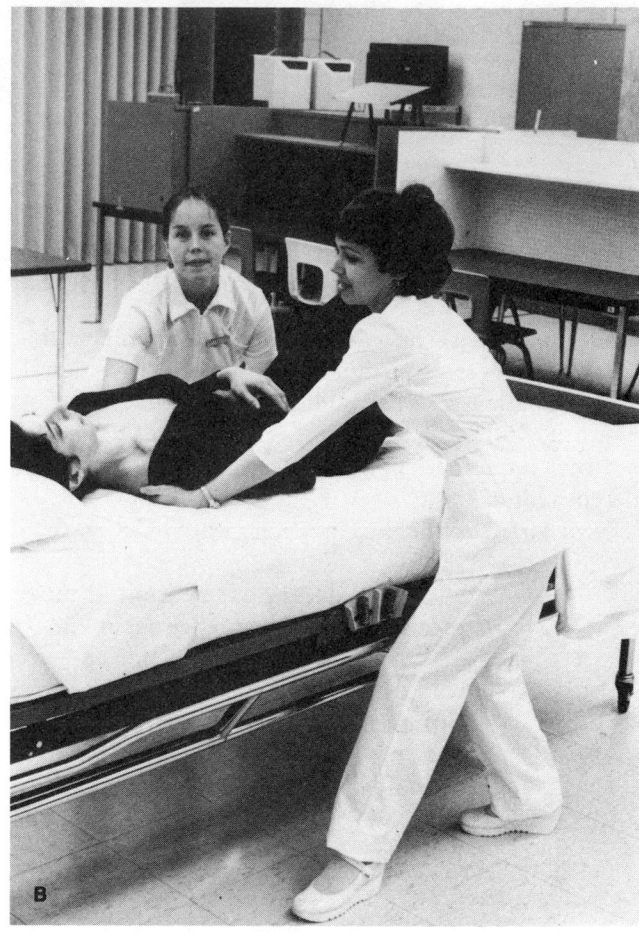

Figure 28–47. **A.** Initial position for moving a patient down in bed. Wide base of support with weight on forward leg. **B.** After move, nurse's weight on rear leg as weight was shifted to help move the load.

rarily out of alignment. (See Nursing Skill 28–3. Nursing Skills 28–4 through 28–8 present additional moving and lifting skills.)

LIFTING OR MOVING AIDS. Mechanical lifters are designed to provide the force for lifting the load with the nurse guiding the action. The maximum capacity on many lifters ranges from 300 to 400 lb. With an extremely obese patient, make sure the weight-lifting limit of the equipment is not exceeded for the patient's safety. The mechanical lifters come with various supporting devices for the patient. A sling provides maximum support for the patient from the head to the knees. A strap, like a playground swing which lifts the patient by the thighs while the patient holds on to the straps, provides minimal support. The type of support the patient will need during lifting depends on the patient's muscle strength, muscle control, and level of consciousness. One nurse is able to move the patient out of bed and into the chair or onto another bed using the me-

chanical lifter. Mechanical lifters are also available for home use operated by the patient or by another person. They help provide independence for patients with impaired mobility.

Roller boards or transfer boards are used to slide the patient from one flat surface to another, as when a patient returns on a cart from surgery. The bed and cart are moved side by side. The sheet under the patient is held on one side of the cart by one or two nurses and held on the other side, across the bed, by the two tallest nurses. The roller or transfer board is under the sheet, bridging the cart and the bed. The patient is then pulled across the board and onto the bed.

Small transfer boards are used to bridge the gap between the bed and chair. The patient then slides across the board, lifting body weight with arm muscles. The bed and chair seat are at the same height, and the arm of the chair near the bed is removed.

Nursing Skill 28–4   **Turning Patient from Supine to Lateral—One Person**

Procedure	Explanation
1. Flex the patient's far knee and put far leg over near leg.	1. Reduces friction of leg dragging over bedding.
2. Place the patient's far arm across the chest. (See Figure 28–48*A*.)	2. Prevents strain and hyperextension of shoulder joint.
3. Position feet wide apart, with front one facing side of bed and back one at a 60 to 90° angle to front foot.	3. Wide base of support for stability; keeps rear foot flat on floor when knees flexed and weight shifted.
4. Place one hand over the patient and under the far shoulder, and the other hand over the patient and under the far hip.	4. Prevents twisting patient's back during turn.
5. Flex knees and press close knee against bed as weight shifted onto back leg and patient pulled over onto side. (See Figure 28–48*B*.)	5. Body weight of nurse used to help turn patient; thigh muscles and biceps used to create force.
6. Put up side rail; go to opposite side of bed; place arms under patient's lower shoulder.	6. Patient in unstable lateral position could roll into prone position and fall off bed if side rail left down.
7. Place feet wide apart with one forward and one back at same angle as above.	7. Same as 3.

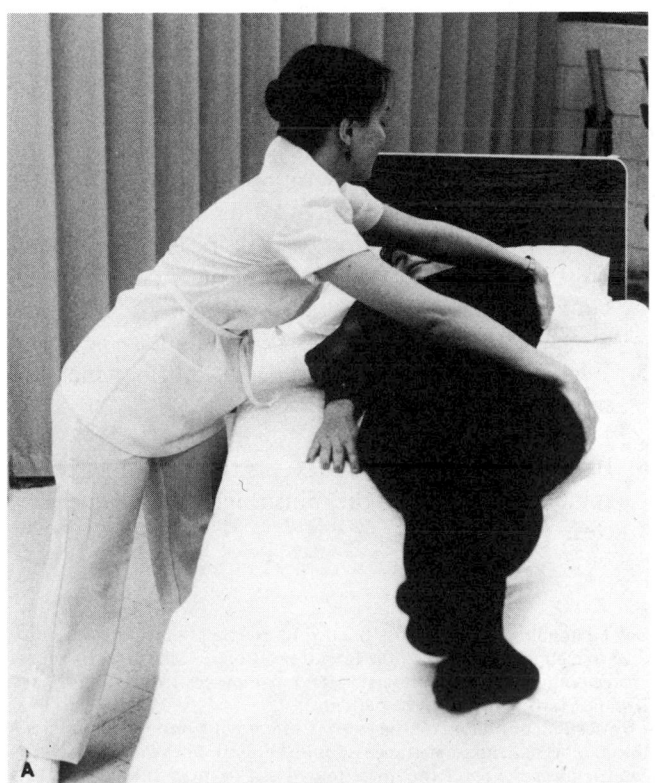 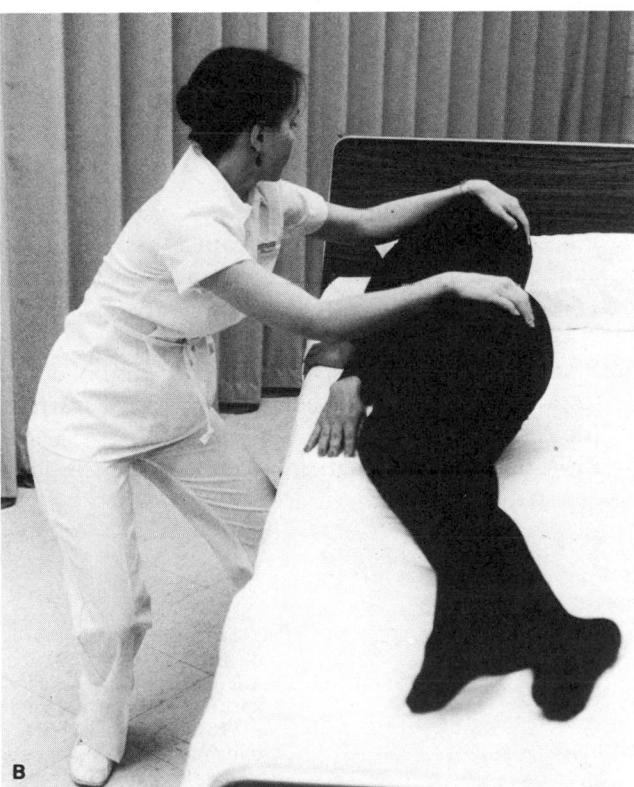

Figure 28–48. Moving a patient into the side-lying position. **A.** Weight of nurse on the front leg. Patient's far arm and leg crossed over body. **B.** Nurses' weight shifted to rear leg to turn patient onto the side.

Procedure	Explanation
8. Shift weight backward while pulling up slightly on patient's shoulder to stabilize on side.	8. Pulling shoulder and hip back stabilizes patient in lateral position and reduces tendency to roll back into supine position.
9. Repeat for hips.	9. Same as 8.
10. Reposition with supports as needed for good alignment.	10. Preservation of joint function in immobile patient.

To turn the patient from lateral to supine, back supports, if used, are removed. The patient's lower shoulders and hips are brought forward, and the patient is allowed to roll over by the force of own body weight. The nurse moves the patient's bottom shoulder and hip with a pulling action and backward shift of weight while facing the patient.

Nursing Skill 28–5   Turning Patient from Supine to Prone Position—One Person

Procedure	Explanation
1. Move the patient to the side of the bed.	1. Prevents patient from being on edge of bed at end of move.
2. Place the patient's far arm close to the body with elbow extended.	2. Patient will roll over this arm so it will not be trapped underneath body following move.
3. Cross the leg near the nurse over the far leg.	3. Reduces friction if leg were to drag across bedding.
4. Place pillows on bed next to patient as needed for abdominal or breast support in prone position.	4. Large breasts or abdomen will receive too much pressure from body weight in prone position unless body weight distributed more evenly by placing pillows above and below breasts or abdomen.
5. Place feet wide apart, (1½ ft), one forward pointing toward side of bed, one behind at 60° angle to front foot.	5. Wide base of support and feet flat on floor increase stability.
6. Place one hand near patient's shoulder and one hand near patient's thigh.*	6. Balanced force on load prevents twisting of patient's spine. Uses body weight, plus thigh and triceps muscles.

---

*The nurse with a short arm span may be unable to reach across the bed to exert a pulling force to move the patient from the far side of the bed in a supine position to the lateral position. In this case, the nurse will use a pushing motion with the force coming from the thighs as the nurse moves from a well-flexed knee position to an upright position, while exerting force on the patient.

The patient may be able to assist by pushing or pulling on the side rails in moving into the lateral position from the prone or supine position. The patient's assistance should be used whenever possible. It makes the patient feel less helpless and reduces the force the nurse must exert to move the patient. It is also a form of exercise for the muscles of the patient's arms.

7. a. Turn patient onto far side by shifting weight forward and pushing on shoulder and hip area.

or

b. After moving patient to side of bed, put up side rail; go to other side of bed; reach across bed; grasp patient behind shoulders and thigh area; shift weight backward and pull patient over onto side.

Continue pulling (7b) or pushing (7a), and allow patient to roll onto abdomen.

7. Uses body weight, plus thigh and triceps muscles.

Uses body weight, plus thigh and biceps muscles.

Uses patient's body weight to reduce force needed for move.

The patient may be turned from a prone to a supine position by reversing the actions used in moving the patient from a supine to a prone position. The patient is first moved to the side of the bed in the prone position. The nurses hold the patient under the shoulder, under the breasts, and under the hip area in moving to the side of the bed. The patient's arm near the nurses is tucked close to the body with the elbow extended. The far leg is crossed over the near leg at the ankles. The nurses move the patient to a lateral position by shifting their weight backward. The patient is allowed to gently roll onto the back from the lateral position by the weight of the body. The patient is then repositioned in the center of the bed.

Nursing Skill 28–6   Total Lift Transfer—Three Person Carry

Procedure	Explanation
1. Patient placed in supine position on flat bed or cart.	**1.** Maintains body alignment during transfer.
2. Cart is positioned at right angle to the bed with head area near foot of bed.	**2.** Requires least lifting time and equal movement by all lifters for smooth transfer.
3. All lifters positioned on same side of bed with one foot forward and one foot back at 60 to 90° angle to front foot. The leg nearest the cart to which the patient will be moved is the front leg. (See Figure 28–49*A*.)	**3.** Wide base of support and both feet on floor provide stability. Allows nurses to turn toward cart without crossing legs.
4. Patient's arms are placed across the chest.	**4.** Protects arms and reduces friction if dragged across bedding.
5. Tallest nurse places one arm under patient's head and shoulders. Second nurse places arms under waist and thighs. Third and shortest nurse places one arm under upper legs and one under lower legs.	**5.** Prevents flexing patient's back or placement in Trendelenburg position during move; distribution of load among lifters.
6. Patient moved to side of bed or cart.	**6.** Load close to lifter's center of gravity to reduce force needed to lift.
7. Nurses rest elbows on bed and roll patient into their arms, supported against their chests. Patient rolled on count of three. (See Figure 28–49*B*.)	**7.** Elbow used as fulcrum with nurses' body weight counterbalancing patient load; load close to center of gravity of lifters.
8. On the count of three, all nurses shift weight to back leg as patient is lifted from the bed.	**8.** Use of thigh muscles and body weight; counting coordinates action.

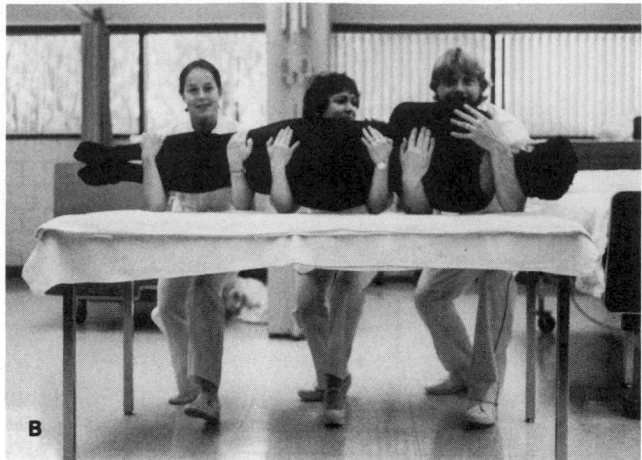

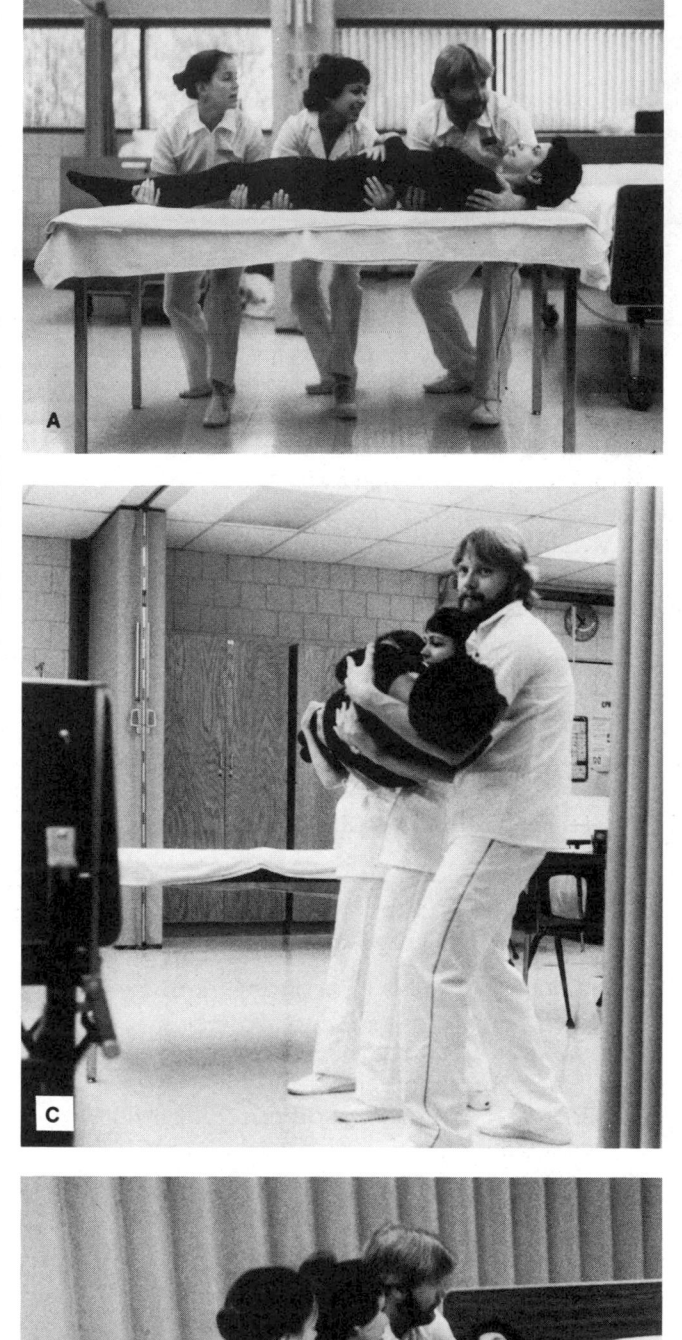

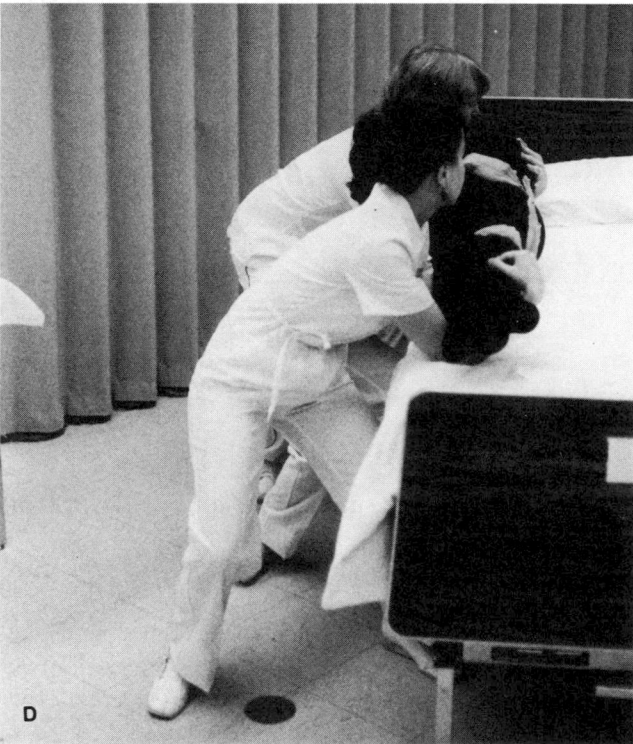

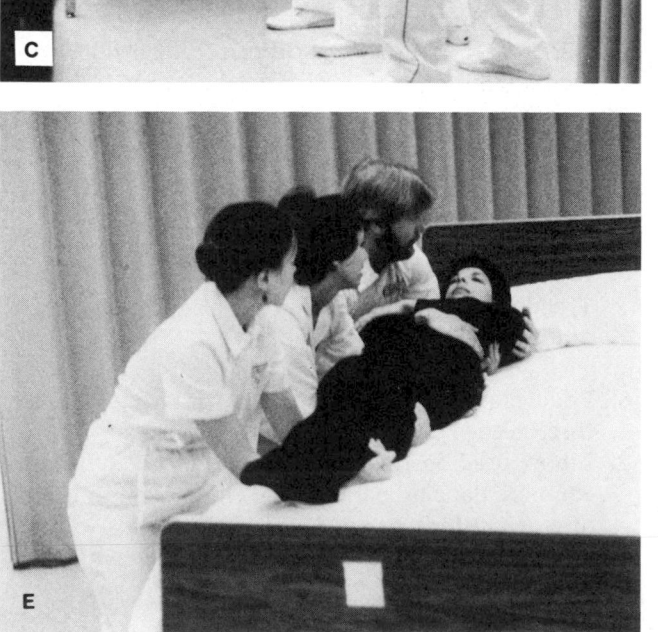

Figure 28–49.   Three-person carry. **A.** All nurses have a wide base of support, with tallest nurse at patient's head. **B.** Patient brought close to nurse's body as weight shifted to rear leg. **C.** Nurses carry patient from table to bed with coordinated stepping movements. **D.** Nurses maintain wide base of support, and use arm and leg muscles to lower patient to bed. **E.** Nurses relax arms and patient rolls into supine position.

Procedure	Explanation
9. As one nurse calls out "step," all nurses move one step backward and take steps forward to reach cart. (See Figure 28–49C.)	9. Coordination of effort.
10. Original foot stance resumed.	10. Wide base of support for stability.
11. Nurses lower elbows to cart by slowly flexing knees. (See Figure 28–49.)	11. Use of thigh muscles with straight back to prevent strain on lifters.
12. On count of three, all nurses relax arms slowly as patient rolls onto the cart in a supine position.	12. Coordinated activity; use of patient's body weight to reduce load on lifters.
13. Nurses remove arms from under patient and position in middle of cart as needed and put up side rails.	13. Patient protected from possible fall if on edge of cart and side rails in down position.

Nursing Skill 28-7   Moving Patient into Sitting Position at Side of Bed—One Person

Procedure	Explanation
1. Move patient to side of bed.	1. Edge of bed will not interfere with flexion of patient's knee while sitting.
2. Elevate head of bed to maximum point, putting patient in a high Fowler's position.	2. Reduces force patient or nurse must exert to achieve move.
3. Assist patient to move legs off side of bed with heels and lower legs dangling.	3. Uses weight of patient's lower legs to counterbalance weight of upper body, reducing force needed to achieve position.

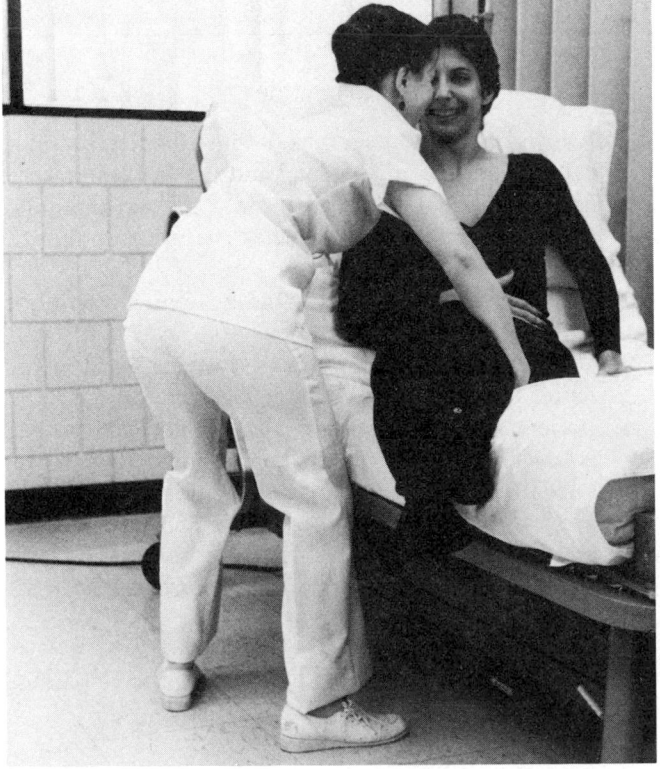

Figure 28-50. Patient being assisted into a sitting position at the side of the bed. Nurse's arms around patient's shoulders and under knees as nurse shifts weight downward to pivot patient into sitting position.

Procedure	Explanation
4. Face head of bed with front foot pointing toward headboard and foot close to bed pointing toward side of bed at 60 to 90° angle from front foot.	4. Wide base of support for stability.
5. Feet placed wide apart (1½ ft).	5. Same as #4.
6. Place far arm around patient's shoulders; arm near bed placed under patient's knees.	6. Distribution of load to prevent twisting patient's back during move.
7. As patient pushes up from bed with one arm (if able), the nurse bends the knees, shifting weight downward and swinging patient's legs down and shoulders up. (See Figure 28–50.)	7. Uses nurse's and patient's weight to reduce load on biceps and triceps of nurse and patient during move.
8. Patient supported at side of bed by shoulders with feet flat on floor.	8. Weakness or dizziness from sudden position change may lead to dizziness and falls if patient unsupported.

To return the patient to a Fowler's position in the bed, the entire process is reversed. This time, the nurse uses the strength of the thigh muscles while rising from a flexed knee position to move the patient's legs and shoulders back onto the bed. The shoulders are simultaneously lowered back down on the bed as the legs come up. The patient is then positioned as needed. The weight of the patient's upper body going back down on the mattress counterbalances the weight of the legs, reducing the nurse's load.

Nursing Skill 28–8   Transfer from Bed to Chair—One Person

Procedure	Explanation
1. Position chair or wheelchair next to bed on patient's strong side, (if patient has weak side).	1. Allows patient to bear weight on strong leg if applicable, reducing nurse's load and risk of falling.
2. Bring patient into a sitting position at the side of the bed.	2. Enables patient participation as much as possible; allows assessment for dizziness before standing to decrease risk of falls.
3. Put transfer belt around patient's waist and secure.	3. Provides safe, balanced hold on patient without stressing joints or limbs.
4. Nurse's feet are wide apart, one foot pointing toward side of bed, the other toward chair.	4. Wide base of support and both feet flat on floor for better stability.
5. Brace patient's close knee with front leg; nurse's other leg is back to create wide base of support.	5. Patient's knee may be unable to hold body weight if leg muscles are weak; bracing knee prevents the knee from flexing which could result in a fall.
6. Patient's arms are positioned on nurse's shoulders.	6. Moves part of load and prevents backward pull of arms if hyperextension of shoulder occurs.
7. Nurse's knees are well flexed with back straight, hands gripping each side of transfer belt.	7. Reduces back strain, use of thigh muscles.
8. On count of three, nurse shifts weight backward and pushes up with thigh muscles as patient exerts effort to stand. The nurse pulls up on the transfer belt to assist the patient's efforts. (See Figure 28–51A, B.)	8. Coordinated efforts of nurse and patient; use of thighs, biceps, and weight of nurse to move patient load.

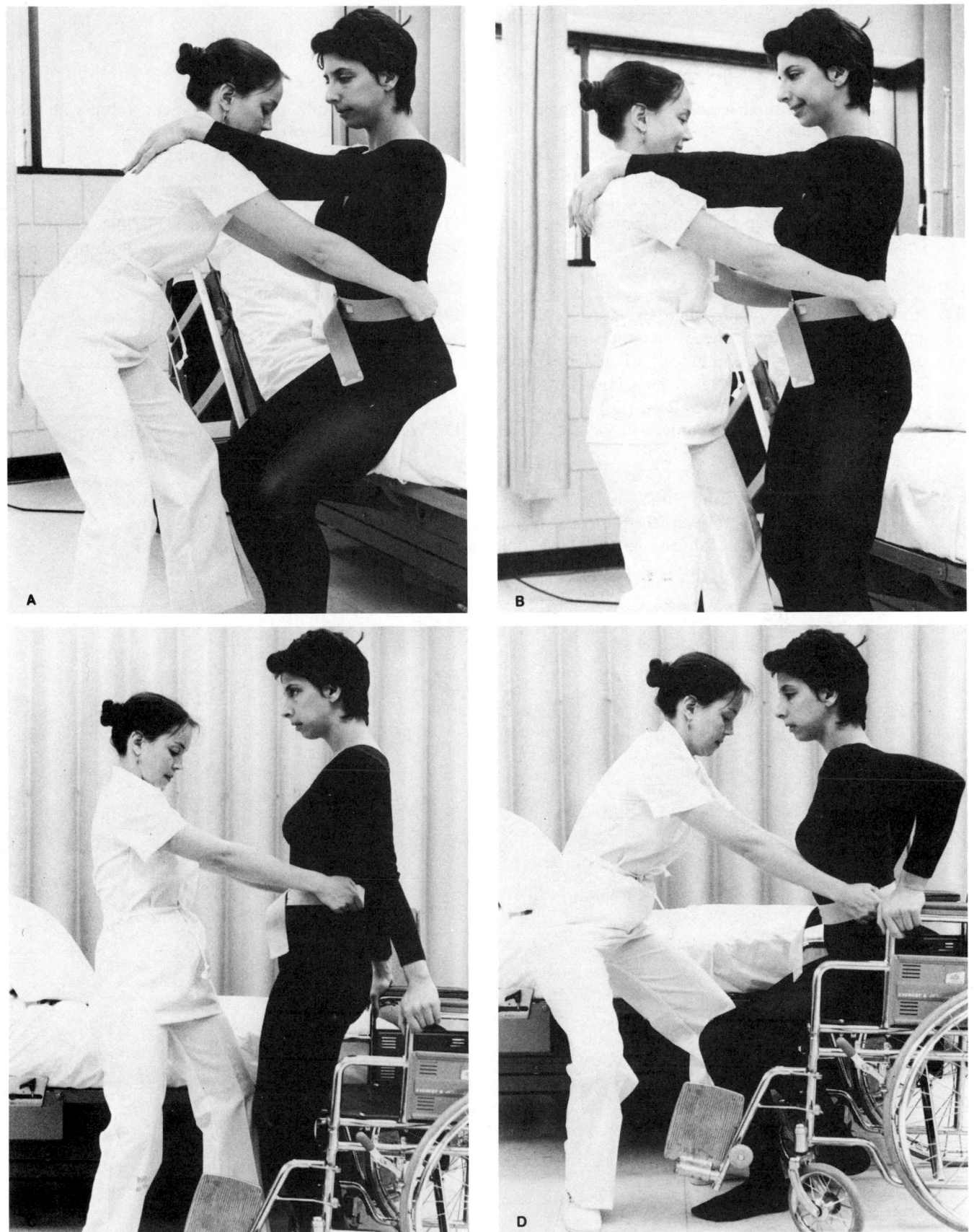

Figure 28–51. Assisting a patient from the bed to a chair (standing pivot transfer). Nurse holds transfer belt, (**A**) braces patient's knee, and shifts weight backward as patient stands. **B**. Nurse supports patient by transfer belt at bedside keeping knee braced. **C**. Nurse and patient pivot turn, and patient uses armrests to lower herself into chair as nurse continues to brace knee. **D**. Nurse keeps back straight with knees flexed and wide base of support as patient sits.

Procedure	Explanation
9. Patient asked to move leg closest to wheelchair forward (if possible).	9. Wider base of support for patient stability and feet in position for pivot turn.
10. Nurse and patient pivot turn so nurse is facing chair and patient's back is toward chair; nurse still holding transfer belt. (See Figure 28–51C.)	10. Least effort for nurse and patient.
11. Patient reaches down and grips armrests; backs of legs touching chair.	11. Use of patient's biceps, when possible, and assurance that chair is in place; use of thigh muscles to lower patient gradually to chair; knee braced prevents forward slipping.
12. As patient eases self into chair using armrests for support, nurse braces one of patient's knees with own knee and nurse's feet block patient's foot from sliding forward. Nurse flexes own knees to lower patient into chair. (See Figure 28–51D.)	12. Same as 11.
13. Patient supported in wheelchair as needed.	13. Weakened patient may fall out of chair or have poor body alignment without support.

To move the patient from the chair to the bed, the entire procedure is reversed. This time, however, the patient's strong side should be positioned closest to the bed, so the wheelchair or chair will have to be placed at the opposite end of the bed or on the opposite side as when the patient got out of bed.

Ambulation

Progressive Ambulation. Early progressive ambulation helps to prevent the development of complications associated with immobility. Patients are often helped to get out of bed the same day as surgery. Patient safety from falls is a primary concern when helping patients ambulate after surgery or after a period of bed rest. Orthostatic hypotension, weakness, pain, and medications all increase the patient's risk of falling. The patient progresses from bed rest to fully ambulatory at an individual pace based on ability.

When the nurse is assisting with ambulation, the following suggestions may be helpful:

1. Timing. Consider when the patient would like to attempt ambulation and your other patient care responsibilities. Ambulating a patient for the first time may be a slow process, and if several other treatments for other patients are due at the same time, the patient and the nurse will feel rushed. If the patient is in a great deal of pain, providing an analgesic medication at least one-half hour prior to ambulating will make the effort less stressful. If two people will be needed to ambulate safely a large or very weak patient, make sure another person is available when choosing a time with a patient.

2. Transfer belts. The use of transfer belts when ambulating a patient provides the nurse with a safe, secure hold on the patient without pulling at the patient's limbs or joints. The transfer belt is secured around the patient's waist and held at each side to help lift and stabilize the patient.

3. Sit the patient with legs off bed before asking patient to stand. By letting the patient sit on the edge of the bed before standing, the nurse can assess the patient for any signs of dizziness or faintness. If these feelings are present and do not clear after sitting for several minutes, the patient is not ready to ambulate because of the risk of falling. Help the patient to lie back down and try again later. The use of elastic support stockings may be helpful in alleviating this obstacle to ambulation. If the patient reports no unusual feelings after sitting for a brief time, begin to ambulate the patient.

4. The patient should stand by the bed before beginning to walk. Again the nurse is assessing the patient for any sign of dizziness or faintness. The bed is close enough for the nurse to sit the patient down should the patient start to faint or fall. If the patient feels fine after standing by the bed for a brief time, walking to a chair in the room is appropriate. If the patient walks to the chair without problems, then walking in the room is planned for the next ambulation. If the patient walks in the room without problems, then walking in the hall is attempted later.

5. Listen to the patient. If patients say they had bet-ter go back to bed, believe them and help them back to bed. If the patient begins to feel faint during the walk, ask someone else to get a wheelchair. Watch the patient's color and ask for data about how the patient is feeling during the walk so signs of fatigue or possible fainting are recognized quickly. Shorter, more frequent periods of walking are more beneficial than infrequent, fatiguing walks. If the patient begins to faint, use the transfer belt to gently lower the patient to the floor.

6. If assistive devices are used by the patient for walking, make sure they are in good repair with nonskid tips. Assess the patent's use of walkers, canes, or crutches for correct technique.

7. Explain to the patient the benefits of early ambulation and that assistance and pain relief are available to make the activity as easy as possible.

8. Protect any tubes from pulling during ambulation.

9. Encourage family or friends to walk with the patient if there is minimal risk of falling. The family may feel more helpful, and it also increases the stimulation in the patient's environment.

10. Have the patient walk in shoes, when possible, rather than in slippers, which are more likely to slip on waxed floors.

Ambulating Patients Needing Assistive Devices. Assistive devices are any type of aid a patient uses when attempting to walk. Crutches, canes, walkers, and braces are common assistive devices. Patients with casts, knee surgery, amputations, and paralysis or muscle weakness in one or both legs will use assistive devices on a temporary or permanent basis. Some patients are afraid of using the equipment for fear of falling. Others may be afraid of becoming dependent on the equipment and never regaining full muscle use. Some people may refuse to use visible assistive devices because it reduces their self-esteem and they are afraid to let other people see them using such equipment. The nurse can listen to the patient's concerns and accept them as important. Yet, the benefits of getting out of bed and rebuilding muscle strength are an important part of the patient's recovery. Patients cannot be physically forced to ambulate against their will, so motivating patients to cooperate is a first step.

Explanation of the device and how it works will be helpful to the patient who is ready to learn assisted ambulation. Seeing others who are successfully walking using the assistive device correctly is also very helpful in learning to use the equipment.

WALKERS. Walkers are held continuously by the patient during ambulation. The walker is lifted, advanced, and set down. The patient then moves the feet until they are up close to the walker. The walker is then

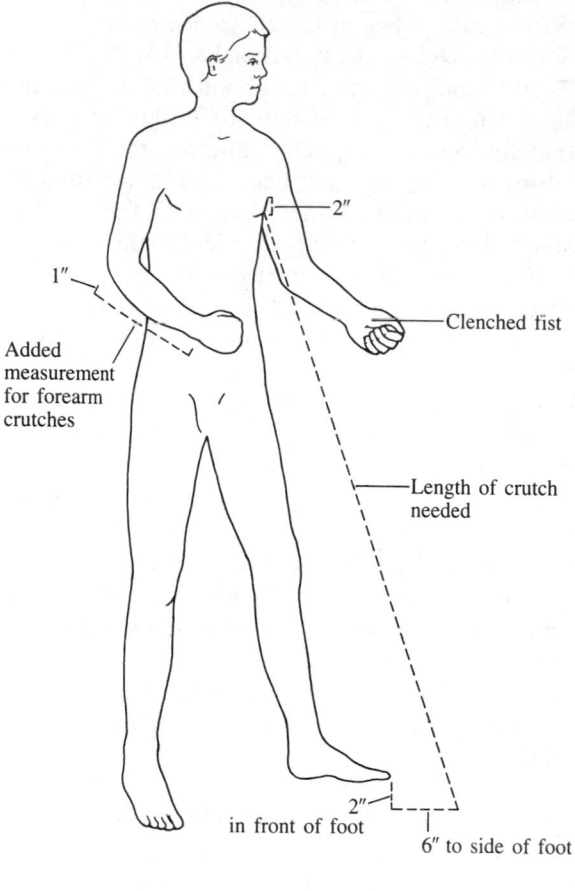

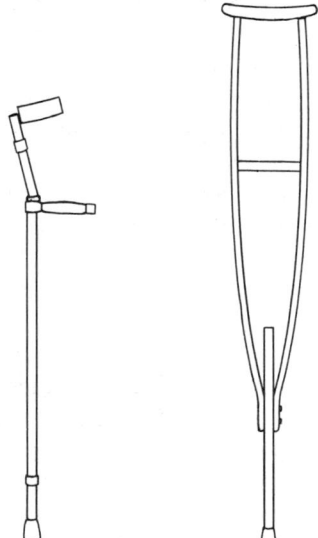

Figure 28–52. Measurements of crutches.

CRUTCHES. Crutches are used to support all or part of the body weight during ambulation. Upper body strength is used to work the action of the crutches. The fit of the crutches depends on the type of crutch being used. One type fits under the patient's axilla. This crutch should be measured from 2 inches under the patient's axilla to 6 inches in front of the toe of the shoe and 2 inches away from the outer border of the shoe. (See Figure 25–52.) The other type of crutch does not come to the axilla but ends just below the elbow. The length is measured in the same way as the other crutches, but the distance from the clenched fist to 1 inch below the elbow is also needed. The handgrips for both types of crutches are measured by having the patient clench the fist and extend the wrist slightly. The elbow is flexed 30 degrees up from full extension to allow the patient to lift body weight by extending the elbows on the crutches. The handgrip is placed at the level of the clenched fist, measured up from the floor position 6 inches in front and to the side of the patient's foot.

Crutch Gaits

THE FOUR-POINT GAIT   (left crutch, right leg, right crutch, left leg). (See Figure 28–53.) This is the safest gait for people using two crutches because it provides the most stability, with a large base of support. The patient requires enough strength to lift the crutch off the floor at the handgrip, while keeping the elbow straight. The patient must also be able to move both feet forward and straighten the knees. There are always three contact points with the floor in this gait, making it stable but slow since the patient makes four separate moves to advance two steps.

1. Start with feet slightly apart with both crutches in front of and to the side of each foot. Weight on both feet and both crutches.
2. Weight shifted off one crutch which is moved forward a small step's distance.
3. Weight shifted onto both crutches and foot on same side as advanced crutch.

Four Point Gait with Crutches

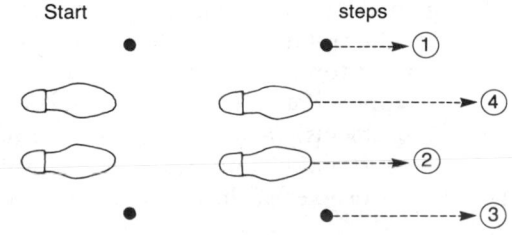

Figure 28–53. Four-point gait with crutches.

picked up and advanced further. The walker has a four-point base for support and stands alone. Walkers are often used by patients who need only slight support or added stability to walk.

4. Opposite foot advanced one step.
5. Weight shifted to both legs and forward crutch.
6. Rear crutch advanced slightly beyond other crutch.
7. Weight shifted to both crutches and forward foot.
8. Rear foot advanced.
9. Steps 2 through 8 repeated.

TWO-POINT GAIT   (right leg and left crutch, left leg and right crutch). (See Figure 28–54.) This type of gait is used by people who have good balance and is a much faster-paced walk. There are only two points in contact with the floor, rather than three as in the four-point gait.

1. Weight on both legs and both crutches to start walking.
2. Weight shifted to one leg and opposite crutch.
3. Opposite foot and crutch are simultaneously advanced one step.
4. Weight shifted to advanced foot and crutch.
5. Back crutch and foot moved ahead of other foot and crutch.
6. Steps 2 through 5 repeated.

THREE-POINT GAIT   (both crutches, step with one leg, both crutches). (See Figure 28–55.) The three-point gait is used by people who cannot bear any weight on one leg but can bear full weight on the other, such as amputees or patients after knee surgery. This type of walk only maintains one or two points on the floor so the patient may be balanced briefly on one leg. More upper body strength is required for this gait compared to the other types, but it is fairly rapid in pace. When the patient steps through the crutches rather than just to them the pace is even more rapid, but more strength is required. The patient often learns to move to the crutches first and later moves through them as performance improves.

Two Point Gait with Crutches

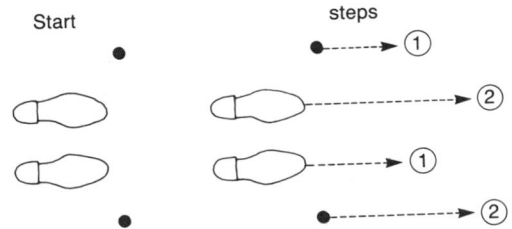

Figure 28–54.   Two-point gait with crutches.

Three Point Gait with Crutches

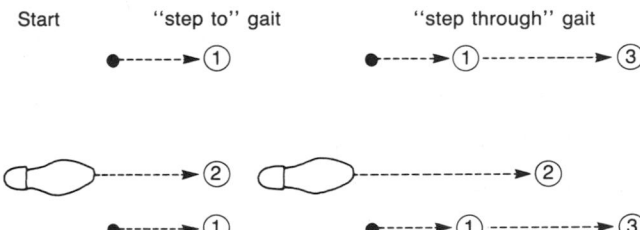

Figure 28–55.   Three-point gait with crutches.

1. Weight on strongest leg and both crutches to start.
2. All weight shifted to strongest leg.
3. Both crutches advanced simultaneously, approximately 5 inches.
4. Weight shifted off leg onto both crutches.
5. Foot on strongest leg advanced to point where toe is even with crutches for the "step to" technique. The foot is advanced until the heel of the foot is several inches ahead of the crutches in the "step through" technique.
6. Weight shifted back to strongest leg to repeat steps 2 through 5.

PARTIAL WEIGHT-BEARING GAIT   (Both crutches and weaker leg, step with normal leg). (See Figure 28–56.) This gait is used by persons who are able to bear some weight on their affected leg but not amounts equal to their strong leg, such as people with casts or joint replacements or those learning to use an artificial leg.

1. Weight mostly on strongest leg, some on affected leg, and crutches at rest.
2. Weight shifted to strongest leg.
3. Both crutches and affected leg advance one step, simultaneously.
4. Weight shifted to crutches and affected leg.
5. Strongest leg takes normal step until heel even with position of crutches.
6. Steps 2 through 5 repeated.

Partial Weight Bearing Gait with Crutches

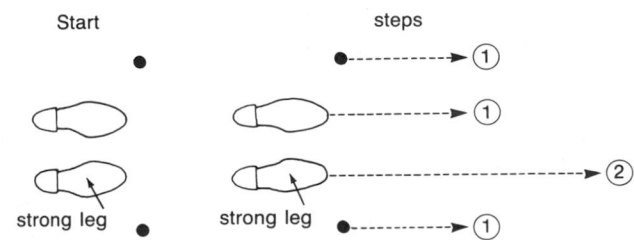

Figure 28–56.   Partial weight-bearing gait with crutches.

Hemiplegic Gait with Cane

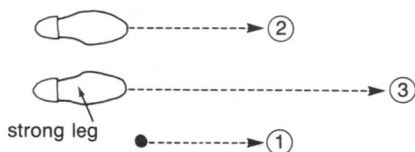

Figure 28–57.   Hemiplegic gait with cane.

In all of the other gaits, the stronger leg is advanced first, followed by the weaker leg, except in the partial weight-bearing gait, where the weak leg is advanced first.

CANES.   Canes are helpful to people who need added balance because canes increase the base of support. Canes are not the best device for people who need help with substantial weight bearing. The length of a cane should extend from the greater trochanter felt at the hip, to the floor. The patient should be able to use the cane to balance by placing the tip about 6 inches to the side of the foot and still having the elbow slightly flexed. The cane is used on the side opposite the involved leg in a hemiplegia patient, because of muscle weakness in the upper extremity as well as the leg.

Cane-Supported Gait (for Hemiplegia) (See Figure 28–57.)

1. Weight on both legs, cane at side for support.
2. Cane moved ahead about 4 inches, but kept to the side.
3. Weight shifted to strong leg and cane.
4. Affected weaker leg steps forward one small step.
5. Weight shifted to affected leg.
6. Strong leg moved forward small step; cane remains stationary.
7. Steps 2 through 6 repeated.

Interpretation and Management of the Environment

Sudden loss of vision, hearing, tactile sense, or mobility is most likely to cause problems for the patient with interpretation and interaction with the environment. Performing activities, communicating with others, and remaining oriented to time and place often depend on the nurse interpreting the environment for the patient. Sights, sounds, equipment, personnel, and activities are communicated to the patient through the nurse. In addition to talking with the patient about the type of help that will be required for normal daily activities, such as eating, washing, and dressing, the nurse has

a role in preserving the patient's sense of time and place. Providing clocks that the patient can see, hear chime, or feel will enable the patient to follow the passage of time without reliance on others. Telling the patient when things will occur, such as mealtime or therapy, will help the patient plan the day. Calendars in the rooms that are marked off each day and discussed with patients in terms of recent past and future events are also helpful in maintaining patients' sense of time. One of the most helpful elements in remaining oriented to time is a window through which the patient can watch the changing activity and light patterns. Exposure to light and dark will help the patient maintain normal circadian rhythms (wake-sleep patterns). Enabling the bed patient to see out the window is also a diversional activity to keep the mind and sense of vision more active. For this reason, rearrangement of room furniture to help meet the patient's stimulation needs would take priority over the institution's standard placement of beds and furniture.

Touching the patient who has tactile sense is another way of increasing the stimulation to the brain and helping the patient remain in contact with reality, when vision, hearing, or mobility are severely impaired. Back rubs and muscle massage not only are soothing but stimulate the senses and tend to increase the level of consciousness. Conversation with the patient during these activities is another form of stimulation.

On entering the room of a patient with impaired vision, verbal communication is used to let the patient know who is there and why. Ask patients if they need any help in locating items in the room, and check the room for any obstacles that may pose a safety hazard. When bringing equipment, food, or other things into the room, explain what they are, where they are in the room, and offer the patient a chance to feel the item, if appropriate. Take the patient's hand and locate the silverware and placement of foods on the tray. Make sure packages are opened on the food tray before leaving. Ask the patient how you can best assist with activities such as eating, walking to the bathroom, and using the bedside appliances such as radio, telephone, and nurse call light.

At times, the nurse may function to reduce the stimuli reaching the patient, if the diagnosis is sensory overload. Reducing the variety of people interacting with the patient is helpful. The patient may then begin to recognize one or two familiar faces, voices, and names. Providing periods of undisturbed rest is also important since fatigue may alter perception and lead to confusion and sensory overload. Necessary physical treatments and assessments can be grouped to provide undisturbed segments of time. Speaking slowly and clearly to the patient in words the patient understands will help reduce sensory overload.

Patients may fear they are going crazy if they are experiencing hallucinations. Explaining to the patient that this is common with sensory deprivation or overload may reduce these specific fears. When patients are frightened because of loss of sensory input, altered level of consciousness, or impaired mobility, holding a hand and staying with the patient will help reduce anxiety. Just being there may calm the patient enough to avoid the need for such things as restraints or sedation.

When the patient is able to wear glasses or hearing aids safely, encourage all personnel working with the patient to assist the patient in using the lenses or hearing aid. Ask family if glasses or hearing aids were used at home, and request for them to be brought to the hospital. A patient may seem confused just because a hearing aid is in the bedside stand instead of in the patient's ear.

Assisting with Satisfaction of Other Needs

During periods of restricted mobility, sensory loss, or perceptual problems, the patient will need some assistance in meeting other needs since normal behavior is difficult or impossible. Some medications that relate to stimulation needs are presented in Table 28–10.

Nutrition and Elimination. Dehydration and weight loss increase the patient's risk of pressure sores, elimina-

tion problems, temperature-regulation problems, and oxygenation problems. When possible, place fluids of the patient's choice where they can be reached. Encourage family to bring in favorite foods. Make eating a social time, whenever possible, so the patient is not eating alone. If the food is not to the patient's liking, make a referral to the dietitian. Make sure in-between meals and snacks are given to patients who need them and not left sitting in the refrigerator for several days.

Incontinence of urine, stool, or both increases the patient's risk of pressure sores and infection. Keep the patient as clean and dry as possible. Consider a bowel-and-bladder-training program to reestablish some of the patient's control. Keep the nurse call light within reach so the patient can obtain help with elimination as needed.

Providing Restraints—A Physical Safety Need. Restraints are used only when the patient is believed to be a danger to self or to others. Confusion alone is not a justified cause for using restraints. Restraints further limit an individual's movement in bed or in a chair and, if used unnecessarily, may be a form of unlawful imprisonment. Consider the following suggestions when using restraints:

1. The patient who requires restraints is often disoriented to time and place, restless, and agitated, doing such things as kicking, biting, and swearing.

Table 28–10. **Classifications of Drugs Related to Stimulation Needs**

Eye, Ear, Nose, and Throat Preparations

Miotics used to reduce intraocular pressure in glaucoma
Mydriatics used to dilate the pupil for examination and in treatment of glaucoma
Carbonic anhydrase inhibitors used in treatment of glaucoma
Anti-infectives used in eye infections, applied topically

Local Anesthetics, General Anesthesia

Alter sensations or eliminate sensations from skin, muscle, tendons, and joints, increasing
  risk of pressure-sore development and disorientation
Decrease spontaneous movements, leading to unrelieved pressure on skin and deeper tissue

Autonomic Drugs

Parasympathomimetic (cholinergic) agents used to treat glaucoma
Skeletal muscle relaxants used to treat spasticity in muscle-nerve disease or trauma

Central Nervous System Drugs

Analgesics reduce perception of sensations
  Make patient more susceptible to pressure-sore development
  May have side effect of causing unusual sensations, impaired coordination and thinking
Tranquillizers, sedatives, and hypnotics alter perception and level of consciousness
  May add to patient's hallucinations from sensory deprivation or overload
  May be needed to prevent harm if patient extremely confused and agitated

2. A physician's order is required to restrain a patient, but in an emergency, when danger to the patient, staff, or other patients is imminent, the nurse can restrain the patient temporarily. The physician's order should be obtained in writing within six hours and renewed every 24 hours, or as indicated by hospital policy.

3. Try to reorient the patient before restraints are necessary. Make sure the patient's environment includes things such as clocks, calendars, and windows so orientation to time is facilitated. Introduce yourself and others involved in caring for the patient. Explain what and why you are doing certain treatments. Encourage position changes, ambulation, and sitting in the hall to stimulate the patient's senses. "Body movement and touching can help your patient reestablish his grip on physical reality" (Misik, 1981). Correct the patient when confusion exists. Use medication such as analgesics and sleeping pills cautiously since these drugs may add to the patient's confusion. Speak slowly and clearly to the patient, and clarify any unusual sights or sounds in the environment.

4. Explain to the patient the reason for restraints and that they will be used only until the patient is able to regain control so injury is prevented. Explain to the family the need for restraints before they see the patient.

5. Use the minimum amount of restraint possible. If only the hands and fingers need restraining to prevent the patient from pulling out tubes, padded mitts may be adequate, rather than restraining the arm movement.

6. When placing a hostile patient in restraints, make sure adequate help is available to prevent injury to the nurse or the patient if a struggle develops.

7. Tie the restraints to the mattress frame, not to the side rails. If the restraint is secured to the bed frame and the patient's bed is elevated or raised into a Fowler's position, the restraints will tighten around the patient and may obstruct breathing. If tied to the side rails, the restraints will become too tight when the side rails are lowered. The patient is able to reach and possibly untie the knot if on the side rail.

8. Use a knot that is easily untied in case the patient develops problems and must have a quick position

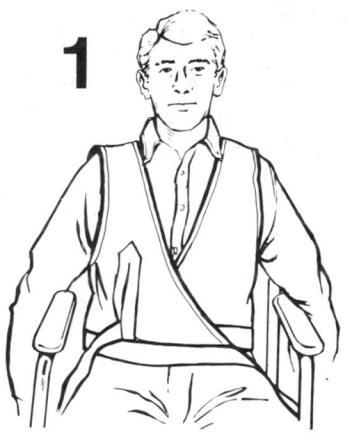

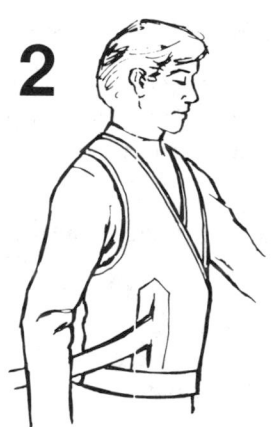

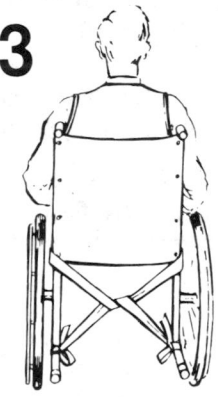

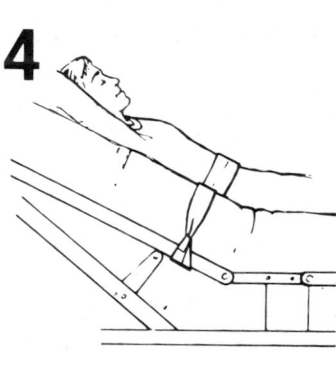

Always put the vest on so the straps criss-cross in front.

Be sure that the vest is the proper size for the patient. The vertical seams under the arm holes should be under the patient's arms. If the seam is in front of the patient's arm, the vest is too large; if in back, the vest is too small. All Posey vests are color-coded by size:

Small
 (90-110 lb., women) ... Red
Medium
 (110-150 lb., men) .. Green
Large
 (150-185 lb.) .... Yellow
Extra Large
 (185-225 lb.) .... Blue

Belts are not color-coded but are sized the same.

When used for a patient in a wheelchair, position the patient's hips at the rear of the seat, and pass vest straps through the slots at the sides of the seat. From behind the wheelchair, draw the straps toward the back, bringing them around the rear legs, crossing over each other, and then secure them to the kick spurs.
IMPORTANT: Be sure that the vest is not too tight. You should be able to place four fingers (with your hand flat) between the patient's abdomen and the bottom of the vest.

When used for a patient in bed, position the patient so that his or her hips are at the center of the bed—where they would be if the bed were elevated. Bring the straps directly over the sides of the bed, wrap once or twice around the bed spring frame, then secure the end of the straps about 6-8" toward the foot of the bed and 6-8" in from the sides of the bed. IMPORTANT: Do not angle the straps toward the head or foot of hte bed. If the patient slides up or down in bed the straps will loosen.

Figure 28–58.   Applying restraints safely. (Courtesy of the J. T. Posey Co., Arcadia, CA.)

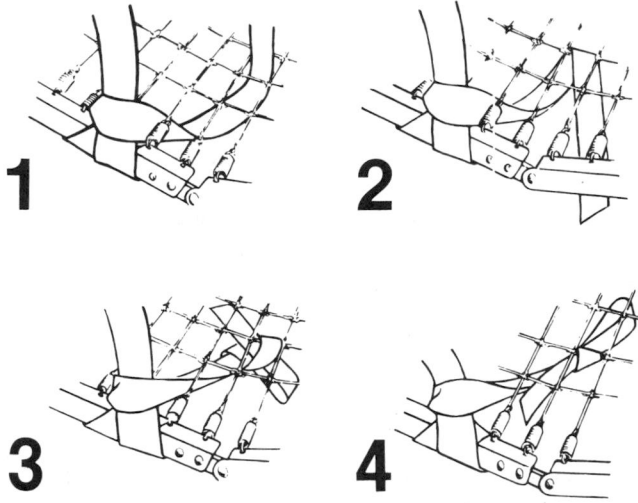

Figure 28-59. A quick-releasing knot for securing restraints. (Courtesy of the J. T. Posey Co., Arcadia, CA.)

change. (See Figure 28-59.) For locked restraints, make sure a key is kept in a visible place in the patient's room. In case of an emergency, the patient's restraint can be unlocked quickly.

9. Restraints should be loose enough to allow several fingers between the patient and the restraint so circulation is not impaired.

10. Patients will need range-of-motion exercises to restrained joints with assessment of the skin for redness or irritation.

11. A patient who has decreased level of consciousness and poor control of secretions in the respiratory tract may aspirate and is restrained in the lateral position so secretions can drain out the mouth.

Promoting Healing of Pressure Sores—A Physical Safety Need. The first step in helping pressure sores heal is to remove the cause of the injury which is pressure, friction, or the shearing force created when someone slips down in bed or in a chair. The patient is not positioned on top of the pressure sore. The patient is not to sit in positions that put pressure on the sore. The frequency of turning and repositioning is increased to every hour or every half hour to prevent formation of additional sores. Attention to adequate nutrition, fluids, and elimination of soiled or damp surfaces contacting the skin receives additional effort. Wound cultures are often taken to check for infection.

To heal, a wound requires oxygen, glucose, and a moist, protein-rich environment of body fluids. This enables epithelial cells to migrate into the damaged area and reproduce. Adhesive, transparent occlusive dressings are now being used to heal pressure sores and show the most promise for facilitating rapid wound healing.

Fluids from the wound are encouraged to accumulate under the transparent tape because they are sealed in by the occlusive dressing. Air and water vapor pass through the dressing. The wound may actually look worse to nurses who prefer clean, dry wounds, but the moist fluids under the dressing serve as a growth medium for healthy epithelial cells.

The tape is placed over the pressure sore after the sore has been cleaned and rinsed well in normal saline. Several inches of tape reach onto healthy tissue all around the wound when the correct-size dressing is applied. The dressing is removed when it begins to fall off naturally. The dressing is not changed routinely several times each day, as was the case with gauze dressings since this destroys the environment of body fluids and cells under the tape. Table 28-11 describes some common techniques for treating pressure sores and identifies some that may interfere with healing rather than facilitate it.

Involving the Patient in Prevention—A Self-Esteem Need. One of the best ways to help patients avoid some of the complications associated with immobility and sensory loss is to actively involve them in prevention of further problems. This gives the patient a greater sense of control over self and the environment. The patient will be able to take responsibility for some areas of recovery. An active, rather than a passive, role in recovery leads to increased self-esteem as a competent partner in establishing a state of maximum health.

The patient may be capable of performing some exercises and position changes without the nurse's help if the reason for these activities is understood. Teaching the patient about pressure sores and how to relieve pressure several times an hour will complement the nurse's

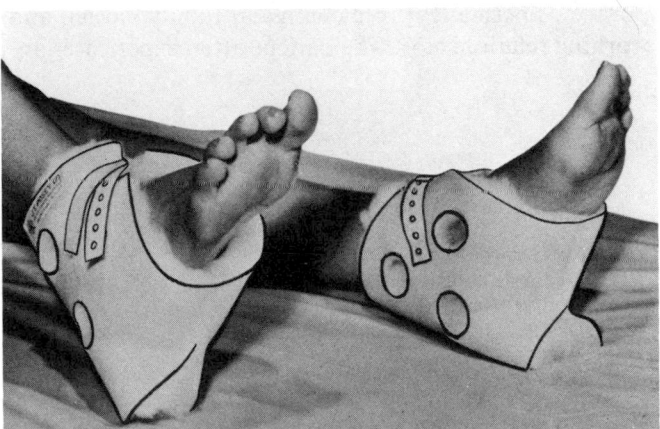

Figure 28-60. Heel protectors. These will decrease friction between the heels and bedding and reduce pressure as a preventive technique for pressure sores. (Photograph courtesy of J. T. Posey Co., Arcadia, CA.)

Table 28–11. **Nursing Interventions Used to Help Pressure Sores Heal**

Adhesive transparent occlusive dressings (OP-SITE) (TAGADERM)	Principle of moist healing; permeable to air and water vapor but seals in body fluids; no dressing change needed until dressing begins to leak or falls off naturally; dressing left in place for several days; may be used even if pressure sore infected; newest treatment showing rapid healing with minimal nursing intervention; healing begins after 6 hours under occlusive dressing, compared to 18 hours under a scab (Torrance, 1981c,d; Ahmed, 1982)
Massage of preulcer area (reddened area of skin caused by unrelieved pressure)	Not recommended; potential for causing further damage to tissues and small capillaries; better healing and decreased pressure-sore formation without massage of area reddened from pressure (Dyson, 1978)
Elimination of pressure	Eliminates the cause of the pressure sore and prevents further deterioration; this technique is combined with other therapies
Blowing air over wound	Not currently recommended; drys the wound and slows healing; forms deeper scab and causes more tissue death with delayed epithelialization (Torrance, 1981c)
Debriding agents (DEBRISAN)	Used to remove necrotic tissue and facilitate regeneration of healthy tissue; prevents scab formation and provides protective layer, sealing in body fluids to facilitate epithelialization (Torrance, 1981d)
Packing wound with sterile gauze	Not recommended; although it may keep wound clean, it may increase pressure on damaged tissue, causing further injury and obstructing local capillary circulation; discourages migration of cells into area for regeneration and healing (Hibbs, 1982); removing the packing also tends to damage the regenerating tissue

intervention of major position changes. Patients in wheelchairs are taught to use their arm muscles to raise themselves up to relieve the pressure on the buttocks many times each hour. Feustal (1982) suggests that patients with upper body control push up from the chair every ten minutes to relieve pressure while sitting as a way of preventing pressure sores of the ischial tuberosities. Many postoperative patients will turn and reposition themselves if they are given encouragement to do so.

Family and Social Interaction—A Love/Belonging Need.   The hospitalized family member is facing a temporary or permanent role change in family, social, and working relationships. The patient often experiences anger and depression over lost physical abilities with sensory or mobility problems. These feelings may be directed at the family or at friends, resulting in avoidance by others. Both the patient and the family may need help to understand and deal with feelings. Loss of mobility, vision, or hearing is often tied to a sense of uselessness by the patient and the family. The patient may not feel worthy of the love of others. The abilities of the patient can be emphasized rather than the inabilities. New ways of communication can be learned to overcome hearing loss. Finding ways for the patient with serious permanent mobility and visual or hearing problems to feel productive in a family and in the larger society is a challenge. Community self-help groups are an excellent resource.

Nursing Care Plan for a Patient with Unmet Stimulation Needs

Assessment

Data.   Mr. John Anderson is a 32-year-old married man with two children who was admitted to the hospital on 9/10 with a possible spinal cord injury following a water accident. He had been sitting on an inner tube and flipped over backward, hitting his head in the sand. He was dazed, under water, and completely paralyzed. Several people helped him to shore. He realized he might have injured his spinal cord because he was a water safety instructor. He kept telling everyone to keep his neck straight with the rest of his back. On admission, he was alert and oriented to time, place, and person and was completely aware of the prognosis of a cervical fracture and the accompanying spinal cord trauma. He was placed on a circle bed. Tongs were inserted into the skull and attached to weights. This was done to keep the neck in traction and perfectly aligned to prevent any further trauma to the spinal cord. His extremities were flaccid, with no sensation of touch or pain. No movement below the shoulders was possible for this patient. He kept repeating, "This can't be happening. I was only in a few feet of water. I didn't hit that hard." His wife was with him from the time of admission. The physician ordered complete bed rest with no twisting of the spine. The patient was to be turned to supine and prone positions only. Elastic stockings were ordered and a Foley catheter was put in place. An IV was started and the patient was NPO for 24 hours. An x-ray of the spine revealed a cervical fracture, but the vertebrae were in good alignment, and there was hope that the cord was not injured but only affected by edema in the area.

Nursing Diagnoses

1. Potential for pressure-sore formation based on paralysis and lack of sensation below shoulders
2. Potential for joint contractures related to paralysis
3. Potential for impaired cognitive functioning related to loss of sensation and immobility
4. Potential for problems related to elimination associated with immobility, NPO status, and positioning restrictions

Planning

Goals of Care

1. Patient will maintain skin integrity during period of immobility.
2. Patient will maintain current range of motion in all joints.
3. Patient will remain oriented to time, place, and person during period of immmobility.
4. Patient will maintain bowel habits while immobile.

Planned Nursing Actions (Interventions)

For Goal 1

1. Explain turning procedure to patient before each turn.
2. Elastic stockings on for all turns.
3. Turn patient prone or supine every two hours.
4. Assess skin every two hours following turning for signs of excess pressure; turn every hour if they develop.
5. Provide general stimulation to the skin by gentle massage to back and shoulders after turning; do not massage area reddened from pressure.
6. Maintain hydration through IV infusion; consult physician in 24 hours for diet order.
7. Change bedding damp with perspiration as needed.
8. Elevate heels off mattress in supine position.

For Goal 2

1. Explain range-of-motion exercises before beginning.
2. Exercise all body joints three times each session at 9 A.M., 1 P.M., 4 P.M., 9 P.M.
3. Position all joints in functional position in supine or prone position.

For Goal 3

1. Approach patient by introducing self and role, length of time you will be with patient, and provide some face-to-face eye contact.
2. Keep room calendar current and in view; provide clock with lighted dial where patient can see it.
3. Position bed so patient can see out the window in the prone position.
4. Adjust mirrors on bed for maximum visual stimulation after changing patient's position.
5. Keep light on in patient's room at night.
6. Offer stimulation such as radio, television, or volunteers to read to patient; avoid use of one medium extensively.
7. Encourage visitors as patient becomes more stable.
8. Share current world events with the patient daily during other treatments.
9. If patient has no preference, give him a roommate.

For Goal 4

1. Assess preinjury bowel habits.
2. Keep hydrated with IV infusion.
3. Explain to patient procedure for having a stool in the supine or prone position, and loss of control and sensation of defecation.
4. Encourage juices and bulk-forming foods in diet as soon as possible.
5. Consult with physician about order for stool softener and laxative as needed.

Evaluation

Goal 1 met, 10/3
Skin has remained intact during immobility. Motor function quickly returning.
Goal 2 met, 10/3
Joint mobility assessed as equal to admission mobility.
Goal 3 not met
On 9/14 patient began hallucinating in the evenings and nights. Disoriented to time and place. Gross, awkward movements began as patient tried to get off circle bed which he said was roof of his camper.
Goal 4 partially met
Patient passing slightly hardened stool every three to four days instead of every other day as was normal pattern.

Reassessment

New Diagnosis.   9/14. Potential for injury related to return of gross movements, hallucinations, and attempts to get off circle bed in neck traction.

New Goal.   Patient will remain in bed in good alignment during periods of disorientation.

NEW ACTIONS

1. Secure patient in restraining body cover during evenings and nights if signs of confusion appear.
2. Provide meaningful stimuli to patient every hour while awake; clear, slow conversation; orient to time, place, and person on evenings/nights.
3. Talk with family about having someone stay with him at night.
4. Omit sleeping medication.

Summary

Stimulation is considered as a basic human need in maintaining normal intellectual functioning and an ability to interact with the environment. Inadequate stimulation of the senses or disuse of the muscles results in disorientation, difficulty thinking, loss of reality, and loss of muscle and joint function. Inadequate sensory input tends to reduce interaction with the environment, leading to less physical movement. Immobility often leads to sensory monotony from a constant pattern of environmental stimulation. Muscle atrophy and loss of joint flexibility begin within a few days of disuse.

The motor unit, consisting of muscle fibers stimulated by one nerve cell, forms the working unit making movement possible. The central nervous system controls the muscles automatically in a constant state of low tension. Muscles move the bones by pulling and are arranged in groups called antagonists, making flexion and extension of body parts possible.

The senses consist of specialized cells or actual afferent nerve endings which are affected either chemically or physically by environmental stimuli. Vision, hearing, taste, smell, touch, and the vestibular senses all depend on transmission of a coded electrical message along nerve pathways and interpretation by special, specific areas within the brain. Damage to the receptor cells, nerves, or areas of the brain will interfere with or eliminate specific sensations. The nervous system is capable of adapting to stimuli from the senses when the stimuli are constant. Changing patterns or stimuli provide more stimulation to the central nervous system.

Sensory overload and sensory deprivation are problems associated with the need for stimulation. Sensory overload occurs when the individual is unable to process all the incoming sensory data. Illness, medication, and altered level of consciousness in a hospital are associated with sensory overload as the person becomes unable to think or act in normal ways. Sensory deprivation is associated with immobility or loss of adequate stimulation. The person loses contact with reality, and hallucinations are common.

Prevention of sensory deprivation, sensory overload, and complications associated with immobility is the focus of nursing interventions. Active and passive exercises and therapeutic positioning preserve joint and muscle function and also provide sensory stimulation to the skin, eyes, ears, and vestibular sense. The nurse's presence also helps to reduce the social isolation experienced by many immobile patients. Progressive ambulation is used to reduce complications of bed rest and provide stimulation from a varied environment. The techniques of walking with assistive aids are discussed.

Management and interpretation of the environment are nursing interventions to increase or decrease the stimuli reaching the patient, depending on the patient's risk of sensory overload or deprivation. Windows, lights, calendars, clocks, movement, and various forms of communication are helpful to the immobile or sensory-deprived patient if stimulation needs are to be met adequately.

Nursing interventions to assist the patient experiencing sensory or mobility loss to meet other needs are discussed. Treatment of pressure sores and the use of restraints protect the patient's physical safety. The patient frequently needs assistance or education in meeting nutritional and elimination needs. Involving the patient in care and prevention of complications is important for the patient's self-esteem. Family and friends of the patient will provide added stimulation and assistance in meeting needs during temporary sensory loss, immobility, or adjustment to a permanent disability.

Terms for Review

active assisted exercises	eversion	joints	quadriplegia
active range of motion exercises	expressive aphasia	load	receptive aphasia
abduction	extension	LOC	retraction
accommodation	flexion	mobility	rotation
adduction	fovea	motor unit	sensory deprivation
analgesia	Fowler's position	muscle tone	sensory monotony
anesthesia	hemiparesthesia	paraplegia	sensory/perceptual overload
antagonist muscle groups	hyperemia	paresthesia	spasticity
aphasia	hyperextension	passive range of motion exercises	stretch reflexes
base of support	intention tremors	perceptual deprivation	supination
clonus	inversion	pronation	supine
contracture	isometric contractions	prone	tension
decubitus ulcer	isotonic contractions	protraction	tetanus

Self-Assessment

Abdominal Muscle Strength

Smith and Feldman (1981) suggest that, in order to protect your back from "patient abuse" while giving nursing care, you should maintain strong abdominal muscles. They feel nurses should be able to perform the following exercise if abdominal muscles are sufficiently strong for moving and lifting patients:

1. A slow, bent-knee sit-up, with hands behind head grasping biceps of opposite arm. The sit-up is held for several seconds and then the nurse goes down slowly. If you are not at "nurse level" with your abdominal muscles, try this slightly easier exercise.
2. A slow, bent-knee sit-up with hands clasping each other behind head. Hold for several seconds and go down slowly. If this is still beyond your range, the following exercise is suggested.
3. A slow, bent-knee sit-up with arms crossed on chest.

If this is also difficult, the arm position is changed to the sides and a slow sit-up is attempted. If you are unable to do a sit-up regardless of the position of your arms, Smith and Feldman feel you will be a likely candidate for low-back pain from muscle strain during your nursing career. They suggest that the nurse or student gradually increase the strength of the abdominal muscles by working at the simplest of the exercises and building up to a safer level.

Exercises to Improve the Nurse's Muscle Strength

Strong abdominal muscles, lower back muscles, good posture, and correct lifting techniques will reduce the nurse's risk of back strain and damage. The buttocks and abdominal muscles are tightened when lifting, and the thighs and biceps are used whenever possible.

Avoid exercises that strain the back. These include straight-leg raises with both legs being raised simultaneously and straight-legged sit-ups. These exercises put the weight of the legs on the lower back and may cause further strain.

The following are some muscle-strengthening exercises for the back and the abdomen (Dilfer, 1981):

1. Pelvic tilt from the supine position with knees flexed. The muscles of the abdomen and buttocks are tightened to flatten the arch in the lower back against the floor. The hips are then slowly raised up several inches off the floor and held for a slow count of 8 to 10. This exercise is repeated four times, several times each day.

2. Leg lifts with one knee flexed. One leg is extended, while the other leg is flexed with the foot flat on the floor. The foot on the extended leg is dorsiflexed as much as possible. The muscles of the abdomen are tightened, and the straight leg is slowly lifted off the floor until both thighs are parallel. This position is held for several seconds, and then the leg is slowly lowered. This exercise is repeated eight or ten times, several times each day, on both legs.

3. Partial sit-ups with knees flexed and feet flat on floor. The hands are clasped behind the neck, abdominal and buttocks muscles tightened, and the head, neck, and shoulders are gradually raised off the floor. The waist area remains in contact with the floor. The up position is held for several seconds, and then the back and head are slowly lowered to the floor. This is repeated eight or ten times, several times a day.

Learning Activities

1. Visit a rehabilitation center and talk with patients about their disabilities.
   How did the initial loss of mobility affect the patient cognitively and emotionally?
   What types of exercises are being used to maintain or restore function?
   What type of assistive devices are being used to increase mobility and independence?
2. Interview someone from local community groups for the prevention of blindness or deafness.
   What services are available to assist people with hearing and vision problems?
   Does technology offer any new hope for preventing or curing blindness or deafness?
   What are the goals of local organizations for the blind or deaf?
3. Place yourself in the patient role and experience moving and turning using circle beds, turning frames, transfer boards or rollers, and hydraulic lifters.
   How did it feel physically?
   Did you have any fears?
4. Plan a nursing laboratory session where students experience blindness or immobility while another student assists them with eating such things as soup, Jell-O.
   What feelings did you have?
   What did your partner do that was helpful or upsetting?
5. Talk with staff nurses on ENT (ears, nose throat) or orthopedics areas about sensory deprivation, patient behavior, and prevention.

Review Questions

1. Inadequate sensory stimulation is associated with which of the following patient data?
   a. Decreased mental alertness, apathy
   b. Improved ability to think and reason
   c. Intention tremors
   d. Increased spontaneous movement
2. Which of the following occurs to maintain normal muscle tone in the body?
   a. Voluntary tightening of muscle groups
   b. Constant contraction of the same muscle fibers
   c. Asynchronous contraction of different muscle fibers
   d. Complete relaxation of flexors and slight contraction of extensors at all body joints
3. What factor controls the duration of a maximum contraction in a muscle fiber?
   a. Length of the muscle fiber
   b. Glycolysis
   c. Supply of ATP
   d. Blood glucose level
4. Isometric exercises have which of the following characteristics?
   a. Muscle fibers shorten.
   b. Utilize high-oxidative muscle fibers.
   c. They are performed without movement of the joints.
   d. They tend to lower the blood pressure.
5. Which of the following activities is an example of isotonic muscle contractions?
   a. A 98-lb nurse straining to move a 180-lb patient
   b. Walking
   c. Muscle-setting exercises
   d. Passive range-of-motion exercises
6. Which of the following is *not* a goal of therapeutic positioning?
   a. Maintaining joint mobility
   b. Distributing body weight over entire supporting surface
   c. Providing stimulation to patient
   d. Increasing muscle strength
7. All of the following are associated with immobility and disuse of the muscles *except*:
   a. Reduced oxygen need
   b. Reduced nutritional need
   c. Increased work load on the heart
   d. Reduced ventilation volumes
   e. Increased heat production
8. Which of the following patient data *decrease* the risk of pressure-sore development?
   a. Alert and oriented
   b. Incontinence
   c. Undernourished
   d. Decreased tactile sensations
   e. Paralysis
9. Which patient-lifting technique places the least strain on the nurse's back?
   a. Shoulder (Australian) life
   b. Three-person carry
   c. Transferring weight backward to move patient up in bed
   d. Keeping the legs straight
   e. Keeping the center of gravity outside the base of support
10. Safe and appropriate use of restraints involves which of the following activities?
    a. Never placing a patient in restraints without a written physician's order to do so
    b. Securing the restraint to the side rail for easy access
    c. Keeping the key for locked restraints locked in the narcotic cupboard in the medication room
    d. Restraining any disoriented patient
    e. Restraining only if there is a risk of physical harm from the patient's behavior
11. Healing of pressure sores is facilitated by which of the following treatments?
    a. Blowing air over the wound
    b. Firmly packing the wound with sterile gauze
    c. Eliminating all pressure on or near the wound
    d. Vigorous massage of skin area reddened from unrelieved pressure

Answers

1. a
2. c
3. c
4. c
5. b
6. d
7. e
8. a
9. a
10. e
11. c

References and Bibliography

Ahmen, M.: Op-site for decubitus care. *Am. J. Nurs.,* **82**:61, 1982.

Allen, S., and Moschak, V.: Step by step. Renew a patient's interest in life with an ambulation incentive program. *Nursing 81,* **11**:56, Aug., 1981.

Arnell, I: Treating decubitus ulcers—two methods that work. *Nursing 83,* **13**:50–55, June, 1983.

Bassett, C.; McClamrock, E.; and Schmelzer, M.: A 10 week exercise program for senior citizens. *Geriatr. Nurs.,* **3**:103, Mar./Apr. 1982.

Brislen, W.: The mecabed. *Nurs. Times,* **78**:1307, Aug. 4, 1982.

Chapman, D.: Human Kinetics: put your back into it! *Nurs. Mirror,* **154**:20, June 10, 1981.

Daws, I: Lifting and moving patients—3. *Nurs. Times,* **77**:2067, Nov. 25, 1981.

Dilfer, C.: Oh, my aching back. *Am. Baby*, **43**:67, Nov., 1981.

Dyson, R.: Bedsores—the injuries hospital staff inflict on patients. *Nurs. Mirror*, **146**:30–32, 1978.

Flaherty, P., and Jurkovich, S.: *Transfers for Patients with acute and Chronic Conditions*. Sister Kenny Institute, Minneapolis, 1970.

Feustel, D.: Pressure sore prevention. *Nursing 82*, **12**:78, Apr., 1982.

Friedman, F.: Clinical controversies: a new decubitus treatment. *RN*, **45**:46, Feb., 1982.

Geden, E.: Effects of lifting techniques on energy expenditures: a preliminary investigation. *Nurs. Res.*, **31**:214, July/Aug., 1982.

Hibbs, P.: Pressure sores: a system of prevention. *Nurs. Mirror*, **155**:25, Aug. 4, 1982.

Jeglum, E.: Ocular therapeutics. *Nurs. Clin. North Am.*, **16**:453, Sept., 1981.

Lentz, M.: Selected Aspects of decondition secondary to immobilization. *Nurs. Clin. North Am.*, **16**:729, Dec., 1981.

Lowthian, P.: A review of pressure sore pathogenesis. *Nurs. Times*, **78**:122, Jan. 20, 1982.

Mangieri, D.: Saving your elderly patient's skin. *Nursing 82*, **12**:44, Oct., 1982.

Minnesota Society for the Prevention of Blindness and Preservation of Hearing: *News for Nurses*. Vol. I, No. I., Sept. 1983.

Misik, I.: About using restraints—with restraints. *Nursing 81*, **11**:50, Aug., 1981.

Mitchell, P., and Laustau, A.: *Concepts Basic to Nursing*. McGraw-Hill, New York, 1981.

Norton, D.: Research and the problem of pressure sores. *Nurs. Mirror*, **148**:65–67, Feb. 13, 1975.

O'Day, J.: Gradual visual loss. *Nurs. Mirror*, Clinical Forum, **155**, Feb. 26, 1981.

Oldham, G.: Back pain: the influence of clothing. *Nurs. Times*, **77**:1038, June 11, 1981.

Porth, C.: *Pathophysiology: Concepts of Altered Health Status*, Lippincott, Philadelphia, 1982.

Riffle, K.: Falls: kinds, causes and prevention. *Geriatr. Nurs.*, **3**:165, May/June, 1982.

Roberts, A.: Nervous system: Testing sensation. *Nurs. Times*, **78**, Center Section, May 5, 1982.

Scholey, M.: The shoulder lift. *Nurs. Times*, **78**:506–507, Mar. 24, 1982.

Smith, O., and Feldman, F.: How to prevent an aching back. *Am. Baby*, **43**:18, July, 1981.

Sorenson, L., and Ulrich, P.: *Ambulation Guide for Nurses*, Rev. ed. Sister Kenny Institute, Minneapolis, 1977. (#707)

Talbot, D.: *Principles of Therapeutic Positioning: A guide for Nursing Action*. Sister Kenny Institute, Minneapolis, 1981. (#701)

Talbot, D., Pearson, V.; and Loeper, J.: *Disuse Syndrome: The Preventable Disability*. Sister Kenny Institute, Minneapolis, 1978. (#712)

Toohey, P., and Larson, C.: *Range of Motion Exercise: Key to Joint Mobility*. Sister Kenny Institute, Minneapolis, 1977. (#703)

Torrance, C.: Pressure sores: medical management and surgical intervention. *Nurs. Times*, **77** (Mar. 19):Center Section, 1981a.

Torrance, C.: Pressure sores: predisposing factors: the "at risk" patient. *Nurs. Times*, Center Section, Feb. 19, 1981b.

Torrance, C.: Pressure sores: physical methods. *Nurs. Times*, Center Section, June 18, 1981c.

Torrance, C.: Pressure sores: topical applications and wound agents. *Nurs. Times*, Center Section, May 7, 1981d.

Vander, A., Sherman, J., Luciano, D.: *Human Physiology: The Mechanism of Body Function*. 3rd ed. McGraw Hill, New York, 1980.

Voke, J.: Not to be sniffed at. *Nurs. Mirror*, Clinical Forum, **154**, Feb. 26, 1981.

Wright, B.: Lifting and moving patients—2. *Nurs. Times*, **77**:2025, Nov. 18, 1981.

Yates, J., and Lundberg, A.: *Moving and Lifting Patients: Principles and Techniques*. Sister Kenny Institute, Minneapolis, 1970. (#720)

CHAPTER 29
THE NEED FOR SECURITY/LOVE/ BELONGING

Objectives

1. Define the needs of security, love, belonging.

2. Explain the relevance of the need for security, love, and belonging to nursing.

3. Describe factors that influence the ability to meet the need for security.

4. Describe factors that influence the ability to meet the need for love and belonging.

5. Describe nursing interventions that decrease unknowns in the patient's environment.

6. Discuss nursing interventions to assist patients to meet their need for love and belonging.

Definition of Love/Security/Belonging Needs

Abraham Maslow states that safety needs emerge once the physiological needs have been met to some degree. Safety needs include security, stability, dependency, and protection; freedom from fear, anxiety, chaos; the need for structure, order, law, and limits (Maslow, 1970). Safety needs may be thought of as operating on two levels. On the physical level, safety is the protection of the organism from bodily harm. An example of physical safety is the correct grounding of electrical equipment in the hospital to prevent electrocution.

Another example is the careful handwashing techniques of the nurse to decrease the transfer of microorganisms. This type of safety is related primarily to survival needs. On a higher level is psychological security, a sense of tranquility and freedom from feelings of fear, anxiety, and apprehension. This also includes a sense of trust in the integrity, reliability, and fairness of other human beings.

Each of the preceding chapters of this text that discussed survival needs (oxygen, temperature maintenance, nutrition, etc.) included a consideration of related physical safety. The focus of this chapter is psychological safety or psychological security.

Security needs are a bridge or transition to higher level needs. If the individual has satisfied security needs, needs for love and belonging arise. Love needs include both giving and receiving love. Love is the understanding and acceptance of others. It is not to be confused with sex. Sex is primarily a physiological need although it may also be a part of love relationships. Maslow (1968) writes, "It would not occur to anyone to question the statement that we need iodine or vitamin C. I remind you that the evidence that we need love is of exactly the same type."

The need for belonging has had little objective scientific research to support its existence. However, everyone has had experiences that demonstrate the need. On the first day in the nursing program, acquaintances were made and groups were quickly formed. That this occurs is evidence of a need to belong. Other illustrations mentioned by Maslow include the neighborhood, one's class, one's gang, one's family.

The Relevance of Safety/Love/Belonging Needs to Nursing

A person who is hospitalized brings all the basic needs to the hospitalization experience. Survival needs are easily identified and receive the attention of most nurses. However, higher level needs, which are just as basic and common to all human beings as are survival needs, are often overlooked. Too often meeting a higher level need is perceived as "something nice to do if you have extra time" or "something only nursing students have time to do." Consider the case of a 64-year-old woman, hospitalized for internal bleeding, who was a constant source of irritation to the nursing staff. This patient made frequent and excessive demands upon the staff. The patient attempted to keep the staff with her constantly by contriving tasks, literally holding on to the staff, and flattering them. The nurse writing about this case notes, "Generally speaking, the demanding patient is lonely, frightened, or anxious" (Robinson, 1972). This patient was clearly demonstrating unmet needs for love and belonging.

The same author also wrote, "Loneliness, it seems to me, is at the core of what the hospital nurse encounters." Upon entering the hospital, patients are separated from friends, family, and relatives. Meals are usually eaten alone or in the company of a stranger who has become a roommate. At a time when a person may most need the comforting touch and caress of a spouse, there is no provision for privacy and intimacy.

Because the mind and the body are inseparable and because they influence each other, nursing care includes a consideration of both the mind and the body. The nurse assists patients in meeting needs for security, love, and belonging just as needs for pain relief and nutrition are met.

Factors Influencing the Ability to Meet Security Needs

Stress

All persons who become patients share the experience of stress, although the particular stressors and the responses to them are highly individualized. Stress interferes with the ability to feel safe and secure. There is physical stress with measurable effects such as elevated blood pressure and pulse rate. There is also psychological stress with its highly subjective interpretation. (See Chapter 2.) Stress-related anxiety may cause one person to withdraw and become irritable, while another person may become jovial and outgoing in an attempt to cover up the emotion.

One cause of stress and decreased feelings of security in hospitalized patients is fear of the unknown. Patients are often admitted to have tests to determine a diagnosis. Often the unspoken fear (but one that the patient worries about) is, "Do I have cancer?" If a diagnosis is determined and the patient is scheduled for surgery, the unspoken question may become, "Will I make it through this? What if something goes wrong?" In less dramatic situations, the patient may fear a certain diagnostic test or procedure. "Will it be painful?" "Will there be an embarrassing lack of privacy?" In teaching hospitals, patients may fear being cared for by students. "Do they know what they are doing?" "Is this the first time the nurse has done this on a real patient?"

Nursing students may also fear the unknown and feel insecure. It is not uncommon for beginning nursing students to be afraid to answer a patient's call light for fear of finding a situation they are unable to handle. Although most of the time a first-year nursing student can handle a patient request either alone or with assistance, the fear of the unknown remains until the student has had sufficient experience to increase personal security in the hospital environment.

Degree of Control of Environment

Adults who enter the health care setting often experience a lack of control over their schedule and environment that is comparable to being a child again. This lack of control of the environment limits a person's ability to meet personal security needs. With the loss of control come increased threats to security. Hospitalized adults are awakened at a time designated by others and served meals on a predetermined schedule. They are assigned roommates (much like children at camp) and informed of the rules: TV off at certain time, showers are available at a certain time, no smoking in your room, and the mode of dress (pajamas or hospital gown) is specified. They are told what to do ("You are having a GI x-ray in the morning.") and how to do it ("You will drink a large amount of barium and will receive a strong laxative after completion of the procedure."). While much of the structure and routine of the health care institution is necessary, it may create negative feelings in patients.

Similarly, nurses may share the feelings of a loss of control and insecurity. For example, staff nurses may complain that they have responsibility for too many acutely ill patients and are not able to give quality nursing care. In contrast is the nurse who can trust that the nursing supervisor will recognize the problem and pro-vide additional help. There is a sense of psychological safety and security in this work environment.

Preventive Measures

Preventive measures taken by an individual can enhance psychological security by reducing the risk of problems occurring in the future or by decreasing the consequence of problems should they arise. People buy hospitalization insurance to assure that if costly health care is needed, they will be able to purchase it for loved ones and for themselves. Seat belts are worn in an effort to prevent fatal injuries resulting from automobile accidents. These and similar measures are taken in an attempt to prevent disastrous results. Having taken these measures gives the individual additional security.

Religion

For some persons, religious practices contribute to a sense of security. Some religious groups, for example, assure members of a life after physical death if they hold certain beliefs and if they follow certain rules of conduct and religious practices. Many people gain a sense of security from following this prescribed behavior. Other religious observances seem to impart a sense of security in and of themselves, apart from the broader significance of the action. Roman Catholic patients, for example, may receive the Sacrament of the Sick, which includes an anointing of the ill person and prayers for the forgiveness of sin and restoration of health. Nurses frequently comment that the patient appears so "at peace" after this practice.

Factors Influencing the Ability to Meet the Need for Love and Belonging

Past Love Relationships

Love experiences begin even before birth for some persons. The fetus may be the object of a great deal of love even while in the uterus. This love is a warm, positive environment that is different from the other, more direct, love that will follow. After birth, the infant receives love in the tangible ways of touch, warmth, food, and physical comfort. Thus, the first step in meeting a love need is being loved by others. The human who has received this love perceives the self as lovable. From this secure base, the individual is able to move out and give love to others. In summary, the sequence of the development of love moves from being loved, to loving self, to loving others. The individual who has not experienced love will probably have difficulty in establishing love relationships with others.

Culture

Although the need for love is common to all human beings, the culture in which people live influences how love is expressed. If, for example, it is not acceptable within the culture for a father to hug and kiss a young son, men learn restraint in demonstrating physical affection with sons. This learned behavior is then passed on over generations. Conversely, if the culture encourages an open demonstration of affection with much hugging and kissing, this is the learned behavior that is passed on.

Illness and Hospitalization

Hospitalization also affects the expression of love. Frequently, the nurse encounters elderly persons who have been married for forty or more years. Out of concern for the spouse of the patient, the nurse may suggest that the person "go home and rest for a while." Often no rest is possible when the spouse is worried about the patient's well-being. It may be harder for the spouse to leave than to suffer the physical exhaustion of staying at the bedside. The need to stay close to the loved one is intense.

It may also be that hospitalization far away from home and loved ones creates a sense of abandonment or loneliness. Often patients who require complex diagnostic or treatment procedures are referred to large medical centers. This institution may be far from the patient's family and home. In such a setting, the patient who has no visitors, while a roommate is visited by many friends, may feel loss of love, whether it is real or not.

Nursing Diagnoses Related to Security/Love/Belonging

The following nursing diagnoses may be seen in patients experiencing unfulfilled security or love and belonging needs. The list is not exhaustive but is intended to give examples:

Fear related to unknown diagnosis
Social isolation related to contagious wound infection
Loss of control of environment associated with paralyzing spinal cord injury

Loneliness associated with separation from family
Fear associated with unknown hospital routine
Anger associated with lack of control of environment
Inadequate information related to specific diagnostic procedures
*Inadequate emotional support related to poor prognosis
*Impaired ability to express love
*Impaired ability to receive love

Nursing Interventions Related to Security

In order to promote psychological security, the nurse plans interventions that reduce or prevent stress by reducing unknowns in the environment and by increasing the patient's control of the environment. The following interventions focus on this goal.

Admission Procedures

Some time ago, admitting patients to the health care facility consisted of filling out brief forms, taking vital signs, and assisting the patient into bedclothes. As such, this task was often delegated to the nurse's aide for it was felt this was not a procedure requiring the skills of a registered nurse. Today, it is usually the registered nurse who admits patients to the hospital. This procedure now includes physical assessment, completion of a nursing history, and initiating a nursing care plan.

At the time of admission, the nurse begins procedures designed to reduce stress and increase predictability for the patient. This begins with an introduction of the nurse and a statement of purpose. This might in-

clude, "Mr. Jones, I am Ms. List. I will be your primary nurse during your hospitalization. I will be responsible for planning the nursing care you receive while you are here. When I am not here, another nurse will follow my plans. Please feel free to ask me any questions you may have or discuss any problems." By such a statement, the nurse has clearly identified the responsible nurse and a source of help and information for the patient.

At some point during the admission procedure, the nurse orients the patient to the facility, pointing out bathrooms, lounge areas, TV controls, call light for the nurse, how to make outgoing telephone calls.

During the admission nursing history, the registered nurse also has the opportunity to do some anticipatory problem solving. The nurse may ask, "Mr. Jones, can you think of any problems you might have while you are in the hospital?" Frequently, patients will be able to anticipate potential problems. Mr. Jones responded,

---

*Campbell, C.: *Nursing Diagnoses and Intervention in Nursing Practice*. Wiley, New York, 1978.

"Well, the last time I was in the hospital, I got all turned around at night when I got up to use the bathroom. That really upset me." This is an example of a potential problem easily resolved by the nurse. The nurse responded, "Do you think it would help if I ordered a small night-light to be kept on both in your room and in the bathroom?" Mr. Jones responded that he would like that solution. This anticipatory problem solving enhances the patient's sense of security.

Maintenance of Home Routine

Although it is not possible to adapt the hospital routine to each individual's preference, many modifications are possible. One such example follows.

Nurse: Mr. Jones, can you tell me something about your routine at home? What is an average day like for you?

Mr. Jones: Well, I get up about 6 A.M. and shower before breakfast. I'm a morning person, even on weekends.

Nurse: Would you like us to waken you at the same time here?

Mr. Jones: Yes, then I could listen to the news with breakfast. Oh, I also have bran cereal and three prunes every day for breakfast. It really helps prevent constipation.

Nurse: Your doctor has ordered a general diet so you may have whatever you choose. I'll make a note of that.

In this example, the nurse has adapted two items to the patient's home routine. It may not always be possible to accommodate to the patient's home routine, but when it is possible, it is another way to increase the knowns in the new environment.

Patient Teaching

One of the most effective ways to decrease the unknown is through patient teaching. A well-known application of this is the natural childbirth method of Dick-Read. He maintained that a fear-tension-pain syndrome exists in childbirth. The fear caused tension which, in turn, caused pain. He believed that education would eliminate the fear and break the cycle. Variations of his method are widely accepted today. The theory can be applied equally well to any area of patient care. Education can reduce fear.

At times, patient education will be as simple as providing information about a medication. (Example: Penicillin is an antibiotic that will treat your skin infection.) At other times, a complex teaching plan may be required, as in teaching self-care to a patient with newly diagnosed diabetes. (See Chapter 9, The Teaching-Learning Process.)

Patient teaching may include both the patient and family members. The patient who is having major surgery requires extensive teaching. Both the patient and the family need to be instructed about what to expect after surgery. The nurse tells them about IVs, a nasogastric tube, a suction machine, a urinary catheter. It may be possible for the nurse to actually show patients the equipment that will be used after surgery. Relatives who do not receive this teaching may be unnecessarily frightened by the sight of the patient after surgery.

Religious Practices

Many patients appreciate the opportunity to maintain religious practices while in the hospital. The nurse may offer to assist the patient by making arrangements for a chaplain to visit, to attend worship services, or by providing privacy and uninterrupted time for prayer or meditation. (See Chapter 30, The Need for Spirituality.)

Discharge Planning

Although most patients are eager to leave the hospital, discharge also presents a new set of problems. Patients frequently express a fear concerning their ability to care for themselves and meet family responsibilities. One patient stated, "I'm worried about how I'll ever manage. Here the nurses provide all my care, meals are served, and all the housekeeping is done. And I'm tired after I just walk the length of the hall a couple of times! What will it be like when I get home and have the children and a house to keep up? It seems overwhelming." The concerns voiced by this patient indicate a lack of security which can be met by discharge planning. The nurse may be able to work with the patient and her family to clarify the physical limitations of the patient and to identify ways in which the family may help. It may be possible to obtain housekeeping help or child care for a temporary period while the patient is unable to handle these tasks. Medications and treatments that will be required after discharge are explained to the patient or responsible family member. At other times, a referral to a public health nurse is necessary. Written discharge instructions are provided for each patient.

The patient to be discharged is also provided with a

telephone number of someone to phone should unanticipated problems or questions arise. This may be for a physician, a public health nurse, or the clinical unit and

the responsible nurse. The patient is thus assured of the availability of help "just in case." All of these measures enhance security.

Nursing Interventions to Meet the Need for Love and Belonging

The Nurse-Patient Relationship

Nursing has been called the "caring" profession, and nowhere is this more apparent than in the nurse-patient relationship. This relationship is characterized by the nurse's attitudes of sensitivity, acceptance, and empathy. The nurse conveys an unspoken (and sometimes spoken!) attitude of, "It matters to me what happens to you." The love that a nurse demonstrates for patients is the caring part of the nursing role. This is demonstrated initially by maintaining eye contact with the patient, by asking how the patient wishes to be addressed, by pronouncing the patient's name correctly. (Some nurses make a note of the phonetic spelling of difficult names on the nursing care plan.)

Nurses also demonstrate love through the use of touch. Nurses can consciously develop a touch that is pleasant and comforting to patients. When the nurse uses the whole hand (rather than only the finger pads) and a firm touch (rather than a tentative brushing motion), patients are more likely to feel the genuine caring of the nurse.

Other nonverbal behavior also demonstrates caring. One intervention is a visit from the nurse when not required by physical care. The nurse may enter the patient's room and say, "I don't have any treatments or pills for you. I'd just like to visit for a few minutes." The nurse may then pull up a chair to the patient's bedside. At other times, the nurse may bring the patient a snack or prescribed nourishment and sit with the patient while it is eaten. Each of these interactions demonstrate caring.

Interaction with Family Members

The nurse not only cares for the hospitalized person but includes family members when planning nursing interventions. On admission, the nurse also orients family members to the hospital environment, including such things as restrooms for their use, the hospital cafeteria and coffee shop (including some approximate prices), and parking facilities. It is also helpful to write down the patient's room number and telephone number (also a telephone number in a waiting area if this will be used) so they may be reached by other family members.

The nurse attempts to make family members as comfortable as possible. Some institutions provide folding cots for relatives who wish to remain near critically ill patients. The nurse may also offer a pillow and a blanket, perhaps a beverage. Although these interventions are done for family members, they assure the patient that loved ones are also important to the nurse.

Patient Groups

Patients with a newly diagnosed condition may feel terribly alone and isolated. They may even doubt the nurse's ability to understand. "How can you understand? You aren't the one with cancer!" Such statements are typical of comments the nurse might hear. These comments reflect an unmet need for belonging. The nurse may encourage this patient to join a support group for patients experiencing similar problems. One example of such a group is "I Can Cope," a group for cancer patients and their families. Another successful group is Alcoholics Anonymous. Membership in such a group offers the patient the support of others who "have been there," who have shared the experience.

One alternative to a group intervention is an interpersonal relationship with a person who has experienced a similar situation. Patients who have experienced a mastectomy (breast removal) may be helped by a volunteer visitor from "Reach to Recovery," an organization of women who have had mastectomies who have volunteered to visit patients after surgery to offer support and information. Patients who are about to begin kidney dialysis are often given the name of another patient on dialysis to obtain "firsthand" information. These interventions decrease the sense of isolation felt by the patient.

Maintenance of Communication

The hospitalized patient may feel cut off from the world outside the hospital. Nurses often observe that patients lose track of the date and day of the week. The nurse may assist the patient in many small ways: commenting on the day and date, providing newspapers, turning on television or radio news for patients or selected TV programs that mark dates for the patient ("I always watch 'Trapper John' on Sunday night.") The door to the patient's room may be left open to encourage the visits of other ambulatory patients. The nurse may offer to look up telephone numbers of the patient who is unable to do so. Nurses in a long-term care facility may offer to write brief letters for patients. (This is based on the premise, "You have to write a letter to get one!") Each of these small interventions helps the patient to maintain contact with a world larger than the hospital room and to maintain the sense of belonging to that world.

Nursing Care Plan for a Patient with Unmet Security/Love/Belonging Needs

Mrs. Janet Lee is a 23-year-old mother of an infant son, who is a first child. She had a normal labor and delivery and is to be discharged on the second post partum day. She has chosen to breastfeed although she states, "None of my family or friends are breastfeeding and they can't understand why I want to. Even my husband isn't too sure it's a good idea."

In her conversation with the nurse, Mrs. Lee has also stated: "How do I know if he's getting enough milk. I mean, won't he get sick if he doesn't nurse well?"

"It really frightens me, going home. Here the nurses watch the babies all night. What if I don't hear him at night and something is wrong?"

"I'm an only child. I've never had any experience at caring for babies and children. I never even babysat. It's really scary! How will I know what to do when he gets sick."

Nursing Care Plan for Mrs. Lee

NURSING DIAGNOSIS	GOAL	PLANNED ACTIONS
1. Lack of support system for breastfeeding	Mrs. L. Will have a support system for breastfeeding by time of discharge.	1. a. Suggest attendance at breastfeeding class on the unit. b. Provide information from La-Leche League, phone number, meeting place, etc. c. Support patient choice to breastfeed.
2. Anxiety related to ability to care for infant	Anxiety will be decreased as evidenced by positive statement from the patient about her ability to care for the child.	2. a. Demonstrate and request return from patient of the following skills: baby bath, cord care, taking rectal temperature, burping, suction with bulb. b. Provide written name and phone number to call for questions—hospital nursing unit may be called 24 hours per day. c. Written discharge instructions for patient. d. Schedule public health nurse visit 4/6/85.

| 3. Inadequate information regarding growth and development of infant | Mother will be able to discuss normal developmental tasks appropriate to son's age. (Evaluate at each clinic visit.) | 3. a. Discuss and illustrate the characteristics of the neonate using Baby Lee. b. Recommend reference books on infant care and encourage Mrs. Lee to browse through those available on the unit. c. Communicate to clinic nurse to continue growth and development instruction. |

Summary

Once survival needs have been satisfied to some degree, higher level needs begin to emerge. Psychological security is a need that is a transition between physiological needs and the need for love and belonging. Security is a feeling of trust in other human beings, as well as a freedom from fear and anxiety. Stress, the degree of control the individual is able to exert over the environment, and the preventive measures an individual is able to take all influence the ability of an individual to meet the need for psychological security. Nursing interventions that help to build psychological security include admission procedures, patient teaching, religious practices, and discharge planning.

The ability to meet the need for love and belonging is influenced by past love relationships, culture, illness, and hospitalization. Nursing interventions to meet the need for love and belonging include the development of the nurse-patient relationship, interaction with family members, and encouraging patient participation in patient support groups.

Self-Assessment

Nurses, like all human beings, have a need for psychological security. Respond to the following questions to assess the measures you have taken to enhance personal psychological security.

1. I have adequate health insurance.
2. My health insurance also covers my dependents.
3. I have disability insurance that will insure me an income if I am unable to work.
4. I have professional liability insurance.
5. I regularly wear seat belts and request that all passengers also do so when I am driving.
6. (If applicable) I have a backup baby-sitter should mine become ill when I am required to be in a clinical laboratory.

If Responsible for the Support of Minors:

5. I have a will that specifies financial arrangements for the care of minors.
6. I have a will that designates a legal guardian for the care of minors.

7. The legal guardian named in the will is aware and has agreed to accept the responsibility for care of minors.

Learning Activities

To increase your personal sense of security within the clinical area of the hospital, go on a "scavenger hunt" and locate the following:

1. Locate the men's and women's public restrooms.
2. Locate the hospital coffee shop and find the price of a hamburger and cup of coffee.
3. Locate the hospital cafeteria and find the price of a dinner that includes meat, green salad, vegetable, dessert, and low-fat milk.
4. Find where extra pillows and blankets are kept on the unit to which you are assigned.
5. Determine where visitors may park and the cost per hour.
6. Locate two public telephones within the hospital.
7. Locate two places where a person may obtain change within the hospital; one must be available after 8:30 P.M.

8. Locate the following items for purchase within two blocks of the hospital:
   - Shaving cream
   - Razor and blades
   - Ms. magazine
   - One red rose
   - Toenail clipper
9. Find the procedure manual on the patient care unit.
10. Find out how to call for help in case of fire and cardiac/respiratory arrest.
11. 10 *extra points* if you can locate a free source of coffee for relatives within the hospital.

Review Questions

1. Which of the following needs are seen as a transition to higher level needs?
   a. Love and belonging needs
   b. Basic needs
   c. Survival needs
   d. Security needs
2. The need for love and belonging is described as
   a. A need for sexual orgasm
   b. The need for understanding and acceptance of others
   c. A need to maintain the self-concept
   d. A need to maintain control of the environment
3. The patient who is excessively demanding may be demonstrating
   a. Needs for love and belonging
   b. Need for relief of severe pain
   c. Need for patient teaching
   d. A problem that may require psychotherapy
4. Which of the following does Robinson believe to be at the core of what the hospital nurse encounters?
   a. Pain
   b. Fear
   c. Anxiety
   d. Loneliness
5. Nursing interventions to meet the need for psychological security have as a goal
   a. The development of a nurse-patient relationship
   b. The reduction or prevention of stress by reducing the amount of the unknown
   c. Enhancing the patient's control of the environment
   d. Meeting the comfort needs of relatives and family members

6. A major intervention designed to assist the patient in meeting the need for love and belonging is
   a. Patient teaching
   b. Providing minimal information so as not to frighten the patient
   c. The nurse-patient relationship
   d. Adequate nutritional intake

Answers

1. d
2. b
3. a
4. d
5. b
6. c

Suggested Readings

Mullins, A., and Barstow, R.: Care for the caretakers. *Am. J. Nurs.,* **79**:1425-26, 1979. The authors recognize the need of nurses for peer support and give several specific ways nurses can give support to each other.

Naugle, E. The difference caring makes. *Am. J. Nurs.,* **73**:1890–91, 1973. A classic article which illustrates nursing interventions to meet the need for security, love, and belonging.

References and Bibliography

Campbell, C.: *Nursing Diagnoses and Intervention in Nursing Practice.* Wiley, New York, 1978.

Flynn, P.: *Holistic Health. The Art and Science of Care.* Robert J. Brady, Bowie, Md., 1980.

Maslow, A.: *Motivation and Personality.* Harper & Row, New York, 1970.

Maslow, A.: *Toward a Psychology of Being.* Van Nostrand, New York, 1968.

Robinson, L.: *Liaison Nursing. Psychological Approach to Patient Care.* Davis, Philadelphia, 1974.

Robinson, L.: *Psychological Aspects of the Care of Hospitalized Patients,* 2nd ed. Davis, Philadelphia, 1972.

Yura, H., and Walsh, M.: *Human Needs and the Nursing Process.* Appleton-Century-Crofts, Norwalk, Ct. 1978.

Yura, H., and Walsh, M.: *Human Needs 3 and the Nursing Process.* Appleton-Century Crofts, Norwalk, Ct., 1983.

CHAPTER 30
THE NEED FOR SPIRITUALITY*

Spirituality as a Higher Need
    Factors Affecting Spiritual Needs

Assessment of Spiritual Needs
    Data Indicating Spiritual Needs
    Nursing Diagnoses Related to Spiritual Needs

Nursing Interventions to Meet Spiritual Needs
    Religious and Cultural Knowledge
    Initiating the Topic
    Establishing Acceptance
    Communication
    Prayer
    Scripture
    Working with Spiritual Leaders
    Special Rituals and Services

Objectives

1. Define the terms "religion," "spiritual," and "spiritual need."
2. Discuss the interrelationship of spiritual and physical needs.
3. Identify the role of the nurse in meeting the needs of a patient and the patient's family.
4. Discuss nursing interventions that can be used to meet the spiritual needs of patient or family related to specific religions: Christian Scientist, Jehovah's Witness, Judaism, Protestant, Roman Catholic.

5. Discuss how the religious or spiritual beliefs of the nurse influence the nursing practice in meeting spiritual needs of a patient and the patient's family.
6. Discuss the components of a patient referral to a chaplain or spiritual leader.
7. Discuss the roles of the nurse and chaplain or spiritual leader working together to meet the patient's and family's spiritual needs.
8. Discuss ways the nurse can maintain spiritual health.

Spirituality as a Higher Need

"Seeking for something, yet not knowing what, coupled with being alone . . ." (Heimler, 1975) is the essence of a spiritual need. One finds it is a need common to all. The following five vignettes are meant to exemplify this need.

    Jerry, a 19-year-old who had recently lost the vision of one eye in an accident was restless. He was unable to sleep and kept saying over and over again, "There has to be some meaning in this." When the nurse inquired if he wanted to talk further, he said, "I've been struggling to figure out what I'm going to do with my life. That job was just temporary. I think the accident has forced me to make some decisions, but I don't know what I want. I didn't think this could happen to me. I'm still in shock. I've got so much time to think. And, I feel so alone . . . and pulled in so many directions." The nurse replied, pulling up a chair, "So many directions . . . would it help to talk?" At

*Written by Delores E. Johnson currently an instructor in nursing at Normandale Community College. Her primary teaching responsibility is in the area of mental health nursing. She is vice president and clinical nursing specialist in mental health at Esse Associates Inc., a private practice for mental health services. She also developed and teaches an elective course, Spiritual Care for Patients and Their Families, at Metropolitan State University, Minneapolis, Minnesota.

the end of the conversation Jerry told the nurse, "Maybe I can put the pieces back together again, but it's tough. Maybe I can rest now. . . ."

Mr. M., a 60-year-old man facing prostate surgery, and his wife were very confident that God would take care of them as they anticipated his surgery. They indicated they were trusting in God in this situation, whatever the outcome. After surgery, the pathologist was not conclusive about the absence of cancer, and many more tests were being done. Waiting for the results was a highly stressful time for the couple. The nurse commented about their discouragement and inquired whether there was anything that could be done to help them. The wife stated that they were very frightened and then asked the nurse to go out into the hallway with her. She told the nurse, "I'm so afraid. Why us? Why now? I can't even pray anymore." The nurse encouraged her to say more by commenting, "Could you tell me more about it?" The patient's wife continued, "I feel I should accept whatever happens, but it's not that easy. I can't even pray or talk to my husband. I told God I'd accept whatever happened, but . . ." and the woman broke into tears. Holding her hand, the nurse asked, "Is there anything I can do?" "Yes," she said, "You can pray with me." The nurse began, "Lord, help Mrs. M. in this difficult situation. Help her to feel the peace and comfort of your love." Softly, Mrs. M. joined in prayer, "Lord, help me trust in your goodness, and give me strength to help my husband." She then went to her husband and shared her feelings with him. Her husband was relieved because he was experiencing the same feelings.

Mrs. T. was dying. When the nursing student entered her room she noted a Bible on her bedside stand. She commented about it. Mrs. T. said, "It was my mother's. I've wanted to read something from it, but I'm just too weak." When the student offered to read it and asked what she'd like to hear, Mrs. T. said, "Choose something you like. I haven't been a very religious woman and don't known very much about the Bible. Now, I find it comforting." The student read the Twenty-Third Psalm ("The Lord is my shepherd").

Mr. and Mrs. D. were concerned that their newborn child be baptized immediately. They had just heard from their physician that their baby would only live for a few hours. The nursing student inquired about who they would like to baptize the baby. The father answered, "It's been so long since we've been to church. I don't want to call our minister." The student told the parents she could call the hospital chaplain if they wished. The parents felt this was a good alternative and found comfort in having the baptism performed immediately.

The P. family was waiting for Mrs. P. to go to surgery. The room was crowded with several family members and their pastor. One of the family members expressed concern about wanting to have a quiet place to pray while her mother was having surgery. The nurse told her about the chapel which was always open and arranged for a volunteer to escort her. The family member then asked if it would be okay if the entire family went to the chapel.

These examples of nursing care suggest that patients are concerned about their *spiritual* as well as their physical health. Since the establishment of health sciences, there has been an awareness of patient needs related to the body and those related to the spirit. Stallwood and Stoll (1975) define *spiritual needs* as "any factors necessary to establish and maintain a person's dynamic personal relationship with God (as defined by that individual)." Spiritual needs are not the same as *religion*, although both may share common elements. Religion is "a belief in the supernatural or divine force that has power over the universe and commands worship and obedience; a comprehensive code of ethics or philosophy." *Spirituality* is a quality broader than religion. It "strives for inspiration, reverence, and awe, even in those who do not believe in any god" (Murray and Zentner, 1975).

In each of these examples, the patient and/or family require support of the element that inspires them to transcend the realm of the material, to go beyond the limits of the physical. An individual or family need in the spiritual area may vary greatly in how it is expressed. In the examples, the needs ranged from a need to pray, to explore the meaning of events, to read religious material (Bible), to practice religious traditions (baptism), to find a quiet place (chapel). These are common expressions of spiritual needs.

Spiritual needs may be strongly or minimally affected by institutionalized religion. Some patients may find their spiritual needs met through the functions of organized religions, while others do not. For many people, institutionalized religion provides a framework to which they can relate their life. It is composed of a set of values and beliefs that aid in daily living.

Factors Affecting Spiritual Needs

Crisis. There are spiritual crises just as there are physical crises in a person's life. For example, when one is facing death or the loss of a loved one, each person's experience is unique, just as it is when a person is facing major surgery or has had a coronary. These situations become a crisis when the usual coping mechanisms don't work anymore. It is a *spiritual crisis* when one's relationship to whatever that person terms "God" is broken. It may be that there is doubt that life has any meaning, doubt that prayers are heard, or doubt that God exists. This is similar to a physical crisis in that one part of the body is not relating to the other parts in the way they were meant to function. Oftentimes, physical crisis and spiritual crisis coincide. The meeting of physical needs can affect the meeting of spiritual needs and vice versa. The longer one examines the body-spirit notion of humankind, the more one becomes impressed with the wholeness of the person. We can examine these two parts, body and spirit, separately for the sake of study, but they are an integrated part of the whole person. When one is giving physical care, one can be giving spiritual care, and the reverse of this process is also true.

Support Systems. Although each person experiences a spiritual crisis in a unique and individualized way, some persons find it is helpful to have others share in that experience to the extent possible. Because the individual in crisis feels very vulnerable, the individual is usually more receptive to help and support at this time. To receive support requires one to be in a dependent position temporarily. For many, this is extremely uncomfortable, perhaps even unacceptable. For others, it is a part of their way of life. Such persons have developed a support system, a network of people who are able to provide support or strength in time of need. Since no one person can meet all of another person's needs, a support system usually involves a number of people. The support system may include family and friends, spiritual leader and members of a congregation, or employer and co-workers. If a support system has been developed, it becomes much easier to add the nurse, physician, chaplain, and so forth to this already existing network of helpers. Some people also identify God in their support system. They feel this provides an added dimension to the strength one gains from people.

Religion. Ideally, one's religious beliefs provide strength, an inner quietness and faith with which to work through life's problems. Religion can provide a framework for living one's life which includes rituals, prayer, spiritual exercises, certain principles of everyday conduct, and so forth. For many Roman Catholics, it is important to participate in Mass on Sunday and to receive the Sacrament of the Sick (Rite for Anointing of the Sick). Families of the Jewish faith keep a bedside vigil when a person is dying. Persons of some faiths (Baptist, Church of Christ, Episcopalian, Mormon) believe in divine healing through the laying on of hands or anointing (Pumphrey, 1977). Each of these religious practices can be a source of strength and support for the ill patient.

Hospitalization During Religious Holidays. Many persons find their faith so much a part of their everyday life that it is upsetting to them to not be able to participate in the celebration of religious holidays. These holidays are usually celebrated with family. A person separated from family at these times may have a higher potential for loneliness, withdrawal, and even depression.

Assessment of Spiritual Needs

Data Indicating Spiritual Needs

A number of questions can be helpful in assessing spiritual needs. Several examples of opening questions are, "What do you think I need to know in order to help you meet your spiritual needs?" "Do you belong to a religious group?" "Would you like to talk about your faith?" "Would you like a chaplain to visit you while you are in the hospital?" These questions often give clues about the patient's concerns. Sometimes the nurse becomes fearful that the answers patients are searching for cannot be answered by the nurse. This is a concern of even very experienced nurses who may feel very uncomfortable discussing spiritual needs. In all of nursing, the nurse's role is to do for the patients what they are not capable of doing on their own at this time. Even when the patient is unable to verbalize needs, it is important to realize that the needs exist. The professional nurse seeks data to determine what that need is.

It is important to assess a patient's spiritual needs in the same systematic way as the patient's physical needs. The nurse may or may not find that a patient's values and beliefs are expressed through religious language or *rituals.* Some patients will gladly discuss their spiritual beliefs and needs, while others feel this area of their life is too private to talk about. The nurse respects the patient's preference. However, it is important to offer the opportunity to a patient to explore the relationship of body and spirit.

Questions that are more directly related to spiritual care were developed by Stoll (1979). Four areas of concern were identified: the person's source of strength and hope, the person's concept of God or a diety, the significance of religious practices and rituals to the person, and the person's perceived relationship between spiritual beliefs and state of health.

A spiritual assessment interview guide is presented in Table 30–1 to provide the nurse with an opportunity to

Table 30–1. **Spiritual Assessment Interview Guide**

1. What does religion mean to you?
2. How does God work in your life?
3. How would you describe God?
4. Are there any religious practices that are important to you? If so, would you tell me about them?
5. Has being sick (or having problems) ever made any difference in your feelings about God? In the practice of your faith?
6. What about your religious faith is most important to you right now?
7. Are you dealing with a crisis or illness at this time?
8. What helps you most when you feel afraid or need help?
9. What kind of spiritual support has been helpful to you in the past?
10. What is your source of strength right now?
11. How can I help you in carrying out your religious practices or in your relationship with God?
12. If you were hospitalized, would you appreciate a visit from you pastor?

Source: Judith Allen Shelly: *Spiritual Care Workbook—A Companion to Spiritual Care: The Nurse's Role.* InterVarsity Press, Downers Grove, Ill.: 1978, pp. 37–38.

develop a style of interviewing that feels most comfortable. These questions need not necessarily be asked in the order written, nor do all of the questions have to be asked at the same time.

Nursing Diagnoses Related to Spiritual Needs

During the procedures of the Fourth National Conference for Classification of Nursing Diagnosis in 1980, one of the accepted nursing diagnoses was spiritual distress (distress of human spirit) (Kim and Moritz, 1983). Several additional diagnoses were suggested by a nursing leader (O'Brien, 1982). They are as follows:

Spiritual pain—alteration in one's relationship with God or whatever one determines to be of highest value; a lack of peace

Spiritual alienation—broken relationship with God or whatever that person considers to be of greatest value

Spiritual anxiety—expressions of fear that God will not be supportive and might be punitive related to one's behavior or fear that the supports one has had in life are no longer available

Spiritual guilt—expressions related to not having lived up to the expectations of God or whatever the person considers to be God

Spiritual anger—expression of frustration toward God or the expression that what has happened to them is unfair

Spiritual loss—expressions of or threatened loss of God's love or feeling emptiness about spiritual things

Spiritual despair—expressions of hopelessness regarding relationship with God or receiving God's care

Nursing Interventions to Meet Spiritual Needs

At this point, the nurse might question, "How can I provide spiritual care when I know so little about religions?" The answer is twofold. First, the nurse can meet spiritual needs without extensive knowledge of religion because all persons have similar spiritual needs, regardless of their religion. Second, it is important to learn about various religions and cultures in order to give effective nursing care.

What is most important is the nurse's openness to assisting an individual or family to express spiritual needs. When people can talk about what they are feeling and thinking about their concerns, it helps them find ways to resolve their problems (Heimler, 1975). This involves the nurse's respecting the ability of the patient to identify needs and possible ways to meet the needs when given opportunity and support.

Religious and Cultural Knowledge

It is also helpful to become acquainted with the religious customs of various faiths. In Table 30–2, there are

Table 30–2. **Practices of Religious Groups that Relate to Health Care**

GROUP	SPIRITUAL LEADER	RELIGIOUS BOOK	BELIEFS, LAWS, CUSTOMS
American Indian	Medicine man Shaman		There are approximately 300 tribes of Indians, each with its own culture and beliefs. Some commonalities are folklore, magic, herbal medicine, protection against disease by supernatural powers. Many Indians are Christian; others hold traditional beliefs.
Church of Christ Scientist (Christian Scientists)	Practitioner	Bible *Science and Health with Key to the Scripture*	Disease is an unreality or an error of the human mind. Healing occurs through the application of natural spiritual law. These persons are rarely admitted to hospitals, and when they are, they prefer the minimum of treatment. The patient may request the practitioner.
Hinduism		*Vedas*—divine revelations *Upanishads*—scriptures	Brahman is the Divine Intelligence, Supreme Reality. The body is the temple for the inner self (*atman*) which is reborn after death. A Hindu reaches God by study, love, work, and meditation. Some illness may be seen as a sign of wrongdoing in a previous life. Veal and beef are not eaten; many are vegetarians.
Islam		*Koran*	God is Allah; Muhammed is his prophet. Belief in heaven and hell and moral life. Prays five times a day facing the East. This requires a prayer rug and water for ritual handwashing. *Ramadan* is a month of ritual fasting from sunup to sunset. Islams do not eat pork, intoxicating beverages, beef. May be vegetarians.
Judaism	Rabbi	*Torah*—first five books of Bible *Talmud*—commentaries on *Torah*	Mandatory circumcision of all but Reform Jews. Kosher is the dietary law kept by many Jews. Jews who keep kosher do not eat pig, horse, shellfish; do not eat milk and meat together. Meat must be slaughtered in a prescribed manner to be acceptable. Jews have a religious obligation to visit the sick and to remain at the bedside of a dying patient. Holidays: *Rosh Hashanah* (New Year) and *Yom Kippur* (Day of Atonement). Day of worship from sundown Friday to sundown Saturday.
Mormons Church of Jesus Christ of Latter-Day Saints	Church priesthood holder	*Book of Mormon* Bible	Disease is seen as a failure to keep health laws, other commandments, not exposure to microorganisms. The day of worship is Sunday. Do not use tobacco, alcohol, or hot drinks such as coffee and tea. The Sacrament of the Lord's Supper. Every Mormon is considered an official missionary.
Protestantism	Minister Reverend Pastor	Bible	There are many denominations, but most share the common belief that no one church has sole authority to interpret God's law. Most believe in baptism marking entry into the church and communion as symbolic of the body of Christ. Sunday is the day of worship. Contact with the religious group is maintained by visits of leader and members. Christmas and Easter are major holy days.
Roman Catholics	Priest (addressed as "Father")	Bible	Belief in death and resurrection of Christ as God. Belief that life on earth is rewarded or punished after death. Infant baptism is mandatory. In an emergency, anyone may baptize. While pouring water on forehead, say, "I baptize you in the name of the Father, and of the Son, and of the Holy Spirit." The Sacrament of the Sick is the anointing of the ill person and prayers for pardon. The nurse calls the priest while the patient is alive. Sunday is a required day of worship, although ill persons are not obligated. The priest may visit in the hospital to bring communion and hear confession, if desired.

Source: R. Murray and J. Zentner: *Nursing Concepts For Health Promotion*, 1975, and J. Pumphrey: Recognizing your patients' spiritual needs. *Nursing 77*, **12**:66–68, 1977.

brief descriptions of a few faiths. After examining the attitudes and requirements of various religious groups, one can readily see that religion influences behavior. Ideally, one's beliefs provide strength, an inner quietness, and faith with which to work through and give meaning to life's problems. It is helpful for the nurse to recognize the struggles involved in working through life's problems so that active support can be given. In instances where the patient holds beliefs that are contrary to the nurse's knowledge and beliefs about health care, it becomes necessary to examine the results of healing the body while injuring the spirit. For example, when a Jehovah's Witness patient chooses to die instead of accepting a blood transfusion or a Christian Science patient delays treatment, nurses may feel angry and find it difficult to care for them. These are situations that the nurse may desire to discuss with the chaplain or spiritual leader in order to resolve personal conflicts related to the priorities chosen by the patient. In many instances, the chaplain or spiritual leader may share the nurse's feelings. When these feelings are shared, it enables each of them better to accept the decision of the patient and then give support and comfort to the patient.

Initiating the Topic

Since religious practices vary from one religious faith to another, a key question for the nurse to ask is, "How can I help you in carrying out your faith?" The response to this question will provide direction for the nurse. It also opens the discussion of spiritual needs for the patient and acknowledges the willingness of the nurse to assist.

It can be both challenging and frightening to be faced with opening oneself up to identifying and meeting spiritual needs of patients. It is challenging because there are many patients who feel very lonely. By exploring with them their spiritual needs there is the possibility of reviving hope. Usually, hope is defined as relating to the feeling that what is desired is also possible, or that events may turn out for the best; however, many times it is less dependent on being cured or getting what one desires than on the feeling that help is available and that active participation in care is encouraged (Buehler, 1975). It is frightening because the human experience is shared. What the nurse sees in the patient, if not resolved in the nurse's life, becomes a reminder, perhaps painful, of the nurse's own need.

Establishing Acceptance

Many people reveal a great deal about themselves when they feel the nurse accepts them as they are with

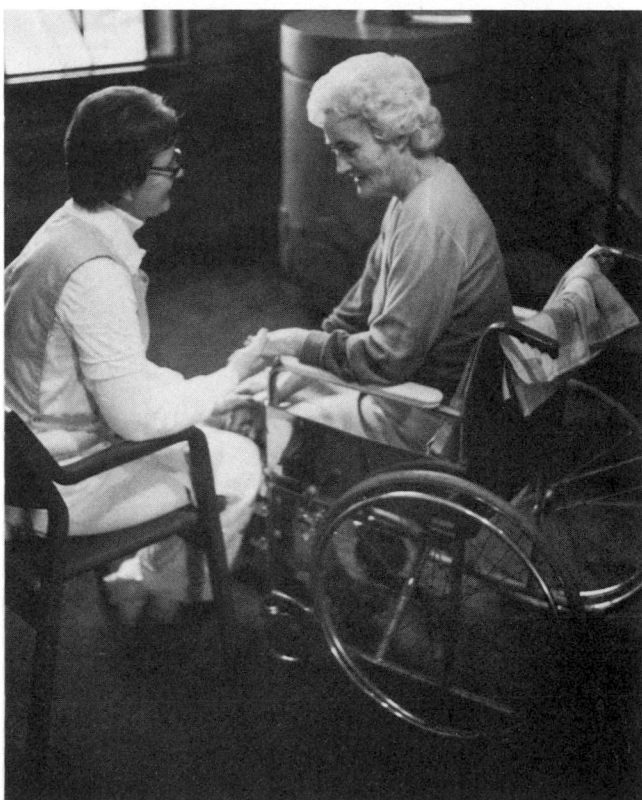

Figure 30-1. A nursing student and a patient discuss spiritual needs in the quiet and privacy of the chapel. (Courtesy of Colleen Spadacinni, Oak Terrace Nursing Home, Minnetonka, MN.)

their strengths and limitations. It is easy to want to change people and then accept them. People are all their strengths and weaknesses. If both cannot be acknowledged, then there is a lack of acceptance of that person. When a person knows acceptance, change is possible. Without acceptance, there is a need to protect self from the hurt of rejection.

Communication

There is much that the nurse can do to assist the patient and family. Often, the patient will want to talk during and immediately after physical care has been given. This is a time when a patient may allow feelings to surface about spiritual needs. Listening intently and encouraging the patient to share both positive and negative feelings help the patient feel accepted. Empathy can be displayed by asking the patient to share how the situation is perceived and then reflecting to the patient what is heard. This helps the patient to develop trust in the relationship and feel more comfortable asking that more intimate desires be met, e.g., prayer and scripture reading.

Prayer

During a period of crisis, a patient may find it difficult to pray or be too weak to pray. The nurse may offer to pray with the patient. (See Figure 30–1.) The nurse can take cues from the patient about the content of the prayer. Patients frequently desire prayer to be able to find comfort and/or deal with the fear about the outcome of their illness. Sometimes, a prayer seeking peace is more potent than sleeping medication. It is generally realistic to pray for strength to cope with the crisis than for an immediate cure. Prayer is not a magic instant answer.

Scripture

The use of scriptures or religious writings is another useful tool for the nurse. Many times, the patient will request a specific passage that is very personally meaningful. At other times, the patient may request the nurse to select something. If the nurse is not able to do so, it may be helpful to find a colleague who is comfortable doing this. This provides an opportunity for nurses to learn from each other in developing their skills in meeting spiritual needs.

Working with Spiritual Leaders

It is important to recognize that there are resources available to assist in providing spiritual care to patients. The chaplain or the patient's own spiritual leader can be of assistance or may even be the primary care-giver. To begin with, it is helpful to develop a working relationship with the chaplain. It is helpful to exchange information about the services each can provide and the criteria for referral. They may also desire to share concerns about ways in which the nurse and chaplain can be mutually helpful to one another in defining and accomplishing their common goal(s) related to spiritual needs.

When the chaplain or spiritual leader comes to see the patient, it is helpful to provide pertinent patient information which includes age, religion, diagnosis, occupation, and any special concerns or nursing observations. The concerns and observations can include a summation of the patient's faith, religious practices the patient finds helpful, sources of hope and strength, and the kinds of spiritual support or assistance that would be helpful (Shelly, 1978).

Special Rituals and Services

Special rituals and services are important to many patients; often Roman Catholic, Jewish, and Protestant services are held in the hospital chapel. For patients who desire to attend the services, the nurse plans the patient's physical care in a manner that encourages participation. Arrangements can also be made for patients who are unable to attend services to participate in meaningful rituals by notifying the chaplain or spiritual leader of the patient's request. Again, planning with the health team to eliminate interruptions is essential. A calendar of religious holidays can be of value in helping nurses to plan for these special observances. The patient's family can also provide information which helps to ensure that the patient's spiritual needs are met in a manner consistent with their usual practices.

Nursing Care Plan for a Patient with Unmet Spiritual Needs

The following patient situation portrays the use of the nursing process when the need for spirituality is not met.

Mrs. H. was a 38-year-old woman being treated by chemotherapy for a recurrence of cancer following treatment for breast cancer four years ago. She had been separated from her husband for several years, had no children, and lived alone. Mrs. H. followed her chemotherapy regimen to the letter, yet she felt nauseated and weak most of the time.

Mrs. H. reported that she was very anxious and wondered aloud, "Why me?" She stated, "It was bad enough to go through this once, but now I can't bear losing hair again." Mrs. H. shared that she had had "faith" but went on to say, "it's much harder this time, especially during the Christmas holidays. I wish I had gone to church more often. Now it's really important to me, but I feel so awful. I wouldn't be able to sit through a service. I'd really like to be able to take communion."

Mrs. H. had many friends who visited her often during her first experience with cancer, but now she wondered, "Won't they get tired of me? I'm always sick. I have to be on chemotherapy for two more years." Mrs. H. commented further, "I've done my time, I've had my share. Everything is falling apart for me. When will it end?"

Nursing Diagnosis	Goal	Nursing Actions
1. Spiritual anger/long illness	1. a. Short term: Patient will verbalize her anger. b. Long term: Patient will state that she accepts her illness and will do what she can to recover.	1. a. Promote warm caring atmosphere. b. Encourage verbalization of anxieties. c. Encourage expression of anger. d. Offer to call chaplain/minister. e. Confer with chaplain.
2. Spiritual loss/long illness	2. Patient will receive communion in her room during the holidays.	2. a. Explain the services of the chaplain, especially communion. b. Assist the patient to identify the times she would like communion. c. Inform chaplain of request. d. Plan nursing care so it will not interfere with communion.

Evaluation	Reassessment
1. a. Short-term goal met. Patient states, "It feels so good just to say what I am feeling. I didn't realize I was so angry. Most of the anger is gone, but I'm still scared. What if I don't make it? How long can I go on like this?" b. Long-term goal met. Patient has talked with chaplain and resumed relationship with her own pastor. She stated, "Now I've found some relief." 2. Goal met. Patient had communion from the chaplain on the Fourth Sunday of Advent and on Christmas day in her room. Patient expresses desire to have communion each Sunday in her room.	1. a. New nursing diagnosis Prone to spiritual anxiety related to recent recurrence of cancer. Continue same nursing actions. b. Continue goal and planned actions. 2. Continue goal and planned actions for Sundays.

Summary

The spiritual dimension of life is a quality broader than religion. Spiritual needs are experienced by all persons. Frequently, a patient becomes acutely aware of these needs during a crisis, e.g., birth, illness, death. The patient's spiritual beliefs can affect the recovery from illness and attitude toward prescribed treatment.

Spiritual needs assessment is done using a systematic approach. A care plan is developed with a patient to meet identified needs. The nursing goals are to assist the patient and the patient's family to identify and meet spiritual needs in a manner acceptable and satisfying to the patient.

The nurse often works in cooperation with the chaplain or spiritual leader. Together, the nurse and spiritual leader try to support beliefs that will help the patient regain health or comfort. The belief system may include rituals related to birth, death, health crisis, diet, and beliefs.

It is important for the nurse to meet personal spiritual needs in order to increase effectiveness in meeting the needs of patients.

Terms for Review

chaplain	ritual	spiritual crisis
religion	spiritual	spiritual need

Self-Assessment

Most nurses anticipate meeting patients' physical needs, but have not given a great deal of thought to meeting the needs of the patients' body and spirit. The word "spiritual" can conjure up many questions. Among them are the following (Fish and Shelly, 1978):

1. Are all religions valid?
2. Is it my religious duty to make converts to my religion?
3. Is there a life after death?
4. What do I believe about sin?
5. Do I believe illness to be a punishment for sin?
6. Why does God permit suffering?
7. Can I meet the patient's spiritual needs if the patient is doing something in conflict with my spiritual values (e.g., abortion, refusing surgery or treatment for a malignancy)?
8. What if the prescribed treatment is in conflict with the spiritual values of the patient (e.g., blood transfusions for an adult or child)?

Questions 1 through 6 are questions faced by all persons, whether one is a nurse or not. These are questions that patients will ask in a variety of ways. The remaining questions are ethical questions that deserve much thought.

Learning Activities

1. Talk with the hospital chaplain about the services offered to hospitalized patients.
2. Talk with the minister (rabbi, or other religious leader) in the community about the ways in which the religious group meets the needs of members who are hospitalized.

Review Questions

Matching Questions
Directions: Match the following terms with the appropriate definition.

1. Spiritual   A. A belief in the supernatural or divine force that has power over the universe and commands worship and obedience; a comprehensive code of ethics or philosophy.

2. Religion   B. Aspects of or pertaining to the spirit as distinguished from the physical nature.

3. Spiritual need   C. A period of time when one's usual coping mechanisms to meet spiritual needs are not working.

4. Spiritual crisis   D. Any factor required to maintain support and viability of the spiritual dimension of life.

Multiple Choice
Directions: Select the best response.

1. An event that is most likely to cause the patient to reevaluate spiritual needs would be
   a. Purchase of a new home
   b. Promotion to assistant manager
   c. Accidental loss of body part
   d. Addition of new member to the family
   e. Move to another state
2. Spiritual assessment of the patient can be done most effectively by doing which of the following?
   a. Excluding family from participating in sharing information about the patient
   b. Referring the patient to the chaplain for assessment
   c. Exploring systematically the patient's spiritual needs and how the patient usually meets them.
   d. Waiting for the patient to verbally indicate a spiritual need
   e. Discussing ways that the nurse can assist the patient to meet spiritual needs.
3. The main goal of nursing intervention in relation to meeting patient's spiritual needs is
   a. Identify spiritual needs
   b. Develop a working relationship with the chaplain
   c. Convert the patient to the nurse's religion
   d. Refer the patient to the chaplain for in-depth counseling
   e. Assist the patient to cope with spiritual distress
4. Which of the following is not considered an acceptable technique in spiritual care intervention?
   a. Providing the patient with information about services of the hospital chaplain
   b. Focusing on what the patient sees as a spiritual need
   c. Diverting the patient away from spiritual concerns in order to concentrate on physical healing
   d. Sharing the responsibility of assisting the patient to meet spiritual needs with the chaplain or spiritual leader
   e. Including the patient's family in spiritual care of the patient when appropriate.

5. In a referral to the chaplain, which of the following sets of information would be most helpful in facilitating communication?
    a. Religion, diagnosis, age, occupation, and special concerns and nursing observations
    b. Religion, marital status, number of children, age, occupation, and hobbies
    c. Diagnosis, age, marital status, attending physician, and occupation
    d. Attending physician, occupation, religion, and name of spiritual leader

Answers

Matching Questions
1. b
2. a
3. d
4. c

Multiple Choice
1. c
2. c
3. e
4. c
5. a

Suggested Readings

Fish, S., and **Shelly, J.**: *Spiritual Care: The Nurse's Role.* InterVarsity Press, Downers Grove, Ill., 1978. This text brings together research, theory, and practice to give specific guidelines to help the nurse define professional responsibilities in spiritual care.

Meyeroff, Milton: *On Caring.* Harper & Row, New York, 1971. This book gives a generalized description of caring and discusses how caring can give comprehensive meaning and order to one's life.

Shelly, J.: *The Spiritual Needs of Children.* InterVarsity Press, Downers Grove, Ill., 1982. This text covers spiritual growth and development, spiritual assessment, and intervention for children and their families.

Bibliography and References

Buehler, J.: What contributes hope in the cancer patient? *Am. J. Nurs.* **75**:1353–56, 1975.

Fish, S., and Shelly, J.: *Spiritual Care: The Nurse's Role.* InterVarsity Press, Downers Grove, Ill., 1978.

Heimler, E.: *Survival in Society.* Weidenfeld and Nocolson, London, 1975.

Kim, M., and Moritz, D. (eds.): *Classification of Nursing Diagnosis: Proceedings of Third and Fourth National Conference.* McGraw-Hill, New York, 1983.

Murray, R., and Zentner, J.: Religious influences on the person. In *Nursing Concepts for Health Promotion*, 2nd ed. Prentice-Hall, Englewood Cliffs, N.J., 1975.

Pumphrey, J.: Recognizing your patients' spiritual needs. *Nursing 77,* **12**:66–68, 1977.

O'Brien, M.: The need for spiritual integrity. In Yura, H., and Walsh, M. (eds.): *Human Needs 2 and the Nursing Process*, Appleton-Century Crofts, Norwalk, Ct., 1982.

Shelly, J.: *Spiritual Care Workbook—A Companion to Spiritual Care: A Nurse's Role.* InterVarsity Press, Downers Grove, Ill., 1978.

Stallwood, J., and Stoll, R.: Spiritual dimensions of nursing practice, In Beland, I., and Pasos, J. (eds.): *Clinical Nursing: Pathophysiological and Psychosocial Approaches*, 3rd ed. Macmillan, New York, 1975.

Stoll, R.: Guidelines for spiritual assessment. *Am. J. Nurs.* **9**:1574–77, 1979.

THE NEED FOR SELF-ESTEEM*

Objectives

1. Define self-esteem and differentiate it from a compensatory security system.

2. Explain the importance of self-awareness to building self-esteem.

3. Describe the steps in developing self-awareness.

4. Explain the physical and emotional consequences of low self-esteem.

5. Describe the relationship between stressful events and the ability of individuals to maintain a positive sense of worth.

6. Describe the two general categories of responses to stressful events and the impact that the use of each has on self-esteem.

7. Identify major esteem-threatening stressors confronted by patients.

8. Identify subjective and objective data indicating satisfaction of esteem needs.

9. Identify subjective and objective data associated with problems of self-esteem.

10. Describe the general goal of nursing interventions in this need area.

11. Discuss the importance of the therapeutic use of self in promoting self-esteem.

12. Describe nursing interventions to increase self-awareness.

13. Describe nursing interventions to enhance self-esteem through promoting a positive perception of and response to stressors.

14. Describe nursing interventions to enhance self-esteem through mobilizing interpersonal resources.

Introduction

Self-esteem is a concept of central importance to nursing. And yet, it is also an idea that is elusive. Just as it is difficult to define what constitutes the self, so it is a problematic task to identify how and what factors contribute to one's sense of self-worth. Recognizing the difficulty of this task, however, does not diminish its im-

*Written by Tom Olson, an Assistant Professor of Nursing at the College of The Virgin Islands, St. Croix campus. His primary responsibility is teaching mental health nursing. Previously, Tom was a clinical nursing specialist in an out-patient mental health setting where he worked with patients in groups as well as individually.

portance, especially to nursing. Bush and Kjervik (1979) convey a feeling of immediacy to this effort in the following quotation:

> It is appropriate and essential that nurses improve their self-image* and take control of their own profession. They need to do this both for themselves as individuals who have chosen to be nurses and for the people whose health is their commitment and concern.

These authors point to a connection between the self-images of nurses and the health of patients. This relationship, which will be explored at several points in the chapter, is based on the belief that the ability of nurses to satisfy their own needs affects their ability to care for the needs of others. Consistent with this idea, this chapter is as much about nurses and prospective nurses as it is about the persons for whom they care.

Defining Self-Esteem

Self-esteem is both a personal feeling and a self-evaluation, or judgment, of one's worth. It refers to how one regards one's self. It is a dynamic concept which involves unique changes for each individual as specific challenges in life are confronted. However simple the concept may seem at first glance, it is in fact a multifaceted phenomenon that influences people's thoughts and behavior in a variety of ways.

Maslow has broken down the need for self-esteem into two sets of esteem-related needs. These groupings include the qualities necessary to feel and believe one is worthwhile, that is, to achieve high self-esteem. In the first, Maslow has included the desires for strength, achievement, adequacy, mastery, competence, confidence, and independence (Maslow, 1954). The feeling and judgment of one's worth in reference to these qualities may come from (within) one's self, as with the inner satisfaction experienced by the student nurse who has mastered giving an IM injection, as well as from a valued person, such as the nursing instructor who praises the success of the student. Clearly, the newly hospitalized patient, thrown into unfamiliar and perhaps even frightening surroundings, may experience threats to these esteem-related needs. Regardless of the condition that precipitated hospitalization, the patient's mastery and control of the environment, and thus self-esteem, will be seriously challenged. In the second set, Maslow has included the qualities of prestige, status, dominance, dignity, and appreciation. In contrast to the first grouping, the satisfaction of these desires requires interaction with others. For example, a nurse's positive self-esteem is reinforced when colleagues are overhead praising the nurse's sensitivity in assisting an elderly man with an amputated limb to work toward acceptance of his loss. In the hospitalized patient, threats in this area

are increased as the individual's contact with significant others is curtailed.

Jean Clarke has offered a brief summary of Maslow's sets of esteem-related qualities in a simple, yet meaningful, definition of self-esteem. She explains that self-esteem is one's assessment of the extent to which one is capable (corresponding to Maslow's first set of qualities) and lovable (corresponding to the second set of qualities) (Clarke, 1978). Clarke has noted that self-esteem is nourished by recognizing one's own lovableness and capabilities, as well as by being recognized as lovable and capable by other people. Thus, the nursing student, for example, grows not only by becoming capable of giving an injection, but also in feeling glad about being a unique and special person. Similarly, the hospitalized patient's self-worth is enhanced not only by mastery of a new environment, but also in continuing to feel appreciated and important as a human being.

Accurate Self-Esteem

It is important at this point to draw a distinction between accurate and inaccurate self-esteem. The latter has been termed a *compensatory security system* (Chrzanowski, 1981). These are very different and opposing ideas, and yet on the surface they may easily be confused with each other. One can begin to clarify these concepts by first taking a look at what constitutes a security system and then, against this background, examining what is meant by accurate self-esteem.

A compensatory security system refers to the projection to others of an image of positive self-worth when, in reality, one's sense of worth is low. The person who has substituted a security system for a valid self-esteem is like Jourard's self-alienated individual who "ignores his tilt signals—anxiety, guilt, fatigue, boredom, pain, or frustration" and essentially pretends to feel good (Jourard, 1971). Such an individual may outwardly project an image of self-confidence in an attempt to hide

---

*Self-esteem may be substituted for self-image in this quotation. The close relationship between these two concepts will be described later in the chapter. Note also that self-esteem, self-worth, and sense of worth are used interchangeably in this chapter.

low self-esteem. The appearance of feeling good about one's self is just that, an appearance. What one sees is actually the person's security system or pseudo-self-esteem. This mask is revealed by the compensatory mechanisms that maintain it, including false pride, conceit, and make-believe or "as-if" performances. Inwardly, this individual is most likely experiencing tension and confusion.

Inaccurate self-esteem can be explained as a self-deception that results from a major clash between the *real self*, who one actually is, and the *ideal self*, who one would like to be. In other words, the person's inner judgment of self is markedly different from actual experience. There are many examples of this in everyday life and patient care situations. For instance, the woman who seems to exude self-confidence and well-being immediately after having experienced a grieving process has most likely substituted a security system in place of an accurate self-esteem. The sharp contrast between her self-portrayal and her actual experience betrays her low self-esteem. The patient has ignored her "tilt signals," probably through excessive use of the defense mechanism of denial (refer to p. 000 for a more complete description of defense mechanisms). What makes this situation particularly problematic in terms of nursing care is that individuals can tolerate only so much inner tension and confusion before serious physical or psychological damage results. Even if this specific patient's security system is strong enough to ward off resulting psychological effects such as depression, her body may register a protest loud enough to be heard in the form of renewed physical illness. Thus, the accuracy of self-esteem is an important issue for the patient and nurse.

Unlike a security system, which basically hides a low self-esteem, an accurate or valid sense of one's worth is based on self-awareness. This means that one is able to value one's self for who and what one really is. The development of self-awareness is part of a process that leads to the formation of a person's self-concept. This, in turn, becomes the foundation for the individual's self-esteem. In order to gain an understanding of how an accurate self-esteem is built, it is necessary to look further at this process and the close interrelationship of these concepts.

Self-Awareness

Self-awareness is a developmental experience which begins at birth. It results in thinking, feeling, acting persons who recognize themselves as playing different roles and consciously displaying different aspects of themselves. Inherent in becoming self-aware is an acceptance of situations, others, and one's own self as they really are. Ideally, self-awareness is a process of continually expanding one's knowledge of self.

The process of self-awareness is symbolized more clearly by considering the self as having four components:

1. The public self, that area of the person readily free and open to one's self and others
2. The semipublic self, that area of which the person is unaware but others perceive
3. The private self, that area known to the person but hidden from others
4. The inner self, that area unknown to the person or others.

Using this representation, the goal of self-awareness has been described in one of the following two ways: first, an enlarging area number one, while reducing the other three; or second, as at least becoming more knowledgeable about and comfortable with areas one, two, and three in order to decrease the need to defend against area four (Stuart and Sundeen, 1979). Regardless of the way it is stated, the aim is still to increase one's awareness of self. Unlike parts of the self that may remain unknown, the steps to accomplish this goal are neither hidden nor mysterious. The steps in developing self-awareness include (1) listening to oneself, (2) listening to and learning from others, and (3) self-disclosure—telling others about oneself.

With the first step, one strives to consciously experience one's thoughts and feelings. This requires the ability to identify and accept varying emotions, such as sadness, joy, and anger. It is often the most difficult step to accomplish for nurses as well as patients. For instance, the nurse who abruptly tries to quiet a crying patient who is grieving the loss of a body part may be reacting more to personal discomfort than to the actual situation. The end result may be further stifling of the nurse's own awareness of inner thoughts and feelings, as well as interference in the patient's experiencing of emotions. This is not to imply that the nurse, confronted with a tearful patient and memories of personal losses, should break down and sob. Rather, it means that in this situation the nurse tries to identify personal feelings and recognize possible causes for them in order to respond to the patient in the most therapeutic manner. For some individuals, this first step may seem insurmountable. Methods such as relaxation training, biofeedback, yoga, and psychotherapy are potentially useful in assisting persons to become more aware of their thoughts and feelings. The second step, listening to and learning from others, may be viewed as opening up area two, the semipublic self, by increasing individuals' awareness of how others perceive them. It may also be a difficult achievement in the process of self-awareness. For instance, student nurses who are told they have done a competent job of transferring a patient may tend to discount this information. In terms of self-awareness, this tendency may interfere with increasing self-knowledge. It is important then, in the process of developing self-awareness, to listen carefully to the critical and positive information about one's self provided by others.

The third step in becoming self-aware involves self-disclosure. Jourard has noted that, "No man can come to know himself except as an outcome of disclosing himself to another person" (Jourard, 1971). In revealing one's self to others, one is better able to acknowledge the real self, with various feelings, strengths, weaknesses, and possibilities for growth. Trust in others is a critical requirement in this part of the process since self-disclosure often means taking a risk, especially as one discloses information from area three, the private self. According to Jourard, the inability to self-disclose results in arrested personal growth and meaningless relationships with people. Nurses are frequently in situations in which patients may share very personal information. For instance, a young man with a disfiguring skin (dermatological) problem shares feelings of sexual frustration with the nurse and reveals a long-standing inability to talk about this problem with anyone. How will the nurse respond?

Nurses who are uncomfortable with their own self-disclosure will tend to discourage such disclosure by others through changing the subject, joking, ignoring patients' statements, or other similar actions. However, in addition to obstructing patients' sharing about themselves, such actions reinforce nurses' self-concealment. In this manner, nursing actions may either lead to increased self-awareness and growth for the nurse and patient, or interventions may compel both to become more hidden from self and others. As pointed out earlier, the steps to developing self-awareness are neither hidden or mysterious. In order to be useful, however, they must be practiced on a regular basis. The result of practicing self-disclosure and carefully listening to one's inner thoughts and feelings, as well as the responses of others, is self-awareness, that is, the ability to be "in touch" with the various aspects of one's self at various points in space and time.

Self-Concept and Its Relationship to Self-Esteem

It is within the process of becoming aware of self that a person's self-concept or self-image begins to emerge. As awareness of one's own being develops, a sense of self made up of the experiences of being and functioning within one's environment is acquired. In this sense, the formation of a person's self-concept is dependent on the process of developing self-awareness.

Self-concept then is the mental picture a person constructs of self based on an awareness of internal and external experiences. Internal experiences include those one has within one's self, such as the feeling of elation accompanying the sudden understanding of a difficult concept, while external experiences involve interactions with other people and one's surroundings. Self-concept includes a person's nonbody-images—such as spiritual, emotional, and intellectual makeup—as well as body-image. *Body-image* is itself a major component of the self-concept. Jourard has accurately described it as the perceptions, beliefs, and knowledge individuals hold in regard to their body's structure, function, appearance, and limits (Jourard, 1963). In short, self-concept is the description used to identify one's self as being unique and different from other individuals. Because each person's experiences within the self and with others and the environment are unique, so each person's self-concept is unique. No two people will ever have identical self-concepts. Moreover, because the self is always changing in response to new experiences, self-concept, like self-esteem, is constantly changing.

A healthy self-concept is a prerequisite for high self-esteem. Accurate self-esteem is a judgment and feeling of self-worth which develops from a healthy self-concept grounded in self-awareness.

Importance of Self-Esteem to Nursing

Self-esteem is more than just a good feeling. The level of one's self-esteem has been shown to influence such diverse phenomena as one's ability to form close interpersonal relationships, as well as one's resistance to psychological and physical illness. With this in mind, the study of self-esteem should be viewed as crucially important to all health care providers, especially nurses.

Individuals with low self-esteem have difficulty in developing and maintaining warm interpersonal relationships. On a very basic level, it seems that if persons are unable to view themselves as worthwhile, they are unable to see value in others and have difficulty believing that others can see value in them. Such individuals exert extreme energy to protect or hide from others those aspects of personality they believe to be the real self. They tend to set themselves apart from people, often resorting to social withdrawal as a defense. In a patient care situation, such patients may appear lonely and depressed. These emotional difficulties, in turn, may complicate the condition for which they initially sought health care assistance.

Depression is related to low self-esteem, both indirectly, as a result of alienation from self and others, as well as more directly, as the consequence of feeling that one is unworthy. One specific aspect of self-esteem that is particularly significant in regard to depression is the absence or presence of the sense of being capable or in control. The loss of control and associated feelings of helplessness are directly related to depression. Using the example given at the beginning of this chapter of problems confronted by the newly hospitalized patient, it is not difficult to understand how the patient's self-esteem, especially as it translates into loss of control, could be threatened during hospitalization and lead to an emotional disturbance such as depression. Depression, though, is far from the only result of low self-esteem specifically as it is related to a feeling of helplessness.

A relationship between loss of control and physical illness has also been shown. For instance, it has been demonstrated that increasing environmental control for those in later life who are institutionalized has a positive impact on both their psychological and physical states (Schulz and Benner, 1977). Murphy (1982) points out that patients' feelings of control may partly determine physical prognosis and psychological reaction to their illness. Other investigators have found a correlation between helplessness and illnesses such as minor viral infections and coronary heart disease (Rahe and Lind, 1971). However, even beyond its relationship to helplessness, self-esteem is an overall critical factor influencing physical and psychological health.

In a general manner, self-esteem can be described as an insulator against stress. For instance, high self-esteem has been found to be associated with low anxiety and fewer psychosomatic symptoms of stress (Coopersmith, 1967). This is of tremendous significance to nurses and patients since stress, or at least the way in which individuals deal with it, has been linked with a multitude of emotional and physical diseases. Pelletier (1977) notes that one standard medical text estimates that 50 to 80 percent of all diseases have their origins in stress. Studies indicate that frequent life changes resulting in high levels of stress may lead to increases in illnesses such as tuberculosis, inguinal hernia, leukemia, nonfatal coronary occlusion, and others (Rahe, 1973; Rahe et al., 1970). Clearly, one's self-esteem is of major importance if it can influence the ability to cope with stress.

Self-esteem is no less relevant to the nurse as an individual than it is to the patient. It has been shown that nurses with high self-esteem were rated as giving better care than nurses who felt less positive about themselves (Dyer et al., 1975). Nurses who are unable to meet their own needs will have difficulty meeting the needs of patients. Clarke (1978) offers a simple yet appropriate summation to this discussion of why self-esteem is important: "positive self-esteem is important because when people experience it, they feel good and look good, they are effective and productive, and they respond to other people and themselves in healthy, positive, growing ways."

Issues in the Development of Self-Esteem

Careful observation of persons—family, work colleagues, classmates, friends—reveals that each communicates something pertaining to how they feel about themselves in a particular time and space. This is conveyed in posture, gait, speech, facial expressions, gestures, silences, assertiveness. How were these assessments of self-worth reached? And, depending on age and other life circumstances, what will the individual be communicating to others about self-esteem in 5, 10, 20 years? These are questions which this section intends to explore by examining some important issues in the development of self-esteem.

Self-Esteem–Building Messages and Recycling

As discussed earlier in this text, one's self-esteem develops within the framework of the individual's overall growth and development. It is interesting to note that at least one researcher has concluded that a primitive sense of self-worth emerges even in infancy (Brissett, 1972). Certainly, the groundwork for a person's self-worth, like so many other aspects of the self, is laid down at a very early age.

Coopersmith (1967) has described four ways to make this foundation strong. He explains that in order to promote a child's self-esteem caring adults need to provide the child with success, instill ideals, encourage aspirations, and help build defenses against attacks of self-perceptions. In describing affirmations for growth, Levin (1974) has taken this one step further by suggesting specific messages adults can send to children to promote self-esteem building. (See Table 31–1.) As Clarke points out in the concept of recycling, everyone may need and benefit from these affirmations at various times in their lives. Recycling, Clarke (1978) explains, is doing early developmental tasks again at an older age and in a more grown-up way. It is the assurance that all persons have more than one chance in life to resolve problems and get what they need in order to feel worthwhile. This is where the concept of self-esteem, in a developmental framework, is most significant and relevant to nursing. Nurses frequently care for persons who have never developed a positive self-esteem and need assistance in affirming the worth of their existence. Even more likely, in the face of new and severe demands, patients may find their well-established sense of worth seriously challenged. Nurses may be in the best position to assist in mobilizing forces around patients, such as family and friends, to support patients' self-esteem. And for nurses themselves, as they confront the rewards and problems of their profession, they will also need to make sure that esteem needs are being met. To be sure, one does not reach an absolute and completed position in terms of achieving self-esteem. Instead, a person's sense of worth may be strengthened or weakened in response to the challenges or stressful events involved in day-to-day living. Consequently, how persons cope with stress-producing situations is an important issue in the development of self-esteem.

Stress, Adaptation, and the Development of Self-Esteem

Self-esteem has been described as an insulator against stress. This may seem to portray stress as primarily a negative reaction. Stress, however, is an essential ingredient of life. Hans Selye, one of the foremost researchers in this area, describes *stress* as the nonspecific response of the body to any demand made upon it (Selye, 1965). The demand, or stimulus, that prompts this response is called the *stressor*. Whether the stressor is primarily physical, such as a change in room temperature, surgery, or an infection, or psychological, such as loss of a loved one or fear of the unknown, the individual is forced to adapt to the situation. Therein lies the greatest significance of this issue in terms of self-esteem and nursing.

Many stressors, some of which will be considered here, seem to have an especially high potential for challenging a person's self-esteem. Illness and hospitalization, being a minority patient in the health care system, and the transition from one developmental stage to another are all stressors that may make extreme demands on the individual, particularly in the area of self-worth. However, how one adapts to the stressful event may mean as much, or even more, in terms of how the individual is affected by it, than the actual event itself! One person's crisis may be to another a zestful life experience. Pelletier (1977) has gone on to conclude that periods of marked stress in a person's life can be times of profound growth. In fact, there is some evidence to consider that adaptation to stress is more predictive of health than the simple absence of stress (Beckman, 1971). What exactly is meant by adaptation?

Adaptation, as White (1974) explains, is an ongoing compromise, a series of exchanges between people and their environments. It means neither complete surrender nor total triumph but rather moving toward a constructive middle point. According to Roy (1974), in order to respond positively to a continually changing environment, individuals must adapt. A person's ability to adapt successfully to stressful events is influenced by a number of factors. Some of these, such as the nature of the stressor itself, one's past experiences, and genetic endowment, the individual may have little or no control over during the actual situation. On the other hand, the person has more control in determining how the stressor and the demands it imposes are perceived, as well as in choosing which coping strategies will be used to deal with it. The focus here is on those aspects over which one has more control, particularly in regard to stressors that threaten self-esteem. Limiting this discussion to those aspects of adaptation most immediately under a person's control is not discounting the significance of factors such as hereditary and past experiences, but rather focusing on those aspects on which it is believed nurses can have their greatest impact. One's perceptions and choice of coping strategies are two such aspects that influence successful adaptation.

Perceptions of Stressors.   One's perception of a stressful situation, provided that it is not grossly unrealistic, is a major determinant in deciding whether one's adaptation is successful and one's sense of worth is maintained or even enhanced. For instance, using an illustration of a relatively low-stress situation, consider two young musicians who attend a piano recital by an accomplished concert pianist. After the recital, one of the youths remarks, "I'm depressed; I'll never be able to play like that." In contrast, the second musician mar-

Table 31-1. **Affirmations to Build Self-Esteem**

People communicate to others how they expect them to behave and feel about themselves by how they affirm them, that is, by what they say to and about them. The following are suggestions for messages that build self-esteem throughout individual's lives:

Affirmations for Being

(Especially 0–6 months, but also important for all people throughout their lives):
I'm glad you are here.
You have every right to be here.
Your needs are okay with me.
I'm glad you are a boy, or, I'm glad you are a girl.
You don't have to hurry.
I like to hold you.

Affirmations for Starting to Do Things on One's Own

(6–18 months, early teens, and everyone else doing things on their own):
I recognize that you are doing things on your own.
You don't have to do tricks (be cute, sick, sad, mad, scared) to get approval.
It's okay to do things (try things, initiate things, be curious) and get support and protection at the same time.

Affirmations for Learning to Think

(18 months–3 years, middle teens, and everyone else who needs to do cause-and-effect thinking):
I'm glad you are growing up.
I'm not afraid of your anger.
You can both think and feel at the same time.
You don't have to take care of me when you think.
You can be sure about what you need.

Affirmations for Discovering One's Identity

(3–6 years, middle teens and all who are striving to fulfill their unique capabilities as persons):
I expect you to start understanding the difference between feelings and actions and to ask in direct ways for your needs to be met.
You can be powerful and still have needs.
You don't have to act scared, sick, sad, or mad to be taken care of.
You can express your feelings straight (it's okay to say you are mad, but not to hit).

Affirmations for Getting Ready to Do Things in One's Own Way

(6–12 years, late teens and early twenties, and everyone else making changes):
I see that you are trying out things in order to be independent and responsible.
You can think before you make that rule your own.
You can trust your feelings to help you know.
You can do it your way.
It's okay to disagree.
You don't have to suffer to get what you need.

Affirmations for Working through Old Problems and Separating from Parents

(Teens and early twenties and everyone else separating from a relationship):
I see that you are going over old needs and problems with an added dimension of sexuality.
It's okay to separate and to assume responsibility for your own needs and feelings and behavior as a person in the world.
You can be a sexual person and still have needs.
It's okay to know who you are.
You're welcome to come home again.
I love you.

Source: Adapted from affirmations featured in P. Levin: *Becoming the Way We Are: A Transactional Guide to Personal Development.* Transactional Publications, Berkeley, Calif., 1974.

vels, "That was beautiful; imagine, that pianist must have started out practicing like us! I can hardly wait to get home and play." The first individual seemed to come away with a decreased sense of self-worth, while the second was inspired. One of the keys to using a situation to grow and enhance one's self-esteem seems to be in developing a positive outlook. The two major requirements of remaining positive are:

1. Defining the world as a relatively positive environment
2. Defining self as capable and worthwhile

For those who tend to take a dim view of themselves and the world around them, it is important to point out that people can work toward altering the way they perceive the challenges of living. By increasing self-awareness and realizing that one can "recycle" through earlier developmental tasks, individuals can change their outlook toward the demands placed on them. Nurses are in an especially unique and significant position to assist patients in making this change. For example, nurses may be able to help the patient in traction to be as independent as possible, thus changing a perception of self as helpless, by encouraging the patient to make decisions regarding health care. It is important to note that such nursing interventions involve recognition rather than denial of the actual nature of the stressor. Their general aim is simply to encourage a positive and hopeful view of the stress-producing event. In addition to encouraging a positive outlook in order to enhance successful adaptation and thus increase self-esteem, the nurse's actions may also influence the individual's choice of coping strategies.

Coping Strategies.   A person's choice of coping strategies in responding to stress-producing situations is another important factor in determining how successfully one adapts to an event and whether self-esteem is maintained, enhanced, or decreased. Reactions to stressful situations that threaten self-worth, such as illness and hospitalization, can be divided into two general categories: task-oriented and defense-oriented responses. Both responses may be adaptive, depending on how and when they are used and in what situations.

Task-Oriented Reactions and Assertiveness. Task-oriented reactions are most readily seen as adaptive. They are conscious, action-oriented responses in which one uses one's cognitive skills to cope with a stressor. In this mode of response, a person reacts initially by making an appraisal of the situation. Questions that are asked in appraising a stressful event include:

What is the nature of the threatening situation and its expected unfavorable consequences?

What is the probability that the threatening event will occur?

If the event materializes, how severe is the possible loss to self?

What alternatives are available for coping with the threat?

What is the probability of success of the varying alternatives?

What is the likely personal cost of using each of the alternatives?

Based on the above, which course of action will most likely succeed at the least cost?

After a realistic appraisal of the event is made, a person then decides on the most effective course of action. Appropriate actions are as varied as the individual and the situation. Such actions might range from talking to a friend to seeking help in an emergency room or crisis center. However, one type of task-oriented response which can be said to be effective in various stress-producing situations that involve interactions with people is the use of assertive behavior.

Assertiveness is a prerequisite for building self-esteem. It is especially important in task-oriented adaptive responses since it is a behavior which expresses the belief that each person is important. Bush and Kjervik (1979) have defined assertiveness as follows:

> *Assertiveness* is thinking and acting in ways in which one stands up for one's legitimate personal rights. It is the act of giving expression to one's positive and negative thoughts in a way that defines one's perspective without subtracting from the legitimate rights of others.

Assertiveness is included here because it is a task-oriented response that enhances self-esteem and enables the person to actively cope with a stressful event. In fact, Petrie and Rotheram (1982) conclude that assertiveness is a subcomponent of self-esteem and that positive self-worth and assertiveness levels are associated with low stress. Still further, one's perception of self as utilizing stress, rather than being a passive victim, increases the likelihood that the personal results of one's response to a stressor will be beneficial (Cassell, 1964). Assertiveness, in particular, and task-oriented behavior, in general, encourage the individual to take control and adapt in a manner that maintains the integrity of the self. Inasmuch as one is able to feel competent and capable in responding to a stressor, one's feeling of self-worth is increased.

Defense-Oriented Responses.   Defense-oriented responses are not necessarily maladaptive or negative in terms of self-esteem. They tend to be used, however, when task-oriented reactions have not been successful in adapting to a stressful situation, and anxiety or related feelings remain high. Certain stressors, such as the death of a loved one, may be severe enough to cause most people to use this type of defense, at least temporarily. The specific coping behaviors that are utilized in this category of responses are called defense mechanisms. (Refer to Table 31–2 for a description of some of the more commonly used ones.) Defense mechanisms operate outside awareness in order to protect a person from feelings of worthlessness and inadequacy. They are legitimate strategies of adaptation which are, in a complicated and often threatening society, regularly used by people to protect their sense of worth. They become problematic when used excessively or otherwise inappropriately. If the entire day is spent being defensive, then the self is not allowing information to enter, which is a crucial factor in adapting to stress. From a nursing point of view, one can understand the importance of carefully assessing whether the patient's use of defense mechanisms is essential to preserving self-image and sense of worth, or whether it is maladaptive, and nursing intervention might offer feasible alternatives to improve functioning.

Table 31–2. **Defense Mechanisms**

Name	Definition	Example
Repression	Widely used mechanism in which unacceptable thoughts and feelings are unconsciously kept out of awareness. Requires considerable energy to keep material repressed.	Mr. K. does not recall having hit his six-year-old child during a disagreement.
Identification	Process by which a person tries to take on the characteristics of another admired individual.	Ms. P., a college student, begins to talk and act like an instructor she admires.
Introjection	One of the earliest mechanisms developed, it is an intense form of identification which involves incorporation of another's qualities or values into one's self. It is most important in the development of one's conscience.	Seven-year-old Sally tells her younger brother, "You must not spill your milk."
Projection	The attribution of one's own thoughts and feelings to another person in an effort to block awareness of their existence in one's self.	Mr. L., unable to admit his own hostile feelings, remarks that other people are always getting angry at him.
Reaction formation	The person disguises unacceptable thoughts and feelings by developing attitudes and behavior patterns that are opposite to what is really felt or believed.	Mrs. B., a staff nurse, has intense feelings of anger toward her head nurse; she covers them up by being extremely polite.
Rationalization	Another commonly used mechanism. It is an attempt to justify unacceptable behavior through the use of socially approved or apparently logical explanations.	Greg fails an examination and blames his "ineffective instructor" rather than his lack of studying.
Denial	The simplest and most primitive defense mechanism. The person ignores or refuses to acknowledge disagreeable or threatening realities.	Ms. O. has recently been hospitalized and diagnosed as having diabetes mellitus. After reviewing with her nurse changes she will need to make in her diet, Mrs. O. calls a friend and states she can't wait to return to her usual home cooking after she leaves the hospital.
Regression	A normal part of growth and development. It is a retreat from excessive stress through specific behavior characteristic of an earlier level of development.	Four-year-old Emily has been toilet trained for about one year. However, when her new baby brother is brought home from the hospital, she begins to wet her pants again.
Displacement	Discharge of feelings on an object or person other than the one to which the feelings rightly belong. This involves shifting emotions toward a safer, less threatening person or object than the actual source of the feelings.	Mrs. A. has had a very difficult day at her job. Her boss has been very critical of her efforts on an important project. Although she did not express her frustration to her boss, when she arrives home, Mrs. A. begins yelling at her husband and children.
Sublimation	The transformation of energy associated with unacceptable urges into socially approved pursuits. This is thought to be one of the more important mechanisms in the process of learning.	John has an extremely aggressive nature. He is able though to transfer energy associated with his aggressive impulses to becoming a star tackle on his high school football team.

In summary, the terms "stress" and "stressor" have been defined, their relationship to self-esteem explored, and ways persons have of adapting to stressful situations examined. It is worthwhile to emphasize again that stress is not an inherently negative quality. In addition, the actual effect of a stress-producing event is largely determined by the individual's response to it. Three examples of esteem-threatening stressors will be discussed to illustrate adaptive and maladaptive responses: (1) developmental stressors, (2) being a minority patient in the health care system, and (3) illness and hospitalization.

Developmental Stressors. Developmental stages, according to Sheehy (1976), are not defined by concrete happenings such as getting or losing a job, they are defined by changes that begin within a person. The impulse toward change seems to be present, especially at certain periods in a person's life. These periods are times of transition or passage during which a person feels more vulnerable. Inasmuch as these passages include change, they also involve stress and necessary adaptive or maladaptive responses from individuals. As used here, adaptive is defined as compromise that is self-esteem maintaining or enhancing. A maladaptive response decreases one's sense of worth. Although every stage of life or time of transition is subject to many stressors, two developmental passages in particular seem to be periods of high potential for significant increases or decreases in one's sense of self-worth. One of these periods is the transition between adolescence and young adulthood. The other is the passage into old age.

PASSAGE TO YOUNG ADULTHOOD. During the passage to young adulthood, the person struggles with major life decisions, such as determining life goals and work. The individual is also deciding what kind of life partner will be chosen. Persons in this transition may long to be independent but may be troubled by self-doubt as they question wither they can really make it on their own. Uncertainty about sex-related roles may continue on from adolescence. It is a traumatic period during which one's status seems to constantly change. Such continual change has an adverse effect on self-esteem and physical health. If one views suicide as the ultimate act of self-rejection, then the self-esteem–threatening nature of this stressful passage is supported by suicide statistics for this age group. In adolescents, it is the fourth leading cause of death, and among college students, it is the second most frequent cause of death (Linden and Breed, 1976). Even more disturbing, Ostrovski (1979) notes that in the past decade there has been a 90 percent increase in suicide among men aged 15 to 24 and a 50 percent increase in suicide among women of the same age. Clearly, this is a transition period where the person's self-worth, one's ability to handle immense

changes, is severely tested. If one uses a positive perspective, it is possible to see that the successful negotiation of this passage, through adaptation to the new stressors, may ultimately result in a greatly increased self-esteem. This is not to say that making this transition eliminates further stress. It means, however, that the period of greatest vulnerability has been passed and that the individual may enter a relatively more stable time of growth. It is also evident, though, that in this currently accelerated society, this passage is becoming more and more difficult for many to make. In caring for persons in this period of transition, nurses may be in a position to assist them in sorting out stressors and maintaining a realistic, yet hopeful, view of their current situation.

TRANSITION TO OLD AGE. Similar to the transition just discussed, it is difficult to pinpoint an exact age range when persons make the transition from middle age to old age. Chronological age is a poor index of aging. In one nationwide survey, for instance, about one-third of the subjects aged 70 to 74 reported that they thought of themselves as middle-aged (Shana, 1968). Individual perceptions are a major factor in responding to developmental stressors. However, regardless of when this transaction is actually made, it is a time of particular vulnerability in the area of self-esteem.

Klopfer (1965) has identified the following self-esteem–threatening stressors to which persons must adapt in making the passage to old age:

1. Conflict between youth and old age
2. Youth worship in our present society
3. Decreased interpersonal relationships due to loss of significant others
4. Lack of resistance or adaptability to major stressors
5. Effects of poor memory, loss of spatial orientation, speed, agility, sensory acuity

Perhaps more than during any other period, a person's sense of worth and ability to adapt is seriously threatened during this time. As with young adults, many older persons do not always successfully negotiate this passage. Although persons over 65 comprise only 10 percent of the population, they account for 25 percent of the suicides (Grace and Camilleri, 1981). Indeed, there is no general agreement about whether self-esteem increases with age. According to some researchers, a person's sense of self-worth seems to increase until middle age and then stabilizes or begins to decline gradually (Lowenthal and Chiriboga, 1972). In any event, as Klopfer's listing shows, this is a period during which those qualities that enable people to feel worthwhile— qualities indentified earlier such as competence, independence, importance, and appreciation—are likely to be threatened. Those who successfully adapt to the new stressors may not only maintain their self-worth, but also enhance it as they are able to gain a renewed appreciation of their uniqueness as human beings. Sheehy (1976) explains that one of the rewards of moving through this period is achievement of what Erikson calls integrity, or that stage "in which one can give a blessing to one's own life." In caring for persons making this passage, nurses may have the opportunity to intervene in ways to affirm the person's uniqueness, to assist them in feeling useful, and to increase their independence. In this manner, the nurse's actions can enhance the person's adaptive skills and thus self-esteem.

Stress, Self-Esteem, and the Minority Patient. Members of minority groups face especially serious esteem-threatening stressors when they become patients. Many health care professionals may neither understand nor appreciate the possibility of cultural differences and similarities among persons for whom they care. Often this is due to the belief that one's own values, beliefs, and ways of life are superior to or more desirable than the life-styles of others (*ethnocentrism*). A nurse responding from an ethnocentric frame of reference ends up, either inadvertently or purposely, "putting down" valued aspects of the patient's self. This not only leads to a diminishment of the person's self-esteem but also, as has been pointed out earlier, jeopardizes physical health. Leininger (1977) points out that there is a challenge to health care professionals to apply an understanding of minority differences and similarities to assist people with their "humanistic, physical, social and psychologic needs in a cultural specific manner." Unfortunately, this challenge is often not met.

Ethnic Minorities of Color. Writing about ethnic minorities of color and health care, White (1977) declares, "to be poor and in need of health care is sad. To be poor, a member of an ethnic group of color, and in need of health care is a disaster." White goes on to explain that within health care institutions patients of color are "often treated in a dehumanizing manner. They are not asked to participate in their treatment and the obstacles they must overcome to get minimal care are almost insurmountable." Whether this is the result of inadvertent or purposeful actions by nurses and other health care providers, the outcomes remain detrimental to patients' physical and psychological health. Since a major part of this problem relates to a lack of understanding of cultural differences, it is useful to take a look at some examples of diverse cultural beliefs that may be very important to the minority patient's sense of self-worth.

American Indian Patients. In the American Indian culture, privacy is particularly valued. Customs of the majority white culture, such as a firm handshake and making eye contact, may be interpreted by American Indians in a way that conflicts with this value. Primeaux (1977) notes that "looking one in the eye is considered disrespectful in many Indian tribes." Primeaux continues that she has heard health care providers remark, "All Indians are shiftless—they won't look at you when speaking to them." Such a remark may be seen as directly attacking the Indian patient's sense of dignity, one of the qualities used by Maslow to describe self-esteem. Similarly, the American Indian patient may withdraw from a vigorous handshake, interpreting it as a display of aggression rather than friendliness.

Many American Indians also have a family system that differs from that of the majority white society. Primeaux (1977) states that "to be really poor in the Indian world is to be without relatives." An Indian child, for instance, may have several sets of grandparents, uncles, cousins, brothers, and sisters, depending on the particular tribal makeup. Consider the effects then of hospital policies that restrict visitors to only immediate relatives or no more than two at a time. Depending on how these rules are applied, they may or may not interfere with maintenance of that part of the patient's self-esteem provided through interaction with significant others. Even these few examples demonstrate the impact that a nurse's understanding or lack of understanding of cultural differences may have on the sense of self-worth of patients from this minority group.

Black Patients. For black patients, illness and hospitalization also present stressors that are unique based on their cultural and physical differences from the majority society. For example, frequently nurses in their initial contact with a patient will use a familiar or first name, without first asking how the individual prefers to be addressed. Although this may be accepted or cause only minimal irritation in the majority white culture, not addressing the black patient by his or her last name, prefaced by "Mr.," "Mrs.," or "Miss," is likely to be regarded as disrespectful. Whether or not a nurse recognizes necessary differences in physical care may also have an impact on the black patient's general level of wellness, including self-esteem. Nurses' awareness that hair care for black patients may be different from their own is especially important in this regard. For instance, if the patient's hair is washed, oil should be applied while it is wet and the hair combed before it dries. Physical assessment of black people also differs from what is the norm for white persons. For instance, in assessing cyanosis (a condition of oxygen deficiency evidenced by bluish, grayish, or dark-purple discoloration of the skin) in black persons, the nurse uses the conjunctiva, lips, and tongue. The black patient who is pale may appear ashen gray rather than white. Also, since redness of the skin may be difficult to observe, the nurse may need to rely more on assessment of pain, warmth, and tenderness. Recognizing these differences in planning nursing care not only protects patients' physical health, but also has a positive impact on self-esteem because it communicates respect for and awareness of their uniqueness as persons.

Hispanic Patients.   Hispanic patients in the health care system also face stressors that differ from those confronted by other groups. Most obvious, if patients speak little or no English, they will have particular difficulty understanding explanations or following instructions. This could lead to feelings of inadequacy and lack of self-confidence. Also, for Mexican-American and Puerto Rican clients, folk medicine may be highly valued (White, 1977). In this regard, the nurse's provision for or discouragement of healing rituals may affect the degree of alienation the minority patient experiences with hospitalization. The recognition of the value and importance of the person through the folk-medicine experience may assist the patient in maintaining a sense of worth. Another important aspect of Mexican-American culture is that the family is often patriarchal. The nurse who is unaware of this and pressures the female patient to make a decision about which the patient feels compelled to consult her husband may be inadvertently challenging the status and importance of various family members.

Although the examples given so far are intended to increase the reader's awareness of self-esteem–threatening stressors facing ethnic minorities of color in the health care system, it is also important to point out that members of less visible minorities also face unique demands when they become patients. One example is the gay or lesbian patient.

GAY AND LESBIAN PATIENTS.   Gay and lesbian patients face specific stressors when seeking health care that are related, at least in part, to the way they are perceived by the larger society. Fears of homosexual patients about receiving less-than-adequate medical care appear grounded in fact. In a sample of a thousand doctors responding anonymously to a questionnaire, three-fourths acknowledged that knowing a male patient was homosexual would adversely affect their medical management (Pauly and Goldstein, 1970). And, if in frustration the patient turns to the nurse for assistance, it does not seem that any more sensitive care will be provided. Lawrence (1975) concludes that "although nursing techniques used in the care of a homosexual patient with a physical illness will not differ from those prescribed for

heterosexual patients, prejudicial attitudes negatively affect the manner in which their care is given." Lawrence goes on to cite several examples where care was negatively affected, such as one ICU patient whose mate of 23 years was not allowed to visit by nursing staff who maintained the mate was not family. More than just having an impact on the homosexual patient's physical condition, the attitudes represented by the altered levels of caring pose a significant threat to the patients' sense of self-worth. These attitudes are stressors associated with increased fear and feelings of worthlessness and helplessness (Martin, 1982; Lawrence, 1975). Through becoming aware of potentially harmful attitudes, the nurse is in a position to affect the self-esteem of gay and lesbian patients in a positive rather than negative manner.

The purpose of this discussion of stress, self-esteem, and minority patients has been to heighten awareness of yet another set of esteem-threatening stressors. The intent has not been to make a comprehensive review of minority health care and self-esteem. Such a review should include Asian-American patients, Amerasian patients, Italian-American, Jewish-American, Anglo-American, and Greek-American patients, and on. Nurses and prospective nurses are strongly encouraged to pursue this exploration independently and extensively. This is essential if nurses are to shatter esteem-threatening assumptions such as the one exemplified by the often-heard phrase, "everybody does it this way." In order for nurses to fully appreciate patients' needs, their knowledge of patients' experiences and points of view must be broad and deep.

Illness and Hospitalization.   Illness and hospitalization confront not only the patient but also the family with tremendous demands. Like other stressors, these may be dealt with in a maladaptive manner, thus further threatening individual and family needs. Or they may be coped with constructively, thus allowing an opportunity for growth, as well as for increasing need satisfaction. Although illness and hospitalization pose threats to all of the individual's basic needs, the focus here is on those that particularly challenge one's sense of self-worth. Moreover, since there seems to be an almost limitless number of variables that may alter persons' responses to these stressors, the discussion will be limited to areas where useful generalizations can be made.

Loss.   Multiple losses are inherent stressors in the process of illness and hospitalization. Moreover, they seem to have a significant impact on individuals' self-esteem. The nature of the illness suffered by the patient may largely determine the extent of loss experienced. All of the following illness-related questions, and no doubt more, are useful in understanding the significance of a particular loss:

Is the illness an acute or chronic condition?
Did it have a sudden or gradual onset?
Is the illness communicable?
What is the prognosis?
Did it result in the loss of a body part, loss of function, or disfigurement?

An illustration may be useful in exploring this issue. According to Rubin, the ability to function with control for time and place is held in personal and social esteem (Rubin, 1968). This idea is emphasized in Jean Werner-Beland's account (1980) of her own reaction to the loss of bowel and bladder function as the result of cervical cord damage in a car accident. Ms. Werner-Beland explains that the act of soiling the sheets because of either involuntary bowel activity or repeated enemas became almost impossible to cope with. In describing the personal reaction to statements from nurses such as, "I don't know why you are so upset, it's just an enema," Ms. Werner-Beland exclaims, "I wanted to scream, I have crapped on my own for 36 years! You just don't understand! I am dead! Some part of me had the audacity to stay alive, but for the most part, I *am dead*!!!" This emotion-filled description provides a vivid look at the relationship between loss of function and loss of self-esteem. The patient's rage over a loss of physical control, and the likely accompanying losses of esteem-related qualities such as adequacy and dignity, culminated in self-rejection, the statement that "I am dead." Indeed, Rubin (1968) reports that "to lose or be threatened with the loss of a complex, coordinated, and controlled functional activity which has been achieved and integrated into the personal system is to lose or be threatened with the loss of self." In essence, loss of control results in a personal judgment of failure. The feelings experienced are those of worthlessness.

The self-esteem–threatening losses associated with other illnesses are also significant. For instance, the person with an amputated limb may lose the role of breadwinner. As a result, the individual may no longer feel important; self-confidence may decrease. Or consider the patient with a communicable disease who is in isolation. Cut off from a familiar network of support, the patient may no longer feel appreciated or loved. Moreover, nurses who do not carefully and adequately explain the reasons for isolation may reinforce fears that there is something personally "wrong" with the patient. In addition to those with infectious diseases, persons with terminal illnesses or disfiguring disorders are also frequently avoided by others. Such avoidance or loss of usual social contacts may have similar self-esteem–lowering results for these individuals. Still, apart from the specific illness, hospitalization, in and of itself, usually means the person will face esteem-threatening losses.

Just as loss of control over one's body functions may lead to lowered self-worth, so loss of control over one's environment may have a similar result. Hospitalization imposes such a loss of control. In the unfamiliar and perhaps frightening hospital environment, the patient is no longer able to experience the usual mastery of surroundings. Others, strangers such as the nurse, now seem to be in control of the patient's world. The issue of relationships with others touches upon other losses associated with hospitalization.

Aside from the loss of usual social contacts associated with certain illnesses, hospitalization itself means that to a large extent the patient is isolated from regular interaction with significant others. One's relationships with people are disrupted. This presents a definite threat to self-esteem since, as was noted earlier, a major portion of one's self-worth develops from interactions with others. In addition to social isolation, the patient may lose, at least temporarily, other roles that provide a sense of competence, importance, and appreciation. For example, hospitalization usually means curtailment of the person's work-related roles. In like manner, the individual may face the loss or alteration of other roles, such as father or mother, son or daughter, husband or wife, sexual partner, choir director, PTA leader and so on. Roles are valued patterns of behavior that are personally adopted or socially assigned. Loss of specific roles through hospitalization means the individual may need to adopt other available roles to satisfy esteem needs or experience a lowered self-worth.

THE SICK ROLE.   The identified role of illness is the sick role. People may give up many roles when they enter the hospital. The one role they tend to assume, however, is the sick role. As with most stressors, the sick role has potential benefits as well as detriments.

On the one hand, the sick role exempts the person from usual work and social responsibilities and allows the person to acknowledge the inability to become well by decision or will. These aspects of the role are important in encouraging the individual to seek medical assistance when it is necessary and to cooperate with health-restoring measures instituted by health care providers. In contrast to these benefits, assumption of the sick role also carries with it potential esteem-threatening demands.

According to Parsons (1951), the sick role is characterized by passivity. The patient is expected to comply with all measures without complaint: invasion of body and privacy, painful and inconvenient procedures and canceling of regular preferences regarding sleeping, eating, and bathing. As Kennedy (1978) explains, "care-givers are permitted to make all the decisions and perform any and all procedures without question.'' Nurses, doctors, and other health professionals see themselves as having the power and sole responsibility for making the patient well. This casts the patient in an extremely passive and dependent role. It is based on this compliance that a person is accorded the label of "good patient." Although to some extent this is useful and necessary behavior on the part of the patient, continuous role playing of the "good patient" may also be esteem damaging.

Weisman and Worden (1976) have found that behaviors associated with this label tend to impair the functioning of people. In their study of cancer patients, they found that those persons who combined confrontation with compliance adapted more successfully than those who remained submissive and passive. Confrontation implies that the individual has taken some control and responsibility in the health-restorative process. Such a patient is actively participating in the treatment process rather than just passively submitting to it. As has been pointed out previously, taking control enables one to feel capable, and this is a primary quality of self-esteem. However, the ability of persons to be more than simply "good patients" may be partially related to how others respond to them.

THE NURSE'S RESPONSE. According to Parsons (1951), the sick role is an institutional expectation. This means that those aspects of the role thus far described are expected by the nurse. Confrontation and the patient's active participation in treatment may not be anticipated. Rather than allowing, or even encouraging, what is likely more healthy behavior on the part of the patient, the nurse' reaction may become another stressor that threatens the patient's sense of self-worth.

This added threat is based in large part on the nurse's own feelings of inadequacy or incompetence because expectations of the patient have not been met. The patient's independence may threaten the nurse's need to be in control! As a result of this occurrence, the nurse may withdraw from the patient. Or, the nurse may become angry and try to force the individual to act the "good patient" role. Still, a third and more positive possibility is that the nurse may reevaluate assumptions and enlist the patient's participation in the treatment plan.

THE FAMILY'S RESPONSE. Just as the nurse's response may help or hinder the satisfaction of an individual's needs, so the response of the family to a member's illness and hospitalization is also important. It should be emphasized that the illness and hospitalization of one family member affect not only that individual but the entire family as well. And families may respond in many ways to the patient.

The family may react in a highly supportive and caring manner to the patient. This can be helpful inasmuch as it facilitates the individual's acceptance of those positive aspects of the sick role. In addition, the family's attention communicates love and regard to the patient. However, continual discouragement of the patient's efforts to become more independent, even as the patient's physical condition improves, may undermine self-confidence and thus have a negative impact on self-esteem. Other families may react with anger or frustration, feeling that they have been abandoned or burdened unfairly with added responsibilities. The patient, in turn, may feel unappreciated or a failure as a family member. In this manner, the family's response may be esteem-enhancing or threatening. The nurse's actions can often play an important part in determining how a family responds to a member's illness and hospitalization.

In summary, stress is not inherently negative. A person's response to a stress-producing event may ultimately lead to either an increase or a decrease in self-esteem. Successful adaptation is the response associated with a heightening of esteem-related qualities such as competence, confidence, and appreciation. This means that one has met whatever the challenge is and has grown as a result. In contrast, maladaptation results in lowering a person's sense of worth. In this case, one has been unable to reach an acceptable compromise and consequently feels less capable or important and less worthwhile. In examining specific stressful situations, this discussion has sought to increase nurses' awareness of how certain stressors may have a higher self-esteem-threatening potential than others. Clearly, it would not be feasible to examine every possible event that might endanger a person's independence, mastery, dignity, recognition, or other esteem-related qualities. Therefore, it is hoped that the reader will use this heightened awareness to evaluate carefully each unique patient situation for its possible impact on the person's sense of self-worth. Before moving to a consideration of nursing care, it is useful to take a brief look at self-worth and the development of the nurse as a health care professional.

Self-Esteem and the Nurse as a Health Care Professional. What has been written thus far about self-esteem applies to the nurse, as a person, just as it does to all people. However, it is also important to look beyond this, to describe those qualities of special significance in the development of the nurse's self-worth as a health care professional.

According to Werner-Beland (1980), the specific foundations of the nurse's self-esteem as a health care professional are knowledge, competence, and independence. Knowledge is, of course, something for which all students are striving to varying degrees. But what happens when one has passed all the tests and there are no more questions from instructors? For the nurse to become a self-confident health care provider, it is necessary to continue to explore and expand knowledge beyond the classroom. Similarly, the nurse needs to work toward an always increasing competency in practicing the art and science of nursing. One does not ever reach an absolute mastery of nursing. Implicit in this idea is the joy of growing in one's work, along with the responsibility of constantly needing to update and improve one's skills. Independence is the third basic quality of the nurse's self-esteem. This means that the nurse has some control over the work situation. Achieving independence often involves becoming more assertive. It is crucial, however, that independence exists along with the ability to be interdependent and dependent. In other words, it is important for the nurse to be able to work with others.

The nurse also faces esteem-threatening stressors which may be seen as unique challenges to the nurse's sense of worth. Being called upon to respond effectively to patient care situations never encountered before, dealing with a difficult health professional, working an inconvenient schedule, intervening in emergency situations, caring for a dying patient are examples of stressful events that regularly challenge the knowledge, competence, and independence of the nurse. Successful adaptation to the demands of nursing and enhancement of one's own sense of worth depend on how solidly the nurse's identity as a health care professional is based on the above qualities.

Nursing Assessment, Diagnosis, and Intervention with Patients Experiencing Problems Related to Self-Esteem

Assessment

People are constantly communicating to themselves and others how worthwhile they feel as persons. Individuals express their sense of worth in a limitless number of behaviors. For instance, one may tell oneself and others that one is important by a direct, purposeful walk and squared shoulders, while another indicates low self-esteem verbally in a statement such as "no one wants to hear what I have to say." The nurse has a wealth of information to evaluate. This makes the task of assessing a patient's self-esteem level a particularly challenging task.

Before describing those behaviors associated with low self-esteem, it may be useful to review briefly the qualities and characteristics upon which one's sense of worth develops. Self-esteem is founded on a self-awareness that enables one to recognize and value oneself for who one really is. Further, it is based on the ability to view the demands of life from a positive perspective and to adapt to these stressors using task-oriented as well as defense-oriented coping strategies. In this manner, the individual comes to be regarded by self and others as capable and worthwhile. Low self-esteem means that this process of developing a sense of worth has been hampered in one of the crucial areas just noted. For instance, perhaps as the result of a lack of early self-affirming messages, the individual never developed a complete awareness of strengths as well as weaknesses. Or possibly having been overwhelmed by stress severely and frequently, the person is unable to view life's challenges as potentially beneficial, thus prompting a retreat into an almost total reliance on defense-oriented coping strategies. No matter where the obstacles have been encountered, the person who has not been able to satisfy esteem needs will express a lack of self-worth both verbally and nonverbally.

Verbal and Nonverbal Expressions of Self-Esteem. Verbal messages may seem to be the most obvious expressions of how people feel about themselves. Verbal communication can convey information about one's sense of worth accurately and efficiently. Patients may make clear statements indicating low self-esteem. Such comments as "I'm no good," or "People don't like me" are readily apparent signs that one does not feel good about one's self. Although nonverbal messages may be less obvious, they can actually be more accurate indicators of one's real meaning than verbal messages.

Nonverbal behaviors such as body posture, facial expression, tone of voice, gestures, movements, general appearance, and response to the nurse tend to be more spontaneous and genuine than verbal behaviors. Moreover, researchers tend to agree that nonverbal communication carries more social meaning than verbal communication (Ekman, 1965). Nonverbal cues help one to judge the reliability of the verbal message. Thus, such behaviors as a patient's stooped shoulders, avoidance of eye contact, apparent lack of attention to hygiene or grooming may give a more accurate picture of the patient's sense of self-worth than what is verbally communicated. The nurse must be careful, however, not to automatically discount what the patient communicates about self, whether this is conveyed verbally or nonverbally. It is important for the nurse to observe closely both verbal and nonverbal clues when assessing the patient's self-esteem. In addition, the nurse will be able to make a more accurate assessment if it is approached in a systematic manner.

Assessment Guidelines.   A systematic approach to the assessment of self-esteem means that even before seeing the patient, the nurse has identified those areas in which it is generally most important to collect data in order to accurately assess the individual's self-esteem. This is not to say that the nurse ignores information that does not fit into the identified framework. It only means that on entering the patient situation the nurse has developed guidelines for assessment in order to avoid inadvertently missing significant information. In addition, having a general plan ensures some uniformity in the assessment. Both of these factors, that is, collecting crucial information and uniformity, increase the accuracy of the assessment. Most important, the more accurate the assessment, the more helpful it is in planning nursing interventions.

Based on what has been presented thus far, five areas of particular significance in assessing self-esteem have been identified. These are simply guidelines which may need to be modified to fit the unique situation in which the nurse is working. The five areas are:

1. Self-awareness
2. Major stressors
3. Perception of and response to stressful situations
4. Interpersonal relationships
5. Other supports

SELF-AWARENESS.   Assessment of the patient's awareness of self is a key to understanding the patient's evaluation of self-worth. The major question is: How accurately does the individual for whom care is provided perceive personal strengths and weaknesses? Does the patient seem to have a realistic self-appraisal, recognizing various personal assets as well as liabilities? Or does the patient seem to either overconcentrate on a particular talent, thus denying other aspects of self, or narrowly focus on a particular disability or shortcoming, similarly blocking out an accurate perception of the total self? This area is important to assess since an accurate view of self is a prerequisite for the development of self-esteem. The two following illustrations describe the behaviors associated with an inaccurate or distorted perception of one's abilities and disabilities. The first example is of an individual whose self-view includes a rigid denial of a major disability.

Mr. O. is a 45-year-old fireman who has recently undergone a below-the-knee amputation. Nursing notes describe his refusal to participate in any part of his rehabilitation process. He angrily yells at the nurse to leave when the nurse begins to explain how to perform stump care and the importance of certain leg exercises. Mr. O. exclaims, "Just leave me alone so I can get out of here and back to fighting fires." He adds, "I expect to be back at my old job in no time at all." As the nurse encourages him to talk about how he is feeling, the patient explains how even as a young boy he had wanted to be a fireman. He states, "Fighting fires is really my whole life, I don't know how to do anything else."

In this situation, the nurse's data collection shows the inaccuracy of the patient's self-view. He has blocked out of awareness the nature and extent of his disability and has narrowly focused on his one role as a fireman. As Mr. O.'s conversation with the nurse reveals, his life has been centered around being a fireman. His present response is likely a defense against feelings of worthlessness as the result of the loss of this role. The patient's reaction in situations such as this is often typified in the setting of unrealistic goals, such as Mr. O.'s plan to be back at work in "no time at all." This becomes a specific nursing care problem in that inaccurate self-assessment interferes with the patient's participation in his care, as noted in Mr. O.'s refusal to learn stump care. This ultimately may impede and lengthen the rehabilitation process.

The second case illustrates a different type of response. It shows an example of behaviors related, not to a denial of a disability, but to an excessive focusing on a particular problem to the extent that the person is unable to identify any personal strengths.

Ms. R. is a 22-year-old woman who works part time as a waitress as she attends modeling school. She has had repeated bouts with ulcerative colitis and one week ago underwent surgery for this condition. She now has a permanent ileostomy. Ms. R. has been very cooperative in her care. The ostomy nurse noted that she asks many questions about her stoma and seems to have quickly learned how to care for this new opening in her bowel. Ms. R.'s primary nurse, however, has observed that the patient seems very preoccupied with her ileostomy. She has refused visits from her many friends. And when the nurse attempts to talk with Ms. R. about topics unrelated to her surgery, the patient turns away and does not respond. Once, when the nurse pressed her to talk about future plans, the patient answered sharply, "I don't have any future plans. Can't you see what has happened to me?" The nurse replied with a statement that Ms. R. has many abilities that she could develop. The patient then began to cry, stating, "I'm no longer good for anything. I don't even know why I should go on living."

In this case, the nurse's data collection again shows a distorted self-view. This time though, the patient seems to define herself almost totally by her disability and is unable to recognize her real assets and strengths. This may become a particular problem in that the patient's feelings of worthlessness may lead to prolonged depression or even the ultimate act of self-rejection, suicide.

Both of these cases illustrate behaviors associated with an inaccurate or distorted self-awareness. The persons described are unable to recognize and accept their strengths along with their limitations. As shown in the examples, this lack of awareness is an important clue to lowered self-esteem. It may be manifested by withdrawal from reality and setting unrealistic goals. Or the nurse might observe that the patient is self-deprecating or overly self-critical. The person may express extreme despair. In both examples, the importance of assessing the patient's awareness of self is emphasized.

STRESSORS. In addition to being directly confronted by the demands of illness and hospitalization, the patient may also be attempting to adapt to many other stressors that challenge self-worth. It is important for the nurse to identify these in order to detect possible esteem-related problems. It is also useful to recall that even positive changes, such as graduating from school or getting married, can bring stress. The following patient situation demonstrates how, at the time of hospitalization, a person may be dealing with numerous stress-producing events.

Ms. M. is a 20-year-old, single, engaged, Native American salesperson who sustained burns over 20 percent of her body. She fell asleep in bed one evening while smoking a cigarette. A fire resulted in which Ms. M. was burned on the thighs, perineum, and abdomen. Consequently, she was hospitalized on the burn unit of a local hospital. Prior to her injury, the patient had made plans to enter the fashion-merchandizing program at an area vocational school.

Consider all of the esteem-threatening stressors in this brief description, and notice how illness and hospitalization may compound their effects. Ms. M.'s engagement is a transition which in and of itself tests her ability to adequately cope with a new role. The stress of engagement has now been complicated as the result of her accident. Ms. M. may fear rejection from her fiance as the result of her burns. As described earlier, being a member of a minority group may also become particularly stressful during hospitalization. The patient may face the concern of whether or not specific cultural practices, important to maintaining her sense of worth, will be allowed and respected by hospital personnel. Beyond this, Ms. M. is now confronted with the question of whether she will be able to resume her duties as a salesperson. Another possible stressor is the feeling of guilt as the result of having fallen asleep with a lighted cigarette. This guilt is a further threat to self-esteem. Finally, the patient had most likely already been coping with stress related to returning to school. Perhaps she had questioned whether she really could succeed in school. Although the challenge of this questioning probably was manageable initially, the stress of her accident and hospitalization may make it unmanageable.

As in the example above, most patients face multiple stressors. The situation of Ms. M. was used to emphasize the importance of the nurse's assessing the major stressors faced by the patient in order to identify problems related to self-esteem. The next area to assess is the patient's perception of and response to stressful situations.

PERCEPTION OF AND RESPONSE TO STRESSFUL SITUATIONS. Adaptation, the development of self-esteem, one's perception of a stressful situation, and one's choice of coping strategies are major determinants in deciding whether one's response to stressors maintains, enhances, or decreases self-esteem. Although a positive, growth-oriented perception of stressful events reinforces self-worth, a tendency to view life's challenges in a hopeless, defeatist manner leads to decreased self-esteem. In addition, a person's choice of coping strategies has an equally important relationship to the satisfaction of esteem needs. Is one's reaction to stressors generally task oriented? Or is one's response usually defense oriented? Although it was previously noted that both types of reactions are necessary, there needs to be some balance between the use of each. For instance, a total reliance on defense mechanisms to adapt to stressors prevents the individual from developing a sense of competence and capability from the use of a problem-solving, task-oriented approach. A case illustration may be useful in pointing out behaviors associated with an esteem-threatening perception of and response to a stressor.

Mr. K. is a 53-year-old, married, certified public accountant who has one daughter who is currently enrolled in medical school. He entered the ER one hour ago complaining of chest pain and saying he thought he was having a heart attack. However, a stat ECG and examination by the emergency room physician revealed anxiety-related symptoms of hyperventilation, tachycardia, and restlessness, but no evidence of cardiac pathology. In attempting to gain a more complete understanding of Mr. K.'s current difficulty, the nurse explores how the patient deals with stress-producing events. It becomes apparent that in the past Mr. K. has tried to avoid stressful situations at all costs. He explains that he is the president of a small accounting firm which has been losing money for nearly two years. In response to these losses, Mr. K. has seemed unable to make decisions which might have saved the firm.

Further, he has repeatedly denied the seriousness of his financial situation as noted in his remarks such as, "There's nothing that a little more time won't fix" and "Everythings going to be all right." Mr. K. tells the nurse that he is now faced with the fact that he'll probably have to declare bankruptcy. He expresses feelings of worthlessness, stating, "I feel so helpless." Mr. K. adds that he sees no hope for the future.

In this situation, the individual's perception of the stressor, that is, increasing financial problems, and his response to it reinforce a low self-esteem. Mr. K. does not meet the demands placed on him but rather attempts to avoid them. When the demands are forced on him despite his avoidance, he consistently reacts in a defense-oriented manner. Thus, he denies the problems even to the point of becoming physically ill. As shown in the examples, several behaviors follow from one's usually viewing stressors as negative influences and continually responding to them with a defense-oriented rather than task-oriented strategy. These include increased feelings of helplessness, ambivalence, and a sense that there is no hope. The individual may also experience increased mental confusion and anxiety as coping strategies fail. This consistently high level of inner tension eventually exacts a physical, as well as an emotional, toll. Mr. K.'s physical pain may have been related, at least in part, to his unsuccessful adaptation to a severe stressor. For others, the increased tension may precipitate or aggravate conditions such as ulcers, bowel disorders, allergies, and arthritis. In any event, as has been described earlier, feelings such as helplessness and indecisiveness are associated with low self-esteem. They are directly opposed to esteem-enhancing qualities such as competence and mastery of one's environment. Consequently, in assessing self-esteem, it is essential to evaluate the way in which the patient perceives and responds to stressors. As in the illustration, this is done not only by observing how the patient reacts to the current stressors of illness and possibly hospitalization, but also by exploring how the person responded to stressful events in the past.

INTERPERSONAL RELATIONSHIPS. Self-esteem derives both from within one's self and from interactions with others. Thus, assessment of a patient's interpersonal relationships, particularly the closeness or distance of them, will provide data about the person's self-esteem. In fact, esteem needs, such as prestige and appreciation, can only be satisfied in an interpersonal setting. A brief illustration demonstrates the importance of this part of the assessment of self-esteem.

Kathy is a 13-year-old, black girl who has been admitted to a pediatric medical-surgical unit for correction of a severe spinal deformity. Treatment of her condition has involved immobilization with traction on a circoelectric bed for the

past week. This is in preparation for possible spinal fusion and immobilization in a body cast. While her physical condition is improving in accord with the treatment plan, the nursing staff has become increasingly concerned about Kathy's emotional well-being. Although she was very talkative on admission, Kathy seldom initiates conversation now and answers questions with only one or two words. In addition, she tends to turn away when others enter the room. Her mother has expressed concern to the nurse about these changes in her daughter and has voiced feeling guilty that she can't visit more frequently. She explains, "Kathy and I used to spend a good deal of the day together; I feel bad that I can't even afford bus fare to visit her every day." Kathy's mother adds, "And I know she misses her school friends." Recently, the primary nurse caring for Kathy heard her crying. She sat quietly next to the patient's bed. Kathy kept repeating, "I'm no good, nobody likes me."

In this situation, the patient has experienced a dramatic change in the frequency and closeness of her interpersonal relationships. Her importance as an individual and her "lovableness," as Clarke terms it, are much less regularly affirmed. Affirming messages are particularly crucial during adolescence when young persons are formulating their identities, although, in general, persons' interactions with others influence their self-esteem throughout their lives. Withdrawn behavior, such as Kathy demonstrated, is a common manifestation of a decreased sense of worth which is associated with a disruption or other problem in a person's interpersonal relationships. In order to fully understand the significance of behavior such as this, it is necessary to assess the patient's usual pattern of relationships. It is important for the nurse to ask who are the valued persons in the patient's life? How close are they—can they exchange thoughts and feelings, what types of things do they do together? Further, does the patient perceive significant others as sources of support and encouragement? How does the patient's appearance change following visits from others—more relaxed, anxious, withdrawn? Perhaps the patient seems never to have had close relationships. In response to the nurse's inquiries, some persons may describe a series of relationships characterized by intense and repeated conflicts. These data are useful in identifying long-term problems of self-esteem. However, just as it is crucial to identify problem areas in relationships, so it is important to become aware of the interpersonal strengths and supports available to the patient. In this manner, the nurse is prepared to intervene not only to resolve current problems but also to assist the patient in mobilizing interpersonal resources to prevent or reduce potential threats to self-worth.

OTHER SUPPORTS. In addition to valued relationships with people, there are other supports that may influence self-worth. Therefore, in assessing the patient's esteem level it is necessary to identify what are the other sources of support in the individual's life, as well as how current stressors, such as illness and hospitalization, have affected them.

For many people, their job may be a primary source of satisfaction of esteem needs. Apart from work-related relationships, the inner satisfaction of accomplishing various tasks reinforces one's judgment and feeling of being capable. Hospitalization and illness may drastically interfere with this reinforcement. A central support of self-esteem for many others may be something as simple as caring for a pet. As Levinson (1969) explains, "A pet can provide, in boundless measure, love and unqualified approval." Levinson goes on to add, particularly in reference to many elderly and lonely people, "Their concepts of themselves as worthwhile persons can be restored, even enhanced, by the assurance that the pets they care for love them in return." Once again, illness and hospitalization may deny the person this source of support. For others, a hobby or some other similar activity may reaffirm their sense of competence or mastery over their environment. It is important for the nurse to ask patients about their interests in order to determine the impact that current stressors may have on them. For instance, patients who collect stamps or knit, depending on their condition, may be able to continue these activities in the hospital. In contrast, for individuals who pride themselves on athletic abilities

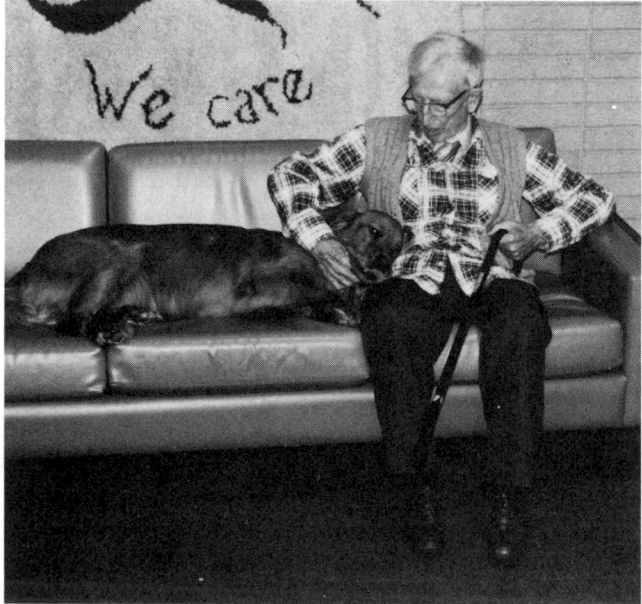

Figure 31–1. For many persons, a pet may be an important source of support for self-esteem. This has been recognized in some nursing homes by including pets in the health care setting, such as the one in which this 93-year-old man is a resident.

such as running or playing tennis, hospitalization poses a more serious threat to satisfaction of esteem needs. Still other persons may experience significant esteem enhancement from a spiritual support. One's relationship with a higher spiritual power can be a crucial source of messages that affirm one's being. Confinement to a hospital or nursing home doesn't necessarily mean that individuals are cut off from this support. As shown in the following illustration, the nurse's attitude and flexibility may be decisive factors in determining the availability of this support to the patient.

Mrs. R. is a 74-year-old, American Indian woman who has been admitted to the medical unit of a rural, county hospital with a persistent high fever of unidentified origin. Since her admission, she has been visited by a steady flow of relatives. On several occasions, she has also been attended to by a medicine man. Most recently, the nursing staff noted that after a brief ritual, the medicine man placed a small bag attached to a necklace around the patient's neck. The nurses have not inquired into the religious and medicinal significance of this item, or the composition of the substance in the bag, although either Mrs. R. or family members could answer these questions. Instead, nurses have complained about the odor from the necklace and have told the patient to "throw out that silly thing." Since given this instruction by nursing staff, Mrs. R. has become increasingly anxious and has tearfully asked her family to take her home.

In this situation, the nurses are unnecessarily interfering with Mrs. R.'s spiritual support and probably increasing the alienation she has already felt as a minority patient in the hospital setting. A more supportive response would have been to ask how long the necklace should be kept around her neck. The question itself is less important than the respect it shows for the item and related ritual as being legitimate. The nurses' reaction in the illustration belittled the significance not only of the religious item, but ultimately of the patient, since she believed in its importance. This demonstrates the need for nurses fully to assess other supports in the individual's life, along with evaluating how current stressors such as hospitalization can affect them.

In collecting data in all of the five assessment areas covered (self-awareness, major stressors, perception of and response to stressful situations, interpersonal relationships, and other supports), the nurse is constructing a picture of the patient's self-esteem, that is, the level of self-worth and how it is maintained. Based on the data, it may become evident that the person has an esteem-related problem. In this case, the nurse will then formulate a problem statement, or nursing diagnosis, about the areas in which the person could benefit from nursing intervention.

Nursing Diagnoses. It is most descriptive and thus useful to express the nursing diagnosis in terms of patient experience. In other words, the formulation of a nursing diagnosis should specify the particular nature of the esteem-related problem and, if possible, any relevant stressors. The following are examples of nursing diagnoses which are based on the illustrations presented so far:

Low self-esteem associated with unrealistic or overly high self-ideals or goals

Social isolation related to alteration in body image

Feelings of worthlessness associated with loss of a valued role

Decreased sense of adequacy associated with illness and hospitalization

Feelings of rejection related to divorce or other similar life change

Depression associated with an unresolved loss

Disturbed body-image related to CVA, amputation, or similar illness

Although this list includes some of the more common esteem-related diagnoses, it is by no means all encompassing. Nurses are constantly encountering new and different patient situations. Their nursing diagnoses should reflect this fact. If they are formulated in this way, as a descriptive statement of problems about a unique patient situation, nursing diagnoses can effectively focus nurses on areas in which intervention is needed.

Planning and Implementation of Nursing Interventions

Regardless of the previous level of one's self-esteem, one's sense of worth is threatened with illness and confinement to a nursing home or hospital. By affirming the patient's being and capabilities during this period of increased vulnerability, the nurse can have a crucial, positive impact on the individual's self-esteem.

Goal-Setting. The general goal of nursing intervention is to improve the patient's feeling and judgment of self-worth by assisting the individual to develop an awareness of strengths and weaknesses, to perceive and respond to stressors in a constructive manner, and to utilize effectively available supports of self-esteem. The nurse's focus, then, in terms of goal setting and planning interventions, is organized around the five areas identified in the section on assessment: self-awareness, stressors, perception of and response to stressful situations, interpersonal relationships, and other supports.

Since self-esteem has been seen to involve such qualities as competency and independence, the patient is encouraged to be an active participant in the formulation and implementation of the treatment plan. The nurse and patient together formulate goals that reflect a positive resolution of the problem and the stressor identified in the nursing diagnosis. The patient's active involvement in this process is necessary in order to identify realistic steps that can be accomplished. In this way, the patient's self-confidence is supported. This, in turn, directly enhances self-esteem. The goals emphasize strengths rather than a pathological condition. Moreover, if they are mutually identified, the patient is more likely to be motivated to be an active part in goal achievement. Research supports this conclusion. It has been found that situations that promote persons' perceptions of competence also increase their inner motivation (Deci, 1971). Patient participation in the planning and achievement of goals fits in this category of competency enhancing events. Following are examples of goals for a patient with a decreased sense of worth associated with a disturbed body-image.

Long-Term and Ongoing Goals

Mr. I. will acknowledge his feelings (e.g., sadness, anger) about his altered body-image after chemotherapy treatment for leukemia by openly expressing these feelings to at least one other person.

Mr. I. will state three positive aspects of his modified body-image within two weeks.

Short-Term Goals

Mr. I. will verbally identify the medications he is receiving by the end of the shift.

Mr. I. will describe the major effects of his medication on his illness and body by the end of the week.

Mr. I. will decide, within appropriate limits, the time of his bath and dressing change by 8:00 A.M. today.

Examples of other goals related to problems of self-esteem are included in the care plan at the end of the chapter.

It is important to point out that, although it may be expedient in terms of explaining concepts and describing nursing care to focus on particular needs such as self-esteem, the individual is viewed as a whole. In addition to esteem needs, the person's physical, safety, and love and belonging needs are also attended to. In defining these categories of needs, Maslow did not intend for them to be rigidly pursued, one after another. Rather, like human development, there is a general order of progression which allows for partial fulfillment for several needs at a time. Thus, nursing interventions in this need area are formulated within the context of the patient's total being, which includes an interrelationship of needs and desires.

Intervention.   Once the goals to be accomplished have been defined by the patient and nurse, a plan of action can be devised. Nursing interventions can generally be organized around the five areas identified in the assessment: (1) self-awareness, (2) major stressors, (3) perception of and response to stressful situations, (4) interpersonal relationships, (5) other supports. The emphasis here is on principles of nursing care that are applicable to various problems of self-esteem. A nursing care plan is presented at the end of this section to illustrate examples of specific nursing interventions. Just as in the assessment of individuals' self-worth, planning nursing actions logically begins with the area of self-awareness.

SELF-AWARENESS AND THE NURSE'S THERAPEUTIC USE OF SELF.   Especially in this area, attention is focused not only on the patient's self-view, but also on the nurse's awareness and acceptance of self. It has been shown, for instance, that nurses who are accepting of themselves and have a high self-esteem are also rated as better care providers than nurses who view themselves less positively (Dyer *et al.*, 1975). In other words, it is important for nurses to have both an accurate understanding as well as acceptance of their own strenghts and weaknesses in order to provide a high level of care to others. This is particularly crucial considering that the primary tool of the nurse when intervening in problems of self-esteem is self!

Therapeutic use of self is a recognition of the fact that there are no special diets, exercises, dressings, or similar treatment measures to improve self-esteem. Instead, the nurse's self, through the verbal and nonverbal messages communicated to patients, is the major means of intervention. Therapeutic use of self requires that nurses be aware of and confront their own thoughts, feelings, and actions. Only with this self-awareness can nurses develop insight into how these factors affect their relationship with the patient. Therefore, the process of intervening is begun with a careful self-assessment (refer to the steps in developing self-awareness included earlier in this chapter). Consider again the nurse who reacts to the crying patient by immediately trying to quiet the patient rather than first attempting to understand the source and meaning of the apparent sadness. The automatic nature of the nurse's response suggests a lack of self-awareness, that is, a lack of understanding and acceptance of the personal significance of crying to the nurse. This is an unfortunate situation for the nurse and patient. One's own feelings are a key to understanding how the patient may be feeling. A lack of self-aware-

ness, including insight into one's own feelings, affects not only the nurse's self-understanding, but also the ability to empathize with patients and to effectively intervene on the basis of patient needs.

Particular emphasis is placed on the importance of nurses being aware of their attitudes toward persons who exhibit cultural, life-style, religious and/or other differences from themselves. Like members of society in general, nurses may tend to react in judgmental and negative ways toward persons who seem very different from themselves. Such reactions can be especially destructive to patients' self-worth when one considers the already increased vulnerability of hospitalized patients. Some examples have been considered earlier in the chapter. For instance, the Caucasian nurse may react to an American Indian's healing ceremony with ridicule. Similarly, a heterosexual nurse may express outrage over seeing a homosexual couple hugging or holding hands. Such responses only serve to increase already present threats to self-esteem. Thus, the prerequisite for therapeutic use of self is self-awareness. Moreover, awareness of one's own thoughts, feelings, and actions is most useful when it is combined with an in-depth knowledge of individual differences. Once nurses have done a careful self-assessment, they can begin to intervene directly in patients' problems of self-esteem.

Nursing intervention is next aimed at assisting patients to increase self-awareness, that is, to assess and accept their own strengths and weaknesses more accurately. Nurses can facilitate this in two ways. The first is through demonstrating an attitude of unconditional positive regard. The second method of promoting persons' self-awareness is through validating their experience of self.

UNCONDITIONAL POSITIVE REGARD.   An attitude of acceptance, or unconditional positive regard, means that one understands and prizes each person's individuality despite possible disagreement with specific behaviors. Positive regard that is unconditional is conveyed to patients by listening with understanding, responding nonjudgmentally, expressing genuine interest, and communicating a sense of caring and sincerity. In this manner, nurses contribute to an increase in patients' freedom to examine the many aspects of themselves, including both positive and negative attributes. What this means in practical terms will differ with each situation since every patient must be viewed as a unique being.

For example, if used appropriately and with sensitive timing, the nonverbal message of touch may alone communicate acceptance to many clients. Touch is particularly important in this regard when nurses care for those with communication problems, such as non-English–speaking persons, those suffering from chronic brain syndrome, aphasia, or speech impediments. In addition, Barnett (1972) notes that the age group most infrequently touched is the 66-to-100-year-old group. Various reasons may explain this finding. It may be that the elderly seem less physically attractive or that they remind people of their own aging or that of their parents. Whatever the explanation, to avoid touching the aged, as well as other groups of clients, reinforces self-doubt or feelings of worthlessness. It is important to point out that different types of touching communicate different things. Burnside *et al.* (1979), for example, have differentiated between task-oriented touching, such as the type of touching nurses do in assisting a patient to ambulate or in giving a bed bath, and nontask-oriented touching, such ask spontaneous, affectionate touch. Caring and acceptance are more likely to be conveyed through spontaneous, affectionate touch rather than touch aimed at accomplishing a task such as ambulating. Touch in the latter instance may only communicate that this is what nurses are supposed to do. This means that, in working with patients who are experiencing lowered self-worth, the nurses may want to spend time with them when there is no physical care required. In addition to touch, there are many other nonverbal ways to convey positive regard. Simply sitting quietly with patients, for instance, might be an especially powerful message of caring and acceptance in certain situations. Of course, positive regard can be communicated through verbal messages also.

Levin's (1974) list of affirmations to enhance self-esteem can be used as a guide in formulating responses to increase a sense of worth (refer again to Table 31-1). For example, explaining that patients have a right to their feelings and can express them in ways that do not harm others may assist patients to accept painful changes. As an illustration, the patient undergoing chemotherapy for cancer may need to express anger about alterations in body-image in order to come to some acceptance of these changes. In order to facilitate this process, the nurse may need to state that it is, in fact, okay for the patient to be angry. In effect, the nurse is saying that the patient is accepted. In all of these messages of positive regard, the goal is to increase patients' security and freedom to understand and accept themselves in all of their many dimensions. The second basic method of promoting persons' awareness of self is through validating their experience of self.

VALIDATION.   The essence of nursing action is validation of human experience. Nurses are in s crucial position to support or verify experiences of persons who may be confronted by major changes in and around themselves. Validation involves affirming the reality of a person's view of self. Invalidation occurs when one receives a message that negates one's experience of self. Nurses send invalidating messages to others when they respond, for example, to the demonstrably anxious pa-

tient by saying, "You're not really worried," or to the patient who is sobbing, "Come now, you can't be all that sad." An invalidating communication has the effect of disconfirming the person, and thus diminishing self-esteem. Nurses may use a variety of nonverbal and verbal techniques to assist patients in this area. However, the essential ingredient in all of them is the therapeutic use of self.

Quietly listening to the patient who has been diagnosed with a terminal illness in many situations may be the most effective way of supporting the patient's apparent request for a verbal verification. The request, at times, may be met best with a concerned silence. For example, the person who asks the nurse, "Is it really as bad as it looks?" may in this question be coming to a personal understanding and acceptance of the situation. In any event, it is essential to avoid attempts to deny the individual's experience. Unfortunately, one often may hear nurses giving pat answers to patients confronted with severe stressors. It is tempting to try to erase the patient's pain and one's own by saying "It's not that bad" or "Everything will be okay," when, in fact, things are bad and getting worse. Such responses impede the process of self-awareness. Moreover, they directly affect the person's ability to achieve acceptance of self.

It is necessary to qualify what has been written thus far about validation by explaining that when validating patients' experiences, it is crucial that nurses take their cues for action from patients. In other words, if patients indicate either verbally or nonverbally that they are not ready to face recent changes, nurses need to respect this by allowing them to accept changes according to their own schedule. For instance, the accident victim may indicate a lack of readiness to accept paralysis by stating, "I plan to go dancing this weekend." Although the nurse does not agree with the patient, it is equally important to refrain from attacking the patient's defenses by trying to contradict or argue. Silence may be the best response in this situation as the patient struggles to cope with the situation based on a personal time clock and individual resources.

Briefly, the primary tool of intervention in problems of self-esteem is the therapeutic use of self. The effective use of this tool depends upon the development of self-awareness by nurses. In the first of the five areas of intervention identified, nurses use the self through validation of human experience and demonstrating unconditional positive regard to increase patients' self-awareness. The therapeutic use of self is also the major means of intervention in the remaining four areas to be discussed.

NURSING ACTION AND MAJOR STRESSORS.   It has been acknowledged earlier in the chapter that stress is a fact of life. Therefore, how an individual learns to manage stress-producing events may be more critical to self-esteem than attempting to avoid such situations. Still, nurses often encounter situations in which attempts to eliminate stressors, or at least reduce their severity, are clearly warranted. In order to understand this idea better and the types of interventions that may be involved in this area, two brief illustrations are presented.

> Mr. A. is a businessman who has had repeated admissions to a medical unit at a local private hospital for problems related to peptic ulcers. Recently, he had a portion of his stomach removed due to perforation of an ulcer. His medical history indicates a close relationship between his physical condition and business pressures. Mr. A. has tried, but to no avail, numerous techniques such as biofeedback and psychotherapy to improve his ability to successfully adapt to work-related stressors. Moreover, during his hospitalizations he expresses increasing feelings of worthlessness and self-doubt about his ability to handle various work and nonwork situations.

Faced with the continuing severity of his physical and emotional condition, the patient may need to consider a career change, a reduction in hours worked, or other similar efforts to decrease the stressors with which he copes. In short, it may no longer be practical for Mr. A. to consider ways to improve his coping abilities without also looking at how he can reduce the number of stressors he regularly encounters. In order to verify this assessment and ensure consistency of care, nursing intervention in this case is begun by consulting with other health care team members, including the physician. Counseling the patient to look at changes he can make in his life-style might only result in confusion for him and frustration for the nurse if other care providers view the situation differently. Once a consistent approach is agreed upon, the nurse can work with the patient to consider ways in which he might reduce the stressors he faces in his life.

The next illustration may also be useful in considering interventions in this area.

> Mrs. Q. is a divorced mother of four, hospitalized with a chronic hepatic condition. During the course of her hospitalization, she has begun to voice suicidal feelings, saying, "What is the point of living if I can't provide for my children?" The nurse has learned that Mrs. Q. is deeply in debt and facing eviction from her apartment because of nonpayment of rent.

In this situation, the patient needs more than just assistance in adapting to poverty-related stressors. The elimination or reduction of the severity of these stressors is at least as important as improving Mrs. Q.'s coping skills. Again, it is crucial that the nurse consults other members of the health team before taking direct action.

However, the nurse here may function most effectively by acting as an advocate for the patient, in suggesting, for example, that the hospital or county social service department work with the patient to find other sources of financial assistance. In any event, the aim of nursing actions in this case, as in the previous one, is to reduce the number and/or severity of major stressors in the patient's life.

Nursing actions here are focused on external events, the stressors themselves, rather than internally, that is, on the person's coping abilities. As suggested in the examples, actions may range from counseling the patient on life-style changes to suggesting that a person meet with a social worker. These actions are useful in situations in which patients are clearly overwhelmed, and the stressful events can be directly eliminated or their severity decreased. However, often this is not possible or even desirable. Nurses cannot change stressful events such as broken limbs or the death of a loved one. Nevertheless, what nurses can do in these and many other similar situations is to promote the abilities of the patients to adapt successfully to such events.

INTERVENTION IN PATIENTS' PERCEPTIONS OF AND RESPONSES TO STRESSFUL SITUATIONS.   In attempting to clarify self-esteem, Brissett (1972) concludes that it involves "experiencing one's self as master of one's activity, of having power over what one does." As discussed earlier in the chapter, hospitalization and illness tend to impede one's ability to control self and surroundings. Faced with such a stressor, even persons with previously high self-esteem may no longer experience themselves as capable and competent individuals who are masters of their environment. As a result, persons may suffer from lowered self-esteem. Therefore, nursing actions in this area are aimed at preserving or even enhancing individuals' control of themselves and their environment through promotion of a positive perception of and response to stressors. Indeed, Rubin (1968) aptly comments that "Enabling another to achieve control of function appropriately in time and space may well be a succinct description of nursing." However, as is apparent in the following discussion, intervening with this objective in mind may involve challenging commonly held beliefs about the nurse-patient relationship.

CHANGING THE SICK ROLE TO A WELL ROLE.   The sick role as described earnlier in this chapter has often been used to define the "good patient." According to this role, patients passively undergo the treatment regimen and suffer any untoward effects silently. Nurses and other health professionals see themselves as having the power and sole responsibility for making patients well. The "bad patient," on the other hand, is often perceived as emotionally unstable. Such a person may be aggressive, impatient, and unconforming to hospital policies and procedures. Through challenging nursing actions and asking difficult questions, this patient may be viewed by nurses as being too independent. The tendency of nurses has been to support the "good patient," who conforms to the sick role, and censure the "bad patient." However, by intervening in this manner, the nursing goal becomes one of controlling the patient rather than promoting health. Although supporting patients' questionings and challenges to routine at times may be uncomfortable for nurses, this intervention may be most effective in promoting self-esteem.

The primary nursing intervention in this area is to facilitate patients' attempts to be capable and competent, that is, to assist patients in gaining an appropriate level of control over self and environment. In this way, even severe stressors can be viewed more positively and seen as opportunities for learning and growth, rather than always being negative events which are merely endured. And with a more positive view and some control, individuals are more able to utilize constructive coping strategies, balancing defense-oriented responses with task-oriented ones. It is through this process that persons' self-esteem is maintained or even enhanced. Nurses can promote this process in several ways.

First, it is important that nurses evaluate their own expectations of patients and , if necessary, modify their view of what constitutes a "good" versus a "bad patient." Then nurses can begin to plan specific interventions. Sometimes, for example, the most helpful intervention in terms of self-worth will be to encourage questioning and challenges. However, as in all of the areas of intervention, specific actions will differ with each changing patient situation.

In general, nurses can teach patients to identify areas of their lives where they can be in control and assist them to exercise control. For instance, one patient may benefit from making choices about dietary items. Another person may be able to maintain a feeling of competence through deciding, within appropriate limits, times to do range-of-motion exercises. As previously indicated, an attempt should be made to include all patients in their goal planning. This may be as simple as working with a patient to establish a schedule of times and distances for ambulating. Involving patients in goal planning reinforces that they are capable persons. This, in turn, increases their motivation for goal achievement which, as objectives are reached, further promotes a sense of competence.

In planning goals with patients, it is important to set objectives that are realistic and that persons can reasonably expect to meet. For example, planning with the hospitalized patient for self-administration of medications when the physician has ordered them to be administered by the nurse would be inappropriate. Similarly unrealistic, and possibly dangerous, would be the formulation of a current goal involving strenuous exercise

for a patient who has recently had a massive myocardial infarction. Aside from potentially being physically harmful, unrealistic goals increase patients' feelings of frustration and helplessness, ultimately threatening self-worth.

Nurses can also support patient self-control in other very simple ways which, nonetheless, are sometimes overlooked. For example, the patient experiencing nausea and vomiting can be helped to control physiological functioning by having an emesis basin and towel placed close to the bed. Another person may be similarly assisted by having a bed pan immediately accessible. For the patient confined to a wheelchair, simply ensuring that the individual is not moved too quickly or unpredictably could be significant in maintaining a sense of being in control.

In promoting patients' healthy attempts to control themselves and their environment, nurses are essentially working toward changing the sick role to a well role. Such interventions enhance patients' sense of competency and capability, and thus, self-esteem.

NURSING ACTION AND INTERPERSONAL RELATIONSHIPS. Self-esteem has been described as being nourished both from within the individual and from without, that is, through being recognized as worthy by others. Interventions in this area focus on mobilizing patients' interpersonal resources, their valued relationships, in order to promote a sense of worth.

It was pointed out in discussing the therapeutic use of self that nurses can be important sources of affirmation and validation for patients. This is especially true in the case of persons who are socially isolated either by choice or by circumstance. For example, in the present highly mobile society, it is not unusual for family members to live at great distances from one another. This means that when one member is hospitalized, it may be economically or otherwise impossible for others to travel in order to lend valuable emotional support and caring to the patient. In these and similar situations, nurses and other health care providers may become the primary source of interpersonal support for patients. In other situations though, significant others may be close by. Nursing actions then are basically concerned with mobilizing this support for patients.

Again, specific nursing actions will differ with the actual patient care situation. For instance, persons with communication disabilities may have difficulty contacting individuals with whom they would like to visit. Nurses can be of use in exploring this possibility and then assisting these patients as needed in contacting family and friends. When significant others do visit, nursing interventions can help maximize the available support to the patient.

In the case of patients who have suffered from severe body-image disturbances, the nurse's preparation of the patient and others may be extremely important in ensuring that interpersonal contacts promote rather than further threaten self-worth. For example, consider the following situation:

> Mr. W. is a 21-year-old college student who has recently been admitted to an intensive care unit with numerous injuries related to a motorcycle accident. He has severe facial lacerations and a compound fracture of his left leg, which is in traction. He has two IVs running and a drainage tube from an abdominal wound. In addition, he is experiencing confusion related to head trauma. Mr. W.'s parents have just come to the nursing desk asking to see their son. This is their first visit. They are referred by the ward secretary to talk first with their son's nurse.

In this situation, the nurse's preparation of the parents, as well as of Mr. W., is critically important in order to maximize the constructive aspects of their visit. Although it is probably not appropriate or necessary to give detailed or in-depth descriptions to the parents, knowing that their son will look different due to his injuries, that he is confused and may tire easily, and that the tubes are temporarily needed for nourishment and drainage may mean the difference between their being able to support their son or being incapacitated themselves by shock. Likewise, Mr. W. is prepared by simply letting him know that his parents are present to visit and that it is okay for him to limit the time they spend together if he becomes very tired. Other information may be provided depending on the actual situation. The nurse can also help by assisting as needed in such things as combing the patient's hair, straightening bed covers, and making sure that chairs are available. Following the visit, the patient and his parents may need the nurse's support as they struggle with their grief and changes in the family structure. The nurse is in a position not only to validate the patient's experience, but also to let family members know that feelings such as sadness and anger are normal and need expression. Other nursing interventions to promote persons' self-esteem through interpersonal relationships may be in much less dramatic situations than the one above. For instance, assisting an aged nursing home resident to write a letter to a family member, or other significant person, may be a crucial yet more ordinary way of increasing the patient's feelings of worth by encouraging continuation of contact with people.

FAMILIES.   In looking more closely at families and self-esteem, particular emphasis is placed on the fact that the entire family is affected by the illness and hospitalization of a family member. Nursing actions that sustain the integrity of the family, such as the simple preparation given to M.W.'s parents and the nurse's follow-up support, benefit the family as a whole, as well

as the patient. If families are able to "pull together" and gain strength in the face of a crisis, they are more able and likely to communicate to members who are ill that they are still important, loved, and cared for. In terms of patients' self-worth, these are very important messages to receive when confronted by the esteem-threatening stressors associated with illness and hospitalization. According to Miller and Janosik (1980), what is most helpful for the family in terms of coping with the stress of illness and hospitalization is a sense of unity and purpose. Nurses can intervene to promote family competence and cohesion by encouraging the family to look for help within itself. Simple actions such as ensuring there is space for visitors, allowing a mother to assist in feeding her sick child, or explaining to the husband of a mastectomy patient that his wife will likely need reassurances that he still loves her are all ways of enhancing the family's sense of unity and purpose. This benefits the esteem of individual family members as well as the family as a whole.

Along with this, it is important to be aware that "family" has a different meaning for different groups of people. For example, the unique kinship system of many American Indians has already been mentioned. This family structure is in direct contrast to the traditional white, middle-class nuclear family consisting of a father, a mother, and children. Or consider the gay or lesbian patient. Their family may include a same-sex partner. These differences demonstrate that, in order for nurses to promote family support, it is necessary to understand the meaning that the patient assigns to "family."

Whether the interpersonal support comes from the nurse, family, friends, or other valued persons, the goal of nursing interventions in this area remains the same. Nursing actions are aimed at mobilizing persons' interpersonal support systems in order to affirm that they are important, loved, and cared for, in short, to promote a sense of worth through drawing on one's interpersonal resources.

NURSING ACTION AND OTHER SUPPORTS.   The final area of nursing intervention includes those supports other than relationships with people. The aim of nursing actions in this area is very similar to the goal of the interventions just discussed. However, instead of mobilizing interpersonal resources to enhance self-esteem, nurses facilitate the use of other supports for the same purpose. As in all of the other areas discussed, interventions here are formulated on the basis of careful assessment. In particular, nursing actions are based on patient data that indicate what other supports are important to self-worth and how current stressors affect these supports.

Other supports may include such things as spiritual

or religious rituals, vocational interests, hobbies or avocations, and a relationship with a pet. These supports may satisfy the need to feel capable or appreciated and thus worthwhile. Especially in this area, nurses are often challenged to be creative in planning actions.

For instance, in one particularly interesting article, a nurse explains how she included two dogs in the emotional care and planning for an elderly woman (Bancroft, 1971). Indeed, Burnside (1979) emphasizes the beneficial aspects of pets in meeting the esteem needs of older people. Thus, an example of a potentially useful nursing intervention in this area might be helping to arrange for the "adoption" of a pet by the residents of a nursing home. For patients whose religious practices affirm self-worth, nursing actions may involve providing for a minister, priest, rabbi, medicine man, or similar religious figure to visit patients. Further, intervention may also include scheduling nursing care to allow for performing religious rituals or ensuring patient privacy to observe specific religious practices. Obviously, nursing actions must not endanger patient health. However, there may be more flexibility in nursing care than is initially seen.

Some nursing interventions may be quite simple, yet easily overlooked. For example, in assessing patients' hobbies and interests, the nurses may identify several things patients could continue to do in the hospital. For example, the suggestion to family members to bring a patients' needlework to the hospital might help to renew the person's sense of accomplishment. This could be especially useful for patients who are expressing feelings of worthlessness. Or perhaps the individual's job is a primary support for self-esteem. Simply scheduling some time to talk with the patient about the job is an uncomplicated, yet potentially useful, intervention to reaffirm the person's inner sense of capability. Individuals whose illness results in a long-term disability that interferes with their functioning on a job, engaging in a hobby, or even performing activities of daily living will need help in adapting to esteem-threatening changes. In addition to providing emotional support and promoting patients' problem-solving abilities, both of which have been discussed earlier, nursing actions may involve reinforcing what patients learn from allied health professionals such as occupational, physical, and speech therapists.

As in all of the areas of intervention, the examples here are included to establish guidelines for nursing actions and to increase the nurse's awareness of the importance of considering these areas in planning care. They are not intended to be exhaustive lists of all possible interventions. Rather, nursing actions must take into account the uniqueness of every patient situation. Still, the overall goal of the interventions remains the same, that is, to promote a positive feeling and judgment of self-esteem. The nurse can refer to the care plan following this section for a more specific illustration of care planning for a patient with a problem of self-esteem.

Nursing Care Plan for a Patient with Unmet Self-Esteem Needs

Mrs. O. is a 48-year-old married woman with three children, ages 21, 18, and 12. Her husband is an executive for an expanding corporate firm and must do a large amount of entertaining. Mr. O. depends on his wife to plan these social events. In addition to social entertaining, Mrs. O. is active in a local tennis club.

Mrs. O. had detected a lump in her breast while bathing. A permanent section confirmed that the lump was cancerous. Subsequently, a modified radical mastectomy was performed which involved the removal of the breast, some fat, and most of the axillary lymph nodes. Mrs. O. is now four days postmastectomy. Her husband has expressed concern to nursing staff that, although his wife has been able to talk about problems in the past, she now seems unwilling to discuss what has happened. Mrs. O. is often tearful and tends to turn away from visitors or nursing staff when they enter her room. On one occasion, she did remark to her nurse, "What good am I to myself or my family? I'm a freak, look at my swollen arm." She continued, "I can't carry out my duties as a wife or mother since this has been done and there is no one who can help me." Mrs. O. has also complained about phantom pain in the missing breast. In addition to physical problems, nurses have identified several present and potential problems of self-esteem.

Nursing Diagnosis	Goals	Interventions
1. Disturbed body-image associated with modified radical mastectomy	**Short term** Mrs. O. will state one positive aspect of her body-image by the end of the shift. Mrs. O. will verbally identify the various types of available breast prostheses by the end of the week. Mrs. O. will demonstrate exercises to decrease lymphedema by her fifth day postmastectomy. **Long term** Mrs. O.'s feminine image will be restored as indicated by her resumption of previous occupational and social activities.	1. a. Assess Mrs. O.'s current body-image and determine what it was prior to surgery. b. Encourage Mrs. O. to express her feelings of shame or embarrassment about her altered body-image. c. Encourage Mr. O. and the children to support Mrs. O.'s verbalizing of concerns about her appearance. d. Assist Mrs. O. as needed in combing hair, dressing, and other ADLs. e. Encourage patient to observe and assist with second dressing change by holding pads in place. (This action must be coordinated with the physician's treatment approach and the woman's emotional readiness to view the scar.) f. Explain that some swelling of the affected arm may occur. g. Describe special arm and hand precautions such as avoiding cuts on affected arm from such things as razors and needles and avoiding wearing articles of clothing that will constrict the arm. h. Encourage patient to practice exercises to decrease edema within limits set by physical therapy department. i. Explain that phantom sensations are normal. j. Check into the possibility of arranging for a Reach to Recovery volunteer to visit Mrs. O. in order to provide emotional support and information about prostheses. (This is another action which must be carefully coordinated with the physician and patient.) k. Encourage Mrs. O. to take an active part in choosing the prosthesis. l. Explain that Mrs. O. will need to wait until her wound is healed before being fitted with a permanent prosthesis.

Nursing Diagnosis	Goals	Interventions
		m. Encourage Mrs. O. to use good posture as a way of enhancing her personal appearance.
		n. Encourage Mr. O. and the children to compliment Mrs. O. on her personal appearance, particularly when she begins to wear her permanent prosthesis.
2. Depression related to loss of breast	Mrs. O. will verbalize feelings about her loss by her fifth day postmastectomy.	2. a. Use reflection and open-ended questions to encourage Mrs. O. to express her feelings of loss, including her sadness and anger.
		b. Spend ten minutes each shift with Mrs. O. when no physical care scheduled; use touch as appropriate; remain with her despite lack of ability to verbalize.
		c. Continue nursing action 1. j.
		d. Encourage Mr. O. and the children not to reprimand her for crying and explain to them the need for her to cry.
		e. Encourage family members to sit with Mrs. O. as she cries and to make body contact by holding her hand or touching her arm.
		f. Explain to Mrs. O. and her family that a period of grieving is normal with a significant loss such as the loss of her breast.
		g. Where appropriate, direct remarks toward the future, even if only to a few hours away.
		h. Encourage Mr. O. and the children to compliment Mrs. O. on accomplishments made when she eventually involves herself in postmastectomy activities.
3. Feelings of worthlessness related to fears of being unable to perform roles as mother and wife	Mrs. O. will make one positive statement of self-worth within twenty-four hours. Mrs. O.'s self-esteem will increase as indicated by her making two statements regarding future plans by her sixth day postmastectomy.	3. a. Encourage Mrs. O. to verbalize feelings about herself.
		b. Share own observations and seek clarification/confirmation.
		c. Continue 2. b.
		d. Maximize choices Mrs. O. can make in her care.
		e. Explain that Mrs. O. will be able to resume usual household responsibilities with the exception of lifting heavy objects.

Nursing Diagnosis	Goals	Interventions
		f. Reassure Mrs. O. that activities such as bedmaking, sweeping, vacuuming, washing, and ironing are a few of the household duties that will enhance arm function on her affected side.
		g. Discuss with Mrs. O. clothing alterations that she feels may be necessary, especially in regard to her entertaining responsibilities and tennis playing.
		h. Continue 1. d, 1. m., and 1. n.
		i. Encourage Mr. O. and the children to be firm yet gentle in encouraging Mrs. O. to gradually resume her previous occupational and social activities after discharge.
4. Prone to feelings of rejection by her husband related to lowered self-esteem	Short term Mrs. O. will verbalize concerns regarding her relationship with her husband by her sixth day post-mastectomy. Long term (ongoing) Reintegrate Mrs. O.'s image of herself as being worthy of her husband's love as evidenced by her and her husband's open discussion of their concerns related to the mastectomy as well as the strengths in their relationship.	4. a. Use open-ended and direct questions to assess Mrs. O.'s current and past thoughts and feelings about her relationship with her husband, including strengths and weaknesses of the relationship.
		b. Encourage Mrs. O. to verbalize her present concerns about the relationship.
		c. Explain to Mr. O. that his reassurances of his love for his wife are especially crucial at this time; encourage him to touch her and verbalize that he loves her and that she is the same woman inside.
		d. Encourage Mr. O. to tell his wife that hesitant responses toward her are not rejection but rather an expression of empathy.
		e. Encourage Mr. O. to express his feelings about viewing the mastectomy scar.
		f. Explain that when Mrs. O. is able to move about with minimal difficulty, she and her husband can resume sexual activities.
		g. Explain that further counseling, on such issues as resumption of sexual activity, is available. (Coordinate any specific referrals with the physician and other members of the health care team.)

Summary

As in other patient care situations, the effectiveness of nursing intervention in problems of self-esteem is measured by the achievement of the treatment goals formulated by nurses and patients. However, the actual impact that achieving these goals has on the self-worth of individuals depends in large measure on the knowledge and experience nurses bring to the patient situation. By understanding what self-esteem means, its importance to all persons, and ways in which it is maintained and enhanced, nurses move closer toward planning and implementing nursing care that has an optimal effect on self-worth. Moreover, in the process of assisting others to feel worthwhile about themselves, it becomes clear that the need for self-esteem is equally important to nurse and patient alike.

Terms for Review

adaptation
assertiveness
body-image
compensatory security system
defense-oriented response
ethnocentrism

real self versus ideal self
self-awareness
self-concept/self-image
self-esteem
sick role

stress
stressor
task-oriented response
therapeutic use of self
unconditional positive regard

Self-Assessment

Self-Esteem Checklist

This self-esteem tool, although not a validated test, can help you assess your self-esteem. Next to each statement below, write the number that describes you best, based on the following scale:

O Never
1 Sometimes
2 About half the time
3 Most of the time
4 All the time

_____ 1. I have warm feelings toward myself.
_____ 2. I do not feel hurt by the opinions of others.
_____ 3. I am free of shame.
_____ 4. I do not feel less than others because they have more money, do things better, or are more popular.
_____ 5. I am happy and relaxed.
_____ 6. I feel good about my accomplishments.
_____ 7. I do not exaggerate what I have done or what my family has or does.
_____ 8. My sense of humor does not include making people laugh by hurting an individual or groups of people.
_____ 9. I speak up for my own needs, wants, and ideas.
_____ 10. I feel good about the good fortune of others.

_____ 11. I do not feel less than others when I lose.
_____ 12. I remain confident of my abilities, even when others disagree with me.
_____ 13. I am comfortable receiving compliments and gifts without having to give something in return.
_____ 14. I do not feel cheated or disappointed by life.
_____ 15. I do not feel inferior to others.
_____ 16. I enjoy being alone.
_____ 17. I am not afraid of letting people see my real self.
_____ 18. I do not feel a need to "put down" or ridicule others.
_____ 19. I do not feel a need to prove myself to others.
_____ 20. I accept others and feel friendly toward them.
_____ 21. I do not need others to agree with me to feel good about myself.
_____ 22. I am open and honest in sharing my thoughts and feelings with others.
_____ 23. I do not feel I have always to please other people.
_____ 24. I am able to admit mistakes without feeling ashamed.
_____ 25. I do not feel a need to defend myself to other people.

Explanation of Scoring

After completing, you can find your self-esteem index by adding all scores. The possible range of scores is from 0 to 100. An index over 90 indicates a solid sense of worth, while under 90 shows that a handicap to self-worth is present. An index less than 70 indicates a more serious problem of self-worth, and below 50 indicates a very low sense of worth which severely diminishes one's feeling of being capable and loved.

Optional:

Make a list of ways you can increase your self-esteem. Discuss in a small group methods of enhancing self-esteem.

Learning Activities

Stressors and the Self-Worth of Nurses

The following is a list of twelve stressors which may be seen as unique challenges to the self-worth of nurses. Rank each according to how stressful you perceive the event to be, with one being the most stressful and twelve being the least stressful.

_____ Intervening during a cardiac arrest or similar emergency
_____ Dealing with the family of a dying patient
_____ Working on an inconvenient schedule
_____ Interacting with a difficult doctor
_____ Working with a demanding patient
_____ Dealing with nonsupportive supervisors
_____ Assuming responsibilities in patient situations never encountered before
_____ Working with unqualified staff
_____ Conflict with co-workers
_____ Performing duties without thanks or recognition
_____ Coordinating ancillary personnel
_____ Caring for a seriously ill patient

Discussion Guide

After ranking the stressors according to your perception of them, divide into small groups and compare your list with those of other group members. Discuss the following questions:

1. What are the possible effects on nurses' self-esteem of the various stressful events (focus on your five most stressful situations).
2. What responses are available to nurses in these situations?
3. How have you reacted, or how might you react, to similar situations?
4. Weigh each response according to its potential to enhance or diminish nurses' self-esteem.

Review Questions

Multiple Choice

1. Self-esteem includes the qualities of
   a. Strength and achievement
   b. Mastery and competence
   c. Dignity and appreciation
   d. All of the above

2. The level of one's self-esteem has been shown to
   a. Eliminate stress
   b. Influence the ability to form close relationships
   c. Have no effect on physical health
   d. All of the above

3. Stress is
   a. Always a negative reaction
   b. An essential ingredient of life
   c. The stimulus that causes a physical response
   d. All of the above

4. Adaptation is an ongoing compromise which is influenced by
   a. Past experience
   b. How a stressor is perceived
   c. Genetic endowment
   d. All of the above

5. Defense-oriented responses
   a. Are conscious, action-oriented reactions
   b. Include acting in an assertive manner
   c. Involve the use of defense mechanisms
   d. All of the above

6. Threats to self-esteem as a result of illness and hospitalization include
   a. Loss of control
   b. Altered relationships
   c. Loss of roles
   d. All of the above

7. The sick role is characterized by
   a. Assertive behavior
   b. Compliance with treatment measures
   c. Patient participation in goal planning
   d. All of the above

8. In contrast to verbal behaviors, nonverbal behaviors tend to
   a. Be less accurate in determining a person's real meaning
   b. Carry less social meaning
   c. Be more spontaneous
   d. All of the above

9. Nurses assist patients to assess and accept their own strengths and weaknesses accurately through
   a. Therapeutic use of self
   b. Unconditional positive regard
   c. Validation
   d. All of the above

10. The aim of nursing action and interpersonal relationships is to
    a. Mobilize patients' interpersonal resources
    b. Provide family psychotherapy
    c. Encourage family members to live close by one another
    d. All of the above

Short Answer

11. List the three steps in developing self-awareness.
12. The nurse's self-esteem as a health care professional is founded on what three qualities?
13. Explain why members of minority groups face especially

serious esteem-threatening stressors when they become patients. Give at least one example.

14. List the five areas that are most important in assessing self-esteem.

15. Describe what is meant by changing the sick role to a well role.

Answers

1. d
2. b
3. d
4. d
5. c
6. d
7. b
8. c
9. d
10. a
11. Listening to one's self, listening to and learning from others, self-disclosure
12. Knowledge, competence, independence
13. Lack of understanding and appreciation of cultural differences by health care providers; examples: direct eye contact as disrespectful in American Indian culture, and so forth
14. Self-awareness, major stressors, perception of and response to stressful situations, interpersonal relationships, other supports
15. Facilitating patients' attempts to be capable and competent

Suggested Readings

Bush, M. A., *and* **Kjervik, D. K.:** The nurse's self-image. *Nurs. Times,* **75**(17):697–701, 1979. The authors describe ways to increase nurses' self-esteem.

Pelletier, K. R.: *Holistic Medicine.* Dell, New York, 1979.

Smoyak, S. A.: Is life the pits. *Imprint,* **3:**34–37+ 1981. Focuses on the importance of perceptions in determining outcomes of stressful situations. Includes a discussion of stress, adaptation, and coping strengths.

White, E. H.: Giving health care to minority patients. *Nurs. Clin. North Am.,* **12**(1):27–40, 1977. Through a discussion of various ethnic groups, this article emphasizes the importance of nurses developing a thorough knowledge and appreciation of cultural differences in order to provide quality health care to minority patients.

References and Bibliography

Bancroft, A.: Now she's a disposition problem. *Perspect. Psychiatr. Care,* 9:96–102, 1971.

Barnett, K.: A survey of the current utilization of touch by health team personnel with hospitalized patients. *Int. J. Nurs. Stud.,* 9:195–209, 1972.

Beckman, B. L.: Life stress and psychological well being. *J. Health Soc. Behav.,* 45:12–35, 1971.

Brissett, D.: Toward a clarification of self-esteem. *Psychiatry,* 35:255–63, 1972.

Burnside, I, M.; Ebersole, P.; and Monea, H. E.: *Psychosocial Caring Throughout the Life Span.* McGraw-Hill, New York, 1979.

Bush, M. A., and Kjervik, D. K.: The nurse's self-image. *Nurs. Times,* 75(17): 697–701, 1979.

Cassell, J.: Social science theory as a source of hypotheses in epidemiological research. *Am. J. Public Health,* 54:1482–89, 1964.

Chrzanowski, G.: The genesis and nature of self-esteem. *Am. J. of Psychother.,* 35(1):38–46, 1981.

Clarke, J. I.: *Self-Esteem: A Family Affair.* Winston Press, Minneapolis, 1978.

Coopersmith, S.: *The Antecedents of Self-Esteem.* Freeman, San Francisco, 1967.

Deci, E. L.: Effects of externally mediated rewards on intrinsic motivation. *J. Pers. Soc. Psychol.,* 18:105–15, 1971.

Dyer, E.; Monson, M.; and Van Drimmelen, J.: *Psychol. Rep.,* 36(1):255, 1975.

Ekman, P.: Communication through nonverbal behavior: a source of information about an interpersonal relationship. In Tomkins, S. S., and Izard, C. E. (eds.): *Affect, Cognition, and Personality.* Springer-Verlag New York, 1965.

Grace, H, K., and Camilleri, D.: *Mental Health Nursing; A Socio-Psychological Approach.* Brown, Dubuque, Iowa, 1981.

Jourard, S. M.: *Personal Adjustment: An Approach Through the Study of Healthy Personality.* Macmillan, New York, 1963.

Kennedy, M. J.: Impact of illness and hospitalization. In Haber, J.; Leach, A. M.; Schudy, S. M.; and Sideleau, B. F. (eds): *Comprehensive Psychiatric Nursing.* McGraw-Hill, New York, 1978.

Klopfer, W. G.: Interpersonal theory of adjustment. In Kastenbau, R. (ed.): *Psycho-Biology of Aging.* Springer-Verlag, New York, 1965.

Lawrence, J. C.: Homosexuals, hospitalization, and the nurse. *Nurs. Forum,* 14(3):304–17, 1975.

Leininger, M.: Cultural diversities of health and nursing care. *Nurs. Clin. North Am.,* 12(1):5–18, 1977.

Levin, P.: *Becoming the Way We Are: A Transactional Guide to Personal Development.* Transactional Publications, Berkeley, Calif., 1975.

Levinson, B.: Pets and old age. *Men. Hyg.,* 53(3): 364–68, 1969.

Linden, L., and Breed, W.: Epidemiology of suicide. In Schneidman, E. S. (ed.): *Suicidology: Contemporary Developments.* Grune & Stratton, New York, 1976.

Lowenthal, M., and Chiriboga, D.: Transition to the empty nest: crisis, challenge, or relief. *Arch. Gen. Psychiatry,* 26(1):8–14, 1972.

Martin, A.: Some issues in the treatment of gay and lesbian patients. *Psychotherapy: Theory, Research and Practice,* 19(3):341–48, 1982.

Maslow, A. H.: *Motivation and Personality.* Harper & Row, New York, 1954.

Miller, J. R., and Janosik, E. H.: *Family-Focused Care.* McGraw-Hill, New York, 1980.

Murphy, S. A.: Learned helplessness: from concept to comprehension. *Perspect. Psychiatr. Care,* 20(1):27–32, 1982.

Ostrouski, M. J.: Young adulthood. In Burnside, I. M.; Ebersole, P.; and Monea, H. E. (eds.): *Psychosocial Caring Throughout the Life Span.* McGraw-Hill, New York, 1979.

Parsons, T.: *The Social System.* Free Press, New York, 1951.

Pauly, I., and Goldstein, S.: Physician's attitudes in treating male homosexuals. *Med. Aspects Hum. Sexual.,* **4:**26–45, 1970.

Pelletier, K. R.: Mind as healer, mind as slayer. *Psychol. Today,* pp. 35–36, Feb., 1977.

Petrie, K., and Rotheram, M. J.: Insulators against stress: self-esteem and assertiveness. *Psychol. Rep.,* **50:**963–66, 1982.

Primeaux, M.: Caring for the American Indian patient. *Am. J. Nurs.,* **77:**91–94, 1977.

Rahe, R. H.: Subjects' recent life changes and their near-future illness reports. *Ann. Clin. Res.,* **4:**1–6, 1973.

Rahe, R., and Lind, E.: Psychosocial factors and sudden cardiac death: a pilot study. *J. Psychosom. Res.,* **15:**19–24, 1971.

Rahe, R.; Mahan, J. L.; and Arthur, R. J.: Prediction of near-future health change from subjects preceding life changes. *J. Psychosom. Res.,* **14:**401–406, 1970.

Roy, S. C.: The Roy adaptation model. In Riehl, J. P., and Roy, S. C. (eds.): *Conceptual Models for Nursing Practice.* Appleton-Century-Crofts, Norwalk, Ct. 1974.

Rubin, R.: Body image and self-esteem. *Nurs. Outlook,* pp. 20–23, June 1968.

Schulz, R., and Benner, G.: Relocation of the aged: a review and theoretical analysis. *J. Gerontol.,* **32:**323–33, 1977.

Selye, H.: The stress syndrome. *Am. J. Nurs.,* **65:**98, 1965.

Shana, E.: A note on restriction of life space: attitudes of age cohorts. *J. Health Soc. Behav.,* **9**(1):86–90, 1968.

Sheehy, G.: *Passages: Predictable Crises of Adult Life.* Dutton, New York, 1976.

Stuart, G. W., and Sundeen, S. J.: *Principles and Practice of Psychiatric Nursing.* Mosby., St. Louis, 1979.

Weisman, A., and Worden, J. W.: The existential plight in cancer: a significance of the first 100 days. *Int. J. Psychiatry Med.,* **1:**7, 1976.

Werner-Beland, J. A.: *Grief Responses to Long-Term Illness and Disability.* Reston, Reston, Va., 1980.

White, E. H.: Giving health care to minority patients. *Nurs. Clini. North Am.,* **12**(1):27–40, 1977.

White, R.: Strategies of adaptation: An attempt at systematic description. In Coelho, G. (ed.): *Coping and Adaptation.* Basic Books, New York, 1974.

THE NEED FOR SELF-ACTUALIZATION*

Objectives

1. Define self-actualization and explain the importance of this need to people.
2. Identify characteristics associated with self-actualization.
3. Describe the impact that satisfaction of basic needs has on the ability of individuals to actualize their potentials.
4. Explain the relationship between crises and self-actualization.
5. Describe how the need for self-actualization is affected by interpersonal relationships.
6. Identify subjective and objective data indicating satisfaction of the need for self-actualization.
7. Identify subjective and objective data associated with obstructed growth.
8. Describe nursing interventions to assist individuals to respond to changes in their personal situations in ways that enhance self-actualization.
9. Describe how nurses can intervene in the teaching role to promote self-actualization.

Introduction

Self-actualization, the development of one's potentials, can be seen as the ultimate goal of human development. As Fromm (1947) declares, "Man's main task in life is to give birth to himself, to become what he potentially is." The urge to express one's capabilities is part of an inner nature which is present in every person. According to Maslow (1968), it has a dynamic force of its own, always pressing for open, uninhibited expression. However, in some persons movement toward self-actualization is obstructed, as a result of growth-discouraging factors (the term "growth" is used interchangeably with "self-actualization" in this chapter) such as fear of changing and ignorance. This drive to self-actualization can become distorted and self-destructive. Maslow

*Written by Tom Olson, an Assistant Professor of Nursing at the College of the Virgin Islands, St. Croix campus. His primary responsibility is teaching mental health nursing. Previously, Tom was a clinical nursing specialist in an out-patient mental health setting where he worked with patients in groups as well as individually.

(1968) terms obstructed growth "human diminution or stunting," and links it to personality disorders and disturbances. The need for self-actualization is important then, both because its expression is sought in all persons and because its obstruction leads to serious difficulties.

In no other need area is it more crucial that nurses view the total or whole being of persons than in responding to the need for self-actualization. The necessity of maintaining and enhancing the unity of the self serves as the dynamic principle for growth. Thus, to view individuals in parts or pieces not only violates their right to be seen as whole functioning persons, but also results in missing or distorting their need for self-actualization. Seeing only parts of people results in treating just kidneys, fractures, lungs, and so on, rather than caring for the whole person. One's need for growth is closely related to the satisfaction of one's other needs. Inasmuch as nursing strives to care for the entire being of patients, this interrelationship with other needs—the requirement of looking at the whole person—makes the needs for self-actualization particularly significant for nursing.

Defining Self-Actualization

Self-actualization is the need to become what one can become—physical, intellectual, emotional, and spiritual growth toward full development of one's unique capacities and potentialities as a human being. It is based on the assumptions that all individuals possess different sets of capacities—promises of what they may become—and that the drive to actualize or fulfill these capacities is present in everyone. Unlike the lower level needs, the need to actualize one's self is often only faintly perceived by individuals. Maslow (1968) recognized that it is the weakest need in that it is "easily overcome, suppressed or repressed." Moreover, generally, before it can be met, each lower level need must be satisfied to some degree. That self-actualization is more a direction than a final destination is best realized in considering it as a process of growth and maturation.

Self-Actualization as a Process of Growth

Growth emphasizes the ongoing process involved in developing one's capacities. In growing, persons begin to realize their potentials. They become more fulfilled, completed, or perfected. However, rather than reaching some absolute state of being, one's growth toward self-actualization is never fully completed. The capacities that persons strive to know and experience are, in large part, ways of thinking, behaving, and becoming. Thus, one is constantly engaged in the process of actualizing one's self. In contrast to Maslow's focusing on the very small percentage of the population that he believes ever become fully actualized, recognizing self-actualization as a process of growth makes it relevant to all persons, at all levels of ability.

Self-Actualization as Maturing

Maturing is the process by which persons become more effectively functioning human beings. This is consistent with the idea of self-actualization. However, maturing adds another dimension to this need. It considers individuals at all age levels in terms of whether or not they are moving toward fulfillment of their potentials. This does not mean that young children would be considered fully mature or self-actualized, but only that one could assess whether or not they are moving in the direction of satisfying this need. Thus, including maturing in this definition opens up the possibility of more completely understanding how persons grow toward actualizing their capacities. Moreover, when considering that persons at all age levels become patients, viewing self-actualization as maturing greatly expands the significance of this need in nursing.

In brief, as used here the meaning of self-actualization has been broadened to recognize that striving to fulfill one's potentials is a process that occurs throughout the entire life span.

Characteristics Associated with Self-Actualization

Various investigators into the process of actualizing one's potentials have proposed lists of characteristics which, based on their studies, they believe describe persons who are farther along the path of fulfilling their capacities than most others. Two such lists are summarized in Table 32–1. The summaries of characteristics of self-actualizing people all describe individuals whose growth is in a direction of satisfying their highest need.

Actualizing Qualities and Nursing. Referring again to Table 32–1, consider the number of characteristics which are also descriptions of qualities that are crucially important in nursing. Both lists refer to the significance that caring for others, and having a purpose beyond one's self, have in terms of growth. To be sure, caring for others is a quality that is synonymous with nursing! Similarly, each summary makes reference in one form

Table 32–1. **Characteristics of Successful Growth**

MASLOW	SHEEHY
1. Realistic perception of world	1. Feeling and belief that one's life has meaning and direction, including involvement with something beyond self
2. Acceptance of self, others, and the world for what they are	2. Handling transitions in a creative manner
3. Spontaneity in behavior	3. Able to use failures as useful experience, including an acceptance of the positive and negative aspects of life
4. Focus of interests on problems outside self	4. Sense of accomplishment from having attained several long-term goals
5. Ability to be objective	5. Satisfaction with one's own growth and development
6. Personal independence; stable in the face of frustrations, criticism from others	6. Deep, mutual loving relationship with another person
7. Freshness of appreciation of people and things	7. Able to build friendships, including a willingness to be open with others
8. Capacity for experiences of happiness and fulfillment	8. Positive outlook on life
9. Feeling of identification and affection for human beings	9. Able to accept criticism or failure without seeing it as an attack on one's solid sense of worth
10. Deep emotional relations with a small circle of friends	10. Absence of major fears
11. Democratic attitudes and values (respect for all persons)	
12. Able to discriminate between means and ends, good and evil	
13. Philosophical rather than hostile sense of humor	
14. Creativeness	
15. Resistance to cultural conformity	

Source: Adapted from A.H. Maslow: Self-actualizing people: A study of psychological health, in *Motivation and Personality*, 2nd ed. Harper & Row, New York, 1954 and 1970; and G. Sheehy: The ten hallmarks of well-being, in *Pathfinders*. Morrow, New York, 1981.

or another to one's interpersonal capacities, including abilities to identify and be open with others and to perceive and accept persons as they are. These are qualities that are directly related to the ability to be empathic, a characteristic which is at the core of effective assessment and intervention. Still further, a positive and stable sense of self-worth is also emphasized as a characteristic of actualizing persons. Confronted on a daily basis with challenges in dealing with patients and colleagues, nurses face becoming overwhelmed by stressors unless they have developed solid self-esteem. If one continues to examine the lists, other qualities also seem to be especially important in nursing.

Maslow includes personal independence, in the sense of being fully in charge of one's self, as a quality associated with growth. Consider the importance of this quality in nursing. Nurses are regularly called on to make critical decisions on their own. Although many of these judgments will later need to be validated by supervisors and/or physicians, particularly in emergency situations nurses may be required to act quickly without the benefit of consulting with others. Especially in these circumstances, the level of nurses' personal independence is ex-

tremely important, although in the case of women who are nurses, this may represent a sharp departure from the traditional stereotype of females as being dependent on males for important decision making.

In a related sense, both lists include creativity, or the capacity to deal with changing stressors in constructive ways. Nurses appear to learn early in their careers that, although guidelines for handling problems are useful, they are no more than simply that—guidelines. For as certain as each patient care situation is guaranteed to differ from the next, so absolute rules fall by the wayside. Nurses are continually challenged to devise alternatives and seek creative solutions to new problems. Clearly, many of the qualities necessary for growth, maturing, self-actualization are of primary importance in nursing! To the extent that nurses develop these qualities in themselves, they can increase not only their personal but also their professional growth. Where such growth is absent or severely diminished, increased complaints of boredom, frustration, and burnout tend to be heard. Moreover, as will be explored further in later sections, the consequences of such problems reach beyond nurses to affect patients as well.

The Process of Self-Actualization: Major Issues and Influences

In examining some of the major factors influencing self-actualization, it is important to keep in mind that growth for one person may not be the same as growth for another. Although certain characteristics, such as

openness, creativity, and independence, may be seen as crucial to all persons engaged in actualizing their potentials, the actual balance of these and other characteristics and the objectives toward which one aims will differ

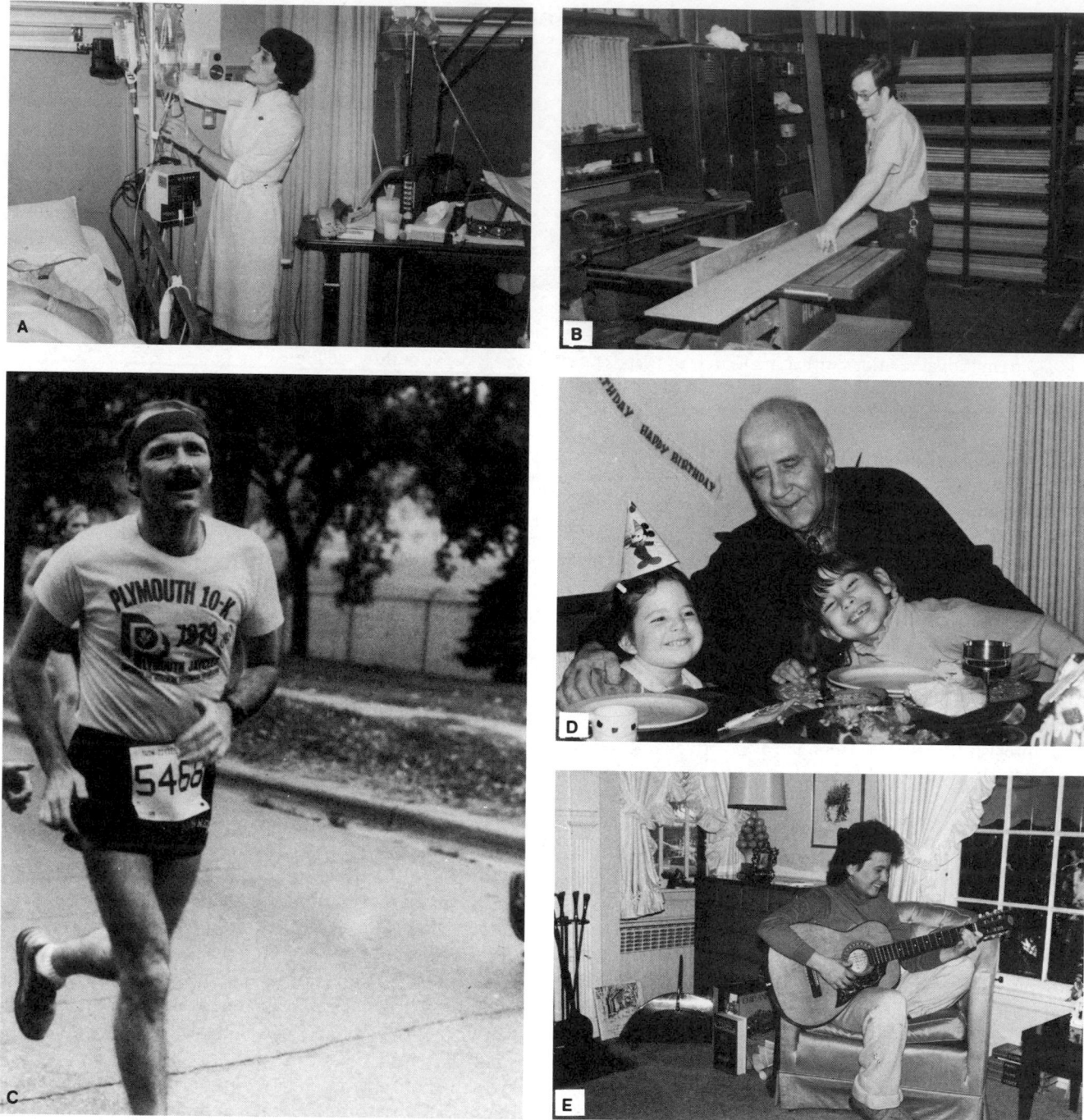

Figure 32–1. Each person has unique potentials to fulfill. For some, as indicated in this illustration, fulfillment may be achieved in part through becoming a nurse, a carpenter, an athlete, a grandparent, or a musician.

with each individual. This is because each person has a unique inner self to actualize. For instance, while one person may show growth by settling down and becoming more conscientious, another demonstrates growth by loosening up, becoming more spontaneous, and worrying less. Similarly, a particular individual moves closer toward fulfilling potentials through becoming a nurse, while for others fulfillment means becoming a musician, mother, or athlete. Thus, the central question is how can one grow toward becoming all that one uniquely is? Three major issues that influence the process of self-actualization will be discussed: satisfaction versus conquest of basic needs, crisis, and interpersonal relationships.

Satisfaction or Conquest of Basic Needs

As a rule, the more adequately lower level needs are being met, the more capable persons are of fulfilling their potentials. For instance, in discussing the newly hospitalized spinal cord–injured patient Starck (1980) explains, "The struggle to meet basic physiological needs consumes such a large proportion of effort and energy that higher level needs satisfaction cannot be sought." In addition to illness, a variety of other factors, such as poverty and lack of education, can interfere with overall need satisfaction in a similar manner. However, when one's life situation is so unfavorable that one's primary energies must be devoted wholly to meeting basic physiological needs, one is likely to experience "feelings of frustration, dissatisfaction, and meaninglessness" (Gale, 1969). In such situations, although basic needs remain only partially satisfied, some individuals may conquer these needs in order to continue their process of growth.

According to Gale (1969), once the need for self-actualization has been awakened in persons, it "may take precedence over the supposedly more basic maintenance needs." Thus, individuals may go without food or sleep, risk their safety, and compromise love needs if actualization stirrings are strong enough. For example, such is sometimes the case with the musical composer who, engaged in a deep expression of self through the manipulation of sounds, at least temporarily ignores hunger, thirst, and other basic needs. Nurses regularly witness similar situations in health care settings, although the deprivation of certain needs may be less voluntary than in the example above. Consider, for instance, the experiences of patients with terminal illnesses who are involved in what Kübler-Ross (1975) terms "the final stage of growth," that is death.

Subjective experience as well as empirical research support the realization that coming to terms with one's mortality accompanies self-actualization (Gamble and Brown, 1981). Kübler-Ross (1975) goes on to quote a patient who, having been diagnosed three months previously with terminal cancer, states, "I have lived more in the past three months than I have during my whole life." Dying persons, as well as other patients, often undertake the search for self—the ultimate goal of growth—under circumstances of extreme deprivation of basic needs. Further, as will be discussed later in this section, nurses are frequently influential participants in this search. In brief, although lower level needs usually take precedence over higher level needs, in many circumstances the growth of individuals occurs despite remarkable physical and psycholgocial deprivation.

Growth Through Crisis

In Chapter 31 the relationship between persons' responses to stressors and self-esteem was explored. Moving one step beyond this, it becomes clear that not only does one's ability to adapt successfully to stressful events influence one's sense of worth, but it also has a profound effect on self-actualization. In particular, this discussion centers on those stressors that are perceived as being so severe that they represent major disruptions or crises in individuals' lives. For just as such a disruption may lead to personal devastation, so it may serve as a catalyst for growth.

A *crisis* is a life turning point, "a crucial period of increased vulnerability and heightened potential" (Erikson, 1968). In times of crisis, individuals' customary coping strategies are no longer adequate. They stand at a fork in the path. One direction leads toward growth, the other toward diminished effectiveness in constructively handling life. Choosing the path that enhances self-actualization requires adapting in new ways which allow persons to find fresh meaning and strength in even the most difficult situations. In fact, crises have been described as an essential condition of growth and psychological change (Bugental, 1965). This realization is important to nurses as human beings as well as health care providers.

Nursing regularly deals with people who are directly encountering crisis and who are thereby potentially embarked on the process of more fully knowing and experiencing themselves. As Sarosi (1968) explains, "Crisis removes the shell that separates the person from his experience." Viewed from this perspective, a crisis becomes a situation from which people may emerge psychologically healthier than prior to the crisis. Moreover, the lives of those who share in the growth of others in crisis are similarly enriched.

Consider the following illustration of a patient who, along with a nurse, encounters a traumatic turning point in life:

Mr. C. is a 46-year-old sales executive who, until his recent hospitalization for complaints of weakness, loss of weight, and abdominal pain, had felt very much in control of his life. He prided himself on still being married after 20 years and in being able to finance college educations for his two children. His ability as an aggressive businessman had brought him considerable financial success. He had carefully nurtured an image of himself as a highly self-sufficient person. And, although at times he had sensed something lacking in his relationships with others, he had quieted these feelings by reminding himself of the outward signs of his success. Initially during his hospital stay, Mr. C. tended to be good-natured and even jovial in his interactions with nursing staff, this despite the uncertainty of illness and continued pain. However, his mood changed drastically following the announcement of a definitive diagnosis. After extensive laboratory tests and a liver biopsy, Mr. C. was told by his doctor that he has widespread cancer of the liver (hepatic carcinoma). It was explained that treatment could help relieve his symptoms but that his illness is terminal.

In the face of this information, Mr. C. appeared depressed and withdrew even from family members. His conversations with nurses were limited to one or two words. Still, the evening shift nurse made a point of asking Mr. C. if he could sit with him for a few minutes, adding that it was okay if he chose not to talk. Mr. C. nodded his head "yes" to this offer. The nurse and patient were silent together for several minutes before Mr. C. began to cry quietly. He went on to explain how he felt so unable to share his vulnerabilities, especially his fear of loss of control, with anyone. He expressed his difficulty over the years in being open with people, adding that he had kept even his relationships with his wife and children on a very distant level. As the conversation continued though, primarily with the nurse listening and Mr. C. talking, he began to think of ways he could get to know his family. However, he also expressed the fear that they might not wish to bother with him since he had taken so little time for them in the past. Their conversation ended with the nurse touching Mr. C.'s shoulder and agreeing to return at a later time.

Like other similar situations, this patient's crisis left him at a fork in the path. One direction could best be described as "throwing in the towel," giving up the possibility of something constructive being achieved in the situation. The other, which Mr. C. seemed to be in the process of choosing, is aimed at turning even huge minuses into partial pluses by finding new meaning and strength in crisis. The overwhelming fact of his illness had cracked the patient's shell and enabled him to recognize more clearly some of the emptiness in his life. Further, he began to see what he could do to enrich his life, to grow. By improving the quality of his interpersonal relationships, Mr. C. also moves closer to becoming all that he can become. This is the essence of self-actualization. In addition, if nurses remain open to the actualizing experiences of patients, they will grow themselves. For example, as Mr. C. shows his struggle toward accepting the fact of his terminal illness, the nurse is also affirmed in coming to terms with the fact of personal mortality. Thus, growth becomes a mutual experience. Indeed, not only do individuals benefit from one another's self-actualization, but the interpersonal relationships of people significantly influence whether or not growth occurs.

Interpersonal Relationships and Self-Actualization

One's relationships with others are worthy of particular note in discussing self-actualization. Psychological research shows that in order to cope with very stressful situations and continue growing, people must have depth relationships in which mutual satisfaction of needs occurs regularly and dependably (Lowenthal and Haven, 1968). Indeed, Clinebell (1979) concludes that impoverishment of one's network of social support produces "emotional malnutrition and diminished growth." In fact, individual growth is most likely to occur within the context of mutually growth-nurturing relationships.

Growth-nurturing relationships are ones in which individuals are allowed and encouraged to fully know and experience themselves. For instance, in such relationships preconceptions about persons' characteristics and potentials are kept to a minimum. This allows individuals to change and to become themselves, rather than having to use their energy to maintain a facade. As Jourard (1968) explains, "If you have a fixed idea of who I am and what my traits are, and what my possibilities of change are then anything that comes out of me beyond your concept, you will disconfirm." In this latter situation, people tend to hide their real selves from others and in turn are less able to actualize their capacities.

Another important aspect of growth-nurturing relationships is that in them individuals are challenged and encouraged by one another to attempt new projects. Persons are supported in their strivings with the idea that, although it is not possible to transcend one's possibilities, people can transcend their *concepts* of what their possibilities might be. In writing a book, climbing a mountain, or entering nursing school, individuals may grow through their discovery of capacities they never before experienced or imagined they had.

Most important, people who keep preconceptions about others to a minimum, along with encouraging the actualizing experiences of others, are better able to appreciate and accept their own unique process of growth. In other words, one can neither appreciate nor encourage the self-actualization of others if one is fearful of fulfilling one's own possibilities. Therefore, mutual growth is the key to growth-nurturing relationships. This is a crucial aspect of all meaningful relationships in which people are involved, relationships such as that of the parent and child, husband and wife, and even nurse and patient.

To illustrate, consider the importance of nurses' comfort with their own growth in the nurse-patient relationship. Jourard (1971) writes, "There is a connection between a nurse's inability or fear to be her real self while on duty and the blocking of patients' self-disclosure." If nurses are ignorant of their own capacities as persons or even afraid to recognize and express these, they are very likely to be threatened by the real-self expressions of patients. Consequently, "a patient might send out a 'trial balloon' concerning what really is on his mind, only to encounter a response from the nurse which effectively squelches him" (Jourard, 1971). And yet, it is precisely through expressing what is really on one's mind that persons more fully understand themselves and thus grow. Return again to the situation involving Mr. C. and imagine how other nurses, less comfortable with genuine self-expression than the nurse in the illustration, might obstruct the patient's growth. For example, rather than really listening to Mr. C., another less growth-oriented nurse might have quickly changed the subject, talked about the weather or attempted to joke, or have quickly made an excuse to leave to do other tasks. However, these inhibiting responses are less likely to occur with nurses who appreciate, accept, and express their capacities and potentials as human beings.

In short, growth-nurturing relationships are of crucial importance in promoting the self-actualizing tendencies of people. These relationships revolve around keeping preconceptions to a minimum and mutual encouragement of growth. Most important, such relationships require that persons appreciate and accept their own movement toward self-actualization.

Nursing Care and Self-Actualization

In no other area of human need is the *art* of nursing emphasized more than in the area of self-actualization. There are no gauges or scales to give an absolute measurement of self-fulfillment; no medications, diet, or other similar treatment measures to promote growth. Nursing care in this area is, at its heart, more a basic orientation toward people than a set of techniques. It is the use of one's self in a growth- and hope-centered way of perceiving, experiencing, and relating to patients.

Assessment

Nursing assessment is organized around areas identified in the previous sections: overall need satisfaction, the uniqueness of each person's development, interpersonal relationships, and the ability to use crises for growth.

Overall Need Satisfaction. In assessing the patient's need for self-actualization, it is particularly important to consider the whole person, recalling that this involves an interrelationship of needs and desires. Although, generally, the more adequately basic needs are met, the more capable persons are of developing their potentials, several needs, including the need for self-actualization, may be partially satisfied at the same time. Thus, the complete hierarchy of needs is surveyed: physiological, safety, love and belonging, self-esteem, and finally, self-actualization.

Consider the following illustration:

R.B. is an 18-year-old high school senior who has had several hospitalizations for Hodgkin's disease, a malignant disorder of the lymph system. He has recently been readmitted to the hospital with a low-grade fever, weakness, and bone pain. Testing has revealed increased bone marrow involvement. To combat the spread of the disease, R.B. is being given chemotherapy. This has produced the side effects of nausea and loss of appetite (anorexia).

R.B. has been receiving numerous cards and visits from family members and friends. Still, at times, he expresses feeling frightened and alone. Initially, the concern shown by others only seemed to make R.B. feel guilty and intensified the natural question, "Why me?" He tended to make self-deprecating remarks about "How skinny I am," remembering how he had once been on the starting line of his high school football team. One evening, after having been visited by a particularly close friend, R.B. remarked as the nurse checked his IV, "I don't think I ever realized before how much some people really care about me." Later, he asked the same nurse, "Do you think I could talk with any of the others on this ward with problems like mine? I wonder if I might be able to help them, maybe give them some support."

In assessing this patient care situation, unmet needs are evident in all five categories of Maslow's hierarchy of needs. Among these are the patient's physiological problems related to nausea, anorexia, possible infection, and pain. His weakness poses a potential safety and security difficulty. The need for love and belonging is threatened by the patient's confinement to a hospital. And his self-esteem is challenged by the loss of his role as an athlete. Unfortunately, nurses often stop at this point in their assessment, reluctant or uncertain about how to include self-actualization in their care planning.

In fact, in this illustration as well as in many actual patient care situations, the patient's struggle to meet basic needs consumes such a large proportion of effort and energy that higher level need satisfaction can be sought only with great difficulty. Moreover, success in nursing care is frequently only measured in terms of physiological accomplishments: Is the patient gaining weight, has the likelihood of infection been decreased, and so on. However, although it is true that more basic needs must often take precedence in planning care, to focus on them exclusively is to ignore caring for the patient as a whole person. Returning again to the case illustration, despite major problems in more basic need areas, R.B. has continued to grow and change. In this process he has recognized his potential for reaching out and caring for others. While his ability to fulfill this potential may be affected by other unmet needs, it is not completely obstructed by them. Indeed, as in the example cited here, it may be as a result of experiences related to hospitalization and illness that growth needs are first recognized and expressed!

Unique Possibilities. The focus of the assessment of self-actualization is on strengths, assets, and potentialities. This is a departure from the tendency to focus mainly on problems, weaknesses, and pathology. Using this point of view, personal limitations are most meaningful in more clearly defining possibilities open to people rather than pointing out options that are closed. It is this perspective that enables Kübler-Ross to describe dying as the last stage of growth, rather than as an end to all development. Or in the illustration involving R.B. (see page 000), illness became an opportunity in terms of self-actualization to reach out to others rather than simply a threat or limitation. Thus, the aim here is to assess patients' capabilities and the values that guide their development.

The most useful questions to ask here revolve around what patients see as their possibilities. This assessment inevitably involves values, since values guide the choices people make and therefore determine their directions of change. For instance, what ambitions or life goals do patients have; what gives life meaning and purpose; what is most important to patients in the present, in the future? Such questions may lead to a variety of responses such as, "I hope to do some traveling"; "My wife and I plan to have another child"; "I'd like to go to college"; "I'm writing a book, but I don't know if I'll be able to finish now." Answers may range from being very helpful to despairing, from being based on actual possibilities to being unrealistic. Nursing interventions related to these varying responses will be discussed in the next section. Most important here is to emphasize the relevance to nursing of asking such questions.

Questions about self-actualization are necessary if nurses are to care for the whole person. Consider, for instance, the mastectomy patient who has sought fulfilment as a fashion model, the patient who aspires to be a professional athlete and who has just had a below-the-knee amputation, or the recent victim of a motorcycle accident whose injuries have ended plans to enter the military. Illness and hospitalization have most likely changed the course of self-actualization for these individuals. However, an alteration in direction doesn't necessarily mean the end of growth. At least, as will be explored with nursing interventions, nurses have an opportunity to exert a positive influence on this change.

Assessment of patients' values and possibilities requires some rapport between patient and nurse, that is, a feeling of connectedness and trust. It is likely that only a feeling of awkwardness and discomfort would be produced if the nurse's first question during the admission interview was "What gives your life meaning?" With the establishment of some relatedness and genuine concern, however, such inquiries may provide information which is useful in planning nursing care. Still, as was seen in the illustration involving R.B., important information about self-actualization may be volunteered by patients. Careful listening then becomes as useful in assessment as remembering to ask specific questions.

The assessment of patients' potentials and values cannot be separated from nurses' evaluation of their own growth process. Understanding one's own personal development also promotes the helping relationship. As Boccuzzi (1979) explains, "The most workable methods for helping others to solve problems and to live their lives more fully can often be found within our own life experiences." It is not expected that nurses' self-assessments should reveal fully self-actualized beings. As a process, growth is always incomplete, for nurses as well as for patients. The unfinishedness of nurses' growth will interfere with facilitating growth in others only if they are unaware of it or pretend to themselves and others that they "have it made." It is as the result of such a lack of self-understanding that persons tend to impose their values, their ideas about growth, on others. In contrast, nurses' awareness and acceptance of their own process of growth allows them to be open to the possibilities of others.

Interpersonal Relationships. The aim of this part of the assessment is to develop an awareness of the role of significant persons in patient's lives. This is primarily to determine whether these relationships tend to encourage or discourage growth. The questions asked here are basic ones, such as who is important in patients' lives, how do patients feel about these relationships, are those involved usually perceived as being helpful and supportive in difficulties such as the present one? Once again, though, careful observation may be just as important as asking questions.

Consider the following illustration:

M.J. is a 21-year-old woman who lives with her parents and works at a part-time job as a receptionist. Three days ago she was admitted to the orthopedic unit of a local hospital with a severe fracture of her left leg. She is currently in traction. Her injuries were the result of a motorcycle accident which also involved her boyfriend. He was treated in the ER for minor injuries and released.

Nursing notes document that, since her hospitalization, M.J.'s appearance has ranged from angry to sad and withdrawn. She has been visited several times by her parents and boyfriend. The latter has seemed supportive, reassuring the patient that she'll soon be up and on her own. During the most recent visit with her parents, the nurse, who was in the process of checking the traction, briefly observed the family members' interactions with one another.

M.J. was quiet as her father exclaimed in a loud voice, "You sure did it this time. What were you doing riding on a motorcycle? You know they're not safe. I doubt you'll ever change; always doing things you shouldn't!" Rather than responding, the patient reached for a book on her bedside stand. However, before she could get it, her mother handed it to her saying, "Dear, you're going to cause yourself another accident; just lie perfectly still." M.J. accepted the book without a word.

Most remarkable in this interaction are the preconceptions ("you'll never change") and the lack of encouragement. And yet, encouragement and a minimum of preconceptions were described as essential to growth-nurturing relationships. Realizing the limitations of nurses in situations such as these—they are not psychotherapists and their time with patients and significant others is usually brief—there are nursing interventions that may be useful in promoting the self-actualizing qualities of relationships encountered in nursing practice. These will be explored in the section on interventions.

Although family relationships tend to be most significant in terms of individuals' growth, because of the long-term and intimate influences they exert, shorter-term relationships may also have important effects on self-actualization. Consider, for example, the nurse-patient relationship. When a severe crisis strikes, such as often is the case with illness and hospitalization, people are challenged to turn to others for support and encouragement, to struggle and learn new coping skills. Nurses are frequently the most available sources of support and encouragement for patients. As a result, they have an opportunity to have a positive impact on patients' growth. Return again to the illustration involving R.B. (page 000). In this situation, it was the nurse to whom the patient turned to reveal his new awareness of how others cared for him. Further, in recognizing his capacity to reach out to others, the patient sought guidance from the nurse. Within brief, yet meaningful, relationships such as these, nurses have the opportunity to influence the growth of others. Therefore, assessment of interpersonal relationships and growth involves developing an awareness of the influences others have on the self-actualization of patients, including significant short-term as well as long-term relationships.

Crisis and Hope. Crises are crucial opportunities for growth. This part of the nursing assessment focuses on the ability of patients to use crises as growth opportunities.

The questions asked here center on how patients have reacted to crises in the past and their ability to utilize realistic hope (the expectation that positive outcomes and personal fulfillment are possible) in their present situation. The past responses of persons are significant because they determine how persons are most likely to respond to present situations. Assessing hope is important because it is the ability to hope that enables persons to continue struggling when growth seems blocked or is very slow, a situation frequently encountered in confronting a crisis.

The first step in assessing past responses is to ask patients if they have ever confronted crises or severe stressors. Next, nurses can ask patients to describe their reactions to these situations. Useful questions include: Did they perceive alternatives or choices in the crisis or did they simply feel trapped? Was there any positive aspect of the experience—did they feel they had changed, gained a different outlook on life, or grown as a result of the crisis?

Patients' ability to hope depends on a variety of factors: their expectation about the future and the meanings it holds for them, the sense of having some power to influence their surroundings and move toward their goals, and the attitudes of significant persons toward them and their future. Therefore, specific questions to ask patients would include: What, if any, future plans do they have? Do they have goals or objectives toward which they aspire? What is their belief about their ability to influence the outcome of their present situation? Are the significant persons in patients' lives hopeful or despairing about the possibility of the patients' gaining something constructive or positive from the current crisis?

In this area, self-assessment is crucial. Nurses' own responses to personal crises will affect their ability to see such events as opportunites for growth and, thus, to convey this impression to patients. Specific nursing actions to promote growth through crises are examined in the section on interventions.

Nursing Diagnosis

Various problems of self-actualization may be encountered by patients and nurses. Nursing diagnoses that recognize these include a brief description of the growth-related difficulty and, if known, the probable cause. Based on the ideas presented in this chapter, some examples of nursing diagnoses associated with self-actualization include:

- Boredom and apathy related to growth-diminishing life-style
- Lack of spontaneity in life associated with disability
- Burnout associated with barriers to career fulfillment
- Dissatisfaction with meaning and purpose of life
- Unresolved anger and hostility related to obstruction of self-actualization

Acknowledged in this list of nursing diagnoses is the importance of self-actualization to all persons. Apathy, unresolved anger, career dissatisfaction, and similar problems related to growth are concerns for nurses and patients alike.

Goal Setting

The primary goal of nursing intervention is to facilitate the maximum development of potentials throughout the life cycle. In addition to approaching the process of self-actualization in unique ways, all persons possess different possibilities of what they may become. In order to reflect this individuality, goals are based on an understanding of each patient's overall need satisfaction, their values and perceptions of their capabilities, the manner in which their growth is affected by those around them, and their response to crisis situations. Following are examples of goals for patients with problems related to self-actualization:

Patient will create one project of her choice in occupational therapy within two sessions of one hour each.
Patient will state one future goal by the end of the shift.
Patient will describe two methods of improving ability to cope with his disability.
Patient will state three realistic alternatives in handling present career conflict within one week.
Patient will identify two athletic activities in which she will be able to participate following discharge from the rehabilitation unit.

Patient will list on paper five highest values in life by the end of the hour.

In examining these goals, it is evident that objectives for growth can be formulated in the same manner as objectives for other needs in Maslow's hierarchy. However, it is important to emphasize here that because self-actualization is an inner-directed process, one in which individuals choose their own directions and set their own pace, it is crucial that patients be actively involved in goal setting. Nurses can assist, but not force, patients to move toward self-actualization.

Nursing Intervention

Nursing intervention to promote self-actualization emphasizes the strengths of patients as persons and their growth potentials. The three nursing roles discussed here include nurses as holistic care providers, as change agents, and as teachers.

Intervention as Holistic Care Providers. Nurses are holistic care providers when their focus is on the total being of patients rather than on only dressings to be changed, calories to be counted, or injections to be administered. In order to promote self-actualization, it is necessary to take into account all need areas. Indeed, intervention to facilitate growth begins with providing for optimum satisfaction of basic, as well as high level, needs. This is less complicated than it may initially seem.

For instance, intervening as a holistic care provider to enhance fulfillment of spiritual potentials may mean planning with the patient to administer pain medication before, rather than after, the patient visits the hospital chapel. Another situation may involve simply offering the patient a bedpan prior to beginning a discussion about current losses and future plans. Or holistic care in the context of promoting self-actualization could include touching an elderly patient's arm—recognizing esteem needs—as a way of supporting the expression of a new self-understanding. Still another example might involve briefly delaying an enema while the patient finishes listening to a favorite symphony on the radio. The key in all of these nursing actions is caring for the entire person.

Caring for the whole persons as a means of enhancing self-actualization does not mean that all needs are perfectly satisfied. This, of course, would be unrealistic. Growth involves both struggle and satisfaction, both pain and joy. Rather, intervening in a holistic manner is an attempt to recognize the interrelatedness of patients' needs and desires and to plan nursing care accordingly.

Intervention as Change Agents.   Nurses regularly come into contact with individuals, patients, whose expectations about themselves are being shattered. The world is no longer the same for the business person who felt invincible until hospitalization for a perforated ulcer, the student who planned to enter college until an accident resulted in a severe and chronic disability, or the parent whose life-style has been permanently altered by a myocardial infarction. Patients are involved in a process of change which is often traumatic. As a result, they are faced with needing to restructure their world. Nurses are in a crucial position to influence the manner in which patients "put the pieces back together again." The aim of nurses' interventions as change agents is to assist persons to respond to alterations in their personal situations in ways that enhance their growth. This is accomplished in two ways: through utilizing an awareness of patients' values and possibilities and by awakening hope.

UTILIZING AWARENESS OF VALUES AND POSSIBILITIES.   Promoting self-actualization through change requires that nurses become aware of patients' values and possibilities. One prerequisite of understanding the values and potentials of patients is establishing a feeling of connectedness and trust in the nurse-patient relationship. Another requirement is careful listening on the part of nurses to patients' communications about what they view as worthwhile and how they perceive their capacities for growth. The importance of these requirements and the significance of this aspect of nursing intervention are emphasized in the following contrasting patient care situations.

Situation 1

K.T. is a 28-year-old, single woman who was recently hospitalized on the Ob-Gyn unit of a large, metropolitan hospital. She has been diagnosed as having invasive cancer of the cervix. Prior to her admission, she had tearfully confided to a friend that she believes her difficulty is related to having been sexually promiscuous. She expressed overwhelming shame and despair, maintaining, despite her friend's reassurances, that her ideal of finding a lifelong marriage partner now would never be fulfilled. The attending physician has just left K.T.'s room after having outlined treatment options with her, including surgery and radiotherapy. She is crying as the nurse enters the room to take routine vital signs. The nurse immediately remarks to K.T., "Don't worry; when you get married, you and your husband can adopt children. I have an adopted child and a biological child, and I love them equally as much." In response to these well-meaning statements, K.T. looks away from the nurse and toward the wall, continues crying, and shakes her head from side to side.

Keeping in mind the importance of developing an awareness of patients' values and their own view of their potentials, contrast the following patient care situation with the one described above.

Situation 2

Mr. C. is a 64-year-old man who was hospitalized three days ago with an obstruction of his trachea. In order to restore his airway, an opening was made into the trachea (tracheostomy). As a result, he is presently unable to speak. While assisting Mr. C. with his bath one morning, the nurse notices that he keeps looking toward his bedside stand. Finally, Mr. C. reaches over to the stand and picks up a book. The nurse notices that it is the patient's Bible. She is behind in completing her morning duties and feels the urge to tell Mr. C. to return the book to the stand immediately so that his bath can be finished. However, remembering that she has often seen the patient holding his Bible in the past, the nurse instead asks if Mr. C. would like to be visited by the chaplain. He shakes his head "no" but holds the book out to the nurse. She asks Mr. C. to write on a piece of paper how she might help him. He writes, "Please read the page with the marker in it." The nurse explains that, although she must first complete several other tasks, she could return in an hour to read the page to him. Mr. C. smiles and nods his head "yes" while returning the book to his bedside stand.

These two very different patient care situations illustrate the importance of nurses being aware of patients' values and their perceptions of their own capacities when intervening to promote self-actualization. In this first situation, the nurse not only fails to assess K.T.'s aspirations, which include becoming married, but also substitutes personal values for the patient's. The nurse mistakenly assumes that K.T. is sad about the possibility of being unable to have children because that is something very important to the nurse. The result is a missed growth opportunity for the patient and the nurse. Not only has a chance been missed to assist the patient to continue to move toward personal fulfillment through learning to cope more effectively with her shame, but the nurse has lost an opportunity to increase self-understanding by learning from the patient's experience. In contrast, the nurse in the second situation does not neglect or confuse the patient's need for spiritual fulfillment because of her need to finish the bath quickly. The result is that the patient's ability to use his present situation for growth is enhanced. In short, in order to help patients respond to changes in ways which promote self-actualization, it is necessary for nurses to base their interventions on self-understanding, as well as an awareness of the values and potentials of patients.

AWAKENING HOPE.   Another aspect of intervening as a change agent is encouraging hope in order to facilitate patients' abilities to make constructive changes, that is, changes that increase their personal development. The key to awakening realistic hope in patients is to believe in their power to grow, even in the face of considerable pain and suffering, and to affirm this power with warmth and caring.

Psychological research has demonstrated that expectations of significant people can be powerful influences on the behavior of others (Rosenthal, 1973). This is important here since nurses, in caring for persons during periods of heightened vulnerability, tend to be viewed by them as significant. Thus, nurses may actually enhance patients' abilities to make constructive changes by believing in their ability to grow, even in times of crisis! For instance, the nurse who truly believes that the patient who has had a stroke can continue to fulfill potentials is more likely to awaken hope in this individual and, consequently, to increase the possibility of growth. In considering this, one is reminded that nursing care to promote self-actualization is more a basic orientation toward people than a specific set of techniques.

Implied in the idea of awakening hope in others, through one's own belief in the ability of persons to continue to actualize themselves even in difficult circumstances, is a view of nurses as being actively involved in providing patient care. In other words, conveying hope to patients requires the establishment of a feeling of warmth and closeness in the nurse-patient relationship. It is not possible to communicate such a deep feeling and belief as a passive or detached observer. Thus, in intervening to promote self-actualization, nurses are faced with a personal choice which may have a crucial impact on patient care. That is, nurses are confronted with choosing between being a spectator or becoming actively involved in caring for patients.

In addition to using one's own growth-oriented beliefs, nurses can encourage hope through affirming efforts of patients to change their situations constructively. For example, in the case of a patient who periodically returns to the hospital for treatment of a chronic kidney problem, the nurse's active listening to the patient's planning of ways in which vocational goals can be pursued, despite the interruptions for treatment, may assist the patient to maintain hope. Similarly, offering encouragement to the paralyzed patient's attempts to become more independent through mastering the use of a specially designed wheelchair may be a simple, yet important, nursing action to awaken hope. Affirming even small efforts of patients to change their situations constructively promotes hopefulness and thus self-actualization.

As nurses help patients to discover that they can change and grow, their hope increases. Actualized hopes foster stronger, more realistic expectations of the future. These new feelings of hope, in turn, provide the energy for further growth.

Intervention as Teachers. Just as the assessment of self-actualization focuses on strengths rather than weaknesses, so the aim of nursing intervention to facilitate growth is to encourage development of potentialities instead of emphasizing opportunities that have been lost. Thus, even dying becomes a final stage of growth (Kübler-Ross, 1975). This is not an attempt to deny the very real pain and suffering experienced by patients, but only to recognize that growth is possible even in very stressful situations. This perspective is most apparent as nurses intervene as teachers to promote self-actualization. Nursing actions here are focused on assisting patients as learners to grow and learn from their experiences within the health care system. Interventions can be divided into two categories: assisting patients to learn that growth is possible through crises, and helping significant persons in patients' lives to learn how they can facilitate the continued development of patients' potentials.

TEACHING GROWTH THROUGH CRISIS. Crises are times when persons are confronted with making choices that will influence their growth. The primary nursing intervention to promote growth through crisis centers on assisting patients to recognize the various alternatives available to them in their situations and to support and encourage choices that lead to greater personal fulfillment. For instance, patients with an opening in their intestinal tract (ostomy), who fear that intimate relationships are no longer possible for them, can be taught about the methods of effectively managing their ostomy, along with explaining that close relationships are not only possible but may even promote their physical and emotional recovery. Similarly, the recently paralyzed patient who in the past highly valued sexual expression, but whose disability has affected sexual response, may be taught about various ways of expressing one's sexuality, emphasizing that sexual expression is as much or more of an emotional response as a physical one. In another illustration, the patient who has become blind as a result of complication from diabetes (usually due to diabetic retinopathy) may benefit from information about community agencies that assist persons with visual impairments and may help the patient in continuing to fulfill career goals. Indeed, a significant aspect of assisting patients to become aware of options and possibilities for growth involves consulting with and providing information about other individuals, groups, and organizations who offer specialized counseling or education aimed at increasing personal development.

In addition to other professional help, such as specialized spiritual, vocational, and psychological counseling, there is an enormous growth resource in the numerous people who have handled crises constructively.

Individuals who have grown as a result of coping effectively with demanding life experiences are potential care-givers and growth-enablers for others going through similar experiences. Thus, Reach to Recovery volunteers may enable mastectomy patients to find new strength and meaning in their situations. Volunteers from Alcoholic Anonymous may awaken hope in chemically dependent patients. Various support groups for patients with cancer, ostomies, multiple sclerosis, and other illnesses may assist others in developing a greater awareness of their own capacities for continued growth. In order to promote self-actualization, it is important that nurses be aware of both professional and nonprofessional growth resources. For example, in caring for a patient in traction who is suffering from long-standing boredom and apathy, the nurse's consultation with the hospital's clinical nursing specialist in mental health may be useful in planning more effective nursing interventions. Or in the case of a patient recently diagnosed with cancer, providing information about community support groups may be a way of encouraging hopefulness and enabling growth.

These interventions also hold personal relevance for nurses. In an occupation which is frequently highly stressful, nurses can also benefit from utilizing available growth resources. The most useful resource will depend upon the specific growth need of the nurse. For some, becoming active in a professional nursing organization may help to renew their sense of purpose. For others, an informal support group, growth group, professional counseling, or taking a course may provide the best opportunity for professional and personal fulfillment. Most important though is the recognition of the relationship between the self-actualization of patients and nurses. Nurses who are comfortable with their own growth are better able to promote the growth of patients.

TEACHING, INTERPERSONAL RELATIONSHIPS, AND GROWTH.   The teaching aspect of nursing is also important in helping family members, friends, or others who are significant in patients' lives to become aware of ways in which they can have a positive influence on the self-actualization of patients. Nursing actions are based on the belief that the ability to develop one's potentials is enhanced within *growth-nurturing relationships*. Therefore, interventions focus on providing information about patients' strengths, as well as limitations, in order to enhance the ability of family and friends to support and encourage growth. Specific nursing actions will differ with each patient care situation.

Consider the following illustration:

Mrs. K. is a 35-year-old woman who has had several hospitalizations for problems related to multiple sclerosis, a neurological disease which affects the brain and spinal cord. On her most recent admission, she has expressed considerable frustration that, as her disease has progressed, her husband has become more and more protective of her, even to the point of hiring another individual to regularly care for their two children, ages 10 and 12. Mrs. K. remarks to the nurse, "I don't know what I'll do if he keeps this up; I think the only thing that really keeps me going is caring for my children."

The nurse is aware that, except during exacerbations of her illness, Mrs. K. is able to care for her children. Therefore, after consulting other members of the health team, the nurse offers to review Mrs. K.'s treatment plans with both her and her husband.

During the brief teaching session with Mr. and Mrs. K., the nurse explains that, although rest is very important for persons with multiple sclerosis, activity is also very necessary. The nurse adds that planning the daily schedule ahead of time may help Mrs. K. to conserve energy for priority activities, thus allowing her to continue to care for their children. As the nurse pauses, Mr. K responds by saying, "I'm always afraid that my wife is going to have a relapse." The nurse acknowledges Mr. K.'s concern and informs Mr. and Mrs. K. of a community-sponsored course which teaches relatives and friends of MS patients how to improve home care.

In this situation, the husband's well-meaning actions have, nonetheless, become obstructions to his wife's fulfillment as a mother. Nursing interventions provide information in an attempt to promote the growth-nurturing aspects of the relationship. In addition to giving information, it may also be useful in some situations for nurses to explain directly to family or friends the need of patients to receive encouragement and support for attempts to develop capabilities. With interventions such as these, nurses promote the self-actualization of patients through growth-nurturing relationships.

Throughout this text, attention has been focused not only on patients but also on nurses. Indeed, the ability of nurses to meet their own needs has a direct effect on their ability to assist in meeting the needs of others. The care plan following this chapter describes difficulties encountered by a nurse.

Nursing Care Plan for a Nurse with Unmet Self-Actualization Needs

Ms. A. is a 29-year-old nurse who has worked on the rehabilitation unit of a suburban hospital for the past five years. As long as she can remember, her ambition had been to be a nurse. She excelled in nursing school and at commencement ceremonies even read a paper she had written on the value of helping others. As a nurse, Ms. A. has achieved a reputation among co-workers as being dependable, cooperative, and always willing to lend a helping hand. Recently, however, other nurses have noticed a change in Ms. A.'s behavior.

Ms. A. has become more irritable and moody. Although she is still quick to help others, her assistance is often prefaced with statements like, "If one more patient needs turning, I think I'll scream." Recently, when a patient pressed a call light for nursing assistance, Ms. A. remarked, "It's just Room 233; all they want is a bedpan."

Following a recent situation in which she was reprimanded by the charge nurse for a mistake made by a colleague, Ms. A. quietly sat down at the nursing station to finish her charting. As she looked at the charts, however, she thought to herself, "Is this what all of my training and experience has led to? I'm tired of always putting others' needs before mine—like canceling my reservations for the nursing conference so that B. could spend the weekend at the cabin. I feel like my career has stagnated. I've been looking out for everybody's needs but my own." As she sat for a few moments longer, she thought to herself, "I need a care plan." She proceeded to write a nursing diagnosis, goals, and interventions aimed at improving her situation.

Nursing Diagnosis	Goals	Interventions
Burnout associated with diminished personal and professional growth	Identify three opportunities for increased personal development and three opportunities for increased professional development (10/29). Increase awareness of personal and professional growth needs as evidenced by requesting to schedule time at work to allow for attending one conference and spending one week of vacation in the next five months.	1. List on paper long-term career objectives and possible methods of achieving these. 2. List on paper goals for personal development and ways to work toward these. 3. Sign up for the assertiveness course sponsored by the hospital. 4. Check into college courses which are available. 5. Join the rehabilitation nurses' group associated with the local nursing organization. 6. Talk to charge nurse about scheduling vacation and time off for the next nursing conference.

Summary

As nurses strive to understand and promote the self-actualization of others, their own need for growth is brought into sharper focus. However, along with this awareness may come the question of how possible it is to fulfill one's potentials in the frequently pressurized and hectic world of nursing. Boccuzzi (1979) answers this question stating, "Nursing, if we take the time to speculate, offers a wealth of experiences that stimulate personal growth, and conversely personal growth offers everything to the practice of nursing." By choosing active involvement over detachment in caring for the needs of others, nurses not only move toward providing more effective patient care, they also open the door to greater personal and professional fulfillment.

Terms for Review

crisis	growth-nurturing relationships	self-actualization
growth	maturing	

Self-Assessment

The Successful "Self-Actualizer"

Researchers have a variety of ideas about which qualities are most crucial to successful growth, maturing, or self-actualization. Based on your life experiences, which human characteristics do you view as most important for self-actualization?

Divide a blank sheet of paper into two columns. On the left side, list at least ten adjectives that describe growth-diminishing qualities. In the other column, list those characteristics which you believe most directly encourage growth.

Examples of both sets of adjectives include:

1. *Growth-diminishing*—rigid, cold, bigoted, empty, fearful, inhibited, insecure, egocentric, self-conscious, depressed, passive, unrealistic, nonrisking, immature, dependent, isolated, self-deprecating, aimless, hostile, dominating.
2. *Growth-encouraging*—active, involved, motivated, creative, helpful, enthusiastic, confident, happy, warm, mature, independent, realistic, kind, direct, spontaneous, friendly, humorous, tolerant, competent, nonthreatened.

After you have finished, reflect on which adjectives best describe you, your friends, and others who are significant in your life. Indicate which adjectives describe yourself by placing an *S* after the term, an *F* for friend, and *O* for significant other. On the basis of your answers, do you consider your relationships to be growth nurturing?

Learning Activities

Potentials Exercise

The purpose of this exercise is to encourage the exploration and use of your own unique growth possibilities.

Divide a blank sheet of paper into three columns. On the left side of the paper, list the major problems, frustrations, pressures, and losses that you are experiencing in your life. In the middle column, list all of your assets, strengths, positive challenges, and new possibilities that life presently holds for you. Now reflect on how you can use the assets and potentials in the middle column to deal with the problems on the left in a constructive and creative manner. With the space on the right, in a brief summary form, list your ideas about what you want to do to develop more of your possibilities in your present life situation.

Optional:
Discuss your responses in a small group.

Review Questions

Multiple Choice
1. The urge to express one's capabilities
    a. Is present in less than 1 percent of the population
    b. Can become distorted and self-destructive
    c. Is dependent on complete satisfaction of basic needs
    d. All of the above
2. Self-actualization is a process which
    a. Involves growth
    b. Occurs throughout the entire life span
    c. Is relevant to persons at all levels of ability
    d. All of the above
3. Characteristics of growth-nurturing relationships include
    a. Maintaining well-established expectations of how others will behave
    b. Being in the upper socioeconomic level of society
    c. Encouraging persons in attempting new projects
    d. All of the above

Short Answers
4. List three actualizing qualities that are particularly important in nursing.
5. Define crisis.
6. Describe nursing interventions to promote self-actualization which involve the nurse in the role of change agent.

Answers

1. b
2. d
3. c

4. Caring for others, abilities to identify and be open with others, and to perceive and accept persons as they are, personal independence, creativity
5. A life turning point, a period of increased vulnerability and heightened potential during which individuals' customary coping strategies are no longer adequate
6. a. Utilizing an awareness of patients' values and potentialities
   b. Encouraging hope

Suggested Readings

Boccuzi, N. K.: **The growth and development of the practicing nurse.** *Matern. Child Nurs. J.,* **4:**71–72 + , 1979.
This is a discussion of how nurses can use their nursing experience to grow personally and professionally. Although directed at maternal-child nurses, it applies as well to those in other areas of nursing.

Kübler-Ross, E.: *Death: The Final Stage of Growth.* Prentice-Hall, Englewood Cliffs, N.J., 1975.
A useful examination of how growth is possible through coming to terms with the fact of personal mortality.

Starck, P. L.: Maslow's needs and the spinal cord injured client. *ARN,* **5:**17–20, 1980
Through discussing the needs of one group of patients, the author illustrates the need to care for all patients in a holistic manner.

References and Bibliography

Beiser, M.; Benfari, R. C.; Collumb, H.; and Ravel, J. L.: Measuring psycho-behavior in cross-cultural surveys. *J. Nerv. Ment. Dis.,* **163:**10–23, 1976.

Boccuzzi, N. K.: The growth and development of the practicing nurse. *Matern. Child Nurs. J.,* **4:** 71–72 + , 1979.

Bugental, J.: The existential crisis in intensive psychotherapy. *Psychotherapy,* **2:**16–20, 1965.

Burnside, I. M.; Ebersole, P.; and Monea, H. E.: *Psychosocial Caring Throughout the Life Span.* McGraw-Hill, New York, 1979.

Cattell, R. B.: The measurement of the healthy personality and the healthy society. *The Counseling Psychologist,* **4:**13–18, 1973.

Clinebell, H.: *Growth Counseling.* Abingdon, Nashville, 1979.

Erikson, E. H.: *Identity: Youth and Crisis.* Norton, New York, 1968.

Frick, W. B.: Conceptual foundations of self-actualization: a contribution to motivation theory. *J. Humanist. Psychol.,* **4:**33–52, 1982.

Fromm, E.: *Man for Himself.* Holt, Rinehart and Winston, New York, 1947.

Gale, R. F.: *Developmental Behavior.* Macmillan, New York 1969.

Gamble, J. W., and Brown, E. C.: Self-actualization and personal mortality. *Omega,* **11**(4):341–53, 1980–1981.

Gardner, J.: *Self-Renewal.* Harper & Row, New York, 1965.

Heath, D. H.: *Maturity and Competence.* Gardner Press, New York, 1977.

Jourard, S. M.: *Disclosing Man to Himself.* Van Nostrand, New York, 1968.

Jourard, S. M.: *The Transparent Self.* Van Nostrand, New York, 1971.

Konopka, G.: Formation of values in the developing person. *Am. J. Orthopsychiatry,* **43**(1):86–96, 1973.

Kübler-Ross, E.: *Death: The Final Stage of Growth.* Prentice-Hall, Englewood Cliffs, N.J., 1975.

Lowenthal, M. F., and Haven, C.: Interaction and adaptation: intimacy as a crucial variable. *Am. Sociolog. Rev.,* **33:**20–30, 1968.

Maslow, A. H.: *Motivation and Personality,* 2nd ed. Harper & Row, New York, 1970.

Maslow, A. H.: *Toward a Psychology of Being,* 2nd ed. Van Nostrand, New York, 1968.

May, R.: Intentionality: the heart of human will. *J. Humanist. Psychol.,* **5:**202–209, 1965.

Monea, H. E.: Ethnicity and sexuality: their impact on caring. In Burnside I. M.; Ebersole, P.; and Monea, H. E. (eds.): *Psychosocial Caring Throughout the Life Span.* McGraw-Hill, New York, 1979.

Rosenthal, R.: The pygmalion effect lives. *Psychology Today,* p. 58, Sept., 1973.

Sarosi, G. M.: A critical theory: the nurse as a fully human person. *Nurs. Forum,* **7**(4):349–63, 1968.

Sheehy, G.: *Pathfinders.* Morrow, New York, 1981.

Starck, P. L.: Maslow's needs and the spinal cord injured client. *ARN,* **5:**17–20, 1980.

Stotland, E.: *The Psychology of Hope.* Jossey-Bass, San Francisco, 1969.

INDEX*

A

*All terms and pages where their definitions appear are indicated by **boldface type.**

errors, patient data and, 208
inputs of, incorrect data and, 193
languages of, 179
learning use of, nurses and, 206
medication and, 192–193
nurses use of, 178–180, 180f
patient charts and, 192–193
patient classification system and, 198
printouts, patient instruction and, 205–206
terminology of, 178–179
user friendly, 179
Conception, cell growth and, 217–218
Condom catheter, use of, 638–639, 638f
Conduction, of body heat, 485
Cone, retina and, 703–704
Confidentiality, of nurse-patient relationship, 133–134
Conflict, resolution of, groups and, 120–125
Consciousness
central nervous system and, 707
unmet fluid need effect on, 574t
Consent, informed, 146
Consolidation, 432
Constipation, 601
causes of, 604
in older adult, 271
treatment of, 632
unmet fluid need effect on, 574t
Constitution, of U.S., lawsuits and, 34
Consumer rights, 32–33
Contamination, 339
IV therapy and, 580–581, 581f
Content, 120
Contraction
isometric, 697
isotonic, 697
Contracture, 701
Contributory negligence, malpractice defenses and, 40
Controller, for IV rate, 590f, 591
Convection
body temperature and, 485–486
wind chill index and, 485, 485t
Cooling blanket, use of, 519–521, 519f
Core temperature, 482f, 483–484
Coronary artery disease, blood flow and, 427
Cough, oxygenation and, 449–453
Counterirritant, disease and, 5
Countersign, 142
Cramp
heat, 495
muscle, unmet fluid need effect on, 574t
Creatine phosphate, ATP and, 696–697
Creativity, self-actualization and, 817
Credibility, 106
Crepitation, 446
Criminal law, 24, 34
euthanasia and, 59
Crisis, 819
as catalyst, for growth, 819–820, 826–827

developmental, 294
dynamics, family and, 294–295
hope and, patient and, 823
nurse and, attitudes towards, 823
situational, 295
spiritual, 773–774
Criticism, context of, 104
Crohn's disease, 546t
Cross-linking theory of aging, 268t
Crutch
four-point gait with, 750–751, 750f
partial weight-bearing gait with, 751–752, 751f
three-point gait with, 751, 751f
two-point gait with, 751, 751f
use of, 750, 750f
Culture, 94
differences in, minority-group patients and, 792–793
dynamics of, groups and, 125
family structure and, 293
food preferences and, 555t
knowledge of, nursing intervention and, 775–777, 776t
love and, expression of, 765–766
sexual attitudes and, 681
stimuli perceptions and, 707–708
Cure role, 15
versus care, 15
Cursor, 185–186
Cystitis, 605

D

Dalton's law, 417
Data
analysis of, 312–313t
patient and, 310–312, 312t
collection of
care plan and, 324
nursing process and, 310–313
patient and, 310, 311t
objective, 87–88
on-line, 180
patient, 18, 20–22, 24
reassessment of, 325
subjective, 87
Data base
limiting access to, coding for, 182, 182f
patient right to privacy and, legal dynamics of, 208
Data processing, nursing service and, liaison between, 197
Dead space, anatomical, 415
Death, 277–278
causes of, 278–279
in adolescents, 251
in United States, 279t
middle adult and, 264
nursing implications of, 279–283
physical changes with, 283–284
understanding of, age groups and, 278t

I

M

education ?

U

V